This book is dedicated to our families
who gave moral support
while we worked on this volume,
and to our patients who
continue to inspire and educate us.

Cancer Therapy

Cancer Therapy

Edited by

DAVID S. FISCHER, M.D., F.A.C.P.
Clinical Professor of Medicine
Yale University School of Medicine

JOHN C. MARSH, M.D., F.A.C.P.
Professor of Medicine and
Lecturer in Pharmacology
Yale University School of Medicine

With the technical assistance of

MARION E. MORRA, M.A.
Communications Manager
Yale Comprehensive Cancer Center
Clinical Instructor
Yale University School of Nursing

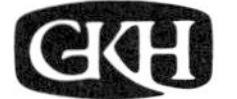
G. K. Hall Medical Publishers
Boston, Massachusetts

G. K. Hall Medical Publishers
70 Lincoln Street
Boston, MA 02111

82 83 84 85 / 4 3 2 1

Fischer, David S.
Cancer therapy.

Bibliography.
Includes index.
1. Cancer—Treatment. 2. Cancer. I. Marsh, John C. II. Morra, Marion E. III. Title.
[DNLM: 1. Neoplasms—Therapy. QZ 266 F519c]
RC270.8.F57 616.99'406 81-13350
ISBN 0-8161-2219-9 AACR2

The authors and publishers have worked to ensure that all information in this book concerning drug dosages, schedules, and routes of administration is accurate at the time of publication. As medical research and practice advance, however, therapeutic standards may change. For this reason, and because human and mechanical errors will sometimes occur, we recommend that our readers consult the *PDR* or a manufacturer's product information sheet prior to prescribing or administering any drug discussed in this volume.

Designed by Carole Rollins
Set in VIP Caslon Old Face by Compset, Inc.

contributors

Richard P. Benton, M.D.
Medical Oncologist and Hematologist
Medical Service
Lawrence and Memorial Hospitals
New London, Connecticut

Joseph R. Bertino, M.D.
American Cancer Society Professor of Medicine and Pharmacology
Co-Chief, Section of Medical Oncology
Yale University School of Medicine
New Haven, Connecticut

Joseph R. Bove, M.D.
Professor of Laboratory Medicine
Yale University School of Medicine
Director, Blood Bank
Yale–New Haven Hospital
New Haven, Connecticut

Ed Cadman, M.D.
Associate Professor of Medicine and Pharmacology
Co-Chief, Section of Medical Oncology
Yale University School of Medicine
New Haven, Connecticut

Francis S. Cardinale, M.D.
Radiation Oncologist
Hospital of St. Raphael
Assistant Clinical Professor of Therapeutic Radiology
Yale University School of Medicine
New Haven, Connecticut

Murray Joseph Casey, M.D.
Professor and Associate Chairman
Department of Obstetrics and Gynecology
University of Wisconsin Medical School
Chairman of Obstetrics and Gynecology
Milwaukee Clinical Campus
Obstetrician – Gynecologist-in-Chief
The Mount Sinai Medical Center
Milwaukee, Wisconsin
Formerly Associate Professor of Obstetrics and Gynecology
University of Connecticut School of Medicine
Farmington, Connecticut

Philip F. Corso, M.D.
Plastic and Reconstructive Surgeon
Senior Attending and Chief of Section of Plastic and Reconstructive Surgery
Bridgeport Hospital and Norwalk Hospital
Bridgeport and Norwalk, Connecticut

Thomas P. Duffy, M.D.
Professor of Medicine
Division of Hematology
Yale University School of Medicine
New Haven, Connecticut

Leonard R. Farber, M.D.
Medical Oncologist
Associate Clinical Professor of Medicine
Yale University School of Medicine
Attending Physician
Yale–New Haven Hospital and the Hospital of St. Raphael
New Haven, Connecticut

David S. Fischer, M.D., F.A.C.P.
Medical Oncologist and Hematologist
Clinical Professor of Medicine
Yale University School of Medicine
Attending Physician
Yale–New Haven Hospital and Hospital of St. Raphael
New Haven, Connecticut
Consultant to Milford Hospital (Milford, Ct.), Griffin Hospital (Derby, Ct.), and West Haven V.A. Hospital.

William H. Greene, M.D.
Associate Professor of Medicine, Infectious Diseases
Yale University School of Medicine
New Haven, Connecticut

Raul E. Isturiz, M.D.
Infectious Diseases Practitioner
Caracas, Venezuela
Former Fellow, Infectious Diseases
Yale University School of Medicine
New Haven, Connecticut

Daniel S. Kapp, Ph.D., M.D.
Assistant Professor of Therapeutic Radiology
Yale University School of Medicine
Attending Physician
Yale–New Haven Hospital
New Haven, Connecticut

Martin E. Katz, M.D., F.A.C.P.
Medical Oncologist and Hematologist
Assistant Clinical Professor of Medicine
Yale University School of Medicine
Attending Physician
Yale–New Haven Hospital and Hospital of St. Raphael
New Haven, Connecticut

Gerard T. Kennealey, M.D.
Assistant Clinical Professor of Medicine
Yale University School of Medicine
Attending Physician
Waterbury Hospital and St. Mary's Hospital
Waterbury, Connecticut

John M. Kirkwood, M.D.
Assistant Professor of Medicine and Dermatology
Yale University School of Medicine
Attending Physician
Yale–New Haven Hospital and West Haven V.A. Hospital
New Haven, Connecticut

Arthur H. Knowlton, M.D.
Radiation Oncologist
Hospital of St. Raphael
Associate Clinical Professor of Therapeutic Radiology
Yale University School of Medicine
New Haven, Connecticut

Ernest I. Kohorn, M.D.
Professor of Obstetrics and Gynecology
Yale University School of Medicine
New Haven, Connecticut

Diane M. Komp, M.D.
Chief, Pediatric Hematology–Oncology
Professor of Pediatrics
Yale University School of Medicine
New Haven, Connecticut

Charles D. Kowal, M.D.
Assistant Professor of Medicine
University of Pittsburgh
Pittsburgh, Pennsylvania
Formerly Post Doctoral Fellow in Medicine (Oncology)
Yale University School of Medicine
New Haven, Connecticut

Hugh F. Lena, M.D.
Senior Attending Surgeon
Lawrence and Memorial Hospitals
New London, Connecticut

Arthur L. Levy, M.D.
Medical Oncologist and Hematologist
Assistant Clinical Professor of Medicine
Yale University School of Medicine
Attending Physician
Yale–New Haven Hospital and the Hospital of St. Raphael
New Haven, Connecticut

Elliot M. Livstone, M.D., F.A.C.P.
Associate Professor of Medicine
Yale University School of Medicine
New Haven, Connecticut

Ivan S. Lowenthal, M.D.
Medical Oncologist
Clinical Instructor of Medicine
Yale University School of Medicine
Attending Physician
Charlotte Hungerford Hospital
Torrington, Connecticut

W. Bruce Lundberg, M.D.
Hematologist and Medical Oncologist
Assistant Clinical Professor of Medicine
Yale University School of Medicine
Attending Physician
Yale–New Haven Hospital and the Hospital of St. Raphael
New Haven, Connecticut

John C. Marsh, M.D., F.A.C.P.
Professor of Medicine and Lecturer in Pharmacology
Yale University School of Medicine
New Haven, Connecticut
Attending Physician
Yale–New Haven Hospital
Consultant, West Haven V.A. Hospital and Uncas-on-Thames Hospital
Norwich, Connecticut

Sue McIntosh, M.D.
Associate Professor of Pediatrics
Yale University School of Medicine
New Haven, Connecticut

William D. Medina, M.D.
Post Doctoral Fellow in Medicine (Oncology)
Yale University School of Medicine
New Haven, Connecticut

J. Scott Nystrom, M.D., F.A.C.P.
Medical Oncologist and Hematologist
Southfield, Michigan
Formerly Assistant Professor of Medicine
University of Connecticut Health Center
Farmington, Connecticut

Bernard Percarpio, M.D.
Assistant Clinical Professor of Therapeutic Radiology
Yale University School of Medicine
New Haven, Connecticut

Jonathan H. Pincus, M.D.
Professor of Neurology
Yale University School of Medicine
New Haven, Connecticut

John L. Pool, M.D.
Associate Clinical Professor of Thoracic Surgery, Emeritus
Yale University School of Medicine
Consultant, Memorial Sloan-Kettering Cancer Center, New York
Honorary Surgeon, Norwalk Hospital
Norwalk, Connecticut

Carol S. Portlock, M.D.
Associate Professor of Medicine
Yale University School of Medicine
New Haven, Connecticut

Leonard R. Prosnitz, M.D.
Professor of Therapeutic Radiology
Yale University School of Medicine
New Haven, Connecticut

David P. Purpora, M.D.
Medical Oncologist
Attending Physician in Medical Oncology
Griffin Hospital
Derby, Connecticut

Paul L. Schulman, M.D.
Chief, Section of Hematology-Oncology
Norwalk Hospital
Norwalk, Connecticut

Peter E. Schwartz, M.D.
Associate Professor of Obstetrics and Gynecology
Director, Gynecologic Oncology
Yale University School of Medicine
New Haven, Connecticut

Frank C. Sparks, M.D.
Surgical Oncologist
Lecturer in Surgery
Yale University School of Medicine
Attending Surgeon
Norwalk Hospital
Norwalk, Connecticut

Richard B. Weininger, M.D.
Medical Oncologist and Hematologist
Hudson, New York
Formerly Assistant Professor of Medicine
Division of Oncology
Yale University School of Medicine
New Haven, Connecticut

Robert M. Weiss, M.D.
Professor of Urologic Surgery
Yale University School of Medicine
Attending Surgeon in Urology
Yale–New Haven Hospital
New Haven, Connecticut

R. Glen Wiggans, M.D.
Medical Oncologist
Assistant Clinical Professor of Medicine
Yale University School of Medicine
Attending Physician
Hospital of St. Raphael and Yale–New Haven Hospital
New Haven, Connecticut

contents

preface

This book is intended as an introduction to modern concepts and practices in cancer therapy for general physicians, house staff, medical students, oncology nurses, and physician's associates. It is not meant to be a definitive treatise for oncologists, as at least two excellent books are available (Holland, J. F., and Frei, E., III. *Cancer medicine,* 2nd edition. Philadelphia: Lea & Febiger, 1982; and Haskell, C. M. *Cancer treatment.* Philadelphia: W. B. Saunders, 1980), and at least two more will be available by the time this book is published (DeVita, V. T., Jr; Hellman, S.; and Rosenberg, S. A. *Principles and practice of oncology.* Philadelphia: J. B. Lippincott, 1982; and Carter, S. K.; Glatstein, E.; and Livingston, R. B., *Principles of cancer treatment.* New York: McGraw-Hill, 1982). Instead, it should prepare others to understand what medical, radiation, surgical, pediatric, and gynecologic oncologists are doing. It may serve some of those specialists when they venture out of their subspecialty into other areas of cancer treatment. A large number of charts, tables, formulae, and compilations of data that were scattered throughout the literature are included for convenience and may be useful to oncologists as well as the groups for whom this book is primarily intended. The emphasis, however, is not on details but on the principles of oncology, such as an understanding of etiology or prevention, the natural history of tumors, and therapeutic approaches, both general and specific. We have also emphasized an understanding of individual drugs, including their mechanism of action, metabolism, and toxicity, so that decisions about chemotherapy, especially combination chemotherapy, can be more rational.

This book grew out of a series of lectures at Connecticut hospitals cosponsored by the Connecticut Oncology Association, the Cancer Coordinating Committee of the Connecticut State Medical Society, the Connecticut Division of the American Cancer Society, the Yale Comprehensive Cancer Center, and the Eastern Cooperative Oncology Group. Physicians were selected for their particular interest and expertise in the topic to be reviewed. They lectured at one of the participating hospitals and were then requested to summarize their remarks with appropriate references, with emphasis on review articles in English. Thirty-six chapters were finally collected from these lecturers, and they form the basis of discussion about individual cancers. It was the original intention to publish just this material. Yet large areas of importance had obviously been omitted. Many of our house officers and senior students on the wards indicated a desire for an introductory volume on cancer and its therapy. We felt that these 36 chapters should be expanded to a more comprehensive treatment in an effort to fill this expressed need. To fill the gaps, 33 additional chapters were written expressly for this volume, one each by Drs. Arthur H. Knowlton, Martin E. Katz, Elliot M. Livstone, and Ernest I. Kohorn, who had lectured and had already submitted a chapter on that basis; one each by Drs. Sue McIntosh and Charles D. Kowal, who had not lectured; and the remaining 27 chapters by ourselves. In all, 17 community-based physicians with academic affiliations and 22 university-based physicians were involved in this collaborative venture.

As with all contributed volumes, the chapters differ somewhat in perspective and in presentation, with inevitable overlapping of material. The individual authors were given great freedom in the handling of their material. Some adhered to the restrictions of space and references, albeit with difficulty; others exceeded those limits. Certain topics warranted more extensive treatment because of their controversial or difficult nature or because they are currently undergoing reappraisal.

We asked each author to stress his or her own approach and conclusions based on the available data and personal experiences. We do not necessarily agree with all the implications of those conclusions, but we exercised editorial control to modify only those that seemed inconsistent with the data. To be as current as possible, many references are to abstracts that appeared in the *Proceedings of the American Association for Cancer Research and the American Society for Clinical Oncology.* We have cited these as either *Proc. Am. Assoc. Cancer Res.* or *Proc. Am. Soc. Clin. Oncol.*, which in 1981 was volume 22. After the page proofs were completed, we learned that the societies are publishing their proceedings separately in 1982: *Proc. Am. Assoc. Cancer Res.* will continue as volume 23, and *Proc. Am. Soc. Clin. Oncol.* will be volume 1.

Every attempt has been made to include the most up-to-date information on cancer treatment. Because the field of oncology is rapidly changing, however, no text can incorporate newer developments from recently published journals. Between submission to the publisher and publication, it is inevitable that some information will be superseded by newer data.

Practitioners in the field of oncology have had much recent success with new modalities of therapy. Failure is all too common, however, and the oncologist must be prepared to deal with it. We have tried to emphasize the ethical and social considerations not only in the chapter devoted to that subject, but in several other places. For example, we have included one hospital's guidelines for a "do not resuscitate" policy.

The practice of medicine requires a lifetime of continuing education. We learn from books, from journals, from our students, our colleagues, and from our patients. We hope that this volume will serve as an introduction to continuing education in cancer as we progress toward curing it in all its forms.

David S. Fischer, M.D., F.A.C.P.
John C. Marsh, M.D., F.A.C.P.

acknowledgments

In addition to the authors of the various chapters, we would like to thank the chairpersons at the following cooperating hospitals for help in arranging the programs at which some of the material in this book was originally presented

Albert Casazza, M.D., Danbury Hospital

Anthony Coscia, M.D., Norwalk Hospital

David Lawler, M.D., Lawrence and Memorial Hospital

Richard Lutes, M.D., Waterbury Hospital

Bhagat Mather, M.D., Uncas on Thames Hospital

J. Scott Nystrom, M.D., University of Connecticut Medical Center

Gerald O'Brien, M.D., and William Whalen, M.D., Windham Memorial Hospital

Stephanie Roth, M.D., Yale–New Haven Hospital

Alfred St. James, M.D., and Videen McGaughey, R.N., Meriden–Wallingford Hospital

Robert P. Zanes, M.D., Hospital of St. Raphael

We are also grateful for the support given by Jack Cole, M.D., director of the Yale Comprehensive Cancer Center; M. Patricia Bergin, R.N., of the Connecticut Division, American Cancer Society; and Robert Brunnel of the Connecticut State Medical Society. For production, proofreading, and secretarial assistance, we thank Patricia Sorrentino, Mary Bridget Jordan, Wendy Shaw, Karen D. Fischer, Francie E. Fischer, Theoria B. Boyd, Barbara Phillips, Barbara Geagan, Marion Hussong, Mary Killion, Ann Bradley, and Marian Kanter. Patricia Wales and Louise E. Fischer helped check references.

part one

General Considerations

one

The Etiologies of Cancer

DAVID S. FISCHER

Because cancer is not one, but a hundred or more diseases, we should not be surprised to find many causes, perhaps hundreds of causes, of the various cancers. The evidence for some of these causes is primarily epidemiologic. For others, it is extrapolation from animal data, and in many cases it is speculation and guess work. Therapy is most rational when etiology is understood, and prevention depends on an understanding of causality.

Whether we like it or not, as physicians and health professionals we are being caught up in the political process in which cancer and carcinogenesis are political gambits. We are asked to support efforts to remove from the market all products that have been shown to produce cancer in any animal species in any dose (the Delaney Amendment to the Food and Drug Act). Can the animal data be extrapolated to humans? Is megadose induction in animals applicable to microdose exposure in people? Are nuclear power plants causing widespread cancer as alleged, or is the danger exaggerated? Is there any danger at all? If so, is the risk acceptable? Are all our foods contaminated with carcinogens so that we must use only organic foods, or is the organic food movement a "rip-off" to get us to pay more for less food? Is tobacco really the single most important cause of preventable cancer, or is the Surgeon General misleading us? Are there genetic predispositions to explain why some individuals exposed to a carcinogen develop cancer and others with similar exposure do not? Is cancer caused by a virus? What are cocarcinogens? These and other questions arise frequently in the political forum and from patients in our offices. Some answers are available; more information is needed.

It has been estimated that 80% to 90% of cancer is environmentally related (Toxic Substances Strategy Committee 1980; Hiatt, Watson, and Winsten 1977). About half of this is associated with our diet, one-quarter is tobacco-related, and 5% or less is occupationally determined (Weisburger 1979) (table 1.1). Most governmental action and appropriations have been for regulation of the occupational exposure, a small amount for education in regard to tobacco, and almost nothing for dietary studies. For many years, abundant research funds were available for studies of viral carcinogenesis, but these funds have diminished recently.

Viral Carcinogenesis

As early as 1908, Ellerman and Bang demonstrated that leukemia could be transmitted to chickens by extracts of tissues that had passed through filters so fine that all bacteria and cells were excluded. Three years later, Rous produced solid tumors in chickens from tumor filtrates and suggested the viral etiology of these sarcomas. For a variety of reasons, the significance of these findings was overlooked for 21 years, and no real progress was made in the field. Then several additional tumors were linked to viruses in rapid succession. Shope demonstrated that fibroma (1932) and papilloma (1933) in rabbits could be transmitted by cell-free filtrates. The following year Lucké reported that carcinoma of the kidney in the frog

Table 1.1. *Causes and Distribution of Human Cancers*

Cause	*Organs Involved*	*Percentage of Total*
High-fat low-fiber, broiled or fried foods(?)	Colon, pancreas, breast, prostate, ovary, endometrium	45 (?)
Tobacco	Lung, pancreas, bladder, kidneys	21
Unknown, possibly radiation and virus	Lymphoma, leukemia, sarcoma, cervix	10–15
Nitrate-nitrite, mycotoxin	Stomach, liver	5
Tobacco and alcohol	Oral cavity, esophagus	5
Tobacco-asbestos; tobacco-mining; tobacco-uranium	Lung, respiratory tract	5
Occupational	Lung, bladder, sinuses, liver, leukemia, kidneys	1–5
Medical radiation, drugs	Leukemia, breast, sarcoma	1

SOURCE: Modified from Weisburger 1979.

could be passed by cell-free extracts. Perhaps the most fascinating of the viral tumors is the mouse mammary carcinoma first described in 1936 by Bittner. The causative agent, referred to as the "milk factor," is a transmissable and filterable substance in the milk of nursing females that induces cancer in their offspring or in foster nurslings. The genetic factors here are of minor significance; the general principle of natural vertical transmission was seen to be an infectious process in which the newborn becomes infected because of lack of an immune response to the virus. At the time, interest in viruses was not sustained, primarily because this form of cancer in chickens and frogs appeared unrelated to that in mammals, and the "milk factor" was regarded as just a special case without general significance (Fischer 1964) (table 1.2).

Subsequent human studies suggest that animal biology is not far removed from human biology. With the observation in mice that the mammary tumor virus was transmitted in the milk, and in some strains, in the ovum or sperm, investigators attempted to demonstrate viral particles in human milk and mammary neoplastic tissue (Schottenfeld 1975).

In studies of the milk of women in the United States with or without a family history of breast cancer, and of Parsi women from Bombay, India, virus-like (type B) particles structurally similar to the mammary tumor virus in mice were noted in 31% of the high-risk American women, 39% of the Parsi women, and only 12% of the low-risk American women (Moore et al. 1971). The Parsi women in Bombay are members of an inbred community of about 80,000 people descended from the Persian Zoroastrians. In contrast to their neighbors, they tend to marry and become pregnant later in life and have fewer children.

The particles isolated from human milk contain the reverse transcriptase enzyme (RNA-directed DNA polymerase). In this circumstance, DNA is synthesized from the template provided by viral RNA. The reverse transcriptase enzyme allows the RNA of a tumor virus to direct the DNA in the host cell, and also allows the RNA virus to remain latent in the cell but capable of vertical transmission through the germ line. In this context, familial aggregation of human breast cancer is compatible with both a viral and a genetic concept of etiology. Ethical considerations prohibit an attempt at fulfilling Koch's postulates to prove causation, if that is the case (Bishop 1980).

Type C viruses cause sarcomas and leukemias in many animal species, and it is unlikely that this is different in humans. A human cancer virus or cocarcinogen seems likely.

In 1958, Denis Burkitt, a British surgeon in Uganda, recognized that a variety of hitherto unrelated tumors of children were different presentations of a single neoplasm called lymphoma. The disease had an exceedingly high incidence relative to other childhood malignancies, affected both black and white children, and seemed to be unrelated to tribal or dietary factors. A striking geographic and climatologic correlation with disease distribution was noted. The disease was rarely encountered at altitudes above 5000 feet at the equator or below 1000 feet in the latitude of Mozambique, suggesting that the limiting factors may be a minimum annual temperature of 60° F and minimum annual rainfall of 20 inches. This circumstantial evidence pointed to an insect-borne agent, probably a virus. So far, the Epstein-Barr virus (EBV) is the foremost contender for the "first human cancer virus." It is the cause of infectious mononucleosis, which has been considered a self-limited leukemia (Henle and Henle 1974). Evidence is mounting for a causative role in Burkitt's African lymphoma and in nasopharyngeal carcinoma; EBV is a lymphotropic herpes virus in humans, and its main

Table 1.2. *Some Important Oncogenic Viruses*

Author/Year	*Virus*	*Major Hosts*	*Nucleic Acid*
Ellerman and Bang 1908	Leucosis	Chicken, turkey	RNA
Rous 1911	Sarcoma	Chicken, turkey	RNA
Shope 1932	Fibroma	Rabbit	DNA
Furth 1933	Lymphomatosis	Chicken	RNA
Bittner 1936	Mammary carcinoma	Mouse	RNA
Lucké 1938	Kidney carcinoma	Frog	DNA
Gross 1951	Lymphoid leukemia	Mouse, rat	RNA
Gross, Stewart, and Eddy 1953–1957	Polyoma	Mouse, hamster, rat	DNA
Friend 1956	Stem cell leukemia	Mouse, rat	RNA
Graffi 1956	Myeloid leukemia	Mouse, rat	RNA
Maloney 1960	Lymphoid leukemia	Mouse, rat, hamster	RNA
Eddy 1960	SV40 (vacuolating)	Monkey, human, hamster	DNA
Trentin 1962	Adenovirus 12	Human, hamster	DNA
Rauscher 1962	Leukemia	Mouse	RNA
Epstein-Barr 1964	Lymphoma	Human	DNA

SOURCE: Modified from Fischer 1964.

target is the human B lymphocyte. Only B lymphocytes have specific EBV receptors and can be transformed by the virus in vitro into permanently growing cell lines (Klein 1975). These can be transplanted into immunologically deficient animals and grow as malignant tumors after heterotransplantation. When reimplanted back to the autochthonous host, they grow progressively and kill the host. Recently, a Yale group reported an in-depth study of a four-year-old child in whom fatal diffuse lymphoma developed during a primary EBV infection that initially appeared to be infectious mononucleosis. The tumor cells were derived from several different populations of B lymphocytes that were transformed in vivo by EBV (Robinson et al. 1980). The question is whether this is an example of a human virus-induced neoplasm, or whether it is simple virus stimulation of polyclonal B lymphocytes in a person with an impaired immunoregulatory system who would develop lymphoma with any similar strong stimulus—viral, chemical, radiation, and so on. Only time and more experience will tell (Schwartz 1980).

Epidemiologic Methods

The epidemiologic approach has been applied extensively in the study of human cancer because people cannot be manipulated like animals in planned experiments. Instead, we study the natural history of the disease and record it under special characteristics, and accumulate data that we call statistics. By means of such statistics, the cancer epidemiologist seeks to discover and exploit variations in occurrence of cancer. These variations are recognized by making comparisons among different time periods, groups of people living widely apart in different areas, and groups of people living closely together but who differ in such characteristics as sex, age, occupation, or habits, for example, smoking. These comparisons are often erroneous and misleading, however, unless the epidemiologists have adhered to stringent criteria of validity.

For the statistics to be valid the diagnosis of cancer must be clearly and uniformly defined, preferably with histologic examination, and the definitions recorded and adhered to. The quality of the diagnostic services should be closely similar for the population groups being contrasted, or allowances made for the differences. There must be uniform and prestated criteria for the data selection and stratification so that they are not manipulated to support a conclusion arrived at before the data are studied. Identical ways of expressing occurrence of cancer must be adopted. The population groups themselves and relevant group characteristics must be adequately defined. After all the epidemiologic information is integrated with experimental and clinical data, the epidemiologist attempts to derive inferences regarding etiologic factors (Lilienfeld, Pedersen, and Dowd 1967).

The most striking epidemiologic feature of most human cancers is that incidence increases geometrically with advancing age. It is so high in old age groups as to suggest that almost all of us would eventually develop cancer. Both total immunity and total avoidance of carcinogenic materials must be rare in itself. On the other hand, only 1 in 1000 people die of cancer before age 15 years, and only 1 in 110 before the age of 45 years. Thus death from cancer typically does not occur until after the end of the usual reproductive period of our species, so susceptibility factors may be transmitted to offspring. Numbers of deaths remain low until after the age at which a large proportion of people in earlier times died of infections and diseases of parasitic etiology (Hammond 1975).

Genetic and Hereditary Influences

An attempt has been made to sort out those factors in cancer causation that are environmental and those that are genetic. The differentiation is not always easily made, which has occasioned a large literature (Goepp 1978; German 1974; Mulvihill, Miller, and Fraumeni 1977; Knudson 1980; Fraumeni 1975).

Nasopharyngeal cancer (NPC) is common in Chinese but rare in whites. The recent finding of a significant association with HLA-A2 and fewer than two antigens at the B locus has suggested a genetic cause. If a racially determined genetic susceptibility exists, however, other evidence suggests that an environmental trigger or cocarcinogen must be present as well (Henderson et al. 1976). Chinese migrants to Hawaii and California have this cancer in decreasing numbers in succeeding generations. Increased risk of NPC was also associated with smoking, chemicals, and foreign birth place. Thus causation is multifactorial. Many disorders and traits are determined by single genes. One such trait is familial polyposis of the colon. By the age of 40 years, one-half of all patients with the mutant gene have colon cancer, and by age 70, nearly all have it (Harris et al. 1980).

Xeroderma pigmentosum is an autosomal recessive disorder that predisposes to skin cancer. There is a known defect of an endonuclease necessary to repair damage to DNA by ultraviolet radiation (Robbins et al. 1974). Here, ultraviolet light is the cocarcinogen. In ataxia telangiectasia, there is an analogous defect in an endonuclease for repairing DNA damage by gamma radiation. This hereditary skin disorder predisposes to leukemia and lymphoma, but is triggered by exposure to ionizing radiation. Other hereditary tumors lack an enzyme and interact with a chemical or hormone to precipitate neoplastic changes.

Cancer may be considered a genetic disease at the cellular level in that evidence from studies of chemical, radiation, and viral carcinogenesis, as well as cytogenetics and hereditary cancers, suggests that irreversible changes in the cellular hereditary material occur in the development of a cancer cell. Hereditary or environmental factors may influence the probability of such changes. A small fraction of human cancers may be attributed to rare hereditary disorders of chromosomal abnormality, mutagenesis, cell growth regulation or differentiation, or immune deficiency. Yet studies of familial cancer suggest that in the absence of such demonstrable abnormalities, predisposition to cancer may follow an autosomal-dominant hereditary pattern, generating tumors that occur at relatively early ages and that may be multiple. The occurrence of hereditary and nonhereditary forms of the same histologic cancer has been attributed to similar genetic changes in germinal or somatic cells respectively. The percentage of tumors arising from germinal mutations varies for each tumor type, but may account for nearly 40% of certain childhood cancers, and a lesser percentage of adult cancers. Study of the interaction of hereditary and acquired risk factors suggests that more than a single genetic change may be necessary for cancer to develop. If a series of mutations is necessary, then those individuals with the inherited mutation present in all cells may be uniquely susceptible to carcinogens. Individuals genetically pre-

Table 1.3. *Some Hereditary Neoplasms*

Type	*Specific Disease*
Colonic adenocarcinomas	Polyposis coli
	Gardner's syndrome
	Gastric and colonic polyps
	Turcot syndrome
	Torre's syndrome
Breast carcinomas	Familial breast cancer syndrome
	Lobular carcinoma in situ
	Familial premenopausal breast cancer
	Familial breast and ovarian cancer
Multiple endocrine neoplasia	Medullary thyroid carcinoma
	Parathyroid adenomas
	Pancreatic islet cell tumors
	Pituitary tumors
	Adrenal cortical adenomas
	Pheochromocytomas
	Thyroid adenomas
	Intestinal ganglioneuromatosis
Miscellaneous	Retinoblastoma
	Nevoid basal cell carcinoma syndrome
	Chemodectomas
	Tylosis with esophageal carcinoma

SOURCE: Compiled from Baylin 1978; Anderson 1978; Fraumeni 1973.

Table 1.4. *Some Hereditary Preneoplastic States*

Type	*Specific Disease*
Hamartomatous syndromes	Neurofibromatosis
	Tuberous sclerosis
	von Hippel-Lindau disease
	Peutz-Jeghers syndrome
Genodermatoses	Xeroderma pigmentosum
	Giant pigmented hairy nevus syndrome
	Kaposi's sarcoma
	Albinism
	Werner's syndrome
	De Sanctis-Cacchione syndrome
	Epidermolysis bullosa dystrophica
Chromosome breakage disorders	Bloom's syndrome
	Fanconi's syndrome
	Louis-Bar syndrome (ataxia telangiectasia)
Immune deficiency syndromes	Di George syndrome
	Wiskott-Aldrich syndrome
	Bruton-type agammaglobulinemia
	Swiss-type agammaglobulinemia
	Chédiak-Higashi syndrome

SOURCE: Compiled from Fraumeni 1973; Lynch and Frichot 1978.

disposed to cancer may be identified through family studies, recognition of associated anomalies, or follow-up of patients with a previous cancer. Appropriate clinical examinations may lead to early detection, and research studies may reveal predisposing genetic markers or early cellular changes (Strong 1977).

Virtually all hereditary cancers and precancerous diseases have early age of onset, a marked excess of bilateral occurrence in paired organs (breasts, kidneys, adrenals, thyroids, acoustic neuromas), multiple primary or multicentric development in increased incidence in nonpaired organs, and vertical transmission in consecutive generations of families with segregation patterns consistent with autosomal-dominant inheritance (Lynch et al. 1979).

Many forms of human cancer tend to occur in families. An interesting chromosomal study of hereditary renal cell carcinoma with inherited karyotypic abnormalities was described in 10 members of one family over three consecutive generations (Cohen et al. 1979). The disease produced symptoms in the proband and six relatives, and was found by screening in three other asymptomatic family members.

Part of the value of understanding hereditary cancers is to devise ways to prevent or cure them. Equally important is to provide genetic counseling to families who know or suspect that there may be a defect in one of their offspring or who want to avoid a pregnancy that will result in tragedy (Lynch and Lynch 1978), or to prevent a person from growing up unaware of an existing or potential hereditary lesion that will become disabling or will be passed genetically. Tables 1.3 and 1.4 provide some background to the range of genetically associated neoplasms.

Tobacco

There is no doubt that the use of tobacco, primarily in smoking cigarettes, is by far the single most important known cause of preventable cancer in the United States today. In spite of the well-financed campaign to the contrary and statements of paid tobacco company medical consultants, evidence is scientifically sound and has been verified by numerous independent investigators from all parts of the world. If I had ever had any doubt about it, the experience of my own practice has convinced me. Of the more than 500 patients with primary cancer of the lung whom I have personally attended, the nonsmokers accounted for less than 5%. Of the more than 60 patients with cancer of the larynx and esophagus seen by me, only 2 were nonsmokers. The conclusion is inescapable.

The consequences of smoking are overwhelming. About 350,000 people in this country die each year from diseases attributable in part or entirely to smoking (Interagency Task Force 1979). Approximately 75% of the excess mortality experienced by cigarette smokers is caused by coronary artery disease, cancer of the lung and other sites, and chronic obstructive pulmonary disease. The evidence suggests a dose-response relationship because excess mortality rises with increasing cigarette consumption and is greatest for those who start at an early age. Hence the effort to reduce or eliminate smoking by adolescents is important (Wynder and Hoffman 1979). The excess mortality for women is less than that for men because there is a 20- to 25-year latent period, but female mortality from lung cancer is rising rapidly. Ironically, the cigarette commercial directed to women has been prophetic: "You've come a long way, baby," from almost no lung cancer (4.4 deaths per 100,000) in 1950 to rapidly accelerating numbers (10.3 per 100,000) in 1975 (Silverberg and Holleb 1975). Estimates for 1980 are 117,000 new cases of lung cancer (85,000 men and 32,000 women) with 101,300 deaths (74,800 men and 26,500 women) (Garfinkel, Poindexter, and Silverberg 1980). The average male cigarette smoker's risk of developing lung cancer is 10 times greater than that of the nonsmoker. In heavy smokers, the risk is 15 to 30 times as great as that of nonsmokers. The risk of developing lung cancer diminishes with cessation of smoking (Holbrook 1977).

When smoking is combined with certain other agents there is a synergistic effect in carcinogenesis. There is a sevenfold increase in lung cancer deaths among asbestos insulation workers who smoke cigarettes (Selikoff, Hammond, and Churg 1968). There is little if any asbestos-induced excess lung cancer among nonsmokers, although asbestos exposure greatly enhances the risk of mesothelioma while smoking does not. Cigarette smoking also increases the risk of lung cancer for uranium miners. It is probable that a large proportion of human cancers have a multiple factorial etiology. The exposure to a cocarcinogen or an agent that inhibits a defense mechanism may make the difference as to whether the disease will or will not occur. Therefore the search for causes cannot be confined to looking for frank carcinogens alone, but must evaluate promoters of many kinds that are called cocarcinogens.

In addition to cancer of the lung, smoking cigarettes, pipes, and cigars is a significant factor in the development of cancer of the oral cavity, pharynx, larynx, and esophagus. Pipe-smoking appears to be causally related to cancer of the lip. The combined exposure to alcohol and cigarettes is associated with an especially high incidence of esophageal, oral, and pharyngeal malignancy. Cancer of the pancreas and bladder are also more common in cigarette smokers than in nonsmokers. Indeed, for neoplasms of the lower respiratory tract, the risk for both sexes is almost double for those who smoked heavily and inhaled. In a study by Cole, Hoover, and Friedell (1971) none of the excess risk of bladder cancer associated with cigarette smoking is explained by any indirect association with occupational experience. We do know from other data that beta-naphthylamine, benzidine, 4-aminobiphenyl, and cyclophosphamide cause bladder cancer in some patients, and beta-naphthylamine is a constituent of cigarette smoke.

Tobacco smoke in the environment may produce significant atmospheric pollution. Although there is no evidence as yet that cancer is induced in nonsmokers by such exposure, there are data to show that under conditions of heavy smoking and poor ventilation, the maximum limit for an eight-hour work exposure (50 ppm) may be exceeded. Air contaminated by cigarette smoke may be especially harmful to persons with coronary artery disease or chronic obstructive pulmonary disease, and the carbon monoxide may reduce exercise tolerance of patients with angina pectoris.

Radiation

The awesome power of nuclear energy was convincingly demonstrated in 1945 at Hiroshima and Nagasaki. Extensive studies by the United States Atomic Bomb Casualty Commission of the survivors of those bombs have been published. They show a causal relationship to the development of acute and chronic myeloid leukemia, acute lymphocytic leukemia, lymphoma, multiple myeloma, and thyroid carcinoma, among others. Some radiation-associated neoplasms are shown in table 1.5.

Table 1.5. *Radiation-Associated Malignancies*

Type	*Circumstance of Illness*
Acute and chronic myeloid leukemia	A-bomb survivors; irradiation for spondylitis or polycythemia vera; thorotrast; radiologists
Acute lymphatic leukemia	A-bomb survivors; thymus or prenatal irradiation
Lymphoma	A-bomb survivors; irradiation for spondylitis
Hodgkin's disease	A-bomb survivors
Multiple myeloma	Radiologists; A-bomb survivors; irradiation for spondylitis
Aplastic anemia and myelofibrosis	A-bomb survivors; radiologists; irradiation for spondylitis and polycythemia vera; thorotrast and radium
Skin squamous cell carcinoma	Radiologists
Osteosarcoma and osteochondroma	Radium ingestion; external irradiation
Thyroid	External irradiation; A-bomb survivors
Lung carcinoma	Uranium and radium miners
Breast carcinoma	External irradiation

SOURCE: Compiled from Upton 1973; Interagency Task Force 1979.

Prominent by virtue of its absence in that table is chronic lymphocytic leukemia. This is significant because the public has become frightened of nuclear power and sometimes perceives dangers that may not exist. A recent example was a three-quarter page story in the New Haven *Register* of November 3, 1980, recounting the misfortune of a World War II veteran whose leukemia was caused by "radiation from atomic bomb tests he was allegedly ordered to observe in 1943 and 1944." Aside from the fact that there is no evidence of any atomic explosion anywhere before July 16, 1945, the story does not reveal until near the end that the patient died from chronic lymphocytic leukemia (CLL). There is no reliable medical or scientific evidence to show an association between ionizing radiation exposure and CLL, yet the reader is left with the impression that this is another victim of nuclear energy exposure.

It is devoutly hoped that there will never be another nuclear explosion to which people are exposed. The discussions about preparing for evacuation of cities and other civilian defense measures seem unrealistic in view of the fact that a nuclear war will not leave enough people alive in the area of detonation to make much difference. Those who do not succumb to the trauma of the blast or the incineration of the fireball that follows, will be debilitated and later die of the excessive radiation exposure with its resulting anemia, leukopenia, thrombocytopenia, and so forth long before they develop cancer.

The real problem is to evaluate the dangers, real or apparent, of low-dose radiation to which we are all exposed. Then we will have a basis for decision making in medical practice and public policy.

Since ancient times, people have been exposed to some radiation, from cosmic rays, emissions from terrestrial stone and water, and ingested isotopes. We measure the dose in rad (radiation-absorbed dose) or rem (roentgen-equivalent-man). Those who live in New York City have an approximate annual background radiation exposure to the gonads of 124 mrem (millirem, one one-thousandth of a rem), while those in Denver have a gonadal exposure of 226 mrem because of the higher elevation (more cosmic ray exposure) and the surrounding mountains (more terrestrial radiation). Radioactive fallout is about the same in the two locales. On the average in the United States, background radiation accounts for a little more than 50% of our exposure, and another 40% is derived from diagnostic x-rays and isotopes. Precise figures are not available and estimates from prestigious sources vary somewhat, as can be seen by comparing tables 1.6 and 1.7.

Nuclear Testing and Energy Plants

Radioactive fallout from nuclear tests creates about 3% of radiation exposure. Most fallout comes from atmospheric weapons testing prior to 1963, but many of the isotopes have long half-lives. China and India are still conducting atmospheric tests of nuclear weapons, and winds carry the fallout all over the world.

The greatest concern about exposure and its consequences followed the March 1979 accident at the Three Mile Island reactor. The available information seems to indicate that there was a negligible release of radioactivity and that there apparently will be no medical consequences. It has been estimated that the two million people in the area may have had an incremental radiation

Table 1.6. *Estimated Annual Average Genetically Significant Dose Equivalents (DE) of Environmental Radiation Exposure*

Source		*DE (mrem/yr)*
Natural radiation		
Cosmic radiation		28
Radionuclides in body		28
External terrestrial		26
	Subtotal	82
Man-made radiation		
Medical and dental x-rays		20
Radiopharmaceuticals		2 to 4
Commercial nuclear power		1 or less
Weapons testing fallout		4 to 5
Consumer products (TV, etc.)		4 to 5
Air travel		0.5
	Subtotal	31.5 to 35.5
	Total (rounded)	120

SOURCE: BEIR III 1980.

Table 1.7. *Estimated Annual Whole-Body Radiation Dose to the United States Population*

Source of Radiation		*Average Dose (mrem/year)*
Natural		
Environmental		
Cosmic		40
Terrestrial		40
Internal radioactive isotopes		20
	Subtotal	100
Man-made		
Environmental		
Global fallout (1975)		4
Nuclear power plants		0.023
Medical		
Diagnostic x-rays		72
Radiopharmaceuticals		1
Occupational		0.8
Miscellaneous		2
	Subtotal	80
	Total	180

SOURCE: American Cancer Society 1980b.

exposure of 1.75 mrem (Gray 1979). Then Secretary of the Department of Health, Education, and Welfare Califano estimated that over the next 20 years this would result in only one additional case of cancer. Shortly thereafter, newspaper headlines indicated that the estimate was off by 50% to 100%. Even if the estimate was incorrect by 1000%, in a population of two million persons with an expected 3800 deaths per year from cancer, how could one detect the incremental difference between 1 or 10 extra deaths among the 76,000 persons who are expected to die from the disease in that period unrelated to the nuclear accident?

Similar problems occur with other reports in the literature of low-level radiation exposure. A study of radioactive fallout in Utah from the Nevada bomb testing suggested that in the period studied, in the counties experiencing high fallout there was greater mortality from childhood leukemia in the high-exposure cohort as compared to the low-exposure cohort (Lyon et al. 1979). The implication is that radioactive fallout caused a temporary rise in mortality from childhood leukemia in the affected areas of the state. A critical editorial (Land 1979) pointed out that in the same time-place frame, that study demonstrated a decrease in mortality from other childhood cancers. It seems unlikely that radioactive fallout caused both an increase in leukemia mortality and a decrease in deaths from other childhood cancers. It is more likely that there is another explanation, probably chance.

A similar report indicates that nine cases of leukemia occurred among 3224 men who participated in military maneuvers during the 1957 nuclear test explosion, "Smoky." This represents a significant increase over the expected incidence of 3.5 cases. They included four patients with acute myelocytic leukemia, three with chronic myelocytic leukemia, and one each with hairy cell and acute lymphocytic leukemia (Caldwell, Kelly, and Heath 1980). The exposure in this report was to one-half rad, and the authors noted the difficulty of reaching conclusions from their data. An accompanying editorial (Bond and Hamilton 1980) pointed out that it is generally agreed that we cannot expect more than a total of one cancer in a population of 10,000 people exposed to 1 rad each. For leukemia, the corresponding figure is about one additional case in 50,000 people exposed to 1 rad. Thus studies with small doses and small populations can shed no clear light on the risk of cancer induction by low-level radiation. Several separate studies, each inadequate to demonstrate quantitative relationships betwee dose and response, do not override the few large, statistically valid studies from which risk estimates are now derived.

In addition to the worries of carcinogenesis from nuclear fallout, the public has been concerned about the consequences of exposure from nuclear power generating plants. There seems to be no evidence of any significant risk from the 75 nuclear energy plants now in operation in the United States as they are now functioning. According to Ahrens and associates (1980), the problem of nuclear waste disposal is a minor technical problem but a major political one.

Diagnostic Procedures

Mammography has been shown to be a valuable diagnostic procedure in the early detection of breast cancer. It was coming into widespread use when a report suggested that more cancer might be induced through mammography than would be found by it (Bailar 1976). Promptly thereafter, use of the procedure declined. Subsequently, it has been realized that exposure doses were far in excess of those produced in modern xeromammography. The concern, however, did serve as a stimulus for a consensus conference (National Cancer Institute 1978). Both the conference and later the American Cancer Society (1980a) agreed that mammography screening below age 50 years did not reduce breast cancer mortality and did produce unnecessary radiation exposure.

The question of carcinogenesis by diagnostic radiation has been difficult to evaluate. As leukemias tend to occur soonest, becoming evident within 2 to 4 years of exposure and reaching a peak within the first 10 years (Upton 1979), it is the logical first place to look for the hazards of diagnostic ionizing radiation. In a study conducted at the Mayo Clinic (Linos et al. 1980), the effect of diagnostic and low-level therapeutic radiation (less than 300 rad to the bone marrow) on the development of leukemia was investigated. During the study, 138 patients with leukemia (representing all known incidence of leukemia in residents of Olmsted County, Minnesota, between 1955 and 1974) were each matched with two controls, and the lifelong experiences of both groups with regard to diagnostic and therapeutic radiation were ascertained. No statistically significant increase was found in the risk of developing leukemia after radiation doses of 0 to 300 rad to the bone marrow when these amounts were administered in small doses over long periods of time, as in routine medical care. Reassuring as this may be, it does not prove that there is no danger from diagnostic radiation. In a critical letter to the editor, Jablon (1980) pointed out that among the 75 cases of lymphocytic leukemia, 46 were CLL and therefore irrelevant.

The problem of estimating cancer risks from low doses of ionizing radiation is far from solved. Disagreements about the somatic risks stem from two difficulties fundamental to the logic of inference from observed data. First, precise direct estimation of small risks requires impracticably large samples. Second, precise estimates of low-dose risks based largely on high-dose data, for which the sample size requirements are more easily satisfied, must depend heavily on assumptions about the shape of the dose-response curve, even when only a few of the parameters of the theoretical form of the curve are known.

Thyroid Cancer and Radiation

An association of thyroid carcinoma with external radiation is now well accepted, but so far there is no convincing evidence that radioactive iodine therapy produces thyroid carcinoma (Holm et al. 1980). Shortly after the turn of the century, treatment with radiation of enlarged thymus glands became popular. Later, radiation was used to treat tonsils and adenoids that were enlarged. The profession was finally alerted to the dangers of this irradiation by a report of 28 cases of cancer of the thyroid in children (Duffy and Fitzgerald 1950), of which 9 were in children who had thymic irradiation between the fourth and eighteenth months of life. In a large series, 2872 patients who had radiation in the general area of the thyroid were compared to their 5005 nonirradiated siblings, and a clear association of cancer with radiation was documented. Of 76 lesions, 24 were found to be malignant in the study group. More than half of these occurred among the 10% treated with much larger than average x-ray dosages by a single radiologist. None was observed in sibling controls (Hempelmann et al. 1975). It is now clear that irradiated patients have an increased incidence of benign adenomas and carcinomas primarily of the papillary and mixed papillary-follicular types. Although not numerous in most studies of irradiated patients, follicular carcinoma is also more common (Stockwell 1979).

Based on the foregoing risk factors, the National Cancer Institute (NCI) (1977) has recommended a follow-up program for patients in three categories:

1. Patients with no visible or palpable abnormalities should be reevaluated every two years.
2. Patients with a discrete nodule or nodules should have them surgically removed.
3. Patients with diffuse enlargement of the gland but without a palpable nodule require additional study.

If thyroid function is normal, a technetium or iodine scan is indicated, and possibly a needle biopsy. If the scan shows no abnormal uptake, thyroid suppressive therapy should be started to shrink the hypertrophied tissue, and the patient should be reexamined in six months. If a nodule is palpable at that time it should be surgically removed. If no nodule is detected, thyroid suppression may be continued indefinitely and the patient reexamined annually. If the scan shows a definite area of no uptake, thyroid suppression may be initiated and the gland reevaluated in six months. If a nodule is detected, it should be surgically removed.

It is now becoming clear that there is always a risk to diagnostic radiation and that it must be kept to the minimum consistent with good medical care, balancing potential risk against potential benefit. When skillfully done, the risk is acceptable. Therapeutic radiation, on the other hand, has a great potential for good or evil, and should be used only for the treatment of malignant disease. There is no place for radiation therapy of dermatologic or inflammatory lesions. In addition, it should be administered only by those trained and skillful in its use.

Chemical Carcinogens

It is a little more than 200 years since Percival Pott described the high incidence of scrotal cancer among the chimney sweeps of London and correctly attributed the cause of the disease to continual contact with coal tar. That description began the field of chemical carcinogenesis, which is probably the major cause of cancer today. The carcinogens are both natural and man-made, but the former do not seem to be increasing, while people are rapidly synthesizing new ones (Heidelberger 1977).

It is important to realize that most chemical carcinogens require metabolic activation by drug-metabolizing enzymes to chemically reactive forms that are the ultimate carcinogens (Miller 1970). In general, these metabolically activated forms are all electrophilic. They seek out negatively charged regions in target molecules and form strong covalent chemical bonds with cellular macromolecules such as DNA, RNA, and proteins. Activation frequently proceeds by N-hydroxylation (aromatic amines) or epoxides (polycyclic hydrocarbons, benzo(a)pyrene, aflatoxin). Of the powerful carcinogenic chemicals, only a few do not require metabolic activation, such as some alkylating agents and nitrosamines.

Some carcinogens are inactive alone and depend on another agent as a cofactor or cocarcinogen to induce neoplasia. This was first demonstrated in murine skin (Berenblum and Shubnik 1949) but has been shown to be a widespread mechanism in many species in a great variety of situations.

Cell culture systems are now available for studies of the cellular and molecular mechanisms of chemical carcinogenesis without the complications of nutritional and immunologic constraints of whole animals. The *Salmonella*-microsome mutagenicity test (Ames, McCann, and Yamasaki 1975) is a quick and promising test for environmental mutagens that correlates fairly well with carcinogens. There is still a need for a validated cell culture-malignant transformation system for the prescreening of environmental carcinogens.

The proliferation of literature on carcinogenesis remains active (Griffin and Shaw 1979; Epstein 1979; Doll 1978; Wynder 1978; Ryser 1971; Miller 1978; Schottenfeld and Haas 1979). In a series of monographs, the various agencies of the federal government have tried to keep abreast of the burgeoning information with valuable general summaries (Toxic Substance Strategy Committee 1980; National Toxicology Program 1980) and also reviews of specific substances like benzene (National Institute for Occupational Safety and Health 1974) and asbestos (Levine 1978). Many additional publications are available. The 18 chemicals pinpointed as carcinogens are shown in table 1.8, and the 8 drugs in table 1.9. Obviously, there are a great many more chemicals and drugs suspected of being carcinogens, but it will take time to confirm or deny the association.

Of the carcinogens listed, only aflatoxin is abundant in nature. It is produced by some types of fungi that grow on food where high temperatures and high humidity favor their formation. Grains, peanuts, cotton seed meal, and oil are among the more common substrates for the growth of these fungi. Meat, eggs, and milk of livestock that consume aflatoxin-contaminated feed may also contain them. Significant levels are found in some parts of Africa and Asia that have a high incidence of liver cancer.

Asbestos is widely used in industry and construction for insulation of various kinds. Not only are the workers at risk, but their families are also exposed by fibers adhering to clothing that is brought home from work. Occupational inhalation of asbestos increases the incidence of lung cancer. As previously noted, the effect is enhanced in those workers who also smoke cigarettes. Asbestos exposure also causes mesotheliomas of the pleural and peritoneal cavities (Selikoff and Hammond 1978).

Benzene is widely used in industry, especially as a solvent and as a base for the manufacture of other chemicals. It is frequently added to gasoline in a concentration up to 4%. Inhalation exposure can lead to aplastic

Table 1.8. *Carcinogenic Substances in Humans*

Chemical	*Target Organ(s)*
Aflatoxins	Liver
4-Aminobiphenyl	Bladder
Arsenic compounds	Skin, lung
Asbestos	Lung and pleura
Auramine	Bladder
Benzene	Bone marrow
Benzidine	Bladder
Bis(chloro-methyl)ether	Lung
Cadmium compounds	Prostate, lung
Chloromethyl methyl ether	Lung
Chromium compounds	Lung
Hematite and iron oxide	Lung
Isopropyl oils	Nasal sinuses, lung
2-Naphthylamine	Bladder
Nickel compounds	Nasal cavity, lung
N, N-bis(2-chloroethyl) 2-napthylamine	Bladder
Soot and tars	Lung, skin (scrotum)
Vinyl chloride	Liver, brain, lung

SOURCE: National Toxicology Program 1980.

anemia, which can not only be fatal in itself, but can go on to leukemia if the patient survives the aplastic state. I have seen three patients with aplastic anemia caused by benzene and all had a stormy course with it but eventually survived. They are now apprehensively waiting to see if they will develop leukemia as a late sequel.

Benzidine has been extensively used in industry, but for many years was also used in clinical laboratories as a test for occult blood. Its use is being phased out both in the dye and chemical industries and in clinical laboratories now that its association with bladder cancer has been fully appreciated.

The carcinogenic drugs are worth a special mention because physicians regulate their use (Weisburger et al. 1975). Chloramphenicol is a simple antibiotic that was synthesized soon after its discovery. It has a broad spectrum of activity. Its propensity to cause aplastic anemia was discovered early but it was widely used by physicians in total disregard of that knowledge. It was heavily promoted by the manufacturer and was frequently used by infectious disease specialists who claimed that they never saw a case of aplastic anemia. As the incidence was 1 in 24,500 to 1 in 227,000 patients, they were probably telling the truth. Curiously, most

Table 1.9. *Carcinogenic Drugs in Humans*

Drug	*Target Organ(s)*
Chloramphenicol	Bone marrow
Cyclophosphamide	Bladder, bone marrow
Diethylstilbestrol	Endometrium, vagina
Melphalan	Bone marrow
Mustard gas	Lung
Oxymetholone	Liver
Phenacetin	Kidney, pelvis
Phenytoin	Lymph nodes

SOURCE: National Toxicology Program 1980.

cases of aplastic anemia did not occur with high-dose parenteral therapy in serious infections, but with low-dose oral or topical therapy for trivial infections. But they did occur, and hematologists saw them — more than 1000 reported cases. I personally saw eight such cases, and only three survived the aplastic anemia to remain at risk for a later leukemia.

Cyclophosphamide is an alkylating agent with a broad spectrum of activity in cancer. It is also immunosuppressive. It and its metabolic products are excreted in the urine and present a danger of sterile cystitis with prolonged exposure. A few cases of bladder carcinoma have been reported. I had one in my practice that I did not report. Many other physicians probably had one and did not report it. Some cases of leukemia have also been reported, as one might expect with an alkylating agent. So far, I have personally seen the development of leukemia in two patients from cyclophosphamide. I think the drug should be used only for cancer or other life-threatening conditions. Its use for the treatment of benign disorders such as arthritis should be reevaluated.

Diethylstilbestrol (DES) is a synthetic estrogenic substance that is widely used both for endocrine effects and in the treatment of breast and prostate carcinoma. At one time it was frequently prescribed for patients with threatened abortion. Many of the female offspring of those patients later developed clear cell adenocarcinoma of the vagina and cervix, with an incidence a little less than 1 per 1000 (Herbst 1980). The data supporting a role for DES in the causation of endometrial carcinoma are suggestive (Weiss and Sayvetz 1980) but not conclusive.

Melphalan is an alkylating agent used in the management of multiple myeloma, and ovarian and breast cancer. Recently there have been several reports of acute myelogenous leukemia associated with its use. After many years of not seeing such a case, I have had three tragedies in my own practice with women who chose to have single-agent adjuvant oral chemotherapy rather than the three- or five-drug regimen recommended, with its frequent intravenous injections. I no longer allow that option in my practice; new patients who insist on melphalan for adjuvant chemotherapy of the breast will have to go to another physician. The role of the agent in ovarian carcinoma is being reevaluated. In multiple myeloma it is presently well established, and is the drug against which all new ones must be compared.

Oxymetholone is an anabolic steroid used widely at one time for the treatment of aplastic anemia. In 1972, the Food and Drug Administration dropped its approval of this indication on the grounds of lack of efficacy. Oxymetholone has been reported to cause malignant liver tumors and blood cysts that could hemorrhage.

Phenacetin was used for many years in combinations for the treatment of pain and fever. It was initially associated with development of nephritis and later, renal pelvic tumors. There seems to be no reason to use it.

Phenytoin was called diphenylhydantoin for many years and is best known by its trade name Dilantin. It is the most widely used drug for the treatment of epilepsy and other seizure disorders. Several case reports and epidemiologic studies have found an increased incidence of malignant lymphomas in epileptics who were treated with this drug. I had one such patient whose biopsy was initially read as pseudolymphoma, but the course of her disease was clearly that of a nodular lymphocytic lymphoma that later progressed to a diffuse histiocytic type and death.

No discussion of carcinogenesis would be complete without mentioning diet (Berg 1976; Wynder 1979). The available data are so far fascinating but inconclusive. They are epidemiologic but sketchy and speculative, except as they involve agents already discussed, such as aflatoxin, DES, or chloramphenicol in food. Even the removal of saccharine from the market has its scientific proponents and detractors (Morrison and Buring 1980; Hoover 1980).

What is the future of regulation for these carcinogens? In the United States, statutes are largely motivated by the ideal of absolute safety at all costs. There is no requirement for risk-benefit assessment. Bias is inherent in the prescribed bioassays. Test findings may have restricted meaning within the specific experiments but cannot be translated into quantitative assessment of human risk. Such data are improperly used in resolving regulatory questions case by case (Gori 1980). Perhaps what we need is a system of relative standards based on tolerable risk or safety compared to anticipated benefits (Dinman 1980). Substances intended for a certain use would then be regulated according to those standards.

We are making progress. We are learning what causes some cancers and what we can do to make changes. We have very much more to learn scientifically and then to translate that knowledge into responsible medical decisions and public policy.

References

Ahrens, R. et al. Radiation risks from nuclear power exaggerated. *N. Engl. J. Med.* 302:1205–1206, 1980.

American Cancer Society. ACS report on the cancer-related health checkup. *CA* 30:194–240, 1980a.

American Cancer Society. Background paper on radiation and cancer (data from A. C. Upton). New York: American Cancer Society, 1980b.

Ames, B. N.; McCann, J.; and Yamasaki, E. Methods for detecting carcinogens and mutagens with *Salmonella*-microsome mutagenicity test. *Mutat. Res.* 51:347–364, 1975.

Anderson, D. E. Familial cancer and cancer families. *Semin. Oncol.* 5:11–16, 1978.

Bailar, J. C., III. Mammography: a contrary view. *Ann. Intern. Med.* 84:77–84, 1976.

Baylin, S. B. The multiple endocrine neoplasia syndromes: implications for the study of inherited tumors. *Semin. Oncol.* 5:35–45, 1978.

BEIR III (Committee on Biologic Effects of Ionizing Radiation). *The effects on populations of exposure to low levels of ionizing radiation.* Washington, D.C.: National Academy of Sciences, 1980.

Berenblum, I., and Shubnik, P. The persistence of latent tumor cells in the mouse's skin by single application of 9,10-demethyl-1,2-benzanthracene. *Br. J. Cancer* 3:384–386, 1949.

Berg, J. W. Nutrition and cancer. *Semin. Oncol.* 3:17–23, 1976.

Bishop, J. M. The molecular biology of RNA tumor viruses: a physician's guide. *N. Engl. J. Med.* 303: 675–682, 1980.

Bittner, J. J. Some possible effects of nursing on mammary gland tumor incidence in mice. *Science* 84:162–163, 1936.

Bond, V. P., and Hamilton, L. D. Leukemia in the Nevada "Smoky" bomb test (editorial). *JAMA* 244:1610, 1980.

Caldwell, G. G.; Kelly, D. B.; and Heath, C. W., Jr. Leukemia among participants in military maneuvers at a nuclear bomb test. *JAMA* 244:1575–1578, 1980.

Cohen, A. J. et al. Hereditary renal-cell carcinoma associated with a chromosomal translocation. *N. Engl. J. Med.* 301:592–595, 1979.

Cole, P.; Hoover, R.; and Friedell, G. H. Occupation and cancer of the lower urinary tract. *Cancer* 29:1250–1260, 1971.

Dinman, B. D. The reality and acceptance of risk. *JAMA* 244:1226–1228, 1980.

Doll, R. An epidemiological perspective of the biology of cancer. *Cancer Res.* 38:3573–3583, 1978.

Duffy, B. J., and Fitzgerald, P. J. Cancer of the thyroid in children: a report of 28 cases. *J. Clin. Endocrinol.* 10:1296–1308, 1950.

Ellermann, V., and Bang, O. Experimentelle leukämie bie hühnern. *Zentbl. Bakt. Parasitkde,* Abt. I. Oori, 46:595–609, 1908.

Epstein, S. S. *The politics of cancer.* Garden City, N.Y.: Anchor Press, 1979.

Fischer, D. S. Viruses and cancer. *Yale Scientific* 39:16–19, 1964.

Fraumeni, J. F., Jr. Genetic factors. In *Cancer medicine,* eds. J. F. Holland and E. Frei III. Philadelphia: Lea & Febiger, 1973, pp. 7–15.

Fraumeni, J. F., Jr., ed. *Persons at high risk of cancer: an approach to cancer etiology and control.* New York: Academic Press, 1975.

Garfinkel, L.; Poindexter, C. E.; and Silverberg, E. Cancer statistics, 1980. *CA* 30:23–38, 1980.

German, J. *Chromosomes and cancer.* New York: John Wiley & Sons, 1974.

Goepp, C. E., ed. Heredity and cancer. *Semin. Oncol.* 5:1–118, 1978.

Gori, G. B. The regulation of carcinogenic hazards. *Science* 208:256–261, 1980.

Gray, J. E. The radiation hazard—let's put it in perspective. *Mayo Clin. Proc.* 54:809–811, 1979.

Griffin, A. C., and Shaw, C. R., eds. *Carcinogens: identification and mechanisms of action.* New York: Raven Press, 1979.

Hammond, E. C. The epidemiological approach to the etiology of cancer. *Cancer* 35:652–654, 1975.

Harris, C. C. et al. Individual differences in cancer susceptibility. *Ann. Intern. Med.* 92:809–825, 1980.

Heidelberger, C. Chemical carcinogenesis. *Cancer* 40: 430–433, 1977.

Hempelmann, L. H. et al. Neoplasms in persons treated with x-rays in infancy: fourth survey in 20 years. *J. Natl. Cancer Inst.* 55:519–530, 1975.

Henderson, B. E. et al. Risk factors associated with nasopharyngeal carcinoma. *N. Engl. J. Med.* 295: 1101–1106, 1976.

Henle, W., and Henle, G. Epstein-Barr virus and human malignancies. *Cancer* 34:1368–1374, 1974.

Herbst, A. L. DES update. *CA* 30:326–332, 1980.

Hiatt, H. H.; Watson, J. D.; and Winsten, J. A., eds. *Origins of human cancer.* Cold Spring Harbor, N.Y.: Cold Spring Harbor Laboratory, 1977.

Holbrook. J. H. Tobacco and health. *CA* 27:344–353, 1977.

Holm, L-E. et al. Malignant thyroid tumors after iodine 131 therapy: a retrospective cohort study. *N. Engl. J. Med.* 303:188–191, 1980.

Hoover, R. Saccharin—bitter aftertaste. *N. Engl. J. Med.* 302:573–575, 1980.

Interagency Task Force. *The health effects of ionizing radiation: report of work group on science.* Washington, D. C.: U.S. Department of Health, Education, and Welfare, 1979.

Jablon, S. Low-dose radiation and leukemia. *N. Engl. J. Med.* 303:814, 1980.

Klein, G. The Epstein-Barr virus and neoplasia. *N. Engl. J. Med.* 293:1353–1357, 1975.

Knudson, A. F., Jr. Genetics and cancer. *Am. J. Med.* 69:1–3, 1980.

Land, C. E. The hazards of fallout or of epidemiological research? *N. Engl. J. Med.* 300:431–432, 1979.

Land, C. E. Estimating cancer risks from low doses of ionizing radiation. *Science* 209:1197–1203, 1980.

Levine, R. J., ed. *Asbestos: an information resource* (NIH) 78-1681. Washington, D.C.: U.S. Department of Health, Education, and Welfare, 1978.

Lilienfeld, A. M.; Pedersen, E.; and Dowd, J. E. *Cancer epidemiology: methods of study.* Baltimore: Johns Hopkins Press, 1967.

Linos, A. et al. Low-dose radiation and leukemia. *N. Engl. J. Med.* 302:1101–1105, 1980.

Lucké, B. A neoplastic disease of the kidney of the frog, *Rana pipens. Am. J. Cancer* 20:352–379, 1934.

Lynch, H. T. et al. Hereditary cancer: ascertainment and management. *CA* 29:216–232, 1979.

Lynch, H. T., and Frichot, B. C., III. Skin, heredity, and cancer. *Semin. Oncol.* 5:67–84, 1978.

Lynch, P. M., and Lynch, H. T. Genetic counseling of high-risk cancer patients: jurisprudential considerations. *Semin. Oncol.* 5:107–118, 1978.

Lyon, J. L. et al. Childhood leukemias associated with fallout from nuclear testing. *N. Engl. J. Med.* 300:397–402, 1979.

Miller, E. C. Some current perspectives on chemical carcinogenesis in humans and experimental animals: presidential address. *Cancer Res.* 38:1479–1496, 1978.

Miller, J. A. Carcinogenesis by chemicals; an overview. *Cancer Res.* 30:559–576, 1970.

Moore, D. H. et al. Some aspects of the search for human mammary tumor virus. *Cancer* 28:1415–1424, 1971.

Morrison, A. S., and Buring, J. E. Artificial sweeteners and cancer of the lower urinary tract. *N. Engl. J. Med.* 302:537–541, 1980.

Mulvihill, J. J.; Miller, R. W.; and Fraumeni, J. F., Jr., eds. *Genetics of human cancer.* New York: Raven Press, 1977.

National Cancer Institute. *Irradiation-related thyroid cancer,* (NIH) 77-1120. Washington, D.C.: U.S. Department of Health, Education, and Welfare, 1977.

National Cancer Institute. National Institutes of Health—National Cancer Institute consensus development meeting on breast cancer screening: issues and recommendations. *J. Natl. Cancer Inst.* 60:1519–1521, 1978.

National Institute for Occupational Safety and Health. *Occupational exposure to benzene,* (NIOSH) 74-137. Washington, D.C.: U.S. Department of Health, Education, and Welfare, 1974.

National Toxicology Program. *First annual report on carcinogens.* Washington, D.C.: U.S. Department of Health and Human Services, 1980.

Robbins, J. H. et al. Xeroderma pigmentosum: an inherited disease with sun sensitivity, multiple cutaneous neoplasms, and abnormal DNA repair. *Ann. Intern. Med.* 80:221–248, 1974.

Robinson, J. E. et al. Diffuse polyclonal B-cell lymphoma during primary infection with Epstein-Barr virus. *N. Engl. J. Med.* 302:1293–1297, 1980.

Rous, P. A sarcoma of the fowl transmissible by an agent separable from the tumor cells. *J. Exp. Med.* 13:397–411, 1911.

Ryser, H. J. P. Chemical carcinogenesis. *N. Engl. J. Med.* 284:721–734, 1971.

Schottenfeld, D. Epidemiology of breast cancer. *Clin. Bull.* 5:135–143, 1975.

Schottenfeld, D., and Haas, J. F. Carcinogens in the workplace. *CA* 29:144–168, 1979.

Schwartz, R. S. Epstein-Barr virus—oncogen or mitogen. *N. Engl. J. Med.* 302:1307–1308, 1980.

Selikoff, I., and Hammond, E. Asbestos-associated disease in United States shipyards. *CA* 28:87–99, 1978.

Selikoff, I.; Hammond, E.; and Churg, J. Asbestos exposure, smoking, and neoplasia. *JAMA* 204:106–112, 1968.

Shope, R. E. A filterable virus causing tumor-like condition in rabbits and its relationship to virus myxomatosum. *J. Exp. Med.* 56:803–822, 1932.

Shope, R. E. Infectious papillomatosis of rabbits. *J. Exp. Med.* 58:607–624, 1933.

Silverberg, E., and Holleb, A. I. Major trends in cancer: 25-year survey. *CA* 25:2–21, 1975.

Stockwell, R. M. Irradiation related thyroid cancer. *Conn. Med.* 43:63–67, 1979.

Strong, L. E. Genetic etiology of cancer. *Cancer* 40:438–444, 1977.

Toxic Substances Strategy Committee. *Toxic chemicals and public protection, a report to the President.* Washington, D.C.: U.S. Government Printing Office, 1980.

Upton, A. C. Radiation. In *Cancer medicine,* eds. J. F. Holland and E. Frei III. Philadelphia: Lea Febiger, 1973, pp. 90–101.

Upton, A. C. Low-level radiation. *CA* 29:306–315, 1979.

Weisburger, J. H. Mechanism of action of diet as a carcinogen. *Cancer* 43:1987–1995, 1979.

Weisburger, J. H. et al. The carcinogenic properties of some of the principal drugs used in clinical cancer chemotherapy. *Recent Results Cancer Res.* 52:1–17, 1975.

Weiss, N. S., and Sayvetz, T. A. Incidence of endometrial cancer in relation to the use of oral contraceptive. *N. Engl. J. Med.* 302:551–554, 1980.

Wynder, E. L. Environmental carcinogenesis. *Clin. Bull.* 8:3–9, 1978.

Wynder, E. L. Dietary habits and cancer epidemiology. *Cancer* 43:1955–1961, 1979.

Wynder, E. L., and Hoffmann, D. Tobacco and health: a societal challenge. *N. Engl. J. Med.* 300:894–903, 1979.

two

Detection and Screening

JOHN C. MARSH

Although research into prevention and therapy undoubtedly has played and will continue to play a significant role in improving survival from cancer, it is clear that a major factor is recognition that early disease has the maximum opportunity for cure, and that as an increased proportion of early lesions is found, the cure rate for a particular type of cancer increases. This has been most convincingly shown for malignancy of the breast and cervix, although studies from colorectal screening are beginning to bear fruit as well, in that increased numbers of early lesions (Dukes' A and B) are being reported in the study populations (Winawer 1980).

Unfortunately, there is no simple blood test that is useful in large-scale screening, although abnormalities in various types of established malignancies are often found. These include carcinoembryonic antigen (CEA), human chorionic gonadotropin (HCG), and alpha-fetoprotein (AFP). Until a useful screening blood or urine test becomes available, early detection of cancer must be based on knowledge of high-risk patients for a particular type of malignancy in the population under study, and use of tests that are safe, effective, and economically feasible.

A distinction has been and should be made regarding the detection of cancer in asymptomatic patients on an individual basis that is carried on typically by the practicing physician, the use of mass screening methods at public expense, and diagnostic methods in the patient with signs and symptoms suggestive of cancer (American Cancer Society 1980a). This chapter focuses on the first of these.

The individual physician, thinking about the problem of detection, should know which cancers have the greatest mortality. They are, in order for the entire population: cancer of the lung, colon and rectum, female breast, prostate, and pancreas; these cause about 60% of all deaths. Uterine cancer (cervix and endometrium combined) is the eighth leading cause of cancer death, ranking behind the five noted above, stomach cancer, and the leukemias (American Cancer Society 1980b).

When considering the individual, these population figures are only guidelines. Factors of age, sex, smoking habits, sexual activity, and family history help to define whether a given patient is in a high-risk or standard-risk category. The best-known example of a high-risk category for a specific malignancy is the habit of cigarette smoking for cancer of the lung.

There is no shortage of recommendations for procedures of early detection. These are in the form of guidelines from the American Cancer Society (1980a) (table 2.1), the Canadian Task Force on the Periodic Health Examination (1979), the Sidney Farber Cancer Institute (Hall and Wood 1979), and various consensus development conferences sponsored by the National Cancer Institute (Beahrs et al. 1977; Brodie 1979; Gordon 1979).

As might be expected, there are differences of opinion regarding the efficacy, safety, and cost-benefit ratio of early diagnostic maneuvers. The recently developed American Cancer Society guidelines (1980a)

Table 2.1. *Summary of American Cancer Society Recommendations for the Early Detection of Cancer in Asymptomatic Persons*

Test or Procedure	Population: Sex	Age	Frequency
Sigmoidoscopy	M, F	Over 50	Every 3–5 years (after 2 negative exams 1 year apart)
Stool guaiac slide test	M, F	Over 50	Every year
Digital rectal examination	M, F	Over 40	Every year
Pap test	F	20–65; under 20, if sexually active	At least every 3 years (after 2 negative exams 1 year apart)
Pelvic examination	F	20–40 Over 40	Every 3 years Every year
Endometrial tissue sample	F	At menopause; women at high risk*	At menopause
Breast self-examination	F	Over 20	Every month
Breast physical examination	F	20–40 Over 40	Every 3 years Every year
Mammography	F	Between 35–40 Under 50 Over 50	Baseline Consult personal physician Every year
Chest x-ray		Not recommended	
Sputum cytology		Not recommended	
Health counseling and cancer checkup†	M, F M, F	Over 20 Over 40	Every 3 years Every year

SOURCE: American Cancer Society 1980a.

*History of infertility, obesity, failure of ovulation, abnormal uterine bleeding, or estrogen therapy.

†To include examination for cancers of the thyroid, testicles, prostate, ovaries, lymph nodes, oral region, and skin.

are perhaps the most controversial because of their changes in long-standing policy with regard to the frequency of Pap smears and chest x-rays. Recommendations regarding the former have already been challenged publicly by the American College of Obstetricians and Gynecologists (1980). Clearly, individual physicians must practice in ways that will serve their patients most effectively according to their best judgments, subject to new information as it becomes available.

Lung Cancer

Bronchogenic carcinoma kills more Americans each year than any other kind of cancer. There is approximately 5% five-year survival, and most patients with any kind of symptoms caused by the disease are already beyond the hope of cure. Accordingly, attention must be focused on the asymptomatic high-risk individual in hopes of detecting the small lesion that is now the only kind of cancer that can be cured. Who is at high risk? Clearly, the majority of patients with lung cancer are cigarette smokers; the correlation has long been known. Pool (chapter 59) has estimated that 90% of lung cancer victims are at least 40 pack-year smokers. (Pack-years equal the product of packs smoked per day times the number of years of smoking.) Although attention has focused on men in screening programs this is no longer appropriate, as the incidence of lung cancer in women is increasing geometrically, probably related to their smoking habits. Lung cancer is fairly uncommon under the age of 40 years, with a peak age incidence at age 55. Other risk factors are urban dwelling, uranium mining, coke manufacturing, and working in the petroleum and asbestos industries; these are relatively insignificant compared to smoking, but seem to increase the risk markedly in smokers (Band et al. 1980).

The only early detection techniques of any potential value and widespread use at present are the chest roentgenogram and sputum cytology. It has been suggested that the two are complementary, as the former can detect peripheral lesions while the latter is better for more central lesions of large bronchi that may not be apparent visually in the early stages (Fontana et al. 1975).

Over 15 years ago, Davies (1966) set the stage for what continues to be empirical wisdom that is as yet unproved by decreases in mortality, when he said:

> *It would behoove male cigarette smokers over age 40, as a minimum, to obtain a cytologic examination of sputum and chest x-rays at alternate six-month intervals and both cytologic and radiographic check-ups semiannually if respiratory symptoms are present. In doing so, an individual might reasonably expect a statistically greater chance of survival if a lesion were found than would be the case if he waited for clear evidence of being ill.*

This advice has been tested in a variety of controlled clinical trials as well as some uncontrolled ones.

The Philadelphia Neoplasm Research Project (Boucot and Weiss 1973) was uncontrolled and nonrandomized. It attempted to screen men with chest x-rays every six months. The overall survival rate for those lung cancers detected was 8% at five years, no different from national figures for unscreened populations. A similar study by the Veterans Administration (Lilienfeld et al. 1966) that used cytology as well as x-ray was also negative with respect to survival rate.

In an uncontrolled nonrandomized study from London (Nash et al. 1968) using semiannual chest x-ray only, the four-year survival rate of detected cases was 18%, estimated to be twice that of the comparable unscreened regional population. Another English study (Brett 1969) was controlled but not randomized. It relied basically on semiannual chest x-rays and was also negative with respect to mortality differences.

A randomized controlled trial was conducted by the Kaiser Foundation using an annual chest x-ray. There was no difference in mortality between the screened and control group from lung cancer deaths (American Cancer Society 1980a).

At the present time there are three American studies that have been in progress for nearly a decade that are randomized, controlled, and use both cytology and chest x-ray. They are being conducted at Johns Hopkins, the Mayo Clinic, and the Memorial Sloan-Kettering Cancer Center. In the Mayo Clinic study, the frequency of cytology plus x-ray is being examined (every four months versus annually), whereas the other two studies are comparing the benefits of cytology plus x-ray to x-ray alone. None of the studies has as yet shown a definitive difference in mortality between screened and control groups, but they are not yet complete.

On the basis of the above data, the American Cancer Society (1980a) has recommended that there be no specific tests for the early detection of lung cancer, but that efforts be made to help smokers stop smoking or switch to low-tar and low-nicotine cigarettes. The costs and risks of screening (particularly of false positive sputum cytologies) are judged not to be worthwhile at present. A similar recommendation has been made by the Canadian Task Force on the Periodic Health Examination (1979).

A Consensus Conference on Screening for Lung Cancer of the National Cancer Institute (Gordon 1979) pointed out that differences in mortality that are developing from the three studies cited might be evident within the next two to three years (from September 1978). It concluded that current studies "do not at present show any evidence of a significant reduction in mortality" and that "until the value of screening . . . by these methods has been demonstrated, mass screening programs should be limited to well designed controlled studies."

Koster (1979) also acknowledges that current screening methods may be ineffective and empirical, but states that annual screening with these tests is a reasonable compromise for physicians "who feel they must follow the heavy smokers among their patients."

The principal investigator of the Mayo Clinic project has written a rebuttal to the American Cancer Society policy (Fontana 1980). He states that the interim results are inconclusive and should not form the basis of a major policy change by the ACS, that the statistics quoted by them are out of date, that the experimental design is misquoted, and that "tentative opinions have been recorded as conclusions and quoted out of context." He states that the intensively screened group at the Mayo Clinic has had more early disease detected with a greater resectability rate and a lower mortality rate, although the difference is not yet statistically significant. While not advocating mass screening at this time, Fontana states that it does not seem appropriate "to withhold the only means of discovering early-stage lung cancer from the asymptomatic patient who seeks a cancer checkup on an individual basis, especially if the patient is in the high-risk group. . . . Failure of proof should not be interpreted as proof of failure."

It is clear that the matter is still controversial and unresolved, although it is likely to be clarified greatly within the next few years. As one who see patients with incurable lung cancer, my own admittedly empirical recommendation is to follow the suggestions of Koster for an annual chest film and cytology in heavy smokers, both men and women, until more data are available.

Colorectal Cancer

Cancer of the large intestine is the most frequent noncutaneous malignancy in the United States and is the number two cause of cancer death. Ninety percent of cases occur in people over age 40 years. The five-year survival rate has remained stable at about 40% over the last three decades, as has the proportion of cancers detected while localized (41%). In contrast to lung cancer, it seems clear that a high percentage of disease can be detected when it is still asymptomatic, and this is very much worthwhile. Winawer (1980) contrasts the survival of localized disease (71%) with nonlocalized (43%), but even more impressive is survival of *asymptomatic* patients (90%).

Of importance for screening is the interesting fact that distribution of these cancers is becoming increasingly proximal; that is, fewer lesions are likely to be detected by rectal examination or by sigmoidoscopy, although clearly these procedures are still of considerable importance for both screening and diagnostic evaluation.

High-risk patients include those with familial polyposis, Gardner's syndrome, ulcerative colitis, a prior history of colonic polyps or carcinoma, or a family history of colorectal cancer.

There are really only three techniques with any practical value for mass screening at the present time: digital examination of the rectum, sigmoidoscopy, and examination of the stool for occult blood.

The Kaiser Health Plan trial of multiphasic screening, employing both periodic rectal examination and sigmoidoscopy (Dales et al. 1979) as well as blood studies for anemia, found three times less mortality from colorectal cancer over an 11-year period in screened patients than in controls who did not choose to avail themselves of examinations on a regular basis. Only about one-third of the screened patients had sigmoidoscopy, so presumably the digital examination played a large role in detection.

In a study conducted at the Strang Clinic in New York (Hertz 1979) offering sigmoidoscopy and a stool guaiac test annually, 58 cancers were found in over 26,000 patients screened. Fifty of these patients were followed at least 15 years, and they had a 90% survival rate.

In a 30-year study at the University of Minnesota with annual sigmoidoscopy, 13 cancers were found in the sigmoid region in over 18,000 patients. All were localized, and with a follow-up of up to 30 years none had died of colorectal cancer (Gilbertsen 1979).

More recent controlled studies using fecal testing for occult blood have provided informative findings. At the University of Minnesota, over 48,000 people have been screened annually or biennially, or have served as controls (Gilbertsen et al. 1980). Of 873 patients with blood in the stool, 74 have been found to have 77 gastrointestinal cancers, 56 in the colon, 16 in the rectum, and the remainder in the stomach or pancreas. More than three-quarters were Dukes' stage A or B. Barium enema done as part of the diagnostic work-up detected only 64% of the colonic cancers. The effect on mortality and comparison with the control group are not yet definitive, but results are most suggestive that early cancers are being found in increased proportion and numbers as a result of screening.

Another controlled trial is in progress at the Strang Clinic–Memorial Sloan-Kettering in New York, in which annual sigmoidoscopy is performed in the control group and the test for occult blood in the study group (Winawer et al. 1980). Of the cancers found in the study group, 66% were Dukes' A, B, or in situ, while only 33% of those in the control group were in these early stages. More follow-up time is needed, but the trend is apparent.

In a large-scale mass screening and public information study in Chicago (Winchester et al. 1980) using one-time Hemoccult testing, 27 cancers were found. Nearly two-thirds of these had Dukes' A or B lesions.

A more sensitive immunochemical test for intact human hemoglobin in feces was recently described by Songster and co-workers (1980). It should not be positive with peroxidase-containing vegetables or meats. Stools of 150 patients with known colorectal cancer were positive in 65% with the immunochemical test and 40% with the Hemoccult test. If confirmed, this may be a valuable technique for future screening programs.

The NIH Consensus Development Conference held in 1978 (Brodie 1979) indicated that no definitive influence on mortality was apparent at that time from screening techniques (and this is still true), and that more time and evaluation were needed before occult blood testing was endorsed for general use. Because of already widespread use and availability, however, it was suggested that it be limited to people over 40 with a meat-free, high-fiber diet during the test, and not used to substitute for sigmoidoscopy.

The current American Cancer Society recommendations (1980a) are that all persons age 40 years and over should have a rectal examination annually, a stool guaiac slide test at and after 50 years annually, and that sigmoidoscopy be performed every three to five years after two initial negative examinations one year apart. People in the high-risk group should be examined earlier and more frequently. This represents a change of policy from the earlier recommendations, which were that all three tests be done annually in anyone over 40.

My own suggestions are in accord with those of the American Cancer Society, which represents a reasonable balance between probable efficacy and practicality.

Osteen (1979) at the Sidney Farber Cancer Institute suggests a rectal examination and Hemoccult test annually in people over 40, with sigmoidoscopy reserved for people with positive occult blood tests. The Canadian Task Force (1979) feels that the value of occult blood testing is supported by "fair evidence" as part of a periodic health examination.

Breast Cancer

Screening methods for this disease include breast self-examination (BSE), physical examination, and mammography. Thermography has been used abroad with claimed effectiveness (Gautherie and Gros 1980) but has not yet achieved wide acceptance in this country.

High-risk women can be identified. They include women with a personal history of breast cancer, a family history of breast cancer particularly in a mother or sister and especially if the cancer in the relative was found in the premenopausal years, demonstrable fibrocystic disease, late pregnancy or nulliparity, and long reproductive life (early menarche before 11 or late menopause beyond 53). Obesity and prior history of endometrial or ovarian cancer also seem to increase the risk (Sadowsky 1979). The effect of birth control pills is still not clear.

It is claimed that this is the one cancer where a single-site, randomized, controlled clinical trial has demonstrated the effectiveness of screening (American Cancer Society 1980a). This is the study of the Health Insurance Plan (HIP) of Greater New York (Shapiro 1977). Women between 40 and 65 were offered annual mammograms and physical examinations, while the control group was simply observed. A definite protective effect from mortality was found in women over 50 years in the study group. One-third of the cancers were found by mammography alone and 22% by both methods.

It is well accepted that survival correlates with tumor size and stage. It was reported that women with cancers found by mammography alone had 78% 10-year survival as contrasted with 58% 10-year survival when detected by physical examination (American Cancer Society 1980a). Another study (Gershon-Cohn cited by Sadowsky 1979) contrasts cancers found by mammography with an average diameter of 1.1 cm and 10% positive axillary nodes, with those found by the patients themselves with an average diameter of 3 cm and 55% positive nodes.

The Breast Cancer Detection Demonstration Projects (BCDDP) suggest that mammography has improved since the HIP study and that the procedure can now detect over 90% of cancers (Beahrs et al. 1977). Caution has been urged concerning its efficacy and particularly radiation risks (Bailar 1976), but it clearly is a useful tool that should be and is being used in routine screening programs as well as in high-risk and symptomatic patients.

Some indication of the value of physical examination alone in screening comes from Gilbertsen (1969). Patients detected through screening by this technique had 95% five-year survival.

Although little is known about the definitive value of BSE, it is clear that the majority of breast cancers are found by patients themselves; it is possible that self-examination may play a major role in detecting early cancers when done in a methodical regular fashion. Several papers are encouraging in this regard (Foster et al. 1978; Greenwald et al. 1978), but there are difficulties with interpretation that have to be addressed (Moore 1978). There are problems with defining the control group, and in one of the studies the yield was actually higher with physical examination than with BSE (Greenwald et al. 1978). The ability of women to detect lumps in breasts (actually, in other women's) has been reported to increase following training with a silicone model (Hall et al. 1980).

The current American Cancer Society recommendations (1980a) are as follows: all women over 20 should practice BSE monthly; women age 20 to 40 years should have a breast examination every three years, and women over 40 annually. This is a change from the previous recommendation for an annual examination for all women from age 20 on.

Mammography is recommended as a baseline between the ages of 35 and 40 years, but if negative it is not to be resumed until age 50, and then on an annual basis. Women under 50 years are urged to consult their physicians for guidance. Women at high risk for breast cancer should have earlier and more frequent examinations.

These recommendations grew out of the National Cancer Institute Consensus Development Meeting (Beahrs et al. 1977), which acknowledged the benefits of the above techniques but recognized the absence of data to show a benefit in women under age 50.

Our Canadian colleagues recommend annual mammography and physical examination for women over 50 (Canadian Task Force 1979).

Sadowsky (1979), a radiologist, suggests mammography as a baseline at some time over age 40 (when the patient is first seen) and then every five years until age 50, and every two to three years if risk factors and physical examination are normal. Moskowitz (1979), also a radiologist, suggests that screening should probably begin earlier than age 50 in asymptomatic women, and in high-risk women the whole screening process should be lowered by 10 years, that is, beginning mammography at age 30.

My own preferences are similar to those of the Cancer Society, but for individualization I would suggest that at age 40 women have mammograms every five years during the next decade and more often if the physical examination becomes positive. Women at high risk (strong family and/or personal history of cancer) should begin the process at age 30 and have annual examinations with mammograms every two years. Clearly, all of these suggestions are only guidelines and await modification as more definitive data become available.

Cancer of the Cervix

Cervical carcinoma is reviewed thoroughly elsewhere in this volume (chapter 48). Screening for this disease is generally accepted as being worthwhile and effective. Invasive cancer seems to be preceded in general by cervical dysplasia and carcinoma in situ (CIS), both of which are thought to have a long quiescent period before transformation and for which some evidence of regression exists, although this is confused by the fact that biopsy may also be excisional and therefore therapeutic. Deaths from the disease have clearly fallen over the last few decades and screening is generally acknowledged to deserve some, if not all, of the credit for this. Controversy exists largely at the level of the appropriate frequency of the Pap smear, without dispute as to its value as a diagnostic tool. Cancer of the cervix is much less important as a cause of death than several other cancers, but because of the apparent efficacy of screening, widespread use of the Pap smear, and the current controversy, the disease assumes a role in this discussion disproportionate to the mortality figures.

It is clear that high-risk women include those with an early history of sexual activity and multiple sexual partners.

While widespread screening has been in force for many years and has produced real benefits, no randomized controlled trial of efficacy has been done and it is unlikely that one will be. The evidence for benefit has come from considerations of the long preinvasive course of CIS, the nearly total cure rate when the disease is found at this stage, and the falling mortality when screened populations are compared with unscreened ones, with a falling rate of invasive disease (American Cancer Society 1980a).

Carcinoma in situ is estimated to remain static (noninvasive) for anywhere from 8 to 30 years, thus raising questions about the need for *annual* screening in either normal or high-risk populations. In addition, the cost of annual tests for the general population is not inconsiderable; one estimate of savings resulting from decreasing the frequency from annually to every three years is one billion dollars a year. The test is clearly not perfect, since there is a significant interobserver variation. Some tips are helpful: two samples should be taken, one from the cervical os by aspiration or cotton swabbing, and the other from the exocervix with a wooden spatula. The vaginal pool sample has a high rate of false negatives (45%) and should probably be abandoned (Richart and Vaillant 1965). Slides should be fixed immediately.

Current American Cancer Society recommendations are as follows: all asymptomatic women over age 20 and those who are sexually active under age 20 should have a Pap smear annually for two negative examinations, and then every three years until age 65. (The peak age for CIS is 38 years, and for invasive cancer is 48.) Women at high risk "may need to be tested more frequently" (American Cancer Society 1980a). This is a marked departure from earlier ACS policy, which had recommended annual screening. The American College of Obstetricians and Gynecologists has continued to recommend that policy (1980) and many patients have been reported to have been diagnosed as having invasive cancer within a short time after a negative Pap smear. The ACS's newest guidelines claim that the test used every three years delivers 97% of the increase in life expectancy delivered by its annual use.

The Canadian Task Force (1979) recommends a test every three years for sexually active women up to age 35 and every five years thereafter, with annual testing for high-risk groups.

The Farber Institute manual (Knapp and Berkowitz 1979) suggests that annual screening is appropriate until better data become available, but if this is not feasible, that annual screening be concentrated on the high-risk group, and that three-year screening after two negative smears could be used in the nonhigh-risk group (the ACS approach).

Clearly, there is no absolute answer, but I am persuaded that the ACS policy is reasonable at this time.

References

American Cancer Society. Guidelines for the cancer-related checkup. Recommendations and rationale. *CA* 30:194–240, 1980a.

American Cancer Society. *Cancer facts and figures*. New York: American Cancer Society, 1980b.

American College of Obstetricians and Gynecologists. Task force on the Pap smear. Cited in the *New Haven Register*, July 24, 1980.

Bailar, J. C., III. Mammography: a contrary view. *Ann. Intern. Med.* 84:77–84, 1976.

Band, P. et al. Potentiation of cigarette smoking and radiation. Evidence from a sputum cytology survey among uranium miners and controls. *Cancer* 45:1273–1277, 1980.

Beahrs, O. H. et al. Report of the working group to review the NCI/ACS breast cancer detection demonstration project. Presented at the National Cancer Institute consensus development meeting on breast cancer screening, September 1977, Bethesda, Md.

Boucot, K. R., and Weiss, W. Is curable lung cancer detected by semiannual screening? *JAMA* 224:1361–1365, 1973.

Brett, G. Z. Earlier diagnosis and survival in lung cancer. *Br. Med. J.* 4:260–262, 1969.

Brodie, D. R., ed. Screening and early detection of colorectal cancer. Consensus development/conference proceedings, Bethesda, Md.: (NIH) 80-2075. National Institutes of Health, 1979.

Canadian Task Force on the Periodic Health Examination. The periodic health examination. *J. Can. Med. Assoc.* 121:3–46, 1979.

Dales, L. G. et al. Evaluating periodic multiphasic health checkups. A controlled trial. *J. Chron. Dis.* 32:385–404, 1979.

Davies, D. F. A review of detection methods for the early diagnosis of lung cancer. *J. Chron. Dis.* 19:819–845, 1966.

Fontana, R. S., Jr. Something old, something new, and something borrowed—the American Cancer Society's report on the cancer-related health checkup. *Mayo Clin. Proc.* 55:459–460, 1980.

Fontana, R. S., Jr. et al. The Mayo lung project for early detection and localization of bronchogenic carcinoma: a status report. *Chest* 67:511–522, 1975.

Foster, R. S., Jr. et al. Breast self-examination practices and breast cancer stage. *N. Engl. J. Med.* 299:265–270, 1978.

Gautherie, M., and Gros, C. M. Breast thermography and cancer risk prediction. *Cancer* 45:51–56, 1980.

Gilbertsen, V. A. Detection of breast cancer in a specialized cancer detection center. *Cancer* 24:1191–1196, 1969.

Gilbertsen, V. A. The detection of colorectal cancers. International symposium on colorectal cancer, March 1979, New York.

Gilbertsen, V. A. et al. The earlier detection of colorectal cancers. A preliminary report of the results of the occult blood study. *Cancer* 45:2899–2901, 1980.

Gordon, R. S., ed. Lung cancer mortality appears unaffected by roentgenographic and sputum screening in asymptomatic persons. *JAMA* 241:1582, 1979.

Greenwald, P. et al. Effect of breast self-examination and routine physician examinations on breast cancer mortality. *N. Engl. J. Med.* 299:271–273, 1978.

Hall, D. C. et al. Improved detection of human breast lesions following experimental training. *Cancer* 46:408–414, 1980.

Hall, D. J., and Wood, M. C., eds. *Cancer screening: when is it worthwhile? A guide for primary care physicians.* Boston: Sidney Farber Cancer Institute, 1979.

Hertz, R. E. L. International symposium on colorectal cancer. March 1979, New York.

Knapp, R., and Berkowitz, R. S. Screening for carcinoma of the cervix. In *Cancer screening: when is it worthwhile? A guide for primary care physicians,* eds. D. J. Hall and M. C. Wood. Boston: Sidney Farber Cancer Institute, 1979, pp. 15–21.

Koster, J. K. Screening for pulmonary carcinoma. In *Cancer screening: when is it worthwhile? A guide for primary care physicians,* eds. D. J. Hall and M. C. Wood. Boston: Sidney Farber Cancer Institute, 1979, pp. 25–27.

Lilienfeld, A. et al. An evaluation of radiologic and cytologic screening for the early detection of lung cancer. *Cancer Res.* 26:2083–2121, 1966.

Moore, F. D. Breast self-examination. Editorial. *N. Engl. J. Med.* 299:304–305, 1978.

Moskowitz, M. Breast cancer: how can we reduce mortality? *Consultant* 19:47–60, 1979.

Nash, F. A. et al. South London lung cancer study. *Br. Med. J.* 2:715–721, 1968.

Osteen, R. Screening for colorectal carcinoma. In *Cancer screening: when is it worthwhile? A guide for primary care physicians,* eds. D. J. Hall and M. C. Wood. Boston: Sidney Farber Cancer Institute, 1979, pp. 21–24.

Richart, R. M., and Vaillant, H. W. Influence of cell collection techniques upon cytological diagnosis. *Cancer* 18:1474–1478, 1965.

Sadowsky, N. Screening for carcinoma of the breast. In *Cancer screening: when is it worthwhile? A guide for primary care physicians,* eds. D. J. Hall and M. C. Wood. Boston: Sidney Farber Cancer Institute, 1979, pp. 8-13.

Shapiro, S. Evidence on screening for breast cancer from a randomized trial. *Cancer* 39:2772–2782, 1977.

Songster, C. L. et al. Immunochemical detection of fecal occult blood. *Cancer* 45:1099–1102, 1980.

Winawer, S. J. Screening for colorectal cancer: an overview. *Cancer* 45:1093–1098, 1980.

Winawer, S. J. et al. Progress report on controlled trial of fecal occult blood testing for the detection of colorectal neoplasia. *Cancer* 45:2959–2964, 1980.

Winchester, D. P. et al. A mass screening program for colorectal cancer using chemical testing for occult blood in the stool. *Cancer* 45:2955–2958, 1980.

three

Diagnostic Approach to the Cancer Patient

DAVID S. FISCHER

The initial suspicion of a malignant tumor is most often raised by the patient or the primary physician, or by a diagnostic imaging technique such as:

I. Radiologic
   A. Plain x-ray
   B. Mammogram
   C. Tomography
   D. Barium contrast
      1. Gastrointestinal series
      2. Enema
      3. Small bowel series
   E. Iodinated liquid contrast
      1. Gall bladder
      2. I.V. Pyelogram
      3. Myelogram
      4. Sialogram
      5. Angiogram
      6. Lymphangiogram
      7. Venogram
      8. Endoscope retrograde cholangiopancreatogram
   F. Computed tomograms
      1. Head
      2. Body
   G. Image-amplifier–directed thin-needle percutaneous biopsy
   H. Digital radiography

II. Isotopic
   A. Bone scan
   B. Liver-spleen scan
   C. Renogram
   D. Thyroid scan
   E. Brain scan
   F. Gallium scan

III. Ultrasound
   A. Uterine
   B. Cardiac
   C. Abdominal
   D. Brain
   E. Eye

The definitive diagnosis is usually established by the surgeon or medical oncologist by providing tissue for histologic examination to the pathologist or hematologist. I cannot emphasize too strongly the importance of the histologic verification of the diagnosis. Several times each year I am asked to give chemotherapy or to recommend radiation therapy for a patient with radiologic or other so-called "obvious" initial evidence of malignancy. On very few occasions I have acceded to such requests and now feel convinced that most of the time it was a mistake. Until new research provides a better technique, the *definitive* diagnosis of cancer must be made through the microscope.

One might easily argue that there are now imaging techniques that are so precise that therapy can be given without such verification. The arteriogram in renal carcinoma is so characteristic that some urologists regard it with the same conviction that histology provides. The computerized tomographic (CT) scan of the brain is so precise that tumors are diagnosed with a high degree of precision. Therapy for tumors is very destructive of tissue, both normal and pathologic, and therefore should not be undertaken without knowing that the tumor is malignant. In general, brain tumors are best removed or debulked surgically before radiation or chemotherapy, and renal cell tumors respond so poorly to either radiation or chemotherapy that there is no justification for their employment without a verified histologic diagnosis. I have personally seen several cases in which the "obvious cancer" turned out to be a benign tumor or a granuloma, and neither would benefit from cytotoxic chemotherapy or radiation. If good medical judgment is not enough to dissuade the clinician from such empirical treatment, recent court decisions with substantial awards to patients for the toxicity and mental anguish of therapy for an unproved malignancy should make anyone pause before treating.

Those of us who are medical oncologists and hematologists have frequently received our initial specialty training in hematology and hence were conditioned personally to review all blood smears and bone marrow specimens before instituting therapy. As a result, I developed the habit early of reviewing the pathology of all tumors whenever possible. Fortunately, I happened to be located where there were excellent pathologists and double-headed microscopes. This provided a one-on-one educational experience that encouraged supplementation by reference to additional summary sources like the fascicles of the *Armed Forces Institute of Pathology,* Willis' *Pathology of tumors,* (1967), Evans' *Histological appearances of tumors* (1966), and Ackerman and del Regato's *Cancer* (del Regato and Spjut 1977). From time to time a patient was referred with a diagnosis of malignancy, but the accompanying histologic material did not really appear to be definitive. On such occasions, we tried to obtain additional material, and if that failed we had a reference pathology consultation. I recall three such cases, and the patients are alive at nine, seven, and six years with no evidence of disease. What a therapeutic triumph it would have been if we had treated them! In each case, the pathologist had some doubts about the material, but misleading clinical data resulted in an uncertain diagnosis of malignancy instead of demonstrating the limitations of both the material and the pathologist's ability to be sure in every case. Of course, we have had the reverse as well—lesions that were initially diagnosed as benign but proved to be malignant. Hence the medical oncologist should review the histologic material with the pathologist whenever possible.

Once a verified diagnosis of malignancy has been established histologically, we are called on to evaluate the possibility of local or distant spread in order to plan therapy. For the evaluation of metastasis we sometimes need histologic confirmation, but often we are on relatively safe ground accepting the probabilities of the various imaging techniques, and the chemical, immunologic, hematologic, and serologic tests with which we are familiar.

There is no point in recapitulating these common techniques. It may be helpful briefly to summarize the experience in our institutions with the use of some of the newer diagnostic methods and indicate their relative reliability, and discuss when multiple tests are indicated and when they represent an unnecessary expense. This is done with due humility, as progress in diagnostic instrumentation in the past 10 years has been greater than that of the preceding millenium, and no one knows precisely what lies ahead, or is totally familiar with the new tools.

Endoscopy

The development of fiberoptic light bundles has revolutionized the field of endoscopy (Shinya and Wolff 1976). The fiberoptic panendoscope can be equipped with an attachment for a camera or a second observer (for teaching), biopsy forceps, cannulas for suction or irrigation, and with a sheathed brush for obtaining cytologic smears. In experienced hands, a correct diagnosis can be made in more than 90% of malignant disease of the stomach, and essentially 100% of cancer of the esophagus. In Japan, where carcinoma of the stomach is extremely common, endoscopy is frequently done as part of a routine diagnostic work-up because the yield is high. Such early diagnosis has led to more cures and greater survival in that country. In the hands of a skilled endoscopist the procedure is relatively simple and atraumatic, and can be done in the office (Winawer et al. 1976). I find myself requesting this examination more and more often to reevaluate a negative gastrointestinal series that I thought should have been positive, or to take a biopsy of a lesion.

A somewhat more difficult test with a lower diagnostic yield is endoscopic retrograde cholangiopancreatography (ERCP). In experienced hands the technique is successful in visualizing the pancreatic duct about 85% of the time (White and Silverstein 1976). A catheter can be passed into the duct and secretions collected for cytologic, biochemical, and enzymatic testing. Contrast material can be injected under image amplification fluoroscopy, and appropriate x-rays taken. The major uses of this technique are to identify strictures, stenosis, and obstruction of the main pancreatic duct, and large cysts. Cholangiography by this technique may reveal pressure deformities or obstruction in the biliary ducts. The diagnosis of carcinoma of the pancreas can frequently be made, but a negative examination does not rule this disease out. I have tended to use ultrasound and CT scanning in preference to ERCP when pancreatic carcinoma is suspected, as the procedures have a similar yield with less discomfort to the patient.

Fiberoptic colonoscopy has extended the area of visualization from 25 cm with the rigid sigmoidoscope, to the entire colon and often the terminal ileum as well. It is more accurate (98%) than the barium enema (BE) (49%) in detecting polyps and tumors, but is a complementary modality and usually follows BE when both are to be used (Shinya and Wolff 1976). The procedure is tedious but usually not painful and can be done in the office. Polypectomy and biopsy can be safely performed by experienced colonoscopists and can lead to more cures from earlier diagnosis. I have found it particularly useful in evaluating iron deficiency anemia in adult men and postmenopausal women without obvious blood loss.

Genitourinary endoscopy is a well established procedure with many improvements made in the cystoscope over the years. The technique of nephroscopy is relatively new and little used, but occasionally is of benefit in evaluating lesions of the renal pelvis and calices (Pfister 1976).

Bronchoscopy has traditionally been performed through a rigid bronchoscope and is uncomfortable for the patient. Fiberoptic bronchoscopy is less traumatic and can yield small biopsies, photographs, brushings, aspirates, irrigation cytologies, and even specimens from transbronchial biopsies. Although many medical respiratory specialists use only the fiberoptic bronchoscope, some experienced ENT and thoracic surgeons feel that both instruments should be used in a complete search for malignancy. The rigid tube is used for examination of the carina and major bronchi and the fiberscope for the segmental bronchi and the subsegmental spurs. Combined, the yield in positive results is quite high and allows diagnosis of more peripheral disease than was formerly possible. I have requested bronchoscopy earlier in diagnostic work-up since the advent of the fiberscope, and have been rewarded with more positive findings. It has proved particularly useful in evaluation of unresolved pneumonias.

Mediastinoscopy or Thoracoscopy

Although bronchoscopy gives a fairly thorough look at the bronchi, much of the drainage of the lung is to the mediastinal lymph nodes. These can be evaluated by chest x-rays and laminograms, but can only be seen and a biopsy specimen taken by making an incision in the thoracic cavity and inserting an endoscopic instrument with its own optics and biopsy forceps. This requires a high degree of skill and experience, but can yield a diagnosis in many cases, and that saves a full thoracotomy (Goldberg et al. 1974; Ash and Manfredi 1974). As our thoracic surgeons have increased their familiarity with this procedure, I have used it more frequently to establish histologic diagnosis, especially to distinguish among lymphoma, lung cancer, sarcoidosis, and granulomatous diseases.

Peritoneoscopy, Laparoscopy, and Culdoscopy

This technique has been used extensively by gynecologists for many years to visualize and take biopsy specimens of pelvic structures, usually by putting the instrument through the rectovaginal septum (culdoscopy) (Donahue, Sciullo, and Knapp 1976). Ovarian tumors can sometimes be diagnosed by the procedure.

In recent years, the peritoneoscope has been used to visualize abdominal lymph nodes and the liver. Directed percutaneous needle biopsies of the liver have been performed with much success, thereby reducing the need for staging laparotomies in early Hodgkin's and non-Hodgkin's lymphomas (Anderson et al. 1977). It has also improved diagnostic accuracy in obtaining biopsies of metastases to the liver. Avoiding laparotomy reduces morbidity and mortality, and allows earlier institution of definitive nonsurgical therapy.

Colposcopy

Gynecologists have recently found that more accurate diagnosis of cervical and vaginal epithelial lesions is possible with the colposcope, a binocular instrument that sharply focuses light on a surface for accurate biopsy. The area of interest is the transformation zone at which columnar and squamous epithelium meet, and where dysplasia and preclinical cancer arise. These targeted biopsies may obviate the need for conization biopsy in some cases.

Radionuclide Imaging

The bone scan is a well-established technique of proved value. Frequently used radionuclides are shown in table 3.1. Technetium Tc 99m pyrophosphate gives good results with a minimal marrow dose (0.1 rad). It is most useful in localizing metastases, especially when pain calls attention to an area. One must be extremely cautious in interpreting bone scans. Uptake of the isotope can be caused by healing fractures, inflammation, growth, degenerative joint disease, or tumor (O'Mara 1976). In some cases of extensive tumor with large lytic

Table 3.1. *Radionuclides Used in Cancer Diagnosis and Therapy*

Radionuclide	*Symbol*	*Physical Half-life*	*Pharmaceutical*	*Indication or Use*
Fluorine 18	^{18}F	1.87 hrs	Sodium fluoride	Bone scans
Phosphorus 32	^{32}P	14.3 days	Sodium phosphate	Eye scans; malignant effusion therapy; P. vera therapy
Chromium 51	^{51}Cr	27.8 days	Cr-red cells	Red cell survival and spleen scans
Gallium 67	^{67}Ga	78 hrs	Gallium citrate	Lymphoma, lung cancer scanning
Selenium 75	^{75}Se	120 days	Selenomethionine	Parathyroid, pancreas, and thymus scans
Strontium 85	^{85}Sr	65 days	Strontium chloride	Bone scans
Strontium 87m	^{87m}Sr	2.8 hrs	Strontium chloride	Bone scans
Technetium 99m	^{99m}Tc	6 hrs	Sodium pertechnetate	Scans of thyroid, kidney, brain
Technetium 99m	^{99m}Tc	6 hrs	Technetium phosphates	Bone scans
Technetium 99m	^{99m}Tc	6 hrs	Technetium sulfur colloid	Scans of liver, spleen, lymph nodes, lung
Technetium 99m	^{99m}Tc	6 hrs	Technetium human serum albumin	Scans of brain, spinal cord, lung
Indium 111	^{111}In	2.8 days	Indium chloride	Lymphoma scanning
Indium 113m	^{113m}In	1.7 hrs	Indium colloids	Liver, spleen, lung scans
Indium 113m	^{113m}In	1.7 hrs	In ferric hydroxide macroaggregates	Pulmonary capillary bed scans
Iodine 123	^{123}I	13.3 hrs	Sodium iodide	Thyroid scans
Iodine 125	^{125}I	60 days	Sodium iodide	Thyroid scans
Iodine 125	^{125}I	60 days	4-(3-dimethylamino-propylamino)-7-radioiodoquinoline	Detection of pigmented melanoma metastases
Iodine 131	^{131}I	8.1 days	Sodium iodide	Thyroid scans, therapeutic ablation

Table 3.1. *Continued*

Radionuclide	*Symbol*	*Physical Half-life*	*Pharmaceutical*	*Indication or Use*
Iodine 131	^{131}I	8.1 days	Sodium orthoiodo-hippurate	Renal scans
Iodine 131	^{131}I	8.1 days	Iodinated aggregated human serum albumin	Liver, lung scans
Iodine 131	^{131}I	8.1 days	Iodinated rose bengal	Liver flow scan
Iodine 131	^{131}I	8.1 days	19-radioiodocholesterol	Adrenal scan
Ytterbium 169	^{169}Yb	32 days	Yb diethylenetriamine pentaacetic acid	Brain, renal scans
Mercury 197	^{197}Hg	2.7 days	Chlormerodrin	Renal scan
Gold 198	^{198}Au	2.7 days	Gold colloid	Liver, lymphoid, lung scans; malignant effusion therapy
Mercury 203	^{203}Hg	47.9 days	Chlormerodrin	Renal scans

SOURCE: Modified from Quinn 1971.

lesions on conventional x-rays, there may be no uptake on bone scan. I have seen this most frequently with myeloma, but occasionally with metastases from breast, kidney, or lung cancer. Thus, although the scan is more sensitive in most cases and will detect bone metastases earlier than the x-ray, the negative study in a patient with pain should be followed by conventional x-rays of the painful area (and if indicated, the spinal areas of its neural innervation).

Occasionally, excessive diagnostic zeal produces more problems than it solves. I have seen two young adult patients who had some local bone pain and underwent scans rather than x-rays on request by their primary physicians. The scans showed increased uptake in the area of pain and in another remote area, and both patients were told that they probably had a metastatic malignancy. After extensive and expensive work-up in and out of the hospital, including conventional x-rays, tomograms, bone marrow aspiration and biopsy, and finally, open orthopedic biopsy of the areas of pain and uptake, no abnormalities were found. Both patients had prolonged disability, loss of employment, and moderate psychiatric problems. One can only guess at the problems of family members. Both patients have remained under observation for several years without any evidence of physical ill health. These experiences reinforce the feeling that bone scans are secondary tests to evaluate spread of proved neoplasia, and are not screening tests for cancer detection.

Tumor scanning with gallium citrate (^{67}Ga) and indium chloride (^{111}In) is a new approach that is yielding some satisfactory results. It was originally hoped that the isotopes would localize only in malignant tumor tissue and yield specificity. Unfortunately, both isotopes localize in areas of inflammation, benign tumors, and in abscesses as well. The large numbers of false positive and negative results with indium chloride so far have cooled the early enthusiasm for it. Gallium citrate has been widely used for localization of lymphomas, hepatomas, melanomas, and lung tumors, especially the small cell carcinoma (DeMeester et al. 1976). Distribution of the isotopic uptake may be a valuable clue to diagnosis (fig. 3.1). Failure of the isotope to accumulate does not suggest the absence of malignancy, just as selective uptake does not necessarily mean tumor. A decrease in uptake on serial studies after therapy would suggest a response, just as an increase or new area of uptake would suggest recurrence or spread. I have been particularly impressed by the specificity of the positive gallium scan when used in a tomographic mode (fig. 3.2). It is also useful in evaluating focal defects in radiocolloid liver scans. Gallium is taken up by a hepatoma or abscess, while the usual liver isotope records an area of nonperfusion in those instances.

Scans are well-established techniques for imaging liver and spleen and detecting areas of inhomogeneity (Spencer 1976). Dynamic scans of the liver depend on the passage of a bolus of intravenous isotope through the liver, initially from the hepatic artery and then from the portal vein. Most tumors have a hepatic artery blood supply but are not perfused by portal vein blood. Static images are usually produced by reticuloendothelial (RE) uptake or radioactively labeled particles, the most popular of which is technetium Tc 99m sulfur colloid. This is accumulated by the normal RE cells so that a tumor, abscess, or cyst is seen as an area of nonperfusion. The incidence of false positive and negative results remains a problem. Increased diagnostic accuracy has been added by the use of gray-scale ultrasonography to evaluate the scan (Taylor et al. 1976), and the combined procedure yields 90% or better reliability on lesions 1.5 cm or larger (Sullivan, Taylor, and Gottschalk 1978).

Radionuclide brain scans are useful for diagnosis and follow-up when positive. If negative, a CT scan is necessary to complete the evaluation. If both are available, I prefer the CT examination and omit the isotopic scan.

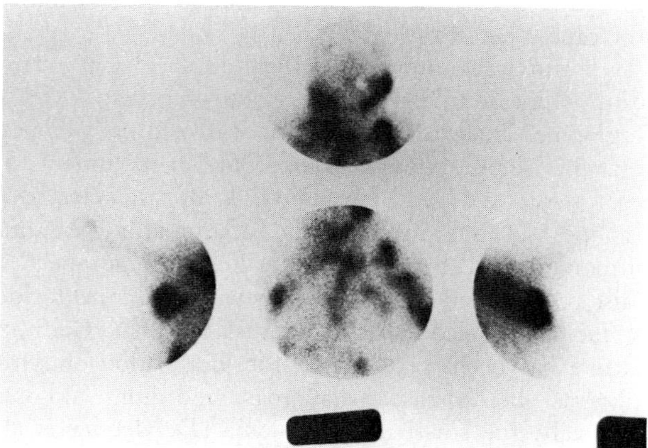

Fig. 3.1. *Conventional gallium scan with anterior and posterior views. In this view, only the anterior films are shown. In this case, a biopsy of the thyroid was interpreted as an anaplastic carcinoma of the thyroid. A gallium scan showing cervical, supraclavicular, mediastinal, axillary, and retroperitoneal nodes led to a re-biopsy and a diagnosis of lymphoma. The patient made a dramatic response to lymphoma therapy. Courtesy of Vincente J. Caride, M.D., Hospital of St. Raphael, New Haven, Conn.)*

Ultrasound

Gray-scale ultrasonography is rapidly finding new uses and has no known adverse side effects (Feimanis 1976; Ferucci 1979). The echoes that are reflected from tumors have different patterns than those from surrounding normal tissues. The method has found considerable use in evaluation of pelvic tumors, abdominal lymph nodes, the liver and biliary tract, the pancreas, spleen (fig. 3.3), and retroperitoneal nodes, the thyroid, kidney, and a midline shift of the brain. To be detected with currently available equipment, a lesion must be 1.5 to 2 cm in size. Techniques are changing rapidly, and it is now possible to do ultrasound-directed percutaneous needle biopsies of the liver and kidney, and kidney cyst aspirations (Rosenfield et al. 1980). The technique will be adapted to examination of other organs in the future.

Ultrasound is desirable in diagnosis in children and in pregnant patients because of the absence of radiation exposure. This advantage also causes it to be used for sequential follow-up of the response to therapeutic modalities. The method has been adapted to radiation therapy planning for delineation of ports and adjustment of the beam (Lee et al. 1980).

Diagnostic Radiology

Of the dozens of procedures and techniques that can be done radiologically to aid in cancer management, five deserve special mention: lymphangiography, arteriography, tomography, computed tomography, and image amplifier-directed percutaneous biopsy.

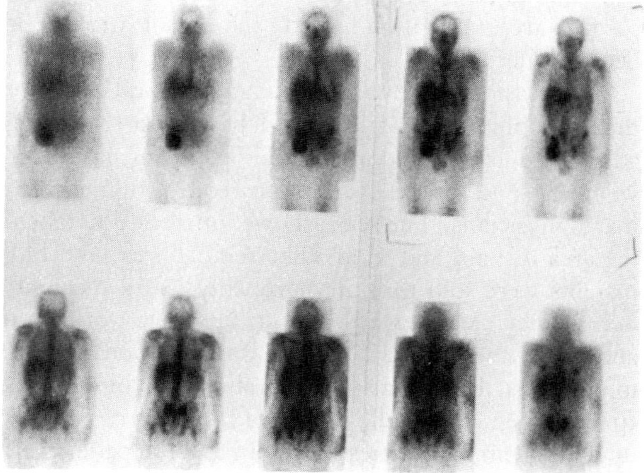

Fig. 3.2. *Tomographic gallium scan showing increased uptake in right inguinal area and retroperitoneal lymph nodes. The advantage of this technique is that it can clarify deep lesions not seen on an ordinary anterior or posterior projection.*

Bipedal lymphangiograms have added to the accuracy of staging in melanoma, Hodgkin's disease, and other lymphomas, as well as testicular, penile, cervical, uterine, vulvar, and ovarian tumors (Koehler 1976). Opacification occurs primarily in the inguinal, lumbar, and paraaortic nodes, but not in the mesenteric, gastric, celiac, splenic, or portal nodes. The contrast material remains in place for about two years so that the radiograph can be used at surgery with a follow-up x-ray on the operating table to check removal of involved nodes at staging laparotomies; with serial studies the response to chemotherapy or radiation can be documented. An initial negative study does not necessarily rule out the presence of disease—it simply fails to demonstrate disease. In spite of gallium and CT scans, which are complementary techniques, I still find the lymphangiogram particularly useful for staging Hodgkin's disease and decreasing the need for a staging laparotomy. In figure 3.4, the lymph nodes are characteristically "foamy" in this case of Hodgkin's disease.

Arteriography became a more generally available diagnostic aid when the percutaneous arterial catheterization method of Seldinger (1953) was introduced and perfected (Reuter 1976). It has been used extensively in vascular surgery, but I have found it useful in evaluating suspected tumors in the kidney, liver, and pancreas. In renal cell carcinoma in particular, demonstration of neovasculature is virtually diagnostic (fig. 3.5). For liver metastases, arteriography can define the blood supply of the tumor for either hepatic artery ligation or cannulation to administer intraarterial chemotherapy. Pancreatic tumors are frequently suspected but difficult to diagnose, and arteriography has occasionally been successful when CT scan, ultrasound, and ERCP failed to define the lesion. A new technique of digital radiography providing, in some instances, an intravenous method of visualizing arterial circulation merits careful observation.

Body section tomograms or laminograms can be made of any section of the body, but have been used primarily in evaluation of the thoracic cavity (Miller et al. 1976). I have found it desirable to get full-lung tomograms before accepting the finding of a solitary metastasis as truly solitary on a PA and lateral chest x-ray. More often than not, the tomogram revealed additional lesions. Recently, a linear "scar" dismissed on

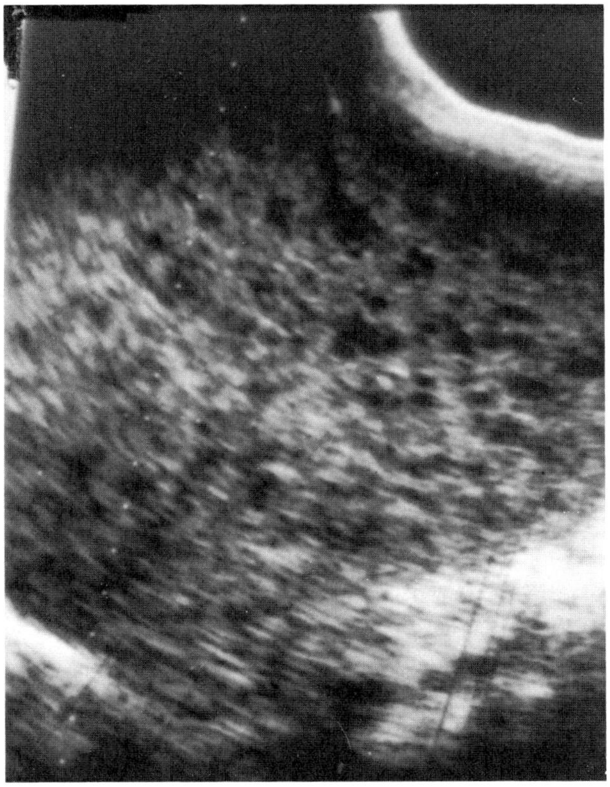

Fig. 3.3. *Ultrasound of the spleen showing multiple defects in a case of Hodgkin's disease.*

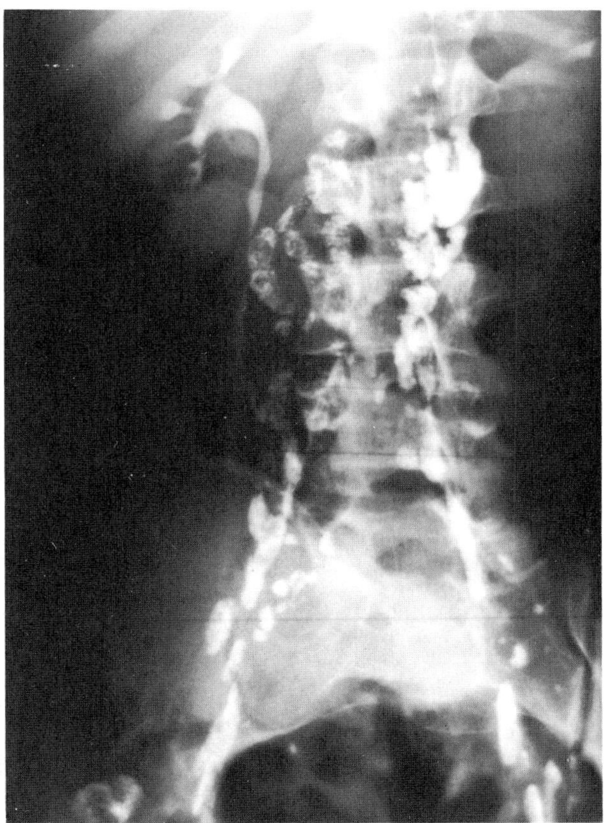

Fig. 3.4. *Lymphangiogram in a case of Hodgkin's disease showing "foamy" lymph nodes that are not enlarged and could be missed on a CT scan. (Courtesy of Gerald Fishbone, M.D., Hospital of St. Raphael, New Haven, Conn.)*

a routine chest film as a "thickened fissure" had the characteristics of a tumor on tomography and on biopsy proved to be an epidermoid carcinoma.

On occasion, the tomographic technique has been successfully adapted to other organs. A patient with severe hip pain had a negative bone scan and a negative conventional x-ray of the hip. Tomograms clearly showed fracture in the surgical neck of the femur.

The development of scans by computed tomography (CT) or computerized axial tomography (CAT) is one of the most significant advances in diagnosis of this generation. Intracranial masses can be safely detected with a sensitivity and precision never before possible by noninvasive techniques (fig. 3.6). To a large extent it has supplanted the isotopic brain scan, the pneumoencephalogram, and cerebral arteriography. In addition, I almost routinely obtain a CT scan of the brain before doing a lumbar puncture in a patient with suspected intracranial mass or the possibility of increased intracranial pressure, to diminish the risk of herniation of the medulla oblongata into the foramen magnum.

Tomographic scanning of other organs has had variable but increasing success with the growth of knowledge and experience. Earlier diagnosis of pancreatic carcinomas has been demonstrated in some cases (Wiggans et al. 1976) (fig. 3.7). I have found it particularly useful in evaluation of thoracic and mediastinal masses (Jost et al. 1978), retroperitoneal masses, pelvic tumors, and urologic malignancies (Riehl et al. 1977).

The use of combined diagnostic modalities such as ultrasound and CT has added another dimension of accuracy in both diagnosis (fig. 3.8) by clinicians and in treatment planning by radiation oncologists.

One of the problems with the CT scan is its relative inaccessability. In view of the high initial purchase cost of the various "generations" of scanners, there has been a clear effort of some governmental agencies by administrative fiat to deny hospitals the opportunity to purchase them. This has occurred in the face of extensive testimony of experienced physicians that the ultimate effect of wise use in referral centers will be cost-saving.

Image amplifier-monitored percutaneous biopsy of deep-seated malignancies has been very successful in my experience. It has provided a histologic diagnosis and thereby saved a major surgical procedure in many cases (Wallace 1976). Recent interventions in my practice include percutaneous biopsies of pancreas, lung, kidney, vertebra, retroperitoneal masses, and thyroid. For the yield to be high and the risk to be low, a team approach is essential. It needs a radiologist skilled in the use of the image intensifier and the biopsy needles, a surgeon either to do the needle biopsy or on standby to handle the rare complication, a pathologist experienced in processing and reading needle biopsies, and an oncologist who will use the diagnostic information to plan a therapeutic program. If the biopsy diagnosis will make no difference in management, it is best not done.

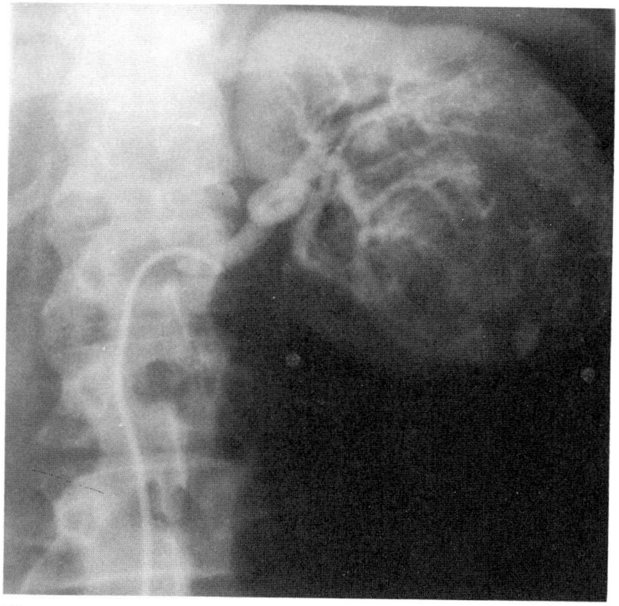

Fig. 3.5. *Renal arteriogram showing characteristic arterial splaying and neovascularity, which is diagnostic of renal cell carcinoma. (Courtesy of Ralph F. Stroup, M.D., Yale–New Haven Hospital, New Haven, Conn.)*

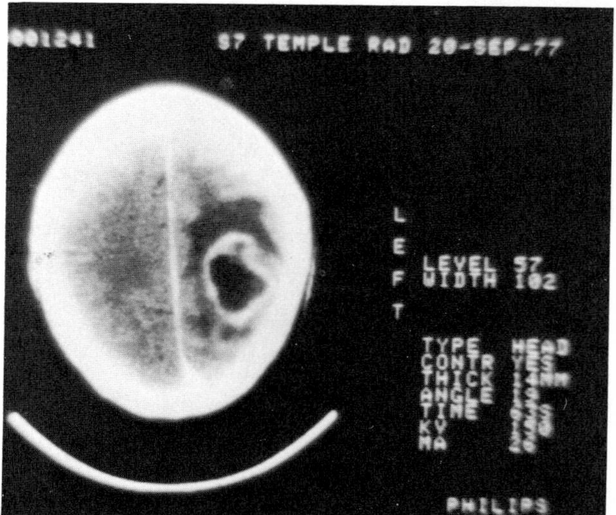

Fig. 3.6. *Glioblastoma multiforme of the left side of the brain seen on CT scan. This provides a new dimension in localization and accuracy preoperatively. (Courtesy of William E. Allen, M.D., Temple Radiology Group, New Haven, Conn.)*

Diagnostic Enzymes

Although a great many enzymes have been used in clinical diagnosis, relatively few (table 3.2) have been consistently useful in cancer diagnosis (Schwartz 1976).

Amylase and lipase are occasionally elevated in pancreatic cancer but only when the tumor is obstructing major ducts, and that is very late in the disease. These enzymes may also be elevated in pancreatitis, perforated ulcers, intestinal obstruction, and renal insufficiency, and are therefore of minimal value in establishing the presence of malignancy.

Acid phosphatase is elevated in about 25% of cases of early prostatic cancer and the majority of cases of metastatic disease when using more specific substrates (Yam 1974). The tartrate inhibition "prostatic fraction" technique has improved diagnostic accuracy only slightly. The use of bone marrow acid phosphatase has been advocated with enthusiasm but I have little personal experience with it so far. The radioimmunoassay for prostatic acid phosphatase appears to enhance diagnostic sensitivity, but I am just beginning to accumulate experience with it.

Lactic dehydrogenase (LDH) is present in liver, heart, muscle, and red blood cells; its isoenzymes are tissue specific. LDH is greatly elevated with liver tumors or metastases but can be elevated with many other causes such as hemolysis.

Alkaline phosphatase is elevated in many diseases of bone and liver. High titers have been recorded with cancer metastatic to bone, osteogenic sarcomas, parathyroid adenomas, and cancer metastatic to liver. In metastatic disease the greatest elevations are seen with osteoblastic lesions to bone and bulky lesions in the liver. Lytic bone lesions will frequently show no elevation, and sometimes significant liver metastases will have a nor-

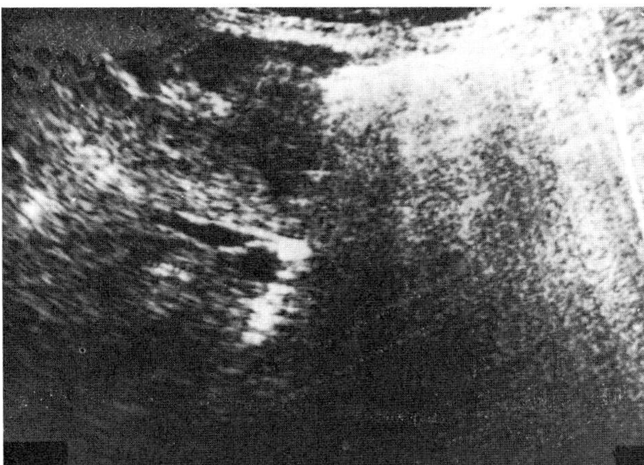

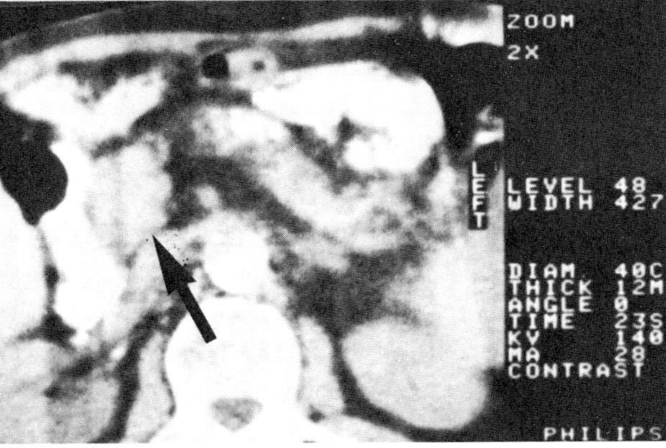

Fig. 3.7. *The CT scan shows an enlarged head of the pancreas* (arrow) *with the tumor impinging on the contrast-filled duodenal sweep. The ultrasound in this case did not visualize the pancreas at all because of overlying gas. (Courtesy of Bruce D. Simonds, M.D., Temple Radiology Group, New Haven, Conn.)*

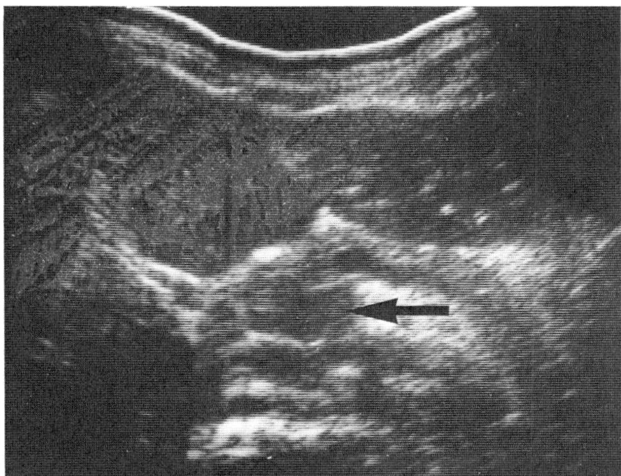

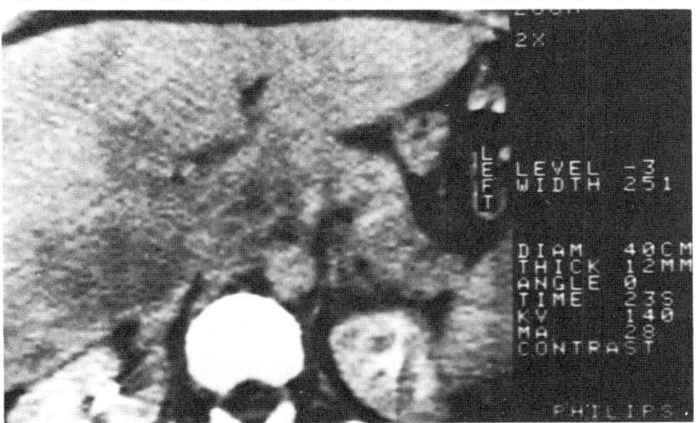

Fig. 3.8. *The CT scan did not visualize the head of the pancreas adequately, possibly because the patient was very thin. The ultrasound clearly shows a small mass* (arrow) *in the uncinate process of the head of the pancreas, which is normal in size. The mass is detectable because of the alteration of the echo consistency of the pancreas by the tumor. (Courtesy of Bruce D. Simonds, M.D., Temple Radiology Group, New Haven, Conn.)*

Table 3.2. *Enzymes Useful in Cancer Diagnosis*

Enzyme	*Tumor*
Amylase	Pancreas
Lipase	Pancreas
Acid phosphatase	Prostate
Alkaline phosphatase	Bone, liver
Lactic dehydrogenase	Liver
5′-Nucleotidase	Liver
Muramidase	Monocytic leukemia

mal value. The 5′-nucleotidase is often elevated in liver metastases even before the alkaline phosphatase is. When the alkaline phosphatase is elevated and liver involvement is suspected in a patient with bone disease, elevation of 5′-nucleotidase would confirm liver involvement. The glutamyltranspeptidase is another enzyme that is not elevated with bone disease but is with liver disease. Unfortunately, it also rises with trivial insults to the liver and has therefore been of limited usefulness.

Muramidase (lysozyme) is elevated in acute monocytic leukemia and myelomonocytic leukemia. It can be elevated in pyogenic infections and abscesses and thus is of relatively limited diagnostic value.

Immunodiagnosis

In recent years, highly sensitive immunologic techniques have been developed (table 3.3) for the detection of very small amounts of proteins, glycoproteins, and peptides (Herberman 1976). In 1965, Gold and Freedman reported finding an antigen in embryonic tissue that was associated with and found in tissue of carcinoma of the colon. Since then the glycoprotein carcinoembryonic antigen (CEA) has been found to be slightly above normal in patients who smoke and those with benign diseases such as bronchitis, inflammatory bowel disease, pancreatitis, cirrhosis, and pulmonary emphysema (Gold et al. 1978). Greatly elevated levels have been found in advanced cancers of the colon, breast, lung, pancreas, stomach, prostate, and many other tumors with liver metastases. Thus CEA cannot be used for screening, but is useful as a baseline in patients with malignant disease if its results are positive. When much of the malignant tissue is destroyed by surgery, radiation, or chemotherapy, the CEA will fall. When it rises, it suggests recurrence, spread, or increased growth of the tumor, and is therefore useful in guiding therapy and estimating (with other factors) prognosis (Minton and Martin 1978). Failure to detect CEA does not rule out malignancy, as the test may be negative even with large tumors with extensive liver metastases.

Table 3.3. *Immunodiagnosis in Cancer*

Test	*Tumor Type(s)*
Carcinoembryonic antigen (CEA)	Colon, breast, lung, stomach, prostate
Gross cystic disease fluid protein (GCDFP)	Breast
Alpha-fetoprotein (AFP)	Liver, stomach, testicle, ovary, choriocarcinoma
Human chorionic gonadotropin (HCG)	Choriocarcinoma, testicle, ovary, breast, stomach, liver

For evaluation of breast carcinoma, Haagensen and co-workers (1977, 1978) have found that the combination of CEA and gross cystic disease fluid protein (GCDFP) is a more accurate and sensitive marker than either alone. A radioimmunoassay has been developed for GCDFP that is identical to a protein present in small amounts in both human milk and saliva but not in human serum. In this series from Duke University, of 216 patients with metastatic breast carcinoma, 50% had abnormal plasma levels of CEA and/or GCDFP. Abnormal plasma levels of CEA were present in 34% of the patients, and abnormal GCDFP levels in 31%. Using both assays, abnormal plasma levels were present in 79% of patients with osseous metastases, 53% of patients with visceral metastases, and 26% with soft tissue metastases. Both assays, when performed serially in patients treated for metastatic breast carcinoma, were found to be useful in monitoring responsiveness. An increasing CEA or GCDFP plasma level indicated disease progression, and a decreasing plasma level indicated regression. The GCDFP is new, and experience is still accumulating.

Another useful fetal antigen is alpha-fetoprotein (AFP), which appears to be elevated in some hepatomas (Chen and Sung 1977), gastric, ovarian, and testicular carcinomas, and choriocarcinoma (Javadpour 1979). As with CEA, it is not useful as a screening test, but its presence may offer confirmation of a diagnosis made histologically; then the AFP titer can be followed to gauge response to therapy.

The peptide hormone human chorionic gonadotropin (HGC) is ordinarily secreted in high titers only in pregnancy. When detected at other times it must be regarded as abnormal. It has proved to be a sensitive marker in gestational trophoblastic tumors such as choriocarcinoma, where therapy is continued to an undetectable titer of the HCG or its beta subunit. Lower titers are found in men when their testicular tumors contain an element of choriocarcinoma. Immunoreactive HCG has been detected in low titers in adenocarcinoma of the ovary, stomach, pancreas, and breast, and hepatomas (Vaitukaitis 1976).

The subject of hormonal activity in the paraneoplastic syndromes is discussed in chapter 6.

References

Anderson, T. et al. Peritoneoscopy: a technique to evaluate therapeutic efficacy in non-Hodgkin's lymphoma patients. *Cancer Treat. Rep.* 61:1017–1022, 1977.

Ash, S. A., and Manfredi, F. Directed biopsy using a small endoscope. Thoracotomy and peritoneoscopy simplified. *N. Engl. J. Med.* 291:1398–1399, 1974.

Chen, D. S., and Sung, J. L. Serum alpha-fetoprotein in hepato-cellular carcinoma. *Cancer* 40:779–783, 1977.

del Regato, J. A., and Spjut, H. J. Ackerman and del Regato's *Cancer: diagnosis, treatment, and prognosis.* St. Louis: C. V. Mosby, 1977.

DeMeester, T. R. et al. Gallium-67 scanning for carcinoma of the lung. *J. Thorac. Cardiovasc. Surg.* 72:699–708, 1976.

Donahue, V. C.; Sciullo, A. J.; and Knapp, R. C. Gynecologic cancer detection and management. *Conn. Med.* 40:443–448, 1976.

Evans, R. W. *Histological appearances of tumors,* 2nd edition. London: Livingstone, 1966.

Feimanis, A. K. Ultrasonic imaging of neoplasms. *Cancer* 37:496–502, 1976.

Ferrucci, J. T. Body ultrasonography. *N. Engl. J. Med.* 300:538–542, 1979.

Gold, P. et al. Carcinoembryonic antigen in clinical medicine. *Cancer* 42:1399–1405, 1978.

Gold, P., and Freedman, S. O. Specific carcinoembryonic antigens of the human digestive system. *J. Exp. Med.* 122:467–481, 1965.

Goldberg, E. M. et al. Mediastinoscopy for assessing mediastinal spread in clinical staging of lung carcinoma. *Semin. Oncol.* 1:205–215, 1974.

Haagensen, D. E., Jr. et al. Evaluation of a breast cyst fluid protein detectable in the plasma of breast carcinoma patient. *Ann. Surg.* 185:279–285, 1977.

Haagensen, D. E., Jr. et al. Comparative evaluation of carcinoembryonic antigen and gross cystic disease fluid protein as plasma markers for human breast carcinoma. *Cancer* 42:1646–1652, 1978.

Herberman, R. B. Immunologic approaches to the diagnosis of cancer. *Cancer* 37:549–561, 1976.

Javadpour, N. The value of biologic markers in diagnosis and treatment of testicular cancer. *Semin. Oncol.* 6:37–47, 1979.

Jost, R. G. et al. Computed tomography of the thorax. *Radiology* 126:125–136, 1978.

Koehler, P. R. Current status of lymphography in patients with cancer. *Cancer* 37:503–516, 1976.

Lee, D. J. et al. The value of ultrasonic imaging and CT scanning in planning the radiotherapy for prostatic carcinoma. *Cancer* 45:724–727, 1980.

Miller, W. E. et al. The evaluation of pulmonary parenchymal abnormalities by tomography. *Radiol. Clin. North Am.* 14:85–93, 1976.

Minton, J. P., and Martin, E. W. The use of serial CEA determinations to predict recurrence of colon cancer and when to do a second look operation. *Cancer* 42:1422–1427, 1978.

O'Mara, R. E. Skeletal scanning in neoplastic disease. *Cancer* 37:480–486, 1976.

Pfister, R. R. Endoscopy and the detection of genitourinary carcinoma. *Cancer* 37:471–474, 1976.

Quinn, J. L., III. Radionuclide imaging procedures in the diagnosis of cancer. *CA* 21:292–301, 1971.

Reuter, S. R. The current status of angiography in the evaluation of cancer patients. *Cancer* 37:532–541, 1976.

Riehl, R. A. et al. Computed tomography in urologic patients. *Urology* 10:529–535, 1977.

Rosenfield, A. T. et al. Ultrasound in the evaluation of renal masses. *Conn. Med.* 44:1–5, 1980.

Schwartz, M. K. Laboratory aids to diagnosis—enzymes. *Cancer* 37:542–548, 1976.

Seldinger, S. I. Catheter replacement of needle in percutaneous arteriography: new technique. *Acta Radiol.* (Stockholm) 39:368–376, 1953.

Shinya, J., and Wolff, W. Flexible colonoscopy. *Cancer* 37:462–470, 1976.

Spencer, R. P. Radionuclide liver scans in tumor detection—current concepts. *Cancer* 37:475–479, 1976.

Sullivan, D. C.; Taylor, K. J. W.; and Gottschalk, A. The use of ultrasound to enhance the diagnostic utility of the equivocal liver scintigraph. *Radiology* 128: 727–732, 1978.

Taylor, K. J. W. et al. Gray scale ultrasound imaging. The anatomy and pathology of the liver. *Radiology* 119:415–423, 1976.

Vaitukaitis, J. L. Peptide hormones as tumor markers. *Cancer* 37:567–572, 1976.

Wallace, S. Interventional radiology. *Cancer* 37:517–531, 1976.

White, T. T., and Silverstein, F. E. Operative and endoscopic pancreatography in the diagnosis of pancreatic cancer. *Cancer* 37:449–461, 1976.

Wiggans, G. et al. Computerized axial tomography for diagnosis of pancreatic cancer. *Lancet* 2:233–235, 1976.

Willis, R. A. *Pathology of tumors.* New York: Appleton-Century-Crofts, 1967.

Winawer, S. J. et al. The role of upper gastrointestinal endoscopy in patients with cancer. *Cancer* 37:440–448, 1976.

Yam, L. T. Clinical significance of the human acid phosphatase. *Am. J. Med.* 56:604–616, 1974.

four

Hematologic Aspects of Malignancies

THOMAS P. DUFFY

The hematologic system constitutes a mirror of the body, reflecting disorders in several organ systems. The "shift-to-the-left" in the leukocyte count is a valuable index of infection in the febrile patient; the presence of microangiopathic red cells is the clue to malignant hypertension in patients with correspondingly high blood pressures. Solid tumors may be highlighted by their direct or indirect impact on the marrow and peripheral blood. Such involvement may facilitate diagnosis but also adds to the morbidity and mortality of these tumors.

This chapter focuses on the many hematologic aspects of solid malignancies; it excludes hematologic tumors, although there is obviously much overlap. The concern is with tumor signals as manifested in the peripheral blood and marrow; recognition of these signals may improve diagnosis, management, and therapy of malignancy.

Anemia

Multiple etiologies exist as potential causes of the anemia frequently present in individuals suffering with malignancies (Crowther and Bateman 1972; Leite and Hoogstraten 1977). Direct involvement of the marrow with metastases occurs in approximately 10% of cases (Anner and Drewinko 1977) and creates hematologic abnormalities through mechanisms that include marrow infiltration, necrosis (Brown 1972; Kiraly and Wheby 1976), fibrosis (Delsol et al. 1979), and cell cytolysis (Zucker and Lysik 1977). Such marrow metastases may be heralded by the presence of nucleated red blood cells and immature white cells in the peripheral blood (Weick, Hagedorn, and Linman 1974). This constellation of findings—a leukoerythroblastic blood picture—occurs in approximately 40% of patients with bone marrow metastases (Delsol et al. 1979). The documentation of leukoerythroblastosis is always good evidence of marrow involvement in patients with known cancer.

Specific tumors have a special predilection for marrow involvement, and aspiration and biopsy should be performed in evaluating such neoplasms. In 19% to 70% of patients with small cell carcinoma, cancer cells have been detected in marrow at the time of initial diagnosis (Ihde et al. 1979). More common tumors such as breast, prostate, and non-small cell lung also frequently (approximately 20%) involve the marrow (Ellman 1976; Leland and MacPherson 1979). Unfortunately, there are no variables other than a leukoerythroblastic blood picture that are highly accurate in predicting marrow metastases (Chernow and Wallner 1978); still the biopsy (especially bilateral trephine biopsy) (Brunning et al. 1975) may establish metastatic disease.

Even in the absence of marrow involvement by tumor, malignancies may frequently contribute to the development of anemia along other paths. Iron deficiency commonly results from blood loss with gastrointestinal tumors. This phenomenon is of such importance that the discovery of iron deficiency anemia in adult men and postmenopausal women dictates a search for occult gastrointestinal malignancy.

Tumors may also create anemia along immunologic pathways. The antibody may be directed against marrow red cell precursors with the production of pure red cell aplasia (Krantz and Kao 1967). Thymomas are present in approximately 50% of patients with selective absence of marrow red cells (Hirst and Robertson 1967). An early red blood cell precursor is the target against which a humoral or cytotoxic and/or suppressor cell injury is directed in pure red cell aplasia. Other antibodies may accompany malignancies and produce an autoimmune Coombs'-positive hemolytic anemia by sensitizing peripheral red cells. Immune-mediated destruction of red cells is not uncommon as a component of lymphoproliferative disorders, but such an anemia, especially in elderly patients, should suggest the rare possibility of carcinoma (Spira and Lynch 1979). Surgical extirpation of the tumor effects hematologic recovery even when such a remission has not been achieved with steroid therapy.

Immune sensitization of red cells abbreviates their survival by extravascular sequestration hemolysis; intravascular hemolysis may occur in malignancies as a result of microangiopathic or traumatic damage to the cells. Fragmentation of the cells may be produced by shearing through pathologically distorted vessels as occurs in giant hemangiomas (Kasabach-Merritt syndrome) or through fibrin strands resulting from intravascular coagulation and laying down of fibrin (Brain et al. 1970; Jacobson and Jackson 1974). Laboratory evidence for intravascular coagulation is often but not universally present when cancer is associated with a microangiopathic process. Its absence has led some observers to attribute a more fundamental role to red cell contact with intraluminal pulmonary embolic tumor cells, rather than fibrin strands, in the production of the red cell fragmentation (Antman et al. 1979). Whatever the pathophysiologic mechanism, the discovery of schistocytes, helmet cells, and microspherocytes in the peripheral smear may be a subtle clue to malignancies (fig. 4.1).

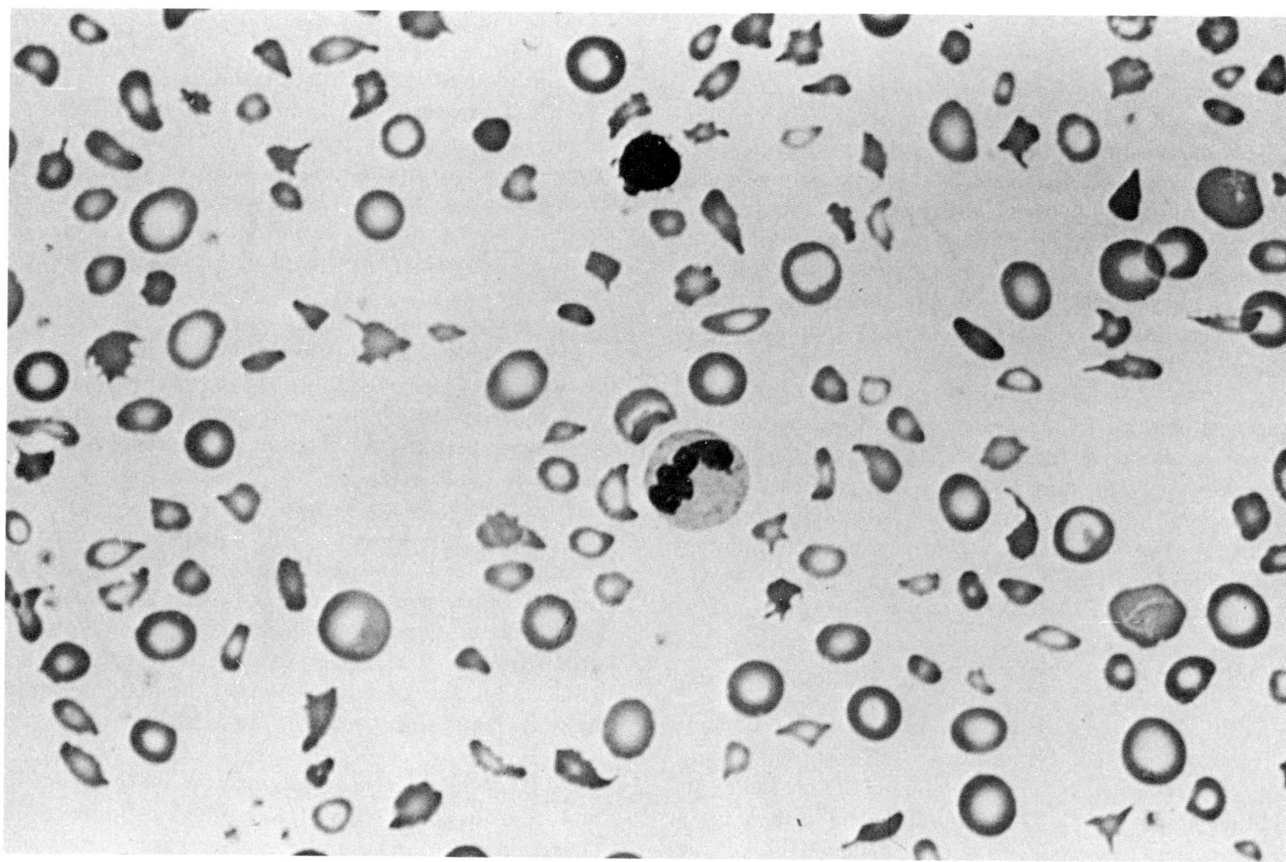

Fig. 4.1. *Example of severe traumatic hemolysis with marked formation of schistocytes, helmet cells, and other red cell fragments.*

The anemias described to this point are complications that may occur in some patients with cancer. In contrast is the more commonplace anemia that accompanies the majority of malignancies independent of marrow involvement, immunologic or other hemolytic insult to the red cells, or deficiency of essential building blocks such as iron. The marrow in the anemia of malignancy appears to participate in a cachexia similar to that involving the remainder of the body, and the mechanism for such anemias is just as clouded as the frequent wasting states. The anemia is usually moderate in degree with hematocrits around 30%; red blood cell morphology is normochromic-normocytic with a tendency toward hypochromia. An extracorpuscular insult, perhaps mediated by an overly avid reticuloendothelial system, imposes a modest abbreviation of red blood cell survival on the peripheral red cells. This premature red cell destruction lacks adequate compensation; reticulocytosis is low relative to the degree of anemia. The marrow does not appropriately increase its output of red cells, a failure that appears to be the major defect in the anemia of malignancy (Cartwright and Lee 1971).

Failure of compensation by the marrow for premature red cell destruction may have many causes, but most have been eliminated as the primary defect. Erythropoietin levels are not uniformly depressed in such patients (Zucker, Friedman, and Lysik 1974; DeGowin and Gibson 1979), and the numbers and response of marrow stem cells committed to erythropoiesis appear comparable to those in normal individuals (DeGowin, Grund, and Gibson 1978). The defect shared by all such patients is the failure to mobilize iron from reticuloendothelial stores; iron is present but not available in adequate amounts for erythropoiesis (Douglas and Adamson 1976). Serum iron levels are low or low normal; serum transferrin levels are in the normal range in contradistinction to the elevated transferrin levels of true iron deficiency.

A possible explanation for this failure of iron transport is the diversion of iron transport proteins to targets other than the red cells. Experiments in the definition of components needed to support growth of tissue cultures have demonstrated the essential role of transferrin in such media (Sato 1977). Growth of certain tumors in serum-free hormone-supplemented media have also documented the need for transferrin in the growth of tumors. Omission of transferrin from a human breast cancer cell line in culture has resulted in rapid cell death of the tumor (Bottenstein et al. 1979).

The explanation for erythropoietin insufficiency in animals and humans with extramedullary tumors may be the diversion of transferrin away from its normal role in erythropoiesis. In the tug-of-war between the marrow and tumor, the cancer is the victor in channeling transportable iron or transferrin to its needs. Erythropoiesis is dampened, with the tumor growing at the expense of the marrow. The only solution to such an anemia is elimination of the tumor, a solution that unfortunately is not frequently available. Since the anemia of malignancy is not severe, it does not require much supportive therapy and usually is not symptomatic. Anemia, however, may be the clue to the presence of the underlying malignancy.

Granulocytosis

Abnormalities in the number and kind of white cells are commonplace in malignancies. Monocytosis (Barrett 1970) and eosinophilia (Isaacson and Rapoport 1946) may be markers of nonhematologic tumors. More common than these alterations in the white cell differential is the occurrence of granulocytosis of varying degree in many neoplasms. The white cell elevation may reach such proportions as to constitute a myeloid leukemoid reaction, defined by Hilts and Shaw (1953) as a white cell count of over 50,000/mm^3. This unusually high leukocyte response has been documented by Fahey (1951) as occurring in 1.8% of 160 cases of lung carcinoma, but it is not restricted to pulmonary malignancies.

The mechanism of tumor-induced neutrophilia remains unexplained. Metastases may be associated with the presence of immature myeloid cells in the peripheral blood, a result of extramedullary hematopoiesis, and/or a breakdown in the normal blood-marrow barrier (Tavassoli 1979). Metastases are not universally present in tumor-induced neutrophilia, however, necessitating some other explanation for any white cell elevation. A granulopoietic factor has been isolated from some animal tumors, but analogous factors in human tumors have not been convincingly demonstrated (Robinson 1974).

The most likely cause of tumor-induced granulocytosis is a nonspecific reaction to tumor necrosis. Using a transplantable mammary tumor in splenectomized mice, Lee and co-workers (1979) demonstrated that tumor necrosis is almost always present in mice with granulocytosis, and concluded that the leukemoid reaction is a nonspecific response of the host to inflammation.

Leukemoid and leukoerythroblastic changes represent reactions to malignancy; further confusion may appear when primary carcinoma cells actually enter the peripheral circulation and create a leukemia-like blood picture. Such metastatic cells have received the designation of carcinocythemia, and their morphologic similarity to leukemia cells requires the use of special histochemical and lysozymal studies to distinguish the entity correctly (Carey et al. 1976). The increasing number of hematologic malignancies superimposed on previously treated tumors makes this differentiation of increasing importance (Casciato and Scott 1979).

Erythrocytosis

An absolute increase in the total red cell mass may be a paraneoplastic manifestation of several tumors (Lange 1976; Altaffer and Chenault 1979). The most common malignancy causing this secondary polycythemia is hypernephroma with 1% to 5% incidence of erythrocytosis. Erythropoietin stimulatory activity has been demonstrated in the serum, urine, and tumor cyst fluid of several patients with this malignancy of the kidney (Hammond and Winnick 1974; Burk et al. 1977).

There is also increasing evidence that the liver is an additional source of extrarenal erythropoietin (Brown et al. 1980), giving some explanation for the 10% incidence of erythrocytosis with hepatomas (Margolis and Homcey 1972). This association provides the clinician with an important marker in the cirrhotic patient, suggesting the added complication of a hepatoma.

Cerebellar hemangioblastomas, large uterine myomas, and pheochromocytomas have also been associated with erythrocytosis. This condition, although a paraneoplastic phenomenon, should not demand a blind tumor search. If polycythemia vera can be excluded on the basis of an absence of any evidence of a panmyelopathy, and if secondary polycythemia due to hypoxic insult is not evident, one is justified in pursuing a renal, hepatic, cerebellar, or uterine tumor as the source of erythropoietin secretion. Removal of the tumor eliminates the secondary polycythemia that may constitute a marker of recurrence.

Thrombocytosis

Modest to extreme elevations of the platelet count have been documented in malignancies in general and lung cancer in particular. Levin and Conley (1964) demonstrated that thrombocytosis is a common accompaniment of cancer, with 40% of patients with malignant disease of all types (excluding carcinoma of the lung) and 38% of patients with lung carcinoma having platelet counts greater than $400{,}000/mm^3$. Bouvenot and associates (1979) claimed the same incidence in their patients with lung cancer, although Silvis, Turkbas, and Doscherholmen (1970) found 60% of their patients with such tumors to have counts outside the normal range.

The mechanism of such platelet elevation is not established. A thrombocyte-stimulating factor has been isolated from hepatoblastoma tissue associated with thrombocytosis (Nickerson et al. 1980). The role of the pulmonary vasculature in platelet kinetics suggests that pulmonary thrombocytosis may represent a specific malfunctioning in the platelet cycle; megakaryocytes are present in the lung under normal circumstances (Kaufman et al. 1965). The explanation for such elevations in platelet count awaits better clarification of the platelet cycle and its control mechanisms.

The elevation in count is usually modest in these circumstances; in Spigel and Mooney's (1977) series of 391 cases, only 7 had counts greater than $1{,}000{,}000/mm^3$. Such elevations are not associated with any significant risks of thrombosis; platelet function is normal with no resulting bleeding. The thrombocytosis is again a marker, frequently of malignancy, with only a tenuous participation in the coagulopathy sometimes seen in malignancy.

Thrombocytopenia

Prior to the ready availability of platelet concentrates, bleeding secondary to thrombocytopenia was a major cause of death in malignancies. Marrow infiltration may create a leukoerythroblastic picture with thrombocytopenia as a prominent component. Splenic metastases may result in a hypersplenic sequestration of platelets. Intravascular coagulation may lead to consumption of platelets with thrombocytopenia as the major abnormality. Solid tumors have been associated with a rare immune-mediated thrombocytopenia, which, analogous to the previously mentioned immune hemolytic anemia, responds to removal of the tumor (Kim and Boggs 1979).

Thrombocytopenia may be a marker of malignancy; its presence complicates the many invasive and surgical procedures used in diagnosis and treatment of tumors. Attention to platelet number and bleeding time will obviate this problem.

Intravascular Coagulation-Fibrinolysis

The vessel wall, platelets, and soluble components of the coagulation cascade are all essential for normal hemostasis; this ability to halt bleeding through thrombus formation is in dynamic equilibrium with the counterforce of fibrinolysis. Any imbalance in this system may result in excessive bleeding or clotting, depending on the site of alteration in coagulation-fibrinolysis. The varying contributions of either to abnormal clotting or bleeding are difficult to interpret because any measurements represent the contributions of both production and destruction; normal levels of a factor may represent relative reduction from pathologically elevated levels or result from adequate compensation for excessive destruction of a factor. It is only by focusing on the dynamic aspects of hemostasis, either by considering the turnover of clotting components or serial measurements, that one can accurately establish the presence of hemostatic imbalance.

Such imbalance is common as an accompaniment of malignancy (Rasche and Dietrich 1977; Weick 1978). The association of thrombosis with malignancy was recognized in 1865 by Armand Trousseau who correctly surmised that "phlegmasia was the consequence of cancerous cachexia." An updating by Sack, Levin, and Bell (1977) expanded the syndrome (the association of thrombophlebitis with malignancy) to include hemorrhage, marantic endocarditis, and arterial emboli. They documented evidence of intravascular coagulation in their patients; hypofibrinogenemia and thrombocytopenia were most common, with the additional findings of increased fibrinogen-fibrin degradation products, microangiopathic hemolytic anemia, cryofibrinogenemia, and reduction in several clotting components. They emphasized that the rate of activation of the cascade and the adequacy of the body's compensatory response both determined the levels of factors in consumptive states. Thrombosis may result from local activation of the cascade; hemorrhage occurs when rapid activation of the cascade results in depletion of the clotting components. The primary role of fibrinolysis in bleeding states is still tenuous although prostatic cancer has been most frequently cited as participating in such disorders (Straub et al. 1967).

The evidence for disordered coagulation with malignancies is compelling, but the pathogenesis is still elusive (Hagedorn et al. 1974; Martens et al. 1974; Sun et al. 1974; Losito, Beaudry, and Valderrame 1977). Cultured human cancer cell lines have been demonstrated to have thromboplastic and fibrinolytic activities (Kinjo et al. 1979); these tumor cell products are thought essential for local and metastatic growth. The hemostatic disorders associated with malignant disease may represent a spillover of these tumor cell products, which also include a factor X-activating procoagulant separate from tissue thromboplastin (Gordon, Frauler, and Lewis 1975). Alterations in platelet glycoproteins have also been described with tumors and have been suggested as possible contributory factors to thrombosis (Scialla et al. 1979).

The appearance of a clotting disorder may be a clue to an occult malignancy. Recurrent thrombosis especially in atypical locations is special cause for concern. Elimination of the clotting disorder is rarely completely attainable because of inability to destroy the underlying tumor. Control is often possible with judicious use of heparin and/or antiplatelet agents (Bick 1978). Coumadin is usually not successful therapeutically in thromboses associated with malignancies. Unfortunately, coagulopathies that occur with cancers may be the harbingers of increased morbidity and early mortality.

References

Altaffer, L., and Chenault, O. Paraneoplastic endocrinopathies associated with renal tumors. *J. Urol.* 122:573–577, 1979.

Anner, R., and Drewinko, B. Frequency and significance of bone marrow involvement by metastatic solid tumors. *Cancer* 39:1337–1344, 1977.

Antman, K. et al. Microangiopathic hemolytic anemia and cancer: a review. *Medicine* 58:377–384, 1979.

Barrett, O. N., Jr. Monocytosis in malignant disease. *Ann. Intern. Med.* 73:991–992, 1970.

Bick, R. Alterations of hemostasis associated with malignancy. *Semin. Thromb. Hemostas.* 5:1–26, 1978.

Bottenstein, J. et al. The growth of cells in serum-free hormone supplemented media. *Methods Enzymol.* 58:94–109, 1979.

Bouvenot, G. et al. Thrombocytose et cancer bronchique. *Sem. Hop. Paris* 55:26–29, 1979.

Brain, M. C. et al. Microangiopathic hemolytic anemia in mucin-forming adenocarcinoma. *Br. J. Haematol.* 18:183–193, 1970.

Brown, C. Bone marrow necrosis: a study of seventy cases. *Johns Hopkins Med. J.* 131:189–203, 1972.

Brown, S. et al. Spontaneous increase in erythropoietin and hematocrit value associated with transient liver enzyme abnormalities in an anephric patient undergoing hemodialysis. *Am. J. Med.* 68:280–284, 1980.

Brunning, R. et al. Bilateral trephine bone marrow biopsies in lymphoma and other neoplastic diseases. *Ann. Intern. Med.* 82:365–366, 1975.

Burk, J. et al. Renal cell carcinoma with erythrocytosis and elevated erythropoietin stimulatory activity. *South. Med. J.* 70:955–958, 1977.

Carey, R. et al. Carcinocythemia (carcinoma cell leukemia). *Am. J. Med.* 60:273–278, 1976.

Cartwright, G., and Lee, G. The anemia of chronic disorders. *Br. J. Haematol.* 21:147–152, 1971.

Casciato, D., and Scott, J. Acute leukemia following prolonged cytotoxic agent therapy. *Medicine* 58:32–47, 1979.

Chernow, B., and Wallner, S. Variables predictive of bone marrow metastasis. *Cancer* 42:2373–2378, 1978.

Crowther, D., and Bateman, C. J. Malignant disease. *Clin. Haematol.* 1:447–473, 1972.

DeGowin, R., and Gibson, D. Erythropoietin and the anemia of mice bearing extramedullary tumor. *J. Lab. Clin. Med.* 94:303–311, 1979.

DeGowin, R.; Grund, F. M.; and Gibson, D. P. Erythropoietic insufficiency in mice with extramedullary tumor. *Blood* 51:33–43, 1978.

Delsol, G. et al. Leukoerythroblastosis and cancer frequency, prognosis, and pathophysiologic significance. *Cancer* 44:1009–1013, 1979.

Douglas, S. W.; and Adamson, J. W. The anemia of chronic disorders: studies of marrow regulation and iron metabolism. *Blood* 45:55–65, 1976.

Ellman, L. Bone marrow biopsy in the evaluation of lymphoma, carcinoma, and granulomatous disorders. *Am. J. Med.* 60:1–6, 1976.

Fahey, R. Unusual leukocyte responses in primary carcinoma of the lung. *Cancer* 4:930–935, 1951.

Gordon, S.; Frauler, J.; and Lewis, B. Cancer procoagulant A: a factor X-activating procoagulant from malignant tissue. *Thromb. Res.* 6:127–137, 1975.

Hagedorn, A. et al. Coagulation abnormalities in patients with inoperable lung cancer. *Medicine* 49:647–653, 1974.

Hammond, D., and Winnick, S. Paraneoplastic erythrocytosis and ectopic erythropoietins. *Ann. NY Acad. Sci.* 230:219–227, 1974.

Hilts, S., and Shaw, C. Leukemoid blood reactions. *N. Engl. J. Med.* 249:434–438, 1953.

Hirst, E., and Robertson, T. The syndrome of thymoma and erythroblastopenic anemia. *Medicine* 46:225–264, 1967.

Ihde, D. et al. Bone marrow metastases in small cell carcinoma of the lung. *Blood* 53:677–686, 1979.

Isaacson, N., and Rapoport, P. Eosinophilia in malignant tumors: its significance. *Ann. Intern. Med.* 25:893–902, 1946.

Jacobson, R., and Jackson, D. Erythrocyte fragmentation in defibrination syndrome. *Ann. Intern. Med.* 81:207–209, 1974.

Kaufman, R. et al. Origin of pulmonary megakaryocytes. *Blood* 25:767–775, 1965.

Kim, H., and Boggs, D. A syndrome resembling idiopathic thrombocytopenic purpura in ten patients with diverse forms of cancer. *Am. J. Med.* 67:371–377, 1979.

Kinjo, M. et al. Thromboplastic and fibrinolytic activities of cultured human cancer cell lines. *Br. J. Cancer* 39:15–23, 1979.

Kiraly, J., and Wheby, M. Bone marrow necrosis. *Am. J. Med.* 60:361–368, 1976.

Krantz, S., and Kao, V. Studies on red cell aplasia. I. Demonstration of a plasma inhibitor to heme synthesis and an antibody to erythroblastic nuclei. *Proc. Natl. Acad. Sci.* 58:493–500, 1967.

Lange, R. Erythrocytosis associated with normal blood gas values. *Adv. Intern. Med.* 21:309–333, 1976.

Lee, M. et al. Kinetics of tumor-induced murine neutrophilia. *Blood* 53:619–632, 1979.

Leite, C., and Hoogstraten, B. Differential diagnosis of anemia and cancer. *CA* 27:88–99, 1977.

Leland, J., and MacPherson, B. Hematologic findings in cases of mammary cancer metastatic to bone marrow. *Am. J. Clin. Pathol.* 71:31–35, 1979.

Levin, J., and Conley, C. Thrombocytosis associated with malignant disease. *Arch. Intern. Med.* 114:497–500, 1964.

Losito, R.; Beaudry, P.; and Valderrame, J. Antithrombin III and factor VIII in patients with neoplasms. *Am. J. Clin. Pathol.* 68:258–262, 1977.

Margolis, S., and Homcey, C. Systemic manifestations of hepatoma. *Medicine* 51:381–391, 1972.

Martens, B. et al. Fibrinolytic split products (FSP) and ethanol gelation tests in preoperative evaluation of patients with prostatic disease. *Mayo Clin. Proc.* 49:642–646, 1974.

Nickerson, H. J.; Silberman, T.; and McDonald, T. Hepatoblastoma, thrombocytosis, and increased thrombopoietin. *Cancer* 45:315–317, 1980.

Rasche, H., and Dietrich, M. Hemostatic abnormalities associated with malignant disease. *Eur. J. Cancer* 13:1053–1064, 1977.

Robinson, W. Granulocytosis in neoplasia. *Ann. NY Acad. Sci.* 230:212–218, 1974.

Sack, G.; Levin, J.; and Bell, W. Trousseau's syndrome and other manifestations of chronic disseminated coagulopathy in patients with neoplasms. *Medicine* 56:1–37, 1977.

Sato, G. H. The growth of HeLa cells in a serum-free hormone supplemented medicine. *Adv. Pathol.* 6:227–232, 1977.

Scialla, S. et al. Alterations in platelet surface sialytransferase activity and platelet aggregation in a group of cancer patients with a high incidence of thrombosis. *Cancer Res.* 39:2031–2035, 1979.

Silvis, S.; Turkbas, N.; and Doscherholmen, A. Thrombocytosis in patients with lung cancer. *JAMA* 211:1852–1853, 1970.

Spigel, S., and Mooney, L. Extreme thrombocytosis associated with malignancy. *Cancer* 39:339–341, 1977.

Spira, M., and Lynch, E. Autoimmune hemolytic anemia and carcinoma: an unusual association. *Am. J. Med.* 67:753–758, 1979.

Straub, P.; Riedler, G.; and Frick, P. G. Hypofibrinogenemia in metastatic carcinoma of the prostate. *J. Clin. Pathol.* 20:152–157, 1967.

Sun, N. et al. Blood coagulation studies in patients with cancer. *Mayo Clin. Proc.* 49:636–641, 1974.

Tavassoli, M. The marrow-blood barrier. *Br. J. Haematol.* 41:297–302, 1979.

Trousseau, A. Phlegmasia alba dolens. *Clinique Medicale de L'Hotel Dieu de Paris 3*. London: The New Sydenham Society, 3:94, 1865.

Weick, J. Intravascular coagulation in cancer. *Semin. Oncol.* 5:203–211, 1978.

Weick, J.; Hagedorn, A.; and Linman, J. Leukoerythroblastosis: diagnostic and prognostic significance. *Mayo Clin. Proc.* 49:110–113, 1974.

Zucker, S.; Friedman, S.; and Lysik, R. Bone marrow erythropoiesis in the anemia of infection, inflammation, and malignancy. *J. Clin. Invest.* 53:1132–1138, 1974.

Zucker, S., and Lysik, R. Cancer-induced cytolysis of normal bone marrow cells. *Nature* 265:736–737, 1977.

five

Neurologic Problems of Cancer and Their Treatment

JONATHAN H. PINCUS

In a number of patients with carcinoma, disorders of the central and peripheral nervous systems and muscles may develop that are independent of metastases. These disorders, which are mostly inflammatory, are called paraneoplastic neurologic syndromes. They are rare and of unknown etiology, and must be distinguished from metastatic disease and from other identifiable forms of nonmetastatic disease. They are outlined as follows:

- I. Metastatic
  - A. Parenchymatous—lung, breast, kidney, thyroid
  - B. Meningeal—breast, lung, lymphoma, stomach (Pressure, cell count, and protein usually elevated; glucose depressed in 40% at first lumbar puncture, 75% ultimately; malignant cells seen in 40% at first lumbar puncture, 80% ultimately)
- II. Nonmetastatic
  - A. Paraneoplastic
    - 1. Inflammatory
      Cerebellum, brain stem, cortex, spinal cord, dorsal root ganglia, peripheral nerves, muscles; syndromes often mixed
    - 2. Non-inflammatory
      Eaton-Lambert
  - B. Intravascular coagulation
  - C. Nonbacterial thrombotic endocarditis
  - D. Metabolic encephalopathy (Inappropriate antidiuretic hormone, Cushing's, hypercalcemia)
  - E. Infection
  - F. Drug toxicity

Several syndromes have been described: cortical cerebellar degeneration, mixed central nervous system involvement with cerebral and brain stem lesions, myelopathy, sensory peripheral neuropathy, mixed peripheral neuropathy (sensorimotor), neuromuscular disorders with myasthenic features, and polymyositis. These paraneoplastic syndromes sometimes are found in pure form, but are more commonly present in combination, with one clinical variety predominating.

The incidence of these disorders is difficult to determine. Wilkinson, Croft, and Urich (1967) found an overall incidence of 6.6%, including patients with mild and limited evidence of neurologic disease. Others (Henson 1970) have estimated that in unselected patients the combined incidence of peripheral neuropathy and encephalomyelitis did not exceed 2% in patients with primary carcinoma of the lung. Although that tumor accounts for about 60% of neurologic problems (Dayan, Croft, and Wilkinson 1965) it is likely that malignant disease of any type may, on occasion, be associated with the development of one of these syndromes. Neurologic symptoms may have their onset months, or unusually, several years before the presence of malignancy can be confirmed despite intensive investigations to demonstrate its existence.

Cortical Cerebellar Degeneration

This condition (table 5.1) is characterized by a widespread degeneration and eventually nearly total disappearance of Purkinje cells in the cerebellar cortex and a

Table 5.1. *Cerebellar Degeneration*

Onset	*Symptoms*	*Association*	*CSF*
Adult, subacute	Ataxia in limbs, nystagmus not prominent, dysphagia, dysarthria, possible mental changes, and peripheral neuropathy	Carcinoma of the lung, ovary	Reflects inflammation
Children, acute	Ataxia in limbs and trunk, opsoclonus, myoclonic jerking of limbs and trunk	Neuroblastoma	Normal

moderate loss of granule cells (Brain and Henson 1958). The spinocerebellar tracts are often degenerated, and meningeal and perivascular lymphocytic infiltrations may be present. There is occasionally an increase in the cells and protein in the cerebrospinal fluid (CSF) with a moderate rise in gamma globulin (IgG). Patients develop an acute or subacute cerebellar disorder with severe ataxia in the limbs. Most have associated dysphagia and dysarthria; nystagmus is seldom prominent. In many there is associated mental deterioration. Although the process may become arrested, remissions seldom occur. Cerebellar degeneration is chiefly associated with carcinoma of the lung and ovary, and the neurologic manifestations often precede those of the tumor.

In children, acute cerebellar ataxia, opsoclonus, and myoclonic jerking of the extremities and trunk may precede the diagnosis of neuroblastoma (Bray et al. 1969). The pathogenesis of this condition is unknown, but excessive catecholamine production does not appear to play a major role (Solomon and Chutorian 1968).

Mixed Form

The lesions in these cases consist of lymphocytic infiltration within the meninges, perivascular cuffing of the blood vessels, degeneration of neurons in Ammon's horn, brain stem nuclei and subthalamic nuclei, and demyelination in the pyramidal tracts and posterior columns of the spinal cord. Intranuclear inclusion bodies have been described.

Patients develop neurologic signs and symptoms correlating with these lesions. Onset can be acute or subacute, symmetric or asymmetric, and both auditory and vestibular manifestations may be present (McGill 1976). In some patients mild cerebellar dysfunction occurs. In most, a severe mental disturbance is present with progressive dementia associated with lesions of temporal lobe limbic structures. Abnormal involuntary movements may become prominent. Eventually, most of these patients develop signs and symptoms of peripheral neuropathy. The CSF is generally negative; there is increased gamma globulin. The association of encephalitis with intranuclear and intracytoplasmic inclusions has raised the possibility of viral etiology, but no virus has yet been isolated. Small cell carcinoma of the lung is the most frequently associated tumor (Corsellis, Goldberg, and Norton 1968).

Other nonmetastatic manifestations of cancer that can cause cerebral neurologic signs include intravascular coagulation and nonbacterial thrombotic endocarditis (Collins et al. 1975; Rosen and Armstrong 1973). Intravascular coagulation appears mainly in women with promyelocytic leukemia or lymphoma, although it also has been described in association with breast cancer. It is manifested by evidence of generalized encephalopathy as well as by focal seizures and hemiparesis. Although all patients with intravascular coagulation have had laboratory evidence of coagulation abnormalities during the course of their illness, these often are not severe when the neurologic symptoms begin. Serial platelet counts and coagulation studies may allow an early diagnosis.

Nonbacterial thrombotic endocarditis is usually seen in association with carcinoma of the lung, pancreas, or prostate. Over half the patients manifest neurologic signs suggesting generalized and fluctuating cerebral dysfunction, as well as focal signs of acute onset.

Other causes of generalized and multifocal brain disease in patients with cancer include opportunistic CNS infections (Chernik, Armstrong, and Posner 1973) and metabolic encephalopathy. The latter includes Cushing's syndrome, which is associated with small cell carcinoma of the lung in most instances, inappropriate antidiuretic hormone (ADH) secretion, and hypercalcemia.

Hypercalcemia causes vomiting and mental disturbance as well as muscle weakness, symptoms that may suggest increased intracranial pressure. Unlike the states of water intoxication resulting from inappropriate ADH secretion, hypercalcemia gives rise to a high blood urea nitrogen. It is most commonly caused by bone metastases, but is sometimes related to the endocrine effects of a tumor. Parathormone is secreted by squamous carcinoma at times, and in such cases hypercalcemia is not suppressed by treatment with steroids. As the condition can induce coma or cardiac death in patients with slowly growing tumors, treatment with calcitonin or mithramycin should be considered if corticosteroids fail (Hills 1977).

Peripheral Neuropathy

In some instances, a predominantly sensory neuropathy develops involving not only the sensory peripheral nerves but also the dorsal roots, dorsal spinal ganglions, and the dorsal columns of the spinal cord. In addition to fiber degeneration, lymphocytic infiltration may be present. The patients experience severe subjective sensory disturbances such as pains and dysesthesias in the extremities, and eventually severe sensory loss causing disabling sensory ataxia. A mixed sensorimotor neuropathy also can occur. This ganglioradiculoneuritis has been considered to be one end of a spectrum of which the other main component is encephalomyelitis associated with carcinoma. In those patients with a primary sensory neuropathy without clinical evidence of encephalitis, sensory signs and symptoms predominate. The cerebrospinal fluid total protein, and particularly the IgG fraction, are often raised. The condition may antedate discovery of carcinoma, usually a small cell carcinoma of the lung, by some months or years; clinical remissions do not occur, because the posterior root ganglion cells are destroyed (Croft 1976).

In some patients the peripheral neuropathy is mixed with both sensory and motor deficits. Carcinoma or lymphoma may be associated with a nonmetastatic peripheral neuropathy (actually a ganglioradiculoneuropathy), which often is present clinically in advance of the discovery of malignancy. The clinical symptoms and signs are usually those of a mixed motor and sensory neuropathy that primarily affects the lower limbs; ordinarily, motor signs predominate. The physical findings are those of a distal neuropathy, and loss of ankle reflexes is an early sign. Onset is usually subacute over a period of weeks to months; acute cases do occur that resemble the Guillain-Barré syndrome. The cerebrospinal fluid protein is often high without a cellular reaction. A few patients with this type of peripheral involvement have shown spontaneous arrest or remission of symptoms. Relapsing and remitting courses have been described. The evidence that steroids can induce a remission is anecdotal. Remission is more likely to occur when the neuropathy is seen in association with tumors other than cancer of the lung, such as Hodgkin's disease, seminoma, and malignant thymoma. In most cases of mixed sensorimotor neuropathy, nerve conduction velocities are normal or near normal (Trojaberg, Frantzo, and Anderson 1969).

Myelopathy

Two forms of myelopathy, both uncommon, may occur. A syndrome similar to amyotrophic lateral sclerosis but with a more benign course has been reported (Brain, Croft, and Wilkinson 1965). This may be associated with bulbar palsy as well. Subacute necrotic myelopathy is even more rare (Mancall and Rosales 1964) and is characterized by ascending paraplegia with sensory deficit and loss of sphincter control. The lesion is a necrotizing one, associated with elevation of CSF protein and pleocytosis.

Neuromuscular Disorder

In association with carcinoma certain patients develop muscular atrophy or weakness, and some have a myasthenic response that is not related merely to general cachexia or to the presence of a polyneuritis.

The myasthenic syndrome of Eaton and Lambert is seen primarily with carcinoma of the bronchus, though occasionally it occurs in the absence of malignant disease (Brown and Johns 1974). Weakness of the proximal muscles occurs initially, more in the lower than the upper extremities. There is often abnormal fatigability on exertion and soreness in the affected muscles. Examination may reveal weakness and wasting of the quadriceps and hip flexors, with diminished or absent knee reflexes. Characteristically, the ankle jerks are retained, which helps to differentiate this syndrome from the peripheral neuropathy described above. Muscle fatigability can be demonstrated after prolonged exercise similar to that seen in myasthenia gravis. After short periods (10 seconds) of voluntary contraction, the power of the muscle contraction may be substantially, although briefly, increased and tendon reflexes that were absent may then be elicited for a short time (Lambert 1966). The electromyographic finding of post-tetanic facilitation with incrementing muscle response to supramaximal stimulation is typical (Eaton and Lambert 1957). Electrical stimulation at slow rates produces low-amplitude potentials gradually decreasing, similar to myasthenia gravis. At a fast tetanic rate an increased facilitatory response is seen.

The main conditions from which this syndrome must be differentiated are myasthenia gravis and peripheral neuropathy (table 5.2). In myasthenia gravis

Table 5.2. *Differences Among Neuromuscular Disorders*

Signs	*Eaton-Lambert Syndrome*	*Myasthenia Gravis*	*Peripheral Neuropathy*
Onset	Subacute	Subacute	Subacute
First symptom	Proximal girdle weakness, especially hip	Bulbar weakness, especially eyes	Distal weakness, especially feet
Soreness	Thighs and calves	None	Calves
Deep tendon reflexes	Diminished	Present	Absent
Tetanic nerve stimulation	Incrementing response	Decrementing response	Normal response or variable
Tensilon test	Negative	Positive	Negative
CSF protein	Normal or mild elevation	Normal	Elevated usually
Guanidine	Improvement	Some improvement	No response

Table 5.3. *Neurologic Complications Associated with Antineoplastic Drugs*

Drugs	*Symptoms*
Alkylating agents	
Nitrogen mustards	
Mechlorethamine (Mustargen) Cyclophosphamide (Cytoxan) Melphalan (Alkeran) Uracil mustard Chlorambucil	Seizures, dementia, nausea, vomiting, cholinomimetic effects including muscular paralysis; herpes zoster, inappropriate antidiuretic hormone
Ethylenimine derivatives	
Alkyl sulfonates (Busulfan)	Impotence
Nitrosoureas	
Carmustine (BCNU) Lomustine (CCNU)	Nausea, vomiting, seizures, delerium
Antimetabolites	
Folate analogues methotrexate (Amethopterin)	Seizures, paraplegia, dementia
Pyrimidine analogues Fluorouracil (5-FU)	Cerebellar degeneration, blindness, oculomotor disturbances; myelopathy with intrathecal use
Cytarabine (Cytosine arabinoside)	Paraparesis, seizures, blindness with intrathecal use

Table 5.3. *Continued*

Drugs	*Symptoms*
Azaribine (Triacetyl-6-azauridine)	Drowsiness, dizziness, tremor, diplopia, dysarthria, aphasia, hyperactive deep tendon reflexes
Natural Products	
Vinca alkaloids Vincristine	Peripheral neuropathy at usual doses, loss of DTR, oculomotor palsies, paralysis of recurrent laryngeal nerves, constipation; CNS toxicity with high doses only (75 μg/kg/1 wk) depression, convulsions, ataxia, athetosis, inappropriate antidiuretic hormone
Cisplatin	Hearing loss, parasthesia, seizures, vomiting, hyponatremia, hypomagnesemia, hypokalemia, hyperuricemia, renal failure

the first muscles to be involved are bulbar, and ptosis and double vision are prominent early symptoms. Conversely, the bulbar muscles are rarely involved in the Eaton-Lambert syndrome. It is rare for proximal weakness of the lower limbs to be the principal symptom in myasthenia gravis. The proximal distribution of weakness helps to differentiate this condition from peripheral neuropathy; however, the incrementing muscle response to stimulation is not specifically diagnostic of Eaton-Lambert syndrome. The same type of response has been reported in acquired myopathies unrelated to carcinoma (Simpson 1976). Also, a similar although quantitatively smaller phenomenon is sometimes seen in myasthenia gravis, usually in muscles that are not clinically affected (Simpson 1974). In contrast to myasthenia gravis, the clinical response to anticholinesterase medications is variable and usually slight. Guanidine is much more effective (Croft 1976). With this syndrome as with myasthenia gravis, patients may have abnormal reactions to muscle relaxants used in anesthesia. Occasional patients are still seen with prolonged and even fatal apnea following the use of muscle relaxants for such procedures as bronchoscopy.

Some patients with carcinoma develop severe proximal myopathy without any clinical or electrical manifestations of myasthenia. Temporary remissions in this syndrome may occur spontaneously. It has been claimed that the onset of symmetrical muscle weakness in men over the age of 50 years is associated with a malignant disorder in 60% of cases; in woman of the same age the incidence of malignant disease is 18% (Shy and Silverstein 1965). Some patients have an associated skin rash and other features leading to diagnosis of dermatomyositis, a rather high proportion of whom are found to have an associated malignancy, with estimates varying from 7% to 34% (Hills 1977).

Neurologic symptoms are sometimes induced by antineoplastic drugs. Intrathecally administered agents or those given in high doses are not surprisingly the most toxic, as most of the antineoplastic drugs do not cross the blood-brain barrier well. The *Vinca* alkaloids quite regularly induce peripheral neuropathy when given systemically at ordinary doses. These data are summarized in table 5.3.

References

Brain, W. R.; Croft, P. B.; and Wilkinson, M. Motor neuron disease as a manifestation of neoplasm. *Brain* 88:479–500, 1965.

Brain, W. R., and Henson, R. A. Neurological syndromes associated with carcinomatous neuromyopathies. *Lancet* 2:971–975, 1958.

Bray, P. F. et al. The coincidence of neuroblastoma and acute cerebellar encephalopathy. *J. Pediatr.* 75: 983–990, 1969.

Brown, J. C., and Johns, R. J. Diagnostic difficulties encountered in the myasthenic syndromes associated with carcinoma. *J. Neurol. Neurosurg. Psychiatry* 37:1214–1224, 1974.

Chernik, M. L.; Armstrong, D.; and Posner, J. B. Central nervous system infections in patients with cancer. *Medicine* 52:563–581, 1973.

Collins, R. C. et al. Neurologic manifestations of intravascular coagulation in patients with cancer. *Neurology* 25:795–806, 1975.

Corsellis, J. A. N.; Goldberg, G. J.; and Norton, A. R. "Limbic encephalitis" and its association with carcinoma. *Brain* 91:481–496, 1968.

Croft, P. Carcinomatous neuromyopathy. *Practitioner* 216:407–413, 1976.

Dayan, A. D.; Croft, P. B.; and Wilkinson, M. Association of carcinomatous neuropathy with different histological types of carcinoma of the lungs. *Brain* 88:501–514, 1965.

Eaton, L. M.; and Lambert, E. H. Electromyography and electric stimulation of nerves in disease of the motor unit: observations of myasthenic syndrome associated with malignant tumors. *JAMA* 163:1117–1124, 1957.

Henson, R. A. Non-metastatic neurological manifestations of malignant disease. In *Modern trends in neurology,* vol. 5, ed. D. Williams. London: Butterworth, 1970, p. 209–225.

Hills, E. A. Unusual manifestations of lung cancer. *Practitioner* 219:648–655, 1977.

Lambert, E. H. Defects of neuromuscular transmission in syndromes other than myasthenia gravis. *Ann. NY Acad. Sci.* 135:367–384, 1966.

Mancall, E. L., and Rosales, R. K. Necrotizing myelopathy associated with visceral carcinoma. *Brain* 87: 639–656, 1964.

McGill, T. Carcinomatous encephalomyelitis with auditory and vestibular manifestations. *Ann. Otol.* 85:120–126, 1976.

Rosen, P., and Armstrong, D. Nonbacterial thrombotic endocarditis in patients with malignant neoplastic diseases. *Am. J. Med.* 54:23–29, 1973.

Shy, C. M., and Silverstein, I. A study of the effects upon the motor unit by remote malignancy. *Brain* 88:515–528, 1965.

Simpson, J. A. Myasthenia gravis and myasthenic syndromes. In *Disorders of voluntary muscle,* 3rd edition, ed. J. Walton. London: Churchill Livingstone, 1974.

Simpson, J. A. Disorders of neuromuscular transmission. *Proc. R. Soc. Med.* 59:993–998, 1976.

Solomon, G. E., and Chutorian, A. M. Opsoclonus and occult neuroblastoma. *N. Engl. J. Med.* 279:475–477, 1968.

Trojaberg, W.; Frantzo, E.; and Andersen, T. Peripheral neuropathy and myopathy associated with carcinoma of the lung. *Brain* 92:71–82, 1969.

Wilkinson, M.; Croft, P. B.; and Urich, H. The remote effects of cancer on the nervous system. *Proc. R. Soc. Med.* 60:683–692, 1967.

six

Paraneoplastic Syndromes

ARTHUR L. LEVY

Paraneoplastic syndromes may be described as disorders of organ functions at a distance from the primary tumor that do not result from space-occupying lesions or metastases (Hall 1974). They are extremely heterogeneous and complicated. Included are syndromes that are clearly due to elaboration of hormones, others that are produced by nonhormonal humoral substances, and finally, a large number of syndromes the etiology of which is not at all clear. Examples of hormonal conditions are the ectopic ACTH, ectopic parathormone (PTH), and Zollinger-Ellison syndromes, inappropriate antidiuretic hormone (IADH) excretion, and erythropoietin production by tumor. Some nonhormonal humoral factors include lactic acidosis, perhaps some types of hypercalcemia, perhaps tumor fever, and probably non–insulin-produced hypoglycemia. Others include the anorexia-cachexia syndromes, and various hematopoietic paraneoplastic syndromes such as coagulopathies, thrombopathies, and leukocytosis.

Classification of Ectopic Hormone-Producing Tumors

It has become possible to classify the hormone-producing tumors based on the observation by Amatruda (1969) and other authors that certain specific types of tumors were likely to elaborate specific types of hormones, and that tumors from similar embryologic anlagen tend to share common endocrine potentials. Grouping of endocrine-producing tumors is as follows:

- Group I (APUD)
  - Bronchial carcinoid
  - Small (oat) cell carcinoma
  - Pancreatic islet cell
  - Pancreatic duct (some)
  - Bile duct (some)
  - Thyroid medullary carcinoma
  - Malignant epithelial thymoma
- Group II (Endodermal and mesodermal)
  - Endodermal
    - Non-oat cell lung
    - Liver
    - Bile duct (some)
  - Squamous
    - Secreting parathormone
  - Mesodermal
    - Retroperitoneal
    - Connective tissue
    - Adrenal cortical
    - Kidney
    - Gonad
- Group III (Transitional)
  - Pheochromocytoma
  - Paraganglioma
  - Neuroblastoma
  - Ganglioneuroma

Group I tumors are in general those that arise from what are called APUD cells (amine content, precursor uptake, and decarboxylation). These cells all arise from the neural crest and travel by way of the endoderm of the gastrointestinal tract, from which some depart as migratory cells to become incorporated into branchial arch derivatives, pancreatic anlage, and the bronchial tree. The hormones produced by these tumors are as follows:

- Group I
  - Insulin
  - Calcitonin
  - ACTH
  - Melanocyte-stimulating hormone
  - Vasopressin
  - Gastrin
  - Glucagon
  - Secretin
  - Biogenic amines
    - Serotonin
    - Histamine
    - Catecholamines
- Group II
  - Parathormone
  - Erythropoietin
  - Erythrocyte-stimulating factor
  - Gonadotropins
  - Human placental lactogen
  - Prolactin
  - Growth hormone
  - Insulin-like activity
  - Renin
  - Thyrotropin
- Group III (overlap I and II)
  - Group I Biogenic amines
    - ACTH
    - Melanocyte-stimulating hormone
    - Insulin
    - Calcitonin
    - Glucagon
    - Secretin
  - Group II Human placental lactogen
    - Insulin-like activity
    - ?Parathormone
    - ?Erythropoietin

Although it is usually the case that one tumor is associated with the production of one hormone, it is important to note that these tumors have multiple endocrine potentials and are capable of producing many, if not all, of the hormones associated with the particular group. Thus while a small cell carcinoma may be recognized to produce ACTH, it may also produce vasopressin, calcitonin, biogenic amines, or any of the other hormones.

The second group of tumors associated with the paraneoplastic production of hormones appears to be a much more heterogeneous group. In fact the unifying factor associated with these is that they are derived from endoderm and mesoderm. This group can be subdivided into three groups: (1) an endodermally derived group consisting mainly of lung tumors (exclusive of small cell and bronchial carcinoid), liver, and bile duct tumors; (2) a small group of squamous tumors that may secrete PTH; (3) a third group, of mesodermal origin, includes retroperitoneal and connective tissue tumors, and tumors of the adrenal cortex, kidneys, and gonads. The hormones produced by these include parathormone, erythropoietin, gonadotropins and human placental lactogen, prolactin, growth hormone, insulin-like activity, renin, and thyrotropin. In addition, these hormones are the ones associated with the fetal antigens such as alpha-fetoprotein and carcinoembryonic antigen, as well as the placental isoenzymes such as Regan isoenzyme of alkaline phosphatase.

It is interesting that corticosteroids, although normal secretory products of some of the parent cells in this group (adrenal cortex, ovary, and testicle), are never ectopically produced. The possible explanation for this may be the large number of enzymatic steps required to permit biologically active steroids to be produced. Tumor cells, being inadequate, would be unable to recapitulate these steps.

The final large group of endocrine-producing tumors is classified as the transitional group. Melanomas may belong here as well, but this is not completely clear. Like group I tumors, these arise from the neural crest and have morphologic and histochemical characteristics of APUD cells. Unlike the cells of group I tumors, these proceed directly from the neural crest to their ultimate location in the adrenal medulla and sympathetic ganglia without traversing the gastrointestinal endoderm. The reason they are classified as transitional is that they secrete hormones that are seen in both group I and group II.

Hyperadrenocorticism and ACTH-Releasing Factor

The association of nonendocrine tumors and hyperadrenocorticism was first noted 45 years ago, before Harvey Cushing described the syndrome named for him. It was not until 1962 that Liddle and associates (Meador et al. 1962; Liddle et al. 1965) demonstrated ACTH-like activity in the nonendocrine tumors of patients with Cushing's syndrome and coined the term ectopic ACTH syndrome. The most common tumors that produce this syndrome are (1) small cell carcinoma of the lung, (2) epithelial thymic tumors, and (3) islet cell pancreatic tumors. Bronchial adenomas, particularly carcinoids, also are frequent causes. Uncommon tumors that have been associated with ectopic ACTH production include pheochromocytoma, medullary carcinoma of the thyroid, parotid tumors, ovarian tumors, prostatic carcinoma, hypernephroma, breast, esophageal, colon, and gallbladder carcinoma, and testicular and uterine tumors.

The diagnosis of ectopic ACTH production may not be clear because major symptoms may be those of the underlying neoplasm. The typical hyperadrenal appearance is often lacking. The tip-off is often unexplained hypokalemic alkalosis and hyperglycemia. The diagnosis may then be made by measurement of plasma cortisol. This determination, however, does not differentiate between ectopic ACTH production and other causes such as true pituitary or iatrogenic Cushing's syndrome due to steroid administration. There are several differentiating features that can be helpful. First, the hyperadrenal appearance is usually present in pituitary Cushing's disease, whereas it is often absent in ectopic ACTH production. Second, hypokalemic alkalosis is often most marked with the ectopic ACTH syndrome. Plasma cortisol, of course, is elevated in all forms of Cushing's syndrome, including iatrogenic and pituitary forms. The diurnal variation in cortisol levels is also lost in all causes of Cushing's syndromes. The most crucial differentiating test is the dexamethasone suppression test. In pituitary Cushing's, the adrenal gland is not suppressed by a low dose of dexamethasone, but is suppressed by a high dose, 2 mg every six hours; in the ectopic ACTH syndrome, even the high dose is not suppressive. Strangely, patients with the ectopic ACTH syndrome may respond to exogenous ACTH or metyrapone. This may be related to the fact that in association with ectopic ACTH production, sometimes there has been reported excess production by the tumor of corticotropin-releasing factor as well. Accordingly, it is possible to continue to have stimulation of the pituitary to produce ACTH even in the presence of high circulating levels of ACTH.

There is some evidence that ectopic ACTH is not identical to pituitary ACTH, as shown by the facts that the quantity as measured by immunoassay exceeds the amount measured by bioassay, and that in sequencing studies, aminoacid composition of the ectopic hormone has been shown to differ from that of pituitary ACTH.

There are several clinical points to remember in the ectopic ACTH syndrome:

1. Cushing's syndrome in a person who smokes is more often due to small cell carcinoma of the lung than to "true" pituitary Cushing's.
2. If careful testing is done, 10% of patients with small cell carcinoma will have evidence of hyperadrenocorticism.
3. A full-blown syndrome is only occasionally seen because of the short life span of patients with ectopic ACTH production who usually die of their malignancy.
4. Presence of hyperpigmentation and/or hypokalemia in a patient with a neoplasm should suggest the ectopic syndrome.

The mainstay of treatment is management of the underlying tumor, whether by surgery, chemotherapy, or radiation. One does not have to cure the tumor. Debulking is often sufficient to reduce ectopic ACTH production enough to diminish the very high circulating levels of cortisol. Failing that, one can use other modalities including potassium replacement, spironolactone, and/or sodium restriction. Mitotane has been used to ablate chemically the adrenal gland and reduce corticosteroid production. In addition, metyrapone and aminoglutethimide (Orth and Liddle 1971) have also been used on occasion, but the efficacy of each of these is limited by its toxicities.

Hypercalcemia

Hypercalcemia is the most common endocrine complication of neoplasia; the most common cause of hypercalcemia is bone resorption secondary to bone metastases. Accordingly, hypercalcemia is seen very frequently in association with carcinoma of the breast, since this is a common malignancy and one with a high predilection to involve bone. It has been recognized, however, that there are patients with neoplasms who do not have evidence for bone metastases, yet who develop hypercalcemia. There is speculation that in these patients the disease may in fact have a humoral cause, such as ectopic PTH production (Sherwood et al. 1967), prostaglandins, particularly prostaglandin E_2, osteoclast-stimulating factor, and perhaps other as yet undiscovered factors. Patients with hypercalcemia may have a variety of symptoms including malaise, fatigue, psychoneurosis, weight loss, pruritus, renal colic, polyuria, polydipsia, constipation, epigastric pain, anorexia, nausea, vomiting, lethargy, muscular weakness, confusion, psychosis, stupor, or coma. There is not a good correlation between the level of calcium and symptoms.

In 1941, Albright described a patient with renal cell carcinoma and metastases to the ileal bone who had hypercalcemia and hypophosphatemia (Albright and Reifenstein 1948). Since one would expect an elevation in serum calcium and either elevated or normal phosphorus with bone metastases, the question of hyperparathyroidism was raised. Exploration of the neck was unremarkable. Accordingly, Albright speculated about the possibility of ectopic PTH production by the tumor. It took 10 years for other authors to report elevated PTH levels in the presence of neoplasia.

The tumors that have been associated with the ectopic PTH syndrome include hypernephroma, epidermoid carcinoma of the lung, and tumors of the bladder, renal pelvis, head and neck, salivary gland, esophagus, penis, vulva, ovary, uterus, pancreas, liver and bile duct, prostate and adrenal, and lymphomas.

The problem with the ectopic PTH syndrome is one of difficulty with the assays. There are several that measure different parts of the molecule, but their reliability is in doubt. In recent years, several investigators have questioned whether the humoral hypercalcemia in most cases is caused by elaboration of PTH by tumors.

In a recent study that raised this question, three groups of patients were investigated. One consisted of patients with malignancies but with normal calcium levels; these were considered a control group. A second group was made up of patients with true hyperparathyroidism due to hyperplasia or adenomas of the parathyroid glands. In the third group were cancer patients with hypercalcemia felt to be from a humoral mechanism. Numerous measurements were evaluated. The first was calcium and the second was the tubular maximum for phosphorus compared to glomerular filtration rate. As expected, the patients with humoral hypercalcemia of malignancy and hyperparathyroidism had both elevated calcium and diminished tubular maximum for phosphorus. In addition, both groups had elevated levels of cyclic AMP. The patients with humoral hypercalcemia of malignancy were shown to have a significantly higher calcium excretion than patients with hyperparathyroidism. This was surprising, since PTH should act on the kidneys by decreasing calcium excretion. Also, the level of 1,25-vitamin D was markedly reduced in patients with humoral hypercalcemia of malignancy, as compared to those with hyperparathyroidism, where it was elevated as expected. Finally, when immunoreactive PTH was measured, it was elevated in the hyperparathyroid group and normal in humoral hypercalcemia of malignancy (Tashjian, Levine, and Munson 1964). This was confirmed with the use of three other antisera. Accordingly, these data suggested that the humoral hypercalcemia of malignancy in a majority of patients was not caused by PTH, but was due to another humoral factor not yet identified that acts primarily on bone rather than on bone and kidney, as does PTH.

The therapy of hypercalcemia in malignancy again rests primarily on the treatment of the underlying neoplasm. One can resort to hydration with saline using furosemide (Lasix) to promote diuresis and calciuria, but not thiazides as they promote calcium retention and can worsen the hypercalcemia. Phosphate preparations such as Neutraphos may be used, particularly when the phosphate level in the blood is low. As long as there is no contraindication, high doses of corticosteroids may be used, but it is the experience of most observers that this is not very efficacious except in diseases such as myeloma, lymphoma, and breast cancer, which may respond. Mithramycin, an antitumor antibiotic, may be useful (Perlia et al. 1970). It acts by inhibiting osteolysis, a mechanism of action distinct from its antitumor activity. The resultant hypocalcemia may be quite durable. Being an antitumor agent, however, mithramycin has hematologic toxicity, particularly thrombocytopenia, which, in a patient who may already be compromised by chemotherapy, may preclude or limit its use. Salmon calcitonin is effective in some cases. Rarely, hypocalcemia has been reported with osteoblastic metastases (Sacknen, Spivack, and Balion 1960).

The Syndrome of Inappropriate Antidiuretic Hormone Excretion

This syndrome (SIADH) is relatively uncommon, seen most frequently in small cell carcinoma of the lung. It is also occasionally seen in undifferentiated lung malignancies other than small cell and rarely in adenocarcinomas of the lung and pancreas. Symptomatology can be quite variable. The patient may be comatose, totally asymptomatic, or just a bit lethargic. The degree of depression of consciousness depends both on the serum sodium level and on the rapidity with which hyponatremia developed.

Diagnosis of SIADH is made on demonstration that the urine osmolarity is greater than the serum osmolarity, despite the abnormally low serum osmolarity. Diagnosis may be difficult in the presence of edema from diuretics.

The mainstay of therapy, again, is treatment of the underlying malignancy with surgery, chemotherapy, or radiation. Particularly in small cell carcinoma of the lung, which is very responsive to chemotherapy and radiation, this may be quite dramatic, and again, one does not have to cure the malignancy to terminate the syndrome, since ablation of a large proportion of the tumor may be completely efficacious. Failing in that, one can effectively manage the SIADH in most cases by fluid restriction, usually to 1 liter a day. Occasionally demeclocycline may be useful because it has an effect similar to that of nephrogenic diabetes insipidus.

Hypoglycemia

Hypoglycemia in a patient with an islet cell neoplasm, which has the potential of producing insulin, is not surprising. There is a form of hypoglycemia not attributable to the production of insulin or a closely related substance (Papaioannai 1966), most commonly caused by large mesenchymal tumors of the chest, abdomen, or pelvis. The mechanism of hypoglycemia in these tumors is not clear (Silverstein, Wakim, and Bali 1964). Several possibilities include: (1) increased insulin-like activity; presumably these tumors may be producing a humoral substance that is not insulin, and which can cause hypoglycemia; (2) increased consumption of glucose by the tumor; (3) chemotherapy; (4) development of an acquired form of glycogen storage disease; (5) inhibition of lipolysis by a humoral substance elaborated by the tumor. None of these mechanisms has been consistently demonstrated.

Lactic Acidosis in Malignancy

Field and co-workers described an association of systemic lactic acidosis with apparently normal tissue oxygenation in several patients with cancer (Field, Block, and Rall 1963; Field 1966). There are many causes of lactic acidosis that can develop as a complication of malignancy, for example, hypoxemia, severe anemia, shock, or one of many other underlying situations. There is a group of patients in whom none of these conditions exist. For the most part, they either have acute leukemia in relapse or lymphomas, particularly Burkitt's lymphoma. It is not uncommon in these situations to see a dramatic resolution of the lactic acidosis with successful treatment of the malignancy. The syndrome appears to be associated with only the most rapidly proliferating neoplasms.

Management requires treatment of the underlying neoplasm. It is often extremely difficult to keep up with the lactic acidosis with bicarbonate infusions, which are usually unsuccessful. Occasionally, hemodialysis may be used, but if the neoplasm cannot be controlled, generally the lactic acidosis also cannot.

Fever

Recurrent unexplained fever is a common manifestation of certain tumors and often cannot be ascribed to coexistent infection or other known causes (Boggs and Frei 1960; Molavi and Weinstein 1970). Malignancies with a particularly high incidence of fever include: (1) lymphomas, especially Hodgkin's disease but also non-Hodgkin's variety, (2) acute leukemia, (3) hypernephroma, (4) bone sarcoma, (5) atrial myxoma, (6) visceral neoplasms, especially gastric carcinoma, and (7) any tumor involvement of the liver, including hepatic metastases.

Unexplained fever that coincides with tumor growth, disappears promptly when the tumor is removed or suppressed, and reappears when the malignancy recurs, can be considered to be tumor-associated. Such an etiology is also probable in other cases in which the fever persists, with uncontrolled tumor activity in the absence of reasonable causes for fever.

In 1948, a pyrogen distinct from endotoxin was reported by Beeson to be present in rabbit leukocytes. This endogenous pyrogen is now thought to be produced by a variety of cell types including monocytes, macrophages, and phagocytic cells from the reticuloendothelial system, but probably not polymorphonuclear leukocytes (Hanson, Murphy, and Windle 1980).

Pyrogen has been reported from hypernephroma tissue in two patients, but not from normal renal tissue from the same patients. This was demonstrated when supernatants from these tissues were injected into test rabbits. Similar studies have been done with spleen and lymph nodes from patients with Hodgkin's disease (Bodel 1974). When the supernatants from incubation of their splenic tissue were injected into rabbits, 11 out of 20 of the specimens caused fever, whereas only 2 out of 17 supernatants obtained from normal splenic tissue did so. Similar activity was observed in lymph nodes. Although the correlation with clinical fever in these cases was not good, there are complicating factors in the intact host that may explain these differences.

References

Albright, F. Acute atrophy of bone (osteoporosis) simulating hyperparathyroidism. *J. Clin. Endocrinol.* 1: 711–716, 1941a.

Albright, F. Case records of the Mass. General Hospital, #2761. *N. Engl. J. Med.* 225:789–791, 1941b.

Albright, F., and Reifenstein, E. C. *Parathyroid glands and metabolic bone disease.* Baltimore: Williams & Wilkins, 1948, p. 93.

Amatruda, T. T. Nonendocrine secreting tumors. In *Duncan's diseases of metabolism,* eds. P. K. Bondy and L.

Rosenberg. Philadelphia: W. B. Saunders, 1969, pp. 1227–1244.

Beeson, P. B. Temperature-elevating effect of a substance obtained from polymorphonuclear leukocytes. *J. Clin. Invest.* 27:524, 1948.

Bodel, P. Tumors and fever. *Ann. N.Y. Acad. Sci.* 230:6–13, 1974.

Boggs, D. R., and Frei, E., III. Clinical studies of fever and infection in cancer. *Cancer* 13:1240–1253, 1960.

Field, M. Significance of blood lactate elevations among patients with acute leukemia and other neoplastic proliferative disorders. *Am. J. Med.* 40:528–547, 1966.

Field, M.; Block, J. B.; and Rall, D. P. Lactic acidosis in acute leukemia. *Clin. Res.* 11:193, 1963.

Hall, T. C., ed. Paraneoplastic syndromes. *Ann. NY Acad. Sci.* 230:1–577, 1974.

Hanson, D. F.; Murphy, P. A.; and Windle, B. E. Failure of rabbit neutrophils to secrete endogenous pyrogen when stimulated with staphylococci. *J. Exp. Med.* 151:1360–1371, 1980.

Liddle, G. W. et al. The ectopic ACTH syndrome. *Cancer Res.* 25:1057–1061, 1965.

Meador, C. K. et al. Cause of Cushing's syndrome in patients with tumors arising from "non-endocrine" tissue. *J. Clin. Endocrinol.* 22:693–703, 1962.

Molavi, A., and Weinstein, L. Persistent perplexing pyrexia—etiology and diagnosis. *Med. Clin. North Am.* 59:379–396, 1970.

Orth, D. N., and Liddle, G. W. Results of treatment in 108 patients with Cushing's syndrome. *N. Engl. J. Med.* 285:243–247, 1971.

Papaioannai, A. Tumors other than insulinomas associated with hypoglycemia. *Surg. Gynecol. Obstet.* 123: 1093–1109, 1966.

Perlia, C. P. et al. Mithramycin treatment of hypercalcemia. *Cancer* 25:389–394, 1970.

Sacknen, M. D.; Spivack, A. P.; and Balion, L. J. Hypocalcemia in the presence of osteoblastic metastases. *N. Engl. J. Med.* 262:173–176, 1960.

Sherwood, L. M. et al. Production of parathyroid hormone by non-parathyroid tumors. *J. Clin. Endocrinol. Metab.* 27:140–146, 1967.

Silverstein, M. N.; Wakim, K. G.; and Bali, R. C. Hypoglycemia associated with neoplasia. *Am. J. Med.* 36:415, 1964.

Tashjian, A. H.; Levin, L.; and Munson, P. L. Immunochemical identification of parathyroid hormone in non-parathyroid neoplasms associated with hypercalcemia. *J. Exp. Med.* 119:467–484, 1964.

seven

Metastasis

DAVID S. FISCHER

Although some cancers kill by local growth in a vital location (e.g., brain tumors), and others do so by local interference with no extension into vital structures (e.g., head and neck tumors), most cause death by distant spread—metastasis. Accordingly, it is important to know the natural history of cancer to plan its management intelligently.

It is clearly illogical to mount a radical surgical or radiologic attack on a tumor with curative intent if there is already evidence of metastasis. Regrettably, we still see this done occasionally. On the other hand, it is clearly not cost-effective or in the interests of the patient with cancer always to obtain bone, liver, brain, and gallium scans, and we also see this done occasionally. One must have an appreciation of the characteristics of the primary tumor, its relative frequency and pathways of metastasis, and its more common target visceral organs (fig. 7.1).

To have some idea of what tumors metastasize frequently and where they are most likely to proliferate, autopsy series have been analyzed as a rough guide (Abrams 1950; Howe and Maniatis 1950; Willis 1952).

Primary tumors with high incidence of metastasis are as follows:

Colon and rectum
Prostate
Lung
Stomach
Breast (stage II or III)
Pancreas
Kidney
Melanoma (depth greater than 2.26 mm)
Primary bone
Childhood tumors
Testis, nonseminoma
Bladder, high-grade, invasive

Breast cancer with one or more positive axillary nodes will be metastatic in 53% of cases, and with four or more positive nodes in 80% of cases within five years (Fisher 1972). For patients with no involvement of axillary nodes at surgery there will be 21% recurrence overall, and less for those with small primary tumors. Primary tumors with a low incidence of metastasis, including stage I breast carcinoma, are listed below. (It must be remembered that "low" is a relative concept.)

Brain
Head and neck
Breast (stage I)
Bladder, low-grade, superficial
Cervix
Melanoma (depth less than 0.76 mm)
Thyroid
Seminoma

As a general principle, very few tumor cells that are released ultimately form metastatic foci in the immunocompetent host (Sugarbaker and Ketcham 1977). The blood stream seems to be a hostile environment for cancer cells shed from a solid tumor. Lymphatics with their slower circulations provide a more suitable environment. Even so, most of the tumor cells are killed in the lymphatic circulation, remain viable and grow in the draining lymph nodes, or are passed through into the venous circulation, either by lymphaticovenous communications or through the thoracic ducts. Thus lymph nodes may serve as a repository for later dissemination. Thoracic duct drainage is into the jugular trunk, then to the superior vena cava, the right heart, the pulmonary arteries, and to the lung. Once a metastasis is established in the lung, it has access to the arterial circulation just as does a primary lung tumor. This is one of the explanations for metastases to the brain, heart muscle, eye, thyroid, skin, and so forth (del Regato 1977). Another suspected pathway is the vertebral vein system that communicates with the caval venous systems, the paravertebral systems to the bones and skull, and through these sinusoidal systems to the arterial circulation without direct access to the heart (fig. 7.2). Thus neuroblastomas can go to the skull from the adrenals, and prostatic metastases to the vertebrae, pelvis, ribs, and long bones.

Serous cavities frequently form a pathway for spread as the proteinaceous fluids float tumor cells to distant parts. Ovarian tumors are often found, as ascitic tumors spread extensively throughout the peritoneal cavity, especially on the under surface of the diaphragm and on the liver surfaces. Pancreatic tumors, appendiceal pseudomyxomas, gastric carcinomas, lymphomas, and endometrial carcinomas can also form as ascites and spread by this route. The thoracic cavity can spread lung, pleural, and breast tumors through the pleural fluid. Some tumors can spread by way of cerebrospinal fluid, including ependymomas, medulloblastomas, lymphomas, melanomas, and neuroblastomas (table 7.1).

Most metastases are ultimately to the lung, liver, or bone (Gilbert 1976). Drainage of the gastrointestinal tract is through the portal system to the liver, and its capillary bed filters out metastases. Secondary metastases from the liver can then go to the lung, and finally, a tertiary metastasis can go from lung to the arterial circulation and thereby to the brain (Weiss, Gilbert, and Posner 1980). Thus in the absence of liver metastases, one would have little reason to perform a CT or brain scan for a patient with gastric, pancreatic, or colonic primary carcinoma. A patient with a lung tumor would have a much higher probability of having brain (Muggia 1974) or bone metastasis (Hansen 1974). The lung as the first major filter after the thoracic duct has a high incidence of metastases from many different primary tumors. The bone gets the most significant proportion of its metastases from the paravertebral venous plexus.

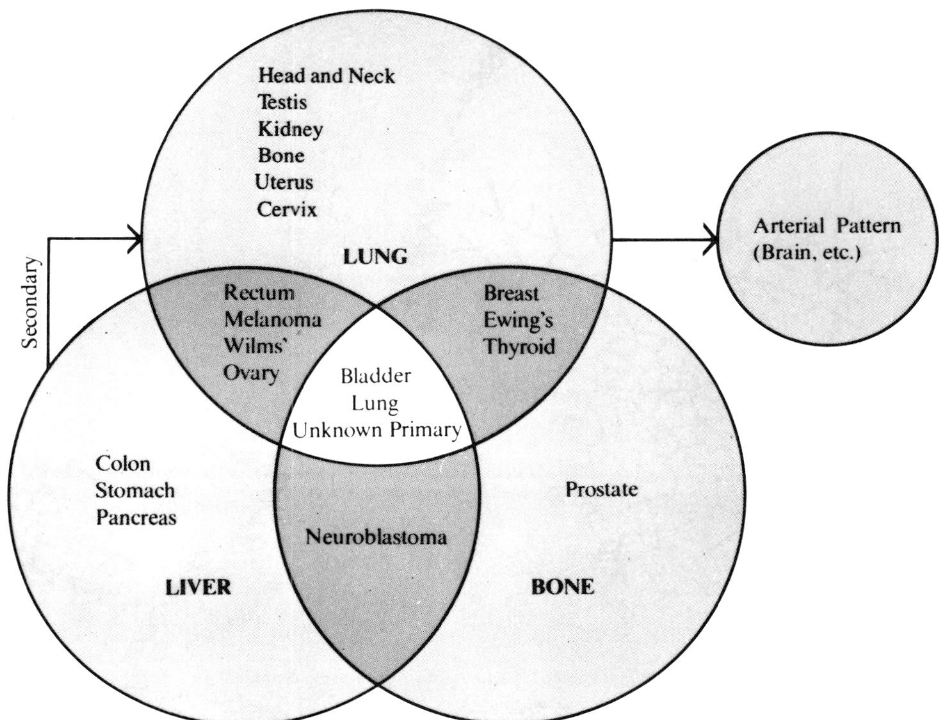

Fig. 7.1. *Primary clinically important metastatic patterns. (Gilbert 1979. Reprinted by permission.)*

Table 7.1. *Tumor Spread through Body Cavities*

Cavity	*Metastasis*
Thoracic	Lung, mesothelioma, breast, lymphoma, melanoma, stomach
Peritoneal	Ovary, pancreas, stomach, appendiceal pseudomyxoma, lymphoma, colon, breast, endometrium
Spinal	Ependymoma, medulloblastoma, lymphoma, melanoma, neuroblastoma

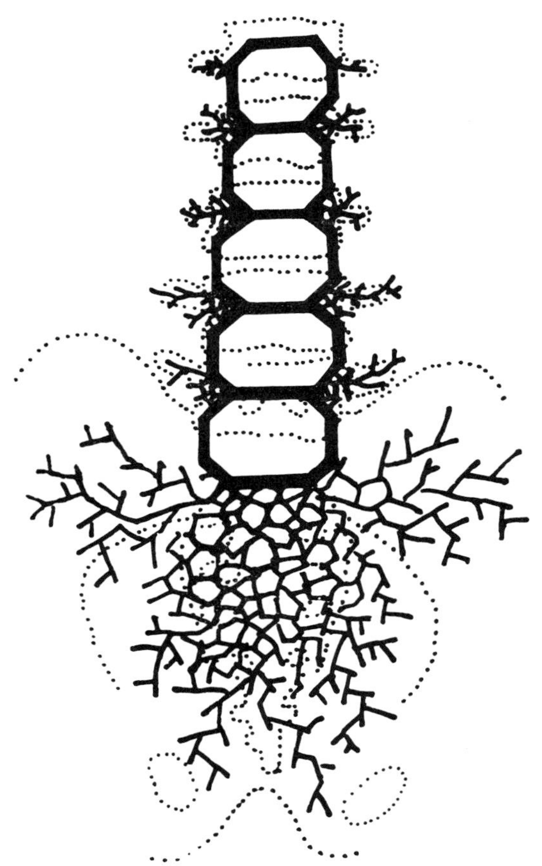

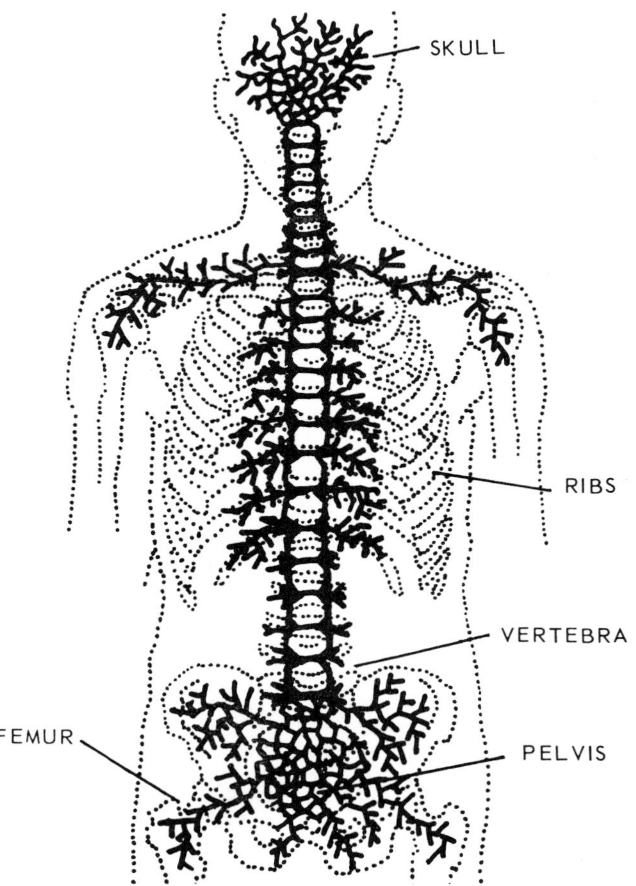

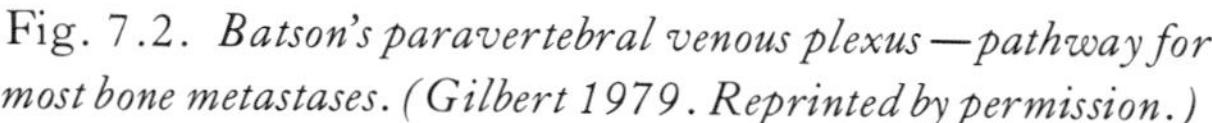

Fig. 7.2. *Batson's paravertebral venous plexus—pathway for most bone metastases. (Gilbert 1979. Reprinted by permission.)*

The sources of liver, lung, bone, and brain metastases are listed as follows:

Liver	**Lung**
Colon	Breast
Stomach	Lung
Pancreas	Ovary
Rectum	Uterus
Melanoma	Bladder
Gallbladder	Kidney
Bladder	Testis
Ovary	Bone
Uterus	Melanoma
Wilms' tumor	Wilms' tumor
Unknown primary	Sarcomas
Lung	Unknown primary
Breast	Cervix
Kidney	Gastrointestinal secondary tumors from liver

Bone	**Brain**
Prostate	Lung
Breast	Melanoma
Ewing's sarcoma	Secondary tumors from lung
Thyroid	
Bladder	
Lung	
Unknown primary	
Neuroblastoma	

There is a group of unusual metastases whose pattern is not clearly defined (Brady, O'Neill, and Farber 1977). Skin metastases have been noted from lung, colon, bladder, kidney, cervix, ovary, and esophagus. Metastases to the gastrointestinal tract tend to come from lung, breast, ovary, cervix, and melanoma. Eye metastases arise from breast, lung, melanoma, and esophagus; myocardial metastases from melanoma, lung, kidney, and leiomyosarcoma; kidney metastases have been documented from lung, breast, melanoma, and esophagus; and thyroid metastases from lymphomas and lung.

If the general principles and patterns of metastasis are understood, unnecessary diagnostic procedures will be avoided, and the patient can be evaluated expeditiously and with maximal safety and minimal expense.

References

Abrams, H. L. Metastases in carcinoma: analysis of 1000 autopsied cases. *Cancer* 1:74–85, 1950.

Brady, L. W.; O'Neill, E. A.; and Farber, S. H. Unusual sites of metastases. *Semin. Oncol.* 4:59–64, 1977.

del Regato, J. Pathways of metastatic spread of malignant tumors. *Semin. Oncol.* 4:33–38, 1977.

Fisher, B. Surgical adjuvant therapy for breast cancer. *Cancer* 30:1556–1564, 1972.

Gilbert, H. *Patterns of metastases.* Columbus, Ohio: Adria Laboratories, 1979.

Gilbert, H. A. Metastasis: incidence, detection and evaluation without histologic confirmation. *Fundamental aspects of metastases,* ed. L. Weiss. Amsterdam: North Holland Publishing Co., 1976, pp. 385–405.

Hansen, J. J. *Bone metastases in lung cancer. A clinical study in 200 consecutive patients with bronchogenic carcinoma and its therapeutic implications for small cell carcinoma.* Munikgaard, Denmark: Christian Christensen & Co., 1974.

Howe, E. R., and Maniatis, W. R. Malignancies and their spread: an analysis of 1330 primary malignancies from 6500 consecutive autopsies at Hartford Hospital 1925–1950. *Hartford Hosp. Bull.* 4:3–26, 1950.

Muggia, F. Lung cancer: diagnosis in metastatic sites. *Semin. Oncol.* 1:217–228, 1974.

Sugarbaker, E. V., and Ketcham, A. S. Mechanisms and prevention of cancer dissemination: an overview. *Semin. Oncol.* 4:19–32, 1977.

Weiss, L.; Gilbert, H. A.; and Posner, J. B., eds. *Brain Metastasis.* Boston: G. K. Hall & Co., 1980.

Willis, R. A. *The spread of tumors in the human body.* London: Butterworth, 1952.

eight

Nutrition and Cancer

DAVID S. FISCHER

"We are what we eat" may be an oversimplification, but it is obvious that we do not live long without some form of nutrition. For the person with cancer this is a very important problem. Cancer in the public mind is almost synonymous with cachexia, or reduced carcass weight. A substantial proportion of people with cancer die *of* or *with* malnutrition. In recent years, it has been suggested that physicians are inadequately trained in nutrition and hence do not effectively use this modality of therapy for their patients, and in particular, for their cancer patients. This neglect may be a contributory cause of patients seeking alternative treatment that we characterize as unorthodox or unproved. Significantly, many involve or have as a central feature, nutritional manipulation. That some achieve a degree of success is not surprising in view of the substantial scientific evidence that nutritional repletion enhances immunocompetence, response to therapy, and survival (Harvey, Bothe, and Blackburn 1979; Copeland 1978; Deitel, Vasic, and Alexander 1978).

Anorexia and Weight Loss

Anorexia is sometimes characterized simply as reduced food intake. In a patient with cancer it should be more precisely defined as food intake that is inadequate to meet the combined needs of the host and the tumor. Thus even if the amount of food eaten remains constant, there could still be loss of carcass weight in a tumor-bearing host (DeWys 1970).

There are many causes of anorexia, and some of them are outlined below:

- I. Anorexia
  - A. Changes in taste
    - 1. Increased recognition of sweet
    - 2. Lessened recognition of bitter
    - 3. Increased threshold for sour and salt
    - 4. Aversion to meat, especially beef and pork
  - B. Changes in odor recognition
  - C. Psychological
  - D. Gastrointestional change
    - 1. Decreased mucosal secretions
    - 2. Mucosal atrophy
    - 3. Muscle atrophy
  - E. Hormonal changes
    - 1. Decreased insulin secretion
    - 2. Increased activity hepatic glucoreceptors
    - 3. Hypothalamic-pituitary changes
  - F. Metabolic
    - 1. Increased lactic acid production
    - 2. Amino acid imbalance
    - 3. Increased lipolysis of triglyceride leading to satiety
- II. Weight loss
  - A. Increased energy expenditure
    - 1. Negative nitrogen balance
    - 2. Excretion of novel proteins and peptides
  - B. Metabolism
    - 1. Hormonal aberrations

2. Enzyme changes
3. Zinc and copper deficiency
4. Selective use of glucose in Cori cycle

C. Obstruction
1. Primary tumor of gastrointestinal tract
2. Metastatic tumor to gastrointestinal tract
3. Pressure on gastrointestinal organs

D. Excess losses
1. Blood loss
2. Protein-losing enteropathy
3. Fistulas
4. Vomiting
5. Secretory losses
6. Diarrhea

E. Malabsorption
1. Inadequate pancreatic enzymes
2. Biliary obstruction
3. Infiltration of bowel by cancer cells
4. Intestinal mucosal changes

Some patients will experience a loss of taste, gastrointestinal changes, and hormonal and metabolic alterations (DeWys 1979). As the patient feels unwell and becomes depressed, food intake is further reduced for psychological reasons, and a vicious cycle begins. In addition, it has been postulated that the tumor elaborates some noxious substances to produce anorexia, but these have not been found. Selective loss of muscle mass rather than just fat depletion seems paradoxical. The tumor cells derive most of their energy from metabolism of glucose to lactate (Cori cycle), rather than from metabolism to carbon dioxide and water (Krebs cycle) that is the major pathway of normal healthy cells. Since fat is metabolized through the Krebs cycle, tumor cells are unable to use fat as an energy source, but must rely on glucose. The conversion of amino acids to glucose draws amino acids from muscle, with resulting atrophy of those tissues (DeWys 1970), often in the presence of adequate amounts of subcutaneous fat. In addition, the tumor burns adenosine triphosphate (ATP) inefficiently as the anaerobic cycle releases only 2 molecules of ATP per molecule of glucose consumed, while the synthesis of glucose from lactate requires 6 molecules of ATP for a net loss (Schein et al. 1975). Thus weight loss must eventually occur although it is often transiently masked by stabilization caused by fluid retention (Theologides 1979).

Once cancer therapy begins, there is a chance of further nutritional deprivation and weight loss due to the treatment itself. Many of these factors are outlined as follows:

I. Surgical treatment
A. Radical resection of oropharyngeal area
1. Dependency on tube feedings
2. Loss of secretions and enzymes

B. Esophagectomy or reconstruction
1. Gastric stasis
2. Fat malabsorption
3. Fistula development
4. Stenosis

C. Gastrectomy
1. Dumping syndrome
2. Malabsorption
3. Hypoglycemia
4. Iron deficiency

D. Intestinal resection
1. Decreased absorption of many nutrients
2. Vitamin B_{12} deficiency
3. Bile salt losses
4. Abnormalities of electrolyte and water balance
5. Blind loop syndrome

E. Pancreatectomy
1. Malabsorption
2. Diabetes mellitus

F. Ureterosigmoidostomy
1. Hyperchloremic acidosis
2. Potassium loss

G. Paracentesis
1. Loss of protein and fluid
2. Potentially improves oral nutrition

II. Radiation therapy
A. Oropharyngeal area
1. Loss of taste and smell
2. Salivary gland injury—dry mouth
3. Periodontal disease
4. Radionecrosis of bone and teeth

B. Chest and mediastinum
1. Esophagitis
2. Esophageal fistulas and stenosis
3. Nausea and vomiting

C. Abdomen and pelvis
1. Nausea and vomiting
2. Diarrhea
3. Malabsorption
4. Bowel damage

III. Chemotherapy
A. Gastrointestinal
1. Nausea and vomiting
2. Diarrhea
3. Mucositis
4. Constipation from vincristine
5. Mucosal damage

B. Metabolic
1. Excess fluid retention or loss
2. Inappropriate antidiuretic hormone
3. Electrolyte imbalance
4. Effect of analgesics and sedatives

Surgical manipulations may lead to loss of nutrients, malabsorption, or secondary problems. Radiation and chemotherapy both have a high incidence of nausea, vomiting, and diarrhea (Lawrence 1979). As a group, patients hospitalized for medical reasons have a 44% incidence of protein-calorie malnutrition, as evidenced by a study in a New England hospital with anthropomorphic measurements (Bistrian et al. 1976). Hospitalized cancer patients had a nearly universal prevalence of protein-calorie malnutrition (Nixon et al. 1980) in a southern hospital. Psychological causes are also important (Schmale 1979).

Nutrition and Metabolic Assessment

While the grossly cachectic patient with reduced carcass weight has always stood out, it is only recently that more attention has been paid to the less obviously depleted patient. Many of these individuals who are afflicted with cancer are really in a poor nutritional state that could adversely affect their prognosis. Nutritional repletion offers hope to these individuals of a better response to therapy. The problem is to identify those who require increased oral and enteral alimentation and parenteral hyperalimentation (Wright 1980) in order to provide the most appropriate nutritional supplementation.

A sophisticated nutritional evaluation program has been devised (Blackburn et al. 1977) based on measurements of height, weight, triceps skin fold, midarm circumference, midarm muscle circumference, total lymphocyte count, serum albumin, total iron-binding capacity, serum transferrin, urinary creatinine, and creatinine height index. Dietitians at the Hospital of St. Raphael, a Yale-affiliated teaching hospital, are seeing selected patients for this assessment and report their results on a summary sheet (appendix 8.1). This is a time-consuming procedure and frequently provides more information than physicians are able to use, but it may be that we physicians have more to learn.

An "instant nutritional assessment" has been proposed (Seltzer et al. 1979) based on the serum albumin and total lymphocyte counts. Abnormalities of these measurements were associated with markedly increased morbidity and mortality in a series of 500 consecutively hospitalized patients. These laboratory reports warned the attending physician of an impending fourfold to twentyfold increased risk of complications at the time of admission. Selected patients were then further evaluated. The weight of the patient should be compared to standard weights for height (appendix 8.2). Lean body mass can be estimated from anthropometric or laboratory determinations. Since creatinine is a product of muscle metabolism, the 24-hour urinary excretion is roughly proportional to the skeletal muscle mass. Ideal creatinine-to-height values are given for comparison in appendix 8.3.

Several measures can be used to assess visceral protein reserve. A serum albumin concentration of less than 3 g/dl in the absence of liver disease indicates protein malnutrition. The normal half-life of albumin is about 20 days. The serum transferrin is also reduced in conditions of protein deficiency. It can be measured directly or derived from total iron-binding capacity. Since the half-life of transferrin is five to seven days, a decrease in the transferrin value in starvation can occur before any significant drop in the level of serum albumin. A total lymphocyte count of less than 1500/mm^3 is also indicative of visceral protein depletion and is commonly associated with cutaneous anergy. Based on these measurements (normal values in appendix 8.4), it is possible to conclude that a patient is not depleted, moderately depleted, or severely depleted. It is also reasonable to plan therapy to correct the deficiency based on the patient's basal energy expenditure (BEE). This may be calculated using the following equation (Rutten 1975):

For men: BEE =
$$66 + (13.7 \times W) + (5 \times H) - (6.8 \times A)$$
For women: BEE =
$$65.5 + (9.6 \times W) + (1.7 \times H) - (4.7 \times A)$$

where W = actual weight in kilograms, H = height in centimeters, and A = age in years. Nutritional therapy may then be calculated using the formulas in appendix 8.5 (Blackburn et al. 1977) to calculate the total caloric and protein requirements. We discuss the needs of other nutritional materials later.

Desirable Nutrition

Most of us think that we know what to eat and can advise our patients. Regrettably, most of us had little formal training in nutrition while in medical school and even less during our postgraduate (internship and residency) years. Many of us do not eat properly and neither do our patients.

Three decades ago, malnutrition was a widespread problem. The recent report of the Senate Select Committee on Nutrition and Human Needs, "Dietary goals for the United States," has stirred much controversy (Hegsted 1979) with its suggestion that Americans eat too much in general, and more specifically, too much meat, fat (especially saturated fat), cholesterol, sugar, and salt. We should eat more fruits and vegetables, grain products, and unsaturated fat. The authors suggest that total fat consumption should be reduced from 40% to 45% of calories in the current diet to about 30% of total calories. The fat should be about one-third saturated and one-third polyunsaturated, and cholesterol intake should be reduced to 300 mg/day. In addition, sugar consumption should be reduced to about 15% of total calories instead of the estimated 15% to 25% in current diets, and salt consumption should be substantially reduced. To replace the sugar and fat there should be an increased use of fruits and vegetables and products providing complex carbohydrates. A comprehensive revision of the Recommended Daily Dietary Allowances was made in 1980 by the Food and Nutrition Board of the National Academy of Sciences–National Research Council (appendix 8.6). It was designed for the maintenance of good nutrition of practically all healthy people in the United States. In view of the extreme interest of some in the need for rare minerals in the diet, a review of the estimated safe and adequate daily dietary intakes of additional selected vitamins and minerals may be of value (appendix 8.7). Recommended energy intake is based on age, sex, and ideal height and weight (appendix 8.8).

The foregoing information is helpful in designing diets for normal individuals. To maintain weight and adequate protein balance in patients with debilitating disease is more difficult, especially if the patient has cancer.

Oral Alimentation

Insofar as possible, it is best to have the patient eat food and supplement the diet with nutritional liquids. A great many diet manuals and cookbooks are available. We have been extremely fortunate to have had early access to the results of a study of 99 cancer patients who live in the New Haven, Connecticut area. Based on interviews with these patients, the study team at Yale–New Haven Medical Center found that most eating problems, regardless of cancer type, fell into five categories:

Nausea and vomiting
Loss of appetite
Mouth soreness and dryness
Tired feeling
Intestinal upset

With the help of the patients and members of the medical center and the Connecticut Division of the American Cancer Society, they formulated suggestions for improved nutrition and provided specific recipes. The manual is called *Eating Hints* (Morra, Suski, and Johnson 1980) and is available free from the Office of Cancer Communications, National Cancer Institute, Bethesda, Md. 20205. We provide a copy to each patient undergoing chemotherapy. The chart of nutritional formulas and preparations is valuable for calculating caloric and protein intake derived from some of the commercially available materials, and is reproduced here as appendix 8.9. A similar resource for parents of children with cancer is available from the same address and is entitled *Diet and Nutrition* (National Cancer Institute 1979).

When patients are unable to maintain their nutrition with food alone, liquid supplements such as those in appendix 8.9 can help to fill the gap. One must measure intake and then calculate the total calories and protein to be sure that both are sufficient. Depending on age, height, and weight, we generally regard 2700 calories and 56 gm of protein as adequate for an adult man, and 2000 calories and 44 gm protein for an adult woman. Men with cancer, however, may require 90 gm protein and women 80 gm protein, and each may require an additional 200 or 300 calories a day.

For patients who are unable to take any food, oral liquid diets are available. These provide complete nutritional maintenance and are suitable for both oral and tube feeding. To be effective, they must be used properly. For example, Ensure provides 106 calories per 100 ml (appendix 8.10, Yale diet formulary abstract), and the usual serving is 8 oz (240 ml) (one can) containing 254 calories and 8.8 gm protein. For adequate protein-caloric nutrition, the patient needs 8 to 12 cans (2000 to 2400 ml) of Ensure per day if it is the sole nutritional source. Relatively few patients take this much even though the material is quite palatable. Alternatively, Precision LR Gelatin can be used, but 8 to 12 servings are required daily.

For those with gastrointestinal diseases that require the lower tract to be at rest (malabsorption, fistula, inflammatory bowel disease, pancreatitis, and so on), fiber-free semisynthetic liquid diets, formerly called elemental diets, are a potential source of complete oral nutrition. They also require 8 to 12 portions of 8 oz each day. They are less palatable and patient acceptance is not as good, so they frequently have to be given by tube.

Enteral Hyperalimentation

Oral feedings can frequently *maintain* the nutritionally depleted patient and prevent further deterioration by providing 2000 to 2700 calories per day and 70% of the recommended daily allowances. To *replete* the starved patient requires hyperalimentation with 2700 to 3500 calories per day and 150% to 300% of the recommended allowances. It is very difficult to give this orally. In the past, large-bore nasogastric tubes were used, but they were poorly and only briefly tolerated. Many physicians then skipped over to intravenous hyperalimentation with central catheters. The advent of small-bore highly flexible catheters and feeding tubes that are well tolerated for long periods revived interest in enteral hyperalimentation, which is easier, more economical, and more physiologic.

Pediatric nasopharyngeal tubes or polyethylene catheters may be passed with the aid of a wire stylet or a Levine tube, which is then withdrawn (Heymsfield et al. 1979). The distal end of the tube should be in the lower esophagus rather than in the stomach, as the latter may be associated with increased reflux, especially when the patient is supine (Shils 1979). The feeding mixture is administered continuously over 24 hours either by a regulated drip or an infusion pump. To prevent aspiration, the head of the bed is kept slightly elevated, even at night.

Although enteral hyperalimentation mixtures can be prepared in the hospital pharmacy according to published formulas, the availability of high-quality commercial preparations makes that unnecessary in the majority of cases. There are three general types available.

1. The monomeric (formerly called elemental diets and now termed fiber-free semisynthetic liquid diets) are well represented by Vivionex, Vivionex HN, and Flexical. They are indicated in situations requiring a low residue, such as chronic diarrheas, enterocutaneous fistulas, inflammatory bowel disease, pancreatic insufficiency, and so forth. They furnish amino acids, oligosaccharides, or monosaccharides, contain little or no triglycerides, and do not require proteolytic or lipolytic activity. They furnish 1 kcal/ml, are hyperosmolar, and moderately expensive.

2. Polymeric mixtures contain protein, fat, and carbohydrate in high molecular weight form, and are lower in osmolality, require normal proteolytic and lipolytic activity, contain about 1 kcal/ml, and are less expensive. Preparations that are lactose-free and low in fat include Citrotein, Precision LR, and Precision HN; those that are simply lactose-free include Isocal, Ensure, Ensure Plus, Precision Moderate N, and Precision Isotonic. They are indicated for patients with a basically normal gastrointestinal tract, normal metabolic rate, and inability to eat because of anorexia, cerebrovascular accident, oropharyngeal or esophageal surgery, and the like.

3. High-density modular preparations are a special group, used for patients who need a high caloric intake like 2 kcal/ml but in a low volume of fluid, because of cardiac, renal, or hepatic disease. These diets are individually prepared by the dietitian in cooperation with the physician, using commercially available mixtures such as Polycose, Controlyte, or Hycal for carbohydrate; Casec, EMF, Citrotein, or Instant Breakfast for protein; and medium-chain triglyceride oil as the source of fat.

Enteral solutions should be prepared or opened freshly each day and put in carefully and clearly marked containers so that they are not mistaken for an intravenous preparation, as they could do great harm if given by that route. About 2500 ml or more is needed each day to provide adequate hyperalimentation. Some patients are unable to manage this volume and need to be supplemented with peripheral venous hyperalimentation. For patients who simply cannot tolerate a nasopharyngeal tube and tend to vomit or cough it out, an esophagostomy, gastrostomy, or jejunostomy may be considered. A tube may be inserted into the esophagus through the pyriform sinus quite easily by those skilled and experienced in the technique. Feedings by this route are easier and aspiration is less of a problem than with a nasopharyngeal tube. Gastrostomy is the time-honored technique and is sometimes initiated at the conclusion of the primary surgery or at a later time. Nurses are experienced in its use and care, and the average patient can be taught to do self-feedings and catheter care. Jejunostomy is reserved for the situation in which there is an obstruction more proximally, as in the pylorus or duodenum. Because digestive opportunities are reduced at this level, medium-chain triglycerides, oligosaccharides, and mixtures of polypeptides and amino acids are used with care to avoid hyperosmolar feedings that could lead to the equivalent of a "dumping syndrome." Sometimes pancreatic extract is given to aid digestion.

With all of its problems, enteral hyperalimentation has advantages for those for whom it is suitable and tolerable. It is safer than central venous hyperalimentation. It is economical, costing only about $30 to $50 per day for a caloric and protein intake that would cost $125 to $150 per day for central or peripheral venous hyperalimentation.

Peripheral Venous Hyperalimentation

For patients who can obtain part of their nutrition naturally but need supplementation, or for those unable to ingest any food, peripheral venous hyperalimentation is a valuable option with fewer risks and potential complications than central venous hyperalimentation. It is indicated for those who are judged to require fewer than two weeks of parenteral supplementation and who are to be maintained in caloric balance, but do not need repletion or weight gain. It should be approached with caution, if at all, in patients with thrombocytopenia (platelet count of less than 50,000), severe liver disease, severe pulmonary disease, persons with a tendency to phlebitis, and patients with a disturbance of normal fat metabolism.

The acceptance of peripheral venous hyperalimentation is more recent than that of central venous hyperalimentation for technical reasons. Peripheral carbohydrate and amino acid solutions simply cannot provide enough calories to maintain nutritional homeostasis (1800 to 2200 kcal/day). In the 1950s, a material known as Lipomul was developed that gave adequate calories but had significant toxicity characterized by fever, sore throat, hepatomegaly, splenomegaly, thrombocytopenia, and hemolytic anemia. These were all reversible, but clearly undesirable, even transiently, in seriously ill patients. The problem at that time was the emulsifier and a tendency to fat embolization, and the product was abandoned.

The introduction of Intralipid in the last few years has made peripheral venous hyperalimentation practical and relatively safe. Intralipid is an intravenous fat emulsion consisting of 10% soybean oil, 1.2% egg yolk phospholipids, 2.25% glycerine, and water for injection, and the solution is adjusted to pH between 5.5 and 9.0 with sodium hydroxide. The soybean oil is a refined natural product consisting of a mixture of neutral triglycerides of predominantly unsaturated fatty acids. The major components of fatty acids are linoleic (54%), oleic (26%), palmitic (9%), and linolenic (8%) acids. Intravenous fat emulsion has an osmolarity of approximately 280 milliosmoles per liter and contains fat particles about 0.5 micron in size, which is very close to the size of chylomicrons that are made by intestinal digestion. Caloric value is 1.1 kcal/ml.

A newer preparation uses safflower oil as the source of fat (Liposyn, 10% fat emulsion), and we employ it interchangeably with Intralipid. Both preparations are supplied in single-dose containers, and no filters are used for administration. The rate of infusion in adults is approximately 1 ml per minute or 60 ml per hour, yielding about 1500 ml per 24 hours. Simultaneously a 4.25% protein (1-crystalline amino acid) solution in 5% dextrose solution is infused at the same rate. Together, these solutions provide 2100 kcal/day. Our protein-glucose solution also contains sodium, 40 mEq/L; potassium, 35.4 mEq/L; calcium, 4.8 mEq/L; magnesium, 8 mEq/L; chloride, 77 mEq/L; phosphate, 21 mEq/L; and acetate, 26 mEq/L. Routine vitamins added each day are MVI, 5 ml; vitamin K, 5 mg; and folic acid, 1 mg. Patients weighing less than 60 kg have their fat emulsion decreased so that the regimen does not exceed 2.5 gm fat/kg/day. If necessary to maintain adequate hydration, the infusion rate of the protein-glucose solution may be increased to compensate for the decreased amount of fat emulsion intake. The infusion rate of the fat emulsion should never exceed that of the protein-glucose solution. Total volume will be 2500 to 3000 ml.

The advantages of peripheral venous hyperalimentation compared to the central venous route are decreased incidence of infection and of surgical complications of tube placement, fewer personnel to maintain an administration team, and greater economy of equipment if not the solutions. This technique is feasible in both small and large hospitals, is easily begun, and easily terminated.

Central Venous Hyperalimentation and Total Parenteral Nutrition

Total parenteral nutrition (TPN) has achieved great popularity recently for nutritional repletion (Copeland and Dudrick 1975; American Cancer Society–National Cancer Institute 1979; Johnston 1978). It has proved of value in increasing survival for patients with burns of significant degree, and those with ulcerative colitis, regional enteritis, pyloric stenosis, enterocutaneous fistulas, massive small bowel resection, acute or chronic pancreatitis, short bowel syndrome, chronic uncontrolled diarrhea, and severe intractable malabsorption syndromes. Other indications include multiple injury syndromes, severe infections with peritonitis, or patients with correctable hypermetabolic states including acute renal failure and acute hepatic failure. More recently, it has been shown to improve survival of patients with cancer by allowing more aggressive radiation therapy, chemotherapy, and even surgery that would have been otherwise too risky (Copeland et al. 1975; Eriksson and Douglass 1980; Hew and Deitel 1979; Dindogru et al. 1980). Leukopenia, anemia, and thrombocytopenia are less severe and of shorter duration with TPN.

The technique consists basically of inserting a large-bore catheter into the subclavian vein directed centrally into the superior vena cava and infusing highly concentrated nutrient solutions continuously through the indwelling catheter. Great care must be exercised when placing the catheter to avoid producing a pneumothorax or hemothorax. We have seen this complication several times, especially in the very cachectic patient who is least able to tolerate it. These patients probably should have the catheter inserted through the jugular vein. They should all be placed by surgeons or physicians who are experienced in the technique; it is not a procedure for the novice to attempt unsupervised.

To minimize complications, we have a hyperalimentation team consisting of a surgeon, nurse, pharmacist, dietitian, and internist with a special interest in metabolic problems. It is desirable for anyone without extensive experience in this field to make use of the services of this team for the benefit of the patient. To remove the economic barrier to such consultation, we fund the team by a surcharge on each liter of TPN solution so that all patients who use the service share the cost (Tanner 1981). The nurse sees every patient at least three times a week and changes dressings. The pharmacist checks the composition of the solutions administered against the results of biochemical tests to see if changes are indicated. Our pharmacy guidelines for TPN are entered into the chart of every patient on the regimen to act as a reminder to the staff (appendix 8.11). There is also a sheet for daily recording of significant biochemical data (appendix 8.12). For adults, we have one special pharmacy order sheet for TPN (appendix 8.13) and a separate pediatric parenteral nutrition form (appendix 8.14). This allows the physician to vary the infusion daily to accommodate to changing body needs.

Once the catheter has been placed in the vein and an x-ray obtained to confirm its correct position in the middle portion of the superior vena cava, aseptic dressings are applied. The site is cleaned at least three times a week and the catheter is used only for hyperalimentation infusions and never for withdrawing blood, central venous pressure, or administering blood, blood products, or any viscid material. Only by keeping the system closed is it possible to avoid the high risk of infection. Some teams use a Millipore filter of 0.22 or 0.45 microns to reduce the possibility of bacterial infections.

The complications of TPN are significant (Paul 1979) and include sepsis, catheter seeding of bloodborne organisms particularly fungus, hyperglycemia, hypoglycemia, nonketotic hyperosmolar states, overhydration, dehydration, metabolic acidosis, azotemia, hyperammonemia, electrolyte imbalances, allergy, and fever.

Indications and Contraindications

Total parenteral nutrition is used in cancer to overcome a temporary obstacle on the road to palliation or cure. It may help a cachectic patient gain enough weight to be an acceptable operative risk or to tolerate radiation therapy or chemotherapy. The improved blood counts often allow higher radiation doses or more aggressive chemotherapy with better therapeutic results.

On the other hand, there is always the temptation to "do something, anything." When there is no acceptable therapeutic option such as surgery, radiation, or chemotherapy, there is probably no role for TPN. An example of this is the patient with intestinal obstruction who is unable to take any food by mouth. If there is some hope that surgery, radiation, or chemotherapy will relieve the obstruction, the patient should be treated with TPN to get over the difficult but temporary period.

If it is clear that the obstruction is totally inoperable and unlikely to respond to radiation or chemotherapy, and if there is no possibility of relieving the obstruction by any modality, there is no reason to use TPN as it will only prolong the agony of dying. We recently saw such an unfortunate patient kept alive by TPN for three extra months at a cost of about $500 per day, or $45,000. The husband of the patient was too upset to consider discontinuing therapy and the physician was afraid or incapable of suggesting that TPN be stopped. Finally, when it was clear that the family had dissipated its savings, used up the children's college funds, and gone into debt, the patient herself requested that the TPN be stopped so that she could die with dignity and without further compromising the future of her family. Even if third party payments cover all expenses, the use of a heroic measure such as TPN to prolong the act of dying should be considered very carefully in terms of the interests of both the patient and of society.

For those patients who need long-term nutritional support while they are receiving treatment with either palliative or curative intent, but do not need hospitalization for an acute condition, programs of home nutrition are available. They are safe and generally preferable to hospitalization, especially if the patient is ambulatory and can receive outpatient radiation or chemotherapy (Ivey et al. 1975; Dudrick et al. 1979; Scribner and Cole 1979). Many of these patients can then go back up the ladder from parenteral to enteral to oral alimentation. For those who must remain on long-term parenteral hyperalimentation, a home-care program is much more economical than hospitalization. Wateska, Sattler, and Steiger (1980) followed patients having home hyperalimentation for a year at an average cost of $19,700, and estimated that the same therapy in the hospital would have cost $73,720. Of course, room and board at $200 per day would be another $73,000 or a total of $146,700.

Oral Care

While chemotherapy or radiation therapy is being given, oral care is frequently neglected. Mucositis and/or stomatitis become troublesome; teeth become loose from periodontal disease; radiation tooth decay causes premature tooth loss with resultant jaw infection and necrosis of bone. Many of these complications can be avoided with good prophylactic oral care. Indeed, for the patient receiving radiation therapy to the head and neck, it is absolutely essential. A regimen for oral health management recommended by Tabachnick (1980) follows.

I. Preradiation therapy
   A. Oral evaluation
      1. Radiologic examination
         a. Panoramic radiograph
         b. Periapical and/or occlusal radiographs as needed
      2. Oral examination
         a. Soft tissue examination
         b. Periodontal status evaluation—loose teeth, pockets, plaque, calculus
         c. Caries activity evaluation—new or recurrent
         d. Endodontic evaluation—involvement of pulp or near exposure
         e. Tooth prognosis—overall—occlusion: traumatic or interferences
   B. Dental treatment
      1. Extraction of nonsalvageable teeth or those with poor prognosis (teeth with gross dental caries, periapical pathology, advanced periodontal disease, and teeth supported by neoplasm)
      2. Scalings—deep, and dental prophylaxis
      3. Restorative and endodontic procedures—perform all presently necessary, and that which will become so within one year
      4. Initiation of oral hygiene regimen (to be followed for rest of patient's life). Highly imperative that the patient perform bacterial plaque removal to prevent caries
         a. Tooth brushing instructions—with soft multitufted toothbrush with rounded nylon bristles—four times a day, and follow each brushing with *oral lavage* and *fluoride rinse*
            1. Modified bass technique—place bristles at junction of tooth and gum
            2. Tilt bristles at 45° angle toward gum
            3. Activate bristles with slight vibratory motion
            4. Brush no more than two teeth at a time
            5. Brush each tooth: inside, outside, and on top
         b. Interproximal cleansing—as important as brushing: dental floss, dental tape, stimudents, water pick twice a day
         c. Disclosing solution—to check successful plaque removal
         d. *Oral lavage instruction*—1 liter of warm water with 1 teaspoon each of NaCl and $NaHCO_3$
         e. *Sodium fluoride rinse instruction*—1 teaspoon 0.05% NaFrinse (OraChem Pharmaceutical) held in mouth 1 minute, then expectorated. This rinse is sometimes discontinued during acute mucositis because of mucosal irritation. Teeth must be clean prior to fluoride rinse, and there should be no eating or drinking for 30 minutes after rinse.
         f. Fluoride treatments daily using a sequential technique with 1.23% acidulated phosphate fluoride gel brushed on clean, dry teeth for two minutes (Sabra Gell, Gell II by Pacemaker Corp.) followed by 0.4% stannous fluoride gel in custom-fitted trays for application on teeth for two minutes (Gel-Kam by Scherer Laboratories). Teeth must be clean and dry before fluoride gel.
         g. Fluoride toothpastes—Colgate, Crest, Aim (not an abrasive, nonfluoride toothpaste)
         h. *No* commercial mouthwashes that contain alcohol, because they dry the tissues.

II. During radiation therapy
   A. Weekly prophylaxis with fluoridated polishing paste
   B. Use of saliva substitute for xerostomia and mucositis
      1. V.A. Oralube
      2. Xerolube
      3. Orex
   C. Pain relievers for mucositis
      1. Systemic analgesics—tablets, capsules, elixirs
      2. Coatings—Oxaine-M
      3. Glycerin/melted butter—topically soothing
   D. Dietary supplements
      1. Nutriment
      2. Sustacal/Sustagen
      3. Meritene, Ensure
      4. Metrecal, Isocal
      5. Carnation Instant Breakfast/Carnation Slender
      6. Include in diet no spicy or hot foods
   E. Antifungal agents *(Candida)* or antibacterial agents as needed
   F. Oral hygiene regimen (B.4. section I) should be continued indefinitely

III. After radiation therapy
   A. Oral hygiene regimen (B.4. section I) should be continued indefinitely
   B. Follow-up visits should be more frequent than for usual dental patients and should be coordinated with oncology and/or radiation therapy recall appointments
   C. Oral, head, and neck examination for detection of recurrent or new neoplastic disease
   D. Dental prophylaxis with fluoridated polishing paste
   E. Restorative and endodontic procedures performed as needed
   F. Any necessary oral surgery to be done under antibiotic coverage with attention to careful management of soft tissues and provision for primary closure of all surgical wounds to avoid osteoradionecrosis
   G. Assess any coagulopathy (especially thrombocytopenia) due to suppression of platelets and of immune system and blood-forming cells and organs prior to any oral surgery in chemotherapy patients (those taking cytoxic drugs, or antimetabolites)

Mention of specific commercial products is for example only. Other similar products may be equally acceptable.

References

American Cancer Society and National Cancer Institute. Proceedings of the National Conference on Nutrition in Cancer. *Cancer* 43:1955–2162, 1979.

Bistrian, B. R. et al. Therapeutic index of nutritional depletion in hospitalized patients. *Surg. Gynecol. Obstet.* 141:512–516, 1975.

Bistrian, B. R. et al. Prevalence of malnutrition in general medical patients. *JAMA* 235:1567–1570, 1976.

Blackburn, G. L. et al. Nutritional and metabolic assessment of the hospitalized patient. *J. Parent. Ent. Nutr.* 1:11–22, 1977.

Copeland, E. M., III. Intravenous hyperalimentation as an adjunct to cancer patient management. *CA* 28:322–330, 1978.

Copeland, E. M., III et al. Intravenous hyperalimentation in patients with head and neck cancer. *Cancer* 35:606–611, 1975.

Copeland, E. M., III, and Dudrick, S. J. Cancer: nutritional concepts. *Semin. Oncol.* 2:329–335, 1975.

Deitel, M.; Vasic, V.; and Alexander, N. A. Specialized nutritional support in the cancer patient: is it worthwhile? *Cancer* 41:2359–2363, 1978.

DeWys, W. D. Working conference on anorexia and cachexia of neoplastic disease. *Cancer Res.* 30:2816–2818, 1970.

DeWys, W. D. Anorexia as a general effect of cancer. *Cancer* 43:2013–2019, 1979.

Dindogru, A. et al. Total parenteral nutrition in leukopenic cancer patients. *JAMA* 244:680–681, 1980.

Dudrick, S. J. et al. New concepts of ambulatory home hyperalimentation. *J. Parent. Ent. Nutr.* 3:72–76, 1979.

Eriksson, B., and Douglass, H. O., Jr. Intravenous hyperalimentation: an adjunct to treatment of malignant disease of upper gastrointestinal tract. *JAMA* 243:2049–2052, 1980.

Harvey, K. B.; Bothe, A., Jr.; and Blackburn, G. L. Nutritional assessment and patient outcome during oncological therapy. *Cancer* 43:2065–2069, 1979.

Hegsted, D. M. Optimal nutrition. *Cancer* 43:1996–2003, 1979.

Hew, L. R., and Deitel, M. Nutrition in the cancer patient and the use of hyperalimentation. *What's New in Cancer* 3:1–4, 1979.

Heymsfield, S. B. et al. Enteral hyperalimentation: an alternative to central venous hyperalimentation. *Ann. Intern. Med.* 90:63–71, 1979.

Ivey, M. et al. Long-term parenteral nutrition in the home. *Am. J. Hosp. Pharm.* 32:1032–1036, 1975.

Jelliffe, D. B. *The assessment of the nutritional status of the community.* WHO monograph 53. Geneva: World Health Organization, 1966.

Johnston, I. D. A., ed. *Advances in parenteral nutrition.* Lancaster, England: MTP Press, 1978.

Lawrence, W., Jr. Effects of cancer on nutrition. *Cancer* 43:2020–2029, 1979.

Morra, M. E.; Suski, N.; and Johnson, B. L. *Eating hints: recipes and tips for better nutrition during cancer treatment.* Bethesda, Md.: National Cancer Institute, 1980.

National Cancer Institute. *Diet and nutrition, a resource for parents of children with cancer,* NIH 80-2038. Bethesda, Md.: National Institutes of Health, 1979.

Nixon, D. W. et al. Protein-calorie undernutrition in hospitalized cancer patients. *Am. J. Med.* 68:683–690, 1980.

Paul, G. J. Total parenteral nutrition: a guide for its use. *Am. J. Gastroenterol.* 72:186–192, 1979.

Schein, P. S. et al. Nutritional complications of cancer and its treatment. *Semin. Oncol.* 2:337–347, 1975.

Schmale, A. H. Psychological aspects of anorexia. *Cancer* 43:2087–2092, 1979.

Scribner, B. H., and Cole, J. J. Evolution of the technique of home parenteral nutrition *J. Parent. Ent. Nutr.* 3:58–61, 1979.

Seltzer, M. H. et al. Instant nutritional assessment. *J. Parent. Ent. Nutr.* 3:157–159, 1979.

Shils, M. E. Enteral nutritional management of the cancer patient. *CA* 29:78–83, 1979.

Tabachnick, T. T. Report of Committee on Oral Health, Connecticut Division, American Cancer Society, Wallingford, Conn., 1980.

Tanner, D. J. Administrative aspects of parenteral nutrition. *Am. J. Intrav. Ther. Clin. Nutr.* 8:28–35, 1981.

Theologides, A. Cancer cachexia. *Cancer* 43:2004–2012, 1979.

Wateska, L. P.; Sattler, L. L.; and Steiger, E. Cost of a home parenteral nutrition program. *JAMA* 244:2303–2304, 1980.

Wright, R. A. Nutritional assessment. *JAMA* 244:559–560, 1980.

Appendix 8.1. *Nutritional Assessment Summary*

Patient ______________ Room ________ Physician ______________ Date ________
Service ______________________ Diagnosis ______________________
Admission weight ________ Height ____________ Ideal weight ________

Parameters	*Patient Values*		*Assessment*	
		> 90% Standard Not Depleted	60–90% Standard Moderately Depleted	< 60% Standard Severely Depleted
Weight/height	kg cm			
Triceps skin-fold (TSF)	mm			
Mid-arm circumference (MAC)	cm			
Mid-arm muscle circumference (MAMC) MAMC (cm) = MAC (cm) − [3.14 × TSF (cm)]	cm			
Lymphocytes, total count	mm^3			
Albumin, serum	g/100 ml			
Total iron binding capacity (TIBC)	mcg/100 ml			
Transferrin Serum transferrin = (0.8 × TIBC) − 43	mg/100 ml			
Urinary creatinine	mg			
Creatinine height index (CHI) $\text{CHI} = \frac{\text{Actual urinary creatinine}}{\text{Ideal urinary creatinine}} \times 100$	%			

Hematocrit ________% Hemoglobin ______ g/100 ml Cellular immunity: ☐ Positive ☐ Negative
Dietary intake evaluation: calories ________ cal/24 hr Protein ____ g/24 hr

Protein Status: nitrogen balance $= \frac{\text{protein intake}}{6.25} - (\text{urinary urea nitrogen} + 4)$ ☐ Positive ☐ Negative

Nutritional status: ☐ Marasmus (M) ☐ Kwashiorkor (K) ☐ Combination M–K ☐ Normal
Proposed nutritional therapy: ____

SOURCE: Blackburn, G. L. et al. Nutritional and metabolic assessment of the hospitalized patient. *J. Parent. Ent. Nutr.* 1:11–22, 1977.

Appendix 8.2. *Ideal Weights for Heights*

Ideal Weight for Height (Men)					
Height (cm)	*Weight (kg)*	*Height (cm)*	*Weight (kg)*	*Height (cm)*	*Weight (kg)*
157	58.6	167	64.6	177	71.6
158	59.3	168	65.2	178	72.4
159	59.9	169	65.9	179	73.3
160	60.5	170	66.6	180	74.2
161	61.1	171	67.3	181	75.0
162	61.7	172	68.0	182	75.8
163	62.3	173	68.7	183	76.5
164	62.9	174	69.4	184	77.3
165	63.5	175	70.1	185	78.1
166	64.0	176	70.8	186	78.9

Ideal Weight for Height (Women)					
Height (cm)	*Weight (kg)*	*Height (cm)*	*Weight (kg)*	*Height (cm)*	*Weight (kg)*
140	44.9	150	50.4	160	56.2
141	45.4	151	51.0	161	56.9
142	45.9	152	51.5	162	57.6
143	46.4	153	52.0	163	58.3
144	47.0	154	52.5	164	58.9
145	47.5	155	53.1	165	59.5
146	48.0	156	53.7	166	60.1
147	48.6	157	54.3	167	60.7
148	49.2	158	54.9	168	61.4
149	49.8	159	55.5	169	62.1

NOTE: These tables correct the 1959 metropolitan standards to nude weight.

SOURCE: Adapted from Jelliffe, D. B. *The assessment of the nutritional status of the community*. WHO monograph 53. Geneva: World Health Organization, 1966.

Appendix 8.3. *Ideal Urinary Creatinine Values (mg), Adults*

*Men**		*Women*†	
Height (cm)	*Ideal Creatinine (mg)*	*Height (cm)*	*Ideal Creatinine (mg)*
157.5	1288	147.3	830
160.0	1325	149.9	851
162.6	1359	152.4	875
165.1	1386	154.9	900
167.6	1426	157.5	925
170.2	1467	160.0	949
172.7	1513	162.6	977
175.3	1555	165.1	1006
177.8	1596	167.6	1044
180.3	1642	170.2	1076
182.9	1691	172.7	1109
185.4	1739	175.3	1141
188.0	1785	177.8	1174
190.5	1831	180.3	1206
193.0	1891	182.9	1240

SOURCE: Blackburn, G. L. et al. Nutritional and metabolic assessment of the hospitalized patient. *J. Parent. Ent. Nutr.* 1:11–22, 1977.

*Creatinine coefficient (men) = 23 mg/kg of ideal body weight.

†Creatinine coefficient (women) = 18 mg/kg of ideal body weight.

Appendix 8.4. *Selected Normal Values for Adults*

Hematocrit (vol % red cells)	
Men	40%–54%
Women	37%–47%
Hemoglobin	
Men	14–17 g/100 ml
Women	12–15 g/100 ml
Lymphocytes, total count	1500–3000/mm^3
Albumin, serum	4.0–5.5g/100 ml
Iron-binding capacity	
total, serum	250–410 mcg/100 ml
% saturation	20%–50%
Transferrin	170–250 mg/100 ml
Creatinine	1.0–1.5 g/24 hr

SOURCE: Blackburn, G. L. et al. Nutritional and metabolic assessment of the hospitalized patient. *J. Parent. Ent. Nutr.* 1:11–22, 1977.

Appendix 8.5. *Nutritional Therapy*

Energy requirements	*Calories required (per 24 hrs)*	
Type of therapy		
Parenteral anabolic	1.75 × BEE*	
Oral anabolic	1.50 × BEE	
Oral maintenance	1.20 × BEE	
Prescriptions for anabolism†	*Protein (g/day)*	*Calories (kcal/day)*
Type of therapy		
Oral protein-sparing	1.5 × weight‡	
Total parenteral nutrition	(1.2 to 1.5) × weight	40 × weight
Oral hyperalimentation	(1.2 to 1.5) × weight	35 × weight

SOURCE: Blackburn, G. L. et al. Nutritional and metabolic assessment of the hospitalized patient. *J. Parent. Ent. Nutr.* 1:11–22, 1977.

*BEE = Basal energy expenditure.

†Levels of protein intake are to be adjusted according to blood urea nitrogen values and nitrogen balance.

‡Weight = actual weight in kg.

Appendix 8.6. *Food and Nutrition Board, National Academy of Sciences—National Research Council Recommended Daily Dietary Allowances,*[a] *Revised 1980. Designed for the maintenance of good nutrition of practically all healthy people in the U.S.A.*

							Fat-Soluble Vitamins			Water-Soluble Vitamins							Minerals					
	Age (years)	Weight (kg)	Weight (lbs)	Height (cm)	Height (in)	Protein (g)	Vitamin A (μg R.E.)[b]	Vitamin D (μg)[c]	Vitamin E (mg α T.E.)[d]	Vitamin C (mg)	Thiamin (mg)	Riboflavin (mg)	Niacin (mg N.E.)[e]	Vitamin B6 (mg)	Folacin (μg)[f]	Vitamin B12 (μg)	Calcium (mg)	Phosphorus (mg)	Magnesium (mg)	Iron (mg)	Zinc (mg)	Iodine (μg)
Infants	0.0–0.05	6	13	60	24	kg × 2.2	420	10	3	35	0.3	0.4	6	0.3	30	0.5[g]	360	240	50	10	3	40
	0.5–1.0	9	20	71	28	kg × 2.0	400	10	4	35	0.5	0.6	8	0.6	45	1.5	540	360	70	15	5	50
Children	1–3	13	29	90	35	23	400	10	5	45	0.7	0.8	9	0.9	100	2.0	800	800	150	15	10	70
	4–6	20	44	112	44	30	500	10	6	45	0.9	1.0	11	1.3	200	2.5	800	800	200	10	10	90
	7–10	28	62	132	52	34	700	10	7	45	1.2	1.4	16	1.6	300	3.0	800	800	250	10	10	120
Males	11–14	45	99	157	62	45	1000	10	8	50	1.4	1.6	18	1.8	400	3.0	1200	1200	350	18	15	150
	15–18	66	145	176	69	56	1000	10	10	60	1.4	1.7	18	2.0	400	3.0	1200	1200	400	18	15	150
	19–22	70	154	177	70	56	1000	7.5	10	60	1.5	1.7	19	2.2	400	3.0	800	800	350	10	15	150
	23–50	70	154	178	70	56	1000	5	10	60	1.4	1.6	18	2.2	400	3.0	800	800	350	10	15	150
	51+	70	154	178	70	56	1000	5	10	60	1.2	1.4	16	2.2	400	3.0	800	800	350	10	15	150
Females	11–14	46	101	157	62	46	800	10	8	50	1.1	1.3	15	1.8	400	3.0	1200	1200	300	18	15	150
	15–18	55	120	163	64	46	800	10	8	60	1.1	1.3	14	2.0	400	3.0	1200	1200	300	18	15	150
	19–22	55	120	163	64	44	800	7.5	8	60	1.1	1.3	14	2.0	400	3.0	800	800	300	18	15	150
	23–50	55	120	163	64	44	800	5	8	60	1.0	1.2	13	2.0	400	3.0	800	800	300	18	15	150
	51+	55	120	163	64	44	800	5	8	60	1.0	1.2	13	2.0	400	3.0	800	800	300	10	15	150
Pregnant						+30	+200	+5	+2	+20	+0.4	+0.3	+2	+0.6	+400	+1.0	+400	+400	+150	h	+5	+25
Lactating						+20	+400	+5	+3	+40	+0.5	+0.5	+5	+0.5	+100	+1.0	+400	+400	+150	h	+10	+50

SOURCE: *Recommended Dietary Allowances,* 9th edition, 1980. Reprinted by permission of the National Academy of Sciences, Washington, D. C.

[a]The allowances are intended to provide for individual variations among most normal persons as they live in the United States under usual environmental stresses. Diets should be based on a variety of common foods in order to provide other nutrients for which human requirements have been less well defined.

[b]Retinol equivalents. 1 retinol equivalent = 1 μg retinol or 6μg β-carotene.

[c]As cholecalciferol. 10 μg cholecalciferol = 400 I. U. vitamin D.

[d]α tocopherol equivalents. 1 mg d-α-tocopherol = 1α T.E.

[e]1 N.E. (niacin equivalent) is equal to 1 mg of niacin or 60 mg of dietary tryptophan.

[f]The folacin allowances refer to dietary sources as determined by *Lactobacillus casei* assay after treatment with enzymes ("conjugases") to make polyglutamyl forms of the vitamin available to the test organism.

[g]The RDA for vitamin B12 in infants is based on average concentration of the vitamin in human milk. The allowances after weaning are based on energy intake (as recommended by the American Academy of Pediatrics) and consideration of other factors such as intestinal absorption.

[h]The increased requirement during pregnancy cannot be met by the iron content of habitual American diets nor by the existing iron stores of many women; therefore the use of 30–60 mg of supplemental iron is recommended. Iron needs during lactation are not substantially different from those of nonpregnant women, but continued supplementation of the mother for two–three months after parturition is advisable in order to replenish stores depleted by pregnancy.

Appendix 8.7. *Estimated Safe and Adequate Daily Dietary Intakes of Additional Selected Vitamins and Minerals*

		Vitamins			Trace Elements*						Electrolytes		
	Age (years)	*Vitamin K* (μg)	*Biotin* (μg)	*Panto-thenic Acid* (mg)	*Copper* (mg)	*Manganese* (mg)	*Fluoride* (mg)	*Chromium* (mg)	*Selenium* (mg)	*Molybdenum* (mg)	*Sodium* (mg)	*Potassium* (mg)	*Chloride* (mg)
Infants	0–0.5	12	35	2	0.5–0.7	0.5–0.7	0.1–0.5	0.01–0.04	0.01–0.04	0.03–0.06	115–350	350–925	275–700
	0.5–1	10–20	50	3	0.7–1.0	0.7–1.0	0.2–1.0	0.02–0.06	0.02–0.06	0.04–0.08	250–750	425–1275	400–1200
Children	1–3	15–30	65	3	1.0–1.5	1.0–1.5	0.5–1.5	0.02–0.08	0.02–0.08	0.05–0.1	325–975	550–1650	500–1500
and	4–6	20–40	85	3–4	1.5–2.0	1.5–2.0	1.0–2.5	0.03–0.12	0.03–0.12	0.06–0.15	450–1350	775–2325	700–2100
Adolescents	7–10	30–60	120	4–5	2.0–2.5	2.0–3.0	1.5–2.5	0.05–0.2	0.05–0.2	0.1–0.3	600–1800	1000–3000	925–2775
	11+	50–100	100–200	4–7	2.0–3.0	2.5–5.0	1.5–2.5	0.05–0.2	0.05–0.2	0.15–0.5	900–2700	1525–4575	1400–4200
Adults		70–140	100–200	4–7	2.0–3.0	2.5–5.0	1.5–4.0	0.05–0.2	0.05–0.2	0.15–0.5	1100–3300	1875–5625	1700–5100

SOURCE: *Recommended Dietary Allowances*, 9th edition, 1980. Reprinted by permission of the National Academy of Sciences, Washington, D.C.

NOTE: Because there is less information on which to base allowances, these figures are not given in the main table of the RDA and are provided here in the form of ranges of recommended intakes.

*Since the toxic levels for many trace elements may be only several times usual intakes, the upper levels for the trace elements given in this table should not be habitually exceeded.

Appendix 8.8. *Mean Heights and Weights and Recommended Energy Intake*

Category	*Age*	*Weight*		*Height*		*Energy Needs (with range)*	
	(years)	*(kg)*	*(lb)*	*(cm)*	*(in)*	*(kcal)*	*(MJ)*
Infants	0.0–0.5	6	13	60	24	kg × 115 (95–145)	kg × .48
	0.5–1.0	9	20	71	28	kg × 105 (80–135)	kg × .44
Children	1–3	13	29	90	35	1300 (900 –1800)	5.5
	4–6	20	44	112	44	1700 (1300–2300)	7.1
	7–10	28	62	132	52	2400 (1650–3300)	10.1
Males	11–14	45	99	157	62	2700 (2000–3700)	11.3
	15–18	66	145	176	69	2800 (2100–3900)	11.8
	19–22	70	154	177	70	2900 (2500–3300)	12.2
	23–50	70	154	178	70	2700 (2300–3100)	11.3
	51–75	70	154	178	70	2400 (2000–2800)	10.1
	76+	70	154	178	70	2050 (1650–2450)	8.6
Females	11–14	46	101	157	62	2200 (1500–3000)	9.2
	15–18	55	120	163	64	2100 (1200–3000)	8.8
	19–22	55	120	163	64	2100 (1700–2500)	8.8
	23–50	55	120	163	64	2000 (1600–2400)	8.4
	51–75	55	120	163	64	1800 (1400–2200)	7.6
	76+	55	120	163	64	1600 (1200–2000)	6.7
Pregnancy						+300	
Lactation						+500	

SOURCE: *Recommended Dietary Allowances,* 9th edition, 1980. Reprinted by permission of the National Academy of Sciences, Washington, D.C.

NOTES: The energy allowances for young adults are for men and women doing light work. The allowances for the two older age groups represent mean energy needs over these age spans, allowing for a 2% decrease in basal (resting) metabolic rate per decade and a reduction in activity of 200 kcal/day for men and women between 51 and 75 years, 500 kcal for men over 75 years, and 400 kcal for women over 75. The customary range of daily energy output is shown for adults in parentheses, and is based on a variation in energy needs of ± 400 kcal at any one age emphasizing the wide range of energy intakes appropriate for any group of people.

Energy allowances for children through age 18 are based on median energy intakes of children these ages followed in longitudinal growth studies. The values in parentheses are tenth and ninetieth percentiles of energy intake, to indicate the range of energy consumption among children of these ages.

Appendix 8.9. *Selected Nutritional Formulas and Preparations Commonly Available*

Product Name/ Company	Sizes Available	Serving Size	Approximate Content per Serving: Calories	Approximate Content per Serving: Protein (Grams)	Special Characteristics	Flavors Available
Liquids						
Ensure*/Ross	8-oz can 32-oz can	8 oz	250	8.8	Lactose and milk-free, contains soy protein	Vanilla, black walnut
Isomil*/Ross	13-oz can concentrate 8, 32-oz can dilute	10 oz	200	6.0	Lactose and milk-free; contains soy protein	
Meritene/Doyle	8-oz can	8 oz	250	14.5	Contains milk	Vanilla, chocolate, eggnog, plain
Mull-Soy*†/Syntex	13-oz can concentrate	10 oz	200	8.5	Milk and lactose-free, contains soy flour	
Neo-Mull-Soy*†/ Syntex	14-oz can concentrate	10 oz	200	5.0	Milk and lactose-free, contains soy protein	
Prosobee*†/Mead Johnson	13-oz can concentrate	10 oz	200	7.5	Contains soy protein	
Sustacal*/Mead Johnson	12-oz can	12 oz	360	21.7	Lactose-free, contains soy protein	Vanilla, chocolate
Powders‡						
Instant Breakfast/ Carnation	Carton of 6, 1.26-oz packets	1 packet	290	16.0	Contains milk and soy protein, high lactose	6 flavors
Citrotein*/Doyle	16-oz can or 1.18-oz packet	1 packet	127	7.7	Egg albumin base, lactose-free	Orange, grape
Meritene/Doyle	1-lb can	1.14 oz measure	277	18.0	Contains milk, high lactose	Vanilla, chocolate, eggnog
Sustacal/Mead Johnson	Carton of 4, 1.9-oz packets	1 packet	360	21.7	Contains milk, high lactose	Vanilla, chocolate

SOURCE: Adapted from Morra, M. E.; Suski, N., and Johnson, B. L. *Eating hints: recipes and tips for better nutrition during cancer treatment*. Bethesda, Md.: National Cancer Institute, 1980.

*Recipes available from the manufacturer.

†Available where infant formulas are sold.

‡Calorie and protein content when prepared as directed on the package.

Appendix 8.10. *Synthetic Fiber-Free Liquid Diets*

	Product		
	Vivonex	*Vivonex HN*	*Flexical**
Calories per 100 ml	100	100	100
Content: 100 ml			
Carbohydrate (gm)	23.0 (90.2%) calories	21.0 (80.96%) calories	15.24 (61.2%) calories
Protein (gm)	2.04 (8.5%) calories	4.38 (18.3%) calories	2.25 (8.75%) calories
Nitrogen (gm)	0.33	0.67	0.4
Fat (gm)	0.15 (1.3%) calories	0.09 (0.78%) calories	3.4 (30.1%) calories
Sodium (mg)	86.0 (3.74 mEq)	77.02 (3.35 mEq)	35.0 (1.52 mEq)
Potassium (mg)	177.0 (2.99 mEq)	70.0 (1.80 mEq)	125.0 (1.57 mEq)
Chloride (mg)	180.3 (5.08 mEq)	185.8 (5.23 mEq)	100.0 (3.20 mEq)
Magnesium (mg)	22.2 (1.85 mEq)	13.3 (1.11 mEq)	30.0 (2.82 mEq)
Calcium (mg)	56.00 (2.8 mEq)	33.0 (1.65 mEq)	60.0 (2.99 mEq)
Vitamin K (mcg)	3.72	2.23	12.50
Osmolality mOsm/kg H_2O (variations depend upon flavor)	550–678	810–920	550.0
Source of:			
Carbohydrate	glucose + glucose oligosaccharides	glucose + glucose oligosaccharides	corn syrup, dextrins, citrate
Protein	crystalline amino acids	crystalline amino acids	hydrolyzed casein + amino acids
Fat	safflower oil	safflower oil	soy oil 80% + MCT oil 20%
Manufacturer	Eaton	Eaton	Mead Johnson
No. of flavors	7	6—vanilla not suitable	4

*Flexical contains both medium chain (MCT) and long chain triglycerides (LCT). Due to the presence of LCT, this product is inappropriate for use in patients with malabsorption disorders.

Appendix 8.10. *Continued*

		Complete Oral Liquid Diets*		
		Ensure	*Isocal*	*Precision LR Gelatin*
Calories following reconstitution:		106/100 ml	106/100 ml	112/100 ml
Content 100 ml				
Carbohydrate (lactose free)	(g)	14.3	13.0	35.6
Protein	(g)	3.7	3.42	3.75
Fat	(g)	3.7	4.46	0.10
Na^+	(mg)	73.0 (3.17 mEq)	53.0 (2.30 mEq)	100.0 (4.35 mEq)
K^+	(mg)	125.0 (3.20 mEq)	132.5 (3.4 mEq)	125.0 (3.20 mEq)
Cl^-	(mg)	104.6 (2.95 mEq)	106.0 (2.98 mEq)	158.30 (4.46 mEq)
Mg^{++}	(mg)	20.8 (1.73 mEq)	21.2 (1.76 mEq)	33.30 (1.37 mEq)
Ca^{++}	(mg)	32.08 (2.60 mEq)	63.6 (3.18 mEq)	83.30 (2.08 mEq)
Vitamin K	(mcg)	99.0	13.25	8.30
Osmolality (mOsm/kg H_2O)		375.0	350.0	700.0

*These oral liquid diets provide complete nutritional maintenance. They are suitable for both oral and tube feeding.

Indications: Nutritional maintenance in patients who have active digestive capability, who cannot eat normally, and who are not in negative nitrogen balance (i.e., facial or maxillary trauma, coma, neuromuscular disorders). Also appropriate for nutritional maintenance of patients who will not eat normally (i.e., anorexia and certain psychological states).

These are complete diets, not supplements to normal dietary intake. Average daily intake is 2000–3000 ml of liquid or 8–12 servings of gelatin.

		Therapeutic Dietary Supplements (High Calorie Liquid and Solid Dietary Supplements)*			
		Citrotein	*Polycose*	*Instant Breakfast*	*Amin-Aid*‡
Calories per 100 gm		63.5	200	Vanilla† 107.7	206
Content: 100 gm					
Carbohydrate	(g)	11.7	50.0	13.5	34.7
Protein	(g)	3.8	—	5.8	1.9
Fat	(g)	0.2	—	3.1	6.5
Na^+	(mg)	70.0	62.0	93.1	12.0
K^+	(mg)	76.0	3.9	273.5	23.0
Cl^-	(mg)	90.0	150.0	—	—
Mg^{++}	(mg)	40.0	—	44.0	—
Ca^{++}	(mg)	100.0	16.0	156.5	—

SOURCE: Yale–New Haven Hospital Formulary 1979–1980.

*Indications: catabolic states (surgery, severe infection, burns), where the ability to consume calories is suppressed by anorexia, pain, fever and/or depressed consciousness.

†Also available in chocolate; contents varies slightly.

‡Amin-Aid is indicated as a complete oral liquid diet or as a supplement in certain cases of advanced or hepatic disease.

Appendix 8.11. *Physician Guidelines for Total Parenteral Nutrition (TPN)–Hyperalimentation*

1. The TPN catheter and line are designed for TPN fluid *only*. The TPN lines should *not* be used for:
   A. Piggy-back infusions
   B. Central venous pressure monitoring
   C. IV bolus injections
   D. Blood withdrawals

2. The Department of Pharmacy Services prepares a standard solution containing necessary amino acids, electrolytes, and additives for most TPN procedures. The standard solution is recommended unless the patient has cardiac or renal failure for which special solutions are available. Total dextrose, electrolytes, protein equivalent, and additives are labeled on each liter of TPN solution.

Central		*Peripheral*	
Adult Standard TPN Solution		*Adult Standard TPN Solution*	
Dextrose	25.0%	Dextrose	5.0%
Protein equivalent	44.0 gm/L	Protein equivalent	44.0 gm/L
Sodium	35.0 mEq/L	Sodium	35.0 mEq/L
Potassium	30.0 mEq/L	Potassium	30.0 mEq/L
Calcium	4.6 mEq/L	Calcium	4.6 mEq/L
Magnesium	5.0 mEq/L	Magnesium	5.0 mEq/L
Chloride	35.0 mEq/L	Chloride	35.0 mEq/L
Phosphate	15.0 mM/L	Phosphate	15.0 mM/L
Acetate	67.5 mEq/L	Acetate	67.5 mEq/L

   In addition, multiple vitamin infusion (MVI concentrate) 2.5 ml, phytonadione injection (Vitamin K, Aquamephyton) 5 mg, and folic acid 1 mg are added to one liter only of TPN solution every day.

   Vitamin B_{12}, 1000 mcg should be injected IM once each month.

   A 24-hour supply of TPN is prepared by the Department of Pharmacy Services every morning between the hours of 8 a.m. and 2 p.m. It is important that orders for TPN be current every 24 hours. The TPN solution must be ordered each day early in the morning to insure continuation of the desired solution.

3. Dressing changes of the catheter insertion site, and routine monitoring of intravenous tubing changes should be performed by a nurse on the division who has been specifically trained in the care of TPN lines and dressings. Dressing changes are recommended on a Monday-Wednesday-Friday schedule.

4. Insulin
   Due to the variation in insulin requirements between patients on TPN therapy, sliding scale subcutaneous insulin coverage may be established according to individual patient response. If necessary, the pharmacy shall add regular insulin to the parenteral nutrition solution to satisfy the specific needs of patients.

5. TPN Team Consultation
   If patient evaluation is desired before instituting therapy and/or during therapy, the attending physician may solicit a TPN team consultation by completing the Yale–New Haven Hospital consultation form and notifying the TPN Service. The patient will be seen by the team physician, pharmacist, and nurse within 24 hours.

Appendix 8.11. *Continued*

6. Physician guidelines for peripheral parenteral nutrition laboratory studies

A. Baseline studies—prior to initiation of therapy

Glucose	Bilirubin	Total protein
BUN	SGOT	Albumin
Creatinine	Alkaline phosphatase	TIBC
Electrolytes (Na, K, Cl, HCO_3)	Hb/Hct	Cholesterol/triglycerides
Calcium/phosphate	PT/PTT	
Magnesium	CBC with differential	(Check NH_3 if liver disease is definite or suspected)

B. Post initiation of therapy

Daily × first week, then 3 times per week	*Mon/Thurs*	*Once each week*
Glucose	BUN	Cholesterol/triglycerides
Electrolytes (Na, K, Cl, HCO_3)	Creatinine	Ca/PO_4
	Intralipid level	Mg
		TP/Alb
		TIBC
		CBC with differential
		SGOT/Alkaline phosphatase
		Bilirubin

7. Physician guidelines for central parenteral nutrition laboratory studies

A. Baseline studies–prior to placement of central catheter

Glucose	Bilirubin	Total protein
BUN	SGOT	Albumin
Creatinine	Alkaline phosphatase	TIBC
Electrolytes (Na, K, Cl, HCO_3)	Hb/Hct	Cholesterol/triglycerides (for patients receiving fat emulsion)
Calcium/phosphate	PT/PTT	
Magnesium	CBC with differential	(Check NH_3 if liver disease is definite or suspected)

B. Stabilization period (7 days)

Daily	*Mon/Thurs*	*Once each week*
Glucose	BUN	TP/Alb
Electrolytes (Na, K, Cl, HCO_3)	Creatinine	CBC with differential
	Ca/PO_4	SGOT/Alkaline phosphatase
	Mg	Bilirubin
		Cholesterol/triglycerides (if patient receiving fat emulsion)

Appendix 8.11. *Continued*

C. Poststabilization period

Three times each week	*Mon/Thurs*	*Once each week*
Glucose	BUN	Ca/PO_4
Electrolytes (Na, K, Cl, HCO_3)	Creatinine	Mg
		TP/Alb
		TIBC
		CBC with differential
		SGOT/Alkaline phosphatase
		Bilirubin
		Cholesterol/triglycerides (if patient receiving fat emulsion)

D. Nursing monitoring parameters

Daily weights, taken at the same time with the same scale
Strict intake and output
Vital signs every 8 hours
Urine glucose and ketones every 6 hours
Admitting height and weight

SOURCE: Yale–New Haven Hospital Formulary 1981–1982.

Appendix 8.12. *Worksheet for Parenteral Hyperalimentation*

Division ______________ Physician(s) ____________ Admission Date __________ Unit ______________

Name ____

Consult __________ Ht ______________ Wt ______________ IBW ____________ Hx wt loss __________

Age __________________ Race ________________ Sex ____________________

Allergies ____

Date start TPN __________

Date stop TPN __________

Reason for D/C __________

Total TPN days __________

Site of line __________

Date	TPN formulation/rate		Date	TPN formulation/rate
1. ____	____________________		6. ____	____________________
2. ____	____________________		7. ____	____________________
3. ____	____________________		8. ____	____________________
4. ____	____________________		9. ____	____________________
5. ____	____________________		10. ____	____________________

Date Rate Intralipid 10%

1. ____ ______ ________ Calorie source ________ FFA deficiency

Week One			*Day One*		*Day Two*		*Day Three*		*Day Four*		*Day Five*		*Day Six*		*Day Seven*	
Labs	K	Na														
	HCO_3	Cl														
	Bun	Cr														
	Glu	Ca														
	PO_4	Mg														
	TP	Alb														
	Nit B	TIBC														
	Wt (kg)															
ADR Metabolic																
Septic																
Technical																
Dietary																
Rate Δ																

Appendix 8.12. *Continued*

Week Two			*Eight*		*Nine*		*Ten*		*Eleven*		*Twelve*		*Thirteen*		*Fourteen*	
Labs	K	Na														
	HCO_3	Cl														
	Bun	Cr														
	Glu	Ca														
	PO_4	Mg														
	TP	Alb														
	Nit B	TIBC														
	Wt (kg)															
ADR Metabolic																
Septic																
Technical																
Dietary																
Rate Δ																

SOURCE: Yale–New Haven Hospital Department of Pharmacy Services.

Appendix 8.13. *Daily Adult Parenteral Nutrition Form (Yale–New Haven Hospital, Department of Pharmacy Services)*

Date to be infused ________________ ________ Renewal Order—Same formula/rate as previous day

________ Initial Order ________ Order Change ________________ MD or TPN team
(Signature)

Send Completed Sheet to Pharmacy before 11 a.m. Daily

Section 1: **Amino Acid — Dextrose Solution**

A. Adult Central—Crystalline amino acids

________ Standard Protein 42 gm — Dextrose 25% per liter

________ Non-standard Protein ________ G/L — Dextrose ________%

B. Adult Peripheral—Crystalline amino acids

________ Standard Protein 42 G/L — Dextrose 5%

________ Non-standard protein ________ G/L — Dextrose ________ %

C. Adult Central—Essential amino acids (Nephramine)

________ Standard Protein 13.5 gm/750 ml — Dextrose 47%

Section 2: **Electrolyte Profile**

		Na	*K*	*Ca*	*Mg*	*Cl*	*PO_4*	*Ac*	*Lac*
A.	________ Standard	40 mEq	34.5 mEq	4.8 mEq	8 mEq	77 mEq	10.5 mM	26 mEq	0.0 mEq
B.	________ Non-Standard/L	________	________	________	________	________	________	________	________
C.	________ Essential A.A.	________	________	________	________	________	________	11 mEq	________

(Fill in additional additives as deemed necessary per 750 ml.)

Section 3: **Vitamins**

Multivitamins	2.5 ml		________ ml
Folic acid	1.0 mg	or	________ mg
Vitamin K	5.0 mg		________ mg

Section 4: **Additives**

(Routinely added to first bottle daily)

	Bottle No.				
________ Trace elements	1	(Zn	Cu	Mn	Cr I)
________ CZI ____ units	1	2	3	4	
________ Other ________	1	2	3	4	

Section 5: **Infusion Rate**

Bottles are scheduled at specific time intervals, determined by Standard rates. The first bottle of every 24-hour time period will be initiated at 2 p.m.

Crystalline A.A. Dextrose Solution

		Liters/Day
A. ____	40 ml/hr	1
B. ____	60 ml/hr	1.5
C. ____	80 ml/hr	2
D. ____	100 ml/hr	2.5
E. ____	125 ml/hr	3
F. ____	150 ml/hr	3.6

Fat Emulsion 10%

		Bottles/Day
A. ____	20 ml/hr	1
B. ____	40 ml/hr	2
C. ____	60 ml/hr	3
D. ____	80 ml/hr	4
E. ____	ml/hr	
F. ____	500 ml/hr infuse over ____ hrs	

Essential A.A.—Dextrose Solution 750 ml

		Bottles/Day
A. ____	30 ml/hr	1
B. ____	60 ml/hr	2
C. ____	90 ml/hr	3
D. ____	ml/hr	

Section 6: **Discontinuation of Therapy**

________ Amino acid/dextrose solution ________ Fat emulsion

SOURCE: Yale–New Haven Hospital Department of Pharmacy Services.

Appendix 8.14. *Daily Pediatric Parenteral Nutrition Form (Yale–New Haven Hospital, Department of Pharmacy Services)*

Date to be infused ________________ ________ Renewal order—same formula and rate as previous day

Initial order ________ Order change ________ ________________ MD or TPN team
(Signature)

Send Completed Sheet to Pharmacy Before 9 a.m. Daily

Section 1: **Crystalline Amino Acid—Dextrose Solution**

For Infants

A. ____ Peripheral ____ Central

B. ____ Standard Protein 20 G/L 2%
____ Non-Standard Protein ______ G/L

C. Dextrose Concentration
____ 10% ____ 12.5% ____ 15%
____ 20% ____ %

For Children

A. ____ Peripheral ____ Central

B. ____ Standard Protein 30 G/L 3%
____ Non-Standard Protein ______ G/L

C. Dextrose Concentration
____ 10% ____ 12.5% ____ 15%
____ 20% ____ 25% ____ %

Section 2: **Electrolyte Profile per Liter**

Infants	____ Stnd	____ Non-Stnd	Children	____ Stnd	____ Non-Stnd
Sodium	24.5 mEq	________	Sodium	35.3 mEq	________
Potassium	23.8 mEq	________	Potassium	36.0 mEq	________
Calcium	*		Calcium	*	
Magnesium	4.8 mEq	________	Magnesium	4.0 mEq	________
Chloride	35.0 mEq	________	Chloride	62.2 mEq	________
Phosphorus	7.8 mM	________	Phosphorus	7.8 mM	________
Acetate	12.0 mEq	________	Acetate	18.7 mEq	________
Lactate	10.0 mEq	________	Lactate	10.0 mEq	________

Vitamin and Trace Element Profile per Liter

Multivitamins	2.5 ml	________	Multivitamins	1.5 ml	________
Folic acid	0.25 mg	________	Folic acid	0.25 mg	________
Vitamin K	0.2 mg	________	Vitamin K	0.2 mg	________
Zinc	2.2 mg		Zinc	3.0 mg	
Copper	150.0 μg		Copper	200.0 μg	
Manganese	110.0 μg		Manganese	150.0 μg	
Chromium	1.5 μg		Chromium	2.0 μg	
Iodine	37.0 μg		Iodine	50.0 μg	

*Peripheral	Central	*Peripheral	Central
Day 1–14 0.0 mEq/L ≥14 days 5.6 mEq/L	11.25 mEq/l	4.7 mEq/L	8.5 mEq/L

Additives

CZI ________________

OTHER ________________

Appendix 8.14. *Continued*

Section 3:

Infusion Rate

First bottle of every 24-hour time period will be initiated at 11:00 a.m.	First bottle of every 24-hour time period will be initiated at 4:00 p.m.	Liters/day			Liters/day
A. ________ ml/hr	A. ____ 40 ml/hr	1	D. ____	100 ml/hr	2.5
	B. ____ 60 ml/hr	1.5	E. ____	125 ml/hr	3
	C. ____ 80 ml/hr	2	F. ____	ml/hr	

Section 4:

Fat Emulsion 10%–500 ml

		No. Units/day			No. Units/day
A. ________ ml/hr	A. ____ 20 ml/hr	1	C. ____	60 ml/hr	3
	B. ____ 40 ml/hr	2	D. ____	ml/hr	

Section 5:

Discontinuation of Therapy

________ Amino Acid/dextrose solution ________ Fat emulsion

SOURCE: Yale–New Haven Hospital Department of Pharmacy Services.

nine

The Oncology Nurse

DAVID S. FISCHER

No cancer update could be complete without a discussion of the revolution in cancer nursing. A little more than a decade ago the role of the nurse seemed to be confined to rubbing backs, passing bed pans, and changing sheets. Without denigrating these essential activities, the horizons have widened so that oncology nurses now participate in chemotherapy planning and administration, patient education, psychosocial support, symptomatic therapy, data collection, protocol monitoring, and community resource coordination, to name only a few activities (Henke et al. 1980; Bouchard and Owens 1976).

The oncology nurse may function in several different situations:

1. Private medical oncology office practice
2. University or hospital medical oncology or radiation therapy outpatient clinic
3. Hospital oncology ward or service
4. Oncology research ward
5. Palliative (symptomatic) chronic care facility
6. Home-care setting

To each of these situations the nurse brings the special skills of the profession. In almost no other illness do patients need personal support as much and as frequently (Proceedings 1974, 1977). They are beset by fear, loneliness, confusion, and depression. The nurse must provide encouragement, understanding, and psychological support to help them deal with these problems (Parsons 1977). They must be taught to achieve the maximum independence possible, but also to live with disability if necessary. The quality of life should be enhanced by imparting the many skills needed to cope with malignant disease and its complications such as ostomy care, dressing changes, decubitus management, skin care, and nutritional supplementation (Peterson and Kellogg 1976; Memorial Sloan-Kettering 1973).

Private Office Practice and Clinic

In the private office, the nurse must first make the patient comfortable and accepting of the environment with as little anxiety as possible. (Although an increasing number of men are entering the nursing profession, the vast majority of nurses are still women, and hence the use of the pronoun "she.") She can ascertain the patient's understanding or lack of information about the disease and emotional reaction to it. She can reassure the patient that help is always available and teach when to call the doctor. She can explain the nature of the patient's disease and the therapeutic regimen and volunteer to answer questions within her domain of understanding and expertise, remembering that neither she nor the physician is really competent to give a prognosis with any degree of certainty (Hellingers 1979; Newton 1979).

In the private office oncology nurses will usually have custody of the drug supplies and will administer them under the supervision of physicians. In our office, the nurses give intravenous drugs by push when appropriate or infusion when necessary. For those drugs that are locally toxic if they extravasate (nitrogen mustard, doxorubicin hydrochloride, daunomycin hydrochloride, dacarbazine, mitomycin, cisplatin, vincristine, vinblastine, dactinomycin, mithramycin, and so on), our nurses set up an IV in the forearm and slowly inject the drug through the side-arm of the rapidly running intravenous in what should be a perfect venipuncture (fig. 9.1) with no leakage (Knopf et al. 1981). They monitor these infusions and injections with extreme care because extravasation may not only be painful, but may lead to a chemical burn with late sloughing of skin and damage to muscles and tendons. They caution patients about after-care of injection sites and warn them to call us if problems develop.

They also instruct the patient in possible side effects of chemotherapy and measures that may be used to cope with these adverse effects. They caution the patients to call early with signs of infection or bleeding, neurologic progression, or evidence of rapid disease spread.

In our office, the nurses apply dressings, remove sutures, do therapeutic pheblotomies, and set up for and assist with bone marrow aspirations and trephine biopsies. They also take EKGs and when things get busy, help the technicians draw blood. They may at times schedule blood transfusions and complex radiologic tests. One of their most important functions is providing emotional support to the patients and serving as a sounding board for concerns, gripes, fears, complaints, and need to ventilate. They also keep the records for protocol studies in which we frequently participate.

In the university or hospital setting, or medical oncology clinic, the nurse has much the same function as in the private office. She may also play a role in lending continuity to the clinic over the course of time, as different staff members work on specific days only and the house staff and fellows change at frequent intervals. In addition, the record- and protocol-keeping may be even more intense, as principal investigators of much research will be the physicians of these clinics. Randomized clinical trials may be a major activity and the collation of collected data an essential continuing activity for all the personnel, but especially for the oncology nurse.

Wards

Many community hospitals have found that an oncology ward is a useful device for training a cadre of nurses and support personnel and giving patients continuity of care. Since many patients return to the hospital periodi-

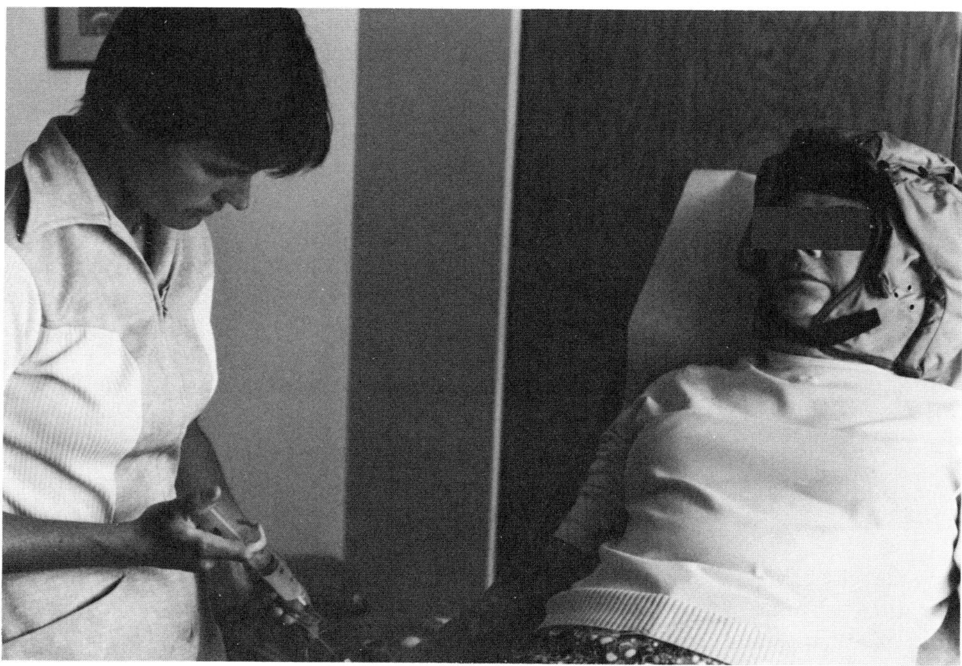

Fig. 9.1. *Patient receiving doxorubicin with oncology nurse pushing the drug through a rapidly running IV. Note that the patient is wearing an ice cap to reduce hair loss.*

cally for chemotherapy or for management of complications of their cancer, it has been worthwhile to have them return to an area that is familiar and to nursing personnel with whom they are already acquainted. Anxiety is diminished and quality of care is improved. Far from being a depressing area, camaraderie and team spirit have made this service in many hospitals the best for patients and for staff.

The oncology ward is a learning experience. Team discussions and planning conferences are held periodically with nurses, house staff, social workers, attending physicians, and when appropriate, psychiatrists, physiotherapists, clergy, pharmacists, and students. Patients' fears and information that may have been given to only one member of the team can be shared with all the health care-givers. In these days of platelet transfusions, total parenteral nutrition, leukocyte transfusions, reverse isolation, and timed-volume delivery pumps, the degree of sophistication is very high, and the need for continuing education absolutely essential (American Cancer Society 1975). The oncology ward has proved to be one of the best educational rotations for house staff and oncology fellows.

An oncology research ward is similar to a regular oncology ward but deals with certain special problems. To a far greater extent, experimental drugs are being used, toxicities of which are not as well known and hence they have to be monitored more intensely. Drug records and administration procedures must be documented more precisely for transmittal to the supervising agency. The potential for unforeseen complications is higher and the need for a greater personnel-to-patient ratio is clear in most instances (Hubbard and DeVita 1976).

Chronic Care Facilities

A variety of facilities exists with varied approaches to terminal care. One of the oldest is Calvary Hospital, a 200-bed facility in Bronx, N.Y., devoted to providing the patient dying with cancer a compassionate environment. In England, St. Christopher's Hospice has set a pattern that is being emulated in several institutions in various parts of the United States. The hospices have endeavored to pay special attention to the relief of pain, creation of a less structured and more home-like atmosphere, and to establishment of understanding and acceptance of the inevitability of the terminal illness. Group participation, discussion, and family involvement are especially encouraged.

A half-century ago, most people died at home in the bosom of the family. As our country became more mobile and families dispersed, the hospital became the place to die. Recently, there has been increased interest by individuals and families to have the inevitable death occur in the familiar surroundings of home and family. Since most physicians are concentrated near hospitals in central cities, neighborhood physicians are in the minority. Hence more and more home services and health supervision are being conducted by nurses. The Visiting Nurse Associations have been doing this for 75 years and now assist with a large proportion of cancer patients. Several other home-care agencies are also in the field. Many hospices have set up programs to assist families to care for the terminally ill at home. Oncology nurses visit and help with the patients and support family in terminal care and later with bereavement.

As oncology nursing has grown, several national conferences have been held, journals of cancer nursing have become popular *(Cancer Nursing)*, and a national organization has been formed known as the Oncology Nursing Society (ONS), which has its own journal *(Oncology Nursing Forum)*. The ONS has formed a liaison with the American Society of Clinical Oncology (ASCO), and they attempt to hold their meetings in proximity both geographically and temporally. The equal partnership of the oncologist (physician) and the oncology nurse is nowhere demonstrated more clearly than in Connecticut where the Connecticut Oncology Association welcomes both equally.

References

American Cancer Society. *A cancer source book for nurses.* New York: American Cancer Society, 1975.

Bouchard, R. and Owens, N. F. *Nursing care of the cancer patient.* St. Louis: C. V. Mosby, 1976.

Hellingers, A. E. Accountability in the health care systems: to whom is the nurse responsible? *Conn. Med.* 43:5–6, 1979.

Henke, C. et al. The nurse oncologist, symposium. *Semin. Oncol.* 7:3–90, 1980.

Hubbard, S., and DeVita, V. Chemotherapy research nurse. *Am. J. Nurs.* 76:560–565, 1976.

Knopf, M. K. et al. *Cancer chemotherapy: treatment and care.* Boston: G. K. Hall & Co., 1981.

Memorial Sloan-Kettering Cancer Center. *Guidelines for comprehensive nursing care in cancer.* New York: Springer Publishing Co., 1973.

Newton, L. H. To whom is the nurse accountable? A philosophical perspective. *Conn. Med.* 43:7–9, 1979.

Parsons, J. Needs of the cancer patient. *Nursing Digest* 5:1–84, 1977.

Peterson, B. H., and Kellogg, C. J. *Current practice in oncology nursing*. St. Louis: Mosby, 1976.

Proceedings of the National Conference on Cancer Nursing. New York: American Cancer Society, 1974.

Proceedings of the Second National Conference on Cancer Nursing. New York: American Cancer Society, 1977.

ten

Ethical and Social Dilemmas in Cancer Care

DAVID S. FISCHER

In addition to the difficult questions of medical, surgical, and radiologic therapy in the management of the patient with cancer, there are many ethical, social, and psychological problems that beset the practitioner. Many of these have been detailed in books and articles by ethicists, social workers, psychologists, psychiatrists, and sociologists, and a partial bibliography of these appears at the end of the chapter. I do not intend to review or comment on all of them, but rather to detail some of the problems, particularly those that have been encountered at the bedside by one clinician in 20 years of practice of hematology and 15 years of oncology. The first person singular pronoun will be used to emphasize that this is one person's experience and opinions, and that the same problems might appropriately be handled differently by another individual. Nonetheless, others may find that they have had similar problems and concerns.

Truth

The question of ethics is a personal one and represents interpretations of what is right and wrong. As such, it is relative; what is right for one person may be wrong for another. In addition, time and place impinge on decisions, and something will seem wrong now that may have been right in a different context. A generation ago American physicians usually lied to patients about a cancer diagnosis and were expected by patients' families to do so. In England, I am told, that is still the expected norm. Today, an increasing number of physicians has come to the conclusion that truth is the best policy. Patients are sophisticated and are not taken in by lies for long. When they discover a lie, the physician loses credibility and effectiveness. Furthermore, patients have the right to know what may be the most important fact in their lives.

A spouse or family member may insist on withholding the truth on the grounds that the patient might commit suicide or be otherwise emotionally unable to handle the fact of having cancer. What has the experience been? In the approximately 3500 patients with cancer I have personally attended, there has not been a single suicide to my knowledge as the result of being told the diagnosis.

I was once confronted by the husband of a patient with breast cancer who wanted me to start chemotherapy but not to tell his wife she had cancer. He insisted that "she couldn't take it." When I asked what she had been told after her mastectomy and again after radiation therapy, he said that she had been told that the tissue was benign but the surgery and radiation were "prophylactic to prevent cancer." As I entered the patient's room and wondered whether she was feeble-minded, and as I pondered what I could say within these constraints, an alert, bright woman greeted me with the statement, "Doctor, promise me you won't tell my husband I have cancer; he couldn't take it." The family cannot give real and compassionate support if they insist on this subterfuge, but fritter away valuable hours denying the obvious. A husband and wife who have shared a lifetime of problems honestly together should not end their relationship with secrecy, deceit, and evasion.

When informing the patient of the diagnosis of cancer, it is important that the physician do so in the company of a close relative or friend of the patient for support. It should be done tactfully, compassionately, and with a positive statement of hope for further help. On occasion, the patient may not be ready for the information and will choose not to hear it. There is no need to press the issue with one who is unwilling or unprepared. On the other hand, some people will accept the fact immediately and deny it late in the course of the illness.

Some years ago I was consulted by a brilliant young professor who came to me and said that he knew he had colon cancer with liver metastases. He indicated that he had reviewed most of the medical literature on the subject and was convinced that the best therapy was single-agent chemotherapy with 5-fluorouracil, and wanted me to administer it. We often talked about his disease and new research in the field. After almost a year of therapy, he developed a cough and I sent him to have a chest x-ray. The radiologist reported a right lower lobe pneumonia. I reviewed the films and felt that it was most likely lymphangitic spread of the carcinoma. When the patient returned he asked me about the x-ray and I let him read the report as was our custom, since he wanted to know everything about his cancer. He inquired about the choice of antibiotics and then took antibiotics and cancer chemotherapy simultaneously. During the several remaining months of his life, however, he never once mentioned cancer or chemotherapy, but chided me frequently for my inability to clear his "pneumonia." He had chosen denial as his defense late in the course and I went along with it. Like so many other patients in my experience, he had not followed the stereotyped five stages of Kübler-Ross in response to terminal illness (in sequence—denial, anger, bargaining, depression, and acceptance). Some patients do, others do not.

Another case of denial had the drama of a soap opera but with tragic and serious consequences for the family. The wife of a 55-year-old man with metastatic carcinoma insisted that her husband not be told his diagnosis. When I pressed the ethical, moral, and legal obligation to tell him, she brought in the family attorney who indicated that there was no legal need to do so, and that even though he had no will probate would be simple because the wife would inherit everything to raise their four minor children. About two months after the patient's death, his wife came in to explain that she could not pay my bill because the estate was tied up in probate. It turned out that the patient had been previously married and had a mentally retarded child by that marriage before it ended in divorce. He had never disclosed this to his second wife or attorney, but had cleverly arranged to send support money on a regular basis and had promised in writing at the time of his divorce to give half of his estate to the first wife for the support of the retarded daughter. At the time of the promise he had no other children. Unaware of his metastatic cancer, he had made no subsequent will or direction for the distribution of his estate. Two years later, when it was finally settled, court and legal fees had dissipated one-third of the estate and each of the wives received one-third for the support of the respective families. A far better outcome would have resulted if the patient had been informed of his diagnosis and motivated to execute a will.

Human Experimentation

There is no doubt that cancer therapy needs to be greatly improved. This can come only through research. As new techniques and drugs are developed they will ultimately have to be tested on humans before being generally accepted or rejected. The question is, what humans and under what circumstances?

There is now general agreement that human investigation should proceed only with informed consent of the subjects on projects carefully screened by a committee of professional and lay persons. Most universities, research institutes, and teaching hospitals have such a human investigation committee (HIC) or equivalent, which attempts to keep their research on an ethical and responsible level. Most of the time this is successful; however, several questions arise in the conduct of HIC activities. How "informed" is informed? If the patient's physician is a member of the research team, will the patient be given an unbiased appraisal? Is such a physician capable of giving an unbiased appraisal, or does the fact of participation taint the attempt? The old specter of "publish or perish" is as real today as it was 20 years ago.

Suppose the physician is a member of the department that has a protocol for treatment. Should a patient be advised to enter the protocol if the physician does not believe it offers the best possible therapy for the patient, but the majority of the department has endorsed it?

Should one recommend a protocol with a placebo arm when standard therapy has a 30% response rate? Suppose a standard drug only has a 10% response rate?

When attempting to obtain consent for a clinical investigation, is it ethical for the researcher to offer to pay for drug therapy if the patient agrees to participate, or for all hospital and outpatient medical expenses if the patient participates? Should the family be asked to make the decision for a competent adult so that the patient does not have to be fully informed? How much pressure (or guilt) should be placed on a sibling to make a white cell, bone marrow, or kidney donation?

These are just a few of the problems that arise every month that must be adjudicated in each physician's own conscience. In addition, the implied or explicit contract with the patient must be remembered. Roughly stated, it is the intention of the patient to place his or her welfare, health, and life in the hands of the physician, and the physician is expected to exercise good judgment to protect the quality and length of life against disease and death. If that can *best* be done with an experimental program in the honest opinion of the physician, the patient should be so advised. If it can best be done with more conventional therapy, then that should be employed. The first priority of the teacher is to education, and of the researcher to research. But the first priority of the physician must be the welfare of the patient.

Allocation of Scarce Resources

Almost every day difficult decisions have to be made as to who gets what. Often, the first decision is who is admitted into the hospital first when there are more requests for admissions than available beds. Should we stick to the rule of "first come, first served"? Should we treat the sickest, that is, emergencies first? Should we triage to treat first those who are likely to benefit the most, for example, the young in preference to the old, and the minimally disabled rather than the severely disabled? The battlefield military tradition is to treat the minimally disabled first because they are likely to return to duty, whereas the most seriously injured are likely to die, and their treatment will require the time of several able-bodied persons. In civilian medicine, our society tends to give priority to those most desperately ill and to give them first call on its resources. When there are not enough resources for all, society will have to reevaluate its priorities.

Recently I observed a septuagenarian receiving daily platelet transfusions while in the terminal throes of illness, at the same time that a more recently admitted teenaged patient of another oncologist needed a few platelet transfusions to recover from chemotherapy-induced thrombocytopenia. The blood bank did not have enough platelets for both. Who should get the platelets? Who should decide?

Most of the time, if several patients need penicillin we can get more by simply ordering more. This is often not true for blood products or organ replacements; we occasionally run out of albumin. We sometimes have more requests for platelets, white cells, and red cells than we can fill, and have to make decisions reflecting the scarcity of resources. The situation becomes particularly difficult when inexperienced physicians order some of these materials simply because their patients' cell counts are a little low.

Should we restrict the freedom of a general physician to order any therapy that he thinks his patient might need? If we do set up restrictions to optimize the use of scarce resources, who makes the rules? Is it ethical for a university-affiliated hospital with a part-time faculty who are also in private practice to restrict the use of expensive or scarce instrumentation to their full-time faculty? As state cost commissions restrict the ability to purchase equipment, monopolistic practices will become more frequent by those fortunate enough to have made the purchases first. It might even be self-defeating by forcing the earliest possible purchase of new equipment when it is most expensive and least well developed. Groups and institutions that wait for the instrumentation to become more refined and cheaper may discover that the state cost commission then blocks its purchase. It would seem that this counter-productive attempt at saving by opposing most purchases forces the hospitals to appeal major acquisitions, budgets, or new construction to the courts. This has made the cost of new equipment prohibitively expensive, because the hospital (and ultimately the patient) pays for both the equipment and the litigation required to purchase it. It seems to me that the result of the cost commission system is that everyone loses—the taxpayer, the doctor, the patient—everyone except the commission staff and lawyers.

Another ethical question one might ask concerns the morality of closed-panel health maintenance organizations (HMOs). These idealistic attempts to provide optimal care at the lowest possible cost often flounder when these two ideals come into conflict. Most HMOs cannot afford to attract first-rate specialists in all areas, and therefore contract with outside providers for these services. Do they contract with the best or the cheapest? Does the patient who has had specialist services, and believes those services to have been the cheapest and not the best, have any recourse? Will the HMO pay for a second opinion? At present, some federal government agencies are promoting second opinions and others are subsidizing HMOs. Most HMOs, however, will not pay for another physician's diagnosis, especially if the patient elects to choose the specialist.

Cost-Benefit Ratios

Even if we have plenty of drugs and ample supplies of blood products, when does it become unwise to treat? When do we stress society's resources beyond their logical limits? As physicians, if we were unrestricted we could probably spend half the gross national product on cancer care and have little left for other purposes. Clearly, decisions have to be made that are difficult and have moral and ethical implications.

Consider a typical problem. An 80-year-old woman with acute leukemia was referred for chemotherapy. One suggestion was to give her transfusions until she reached a comfortable level, and let her go home to live out her life with supportive care. The other was to put her on our protocol with daunorubicin, cytarabine, and thioguanine and try to induce a remission and support her until recovery. The family and some of our staff agreed on aggressive chemotherapy. Shortly after therapy she became leukopenic, neutropenic, anemic, and thrombocytopenic. She developed a bacterial and an *Aspergillus* pneumonia. She was admitted to the ICU where she had a respiratory arrest and was resuscitated. Endotracheal intubation was performed, and she was supported by a respirator for a week. She then had a tracheostomy. The aspergillosis of the lung was treated with amphotericin. She developed hypotension and was given steroids several times, together with dopamine. Her bone marrow was normal at 60 days but she was still dying of respiratory problems. After 75 days of ICU care and hyperalimentation, she died. Autopsy permission was refused. Estimated cost of care was in excess of $100,000. Was the decision to treat her aggressively a wise one? Was it in the patient's best interests? Was it in society's best interests?

As new drugs and procedures are developed, the costs of therapy become increasingly high. Drugs like doxorubicin (Adriamycin), bleomycin (Blenoxane), mitomycin (Mutamycin), and cisplatin (Platinol) have added a cost dimension never imagined when third party insurance began. Few individuals could afford chemotherapy costing $300 to $400 every three to four weeks for palliation of advanced malignancies. When I began practice, drug costs for chemotherapy were seldom more than $10 per month but the individual or the family paid for it. They would often decide against chemotherapy because it was not worth it in view of the prognosis. With total coverage by third party payers, many families have adopted the philosophy, "We demand the best regardless of what it costs, for as long as it takes." Under this circumstance, oncologists are frequently put in the difficult position of initiating excessively costly therapeutic programs involving prolonged hospitalizations that have only the remotest possibility of producing significant benefit. At present, each oncologist handles the situation with the best judgment possible. Someday, society will have to address this problem.

Termination of Support Systems

There comes a time in many cases of cancer when the quality of life begins to deteriorate. The choice of therapeutic options may become a selection of lesser evils. How heroic should the physician be? Should each physician make the decision alone in each case? Should the health care team be polled? Should the family, especially the next of kin, be consulted? Should the patient participate in the decision?

Depending on the situation, different answers seem appropriate. For a young individual with stage III Hodgkin's disease and a complicating infection, heroic therapy is probably strongly indicated. With current medical regimens, cure of the infection can reasonably be expected, and there is a high likelihood of long-term survival with therapy for the Hodgkin's disease. The patient with pancreatic carcinoma with liver metastases has a poor prognosis with current modalities of therapy. If there is no response to reasonable chemotherapy, heroic therapy is probably not indicated. I personally would not intubate such a patient, or use a respirator, or attempt a resuscitation unless specifically requested to do so by the patient or next of kin. It would not be to the patient's benefit.

While it seems entirely ethical to me not to resort to heroic therapy for a patient with terminal cancer, but to allow nature to take its course, it is an entirely different matter to attempt euthanasia—the practice of actively putting a patient to death. The distinction is clear. Where it becomes blurred is when someone has thoughtlessly initiated extra therapy such as a respirator for a terminally ill patient, soon after which a decision has to be made to turn off the life-support system. Should only the physician do it? Should one insist on the consent of other physicians, lawyers, judges, clergy, family, or of the patient?

In recent years there has been an increasing trend for physicians not to expose themselves to this decision, but to petition judges for a court order. I personally regard this as a failure on the part of the physician or medical team. The physician who has good rapport and the trust of the patient knows whether the patient wants this extreme of therapy. In many cases, I discuss it with the patient quite explicitly, and in most instances the choice is clearly against these measures. Some have even signed so-called living wills early in the course of illness (appendix 10.1). If the patient's choice is not to undergo such treatment and if this decision is reasonable in the light of known facts, it should be honored and a "do not resuscitate" order written so that the entire staff is aware of the preferred course. When the patient is unprepared or unable to discuss this decision, it should be presented to the next of kin together with all the available facts. Most of the time a caring family will recognize the inevitable and request that nothing be done to prolong the act of dying, and that the patient be given compassionate, supportive care to ensure comfort until the time of dignified death. Again, a "do not resuscitate" order should be written and care adjusted. Spiritual support and psychic comfort should be provided. Sometimes this can best be done at home, sometimes in a hospice. The guidelines for the "do not resuscitate" policy have been formalized in several publications. As an example, we append the report of one of our committees with which we concur (appendix 10.2).

Rights of the Cancer Patient

To considerate and respectful care

To full confidentiality of records

To the best curative or palliative therapy available

To know the true diagnosis if desired

To have relief of pain to the extent it is safe

To be fully informed of therapeutic alternatives if desired

To be fully informed of the risks of therapy

To be fully informed of experimental therapy before consent is requested

To continuity of care

To have the freedom to refuse any or all therapy

To employment opportunities commensurate with ability

To have the maximal quality of life the disease permits

To have spiritual or religious support if desired

To have an appropriate death with dignity

To have hope.

References

Abrams, R. D. *Not alone with cancer.* Springfield, Ill.: Charles C. Thomas, 1974.

Alfidi, R. J. Informed consent: a study of patient reaction. *JAMA* 216:1325–1329, 1971.

Bahnson, C. B. Psychological and emotional issues in cancer: the psychotherapeutic care of the cancer patient. *Semin. Oncol.* 2:293–308, 1975.

Beecher, H. K. Ethics and clinical research. *N. Engl. J. Med.* 274:1354–1360, 1966.

Black, M. P. Brain death: I, II. *N. Engl. J. Med.* 299:338–344; 393–401, 1978.

Boks, S. The ethics of giving placebos. *Sci. Am.* 2317:17–23, 1974.

Boks, S. Personal directions for care at the end of life. *N. Engl. J. Med.* 295:367–369, 1976.

Childress, J. Ethical issues in the experimentation with human subjects. *Conn. Med.* 43:26–31, 1979.

Creech, R. H. The psychological support of the cancer patient: a medical oncologist's viewpoint. *Semin. Oncol.* 2:285–292, 1975.

Dunphy, J. E. On caring for the patient with cancer. *N. Engl. J. Med.* 295:312–319, 1976.

Fiore, N. Fighting cancer—one patient's perspective. *N. Engl. J. Med.* 300:248–287, 1979.

Fitts, W. T., and Raudin, I. S. What Philadelphia physicians tell patients with cancer. *JAMA* 153:901–904, 1953.

Fletcher, J. *Morals and medicine.* Boston: Beacon Press, 1954.

Freireich, E. J. Ethical consideration in the prolongation of life. *Proceedings of the Second National Conference on Cancer Nursing.* New York: American Cancer Society, 1977.

Halper, T. Ethics and medical experimentation: some unconfronted problems. *Conn. Med.* 43:24–25, 1979.

Harvard Medical School. Report of the ad hoc committee: a definition of irreversible coma. *JAMA* 205:337–340, 1968.

Hiatt, H. H. Protecting the medical commons: who is responsible? *N. Engl. J. Med.* 293:235–241, 1975.

Jakobovits, I. *Jewish medical ethics.* New York: Bloch, 1975.

Jonsen, A. R.; Cassel, C. L. B.; and Perkins, H. S. The ethics of medicine: an annotated bibliography of recent literature. *Ann. Intern. Med.* 92:136–141, 1980.

Konior, G. S., and Levine, A. S. The fear of dying: how patients and their doctors behave. *Semin. Oncol.* 2:311–316, 1975.

Kübler-Ross, E. *On death and dying.* New York: Macmillan, 1970.

Lo, B., and Jonsen, A. R. Ethical decisions in the care of a patient terminally ill with metastatic cancer. *Ann. Intern. Med.* 92:107–111, 1980.

Novack, D. H. et al. Changes in physicians' attitudes toward telling the patient. *JAMA* 175:897–900, 1979.

Okan, D. What to tell cancer patients: a study of medical attitudes. *JAMA* 175:1120–1128, 1961.

Pattison, E. M. *The experience of dying*. Englewood Cliffs, N.J.: Prentice-Hall, 1977.

Potter, J. F. A challenge for the hospice movement. *N. Engl. J. Med.* 302:53–55, 1980.

Rabkin, M. T.; Gillerman, G.; and Rice, N. R. Orders not to resuscitate. *N. Engl. J. Med.* 295:364–366, 1976.

Relman, A. S. The Saikewicz decision: judges as physicians. *N. Engl. J. Med.* 298:508–509, 1978.

Rosenbaum, E. H. *Living with cancer*. New York: Praeger, 1975.

Roy, W. R. An agenda for physicians and legislators. *N. Engl. J. Med.* 295:589–596, 1976.

Schwartz, W. B., and Joskow, P. L. Medical efficacy versus economic efficiency: a conflict of values. *N. Engl. J. Med.* 299:1462–1464, 1978.

Simonton, O. C.; Simonton, S. M.; and Creighton, J. *Getting well again*. Los Angeles: J. P. Tarcher, 1978.

Spencer, S. S. "Code" or "no code": a nonlegal opinion. *N. Engl. J. Med.* 300:138–139, 1979.

Spiro, H. Constraint and consent—on being a patient and a subject. *N. Engl. J. Med.* 293:1134–1135, 1975.

Veatch, R. *Death, dying, and the biological revolution: our last quest for responsibility*. New Haven: Yale University Press, 1976.

Appendix 10.1. *Sample Living Will*

To My Family, My Physician, My Lawyer, and All Others Whom It May Concern

Death is as much a reality as birth, growth, maturity, and old age—it is the one certainty of life. If the time comes when I can no longer take part in decisions for my own future, let this statement stand as an expression of my wishes and directions, while I am still of sound mind.

If at such a time the situation should arise in which there is no reasonable expectation of my recovery from extreme physical or mental disability, I direct that I be allowed to die and not be kept alive by medications, artificial means, or "heroic measures." I do, however, ask that medication be mercifully administered to me to alleviate suffering even though this may shorten my remaining life.

This statement is made after careful consideration and is in accordance with my strong convictions and beliefs. I want the wishes and directions here expressed carried out to the extent permitted by law. Insofar as they are not legally enforceable, I hope that those to whom this Will is addressed will regard themselves as morally bound by these provisions.

Signed ______________________

Date ______________________

Witness ______________________

Witness ______________________

Copies of this request have been given to ______________________

____

____

____

SOURCE: Adapted from material from the Concern for Dying, New York, New York

Appendix 10.2. *Recommendations of the Committee on Policy for "Do Not Resuscitate" Decisions*
Department of Internal Medicine
Yale University School of Medicine
Robert J. Levine, Chairman of Human Investigations Committee
April 1979

This document sets forth the recommendations of the Committee for consideration by the Department of Medicine. These recommendations are abstracted from the Report of the Committee (March 1979); those who are interested may obtain copies from Dr. Thier's office. Members of the Department are invited to address their comments on these recommendations to Dr. Robert J. Levine, Chair of the Committee; these comments will be considered in the development of final Departmental policy.

In its Report, the Committee concluded that faulty communication is the most important obstacle to the making and implementation of decisions on withholding cardiopulmonary resuscitation (as well as other decisions germane to the management of those who are—or appear to be—terminally ill). These recommendations are designed to eradicate—or at least to minimize—the barriers to communication identified by the Committee. There are no guidelines for determining what medical conditions are to be considered grounds for withholding resuscitation or other life-sustaining therapy. Rather, it identifies the personnel who should be held accountable for ensuring that such decisions are made and the procedures that they should employ to facilitate clear and unambiguous communications relevant to these decisions.

The recommendations are presented in the following order:

I. Identification of the responsible physician
II. Communications between health care professionals
III. Classification of approaches to management of the terminally ill
IV. Communications with the patient and the family
V. The mechanics of writing Do Not Resuscitate orders and classification notes
VI. Glossary

I. Identification of the Responsible Physician

The "Policies Governing Responsibility for Care of Patients" in Yale–New Haven Hospital specify that all patients admitted to Yale–New Haven Hospital are to be under the care of a member of the hospital staff who is designated the "responsible physician." The responsible physician has the overall responsibility, both medically and legally, for the patient's care.

In the care of patients who are terminally ill, clear identification of the responsible physician is of paramount importance. If at any time the identity of the responsible physician is unclear to any member of the health care team, he or she should ask the house officer to identify the responsible physician. If the house officer is unable to do so, he or she should contact the chief medical resident who has the obligation to provide prompt identification of the responsible physician.

The obligations of the responsible physician in the care of terminally-ill patients—in addition to those specified in the March 1978 version of the YNHH *Policies*—are elaborated in each of the subsequent sections.

II. Communications Among Health Care Professionals

When it becomes apparent to the responsible physician that a decision must be made about management classification of a terminally-ill patient, he or she should signal to all members of the health care team the intention to make such a decision by writing a note to that effect in the patient's chart. Such a note might be worded: "The condition of this patient is deteriorating and it is necessary to formulate plans with regard to future management. This will be done at (specify a time and place; e.g., tomorrow at work rounds)."

Such a note should alert all parties (e.g., physicians, nurses, social workers, chaplains, students, and so on) that a management classification decision is about to be made. Thus they may contribute any information they consider relevant either by speaking directly with the responsible physician or by planning to be present at the designated time for making the decision.

Any member of the health care team who considers that the management classification for a patient is inappropriate (or, in some cases, when there is no management classification, that there should be one) should report this opinion to the responsible physician; any health care professional holding such an opinion should consider it an obligation, not merely a prerogative, to report such an opinion to the responsible physician. Further, it is the obligation of the responsible physician to act upon such communications. The responsible physician has the right and the obligation to make *final* judgments with regard to the medical reversibility (Section VI) of the patient's condition; in the event of irreconcilable disagreements between health care professionals, suitable consultation should be obtained. If the disagreements cannot be resolved with the aid of a consultant, the matter should be referred to the Chief of Service for arbitration or mediation.

In many instances, the physician having the best relationship with the family or the patient may be a member of the house staff and not the responsible physician. Therefore, discussions with the patient or family that ultimately lead to a change in management classification may be conducted by that house officer. However, these discussions should first be approved by the responsible physician; delegation of authority to conduct such discussions must be explicit.

In general, health care personnel should refrain from initiating discussions with the patient or the family that seem to reflect a consensus on management classification until such a consensus is reached through appropriate discussions among members of the health care team.

The authority to write a Do Not Resuscitate order may not be delegated; it must be written personally by the responsible physician. However, house officers have the authority to cancel Do Not Resuscitate orders as appropriate. For example, such orders should be cancelled at the request of the patient, or duly authorized member of the family (Section IV). Further, an unexpected finding that suggests that the prognosis for medical reversibility has been substantially underestimated should signal the need for such cancellation. In the latter case, the order should be suspended temporarily while the house officer attempts to discuss the unexpected finding with the responsible physician.

In the absence of a house officer, nurses may be called upon by family members to perform cardiopulmonary resuscitation on patients for whom Do Not Resuscitate orders have been written. Under these circumstances, the nurse should contact either the house officer or the responsible physician as soon as possible. In the event the request to disregard a Do Not Resuscitate order is made during cardiopulmonary arrest, and no physician is available, the nurse is authorized to proceed with cardiopulmonary resuscitation. However, all professionals should be aware that—at the moment of cardiopulmonary arrest—members of the family who have previously carefully thought through decisions to authorize Do Not Resuscitate orders may respond to the immediate situation by saying, "Do something." Professionals who are experienced at working in intensive care units can ordinarily distinguish this reaction from a determination to reverse a previously well thought out decision.

III. Classification of Approaches to Management of the Terminally Ill

The purpose of this classification system is to provide an easily accessible reference for those health professionals who might be called upon to make judgments about implementation of various therapeutic maneuvers when the responsible physician is not available for timely consultation. Definitions of terms marked with an asterisk are provided in the Glossary (Section VI).

Class A

The general presumption in this Class is that patients are to receive all curative* and functional maintenance therapies* as indicated. The primary goal is to achieve arrest, remission, or cure of the basic disease process*. The aims of curative therapy take priority over those of functional maintenance which, in turn, hold a higher priority than those of comforting therapy*.

Class B

The general presumption in this Class is that any curative therapy in progress (if any) will be continued until its outcome has been determined and, further, that no new curative therapy will be implemented. The goals of functional maintenance therapy take priority over the goals of comforting therapy. The responsible physician should specify limits—if any—to be imposed on functional maintenance therapy: for example, if sepsis occurs, should it be treated with antibiotics?

Class B is further subdivided as follows:

B1: In the event of cardiopulmonary arrest, the patient is to be resuscitated.

B2: Do Not Resuscitate order is written.

Class C

The goals of therapy are to comfort the patient as he or she is dying. A Do Not Resuscitate order is written, and comforting therapy dominates the approach to medical care. The limits of functional maintenance therapy should be specified.

The general presumption is that all patients are in Class A unless otherwise specified. Patients are to be classified according to this system only when there exists some legitimate cause to suspect that a patient should be in either Class B or C. Writing in the chart that a patient is in Class A should be done only to signal the fact that the health care team has—with due deliberation and consultation—rejected classifying the patient as either B or C.

Patients should be classified in Class B only when there is a very low probability of achieving any consequential remission. In general, reasonable curative therapies have been tried and failed or have been rejected for good cause. For example, the patient may have refused some potentially curative therapies. For some patients in this Class a curative therapy may be in progress but there is little likelihood of success.

Class B is, in general, to be considered a temporary classification. Some of these patients will show surprising responses to curative therapy in which case they will be transferred to Class A. Most of them, however, will become suitable candidates for Class C.

IV. Communications with the Patient and Family

When the responsible physician—with due consultation with other health care professionals—has reached a decision regarding the medical reversibility of a patient's condition, a discussion should be initiated with the patient and/or the family with the aim of defining the overall management objectives. The ultimate authority to determine the overall management objectives resides with the patient and/or the family.

If the patient is conscious and competent, he or she has the clear right to refuse any treatment (including resuscitation) even if the consequences of such refusal may be death. Thus, if the patient, after discussion of the alternatives, is capable of understanding the situation and wishes not to be resuscitated, the physician is entitled to rely on such a decision; this entitlement obtains even when the decision is opposed by one or more of the patient's relatives. In general, if a competent adult patient refuses any therapy, that therapy may be given only when authorized by a court order. It should be noted, however, that in cases of attempted suicide, it is customary and legal to oppose the expressed wishes of the patient to refuse life-saving therapy.

If a legally competent patient is steadfast in refusing any type of therapy and if in the judgment of the responsible physician, such refusal seems irrational, the Chief of Staff or Hospital Counsel should be consulted. The Hospital will almost never initiate incompetency proceedings based solely on the fact that a patient is refusing treatment.

If the patient is comatose or incompetent and a legal guardian (known in Connecticut as the conservator of the person) has been appointed, the conservator of the person has the right to make such decisions. Only a patient who has been so adjudicated by a court is legally incompetent; all other patients are to be considered competent as a matter of law. Ideally, the family should be urged to obtain a court order appointing a conservator prior to the time such decisions are to be made if the patient seems incapable of speaking for himself or herself; however, in many cases this is impractical.

Decisions to discontinue life-saving therapies or to withhold resuscitation must be authorized by the patient or, when appropriate, the guardian. Failure to secure such authorization (Glossary) may impose legal liability on the physician. Consequently, when such decisions are contemplated in the course of management of comatose or incompetent patients, every effort should be made to contact an individual who is entitled to provide such authorization. If such a person cannot be located, the Chief of Staff and Hospital Counsel should be notified.

If the patient is comatose or legally incompetent, the following order of decision-making should be followed: The spouse, if present and competent, has the clear paramount right over adult children to be appointed conservator of an incompetent patient and, even if not appointed, to make decisions about treatment. Where there is no spouse but there are adult offspring, in situations where there is consensus, any one sibling may act for all. If there is disagreement, Hospital Counsel should be called.

When the authority to make a decision resides in a group (e.g., of siblings), it is legally perilous to discontinue therapy while there is conflict among members of the group. At times, it may be necessary to resuscitate the patient, perhaps several times, while awaiting consensus to develop.

Some legally incompetent patients may be capable of expressing their wishes about their management. When there are conflicts between the conservator and the patient, no decision to withdraw curative or functional maintenance therapies or to write Do Not Resuscitate orders should be made without authorization from the Chief of Staff and the Hospital Counsel.

In any case in which the physician believes there is a reasonable possibility of medical reversibility of the basic disease process and the patient is comatose or incompetent, the physician has the legal authority to treat the patient over the family's objection. In the event a family member is adamant in opposing a physician's plans to continue life-sustaining therapy, Hospital Counsel should be consulted.

In some cases in which the responsible physician and the patient and/or family are in irreconcilable conflict about the appropriate course of management, the physician may offer to withdraw. In these circumstances the responsible physician should also offer assistance in identifying and contacting another who will assume the role of the responsible physician.

In the event a patient meets the criteria for "brain death," the patient may be pronounced dead and then all therapeutic maneuvers discontinued notwithstanding any expressions of wishes to do otherwise. (See Black, P. M. Brain death. *N. Engl. J. Med.* 299:338–344 and 393–401, 1978.)

V. Mechanics of Writing Do Not Resuscitate Orders and Classification Notes

Decisions to withhold resuscitation in the event of cardiopulmonary arrest are to be written on the *order sheet.* They should be spelled out; the abbreviation DNR is not to be used. Also not to be used are such euphemisms as "no code" or "in case of CPA, page house officer, stat." Only the responsible physician may write the Do Not Resuscitate order; verbal orders are not permitted. It is presumed that Do Not Resuscitate orders will be reviewed at least once daily and commonly more frequently.

The responsible physician should also write on the *order sheet* a notification that a management classification note has been written in the progress notes. This should indicate the date on which it was written and identify the individual who wrote it. Substantive changes in the management classification should similarly be noted on the order sheet. In all cases in which a Do Not Resuscitate order is written, a management classification note is mandatory.

In the Kardex, the nurse should note prominently that a Do Not Resuscitate order has been written. In close proximity to that notation there should be an additional notation of when the most current management classification note was written in the progress notes. When applicable, there should also be a list of limitations of such things as functional maintenance therapies.

Progress notes

Management classification notes should provide a clear account of the rationale for the determination of the objectives of management. There should be an identification of the basic disease process(es) and an estimation of the probability and magnitude of its medical reversibility. There should be a statement as to whether the management objectives are those of Class A, B (1 or 2), or C. Limitations, if any, on functional maintenance therapies (or other therapies) that have been agreed upon with the patient are to be identified. Further, there should be a statement on the extent to which the objectives of comforting take priority over those of functional maintenance.

Finally, there should be a statement as to who authorized this approach to management—either the patient or the appropriate relative(s) or guardian. This statement should include a brief account of the information that was conveyed to the patient and/or family that formed the basis of the authorization.

Occasionally it is necessary to ask either the patient or a member of the family to sign an authorization note for a Do Not Resuscitate order. These are situations in which either (1) there is irreconcilable disagreement between the person having the legal authority to make the decision and one or more members of the family, or (2) strong disagreements between equally entitled siblings have been resolved recently. In these cases, the member of the family who takes responsibility for authorizing a Do Not Resuscitate order should be asked to sign (or, if they prefer, write) an authorization note in the medical record (progress notes). This should be a brief note indicating that the responsible person(s) understands and agrees to the Do Not Resuscitate order. The note should include the fact that the condition of the patient is terminal, that discussions have been held with the family (and, if appropriate, the patient) and that a decision has been made not to resuscitate the patient in the event that breathing or the heart stops. While no set form for such a note is suggested by the Committee, each one should include a reasonably full statement of the rationale for the decision and a summary of the discussions with the patient and/or family. Those who prefer not to sign such notes should not be coerced to do so; in such cases the physician should record the fact that the individual(s) preferred not to sign; the reasons for this preference, if known, should also be recorded.

A copy of a "living will" may be entered in the medical record if the patient authorizes this entry; the date of such authorization should be noted in the progress notes.

When patients for whom Do Not Resuscitate orders are written are transported outside the patient care unit to other parts of the Hospital, it is the obligation of the responsible physician (or the house officer to whom he or she delegates such responsibility) to communicate clearly with the personnel of the department (e.g., Radiology) to which the patient is being transported that there is a Do Not Resuscitate order. Ideally, a professional from the patient care unit should accompany the patient to see to it that—among other things—Do Not Resuscitate orders are respected. However, at times when this is not feasible, the responsible physician—or his or her delegate—should communicate clearly on this matter with a health professional in the department to which the patient is being transported that there is a Do Not Resuscitate order. The individual on the receiving end of this communication should be one who will be responsible for seeing to it that this order is respected while the patient is in his or her department.

VI. Glossary

Basic disease process

This is the disease process that plays the dominant role in determining whether the patient's illness is "medically reversible" *(infra)*. In some patients there may be two (or rarely more) basic disease processes.

Medical reversibility

The medical reversibility of a basic disease process is strictly a technical judgment. In the hospital setting the personnel who are most qualified to render such a judgment are physicians. Judgments with regard to medical reversibility should include statements both of its probability and of its magnitude. A characteristic technical statement of medical reversibility is: If we implement therapy X there is about a 10% chance of inducing a 50% reduction in, for example, the size of the tumor. In order to translate this technical statement into language that is of use to a patient and his or her family an elaboration is ordinarily required. For example, if we implement therapy X there is about a 10% chance that it will work. If it does, we might hope to see a substantial return of, for example, the ability to communicate.

Curative therapy

These are therapies that are directed at the basic disease process for the purpose of either arresting or reversing its progress, with the aim of inducing a partial or total remission. Implementation of a curative therapy presupposes that a judgment has been made that the basic disease process is potentially medically reversible.

Functional equilibrium

This term refers to a physiologic status of the patient that is compatible with biological survival. In general, a patient is said to be in functional equilibrium if there is adequate ventilation, nutrition, perfusion of vital organs, excretory function, and so on. Impairments of any of these functions may be caused by a variety of phenomena which may or may not be labelled appropriately as diseases. For example, impairments in respiratory function might be caused by obstruction to the airways either by excessive secretions or by tumors. They may also be caused by pneumonia or by paralysis of respiratory muscles. Actions directed toward removing these detriments to respiratory function are performed in the interests of maintaining functional equilibrium, notwithstanding the status of the detriment as a disease or some other thing.

Pneumonia, for example, may be viewed as either a basic disease process or a detriment to functional equilibrium. Its status is determined by virtue of its role in making global determinations of the potential reversibility of the patient's medical illness. Thus, in a patient having a basic disease process—for example, a metastatic solid tumor—that has rendered him or her totally incapacitated and which—in the considered judgment of the health care team—is nearly devoid of potential for medical reversibility, treatment of pneumonia may be considered functional maintenance therapy. A decision to treat pneumonia in such a patient has much more in common with a decision to use a respirator than it does with a decision to administer "curative" therapy.

Functional maintenance therapy

These are therapies designed to achieve or maintain functional equilibrium.

Comforting therapy

These are therapies designed to achieve or maintain the patient's comfort.

Determinations of what constitutes functional equilibrium lie nearly exclusively in the domain of the physician. By contrast, when the patient is capable of communicating, determinations of what constitutes comfort lie exclusively in his or her domain. Often, therapies designed to be curative or to maintain functional equilibrium (e.g., endotracheal tubes) will produce discomfort. Similarly, therapies designed to produce comfort may induce functional dysequilibria, (e.g., morphine given for purposes of producing comfort may inhibit respiratory function or induce ileus). Thus, it is necessary to make clear statements as to whether producing comfort takes priority over maintaining functional equilibrium.

Although the patient or the physician may be most competent to make judgments as to what constitutes comfort or functional equilibrium, respectively, such judgments are to be distinguished from decisions to take action. Decisions to take actions—for example, implementation or withholding of various therapeutic maneuvers—are to be done in accord with agreements reached through appropriate discussions between all concerned parties—health care professionals and patients and/or their families.

Authorization

According to YNHH policy, therapeutic procedures may be implemented only with the *informed consent* of the patient. The agreements reached between physicians and patients and/or their families that result in management classifications with or without Do Not Resuscitate orders may, at times, be based upon discussions that can truly be considered as resulting in a condition known as "informed consent." In general, this term can be properly applied in cases where the discussions are begun several weeks or months before a Do Not Resuscitate order might be implemented. In such cases the negotiations for informed consent may result in a document known as a "living will." The Committee strongly encourages the early initiation of such discussions and the development of living wills. Such documents provide the most clear and unambiguous expressions of the patient's values rendered at times when the patients are relatively rational and autonomous and when there is time for due deliberation; their situations are substantially and relevantly different from what they will be in the ICU.

When discussions are initiated by physicians under circumstances in which it seems appropriate to enter a patient in management Class B or C, it is rarely possible to achieve the informed consent. Ordinarily, the physician approaches the patient and/or family with a statement that there is no reasonable chance of medical reversibility; accordingly, they are asked to "authorize" a shift in management objectives to Class B or C. The Committee recommends that the term *authorization* be used to refer to such agreements. As much time and support should be given as is necessary for the patient and/or family to reach a decision and to seek consultation with such advisors as they may choose, medical and otherwise. In these cases, what is sought is the authorization of the patient or the family to a particular plan of management based upon the estimation of the health care professionals as to what medicine can and cannot achieve. However, the patient and/or family have the legal authority to require that a patient be managed according to Class B1 even when the physician believes that Class C management would be more appropriate; the physician is obliged to proceed according to these wishes.

eleven

Follow-up of Cancer Patients

DAVID S. FISCHER

The goal of cancer therapy is cure, not "five-year survival." By cure we now mean that the person afflicted will have an actuarial survival equal to that of an age-matched cohort free of cancer. Even to begin to approach this goal we need early diagnosis, definitive therapy, and a system of follow-up to detect recurrences while they are still curable or at least treatable.

Physicians have spent much time and effort in sharpening their diagnostic and therapeutic skills. Somehow, though, it came to be regarded as crass and commercial for physicians to recall these patients for follow-up, although dentists do it routinely.

On April 5, 1973, the Council of the Connecticut State Medical Society (CSMS) resolved that ". . . it is both proper and advisable for the attending physician to call patients back for appropriate follow-up examination . . . this is not an unethical practice but, in fact, quite the contrary." It urged that physicians, hospitals, and the public be so informed, and that the cooperation of the Connecticut Division of the American Cancer Society (ACS) be enlisted in pointing out to the public "its value to patients" [of such practice] in the treatment of malignant disease.

As a result of this impetus, a cooperative effort was begun in 1973 by the Cancer Coordinating Committee of CSMS, the Connecticut Division of ACS, and the Connecticut State Department of Health to write a handbook for physicians. In 1974 a pamphlet was published entitled *Follow-up of cancer: a handbook for physicians* with E. Tremain Bradley as editor and the late Harold S. Barrett as co-editor. The 13-member editorial committee sought the advice and expertise of 44 other physicians and came up with guidelines (not standards) to assist in the follow-up of cancer of 11 major sites.

In 1976, the Commission on Cancer of the American College of Surgeons published *The patient with cancer: guidelines for follow-up* based on the Connecticut manual but expanded to cover 26 sites. The booklet was unbound and fastened so that it could easily be disassembled to allow any page to be removed to be duplicated and placed in a patient's chart. In 1977, some of the charts from the Connecticut manual were used in *Clinical oncology* by J. Horton and E. J. Hill.

In the seven years since the original publication, new information and new tests have become available. Hence I have tried to update the handbook, having received permission of the Cancer Coordinating Committee of CSMS at a vote on July 1, 1980. All final decisions have been my own; although the committee made many excellent suggestions, it is in no way responsible for errors of judgment or fact in this update.

How often should cancer patients be recalled? What should be done at each visit? It is often difficult to remember each procedure or examination that might be done and then to decide which is important and which unnecessary. Data from the Connecticut Tumor Registry directly and from other programs, in some of which the Tumor Registry participated, constitute a significant part of the basis for these conclusions.

There are two phases to follow-up: continued assessment of the malignant disease is, of course, vital and largely scientific, but follow-up of the patient as a person is just as important. Whether or not the physician who administered the definitive treatment continues to see the patient periodically, the family physician is urged to maintain a strong supportive relationship with the patient and the family. Emotional support is essential. The physician can often aid in job rehabilitation.

Disaster may result from patients being "lost to follow-up." To avoid such tragedy, and to make important statistical analyses valid, careful cooperation is necessary between the family physician and the physician responsible for definitive therapy, lest each assume the other to be following the patient and neither is seeing the patient. They should be specific with each other and with the patient. In fact, the patient must be an active partner in follow-up, should be impressed with the importance of keeping recall appointments, and should be urged to report early and promptly any significant signs or symptoms.

The risk of a second primary tumor in the same or a different organ is higher in individuals who have already had one cancer. Attention during follow-up is therefore also directed toward early detection of new disease. Routine pelvic examination with Pap smear is recommended for women, with frequency dependent on age, sexual activity, and endocrine history. Men and women should have sigmoidoscopy every two years when they have reached the age of 50 and a test for occult blood in the stool annually. It is assumed that good follow-up includes these principles, and they will not be mentioned again in the appendixes dealing with individual sites of primary disease.

It should be emphasized that the *guidelines* that follow in appendixes 11.1 – 11.21 are for patients who have had definitive (curative intent) therapy with no obvious evidence of residual disease. These are *guidelines* to help remind, suggest, and assist, but in no way limit or direct the physician. They are *not standards* of minimum or optimum care. Each patient deserves a tailor-made personalized follow-up. Recommendations are the somewhat arbitrary preferences of one physician, and while considered appropriate in many cases, will, of course, be modified in consideration of stage and histologic type as well as other individual features. The guidelines do not address the matter of therapy but are restricted to follow-up of previous, and the detection of additional, malignant neoplasms. Clearly, patients with known residual cancer should be under the care of an oncologist and seen more frequently.

Patients who fail to keep an apointment should be called, because often they are too sick to come in and actually should be seen. Variations, innovations, developments, and obsolescences must be taken into account as medical science progresses. Suggested dates for follow-up are from time of completing and following the effects of treatment. Obviously, the times are arbitrary, and longer or shorter intervals will be appropriate for individual patients and their physicians. Suspicious findings may well require further investigation that could lead to additional therapy. On the other hand, some malignancies rarely have late recurrences. Patients with Hodgkin's disease and testicular carcinoma are probably cured if there has been no recurrence after four years, whereas patients with breast carcinoma are at risk for the rest of their lives.

References

Bradley, E. T., and Barrett, H. S., eds. *Follow-up of cancer: a handbook for physicians.* New Haven, Conn.: Connecticut State Medical Society, 1974.

Commission on Cancer. *The patient with cancer: guidelines for follow-up.* Chicago: American College of Surgeons, 1976.

Horton, J., and Hill, E. J. *Clinical oncology.* Philadelphia: W. B. Saunders, 1977.

Appendix 11.1. *Bladder, Ureter, Renal Pelvis: Follow-up Procedure Suggested*

		First Year				*Second to Fifth Year*		*Thereafter*
		Months				*Months*		*Months*
		3	6	9	12	6	12	12
History	Complete				x		x	x
	Hematuria	x	x	x		x		
	Dysuria	x	x	x		x		
	Frequency	x	x	x		x		
Physical	Complete				x		x	x
	Abdomen	x	x	x		x		
	Rectal	x	x	x		x		
	Stoma (if any)	x	x	x		x		
	Lymph Nodes	x	x	x		x		
	Cystoscopy		x		x	x	x	x
	Pelvic (female)		x		x	x	x	x
Tests	Chest x-ray				x		x	x
	CBC		x		x		x	x
	Urine	x	x	x	x	x	x	x
	BUN, alkaline phosphatase		x		x		x	x
	IVP				x		x	
	Urine cytology		x		x		x	

Appendix 11.2. *Bone and Soft Tissue Sarcoma: Follow-up Procedure Suggested*

		First Year				*Second to Fifth Year*		*Thereafter*
		Months				*Months*		*Months*
		3	6	9	12	6	12	12
History	Complete				x		x	x
	Pain	x	x	x				
	Lumps	x	x	x		x		
	Appetite—weight	x	x	x		x		
	Respiratory symptom	x	x	x		x		
	CNS Symptoms	x	x	x		x		
Physical	Complete				x		x	x
	Primary site	x	x	x		x		
	Lymph nodes	x	x	x		x		
	Chest	x	x	x		x		
	Abdomen	x	x	x		x		
	Liver	x	x	x		x		
	Neurologic	x	x	x		x		
Tests	Chest x-ray	x	x		x	x	x	x
	CBC	x	x		x	x	x	x
	Alkaline phosphatase, bilirubin				x		x	x
	LDH, Ca				x		x	x
	Liver, bone scan	As indicated						

Appendix 11.3. *Brain: Follow-up Procedure Suggested*

		First Year				*Second to Fifth Year*		*Thereafter*
		Months				*Months*		*Months*
		3	6	9	12	6	12	12
History	Complete				x		x	x
	Headache	x	x	x		x		
	Seizures	x	x	x		x		
	Mental changes	x	x	x		x		
	Motor deficit	x	x	x		x		
	Speech changes	x	x	x		x		
	Balance problems	x	x	x		x		
Physical	Complete				x		x	x
	Cranial nerves	x	x	x		x		
	Motor exam	x	x	x		x		
	Sensory exam	x	x	x		x		
	Gait	x	x	x		x		
	Fundi	x	x	x		x		
Tests	Chest x-ray				x		x	x
	CBC				x		x	x
	CT scan (brain)		x		x		x	
	EEG	As indicated						
	Skull x-ray	As indicated						

Appendix 11.4. *Breast: Follow-up Procedure Suggested*

		First Year				*Second to Fifth Year*		*Thereafter*	
		Months				*Months*		*Months*	
		3	6	9	12	6	12	6	12
History	Complete				x		x		x
	Lumps	x	x	x		x		x	
	Cough or dyspnea	x	x	x		x		x	
	Bone or chest pain	x	x	x		x		x	
	Weight—appetite	x	x	x		x		x	
	Breast self-exam	x	x	x		x		x	
Physical	Complete				x		x		x
	Mastectomy area	x	x	x		x		x	
	Remaining breast	x	x	x		x		x	
	Lymph nodes	x	x	x		x		x	
	Abdomen, liver	x	x	x		x		x	
	Chest	x	x	x		x		x	
	Bones	x	x	x		x		x	
	Pelvic	x	x	x		x		x	
Tests	Chest x-ray		x		x		x		x
	CBC	x	x		x		x		x
	Ca, LDH, alkaline phosphatase				x		x		x
	CEA				x		x		x
	Mammogram— remaining breast				x		x		x
	Liver and bone scan	If indicated by history and physical							

Appendix 11.5. *Cervix, Vulva, and Vagina: Follow-up Procedure Suggested*

		First Year				*Second to Fifth Year*		*Thereafter*
		Months				*Months*		*Months*
		3	6	9	12	6	12	12
History	Complete				x	x	x	x
	Vaginal bleeding	x	x	x		x		
	Bone pain	x	x	x		x		
	Leg edema	x	x	x		x		
	Vaginal discharge	x	x	x		x		
	Weight–appetite	x	x	x		x		
	Bowel function	x	x	x		x		
	Bladder function	x	x	x		x		
Physical	Complete				x		x	x
	Lymph nodes	x	x	x		x		
	Pelvic exam	x	x	x		x		
	Abdomen	x	x	x		x		
	Breast	x	x	x		x		
	Rectal	x	x	x		x		
Tests	Chest x-ray				x		x	x
	CBC		x		x	x	x	x
	Pap smear		x	x	x	x	x	x
	Urine	x	x		x	x	x	x
	Stool for blood	x	x		x	x	x	x
	IVP				x			

Appendix 11.6. *Colon, Rectum, and Anus: Follow-up Procedure Suggested*

		First Year				*Second to Fifth Year*		*Thereafter*
		Months				*Months*		*Months*
		3	6	9	12	6	12	12
History	Complete				x		x	x
	Appetite–weight	x	x	x		x		
	Bowel function	x	x	x		x		
	Abdominal pain	x	x	x		x		
	Jaundice	x	x	x		x		
	Urine color	x	x	x		x		
Physical	Complete				x		x	x
	Abdomen	x	x	x		x		
	Liver	x	x	x		x		
	Rectal or stoma	x	x	x		x		
	Jaundice	x	x	x		x		
	Lymph nodes	x	x	x		x		
	Sigmoidoscopy		x		x	x	x	x
	Colonoscopy	As indicated						
Tests	Chest x-ray				x		x	x
	CBC	x	x	x	x	x	x	x
	Bilirubin–alkaline phosphatase		x		x	x	x	x
	CEA		x		x	x	x	x
	Stool for blood	x	x	x	x	x	x	x
	Barium enema				x		x	x
	Liver scan	As indicated						

Appendix 11.7. *Endometrium: Follow-up Procedure Suggested*

		First Year				*Second to Fifth Year*		*Thereafter*
		Months				*Months*		*Months*
		3	6	9	12	6	12	12
History	Complete				x		x	x
	Vaginal bleeding	x	x	x		x		
	Pelvic pain	x	x	x		x		
	Abdominal size	x	x	x		x		
	Hormonal medication	x	x	x		x		
	Leg edema	x	x	x		x		
Physical	Complete				x		x	x
	Pelvic exam	x	x	x		x		
	Abdomen	x	x	x		x		
	Lymph nodes	x	x	x		x		
	Breast	x	x	x		x		
	Rectal	x	x	x		x		
Tests	Chest x-ray				x		x	x
	CBC		x		x		x	x
	Pap smear		x	x	x	x	x	x
	Stool for blood	x	x		x	x	x	x
	Urine	x	x		x		x	x

Appendix 11.8. *Esophagus: Follow-up Procedure Suggested*

		First Year					*Second to Fifth Year*			*Thereafter*	
		Months					*Months*			*Months*	
		1	3	6	9	12	4	8	12	6	12
History	Complete					x			x		x
	Dysphagia	x	x	x	x		x	x		x	
	Substernal distress	x	x	x	x		x	x		x	
	Appetite–weight	x	x	x	x		x	x		x	
	Cough, hoarseness	x	x	x	x		x	x		x	
	Lumps	x	x	x	x		x	x		x	
	Bowel function	x	x	x	x		x	x		x	
Physical	Complete					x			x		x
	Lymph nodes	x	x	x	x		x	x		x	
	Chest	x	x	x	x		x	x		x	
	Abdomen, liver	x	x	x	x		x	x		x	
	Nutrition	x	x	x	x		x	x		x	
Tests	Chest x-ray	x	x	x		x	x	x	x	x	x
	CBC	x	x	x		x	x	x	x	x	x
	Barium swallow		x	x		x			x		x
	Stool for blood	x	x	x	x	x	x	x	x	x	x
	Esophagoscopy	As indicated									

Appendix 11.9. *Hodgkin's Disease: Follow-up Procedure Suggested*

		First Year					*Second to Fifth Year*			*Thereafter*
		Months					*Months*			*Months*
		1	3	6	9	12	4	8	12	12
History	Complete					x			x	x
	Appetite–weight	x	x	x	x		x	x		
	Fever	x	x	x	x		x	x		
	Itching	x	x	x	x		x	x		
	Pain (including alcohol-induced)	x	x	x	x		x	x		
	Lumps	x	x	x	x		x	x		
	Night sweats	x	x	x	x		x	x		
	Respiratory symptoms	x	x	x	x		x	x		
Physical	Complete					x			x	x
	Lymph nodes	x	x	x	x		x	x		
	Abdomen	x	x	x	x		x	x		
	Liver–spleen	x	x	x	x		x	x		
	Skin	x	x	x	x		x	x		
	Oropharynx	x	x	x	x		x	x		
	Chest	x	x	x	x		x	x		
Tests	Chest x-ray		x	x	x	x	x	x	x	x
	CBC		x	x	x	x	x	x	x	x
	Alkaline phosphatase, LDH		x			x			x	x
	Bilirubin, SGOT		x			x			x	x
	Urine		x			x			x	x
	Serum copper		x			x			x	x

Appendix 11.10. *Kidney (Renal Cell): Follow-up Procedure Suggested*

		First Year				*Second to Fifth Year*			*Thereafter*
		Months				*Months*			*Months*
		3	6	9	12	4	8	12	12
History	Complete				x			x	x
	Hematuria	x	x	x		x	x		
	Dysuria	x	x	x		x	x		
	Appetite–weight	x	x	x		x	x		
	CNS symptoms	x	x	x		x	x		
	Respiratory symptoms	x	x	x		x	x		
	Back pain	x	x	x		x	x		
Physical	Complete				x			x	x
	Abdomen	x	x	x		x	x		
	Liver	x	x	x		x	x		
	Lymph nodes	x	x	x		x	x		
	Neurologic	x	x	x		x	x		
	Chest	x	x	x		x	x		
Tests	Chest x-ray		x		x			x	x
	CBC	x	x	x	x	x	x	x	x
	BUN, alkaline phosphatase		x		x			x	x
	Urine	x	x	x	x	x	x	x	x
	IVP				x			x	
	Bone, liver scan	As indicated							

Appendix 11.11. *Liver, Gall Bladder, and Bile Ducts: Follow-up Procedure Suggested*

		First Year				*Second to Fifth Year*			*Thereafter*
		Months				*Months*			*Months*
		3	6	9	12	4	8	12	12
History	Complete				x			x	x
	Appetite–weight	x	x	x		x	x		
	Jaundice–itching	x	x	x		x	x		
	Nausea–vomiting	x	x	x		x	x		
	Abdominal pain	x	x	x		x	x		
	Urine color	x	x	x		x	x		
	Bowel function	x	x	x		x	x		
Physical	Complete				x			x	x
	Abdominal mass	x	x	x		x	x		
	Liver	x	x	x		x	x		
	Jaundice	x	x	x		x	x		
	Ascites	x	x	x		x	x		
	Rectal	x	x	x		x	x		
Tests	Chest x-ray				x			x	x
	CBC	x	x	x	x	x	x	x	x
	Bilirubin, alkaline phosphatase	x	x	x	x	x	x	x	x
	CEA		x		x			x	x
	Alpha-fetoprotein		x		x			x	x
	Urine for bile	x	x	x	x	x	x	x	x
	Liver scan	As indicated							

Appendix 11.12. *Lung: Follow-up Procedure Suggested*

		First Year					*Second to Fifth Year*			*Thereafter*	
		Months					*Months*			*Months*	
		1	3	6	9	12	4	8	12	6	12
History	Complete					x			x		x
	Cough, dyspnea	x	x	x	x		x	x		x	
	Chest pain	x	x	x	x		x	x		x	
	Appetite–weight	x	x	x	x		x	x		x	
	Hemoptysis, wheezing	x	x	x	x		x	x		x	
	CNS symptoms	x	x	x	x		x	x		x	
	Hoarseness	x	x	x	x		x	x		x	
	Swelling face and arms	x	x	x	x		x	x		x	
Physical	Complete					x			x		x
	Lungs	x	x	x	x		x	x		x	
	Lymph nodes	x	x	x	x		x	x		x	
	Heart	x	x	x	x		x	x		x	
	Neurologic	x	x	x	x		x	x		x	
	Liver	x	x	x	x		x	x		x	
	Bronchoscopy	As indicated									
Tests	Chest x-ray		x	x	x	x	x	x	x	x	x
	CBC			x		x			x		x
	Urine			x		x			x		x
	CEA			x		x			x		x
	Sputum cytology		x	x		x			x		x
	Ca, cortisol	As indicated									
	Bone, liver scan	As indicated									
	CT scan (brain)	As indicated									

Appendix 11.13. *Melanoma: Follow-up Procedure Suggested*

		First Year				*Second to Fifth Year*			*Thereafter*	
		Months				*Months*			*Months*	
		3	6	9	12	4	8	12	6	12
History	Complete				x			x		x
	Skin	x	x	x		x	x		x	
	Lumps	x	x	x		x	x		x	
	GI symptoms	x	x	x		x	x		x	
	CNS symptoms	x	x	x		x	x		x	
	Pain	x	x	x		x	x		x	
	Respiratory symptoms	x	x	x		x	x		x	
Physical	Complete				x			x		x
	Primary site	x	x	x		x	x		x	
	Lymph nodes	x	x	x		x	x		x	
	Chest	x	x	x		x	x		x	
	Abdomen	x	x	x		x	x		x	
	Liver	x	x	x		x	x		x	
	Neurologic	x	x	x		x	x		x	
Tests	Chest x-ray				x			x		x
	CBC	x	x	x	x	x	x	x	x	x
	Stool for blood	x	x	x	x	x	x	x	x	x
	Urine for bile, melanin	x	x	x	x	x	x	x	x	x
	Liver, bone scan	As indicated								
	CT scan (brain)	As indicated								

Appendix 11.14. *Non-Hodgkin's Lymphoma: Follow-up Procedure Suggested*

		First Year					*Second to Fifth Year*			*Thereafter*
		Months					*Months*			*Months*
		1	3	6	9	12	4	8	12	12
History	Complete					x			x	x
	Appetite–weight	x	x	x	x		x	x		
	Fever	x	x	x	x		x	x		
	Pain	x	x	x	x		x	x		
	Lumps	x	x	x	x		x	x		
	Respiratory symptoms	x	x	x	x		x	x		
	GI symptoms	x	x	x	x		x	x		
	CNS symptoms	x	x	x	x		x	x		
Physical	Complete					x			x	x
	Lymph nodes	x	x	x	x		x	x		
	Chest	x	x	x	x		x	x		
	Abdomen	x	x	x	x		x	x		
	Liver–spleen	x	x	x	x		x	x		
	Oropharynx	x	x	x	x		x	x		
	Skin	x	x	x	x		x	x		
	Neurologic	x	x	x	x		x	x		
Tests	Chest x-ray		x	x	x	x	x	x	x	x
	CBC		x	x	x	x	x	x	x	x
	Alkaline phosphatase, LDH		x			x			x	x
	SGOT, bilirubin		x			x			x	x
	Urine		x			x			x	x
	GI and small bowel x-ray	x				x	If diffuse histiocytic			

Appendix 11.15. *Ovary: Follow-up Procedure Suggested*

		First Year				*Second to Fifth Year*		*Thereafter*
		Months				*Months*		*Months*
		3	6	9	12	6	12	12
History	Complete				x		x	x
	Abdominal size	x	x	x		x		
	Pelvic pain	x	x	x		x		
	Vaginal bleeding	x	x	x		x		
	Masculinizing signs	x	x	x		x		
	Leg edema	x	x	x		x		
Physical	Complete				x		x	x
	Pelvic exam	x	x	x		x		
	Abdomen	x	x	x		x		
	Lymph nodes	x	x	x		x		
	Breast	x	x	x		x		
Tests	Chest x-ray				x		x	x
	CBC		x		x	x	x	x
	Pap smear		x		x	x	x	x
	Stool for blood		x		x	x	x	x
	Urine		x		x		x	x
	CEA				x		x	x

Appendix 11.16. *Pancreas: Follow-up Procedure Suggested*

		First Year					*Second to Fifth Year*			*Thereafter*
		Months					*Months*			*Months*
		1	3	6	9	12	4	8	12	12
History	Complete					x			x	x
	Appetite–weight	x	x	x	x		x	x		
	Diarrhea	x	x	x	x		x	x		
	Nausea–vomiting	x	x	x	x		x	x		
	Jaundice–itching	x	x	x	x		x	x		
	Abdominal pain	x	x	x	x		x	x		
	Urine color	x	x	x	x		x	x		
	Bowel function	x	x	x	x		x	x		
Physical	Complete					x			x	x
	Abdominal mass		x	x	x		x	x		
	Liver	x	x	x	x		x	x		
	Ascites	x	x	x	x		x	x		
	Rectal		x	x	x		x	x		
	Jaundice	x	x	x	x		x	x		
Tests	Chest x-ray					x			x	x
	CBC	x	x	x	x	x	x	x	x	x
	Bilirubin, alkaline phosphatase	x	x	x		x	x	x	x	x
	Urine for bile	x	x	x		x	x	x	x	x
	Stool for blood	x	x	x		x	x	x	x	x
	CEA		x	x		x			x	x

Appendix 11.17. *Penis and Scrotum: Follow-up Procedure Suggested*

		First Year				*Second to Fifth Year*		*Thereafter*
		Months				*Months*		*Months*
		3	6	9	12	6	12	12
History	Complete				x		x	x
	Urinary symptoms	x	x	x		x		
	Pain	x	x	x		x		
	Leg swelling	x	x	x		x		
	Appetite–weight	x	x	x		x		
Physical	Complete				x		x	x
	Lymph nodes	x	x	x		x		
	Operative site	x	x	x		x		
	Abdomen	x	x	x		x		
	Leg edema	x	x	x		x		
	Rectal		x			x		
Tests	Chest x-ray		x		x		x	x
	CBC				x		x	x
	Urine	x	x	x	x	x	x	x
	IVP				x			
	Stool for blood	x	x	x	x	x	x	x

Appendix 11.18. *Prostate: Follow-up Procedure Suggested*

		First Year				*Second to Fifth Year*			*Thereafter*
		Months				*Months*			*Months*
		3	6	9	12	4	8	12	12
History	Complete				x			x	x
	Pain	x	x	x		x	x		
	Urinary symptoms	x	x	x		x	x		
	Cardiac symptoms	x	x	x		x	x		
Physical	Complete				x			x	x
	Wound	x	x	x		x	x		
	Meatus	x	x	x		x	x		
	Rectal	x	x	x		x	x		
	Bladder residual	x	x	x		x	x		
	Lymph nodes	x	x	x		x	x		
Tests	Chest x-ray				x			x	x
	CBC		x		x			x	x
	Acid and alkaline phosphatase		x		x			x	x
	Pelvic x-ray				x			x	x
	Urine	x	x	x	x	x	x	x	x
	Bone scan, IVP	As indicated							

Appendix 11.19. *Stomach and Small Intestine: Follow-up Procedure Suggested*

		First Year				*Second to Fifth Year*		*Thereafter*
		Months				*Months*		*Months*
		3	6	9	12	6	12	12
History	Complete				x		x	x
	Appetite–weight	x	x	x		x		
	Abdominal pain, size	x	x	x		x		
	Dysphagia	x	x	x		x		
	Heartburn	x	x	x		x		
	Nausea–vomiting	x	x	x		x		
	Jaundice	x	x	x		x		
	Bowel function	x	x	x		x		
Physical	Complete				x		x	x
	Lymph nodes	x	x	x		x		
	Chest	x	x	x		x		
	Abdomen, masses	x	x	x		x		
	Liver	x	x	x		x		
	Rectal	x	x			x		
Tests	Chest x-ray		x		x		x	x
	CBC	x	x	x	x	x	x	x
	GI series				x		x	x
	Stool for blood	x	x	x	x	x	x	x
	CEA		x		x		x	x
	Panendoscopy	As indicated						

Appendix 11.20. *Testis: Follow-up Procedure Suggested*

		First Year				*Second to Fifth Year*			*Thereafter*
		Months				*Months*			*Months*
		3	6	9	12	4	8	12	12
History	Complete				x			x	x
	Abdominal pain	x	x	x		x	x		
	Cough	x	x	x		x	x		
	Leg swelling	x	x	x		x	x		
	Appetite–weight	x	x	x		x	x		
	Respiratory symptom	x	x	x		x	x		
Physical	Complete				x			x	x
	Remaining testis	x	x	x		x	x		
	Lymph nodes	x	x	x		x	x		
	Abdomen	x	x	x		x	x		
	Chest	x	x	x		x	x		
Tests	Chest x-ray	x	x	x	x	x	x	x	x
	CBC	x	x	x	x	x	x	x	x
	Urine	x	x	x	x	x	x	x	x
	Human chorionic gonadotrophin	x	x	x	x			x	
	Alpha-fetoprotein	x	x	x	x			x	
	IVP				x				

Appendix 11.21. *Thyroid: Follow-up Procedure Suggested*

		First Year			*Second to Fifth Year*		*Thereafter*
		Months			*Months*		*Months*
		1	6	12	6	12	12
History	Complete			x		x	x
	Cough	x	x		x		
	Hoarseness	x	x		x		
	Lumps	x	x		x		
	Bone pain	x	x		x		
	Muscle spasm	x	x		x		
	Thyroid symptoms	x	x		x		
Physical	Complete			x		x	x
	Operative site	x	x		x		
	Neck	x	x		x		
	Chest	x	x		x		
	Abdomen	x	x		x		
	Laryngoscopy	x	x			x	x
Tests	Chest x-ray	x	x	x		x	x
	CBC	x	x	x		x	x
	Thyroid scan	x		x			
	Bone scan	x	If indicated by pain				
	Special endocrine	For medullary carcinoma					

twelve

Unproved Methods of Treatment

DAVID S. FISCHER

Why are tens of thousands of people who have cancer going to quacks? Whenever the available modalities of treatment in any disease are less than curative in the majority of cases, there is need for improvement. Over the centuries, the best technique that has evolved has been the carefully controlled scientific experiment. Every day physicians, scientists, and research teams conduct such studies at hospitals, clinics, and private offices as part of the search for knowledge and improved therapy. Whenever any promising information becomes available, reputable investigators share it with their colleagues as formal presentations at scientific or medical meetings and in the pages of hundreds of professional journals. Those who fail to present their data for peer review but go directly to the public through the media will have their motives and data under suspicion by their colleagues.

Unproved methods of management differ from *experimental* methods in that the proponents of the former do not submit their data for scientific evaluation by the profession. Although some of these advocates are honest but misguided, and a rare individual may be a prophet before his time, the great majority appear to be crooks and chiselers who just want to separate the "suckers" from their money even if it means increased suffering and premature death for those suckers. Unfortunately, the people who are taken in are usually victims of a disease regarded by many as incurable, such as cancer and arthritis. These desperate individuals and their families may become disillusioned with the inadequacies or side effects of standard treatment and seek what they believe are simpler, cheaper, and more effective "cures." They are neither cheap nor effective, and together, they literally steal more than two billion dollars a year.

To an extent, the cancer quack is the beneficiary of what the American Cancer Society (1979) calls "the overworked, the incompetent, the disinterested, the brusque professional and orthodoxy's misuse and overuse of drugs, the 'no time to listen or explain' syndrome, therapy that is often prolonged and unpleasant, the fear of mental or physical incapacity, and the 'what have I got to lose' attitude."

While cure is often not possible, palliation usually is, and compassionate care to keep the patient comfortable should always be available together with psychological support for the patient and the family. All too often, the family is overlooked and the resort to cancer quackery occurs to fulfil family members' needs rather than the patient's.

The cancer quacks are a diverse group (table 12.1), but they have a few characteristics in common: (1) they claim that physicians, the AMA, the American Cancer Society, and the United States government are in collusion to suppress cancer cures in general and theirs in particular; (2) they are generally isolated from the medical and scientific communities; (3) their records are usually scanty or nonexistent; (4) they rarely publish results, but when they do, it is usually in "fringe" journals and their articles are devoid of data; (5) their

Table 12.1. *Some Unorthodox Methods of Therapy*

Era	*Method of Therapy*
Ancient	Arsenic
	Boiled barley
	Hot pokers
	Witch doctors
Medieval	Crab powder
	Exorcism
	Potable gold
	Powdered mummy
	Royal touch
	Snake venom
	Spices and herbs
	Tartar emetic and lemon
	Unicorn horn
Modern	Chapparal tea
	Fresh cell therapy
	Gerson dietary method
	Grape cure
	Hoxey method
	Immunological Research Center
	Kelley ecology therapy
	Koch antitoxin
	Krebiozen
	Laetrile
	Rand coupled fortified antigen
	Vitamin C

methods of treatment are secret or available only from them, or they sell the materials needed; (6) they rarely document the presence of cancer by biopsy, and their successes are usually in patients with no evidence of initial or residual cancer; (7) their chief supporters tend to come from all walks of life, but are rarely persons trained in the care of patients with cancer or in scientific methodology.

To protect patients from being exploited by proponents of these unproved methods, physicians should be familiar with the more common modalities being offered. Specific information can be obtained from the American Cancer Society, Inc. A few of the more common or more interesting ones are reviewed here.

Krebiozen

This material is of particular interest to me because it was the first unproved cancer drug I was personally asked to administer as a resident physician in 1957. The attending physician was a gastroenterologist and had no particular expertise or interest in cancer. I refused to administer the drug because I knew nothing about it, and then decided to find out what I could.

Krebiozen was introduced into the United States in 1949 by Steven Durovic, a Yugoslavian physician who originally made it in Argentina as an extract of the blood of 2000 horses. A major sponsor was A. C. Ivy, M.D., a gastroenterologist and physiologist, and a professor at the University of Illinois School of Medicine. The drug was made in Chicago by Promak Laboratories, Inc. and distributed by the Krebiozen Research Foundation (KRF), a nonprofit corporation in Illinois. Physicians requesting it were asked to have their patients make a voluntary contribution to Promak Laboratories before receiving the drug. The evidence for the activity of Krebiozen was scant.

Subsequently, 504 case records were submitted to the National Cancer Institute by KRF and reviewed by 24 scientists. After extensive examination of those abstracts, the original charts and x-rays, and so on, it was concluded that there was no evidence of efficacy to justify a clinical trial. In September 1963, the Department of Health, Education, and Welfare announced that both government and independent scientists had identified the Krebiozen powder given to a Food and Drug Administration (FDA) inspector in July 1963 as creatine, a cheap and easily available amino acid. In spite of pressure exerted by Senator Paul H. Douglas, the FDA refused to license the drug and it fell out of favor even with the proponents of unproved methods.

Laetrile

At this writing, the most popular unproved method—or the quack drug of the year—is Laetrile. It is available under a variety of names including amygdalin, vitamin B_{17}, nitriloside (which is really a class of cyanide-type substances), and commercially as Cyto-H3, Kemdalin, and other names. It is promoted variously as a new "cancer cure," a "cancer preventative," or as "an essential vitamin" (Culbert 1974; Kittler 1963; Westover 1973; Richardson and Griffin 1977). What are the facts?

Laetrile is hardly a new drug. Its story really began about 1920, when Ernest T. Krebs, Sr., a California physician, was looking for a substance to improve the flavor of bootleg whisky (Culbert 1974). He developed a crude extract of apricot pits and noted that it had an antitumor effect in rats. It soon proved to be too toxic for humans and was abandoned.

In 1949, Ernest T. Krebs, Jr., a biochemist and medical school drop-out, began the isolation and purification of the apricot pit extract developed by his father. In 1952, he announced the isolation of a laevorotatory mandelonitrile and combined the first and last syllables to derive the name Laetrile for this chemical, also called amygdalin. In 1959, he announced that the compound contained benzaldehyde, glucuronic acid, and hydrocyanic acid. Hence it was also called 1-mandelonitrile-beta-glucuroniside. The theory was that as soon as it came in contact with the enzyme beta-glucuronidase in the tumor, hydrocyanic acid would be liberated and all tumor cell activity would cease.

Unfortunately, the enzyme beta-glucuronidase is no more active in tumor tissue than in normal tissues, and Laetrile just does not kill cancer cells. When this became obvious, the younger Krebs stopped claiming cures and began to claim that Laetrile may slow down the spread of cancer and make the patient feel better. When even this failed to occur and the FDA began to investigate Laetrile, Krebs "discovered" in 1970 that it was vitamin B_{17} and suggested that everyone needed it to avoid cancer. This clever falsehood served two purposes: (1) it tried to avoid FDA regulation since vitamins are exempt from FDA supervision, and (2) it enlarged the potential market from just people with cancer to everyone, with an enormously greater profit potential.

Of course, there is no evidence that Laetrile is a vitamin (Herbert 1978; Greenberg 1980) just as there is some doubt that Krebs is a biochemist. (His doctorate is reported to be an honorary degree from American Christian College in Tulsa, Oklahoma.) Along with Krebs, Andrew McNaughton has spread the interest in Laetrile. McNaughton established the nonprofit McNaughton Foundation to study odd scientific theories and made the drug his major interest. In addition to the profits from making and selling Laetrile, the McNaughton Foundation also accepts tax-free contributions. Andrew McNaughton himself was convicted in Canada of conspiracy to misrepresent the value of a money stock and had a year in jail and a $21,000 fine. He was also charged in Italy with swindling investors in a plant to produce Laetrile (Clark 1977).

Now support for Laetrile has abandoned any scientific claims and is being promoted politically by a number of fringe groups as a crusade for "freedom of choice." These include such benign-sounding groups as the National Health Federation (a promoter of health foods), the International Association of Cancer Victims and Friends, the Cancer Control Society, and the Committee for Freedom of Choice in Cancer Therapy. They have been quite successful in getting more than 20 states to legalize Laetrile therapy. They convinced Federal District Court Judge Bohanon that Laetrile is safe and should be available to anyone who wanted it. His order blocked FDA attempts to regulate Laetrile until it was overturned by the United States Supreme Court in 1979 (*United States* vs *Rutherford et al.* 1979). In spite of the difficulty in obtaining Laetrile in this country, it is estimated that 50,000 to 75,000 Americans have used it.

The claim that the agent is harmless is belied by the reports of toxicity and death now in the literature (Humbert 1977; Smith et al. 1978). The major danger, however, is that patients who might have significant palliation or possibly a cure with conventional medical therapy may waste their precious time and resources on unproved methods like Laetrile until it is too late to benefit from the standard therapy (American Cancer Society 1977; FDA 1977a, 1977b; Schultz and Lindeman 1973). Of the six patients who I have attended who took Laetrile, all died shortly after starting Laetrile. Two of them had been doing very well on chemotherapy when they were treated by Dr. Ernesto Contreras in Tijuana, Mexico. When they returned, they were both moribund and their families were financially destitute. This is the tragedy of Laetrile, the promise and the deception (fig. 12.1).

The National Cancer Institute's (NCI) controlled clinical trial of Laetrile began in July 1980 at the Mayo

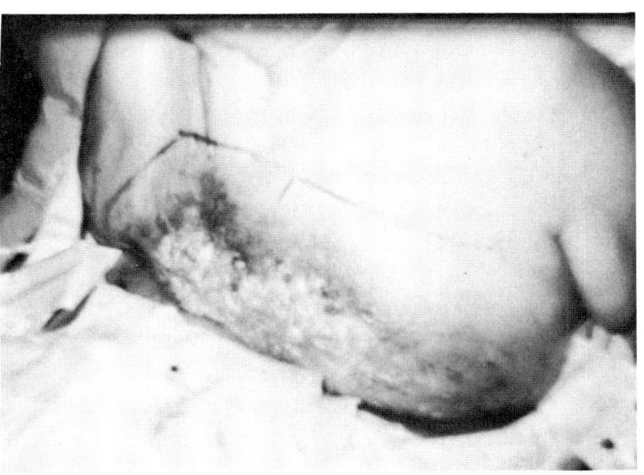

Fig. 12.1. *This patient had a mass of 1 cm detected in the breast on a routine exam and confirmed by mammography and biopsy. She refused a mastectomy and had Laetrile treatment instead. This ulcerating lesion became worse, resulting in her death.*

Clinic, Memorial Sloan–Kettering Cancer Center in New York City, the University of California in Los Angeles, and the University of Arizona in Tucson. Only patients who had measurable malignant tumors and for whom no established treatment had been effective, or who were no longer responding to conventional drugs, were considered for the study. Of 156 patients treated, only one had even a brief response (Moertel et al. 1981).

Hydrazine Sulfate

Classification of hydrazine sulfate as an unproved method of cancer treatment is very difficult. It does not fall into the usual pattern previously described, and there appears to be no profit motive involved.

Hydrazine sulfate is an inexpensive common chemical, commercially available for use in chemistry, photography, explosives, rocket fuel, and so on. Joseph Gold, a general practitioner and director of the Syracuse Cancer Research Institute, has been the major proponent of its use in cancer therapy. He describes it as an inhibitor of gluconeogenesis at the phosphoenolpyruvate carboxykinase level. He postulates that it can inhibit cancer cell-stimulated gluconeogenesis, which is responsible for energy loss and cachexia in patients with cancer. He began describing animal and human results in a series of reports at prestigious oncologic society meetings and in scientific papers beginning in 1971. These reports received great prominence in the lay press. In a series of 85 evaluable cases in an uncontrolled phase I study, 34% of patients had no improvement, 52% had subjective improvement only, and 14% had objective improvement. Subjective improvement was principally an increase in appetite and/or weight gain, improved performance status, and a decrease in pain. Side effects were described as mild, and there was no evidence of hematopoietic depression or immunosuppressive effects (Gold 1968, 1971, 1974a, 1974b, 1975).

Based on these reports, Dr. William Regelson of the Medical College of Virginia filed an investigational new drug (IND) application with the FDA that was then used as the basis for cross-filing by Memorial Sloan-Kettering Cancer Center (MSKCC) and Cal-Biochem in San Diego, which became the provider for a large number of clinicians testing the drug throughout the country. Ochoa and co-workers (1975) reported the results from MSKCC. In 29 patients adequately treated with hydrazine sulfate, there were no significant subjective or objective responses. In contrast, significant toxicity, particularly neurologic impairment, was evident.

Several reports from the Soviet Union have been cited in support of the use of hydrazine sulfate. One of the most favorable was by Gershanovich and associates (1976) and indicated that subjective improvement was striking, with mood elevation and even euphoria right up to the time of death. Objective responses of 50% or greater were seen in only 3 of 95 evaluable patients and of 25% or greater in only 3 additional patients.

Publicity in the lay press has been extensive, with charges that the American Cancer Society and other "establishment" agencies were blocking the use of this miracle drug. In August 1973, Dean Burk, former head of the cytochemistry section of NCI, issued a monograph on official HEW memorandum paper to "Interested Parties" describing dramatic results with hydrazine sulfate. In the Spring 1974 issue of *New England Natural Food Associates Bulletin* (Burk 1974) he extolled the virtues of Laetrile, pangamic acid, and hydrazine sulfate, and reiterated the conspiracy theory against the cancer cure, sensationalized later by *Penthouse* magazine. At press time, we were informed that an IND had been submitted by Solomon Garb of the American Medical Center, Denver, Colorado.

In summarizing the extensive studies at the Medical College of Virginia, Regelson (1980) entitled his commentary "The 'grand conspiracy' against the cancer cure." In 66 patients with advanced cancer, they found no effect on survival. As part of a randomized double-blind study, 15 patients received hydrazine sulfate and 14 received placebo. No patient showed a substantial objective tumor response that could be ascribed to hydrazine, and the brief subjective responses were not distinguishable from placebo effect (Spremulli et al. 1979; Lerner and Regelson 1976). Regelson concluded, "Hydrazine, despite its scientific rationale, on review of our experience, had minimal if any value subjectively or objectively. There is no plot on the part of cancer therapists to avoid finding a cure, and Dr. Gold should seek for better compounds."

Immunology Researching Foundation

After extensive newspaper, tabloid, and magazine publicity, the Immunology Researching Foundation, Inc. (IRF) hit it big by being featured with Harry Reasoner on the *60 Minutes* television show on Sunday, May 18, 1980. Claims have been made that more than 50% of people with cancer could be cured by their treatments. Not surprisingly, there are no scientific reports of their activities over the past seven years of their existence.

The IRF was established in 1973 in Great Neck, Long Island, N.Y. "to investigate and stimulate immunological research for the ultimate control of cancer through the victim's own immune defense mechanism."

In 1974, the NCI offered to test and attempt to confirm the claims by Lawrence Burton and Frank Friedman, but the offer was not accepted. In December 1974, an investigational new drug application (IND) was submitted to FDA but *not* approved pending a request for additional information. The IRF was advised to "continue to withhold the use of their products from human subjects until responses to our questions and comments had been received and acknowledged to be satisfactory." Apparently in an effort to avoid FDA regulation, the IRF moved to Freeport, Grand Bahamas Island in July 1975, and has operated from there ever since.

Because no scientific data have been published, information is sketchy and we must rely on reports of patients and visitors. The IRF claims to treat everybody free of charge, but a 1977 leaflet required a "free-will donation" of $5000 before a patient would be accepted for treatment. According to several people, inflation has now raised the required "donation" to $7500, although an IRF brochure now lists fees for consultation and treatment.

The theory behind the IRF clinical approach (Terry 1978) is based on the belief that

> *Every healthy animal has in its blood serum certain complex bodies which can protect against cancer by destroying malignant cells. There exist also in the animal's blood chemical agents which can nullify the defense mechanism (blocking agents) and thus permit the growth of cancer cells. These blocking agents, which are closely associated with a growing tumor, operate by inhibiting two or three other substances, probably protein in nature (deblocking protein) which are associated with tumour destruction, i.e. the defense mechanism. Two of these deblocking proteins have, by a trial and error method, been isolated by IRF's scientists, from tumour-free individuals. When these deblocking proteins are introduced into a tumourous animal, they reduce the concentration of blocking agents, thus allowing the natural anti-cancer defense mechanism to destroy the tumour.*

In early reports, IRF claimed that of 50 patients with terminal cancer, 21 showed definite improvement, 22 showed arrest of the disease, and 7 died after showing some improvement.

The only public or quasi-public reports by a trained scientist are several statements based on a site visit by William Terry, Associate Director, Immunology Program, NCI (Terry 1978). He states that in reviewing case histories there, several patients had limited disease susceptible to conventional treatment. Some had no histologic proof of malignancy. The material being used in treatment is a totally unknown quantity except that it is prepared from human serum. Baseline studies were rarely done, and tumor measurements, when done, were very vague.

Terry (1978) concluded:

> *There are many reasons why this trial is not evaluable. A consecutive series of patients is not being studied; rather all patients with the worst prognoses are excluded. This includes those not accepted in the first place, as well as those who are accepted and who have rapid growth of tumor and are then dropped. The only patients maintained on treatment are those who will be expected to do relatively well even if they receive no treatment. It will not be possible to compare their aggregate survival with any other group of patients—there is no appropriate comparison group. Moreover, the quality of medical evaluation prior to the acceptance onto the protocol, the quality of medical evaluation while the patients are in the Bahamas are all so poor and inadequate that even assessment of single patients for "unexpected" results will be unrevealing.*
>
> *No evidence was presented at this site visit that convinced me that the treatments being given were of any value to patients with cancer. . . . The use of an unproven remedy for cancer under circumstances where its efficacy cannot be evaluated, especially if this involves patients who may actually be responsive to conventional treatment, constitutes, in my opinion, ethical misconduct. Patients should not be referred to the Immunology Researching Center [another name for IRF].*

Vitamin C and the Orthomolecular Approach

There has been a large media exposure of and hence public interest in various aspects of the nutritional approach to cancer treatment. We have noted its relationship to the Laetrile and pangamic acid proponents (Burk 1975), but the emphasis on vitamin C and orthomolecular therapy has had a different genesis. The recognized leader of this movement is Linus Pauling, Nobel laureate in Chemistry (1954) and Peace (1962), and Professor of Chemistry Emeritus, Stanford University, and Director of the Institute of Orthomolecular Medicine. With his demonstration of the distinct electrophoretic mobility of hemoglobin S as compared to hemoglobin A, and the suggestion that the sickling phenomenon was due to molecular interaction between the abnormal proteins, Pauling is generally regarded as the father of the concept of molecular diseases. His major co-worker in the espousal of vitamin C in the treatment of cancer has been Ewan Cameron, a surgeon in Dunbartonshire, Scotland, who has treated a large number of people with terminal cancer with vitamin C and reported in detail results of his uncontrolled studies (Cameron, Pauling, and Leibovitz 1979).

Proponents define orthomolecular medicine as the preservation of good health and treatment of disease by varying the human body's concentrations of substances that are normally present and are required for health. They regard the vitamins as especially important and vitamin C as a substance whose importance has been underestimated (Cameron and Pauling 1973).

Their hypothesis is that natural body defenses determine the outcome in cancer, and vitamin C (ascorbic acid) is an essential component of that defense. It is suggested that cells are normally restrained from proliferating by the highly viscous nature of the intercellular glycosaminoglycans. To proliferate, cells must escape from this restraint by depolymerizing the glycosaminoglycans in their immediate vicinity. This is accomplished by the release of the enzyme hyaluronidase and is kept in check by physiologic hyaluronidase-inhibitor (PHI). It is suggested that PHI is an oligoglycosaminoglycan that requires ascorbic acid for its synthesis and/or incorporates residues of ascorbic acid. This would explain the pathogenesis of scurvy and the supposed increased requirement for ascorbic acid that occurs in many cell-proliferative diseases, including cancer (Cameron and Pauling 1974).

Originally (Cameron and Campbell 1974), ascorbic acid therapy was begun in all patients intravenously, usually at 10 gm per day or more, and later changed to an oral liquid preparation. In patients able to take oral medication, they now advocate this route and give 2.5 gm ascorbic acid 4 times a day after meals. Responses were categorized as (1) no response, (2) minimal response, (3) growth retardation, (4) cytostasis (or standstill effect), (5) tumor regression, and (6) tumor hemorrhage and necrosis. In the last category, the response in patients with rapidly proliferating and widely disseminated tumors was so brisk as to precipitate tumor hemorrhage and necrosis with disastrous consequences such as ulcerations, sloughs, convulsions, coma, and death. Clinical descriptions of some cases in each of these categories are given in the cited literature. The authors seem certain that with greater experience they can achieve better results with ascorbic acid and produce (1) relief of pain from skeletal metastases, (2) reduction of narcotic dosage, (3) diminution of high urinary hydroxyproline, (4) objective tumor regression, and (5) prolongation of life. They expect to do all this with little or no toxicity.

Effects of ascorbic acid on cancer have been demonstrated independently (DiPalma and McMichael 1979). It has been shown that vitamin C or L-cysteine added to hamster lung cultures protects them against the abnormal growth and malignant transformation induced by exposure to smoke from tobacco or marijuana cigarettes (Leuchtenberger and Leuchtenberger 1977). Decreases of DNA synthesis and neoplastic cell proliferation have been observed for ascorbic acid in tumor cell lines in culture (Bishun et al. 1978).

When taken in daily gram amounts for prolonged periods, vitamin C can be toxic. It depresses serum B_{12} levels and can lead to bone marrow changes (Herbert and Jacob 1974). In patients receiving radiation therapy, ascorbic acid can react with radiation-induced free radicals, and the resulting additional oxygen consumption may produce a greater degree of hypoxia and subsequent radioprotection. Drugs such as metronidazole and misonidazole cause reoxygenation of tumor tissue and thereby increase radiosensitivity. Patients taking large amounts of ascorbic acid are subject to an inhibiting interaction with radiosensitizing drugs (Biaglow and Jacobson 1977).

In their review of 50 patients with terminal disease treated with high-dose vitamin C, Cameron and Campbell (1974) were unable to remove so-called placebo bias, but addressed the problem and tried to minimize it. A recent Mayo Clinic trial approached this problem more successfully (Creagan et al. 1979). They entered 128 terminally ill patients with histologic proof of malignant disease into a double-blind study of the efficacy of high-dose vitamin C. All patients selected were deemed unsuitable for or had already failed standard therapy. By the technique of dynamic randomization, patients were assigned to one of two programs: vitamin C, 10 gm/day orally in 4 divided doses, or a comparably flavored lactose placebo in identical capsules. Both were dispensed in coded bottles. Treatment was continued until death or until the patient could no longer take oral medication. Symptomatic status was evaluated at two-week intervals by questionnaire. The groups were comparable by age, sex, tumor site and grade, performance status, and exposure to prior chemotherapy.

In the 102 evaluable patients, no significant side effects could be demonstrated for those treated with vitamin C compared to placebo. There was also no substantive difference with regard to changes in symptoms, performance status, weight, or appetite. The estimated median survival for each group was six weeks with survival curves that essentially overlapped. No therapeutic benefit for vitamin C was discernible.

No objective responses were seen in a group of 28 patients with evaluable non-small cell lung cancer treated in a cooperative group trial with vitamin C in doses of 3 to 5 gm/m^2 daily. Three had no change while 25 had progressive disease (Mehta and Cohen 1980).

At the present time there is no convincing evidence that vitamin C or orthomolecular diets improve the outcome of people with cancer (Herbert 1980). Studies will no doubt continue, but the burden of proof is on those who wish to introduce the new modality. It remains unproved.

Conclusions

In addition to those few we have reviewed here, there is a multitude of additional unproved methods. Most of them are worthless. Some are exploited by unscrupulous individuals for private profit. Some are espoused sincerely but in ignorance. A few may go on to be documented scientifically and enter the mainstream of therapy.

One modality in the last category is Coley's toxin. In 1893, Dr. William B. Coley of Memorial Hospital in New York City published the first of many papers on the use of repeated inoculations of extracts of streptococcal strains and other bacterial products in the treatment of malignant tumors. In spite of some published successes, the method fell into disrepute. In 1953, Helen Coley Nauts founded the New York Cancer Research Institute, Inc. (changed to Cancer Research Institute, Inc. in 1973) to reexplore the techniques pioneered by her father and to expand immunologic research in cancer. While the use of streptococcal extracts has not yet proved to be clinically useful, streptokinase is being studied with great interest. There are ongoing studies of staphage lysate, *Corynebacterium parvum,* BCG and its derivatives, as well as the effects of hyperthermia (Nauts 1978). In a roundabout way, these may be the fruits of Coley's pioneering investigations, which were ahead of the methodology of the time.

Such may be the problem of other unproved methods. The essence of the matter, however, is how the investigations are pursued and how, where, and to whom the data are reported. While we are aware of occasional attempts at suppression of reports by scientific and medical journals for misguided reasons, perseverence eventually is successful and the truth becomes known. It is always best to present new information in the scientific marketplace to one's peers for review and critique. If this is done, there will be fewer unproved therapies regarded with disapprobation.

References

American Cancer Society. *Laetrile background information.* New York: The American Cancer Society, 1977.

American Cancer Society. *Unproven methods of cancer management.* New York: The American Cancer Society, 1979.

Biaglow, J. E., and Jacobson, B. The reaction of hypoxic cell radiosensitizing drugs with vitamin C. *Br. J. Radiol.* 50:844–846, 1977.

Bishun, N. et al. The effect of ascorbic acid (vitamin C) on two tumor cell lines in culture. *Oncology* 35:160–162, 1978.

Burk, D. New approaches to cancer therapy. *N. Engl. Natural Food Assoc. Bull.,* Spring 1974.

Burk, D. A brief on foods. Vitamins, vitamin B-17 (amygdalin, nitriloside, laetrile), vitamin B-15 (pangamate) and vitamin B-13 (orotate). Sausalito, Calif: Science Press International, 1975.

Cameron, E., and Campbell, A. The orthomolecular treatment of cancer. II. Clinical trial of high-dose ascorbic acid supplements in advanced human cancer. *Chem. Biol. Interact.* 9:285–315, 1974.

Cameron, E., and Pauling, L. Ascorbic acid and the glycosaminoglycans: an orthomolecular approach to cancer and other diseases. *Oncology* 27:181–192, 1973.

Cameron, E., and Pauling, L. The orthomolecular treatment of cancer. I. The role of ascorbic acid in host resistance. *Chem. Biol. Interact.* 9:273–283, 1974.

Cameron, E.; Pauling, L.; and Leibovitz, B. Ascorbic acid and cancer: a review. *Cancer Res.* 39:663–681, 1979.

Clark, M. Laetrile and cancer. *Newsweek* 89:48–56, 1977.

Creagan, E. T. et al. Failure of high-dose vitamin C (ascorbic acid) therapy to benefit patients with advanced cancer. *N. Engl. J. Med.* 301:687–690, 1979.

Culbert, M. L. *Vitamin B-17, forbidden weapon against cancer.* New Rochelle, New York: Arlington House, 1974.

DiPalma, J. R., and McMichael, R. The interaction of vitamins with cancer chemotherapy. *CA* 29:280–286, 1979.

Food and Drug Administration. Laetrile: the making of a myth. *FDA Consumer* 10:5–9, 1977a.

Food and Drug Administration. Update on Laetrile. *FDA Drug Bull.* 10:2–4, 1977b.

Gershanovich, M. L. et al. Clinical data on the antitumor activity of hydrazine sulfate. *Cancer Treat. Rep.* 60:933–935, 1976.

Gold, J. Proposed treatment of cancer by inhibition of gluconeogenesis. *Oncology* 22:185–207, 1968.

Gold, J. Inhibition of Walker 256 intramuscular carcinoma in rats by administration of hydrazine sulfate. *Oncology* 25:66–71, 1971.

Gold, J. Cancer cachexia and gluconeogenesis. *Ann. NY Acad. Sci.* 230:103–110, 1974a.

Gold, J. Use of hydrazine sulfate in advanced cancer patients: preliminary results. *Proc. Am. Assoc. Cancer Res.* 15:83, 1974b.

Gold, J. Use of hydrazine sulfate in terminal and preterminal cancer patients: results of investigational new drug (IND) study in 84 evaluable patients. *Oncology* 32:1–10, 1975.

Greenberg, D. M. The case against Laetrile, the fraudulent cancer remedy. *Cancer* 45:799–807, 1980.

Herbert, V. The nutritionally unsound, nutritional and metabolic antineoplastic diet of Laetrile proponents. *JAMA* 240:1139–1140, 1978.

Herbert, V. The vitamin craze. *Arch. Intern. Med.* 140:173–176, 1980.

Herbert, V., and Jacob, E. Destruction of vitamin B_{12} by ascorbic acid. *JAMA* 230:241–242, 1974.

Humbert, J. R. et al. Fatal cyanide poisoning. Accidental ingestion of amygdalin. *JAMA* 239:479, 1977.

Kittler, G. D. *Laetrile (the anticancer drug) control for cancer.* New York: Warner Paperback Library, 1963.

Lerner, H. J., and Regelson, W. Clinical trial of hydrazine sulfate in solid tumors. *Cancer Treat. Rep.* 60:959–960, 1976.

Leuchtenberger, C., and Leuchtenberger, R. Protection of hamster lung cultures by L-cysteine or vitamin C against carcinogenic effects of fresh smoke from tobacco or marijuana cigarettes. *Br. J. Exp. Pathol.* 58:625–634, 1977.

Mehta, C., and Cohen, M. *Final reports of terminated studies, Eastern Cooperative Oncology Group,* vol. 2. Madison, Wisc.: ECOG, 1980, pp. 338–393.

Moertel, C. et al. A phase II trial of amygdalin (Laetrile) in the treatment of human cancer. *Proc. Am. Soc. Clin. Oncol.* 22:383, 1981.

Nauts, H. C. Bacterial vaccine therapy of cancer. In *Proceedings of a symposium on biological preparations in the treatment of cancer.* Basel and New York: S. Karger, 1978.

Ochoa, M. et al. Trial of hydrazine sulfate in patients with cancer. *Cancer Chemother. Rep.* 59:1151–1154, 1975.

Regelson, W. The "grand conspiracy" against the cancer cure. *JAMA* 243:337–339, 1980.

Richardson, J. A., and Griffin, P. *Laetrile: case histories.* New York: Bantam Books, 1977.

Schultz, T., and Lindeman, B. The victimizing of desperate cancer patients. *Today's Health* 51:28–33; 51–53, 1973.

Smith, F. P. et al. Laetrile toxicity: a report of two patients. *Cancer Treat. Rep.* 62:169–171, 1978.

Spremulli, E. et al. Clinical study of hydrazine sulfate in advanced cancer patients. *Cancer Chemother. Pharmacol.* 3:121–124, 1979.

Terry, W. *Summary of Site Visit to the Immunology Researching Center, Ltd., Freeport, Grand Bahamas Island, Bahamas, Jan. 1978.* New York: American Cancer Society, 1978.

United States vs *Rutherford et al.,* Supreme Court of United States 78-605, June 18, 1979.

Westover, W. *Physicians' handbook of vitamin B-17 therapy.* Sausalito, Calif.: Science Press International, 1973.

part two

Research and Advances

thirteen

Clinical Research in Oncology

DAVID S. FISCHER

Although we tend to think of cancer chemotherapy as an established technique now that oncology is a recognized subspecialty, in fact, the entire field encompasses barely 35 years. The treatment of some cancers has now become somewhat routine with so-called standard protocols, but even with therapy of those few tumors that respond well there is room for improvement. For the majority of cancers, results are far from satisfactory, and the treatment of each and every patient is in the nature of a clinical trial. Some of these trials are formalized as investigative procedures in research institutions or cooperative group studies. Others are simply individual observations of a skilled physician treating the patient. In either case, careful, complete records are important.

To evaluate a response to therapy, there must be some consistency in describing the extent of the neoplastic diseases of different anatomic systems and organs. Appropriate classification and staging are also helpful in the selection of therapy. In early stages of Hodgkin's disease radiation alone may be curative, whereas in advanced disease multiple-drug chemotherapy alone or in combination with radiation is more likely to achieve long-term survival free of disease.

Obviously, staging is not an exact science. A variety of methods is in use while national and international bodies try to reach consensus. The TNM classification (1974) was developed by the International Union Against Cancer (UICC) and is widely used. It is based on the observation that prognosis is related to tumor size (T), to the extent of involvement of the regional (draining) lymph nodes (N), and the presence or absence of metastatic disease (M). A grouping of the T, N, and M from retrospective or prospective studies can be used to devise a classification with prognostic significance. Staging based solely on physical examination and laboratory and nonsurgical diagnostic techniques is called clinical staging. After surgery and histologic examination of tissues it is possible to have somewhat more precise evaluation called pathologic staging. The significance of the markers T, N, and M may be different in the natural history and evolution of different tumors. Hence a dissimilar grouping of the three characteristics may yield similar or identical staging. For some tumors, the system has not been found useful and others have been devised, such as the Ann Arbor modification of the Rye staging system for Hodgkin's disease. In the United States, the most widely accepted method is that of the American Joint Committee for Cancer Staging and End-Results Reporting (1978). Prognosis may also be related to histopathologic grade. The generally accepted grading is:

- G1 well-differentiated
- G2 moderately well-differentiated
- G3 poorly differentiated
- G4 very poorly differentiated (anaplastic)

The higher the grade in general, the more likely is metastasis.

Another prognostic postoperative determinant is the extent of residual tumor (if any) left behind after

Table 13.1. *Criteria of Performance Status (PS) (Karnofsky)*

Level of Performance	%	*Status*
Able to carry on normal activity; no special care is needed	100	Normal; no complaints; no evidence of disease
	90	Able to carry on normal activity; minor signs or symptoms of disease
	80	Normal activity with effort; some signs or symptoms of disease
Unable to work; able to live at home; cares for most personal needs; a varying amount of assistance is needed	70	Cares for self; unable to carry on normal activity or to do active work
	60	Requires occasional assistance but is able to care for most needs
	50	Requires considerable assistance and frequent medical care
Unable to care for self; requires equivalent of institutional or hospital care; disease may be progressing rapidly	40	Disabled; requires special medical care and assistance
	30	Severely disabled; hospitalization is indicated, although death not imminent
	20	Very sick; hospitalization necessary; active support treatment necessary
	10	Moribund; fatal processes progressing rapidly
	0	Dead

SOURCE: Karnofsky et al. 1948.

surgery. This is not used for staging of all tumors but is prognostically significant and is frequently recorded as:

R0 no residual tumor

R1 microscopic residual tumor

R2 macroscopic residual tumor (site and extent specified when possible)

In addition to the size of the primary tumor, its nodal and distant spread, histopathologic grade, and the extent of residual tumor, the patient's physical state before treatment (performance status, or PS) is a major determinant of prognosis. With a variety of tumors, all other values being equal, the patient with a good PS seems to live significantly longer than one with a low PS. A classification of the criteria for evaluating PS was devised by Karnofsky and associates (Karnofsky et al. 1948; Karnofsky and Burchenal 1949; Karnofsky 1965) and is still widely used (table 13.1). Its validity and reliability have been evaluated (Yates, Chalmer, and McKegney 1980). A simplification was developed by the Eastern Cooperative Oncology Group (ECOG), known as the ECOG PS or Zubrod PS (Zubrod et al. 1960), and is used by several cooperative groups. It is compared to the Karnofsky PS in table 13.2.

Formal Clinical Trials

Because the result of most cancer therapy leaves room for improvement, and since new drugs must be tested in a manner to yield reproducible answers, formal clinical trials have been devised. Much or most of those in the United States have been influenced by the National Cancer Institute (NCI) and its guidelines. An outline for a clinical protocol follows:*

1. Introduction and scientific background
2. Study objectives
3. Ethical justification; human investigation committee approval
4. Selection of patients
5. Study design (including schematic diagram)
6. Randomization
7. Treatment programs
8. Study values
9. Procedure in event of response, no response, or toxicity
10. Required clinical and laboratory data

*Modified from Carter 1977.

Table 13.2. *ECOG Performance Status*

Grade	Level of Performance
0	Fully active, able to carry on all predisease performance without restriction (Karnofsky 90–100)
1	Restricted in physically strenuous activity, but ambulatory and able to carry out work of a light or sedentary nature, i.e., light house work, office work (Karnofsky 70–80)
2	Ambulatory and capable of all self-care, but unable to carry out any work activities, up and about more than 50% of waking hours (Karnofsky 50–60)
3	Capable of only limited self-care, confined to bed or chair more than 50% of waking hours (Karnofsky 30–40)
4	Completely disabled, cannot carry on any self-care, totally confined to bed or chair (Karnofsky 10–20)

SOURCE: Zubrod et al. 1960.

11. Criteria for evaluating response
12. Statistical considerations
13. Informed consent
14. Records to be kept (forms)
15. References and bibliography
16. Study coordinator(s) and telephone number(s)

Many of the guidelines that seemed simple at one time have become complex. There is much controversy over the ethical basis of clinical research—its need, its costs, and its monitoring (DeVita 1978; Kass 1980; Sedransk and Carter 1980; Gibson 1980). Should the patient be fully informed or will to much information frighten and confuse (Miller 1980; Cousins 1980; Fries and Loftus 1979)?

There are differing views among leaders in the field over the necessity for double-blind, prospective randomized trials in preference to the use of historical controls (Gehan and Freireich 1974; Chalmers, Block, and Lee 1972; Livingston et al. 1976). Any valid evaluation of the findings must begin with definition of the statistical criteria for significance, include the appropriate number of subjects, and define what is accepted as a difference (Mike and Shottenfeld 1972; Gehan and Schneiderman 1973). Statistical analysis of the final data must be performed by the prestudy criteria and not manipulated later to fit one of the many possible statistical models to achieve some degree of significance, and hence credibility. If the trial was a failure, it should be so stated, but a useful therapy should not be lost because of poor study design, inadequate sample size, and inappropriate counting criteria (Freiman et al. 1978; Sackett and Gent 1979). Attention to statistical detail is clearly important, and failure to appreciate this has doomed many studies to be wasted efforts.

Phase I, II, III, and IV Drug Trials

As an introduction to drug trials, the following is an outline of the four phases of these evaluations modified from guidelines of the NCI and FDA.

Phase I. Clinical pharmacology in patients with advanced cancers with or without measurable lesions
1. Establish maximally tolerated dose
2. Establish limits of toxicity
3. Pharmacologic evaluation, absorption, distribution, metabolism, excretion
4. Antitumor activity not required

Phase II. Survey for clinical activity in patients with measurable or evaluable disease
1. Nonrandomized studies
2. 15 to 20 patients in 7 signal tumors
   A. Adenocarcinoma of colon
   B. Bronchogenic carcinoma
   C. Adenocarcinoma of breast
   D. Undifferentiated lymphosarcoma
   E. Acute myelocytic leukemia
   F. Acute lymphocytic leukemia
   G. Melanoma

Phase III. Definitive studies to establish role in cancer therapy
1. Controlled clinical trials
2. Combination studies

Phase IV. Commercial availability and multimodality trials

Once a drug has been shown to be an effective antineoplastic agent in cell culture and its toxicity evaluated in a variety of animal studies, it is ready for a phase I clinical trial. This is a small study with patients who have either failed all other chemotherapy or who have no other therapeutic options with any reasonable chance of response. They are treated in a nonrandom mode to ascertain the toxicity of the drug in humans, its maximal tolerated dose, and its pharmacokinetics.

After a phase I trial has established a drug's relative safety and defined a tolerated dose, phase II studies are initiated in the seven so-called signal tumors to ascertain the cancers that will respond. This early phase II study is also nonrandomized and requires a moderate number of patients for adequate testing.

A disease-oriented phase II study can be protected to some extent from conscious or unconscious bias by randomization and stratification. Patients entering the study are categorized by sets of known important prognostic factors, and the individuals falling within each set form a group or stratum. The patients in each group are separately randomized to the treatment programs. This avoids a young, good-risk patient with early disease being compared to an elderly patient with end-stage disease who is unlikely to respond. Simple randomization to treatment programs would not necessarily ensure an approximately equal distribution of important prognostic factors in the relatively small groups used in phase II studies (Carter 1977).

When a drug has been found to have acceptable toxicity in phase I and some demonstrated activity in a particular neoplasm in phase II studies, it is ready to proceed to phase III to try to establish its role in therapy of a specific cancer. For this, larger numbers of patients are needed, especially if the drug is only moderately active and not spectacularly and rapidly effective. Here, a randomized, prospective, double-blind study is desirable because it removes the bias of the investigators, compensates for the placebo effect, and yields a more statistically sound result. The defenders of the use of historical controls emphasize the limited number of suitable patients available for study, and hence the need to use all available subjects in the test to compare against matched individuals treated in the past, especially if the results were consistent. In such a trial, it is very important to adhere strictly to protocol. The generally accepted criteria for complete response (CR), partial response (PR), progression (prog), and all the others between, are shown below. Studies may be of the single agent or combination chemotherapy.

Complete response (CR): complete disappearance of all objective evidence of tumor, also designated no evidence of disease (NED)

Partial response (PR): a 50% or greater decrease in the sum of the products of the diameters of the tumors and no progression in other areas

Improvement (IMP): some reduction in tumor size, but less than 50%

Stabilization (stable): lesions stable or with growth arrest after initiating therapy and with improvement in symptoms

No change (NC): increase of less than 25% or decrease of less than 50% in the sum of products of diameters

Progression (prog): greater than 25% increase of any measured lesion, or development of new lesions

Progression after a response: new lesions or a 50% or greater increase in product of diameters over minimal size

Duration of response
PR: Time of 50% decrease to relapse
CR: Time of NED to relapse

A drug that has successfully completed phase III studies is ready to be recommended for approval by the Food and Drug Administration for commercial distribution. A new concept that is being accepted is the inclusion of new drugs in multimodality protocols combining surgery, radiation, and chemotherapy; some people designate these studies as phase IV (Carter and Soper 1974; Muggia 1978). With increasing experience some of these trials are being run in humans relatively early, that is, after limited animal experience. One of the biggest problems is patient accrual. University hospitals and research institutes are not seeing as many suitable patients as in former years. An entire cadre of young oncologists (medical, pediatric, gynecologic, surgical, and radiation) has been trained and sent out into the community hospitals. They feel qualified to treat the patients there, and if research is to be done it will have to be in cooperation with some of the cooperative groups working with oncologists based in these institutions (Carter 1978; Dugan et al. 1979; Lee, Marks, and Simpson 1980). The recent demonstration that elderly patients are not unduly predisposed to toxicity from most cancer chemotherapy agents may add impetus to the inclusion of senior citizens in research protocols (Begg, Cohen, and Ellerton 1980).

The progress in cancer chemotherapy in the United States in general, and the success of clinical trials in particular, is due to a large extent to the Cooperative Clinical Trials Program of the NCI (Weiss and Jacobs 1979; Hoogstraten 1980). New drugs have been tested and proved to be of value, and the entire concept of combination chemotherapy has been largely tested in cooperative groups. From early exclusivity with limitations to major research institutes, they have now broadened their base and welcome the participation of well-trained community oncologists working through a member institution. The major cooperative groups and

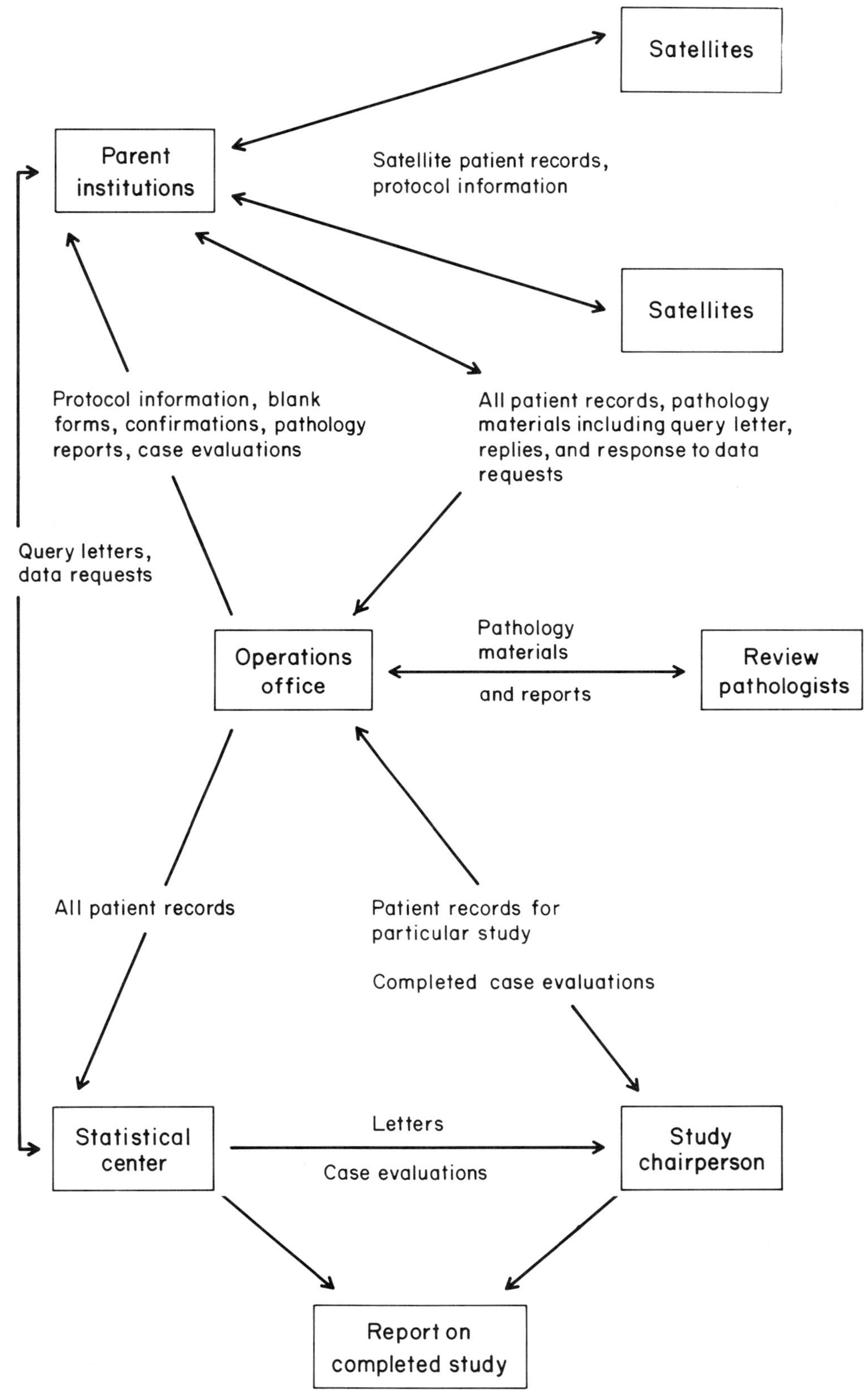

Fig. 13.1. *Flow of data in ECOG. (Eastern Cooperative Oncology Group* 1979.)

Table 13.3. *Examples of Dose Modification*

A. Determination based on white cell and platelet counts just prior to next dose.
Hematologic toxicity (WBC and platelets to be obtained before *each* dose)*

WBC	*Platelets*	*Dose Modification (In Absence of Other Toxicity)*
≥ 4000	≥ 100,000	Full protocol dose
3001–3999	75,000–99,999	Reduce dose 50%; reduce 10% for next dose
1999–3000	50,000–74,999	Withhold dose; reduce 25% for next dose
1000–1999	25,000–49,999	Withhold dose; reduce 50% for next dose
< 1000	< 25,000	Withhold dose; no further therapy

*In the event that unusual life-threatening or fatal toxicity is encountered, the study chairperson must be notified in writing within 10 days and by telephone.

B. Determination based on granulocyte and platelet count just prior to next dose in a combination protocol using cyclophosphamide (Cytoxan), doxorubicin (Adriamycin), and vincristine (Oncovin).

Hematologic tolerance

Granulocytes	*Platelets*	*Chemotherapy*
> 2000	> 150,000	Full dose
1500–2000	100,000–150,000	Decrease doses of CTX, Adriamycin by 50%
< 1500	< 100,000	Hold therapy, reassess one week later

Adriamycin will be reduced for bilirubin elevation as follows:

Bilirubin	*Decrease in Adriamycin Dosage*
> 1.5–3mg%	50%
> 3mg%	70%

C. Determination based on nadir white cell and platelet counts using a protocol with a long-acting (6- to 8-week) drug such as mitomycin-C.

WBC	*Platelets*	*Dose Reduction*
Early (2–3 weeks) 2000		5-FU by 25%
Late (4–5 weeks) 1500–2500		Mito-C by 25%
< 1500		Mito-C by 50%
	50–75,000	Mito-C by 25%
	< 50,000	Mito-C by 50%

Table 13.3. *Continued*

D. Determination based on white cell and platelet counts just prior to next dose with a drug administered weekly and with planned dose escalation.

Complete blood counts must be obtained once weekly and the dose modified as follows for cytopenia.

		Platelet count/mm³		
		100,000 or more	75,000–99,999	Less than 75,000
WBC count (cells/mm³)	4000 or more	100%	50%	0
	2500–3999	50%	50%	0
	Less than 2500	0	0	0

If there is no hematologic toxicity during any period of four consecutive weeks of therapy (WBC 4000, platelets 100,000) then the dose should be escalated 10%. If no toxicity is produced in the succeeding 4-week period, a second escalation should be accomplished by 20%.

their addresses are included in appendix 13.1. A flow diagram of data for one major cooperative group is shown in figure 13.1. Common problems in the use of cooperative group protocols are listed below:*

1. Incompleteness (blanks and/or partial answers)—any indication that the information is unavailable or unknown would suffice
2. Inconsistency between forms, i.e., "measurable area of disease"
3. Treatment assigned varies from treatment given
4. Missing surface area or height and weight (on-study form)
5. Flow sheets—incomplete, scant, dosage omitted, dates of administration omitted, lab values omitted, overlapping steps of treatment
6. Missing or unclear measurements. No initial measurements (measurement form)
7. Objective response does not comply with the protocol definition
8. Date of response is not documented
9. Response section is blank
10. Response is claimed on day 1 of treatment
11. Toxicities are not documented or those appearing on flow sheets are not on summary form
12. Date treatment ended is not date of last dose of last course
13. Combined summary for more than one step of treatment
14. Sequence number missing on forms or wrong sequence number used
15. Illegibility of writing and/or the use of blue ink (not easily reproduced)

Many of the drugs studied by the cooperative clinical groups have gone from experimental to commercial status. Along the way they were known by National Service Center (NSC) numbers, chemical abbreviations, or a manufacturer's designation. As they approach clinical usefulness they are assigned a nonproprietary name by the United States Adopted Names (USAN) Council, which is sponsored by the American Medical Association (AMA), the American Pharmaceutical Association (APHA), and the U.S. Pharmacopeial Convention, Inc., in cooperation with the respective pharmaceutical manufacturers. The designation USAN distinguishes these formally adopted nonproprietary names from other names. Adoption of USAN does not imply endorsement of the claims or products by the AMA, APHA, or the *U.S. Pharmacopeia*. In some instances, the drugs listed are available only from the manufacturer to properly qualified investigators for clinical study.

Currently, distribution of most investigational drugs is conducted by the Division of Cancer Treatment (DCT) of the NCI. The latest listing of the drug groups and the drugs is shown in appendix 13.2, and includes tetrahydrocannabinol (THC) (Henney 1980).

Bone marrow, liver, and kidney toxicity may occur when using combination chemotherapy protocols. To avoid permanent damage to these organs, dose reduction schedules are tailored to the specific protocol and based on the nature of the drugs being used. Examples of four such schedules are shown in table 13.3.

Throughout the practice of oncology, the principles developed in the clinical trials will recur again and again. The clinical trials program has been both a successful research venture and an excellent educational experience.

*From *Eastern Cooperative Onocogy Group* 1979.

References

American Joint Committee for Cancer Staging and End-Results Reporting. *Manual for staging of cancer, 1978*. Chicago: Whiting Press, 1980.

Begg, C. B.; Cohen, J. L.; and Ellerton, J. Are the elderly predisposed to toxicity from cancer chemotherapy? An investigation using data from the Eastern Cooperative Oncology Group. *Cancer Clin. Trials* 3:369–374, 1980.

Carter, S. K. Clinical trials in cancer chemotherapy. *Cancer* 40:544–557, 1977.

Carter, S. K. Clinical research and community involvement. Editorial. *Cancer Clin. Trials* 1:79–82, 1978.

Carter, S. K., and Soper, W. T. Integration of chemotherapy into combined modality treatment of solid tumors. I. The overall strategy. *Cancer Treat. Rev.* 1:1–13, 1974.

Chalmers, T. C.; Block, J. B.; and Lee, S. Controlled studies in clinical cancer research. *N. Engl. J. Med.* 287:75–78, 1972.

Cousins, N. A layman looks at truth telling in medicine. *JAMA* 244:1929–1930, 1980.

DeVita, V. T., Jr. The evolution of therapeutic research in cancer. *N. Engl. J. Med.* 198:907–910, 1978.

Dugan, W. M. et al. Clinical oncology program: a community cancer control model. *CA* 29:300–305, 1979.

Eastern Cooperative Oncology Group. Data manager manual. Madison, Wisc.: ECOG, 1979.

Freiman, J. A. et al. The importance of beta, the type II error and sample size in the design and interpretation of the randomized control trial. *N. Engl. J. Med.* 299:690–694, 1978.

Fries, J. F., and Loftus, E. F. Informed consent: right or rite. *CA* 29:316–318, 1979.

Gehan, E. A., and Freireich, E. J. Non-randomized controls in cancer clinical trials. *N. Engl. J. Med.* 290:198–203, 1974.

Gehan, E. A., and Schneiderman, M. A. Experimental design of clinical trials. In *Cancer medicine,* eds. J. F. Holland and E. Frei, III. Philadelphia: Lea & Febiger, 1973, pp. 499–519.

Gibson, W. C. The cost of not doing medical research (if you think medical research is expensive, try disease). *JAMA* 244:1817–1819, 1980.

Henney, J. Investigational drug distribution—update. *DCT Bulletin,* September 1980.

Hoogstraaten, B., ed. *Cancer research. Impact of the cooperative groups.* New York: Masson, 1980.

Karnofsky, D. A. Problems and pitfalls in the evaluation of anticancer drugs. *Cancer* 18:1517–1528, 1965.

Karnofsky, D. A. et al. The use of the nitrogen mustards in the palliative treatment of carcinoma with particular reference to bronchogenic carcinoma. *Cancer* 1:634–656, 1948.

Karnofsky, D. A., and Burchenal, J. H. The clinical evaluation of chemotherapeutic agents in cancer. In *Evaluation of chemotherapeutic agents,* ed. C. M. Macleod. New York: Columbia University Press, 1949, pp. 191–205.

Kass, L. R. Ethical dilemmas in the care of the ill. *JAMA* 244:1811–1816; 1946–1949, 1980.

Lee, J. Y.; Marks, J. E.; and Simpson, J. R. Recruitment of patients to cooperative group clinical trials. *Cancer Clin. Trials* 3:381–384, 1980.

Livingston, R. B. et al. Design and conduct of clinical trials. In *Cancer patient care at M. D. Anderson Hospital and Tumor Institute,* eds. R. L. Clark and C. D. Howe. Chicago: Year Book, 1976.

Mike, V., and Schottenfeld, D. Observations on the clinical trial. *Clin. Bull.* 2:130–135, 1972.

Miller, L. J. Informed consent. *JAMA* 244:2100–2103; 2347–2350, 1980.

Muggia, F. M. Clinical trials in cancer: general concepts and methodologies. *Cancer Clin. Trials* 1:139–144, 1978.

Sackett, D. L., and Gent, M. Controversy in counting and attributing events in clinical trials. *N. Engl. J. Med.* 301:1410–1412, 1979.

Sedransk, N., and Carter, S. K. Proceedings of the symposium on designs for clinical cancer research. *Cancer Treat. Rep.* 64:361–538, 1980.

TNM classification of malignant tumors, 3rd edition. Geneva: International Union Against Cancer (UICC), 1974.

Weiss, R. B., and Jacobs, E. M. The National Cancer Institute cooperative clinical trials program. *CA* 29:287–290, 1979.

Yates, J. W.; Chalmer, B.; and McKegney, F. P. Evaluation of patients with advanced cancer using the Karnofsky performance status. *Cancer* 45:2220–2224, 1980.

Zubrod, G. C. et al. Appraisal of methods for the study of chemotherapy in man: comparative therapeutic trial of nitrogen mustard and triethylene thiophosphoramide. *J. Chron. Dis.* 11:7–33, 1960.

Appendix 13.1. *Clinical Trials Groups and Institutional Projects Administrative Information*

Brain Tumor Chemotherapy Study Group

David A. Pistenma, M.D., Chairman
Landow Building, Room 4A22
National Cancer Institute, NIH
Bethesda, MD 20205
310-496-9361

Operations Office
Thomas A. Strike, Ph.D., Administrator
Landow Building, Room 4C33
National Cancer Institute, NIH
Bethesda, MD 20205
301-496-5297

Statistical Office
Sylvan B. Green, M.D.
David P. Byar, M.D.
Landow Building, Room 509C
National Cancer Institute, NIH
Bethesda, MD 20205
301-496-4208

Cancer and Leukemia Group B

Emil Frei III, M.D., Chairman
Sidney Farber Cancer Institute
49 Binney St.
Boston, MA 02115
617-732-3555

Operations Office
Janice M. Gray, Ph.D., Administrator
Two Overhill Rd., Suite 208
Scarsdale, NY 10583
212-650-6363

Statistical Office
Oliver Glidewell, Group Biostatistician
Two Overhill Rd., Suite 208
Scarsdale, NY 10583
914-472-0710

Gastrointestinal Tumor Study Group

Douglas Holyoke, M.D., Chairman
Roswell Park Memorial Institute
666 Elm St.
Buffalo, NY 14263

Philip Schein, M.D., Co-Chairman
Georgetown University Medical Center
Room 2230
3800 Reservoir Rd., NW
Washington, DC 20007
202-652-7081

Operations Office
Philomena Grifone, Administrator
850 Sligo Ave., Suite 601
Silver Spring, MD 20910
301-585-4844

Statistical Office
Joel W. Novak
EMMES Corporation
Suite 206
7825 Tuckerman Lane
Potomac, MD 20854
301-299-2484

Gynecologic Oncology Group

George C. Lewis, Jr., M.D., Chairman
Gynecologic Group Headquarters
1234 Market St., Suite 430
Philadelphia, PA 19107
215-854-0770

Operations Office
John R. Kellner, Group Manager
1234 Market St., Suite 430
Philadelphia, PA 19107
215-854-0770

Statistical Office
John Blessing, Ph.D.
Roswell Park Memorial Institute
Towers Apartments, 2nd Floor
666 Elm St.
Buffalo, NY 14263
716-854-5702

Children's Cancer Study Group

Denman Hammond, M.D., Chairman
University of Southern California
2025 Zonal Ave.
Keith Administration Building, Room 509
Los Angeles, CA 90033

Operations Office
Richard Honour, Ph.D., Administrator
University of Southern California
School of Medicine
1721 Griffin Ave.
Los Angeles, CA 90031
213-223-1373

Statistical Office
Harland Sather, Ph.D.
University of Southern California
School of Medicine
Barracks A
2025 Zonal Ave.
Los Angeles, CA 90033
213-222-7151

Clinical Trials for Breast Cancer

Umberto Veronesi, M.D., Principal Investigator
Gianni Bonadonna, M.D., Co-Principal Investigator
Istituto Nazionale per le Studio e la Cura Dei Tumori
Via Venezia 1
20133 Milano, Italy

Eastern Cooperative Oncology Group

Paul Carbone, M.D., Chairman
Wisconsin Clinical Cancer Center, Room K4-614
600 Highland Ave.
Madison, WI 53792
608-263-8610

Operations Office
Barbara Miller, Administrator
Medical Science Center
Room 4765
420 No. Charter Street
Madison, WI 53706
608-263-7837

Statistical Office
Colin B. Begg, Ph.D.
Marvin Zelen, Ph.D.
Kenneth Stanley, Ph.D.
Sidney Farber Cancer Institute
44 Binney St.
Boston, MA 02115
617-732-3012

Head and Neck Contracts Program

Bimal Ghosh, M.D.
Landow Building, Room 4A04
National Cancer Institute, NIH
Bethesda, MD 20205
301-496-6056

Operations Office
Philomena Grifone, Administrator
850 Sligo Ave., Suite 601
Silver Spring, MD 20910
301-585-4844

Statistical Office
Richard Simon, Ph.D.
Building 10, Room 3B16
National Cancer Institute, NIH
Bethesda, MD 20205

Intergroup Testicular Studies

William DeWys, M.D., Project Officer
Landow Building, Room 4A04
National Cancer Institute, NIH
Bethesda, MD 20205
301-496-4505

Operations Office
Philomena Grifone, Administrator
850 Sligo Ave., Suite 601
Silver Spring, MD 20910
301-585-4844

Statistical Office
Sylvan B. Green, M.D.
Landow Building, Room 509C
National Cancer Institute, NIH
Bethesda, MD 20205
301-496-2522

Lung Cancer Study Group

John Y. Killen, Jr., M.D., Project Officer
Landow Building, Room 4A16
National Cancer Institute, NIH
Bethesda, MD 20205
301-496-2522

Operations Office
Philomena Grifone, Administrator
850 Sligo Ave., Suite 601
Silver Spring, MD 20910
301-585-4844

Statistical Office
Mitchell H. Gail, M.D., Ph.D.
Landow Building, Room 509C
National Cancer Institute, NIH
Bethesda, MD 20205
301-496-4208

National Surgical Adjuvant Project for Breast and Bowel Cancers

Bernard Fisher, M.D., Chairman
914 Scaife Hall
3550 Terrace St.
Pittsburgh, PA 15261
412-624-2671

Operations Office
Norman Wolmark, M.D., Executive Medical Officer
914 Scaife Hall
3550 Terrace St.
Pittsburgh, PA 15261
412-624-2666

Statistical Office
Carol Redmond, Sc.D., Director, Statistical Unit
Graduate School of Public Health
318 Parran Hall
130 DeSoto St.
Pittsburgh, PA 15261
412-624-3027

Madeline Bauer, Ph.D., Coordinating Statistician
3515 Fifth Ave., Suite 730
Pittsburgh, PA 15213
412-624-2666

National Prostatic Cancer Project

Gerald P. Murphy M.D., Project Director
Roswell Park Cancer Project
666 Elm Street
Buffalo, NY 14263
716-845-5770

National Wilms' Tumor Study Group

Giulio D'Angio, M.D., Chairman
Children's Cancer Research Center
34th & Civic Center Blvd.
Philadelphia, PA 19104
215-287-5518

Operations Office
Juanite Guagenti, Administrator
Children's Cancer Research Center
34th & Civic Center Blvd., Room 90975
Philadelphia, PA 19104
215-596-9614

Statistical Office
Norman Breslow, Ph.D.
Fred Hutchinson Cancer Research Center
1124 Columbia St.
Seattle, WA 98104
206-292-2226

North Central Cancer Treatment Group

James M. Ingle, M.D., Chairman
Department of Medical Oncology
Mayo Clinic
200 First St., SW
Rochester, MN 55901
507-284-2511

Operations Office
Christopher Batchelder, Administrator
Administrative Services
Mayo Clinic
200 First St., SW
Rochester, MN 55901
507-284-2072

Statistical Office
Judith R. O'Fallon, Ph.D.
Department of Oncology
Mayo Clinic
200 First St., SW
Rochester, MN 55901
507-284-2511

Northern California Oncology Group

Stephen K. Carter, M.D., Chairman
1801 Page Mill Rd.
Building B, Suite 200
Palo Alto, CA 94304
415-497-7431

Operations Office
Susan Hesse, Administrative Assistant
1801 Page Mill Rd.
Building B, Suite 200
Palo Alto, CA 94304
415-497-7512

Statistical Office
Byron W. Brown, Jr., Ph.D.
Department of Biostatistics
Stanford University Medical Center
Stanford, CA 94305
415-497-5687

Phase I/II Studies of New Anticancer Drugs (Phase I/II Working Group)

Daniel Hoth, M.D., Project Officer
Cancer Therapy Evaluation Program
Landow Building, Room 4C17
National Cancer Institute, NIH
Bethesda, MD 20205
301-496-5223

Phase II/III Studies in Patients with Disseminated Solid Tumors

John Y. Killen, M.D., Coordinator
Landow Building, Room 4A16
National Cancer Institute, NIH
Bethesda, MD 20205
301-496-2522

Phase II Trials in Gastrointestinal Carcinoma

Gary Witman, M.D., Project Officer
Landow Building, Room 4A18
National Cancer Institute, NIH
Bethesda, MD 20205
301-496-2522

Polycythemia Vera Study Group

Louis R. Wasserman, M.D., Chairman
Mt. Sinai Hospital
19 East 98th St.
New York, NY 10029
212-876-2734

Operations Office
Paul B. Donovan, M.D., Executive Officer
Helen Walton, Administrator
19 East 98th St., Room 4C
New York, NY 10029
212-876-2734

Statistical Office
Judith Goldberg, Sc.D.
Mt. Sinai Medical School
19 East 98th St.
New York, NY 10029
212-650-5851

Radiation Therapy Oncology Group

Luther W. Brady, M.D.
Hahnemann Medical College and Hospital
230 North Broad St.
Philadelphia, PA 19102
215-928-6700

Operations Office
Lawrence Davis, M.D., Associate Chairman
Meg Keiser, Coordinator
925 Chestnut St.
Philadelphia, PA 19107
215-574-3176

Statistical Office
Marcello Pagano, Ph.D.
Sidney Farber Cancer Institute
44 Binney St.
Boston, MA 02115
617-732-3012
617-732-3601

Radiotherapy Hodgkin's Disease Group

George B. Hutchison, M.D., Chairman
Harvard University
School of Public Health
Department of Epidemiology
677 Huntington Ave.
Boston, MA 02115
617-732-1050

Statistical and Operations Office
George B. Hutchison, M.D., Administrator
Harvard University
School of Public Health
677 Huntington Ave.
Boston, MA 02115
617-732-1050

Southeastern Cancer Study Group

John R. Durant, M.D., Chairman
Comprehensive Cancer Center
University of Alabama School of Medicine
University Station
LBWTI-214
Birmingham, AL 35294
205-934-5077

Operations Office
Rosalie Avent, Administrator
University of Alabama School of Medicine
University Station
LBWTI-215
Birmingham, AL 35294
205-934-5270

Statistical Office
Alfred Bartolucci, Ph.D.
University of Alabama School of Medicine
University Station
LBWTI-G01
Birmingham, AL 35294
205-934-4340

Southwest Oncology Group

Charles Coltman Jr., M.D., Chairman
Cancer Therapy and Research Center
4450 Medical Drive
San Antonio, TX 78229
512-690-1111

Operations Office
Cherry Reynolds, Administrator
3500 Rainbow Blvd., Suite 100
Kansas City, KS 66103
913-588-5996

Statistical Office
Edmund Gehan, Ph.D.
M.D. Anderson Hospital and Tumor Institute
6723 Bertner Drive
Houston, TX 77030
713-792-3320

Pediatric Oncology Group

Operations Office
Julie Myers, Administrator
4386 Lindell Ave.
St. Louis, MO 63108
314-535-5660

Total Parenteral Nutrition Studies

William DeWys, M.D., Project Officer
Landow Building, Room 4A04
National Cancer Institute, NIH
Bethesda, MD 20205
301-496-6056

Operations and Statistical Office
Lloyd Lininger, Ph.D., Administrator and Statistician
Information Management Services
4853 Cordell Ave., Suite B10
Bethesda, MD 20014
301-986-0030

Uro-Oncology Research Group

David F. Paulson, M.D., Chairman
P.O. Box 2977
Duke University Medical Center
Durham, NC 27710
919-684-5057

Operations Office
Judy Reich, Administrator
VA Hospital
508 Fulton St.
Durham, NC 27705

Veterans Administration Surgical Oncology Group

George A. Higgins, M.D., Chairman
Chief, Surgical Service
VA Hospital
50 Irving St., NW
Washington, DC 20422
202-389-7266

Operations Office
Melinda Smith, Administrator
VA Hospital
50 Irving St., NW
Washington, DC 20422
202-389-7266

Statistical Office
Robert J. Keehn, MFUA/JH616
National Research Council
2101 Constitution Ave.
Washington, DC 20418
202-389-6467

Coordinating Center for Clinical Study of Melanoma

Istituto Nazionale per le Studio e la Cura Dei Tumori
Via Venezia 1
20133 Milano, Italy

Umberto Veronesi, M.D.
Gianni Bonadonna, M.D.
Natale Cascinelli, M.D.
Sergio Orefice, M.D.
Maurizio Vaglini, M.D.

European Organization for Research on Treatment of Cancer

Institut Jules Bordet
rue Heger-Bordet 1
1000 Brussels, Belgium

Henri J. Tagnon, M.D., President
Maurice J. Staquet, M.D., Director, Coordinating and Data Center

NCI-PAHO Collaborative Cancer Treatment Research Program

Pan American Health Organization
525 23rd St., NW
Washington, DC 20037
202-861-3332

Jorge Litvak, M.D., Program Director
Rodrigo Prado, M.D., Medical Director
Magaly Henson, Administrator

National Cancer Institute, NIH
Bethesda, MD 20205

Franco Muggia, M.D., NCI Coordinator, 212-340-7227
Elise W. Mackie, Administrator, 301-496-6056

SOURCE: *Membership Roster, Cancer Clinical Trials Groups and Projects.* Cancer Therapy Evaluation Program, Division of Cancer Treatment, National Cancer Institute, Department of Health and Human Services, September 1981.

Appendix 13.2. *Investigational Drug Distribution Update (September 1980)*

In July 1979, the *DCT Bulletin* reported an updated listing of investigational drugs classified according to one of three categories that correlate with specific development objectives and distribution procedures. The current system was designed in 1977 to comply with FDA regulations and to maximize the amount of information obtained from studies of drugs under IND sponsorship by DCT. The bulletin will continue to report a current listing of drugs of investigational status within each category on a yearly basis, with summaries of status changes in the interim editions. A brief description of each category of drugs follows with a current listing of all drugs in each category.

Group A Drugs

This group includes drugs in phase I clinical trials and phase II clinical trials in specified signal tumors. Protocol acceptance and drug distribution are limited to intramural investigators, members of the phase I and II working group, cancer therapy evaluation program contractors, and cooperative groups designated to carry out these phase I and II studies.

Group A_1 (Phase I)

αTDGR (NSC 71851)
AT-125 (NSC 163501)
Heroin (NSC 302357)
Amygdalin D (NSC 15780)
Amygdalin DL (NSC 251222)
Aminothiadiazole (NSC 4728)
BUdR (NSC 38297)
Aclacinomycin (NSC 208734)
Dichloroallyl-Lawsone (NSC 126771)
AZQ (NSC 182986)
Misonidazole (IV) (NSC 261037)
2′-deoxycoformycin (Pentostatin) (NSC 218321)

Group A_2 (Phase II)

DON (NSC 7365)
Gallium nitrate (NSC 15200)
Methyl-G (NSC 32946)
Indicine-N-oxide (NSC 132319)
ICRF-187 (NSC 169780)

Chlorozotocin (NSC 178248)
Thioguanine (IV) (NSC 752)
Cycloleucine (NSC 1026)
F3TDR (NSC 75520)
PCNU (NSC 95466)
Diglycolaldehyde (NSC 118994)
Cyclocytidine (NSC 145688)
Alanosine (NSC 153353)
Thymidine (NSC 21548)
PMM (NSC 118742)
3-Deazauridine (NSC 126849)
Zinostatin (NSC 157365)
Bruceantin (NSC 165563)
PALA (NSC 224131)
Mitoxantrone (NSC 301739)
Misonidazole (oral) (NSC 261037)

Group B Drugs

This group includes drugs tested in initial phase II studies and deemed of clinical interest in the new drug liaison meetings and by the cancer therapy evaluation program staff. Protocol acceptance and drug distribution are extended to include cooperative groups, NCI contractors, and cancer centers through the new drug studies mechanisms.

Group B_1—Drugs for the New Drug Studies Mechanism, DCT Contractors, and Cooperative Groups

DMSO (NSC 736)
ICRF-159 (NSC 129943)
TMCA (NSC 36354)
Dibromodulcitol (NSC 104800)
Dianhydrogalctitol (NSC 132313)
Piperazinedione (NSC 135758)
Melphalan IV (NSC 8806)
VM-26 (NSC 122819)
AMSA (NSC 249992)

Group B_2—Drugs Available Only to DCT Contractors and Cooperative Groups

Methotrexate (NSC 740)
Calcium leucovorin (NSC 3590)
Isophosphamide (NSC 109724)
BCG-Tice (NSC 116327B)
BCG-Pasteur (NSC 116328B)
BCG-Connaught (NSC 116341B)
BCG-MER (NSC 143769)
Levamisole (NSC 177023)
C. parvum (NSC 220537)

Group B_3—Drugs Available Only for Existing Studies

6-Mercaptopurine (IV) (NSC 755)
Procarbazine (IV) (NSC 77213)
TIC-HN_2 (NSC 82196)
Yoshi-864 (NSC 102627)
Ftorafur (NSC 148958)
Anguidine (NSC 141537)
Pyrazofurin (NSC 143095)
Maytansine (NSC 153858)
Dichloromethotrexate (NSC 29630)
Streptonigrin (NSC 45383)
Azapicyl (NSC 68626)
Nafoxidine (NSC 70735)
β-TGDR (NSC 71261)
Phenestrin (NSC 104469)
Triazinate (NSC 139105)

Group B_4—Existing INDs Will Be Closed

IMPY (NSC 51143)
Camptothecin (NSC 100880)
Rubidazone (NSC 164011)
Azaguanine (NSC 749)
Tubercidin (NSC 56408)
Thalicarpine (NSC 68075)

Group C Drugs

Group C includes drugs that demonstrate efficacy within a tumor type in more than one study, alter the pattern of care of the disease in question, and are safely administered by properly trained physicians without requiring specialized supportive care facilities. This classification includes:

Streptozotocin (NSC 85998)—for islet cell carcinoma of the pancreas, carcinoid

MeCCNU (NSC 95441)—for carcinoma of the colon and stomach, melanoma

Azacytidine (NSC 102816)—for refractory AML

Erwinia asparaginase (NSC 106977)—for ALL inpatients sensitive to *E. coli* L-asparaginase

Hexamethylmelamine (NSC 13875)—for ovarian carcinoma

VP-16-213 (NSC 141540)—for small cell carcinoma of the lung

THC* (NSC 134454)—for patients who have nausea and vomiting due to chemotherapy that is refractory to marketed antiemetics.

Group C drugs are also available for research protocol study as Group B_1 drugs. The procedure for drug distribution of Group C drugs (except THC*) is:

1. A physician must be registered with the National Cancer Institute as an investigator by having completed an FD-Form 1573.
2. A written request for the drug, indicating the disease to be treated, must be submitted.
3. The use of the drugs shall be limited to indications outlined in the guidelines that will be provided to the investigator.
4. All adverse reactions must be reported to the Investigational Drug Branch.

*In contrast to the usual procedures for obtaining Group C drugs, THC will be distributed by hospital pharmacies registered with NCI as designated distribution facilities. At this time, more than 300 pharmacies are registered with NCI to participate in the program. Physicians requiring information on particular pharmacies in their local areas should contact the Office of the Chief, Investigational Drug Branch, CTEP, DCT, National Cancer Institute, Building 37, Room 6E20, Bethesda, Maryland 20205.

fourteen

Hyperthermia

CHARLES D. KOWAL

One of the emerging cancer therapies of this decade will be hyperthermia, or heat. Interest in this form of therapy has grown substantially during recent years. Extensive reviews (Cavaliere et al. 1967; Field and Bleehen 1979) are available, including in vitro tissue culture and animal studies. There are also lists of references (Atkinson 1979) and abstracts (Barlogie 1979).

Reports on the use of hyperthermia in cancer treatment are actually quite old, one of the earliest reports having appeared in about 1866. The patient with a histologically proved facial sarcoma had complete disappearance of tumor following two attacks of erysipelas associated with high fever, and remained free of disease two years later. Numerous additional reports subsequently reinforced the observation that a substantial proportion of patients with cancer who experienced high fevers associated with infection had complete disappearance of their tumor. These studies led to the deliberate infection of patients with cancer using mixed bacteria (Coley's toxin) to induce fever. Use of such toxins to produce a heat state for cancer therapy confuses our understanding of the contribution of heat itself to the destruction of tumors. Introduction by toxin of components with vasoactive and immunologic properties is one area of uncertainty. The effect of heat alone on tumor destruction remains obscure.

Crile (1963) implanted sarcoma (S 180) cells in the legs of mice and immersed their limbs in water of various temperatures for different lengths of time. Two important observations were made from this study. First, it was learned that a majority of animals could be cured of their tumors by hyperthermia treatments of various duration and intensity. The relationship between temperature duration and intensity was observed to be an inverse one. Thus therapy with higher temperatures for shorter periods of time is as effective as that at lower temperatures for longer periods of time, at least within limits. The second important observation was that treatment at 43° C for 70 minutes killed the tumor and cured a majority of the animals. More than five times longer duration of exposure at the same temperature was required to cause necrosis of normal tissues. The significance of this was the notion that tumor cells are more sensitive to heat than normal cells.

In a pioneering study, Cavaliere and co-workers (1967) gave intraarterial regional hyperthermia perfusions using heated blood to 22 patients with cancers of the limbs. Patients were given treatments of 41.5° to 43.5° C for one to six hours. Although toxicity was significant, 50% of the patients showed complete disappearance of their disease. This study unequivocally demonstrated that hyperthermia can be effective in eradicating tumors.

Since the time of this study, many subsequent ones have extended some of the early observations with important results.

1. Tumor cells are intrinsically more heat-sensitive than normal tissues at temperatures in the range of 40° to 45° C. This difference allows for a measure of specificity in the treatment of cancer,

whereby tumor cells are selectively killed and normal cells are not.

2. The sensitivity of tumor cells to hyperthermia may be markedly increased by the cellular environment. The conditions that produce sensitivity over baseline values are low pH, low oxygen tension, and diminished nutrient supply. Significantly, these are the conditions that are present in solid tumors, suggesting that they may have greater heat sensitivity than cell suspensions.

3. Solid tumors have significantly less blood flow, and therefore significantly less ability to dissipate heat than normal tissues. This has led some to suggest that differences in blood flow-related heat dissipation will further add to the selective effects of heat on cancer. Additionally, some recent studies have shown that hyperthermia leads to a reduction in tumor blood flow, which may further augment the effects of cellular environment toward increased tumor cytotoxicity.

4. Hyperthermia appears to be synergistic with radiation therapy. Significantly lower doses of radiation may be used in combination with heat to achieve the same degree of tumor cell kill as with radiation alone at 37° C. Additionally, hyperthermia has been shown to be more lethal to hypoxic tumor cells than to oxygenated tumor cells, whereas radiation therapy is known to be more lethal to oxygenated tumor cells. On this basis the two treatment modalities are quite complementary.

5. Hyperthermia also appears to be synergistic with many chemotherapeutic agents, as listed below.

Cisplatin
Cyclophosphamide
Mechlorethamine
Melphalan
Thiotepa
Mitomycin
5-Fluorouracil
Dactinomycin
Doxorubicin
Bleomycin
Nitrosoureas: carmustine (BCNU), lomustine (CCNU), and semustine (MeCCNU)

Extensive systematic studies with all of these drugs have not been done, and other agents have been studied only briefly. Bull and associates (1979) studied doxorubicin and a nitrosourea in humans with whole-body hyperthermia. Barlogie and colleagues (1979) used etoposide (VP-16), and at the Baltimore Cancer Research Center cyclophosphamide is under study in conjunction with whole-body heating.

As discussed by Kowal and Bertino (1979), the potential benefits of hyperthermia added to chemotherapy may be substantial. The degree of synergism between the modalities is in the range of several additional logs of cell kill, and at temperatures that are achievable clinically. The use of hyperthermia and chemotherapy may allow for an improvement in response with tumors that are now relatively unresponsive to drugs, for example, colon or pancreatic carcinomas. Alternatively, hyperthermia may be used to reduce the amount of chemotherapy necessary to achieve a given degree of tumor reponse, as has been done with thiotepa for bladder tumors.

The mechanism by which hyperthermia potentiates the cell kill of a given chemotherapeutic agent remains to be elucidated. Hahn, Braun, and Har-Kedar (1975) have looked at bleomycin uptake in Chinese hamster ovary (CHO) cells at normal and elevated temperatures. This agent is quite synergistic with hyperthermia and results in a significant tumor cell kill. Surprisingly, less bleomycin uptake occurs at elevated temperatures where there is synergistic cell kill, than that occurring at 37° C. Little additional work with the drug has been done to explain this observation. We do not know whether synergism between hyperthermia and chemotherapy is the same for all drugs, or whether it is different for each class of agent. Although the mechanism is not known, the important fact remains that it exists.

This is not the case with all drugs at all the temperatures that have been used. Bleomycin, for example, shows little synergism with hyperthermia at temperatures below 42° C. Since whole-body hyperthermia is generally limited to temperatures at or below this temperature, Hahn has suggested that certain drugs may be useful only for local heating, where temperatures well above 42° C can be achieved. The implications of this are important. The observation of a temperature threshold for bleomycin synergism has only been made in CHO cells, however, not in other cell lines, and not in animals.

Weinstein and co-workers (1979) have used local hyperthermia to study methotrexate uptake from liposomes in Lewis lung tumors transplanted in mice. The lipid composition of the liposomes had a transition temperature (Tc) of 42° C. The authors claim to have heated the tumors to 43° C using a microwave apparatus. They felt that local heating of the tumor above the Tc of liposomes would lead to increased methotrexate concentrations in the tumor as the liposomes passed into the heated field and released their drug. They observed a 360% increase of tritiated methotrexate in tumors as compared to appropriate controls following exposure of drug-laden liposomes to local hyperthermia. This result is quite intriguing, and has significance for drug delivery systems and for hyperthermia.

Methods for Producing Hyperthermia

Heat treatments may be given in several ways, and can be conveniently divided into whole-body and local heating categories.

- Systemic or whole-body heating
  - Mixed bacteria (Coley's toxin)
  - Radiant heat
  - Beeswax encapsulation
  - Radiofrequency
  - Water blanket
  - Extracorporeal blood heating
- Localized heating
  - Ultrasound
  - Radiofrequency
    - a. Microwave region
    - b. Low megahertz region
  - Limb immersion
  - Perfusion of limb
  - Forced air
  - Radiant heat

We shall consider only those techniques applicable to treating humans.

Whole-Body Heating

Because of limited tolerance to systemic temperature elevations, whole-body hyperthermia is limited to temperatures in the 41.8° to 42.0° C range. It would appear to be more suitable as therapy for patients with widely disseminated tumors. The technique in humans has been studied in several centers.

One of the first efforts at introducing systemic hyperthermic states directly to patients has been by Pettigrew and colleagues (1974). Their technique insulates against heat loss by encapsulating the patient in beeswax. It introduces additional heat other than by metabolism from the latent heat of fusion obtained from the change of state of the beeswax, and from warmed dry respiratory gases. Their report indicates that 272 treatment sessions with over 665 treatment hours at core body temperatures over 40° C had been performed. There were 4 deaths within 48 hours of hyperthermia from a sample of 82 patients. Toxicity included circumoral herpes simplex in 50%, occasional sore throats, and a few instances of superficial burns or pressure sores. Over 150 patients have now been treated using this technique. It has been found to be a relatively safe procedure, provided that esophageal temperatures are limited to 41.8° C.

The technique of Larkin, Edwards, and Smith (1976) involved heating patients by wrapping them in a plastic water blanket. The temperature of the water was adjusted to yield a body temperature of 41.9° C. The patients were intubated under light general anesthesia. They treated over 77 patients, with over 170 treatments, and more than 580 hours at core body temperatures at or above 41.5° C. They reported no deaths during treatment, although five patients with advanced disease did die in the days following hyperthermia. Several of these patients had massive hepatic tumors. The authors felt that by proper selection, deaths attributable to the procedure should be avoidable. Other toxicity includes mild metabolic acidosis, dilutional hyponatremia, mild hypocalcemia, hypokalemia, hypomagnesemia, hypophosphatemia, leukocytosis, and mild thrombocytopenia. All of these changes occurred during therapy and were corrected with cessation of treatment. No signs of pulmonary, renal, or central nervous system dysfunction were seen, nor was there any evidence of persistent or subsequent marrow toxicity.

Parks and Smith (1980) have used an extracorporeal blood-warming device that involved surgical intervention with the patient's arteriovenous system. Heated blood was circulated from the machine to the patient, and fluid could be easily added to the vascular space. Although they claimed lower morbidity than with other techniques using heated perfusate in a limb, no complete data are as yet available. Extracorporeal blood heating may offer some advantages over other methods for whole-body hyperthermia because there is some suggestion that increased tumor cell kill may be obtained when the patient's temperature is raised to 41.8° C in a relatively short time. Extracorporeal heating can raise a person's temperature from 37° C to 41.8° C in about 30 minutes, whereas other techniques, such as those used by Bull or Larkin, require approximately 120 to 360 minutes to reach 41.8° C.

The technique used by Bull and colleagues (1979) initially involved the use of a NASA hot-water space suit to heat patients to 41.9° C for four hours. This suit was expensive and cumbersome. Bull also used plastic water-heating blankets to raise temperatures. The patients were lightly anesthetised, but were not intubated and breathed room air without assistance. Toxicity appeared to be minimal. It consisted primarily of fatigue, decreased appetite, nausea, diarrhea, posttreatment fever, and transient neuropathy, but in only some of the patients. The duration of these symptoms was relatively short. No CNS or persistent marrow toxicity or major electrolyte disturbances were seen, nor have there been any deaths during treatment or within a seven-day period following treatment. Of all of the techniques for whole-body hyperthermia, this one would appear to be the safest and least invasive.

Results of Clinical Studies

Pettigrew and co-workers (1974) have treated patients with whole-body hyperthermia alone and in combination with either chemotherapy or radiotherapy. Hyperthermia was achieved by beeswax encapsulation. Objective responses were seen in 22 of 49 with hyperthermia alone, 12 of 15 with hyperthermia and chemotherapy, and 3 of 3 with hyperthermia and radiotherapy. The nature of the chemotherapy was not specified. Inasmuch as there was no group treated with chemotherapy alone, the contribution of either heat or drug cannot be assessed. Nevertheless, the results for patients who have failed conventional therapy are promising. High response rates were seen in soft tissue sarcomas and neuroblastomas, with moderately high response rates in cancer of the colon and lung, and melanomas.

Larkin, Edwards, and Smith (1976) treated 77 patients with whole-body hyperthermia with a 43% objective response rate to heat alone, and with 6% of patients showing complete disappearance of disease. Three of these patients had melanoma. Many had a marked reduction in pain.

In the series of Bull and co-workers (1979), 38% of patients had disease progression during treatment; however, 31% showed stabilization of disease, and an additional 31% showed a response to heat alone. These authors observed objective responses in one patient each with melanoma, colon, rectal, and adrenal tumors.

Barlogie's group (1979) failed to obtain any partial or complete responses to treatment with heat alone. Four of eleven patients did show objective regression of tumor. They found significant toxicity, including seizures, in 6 of 11 patients, which prevented these patients from receiving further therapy. The use of nitrous oxide anesthesia during treatments may be a contributing factor in toxicity.

Whole-body hyperthermia is now under study at a number of institutions. Some trials are addressing the question of which technique is the best, and others are looking at the combination of heat and chemotherapy.

Local Hyperthermia

Delivery of heat to a portion of the body is more suitable for clinical situations involving tumors that are not widespread, or where only a portion of the body needs to be treated. Because more heat-sensitive organs such as liver or brain are usually outside the heated field, higher temperatures may be used in local hyperthermia than can be used in whole-body therapy. Because the use of higher temperatures means more tumor cell kill, this advantage is likely to be of clinical importance. Several techniques have been used to produce local heating in humans.

Radiofrequency heating. Two types of radiofrequency heating have been used—capacitatively coupled, and inductively coupled. In the former, the tissue is placed between two applicators or electrodes, and heat is given. Heating depends on tissue resistance and current flow. Tissues containing fat are more easily heated than those containing water. More energy is deposited on surface tissues than on deeper tissues, and despite water-cooling of the electrodes, skin burns have occurred.

Inductive radiofrequency heating depends mainly on tissue-magnetic properties and the induction of current flow by the generation of a locally intensive magnetic field. Both kinds of devices have used frequencies of 13.56 MHz or in the range of 20 to 30 MHz. At these frequencies the radiofrequency wave will penetrate the body.

Microwave heating. Numerous investigators have used microwaves to generate local heat. Heating depends on electrode power output, applicator radiation pattern, and tissue absorption of microwave energy. Absorption is dependent on the dielectric properties of the tissues, and results primarily from excitation of rotational states. Penetration of microwaves into tissues is less than that of lower-frequency radiofrequency waves. Needles inserted into tumors have been used by some as microwave antennae, generating heat from within the tumor.

Ultrasound. Electrical excitation of piezoelectric crystals ranging from 1 to 3 MHz results in the generation of pressure waves that may be transmitted to tissue through a coupling medium and dissipated as heat. The rate of energy transfer depends on absorption coefficients of the tissue. For example, bone absorbs more than skin, with muscle showing moderate absorption, and fat showing the least. The range of frequencies used for hyperthermia, 1 to 3 MHz, was derived when it was shown that higher frequencies do not readily penetrate body tissue, and that lower frequencies do not generate as much heat. Ultrasound has been shown to destroy tumor tissue in human neoplasms. Unlike radiofrequency heating, ultrasound heating does depend on the presence of a coupling medium, and cannot penetrate through air without significant loss of power. It is not suitable for treating lung neoplasms, for example, that are surrounded by parenchyma containing air. Of significant advantage is the fact that ultrasound heating may be focused to concentrate its energy for deposition into very small volumes.

Limitations

Regional perfusion of limbs with heated blood and chemotherapy, such as that used by Cavaliere and associates (1967), requires invasive surgery associated with significant morbidity. It is only suitable for those few situations in which a patient's tumor is confined to a distal portion of an extremity, and not for cranial, thoracic, or abdominal tumors.

Most of the disadvantages and limitations have to do with inability to heat a volume of tissue with minimal toxicity, and difficulties with dosimetry. With radiofrequency and microwave heating, it is not possible to use conventional, clinically applicable, temperature-sensing devices such as thermistors or thermocouples. This is because they will be affected by the radiofrequency field, and the temperature measurement will be distorted. Although there are nonperturbing temperature probes, they are not yet widely available and their cost is so prohibitive as to make them essentially unsuitable for clinical use. The difficulty in measuring temperature with radiofrequency and microwave devices means that the configuration of the heated volume produced by the device is difficult or impossible to define accurately. Accuracy is important, as a variation of as little as 0.5° C can make a significant difference in the amount of cell kill.

LeVeen and co-workers (1976) reported some benefit using radiofrequency hyperthermia on human patients; however, their study was poorly controlled. Marmor and associates (1979) have used unfocused ultrasound to treat patients with surface tumors that have failed prior treatment with radiation and chemotherapy. They report an objective response rate of 66%, with 52% partial responses and 14% complete responses in a group of 21 patients. A subgroup of patients with squamous cell carcinoma showed a higher response rate, with 80% (8 of 10) partial responses, and 10% (1 of 10) complete responses. Toxicity was superficial burns (19%), central tumor necrosis (15%), and pain (38%).

Lele and colleagues (1980) have treated 43 patients with advanced disease using focused ultrasound. About half of the patients had squamous cell cancers of the head and neck. All received six weekly treatments consisting of 42.5° to 43° C for 20 minutes. Response was excellent, with 10% of the patients having complete disappearance of disease, and approximately 70% showing a partial response. In contrast to other studies using unfocused ultrasound, no skin burns, pain, or central tumor necrosis was observed. In effect, the treatments were nontoxic. Because of the nature of this multiinstitutional trial, little can be said about the duration of responses. With these and other studies there now is no doubt that hyperthermia can eradicate tumors. Just what human tumors are the most heat-sensitive, and just what are the best combinations of duration and temperature remain to be elucidated. In all probability, hyperthermia will be most effective when combined with either radiation or chemotherapy, or both.

In general, the results of many studies appear to suggest that there is benefit from a combination of hyperthermia and radiation. Extensive prospective randomized trials, however, have not been done. Kim, Hahn, and Tokita (1978) showed that this combination in patients with melanoma resulted in 79% CRs versus only 22% CRs for radiation alone. Bicher, Sandhu, and Hetzel (1980) have used a regimen consisting of four microwave hyperthermia treatments, 45° C for 90 minutes every three days, followed after an interval of one week by four treatments of combined hyperthermia and radiation. For the combined modality the hyperthermia was given as before, and radiation consisted of 1600 rad given with hyperthermia every three days in 400-rad fractions. This study has now accumulated over 100 patients who had already failed curative radiation therapy. Complete responses were seen in about 60%, and partial responses in about 35%. It is still too early to completely assess duration of response, with the follow-up period ranging from 2 to 12 months. Similar promising results with a smaller group have been seen by Arcangeli and associates (1980) using combined radiation and hyperthermia. Misonidazole, a hypoxic-cell sensitizer, plus radiation therapy and hyperthermia added nothing in this study.

Li and colleagues (1980) have studied the use of intraluminal microwave hyperthermia alone and in combination with radiation therapy in esophageal cancer. Combined modality treatments consisted of one to six heat treatments, 44° to 46° C for 30 minutes, plus radiation of 4000 rad over four weeks. Of 93 patients, 11 had subsequent surgical resection of their tumor. These patients were compared to other similar-sized groups of patients with esophageal cancer who had surgical resection following treatment with heat only, radiation therapy only (6000 rad/4 weeks), and controls receiving no treatment. Three of eleven patients given combination therapy had no histologic evidence of tumor at the time of surgery, whereas all patients in the other groups had evidence of residual tumor at surgery. Six-month survival was 63% for patients given "curative" radiation (6000 rad/4 weeks) alone, as compared to 86% for heat plus lower-dose radiation (4000 rad/4 weeks). Longer-term evaluation of survival is now in progress.

A few studies in humans have been done with a combination of local hyperthermia plus chemotherapy. One interesting study (Arcangeli et al. 1979) used either doxorubicin (Adriamycin) or bleomycin, alone or in combination with microwave local hyperthermia, in patients with head and neck squamous cell carcinomas metastatic to the neck. Drug treatments were given twice daily every other day alone or with hyperthermia, 43° to 45° C for 45 minutes. Complete responses to drug only were in the 0% to 15% range, and adding partial responses (PR) brought overall response rates to about 30% for each of the two drug groups. Combined drug and local hyperthermia, however, produced about 40% CR and 60% PR in both drug groups. Toxicity was noted to be minimal and mild.

References

Arcangeli, G. et al. Enhanced effectiveness of Adriamycin and bleomycin combined with local hyperthermia in neck node metastases from head and neck cancers. *Tumori* 65:481–486, 1979.

Arcangeli, G. et al. Multiple daily fractionization (MDF) radiotherapy in association with hyperthermia and/or misonidazole. Experimental and clinical results. *Cancer* 45:2707–2711, 1980.

Atkinson, E. R. Assessment of current hyperthermia technology. Cancer Res. 39:2313–2324, 1979.

Barlogie, B. Selected abstracts on hyperthermia as a modality for cancer therapy. In *International cancer research data bank monograph*. Bethesda, Md.: National Cancer Institute, 1979.

Barlogie, B. et al. Total-body hyperthermia with and without chemotherapy for advanced human neoplasms. *Cancer Res.* 39:1481–1489, 1979.

Bicher, H. I.; Sandhu, T. S.; and Hetzel, F. W. Clinical thermoradiotherapy. *Henry Ford Hospital Medical Journal* 29:10–15, 1981.

Bull, J. M. et al. Whole-body hyperthermia: a phase-I trial of a potential adjuvant to chemotherapy. *Ann. Intern. Med.* 90:317–323, 1979.

Cavaliere, R. et al. Selective heat sensitivity of cancer cells. *Cancer* 20:1351–1381, 1967.

Crile, G. The effects of heat and radiation on cancers implanted on the feet of mice. *Cancer Res.* 23:372–380, 1963.

Field, S. B., and Bleehen, N. M. Hyperthermia in the treatment of cancer. *Cancer Treat. Rev.* 6:63–94, 1979.

Hahn, G. M.; Braun, J.; and Har-Kedar, I. Thermochemotherapy: synergism between hyperthermia (42-43° C) and Adriamycin (or bleomycin) in mammalian cell inactivation. *Proc. Natl. Acad. Sci.* 72:937–940, 1975.

Kim, J. H.; Hahn, E. W.; and Tokita, N. Combination hyperthermia and radiation therapy for cutaneous malignant melanoma. *Cancer* 41:2143–2148, 1978.

Kowal, C. D., and Bertino, J. R. Possible benefits of hyperthermia to chemotherapy. *Cancer Res.* 39:2285–2289, 1979.

Larkin, J. M.; Edwards, W. S.; and Smith, D. E. Total-body hyperthermia and preliminary results in human neoplasms. *Surg. Forum* 27:121–123, 1976.

Lele, P. P. et al. Treatment of advanced squamous cell cancers of the head and neck region by local hyperthermia by focused ultrasound. Presented at the International Head and Neck Oncology Research Conference, September 8–10, 1980, Roslyn, Virginia.

LeVeen, H. H. et al. Tumor eradication by radiofrequency therapy. *JAMA* 235:2198–2200, 1976.

Li, D. J. et al. Intraluminal microwave hyperthermia in the combined treatment of esophageal cancer. A preliminary report on 103 cases. Presented at the Third International Symposium on Cancer Therapy by Hyperthermia, Drugs and Radiation, June 22-26, 1980, Fort Collins, Colorado.

Marmor, J. B. et al. Treatment of superficial human neoplasms by local hyperthermia induced by ultrasound. *Cancer* 43:188–197, 1979.

Parks, L., and Smith, G. Whole-body hyperthermia by means of extracorporeal heating. Presented at the Third International Symposium on Cancer Therapy by Hyperthermia, Drugs, and Radiation, June 22–26, 1980, Fort Collins, Colorado.

Pettigrew, R. T. et al. Clinical effects of whole body hyperthermia in advanced malignancy. *Br. Med. J.* 4:679–682, 1974.

Weinstein, J. N. et al. Liposomes and local hyperthermia: selective delivery of methotrexate to heated tumors. *Science* 204:188–191, 1979.

Additional Readings

Conference on Hyperthermia in Cancer Treatment, American Cancer Society, San Diego, California, September 15–16. *Cancer Res.* 39:2231–2340, 1979.

Jain, R. K., and Gullino, P. M., eds. Thermal characteristics of tumors: applications in detection and treatment. *Ann. NY Acad. Sci.* 335:1–542, 1980.

Proceedings of the International Symposium on Cancer Therapy by Hyperthermia and Radiation, April 28–30, 1975, Washington, D.C., American College of Radiology.

Proceedings of the Second International Symposium on Cancer Therapy by Hyperthermia and Radiation, eds. C. Streffer et al. Essen, Germany: Urban & Schwarzenberg, 1978.

The Third International Symposium on Cancer Therapy by Hyperthermia, Drugs, and Radiation, June 22–26, 1980, Fort Collins, Colorado.

fifteen

Immunotherapy

JOHN C. MARSH
DANIEL S. KAPP

The past decade has seen great interest in the clinical immunotherapy of cancer. As Terry (1980) has pointed out, this has been due largely to the assumptions that (1) human cancer cells have antigens that persist from the time the malignant cells develop until the cancer is clinically apparent; (2) these antigens are recognizable by the human immune system; (3) they are capable of eliciting an effector response by cellular or humoral components of the immune response; and (4) the antigens must serve as a site for antibody- or cell-mediated damage to tumor cells. Antigens with all these characteristics have not yet been found on any human cancer cells.

Immunotherapy is not yet established as an effective mode of anticancer treatment and should not become part of standard practice. The results of many clinical trials have led to the generation of more trials; in general they have been negative when well controlled and randomized, in contrast to some positive trials when historical controls or nonrandomized techniques are used. Similarly, it is possible to see positive results from the early analysis of trials with small numbers, while those continuing for a longer time with larger numbers of patients are often negative.

Clinical trials using immunotherapy will continue, but once again, as Terry (1980) has indicated, more knowledge about the surface membranes of malignant cells and the ability to develop highly specific antibodies capable of reacting with unique antigens or antigens present in high concentration may be the most fertile directions for immunotherapy, rather than generalized stimulation of the immune system. Some theoretically possible (and experimentally demonstrable) types of immunotherapy are outlined below.*

I. Non-specific
    A. BCG (or methanol-extractable residue (MER))
    B. *Corynebacterium parvum*
    C. Levamisole
II. Specific-active
    A. Immunization by tumor cells, either intact, killed, or altered by enzymes or virus
III. Specific-passive
    A. Transfer of immune cells
    B. Transfer of subcellular fractions
        1. RNA
        2. Transfer factor
    C. Transfer of antitumor antibodies

This chapter summarizes the current status of clinical immunotherapy in certain malignant diseases.

Melanoma

Perhaps of all cancers, melanoma has attracted the greatest interest in the potential of immunotherapy. This is related to the ability to predict patients at high risk of

*Adapted from Goodnight and Morton 1978.

recurrence (thickness and/or anatomic depth of skin involvement, involvement of regional nodes), the rather long disease-free interval in some patients before recurrence, and the impressive incidence of spontaneous regression, both of primary tumors and even of metastases. The development of halo nevi and vitiligo has been interpreted to mean an active host-immune response, with the intradermal location of melanoma being "ideal for the induction of cellular immune reactivity, which could be enhanced by immunotherapy" (Spitler and Sagebiel 1980). The ability of BCG to induce regression of intradermal lesions of melanoma when injected into them has been well documented (Morton et al. 1974). This phenomenon has led to numerous therapeutic trials with BCG given as an adjuvant both to surgery in primary disease and to chemotherapy for metastatic disease. The trials have been controlled and noncontrolled, randomized and nonrandomized, injected near the original lesions, and injected at many different sites (fig. 15.1). There have been numerous schedules, methods of administration, doses, sources of BCG, and different strains used, so that it is possible to raise objections to nearly every study that has been done. One may summarize them by saying that several early uncontrolled or nonrandomized studies have shown an apparent beneficial effect when BCG is used as a surgical adjuvant, but that controlled randomized studies have not shown any effect that is statistically significant.

A study by Gutterman and co-workers (1978b) from M. D. Anderson Hospital using historical controls indicated a positive effect for high-dose, but not low-dose, Tice BCG in terms of disease-free interval and survival when the agent was given postoperatively. The positive effect was seen in patients with melanoma of the trunk in whom the regional lymphatics were exposed to BCG, but not in head and neck disease in which the lymphatics were not exposed, and it was suggested that a regional effect of BCG is required.

The UCLA group initially found a positive effect of BCG in a "simultaneously controlled but nonrandomized" study (Eilber et al. 1976). A more recent randomized controlled trial with 94 patients using BCG, BCG plus tumor cells, or no therapy following surgery shows a trend in favor of the immunotherapy (disease-free interval and survival) but has not achieved statistical significance (Morton et al. 1978).

A large cooperative group study (Cunningham et al. 1978) showed no activity for BCG as a surgical adjuvant and no difference between BCG or BCG plus DTIC in the subgroup of patients with melanoma of the trunk and positive lymph nodes.

BCG had no activity as a surgical adjuvant in a controlled study (Pinsky et al. 1978b). In a European study, a trend was developing for some beneficial effect of BCG, DTIC, or the combination, as compared to a control group treated by surgery alone, but significance had not been determined at the time of reporting (Beretta et al. 1978).

The combination of BCG with DTIC was more effective in preventing recurrence than either agent used alone as reported in a surgical adjuvant study in a small randomized trial from the Massachusetts General Hospital (Wood et al. 1978). Preliminary results from a large World Health Organization trial found this combination to be of no value (cited by Terry 1980). A controlled trial using levamisole was negative overall, although there was a trend at borderline statistical significance favoring the drug in patients with stage I, but not stage II, disease (Spitler and Sagebiel 1980).

Advanced metastatic disease has also been treated with various types of immunotherapy, usually in addition to chemotherapy. In a randomized trial from the Southwest Oncology Group, BCG did not improve the response rate with either DTIC or the combination of DTIC, hydroxyurea, and BCNU (Costanzi 1978).

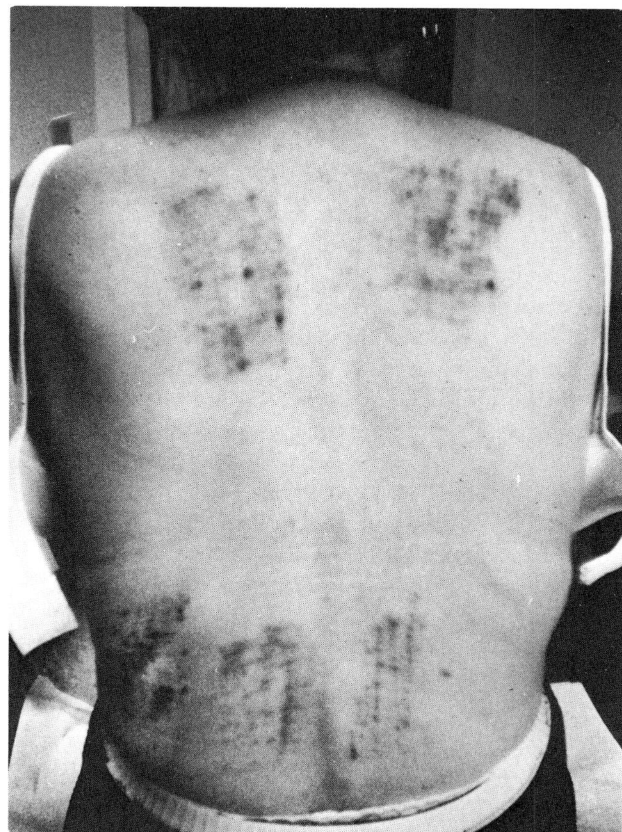

Fig. 15.1. *Patient with melanoma treated with dacarbazine and BCG applied by template. Rash and reaction are seen in each of the template sites.*

The response rate to methyl-CCNU was also not improved by BCG and killed melanoma cells (Mastrangelo et al. 1978).

Gutterman and associates (1978b), using historical controls, reported that BCG added to DTIC improved the survival of patients so treated but did not improve the response rate.

Corynebacterium parvum intravenously did not improve the results with DTIC and cyclophosphamide (Presant et al. 1978).

BCG with neuraminidase-treated autologous cells did not show benefit as either a surgical adjuvant or when added to DTIC in advanced disease (Simmons et al. 1978).

The preliminary results of a randomized controlled trial using BCG and plasma containing so-called "unblocking" activity (from black donors) showed no benefit compared to the use of plasma from white donors or, indeed, to no immunotherapy at all (Wright et al. 1978).

In summary, although there are suggestive pieces of information that indicate a small effect of immunotherapy in melanoma, no controlled study has yet shown clear benefit to the point where immunotherapy can be recommended as standard therapy.

Breast Cancer

One of the more encouraging studies is in inoperable (stage III) breast cancer treated with local radiotherapy with and without levamisole after completion of radiation (Rojas et al. 1978). The group taking levamisole had a superior disease-free interval (DFI) (median of 22.5 months vs 9 months) and survival (41.5 months vs 22 months) compared to the controls who were not given the drug. The patients (20 and 23 in the groups) were well matched with respect to TNM status and the control group resembled earlier historical controls in TNM distribution, DFI, and survival. Some patients taking levamisole had improvement in their ability to react to a dinitrochlorobenzene (DNCB) skin test; these patients did better as a group. The drug was given 150 mg for three days every other week. Toxicity was negligible. A second group of 93 such patients has been studied in an identical fashion with virtually identical results (Olivari et al. 1980).

In a controlled study that evaluated the addition of levamisole to CMF adjuvant chemotherapy for breast cancer, no advantage has been shown over CMF alone. The study is incomplete (mean follow-up time is 27.6 months) and not yet definitive (Forastiere et al. 1980).

The addition of *C. parvum* to combination chemotherapy of patients with advanced metastatic disease did not markedly improve the response rate or overall survival, but did significantly improve the survival of responders receiving *C. parvum* as compared to those on chemotherapy (Pinsky et al. 1978a). The *C. parvum* was given weekly, 4 mg subcutaneously.

Another smaller study that evaluated the effect of subcutaneous *C. parvum* added to combination chemotherapy in advanced disease has shown no benefit (Haskell et al. 1980).

BCG given by scarification on 3 days of a 21-day treatment cycle was added to combination chemotherapy in a noncontrolled study (Hortobagyi et al. 1978). The response rate was not increased compared to that with historical controls treated with only the same chemotherapy, but those receiving immunotherapy did have an increased remission duration and survival, with a survival gain of about six months. The usual cautions about historical controls apply.

Colorectal Cancer

The effects of immunotherapy with MER (methanol-extractable residue of BCG) combined with chemotherapy have been compared with chemotherapy alone at the Mayo Clinic (Moertel et al. 1978). In 181 patients with advanced disease treated with three chemotherapy regimens, MER did not improve the response rate, duration of remission, or survival. When given early with the chemotherapy, MER was associated with an increase in the severity of leukopenia.

Weekly BCG given with 5-FU produced no improvement in response rate or overall survival, but was associated with a somewhat longer duration of remission in that portion (34%) of patients who responded. This study contained a total of 47 patients (Engstrom et al. 1978).

Immunotherapy has been used alone and with chemotherapy as an adjuvant in colorectal cancer. The study of McPherson and colleagues (1980), not yet complete in 148 patients, shows no beneficial effect with oral BCG as compared to controls. There was an apparent improvement in DFI in patients with Dukes' B2 disease and worsening in those with Dukes' C cancer when oral BCG is combined with 5-FU and methyl-CCNU chemotherapy.

In a study using historical controls, patients with Dukes' C colorectal cancer were treated with oral 5-FU and BCG by scarification or BCG alone. Both groups were reported to have an increased DFI and survival compared to controls (Mavligit et al. 1978).

The Gastrointestinal Tumor Study Group trial of adjuvant chemotherapy and chemoimmunotherapy, and immunotherapy with MER currently in progress has shown no significant difference in DFI or survival in any of the groups as compared to controls after analysis of 566 patients (Lokich 1979).

Thus controlled randomized clinical trials in colorectal cancer have not defined a place for immunotherapy, either in the treatment of advanced disease or as adjuvant therapy.

Very recently, two positive trials using levamisole have been reported to the Second International Conference on Immunotherapy sponsored by the National Cancer Institute (NCI). My only specific source at this writing is *Oncology News,* vol. 6, no. 5, September–October 1980. As reported there, Borden and colleagues found a positive effect on survival when levamisole was added to 5-FU compared to 5-FU alone in advanced disease, while results with these therapies were no different when used as adjuvant treatment. These results are alluded to in a later abstract (Borden, Groveman, and Wolberg 1981). At the same conference, Verhaegen from Belgium reported that levamisole as adjuvant therapy improved the DFI as compared to a matched control group.

These studies with levamisole in colorectal cancer will need to be evaluated in more detail and extended, but use of that drug appears more promising than the use of BCG or MER as immunotherapy.

Acute Lymphoblastic Leukemia

A major step forward in the therapy of ALL seemed to have been taken when Mathé and co-workers (1969) reported that BCG and allogeneic leukemia cells could prolong remission after first induction, compared to unmaintained controls. A recent follow-up (Mathé et al. 1978) states that all of 10 controls relapsed within 4 months, while 7 of 20 in the immunotherapy group are still in their first complete remission 10 to 13 years later. Unfortunately, further attempts by many other groups and by the original group as well to confirm this have not been successful, and one must regretfully conclude that a place for immunotherapy in ALL has not yet been demonstrated, with the possible exception of levamisole.

A European group (Andrien et al. 1978) found that BCG and allogeneic cells did not prolong remission compared to maintenance chemotherapy after remission induction, consolidation for one year, and CNS prophylaxis. It might be argued that most of the important antitumor therapy has already been given by the time immunotherapy has started, but in this context it is at least as good as chemotherapy, but no better in maintaining remission.

In a large British trial (Kay 1978) patients were randomized after induction and CNS prophylaxis (21 weeks after beginning therapy) to receive no further treatment, BCG, or methotrexate. Duration of remission for patients in the last group was significantly superior to that with patients receiving BCG and no treatment (which were not different).

In a study from the NCI (Poplack et al. 1978) BCG plus allogeneic cells were compared to methotrexate as part of a complex cycling multidrug maintenance program following induction, consolidation, and CNS prophylaxis. It was designed to expose patients to immunotherapy early, but the results show no difference in relapse rates or remission duration.

In a large study with over 500 children, the Children's Cancer Study Group (Heyn et al. 1978) found that BCG or no treatment was equally inferior to chemotherapy in maintaining primary or secondary remission.

Levamisole has been reported to prolong the duration of chemotherapeutically maintained remission in low-risk (white blood cell count less than 50,000) children with ALL, but not to be effective in high-risk children or adults (Pavlovsky et al. 1980).

Acute Myeloblastic Leukemia

Attempts to use immunotherapy in AML have primarily involved BCG or other more specific putative immunostimulants such as allogeneic leukemia cells, sometimes altered by enzyme treatment or viral infection, to maintain remissions that have been accomplished by chemotherapy. Questions of dose, schedule, and type of BCG have complicated interpretation of these studies, as BCG is viable, may be unstable on storage, and a specific dose is hard to measure since proliferation of the organism may occur in the host after administration. Nevertheless, it is fair to say that some encouraging positive results have been found with this type of therapy in AML, much more so than is the case with ALL.

One of the best-known studies is that of Powles and co-workers (1973, 1978) from St. Bartholomew's Hospital, London, using weekly intradermal BCG and irradiated allogeneic leukemia cells given subcutaneously during maintenance chemotherapy. The median survival was significantly better than that of those receiving chemotherapy alone (510 days vs 210 days), although the duration of the first remission was not significantly longer. The frequency of a second chemotherapy-induced remission was higher in the immunotherapy group. It has been postulated that normal hematopoiesis might have been stimulated by the immunotherapy so that at relapse, tolerance for chemotherapy necessary to induce remission might be relatively greater.

Another study from Sweden and Austria (Reizenstein et al. 1978) with both randomized and nonrandomized patients had essentially the same results, using BCG and *viable* leukemic cells added to chemotherapy in the maintenance phase.

The Medical Research Council (MRC) in England attempted to duplicate the St. Bartholomew's study. With a somewhat larger number of patients, no benefit could be ascribed to immunotherapy (Peto 1978). All groups in this study did about as well as the superior immunotherapy group of Powles. The latter group was from an earlier time, and chemotherapy or better host-prognostic factors may have improved the later results of the MRC.

The results of a Southeastern Group study (Vogler et al. 1978), although positive, are different from the studies cited. Here BCG was given with methotrexate during remission maintenance; no significant benefit was observed on survival, but there was a modest improvement in the duration of the first remission.

When BCG was added to OAP (vincristine, cytarabine, prednisone) at the M. D. Anderson Hospital (Gutterman et al. 1978a) using historical controls, the results were similar to those of the early British study; that is, there was insignificant improvement in the duration of first remission but improvement in survival. A larger, properly randomized, controlled study done by the Southwestern group using the same chemotherapy and BCG was negative (Hewlett et al. 1978). The dose of BCG was, however, about one-third of that used in the M. D. Anderson study.

A study from Cardiff, Wales (Whittaker and Slater 1978) using intravenous BCG in addition to chemotherapy in a controlled trial showed a beneficial effect on survival but not on duration of remission.

It has been reported that allogeneic leukemia cells treated with neuraminidase extended remission duration in patients receiving chemotherapy, but that the same treatment combined with MER therapy as well was of no benefit (Holland and Bekesi 1978).

Use of allogeneic cells infected with a murine myxovirus did not show evidence of activity when combined with chemotherapy in the maintenance phase of AML (Sauter et al. 1978).

The interferon inducer, poly I:poly C was also inactive as an adjunct to maintenance chemotherapy in a cooperative group study (McIntyre et al. 1978).

When given both as an adjunct to induction therapy and to maintenance chemotherapy, MER is showing some suggestive benefit, but the study is still too early and the differences too small to be declared significant (Cuttner et al. 1978).

There is also suggestive benefit in terms of remission duration in patients given *Pseudomonas aeruginosa* vaccine during remission induction and consolidation. Remission rates were not enhanced. This vaccine was originally given in the hope that it might prevent *Pseudomonas* infections in AML, which it did not (Gee et al. 1978).

Osteosarcoma

The adjuvant therapy of osteogenic sarcoma, both immunotherapy and chemotherapy, has been complicated by disputes over the proper prognostic factors, the type of therapy, and the adequacy of historical controls. Although an uncontrolled study at Memorial Sloan–Kettering Cancer Center showed a trend in favor of the efficacy of a lysed autologous tumor cell vaccine, the differences were not statistically significant. A whole-cell vaccine did not show any activity (Miké and Marcove 1978). Transfer factor has also been tried as an adjuvant therapy without success (Ritts et al. 1978); BCG combined with allogeneic sarcoma cell vaccine was also unsuccessful in the adjuvant setting (Eilber et al. 1978).

Lymphoma

A cooperative group study in Hodgkin's disease testing the ability of BCG to prolong chemotherapy-induced complete remissions failed to show any significant benefit when the BCG was given at one, two, four, and six months, and every three months until relapse (Bakemeier et al. 1978). Uncontrolled studies have shown an apparent advantage for BCG in patients with early stage of lymphoma when it was added to radiotherapy (Sokal et al. 1974). Preliminary results in a trial of BCG added to combination chemotherapy in patients with advanced non-Hodgkin's lymphoma suggest that BCG increases the total, although not the complete, remission rate (Jones et al. 1978). Remission duration was not improved with BCG, but the survival of patients with nodular histology appeared to be.

Lung Cancer

BCG Trials

Although the use of chemotherapy in the treatment of small cell cancer of the lung is quite exciting, adjuvant chemotherapy has failed in its promise to aid us significantly in the treatment of non-small cell cancers of the lung. A recent review of adjuvant chemotherapy in lung cancer by Legha and colleagues (1977) presented the disappointing results from 15 trials in non-small cell tumors. (See chapter 61 for further discussion of chemotherapy of non-small cell cancer of the lung.) There is, however, a ray of hope on the horizon for the treatment of these patients. In recent years several studies on the use of adjuvant immunotherapy have resulted in dramatic preliminary responses.

In the early 1960s, several investigators noted the sometimes dramatic and prolonged survival of patients who developed postoperative empyema following resection for lung cancer. All of the subsequent retrospective analyses, except those by Cady and Cliffton (1967) and Minasian and co-workers (1978), demonstrated a significant improvement in survival in these patients, with five-year rates as high as 54% being reported. Takita (1970) reviewed the records of 192 patients who underwent pulmonary resections for lung cancer and compared 14 patients who developed postoperative empyema with the 178 who did not. The five-year survival rate in patients who developed empyema was 54% compared to 27% in those who did not have postoperative infections. Similarly, Ruckdeschel and associates (1972) reviewed the records of 489 patients and reported similar results, with the most dramatic improvement in survival in patients whose cancer was either localized to the lung alone or to the lung and the regional draining nodes.

McKneally and colleagues (1976) felt that the empyema served as a nonspecific immunostimulant that aided the body in destroying residual tumor. Shortly thereafter they set out to reproduce the natural experiment in a randomized controlled trial by employing intrapleural BCG instillation after pulmonary resection for lung cancer. They used a surgical staging system in which patients with stage I disease were those who had tumors less than 3 cm in diameter with positive or negative hilar nodes, or tumors greater than 3 cm in diameter without the involvement of adjacent structures or hilar lymph nodes. Stage II disease was tumor greater than 3 cm in diameter with positive hilar nodes, and stage III tumors involved the mediastinal structures or chest wall, or mediastinal lymph nodes. The study consisted of 100 patients with non-small cell carcinoma of the lung. They were subsequently randomized to receive 10^7 colony-forming units of Tice strain BCG intrapleurally on postoperative days four to six. The side effects of the BCG, including malaise and chills, were relatively well tolerated, although significant fevers (maximum temperature 104° F) often developed. It is interesting to speculate on the role that hyperthermic response may have had in the favorable outcome of this study. Patients with stage I cancer had a significant reduction in the incidence of tumor recurrence (only 1 of 30 patients treated with BCG died of metastatic lung cancer) versus 11 of 33 recurrences in the control group. Those with stage II and stage III disease demonstrated no benefit from the BCG. The patterns of recurrence were similar to those in other series, and interestingly, skin test reactivity and lymphocyte cytotoxicity tests *did not* reflect or predict the clinical course.

A similar study was undertaken by Pines (1976) employing BCG vaccination in conjunction with radiation therapy in inoperable lung cancer. Forty-eight patients with advanced squamous cell carcinoma with disease confined to the chest had radiation therapy (4000 to 6000 rad in four to five weeks) and then were randomized to no further treatment or to BCG vaccination (25 to 125 million organisms [Glaxo] per application every two to four weeks). At one year an increased survival was noted in those treated with BCG (80% vs 57%), and the only survivors at five years were three BCG-treated patients (12%). The BCG was noted to have prevented or suppressed metastases ($P = 0.02$) but did not decrease the incidence of local recurrences.

A recent study by Jensen and co-workers (1978) used BCG scarification postoperatively (165 million viable microorganisms weekly for six weeks, and then every two to three months) in squamous cell carcinoma of the lung. This study also demonstrated an increased disease-free survival rate of 31% at 18 months for those treated with BCG, versus 0% for the control group. Furthermore, Yamamura and associates (1979) have demonstrated the benefit of adjuvant immunotherapy in the treatment of lung cancer using a BCG cell wall skeletal extract administered following conventional therapy of surgery, radiation therapy, and/or chemotherapy. In patients receiving immunotherapy, the 50% survival time was 13.5 months as opposed to 8.5 months for historical controls. The most significant improvement was noted in the small cell carcinomas and in stage III squamous cell carcinomas and adenocarcinomas. Other studies, such as that by Anthony and colleagues (1978) employing postoperative intradermal BCG (Glaxo, 0.1 ml intradermally every month for seven months) failed to show a significant prolongation of survival. Nonetheless, these workers noted a prolongation of general health in those patients treated with BCG.

The strain of BCG, the numbers of viable and of nonviable organisms injected, the extent and duration of febrile response, and the route and frequency of administration, may all be important in the therapeutic effectiveness of BCG adjuvant therapy in lung cancers. Certainly, additional carefully controlled studies are warranted.

Levamisole

An alternative approach in the use of immunoadjuvants for the treatment of bronchogenic carcinoma involves the use of levamisole, an imidazothiazole derivative that is a widely used antihelminthic agent. This drug has been shown to restore ineffective host-humoral and cell-mediated immunoresponsiveness (Symoens 1978). It has also been an effective adjuvant in the treatment of breast cancer (Rojas et al. 1976) and in head and neck tumors (Wanebo et al. 1978).

The use of levamisole as an adjuvant in resectable lung cancer has been studied extensively by Amery (1975). Two hundred eleven patients with surgically resectable lung cancer were randomized preoperatively to placebo or levamisole, administered 50 mg three times daily orally for three days every two weeks, starting three days prior to surgery and continuing for a total of two years or until evidence of relapse. The drug was well tolerated and only 2% of the levamisole-treated patients failed to complete this study because of side effects (predominantly gastrointestinal). Aside from a slight increase in nervous system symptoms or sleep disorders, those receiving levamisole showed no significant drug-related side effects when compared to the control (placebo-treated) group. Levamisole was shown to increase both overall survival and DFI in patients who received greater than 2 mg/kg. This was seen for all histologic subgroups and in both good and poor responses to skin tests. In contrast to the results of the McKneally BCG studies (which showed significant improvement only in those patients with stage I disease), the benefit of levamisole was found primarily in patients who had more advanced cancers at the time of surgery.

Current BCG-Levamisole Trial

The very promising results of these studies with BCG and levamisole as immunoadjuvants in lung cancer have stimulated members of the surgery, pulmonary medicine, and radiotherapy departments at Yale to institute a randomized trial using the combination of levamisole and intratumoral BCG in conjunction with radical radiation therapy, in the treatment of locally advanced, surgically unresectable, non-small cell cancers of the lung. The use of intralesional BCG was shown to be locally effective in the treatment of several malignancies (Bast et al. 1974). At our institution BCG has been administered to over 40 of these patients with relatively low risk of significant complications.

Our clinical trial consists of combining intratumoral BCG, radiation therapy, and levamisole in the belief that (1) radiation will reduce the tumor burden sufficiently to permit the BCG to be effective in stimulating the immune system locally, regionally, and perhaps systemically; (2) the addition of levamisole may aid in restoring any depression of immune responses secondary to the malignancy; and (3) levamisole may also protect against the possible deleterious effects of radiation therapy on the immune system. All patients with previously untreated, advanced, unresectable non-small cell carcinoma of the lung with disease limited to the hemithorax and supraclavicular nodes, and patients with resectable disease who are poor surgical risks or who refuse surgery, will be eligible for this study. They will be randomized to radiation therapy alone, levamisole plus irradiation, and levamisole, radiation therapy, and intratumoral BCG. The radiation therapy is administered by our usual split-course technique.

References

Amery, W. Immunopotentiation with levamisole in resectable bronchogenic carcinoma: a double-blind controlled trial. *Br. Med. J.* 3:461–464, 1975.

Andrien, J. M. Immunotherapy versus chemotherapy as maintenance treatment of acute lymphoblastic leukemia. In *Immunotherapy of cancer: present status of trials in man,* eds. W. D. Terry and D. Windhorst. New York: Raven Press, 1978, pp. 471–480.

Anthony, H. M. et al. A stratified randomized study of intradermal BCG in patients with carcinoma of the bronchus. *Cancer* 42:1784–1792, 1978.

Bakemeier, R. F. et al. BCG immunotherapy following chemotherapy-induced remissions of stage III and IV Hodgkin's disease. In Terry and Windhorst, eds., 1978, pp. 513–517.

Bast, R. C. et al. BCG and cancer. *N. Engl. J. Med.* 290:1413–1420, 1458–1469, 1974.

Beretta, G. et al. Controlled study for prolonged chemotherapy, immunotherapy and chemotherapy plus immunotherapy as adjuvant to surgery in stage I-II malignant melanoma: preliminary report, International Group for the Study of Melanoma. In Terry and Windhorst, eds., 1978, pp. 65–72.

Borden, E. C.; Groveman, D.; and Wolberg, W. H. Effects of levamisole on monocyte chemotaxis in colorectal carcinoma. *Proc. Am. Assoc. Cancer Res.* 22:279, 1981.

Cady, B., and Cliffton, E. E. Empyema and survival following surgery for bronchogenic carcinoma. *J. Thorac. Cardiovasc. Surg.* 53:102–108, 1967.

Costanzi, J. J. Chemotherapy and BCG in the treatment of disseminated malignant melanoma. In Terry and Windhorst, eds., 1978, pp. 87–93.

Cunningham, T. J. et al. A controlled study of adjuvant therapy in patients with stage I and II malignant melanoma. In Terry and Windhorst, eds., 1978, pp. 19–25.

Cuttner, J. et al. Chemoimmunotherapy of acute myelocytic leukemia with MER. In Terry and Windhorst, eds., 1978, pp. 405–412.

Eilber, F. R. et al. Adjuvant immunotherapy with BCG in treatment of regional lymph node metastases from malignant melanoma. *N. Engl. J. Med.* 294:237–240, 1976.

Eilber, F. R. et al. Adjuvant immunotherapy of osteosarcoma with BCG and allogeneic tumor cells. In Terry and Windhorst, eds., 1978, pp. 299–303.

Engstrom, P. F. et al. Fluorouracil versus fluorouracil + BCG in colorectal adenocarcinoma. In Terry and Windhorst, eds., 1978, pp. 587–595.

Forastiere, A. A. et al. CMF ± levamisole breast adjuvant therapy: analysis of results after 3.5 years. *Proc. Am. Assoc. Cancer Res.* 21:402, 1980.

Gee, T. S. et al. Evaluation of *Pseudomonas aeruginosa* vaccine for prolongation of remissions in adults with acute nonlymphoblastic leukemia treated with the L-12 protocol: a preliminary report. In Terry and Windhorst, eds., 1978, pp. 415–422.

Goodnight, J. E., Jr., and Morton, D. L. Immunotherapy for malignant disease. *Ann. Rev. Med.* 29:231–283, 1978.

Gutterman, J. U. et al. Chemoimmunotherapy of acute myeloblastic leukemia: four-year follow-up with BCG. In Terry and Windhorst, eds., 1978a, pp. 375–381.

Gutterman, J. U. et al. Postoperative immunotherapy for recurrent malignant melanoma: an updated report. In Terry and Windhorst, eds., 1978b, pp. 35–55.

Haskell, C. M. et al. Failure of *Corynebacterium parvum* to benefit metastatic breast cancer treated with doxorubicin plus cyclophosphamide in a randomized trial. *Proc. Am. Assoc. Cancer Res.* 21:413, 1980.

Hewlett, J. S. et al. Remission maintenance in adult acute leukemia with and without BCG. A Southwest Oncology Group study. In Terry and Windhorst, eds., 1978, pp. 383–390.

Heyn, R. M. et al. BCG in the treatment of acute lymphocytic leukemia. In Terry and Windhorst, eds., 1978, pp. 503–512.

Holland, J. F., and Bekesi, J. G. Comparison of chemotherapy with chemotherapy plus VCN-treated cells in acute myelocytic leukemia. In Terry and Windhorst, eds., 1978, pp. 347–352.

Hortobagyi, G. N. et al. Chemoimmunotherapy of advanced breast cancer with BCG. In Terry and Windhorst, eds., 1978, pp. 655–663.

Jensen, H. M. et al. Adjuvant immunotherapy with BCG in squamous cell bronchial carcinoma. Immunoreactivity in relation to immunostimulation (preliminary results in a controlled trial). *Thorax* 33:429–438, 1978.

Jones, S. E. et al. Chemoimmunotherapy of non-Hodgkin's lymphoma with BCG: a preliminary report. In Terry and Windhorst, eds., 1978, pp. 519–527.

Kay, H. E. M. Acute lymphoblastic leukemia: 5-year follow-up of the Concord trial. In Terry and Windhorst, eds., 1978, pp. 493–496.

Legha, S. S. et al. Adjuvant chemotherapy in lung cancer. Review and prospects. *Cancer* 39:1415–1424, 1977.

LeRoux, B. T. Empyema thoracis. *Br. J. Surg.* 52:89–99, 1965.

Lokich, J. J. Adjuvant therapy for surgically curable colon cancer: a controlled study of chemo- and immunotherapy. Gastrointestinal Tumor Study Group. *Proc. Am. Assoc. Cancer Res.* 20:423, 1979.

Mastrangelo, M. J. et al. A randomized prospective trial comparing methyl-CCNU + vincristine to methyl-CCNU + vincristine + BCG + allogeneic tumor cells in patients with metastatic malignant melanoma. In Terry and Windhorst, eds., 1978, pp. 95–102.

Mathé, G. et al. Active immunotherapy for acute lymphoblastic leukemia. *Lancet* 1:697–699, 1969.

Mathé, G. et al. Chemotherapy followed by active immunotherapy in the treatment of acute lymphoid leukemias for patients of all ages: results of ICIG protocols 1, 9, and 10, prognostic factors and therapeutic indications. In Terry and Windhorst, eds., 1978, pp. 451–468.

Mavligit, G. M. et al. Systemic adjuvant immunotherapy and chemoimmunotherapy in patients with colorectal cancer (Dukes' C class): prolongation of disease-free interval and survival. In Terry and Windhorst, eds., 1978, pp. 597–604.

McIntyre, O. R. et al. Polyriboinosinic: polyribocytidylic acid as an adjunct to remission maintenance therapy in acute myelogenous leukemia. In Terry and Windhorst, eds., 1978, pp. 423–431.

McKneally, M. F. et al. Regional immunotherapy of lung cancer with intrapleural BCG. *Lancet* 1:377–379, 1976.

McPherson, T. A. et al. Adjuvant chemoimmuno- and immunotherapy in B_2 and C colorectal cancer. *Proc. Am. Assoc. Cancer Res.* 21:402, 1980.

Mike, V., and Marcove, R. C. Osteogenic sarcoma under the age of 21: experience at Memorial Sloan–Kettering Cancer Center. In Terry and Windhorst, eds., 1978, pp. 283–292.

Minasian, H. et al. Influence of postoperative empyema on survival after pulmonary resection for bronchogenic carcinoma. *Br. Med. J.* 2:1329–1331, 1978.

Moertel, C. G. et al. A controlled evaluation of combined immunotherapy (MER-BCG) and chemotherapy for advanced colorectal cancer. In Terry and Windhorst, eds., 1978, pp. 573–584.

Morton, D. L. et al. BCG immunotherapy of malignant melanoma: summary of a seven-year experience. *Ann. Surg.* 180:635–643, 1974.

Morton, D. L. et al. Adjuvant immunotherapy of malignant melanoma: preliminary results of a randomized trial in patients with lymph node metastases. In Terry and Windhorst, eds., 1978, pp. 57–64.

Olivari, A. J. et al. Six-year follow-up in levamisole treated stage III breast cancer patients. *Proc. Am. Assoc. Cancer Res.* 21:362, 1980.

Pavlovsky, S. et al. Chemoimmunotherapy with levamisole during maintenance of remission in acute lymphoblastic leukemia. A four years' report. *Proc. Am. Assoc. Cancer Res.* 21:436, 1980.

Peto, R. Immunotherapy of acute myeloid leukemia. In Terry and Windhorst, eds., 1978, pp. 341–346.

Pines, A. A five-year controlled study of BCG and radiotherapy for inoperable lung cancer. *Lancet* 1:380–381, 1976.

Pinsky, C. M. et al. *Corynebacterium parvum* as adjuvant to combination chemotherapy in patients with advanced breast cancer: preliminary results of a prospective randomized trial. In Terry and Windhorst, eds., 1978a, pp. 647–654.

Pinsky, C. M. et al. Surgical adjuvant immunotherapy with BCG in patients with malignant melanoma: results of a prospective, randomized trial. In Terry and Windhorst, eds., 1978b, pp. 27–34.

Poplack, D. G. et al. Treatment of acute lymphatic leukemia with chemotherapy alone or chemotherapy plus immunotherapy. In Terry and Windhorst, eds., 1978, pp. 497–502.

Powles, R. L. et al. Immunotherapy for acute myelogenous leukemia. *Br. J. Cancer* 28:365–376, 1973.

Powles, R. L. et al. Immunotherapy for acute myelogenous leukemia: analysis of a controlled clinical study two and one-half years after entry of the last patient. In Terry and Windhorst, eds., 1978, pp. 315–326.

Presant, C. A. et al. Effect of *Corynebacterium parvum* on combination chemotherapy of disseminated malignant melanoma. In Terry and Windhorst, eds., 1978, pp. 113–122.

Reizenstein, P. et al. Effect of immunotherapy of survival and remission duration in acute nonlymphatic leukemia. In Terry and Windhorst, eds., 1978, pp. 329–339.

Ritts, R. E., Jr. et al. Transfer factor versus combination chemotherapy: an interim report of a randomized postsurgical adjuvant study in osteogenic sarcoma. In Terry and Windhorst, eds., 1978, pp. 293–298.

Rojas, A. F. et al. Levamisole in advanced human breast cancer. *Lancet* 1:212–215, 1976.

Rojas, A. J. et al. Levamisole action in breast cancer stage III. In Terry and Windhorst, eds., 1978, pp. 635–645.

Ruckdeschel, J. C. et al. Postoperative empyema improves survival in lung cancer. Documentation and analysis of a natural experiment. *N. Engl. J. Med.* 287:1013–1017, 1972.

Sauter, C. et al. Viral oncolysis: its application in maintenance treatment of acute myelogenous leukemia. In Terry and Windhorst, eds., 1978, pp. 355–362.

Sensenig, D. et al. Results of the surgical treatment of bronchogenic carcinoma. *Surg. Gynecol. Obstet.* 116:279–284, 1963.

Simmons, R. L. et al. Active specific immunotherapy for advanced melanoma utilizing neuraminidase-treated autochthonous tumor cells. In Terry and Windhorst, eds., 1978, pp. 123–134.

Sokal, J. E. et al. Delay in progression of malignant lymphoma after BCG vaccination. *N. Engl. J. Med.* 291:1226–1230, 1974.

Spitler, L. E., and Sagebiel, R. A randomized trial of levamisole versus placebo as adjuvant therapy in malignant melanoma. *N. Engl. J. Med.* 303:1143–1147, 1980.

Symoens, J. Treatment of the compromised host with levamisole, a synthetic immunotherapeutic agent. In *Immune modulation and control of neoplasia by adjuvant therapy,* ed. M. A. Chirigos. New York: Raven Press, 1978.

Takita, H. Effect of postoperative empyema on survival of patients with bronchogenic carcinoma. *J. Thorac. Cardiovasc. Surg.* 59:642–644, 1970.

Terry, W. D. Immunotherapy of malignant melanoma. *N. Engl. J. Med.* 303:1174–1175, 1980.

Terry, W. D., and Windhorst, D., eds. *Immunotherapy of cancer: present status of trials in man.* New York: Raven Press, 1978.

Vogler, W. R. et al. A randomized clinical trial of BCG in myeloblastic leukemia conducted by the Southeastern Cancer Study Group. In Terry and Windhorst, eds., 1978, pp. 365–373.

Wanebo, H. J. et al. Randomized trial of levamisole in patients with squamous cancer of the head and neck: a preliminary report. *Cancer Treat. Rep.* 62:1663–1669, 1978.

Whittaker, J. A., and Slater, A. J. Immunotherapy of acute myelogenous leukemia using intravenous BCG. In Terry and Windhorst, eds., 1978, pp. 393–404.

Wood, W. C. et al. Randomized trial of adjuvant therapy for "high risk" primary malignant melanoma. *Surgery* 83:677–681, 1978.

Wright, P. W. et al. Serotherapy of malignant melanoma. In Terry and Windhorst, eds., 1978, pp. 135–142.

Yamamura, Y. et al. Adjuvant immunotherapy of lung cancer with BCG cell wall skeleton (BCG-CWS). *Cancer* 43:1314–1319, 1979.

sixteen

Interferon

DAVID S. FISCHER

Why bother with a whole chapter on interferon? Isn't it just another drug in short supply, of unproved value, obtainable only at a few research centers? Why wasn't it discussed with miscellaneous chemotherapy agents or better yet, in the chapter on unproved methods of cancer treatment?

Interferon is best described as a biologic modifier rather than a chemotherapeutic agent. In the past year (1980), for better or for worse, hardly a day went by without a patient or family asking me about interferon. It wasn't "just another drug," it was "the drug of the year." How many other drugs were spelled out in large letters on the cover of a national weekly magazine (*Time*) (Toufexis and Jucius 1980) with a readership greater than all the medical journals in the world? Newspapers, lay magazines, radio, and television have been the major sources of information about interferon. Nonetheless, there is substantial medical-scientific literature on this "new drug" first described more than two decades ago (Isaacs and Lindenmann 1957). There is documented scientific evidence for both antiviral and anticancer activity. The question is, how much and at what cost? To answer this in a reputable scientific manner, controlled prospective trials are being carried out. Some are being sponsored by the American Cancer Society (ACS), which has committed $6.8 million, and some by the National Cancer Institute (NCI), which has earmarked $13.5 million to the study of biologic modifiers, but primarily interferon. This kind of money makes news. Smaller in-house projects are also being conducted independently by several institutions including the M. D. Anderson Hospital and Tumor Institute in Houston, Memorial Sloan–Kettering Cancer Center in New York City, the Wadley Institutes of Molecular Medicine in Dallas, and Roswell Park Memorial Institute in Buffalo.

Interferon is not a single substance but rather a group of inducible secretory glycoproteins produced by eukaryotic cells in response to viral infections or other stimuli (table 16.1). They do not act on viruses directly but bind to specific cell surface receptors and induce the cell to produce an antiviral protein. Hence the interferons have been called "inducible inducers."

There are at least three types of interferon that are induced by viruses, and diffuse out of the cell to act as messengers to cells that have not yet been infected. The interferon induces those unaffected cells that it contacts to elaborate antiviral protein for protection. Most of what is elaborated by infected cells we call fibroblast interferon because it has been studied as a product of human fibroblasts, primarily from foreskins, grown in tissue culture and harvested. Another type is lymphoblastoid, which is virus-induced in lymphoblasts previously transformed by Epstein-Barr virus and grown in broth suspensions. Although interferon has been generally considered species-specific, so animal material has not been used in humans, there is some evidence that this specificity is not as rigid as previously thought. Human interferon has been shown to have antiviral activity in rabbits, and monkey interferon works with

Table 16.1. *Physical Properties of Interferons*

Derivation	*Type*	*pH-2*	*Molecular Weight*	*SDS-PAGE**	*Iso-electric Point*
Leukocyte	I	stable	36,000	2 peaks	5.5–6.6
Fibroblast	I	stable	20,000	1 peak	6.8–7.8
Lymphoblast	I	stable	40,000	2 peaks	5.0–6.5
Immune	II	labile	—	—	—

SOURCE: Compiled from Priestman 1979 and Krim 1980.

*SDS-PAGE = sodium dodecyl sulfate–polyacrylamide gel electrophoresis.

human cells in culture. Nevertheless, it is unlikely that animal sources will be used for clinical material.

The interferon being used in the majority of clinical trials up to this time is leukocyte interferon, or leukocyte interferon type I. The latter designation is relatively recent and is used to clarify differences among subgroups of interferons. Type I interferons are glycoproteins produced by vertebrate cells following invasion of a virus. Type II interferons are produced by lymphocytes following stimulation by a specific antigen, virus-infected cell or tumor cell. A variety of natural and synthetic inducers exist, for these two types. Type I interferon has been induced by viruses, by double-stranded RNA, by synthetic double-stranded RNAs such as polyriboinosinic acid: polyribocytidylic acid (poly-I:C), and more recently with the introduction of poly-L-lysine into the conjugates, by poly-ICL stabilized in carboxymethyl cellulose (ICLC). Type II (immune) interferon has been induced in cultures of human T and B lymphocytes by phytohemagglutinin, concanavalin-A, pokeweed mitogen, antilymphocyte sera, and *Corynebacterium parvum*. The resulting protein differs both physically and antigenically from virally induced material. It has recently been shown to have a more potent tumor inhibitory effect than type I material in two mouse tumor models. The studies are very early and limited, but have great implications as all data supporting antitumor action are derived from studies with type I protein.

Most clinical studies use leukocyte interferon type I prepared by the technique of Dr. Kari Cantell of the Finnish blood transfusion service. The blood donated to the Finnish Red Cross is spun to separate the red cells, buffy coat (containing leukocytes), and the plasma. The red cells and plasma are used for the usual transfusion and fractionation purposes. The buffy coat of white cells is infected with Sendai virus and incubated at 37.5° C (99.5° F) for 24 hours. The material is centrifuged to remove the white cells and further purified to destroy the virus. The resulting solution contains about 0.1% interferon and is made available for clinical investigators to purchase. The material contains up to 4×10^6 units interferon per milligram of protein. One unit of activity is defined as the reciprocal of that dilution of an interferon preparation that inhibits virus plaque formation by 50%. When calibrated against an international reference standard, the titer of interferon preparations can be expressed in international units (IU). Although the Finnish interferon is among the purest used so far for clinical studies, by most scientific standards it is quite impure and heterogeneous. It has even been suggested that any effects seen are caused by the impurities, but this is unlikely because preparations containing 10×10^8 units per milligram of protein have been produced and yield the same effects unit for unit that are seen with the impure solutions.

There are extensive reviews of the literature that include most of the animal viral and animal tumor studies reported (Priestman 1979; Krim et al. 1980; Krim 1975, 1980a, 1980b; Gresser 1980; Vyas, Cohen, and Schmidt 1978; Stewart 1977, 1979). One of the exciting observations has been that the combination of interferon and a cytotoxic chemotherapeutic agent has resulted in synergistic tumor responses in several animal model systems with several different drugs.

Human studies began as early as 1962, with topical application that was shown to inhibit "takes" in volunteers vaccinated against smallpox, and then vaccinial keratitis was treated effectively. Controlled trials of interferon in patients with cancer with herpes zoster (shingles) have been encouraging. Merigan and coworkers (1978a) in a prospective randomized trial showed that with interferon therapy, acute herpetic neuralgia subsided faster, cutaneous dissemination of lesions was lessened, and visceral complications and resulting mortality were reduced. In immunosuppressed patients with renal transplants a double-blind, placebo-controlled study showed that with leukocyte interferon, the incidence of virus excretion and viremia with cytomegalovirus, herpes simplex, and Epstein-

Barr viruses was significantly reduced (Cheeseman et al. 1979).

Human antitumor effects have been demonstrated with fibroblast interferon in superficial nodules of melanoma, breast carcinoma, and prostate cancer (Nemoto et al. 1980; Horoszewicz et al. 1978). Systemic responses to parenteral injection with fibroblast interferon have been reported with colon cancer and leukemia (McPherson and Tan 1979), and in one patient with Hodgkin's disease with disappearance of bone infiltration (Dunnick and Galasso 1979).

The first trial with leukocyte interferon type I in cancer was begun in 1972 and is ongoing at the Karolinska Hospital in Sweden in patients with osteogenic sarcoma (Strander 1977). Consecutive patients are included who have a primary tumor in the long bones or pelvis, a normal chest x-ray, and histologic proof of the tumor. Treatment begins before surgery and continues with daily injections of interferon for one month after surgery, then three times a week for 17 additional months after which it is stopped. Chest x-rays are performed every two months on the treated patients and every five months on the contemporary controls. So far, Strander reports 5 of 10 interferon-treated patients have remained alive and disease-free for 5 years, while only 5 of 21 contemporary controls have been as fortunate (Krim et al. 1980b). The results suggest a beneficial effect of interferon, but they are far from conclusive.

At the Karolinska Hospital, of 12 patients with previously untreated multiple myeloma given 3×10^6 units intramuscular leukocyte interferon type I daily, 4 had partial remissions, 1 showed no change, 3 had complete remissions, and 4 progressed. Among four additional interferon-treated patients who had received prior chemotherapy and were resistant, one had a clear partial remission (Mellstedt et al. 1979).

In studies at M. D. Anderson Hospital, of nine evaluable patients with multiple myeloma, five responded (Gutterman et al. 1979). In the ACS-sponsored study, 11 patients were treated and disease regression was noted in 3, and stabilization in 2. When interferon was discontinued in the stabilized patients they both relapsed (Osserman et al. 1980). The material used had been lyophilized, and investigators doubted that the reconstituted material had the activity claimed on the labels of vials supplied to them. They suggested that much larger amounts of much purer material would have to be supplied to clarify the efficacy of interferon in multiple myeloma.

There have been a few encouraging reports of responses to interferon in leukemia (Ahstram et al. 1974; Hill et al. 1979, 1980), but they are small in number and primarily anecdotal. The same situation applies to Hodgkin's disease (Blomgren et al. 1976).

Non-Hodgkin's lymphoma was studied in six patients by Merigan and associates (1978b). The three patients with diffuse histiocytic lymphoma did not respond at all. The three with indolent nodular lymphocytic poorly differentiated (NLPD) lymphoma all responded with dramatic regression of peripheral and/or retroperitoneal lymph nodes, and one had normalization of previously involved bone marrow. In the study by Gutterman and colleagues (1979), among eight evaluable patients regressions were seen in two of three with chronic lymphocytic leukemia, three of four with NLPD, and the one patient with histiocytic lymphoma.

Results in non-small cell carcinoma of the lung have been disappointing. Twelve patients (ten with adenocarcinoma and two with epidermoid carcinoma) were treated with 3×10^6 units per day intramuscularly for 30 days. No objective tumor regression was seen (Krown et al. 1980).

Breast cancer is probably the most extensively studied tumor with interferon so far. Of 18 patients treated by Gutterman and co-workers (1979), 12 received low-dose interferon (3×10^6 units daily) and 6 received high-dose (9×10^6 units daily). Of the 12 women receiving the lower dose, 5 responded, as did 2 of the 6 receiving the higher dose. Regressions were seen in soft tissue, bone, and marrow infiltration. In the ACS-sponsored trial reported by Borden and associates (1980), 5 of 16 patients had a partial response and 2 additional patients had a reduction in tumor size not sufficient to meet PR criteria. Responses ranged from 14 to 121 days.

An early compilation of responses to interferon from abstracts and committee reports is given in table 16.2.

Toxicity of interferon is still being evaluated. In the short term, myelosuppression is seen 90% of the time and is usually apparent within a few weeks of starting treatment. White blood cell counts tend to fall to the 2000 to 3000 range but seldom go below 1000, and infection is a rare complication. Thrombocytopenia in the range of 100,000 to 125,000 is common, but less than 100,000 is rare; abnormal bleeding has not been a problem. Fever is seen almost universally but rarely exceeds 102° F for long. Malaise is a common complaint. Weight loss has been documented in about half the patients treated. Pain at the local site of injection occurs in about one-third of patients. Severe headaches and/or skin rash have been problems in some 10% of cases. A few patients have abnormal liver function tests while on therapy, but the incidence of this and its significance are unknown. How much of the toxicity is from the interferon and how much from impurities is also unknown, but in general it is tolerable and less than that with cytotoxic chemotherapy.

Table 16.2. *Early Clinical Responses to Leukocyte Interferon (3 to 9 × 10⁶ units/day)*

	Number of Cases			
	Complete Remission	*Partial Remission*	*No Change (stable)*	*No Response*
Breast cancer	0	11	3	19
Multiple myeloma	3	5	10	20
Malignant lymphoma	4	3	2	8
Lung cancer	0	0	5	4
Chronic lymphocytic leukemia	0	3	6	0
Malignant melanoma	0	6	7	22
Ovarian cancer	0	0	4	9

NOTE: Collected from multiple abstracts of preliminary reports to illustrate results with material 1% pure.

Oral interferon in adult animals is apparently degraded as any other protein would be. In suckling mice, it has been detected in the blood after nursing from interferon-treated mothers. In humans, all interferon has been given topically or systemically, usually intramuscularly. Following injection, peak blood levels are achieved in two to four hours and maintained for a further four to six hours before gradually declining. In general, a dose of 100,000 units/kg of leukocyte interferon type I should give a mean blood level of 50 units/ml over 12 hours. By contrast, circulating levels of fibroblast interferon are minimal in most studies following intramuscular injection, suggesting that the material is tightly bound locally or unstable in muscle. There have been no studies reported as yet on the pharmacokinetics of lymphoblastoid or leukocyte type II (immune) interferons.

The mechanism of antitumor activity is unknown. Interferon was originally tried as an antitumor agent based on its demonstrated action against viruses and the large number of well-documented virus-induced animal cancers. This may be one modality of activity, but chemically-induced and radiation-induced tumors also seem to respond. Hence other mechanisms have been suggested. Interferon has a direct cytostatic effect on both tumor and normal cell lines in vitro. It is able to delay or arrest cell division and may be cell cycle phase-specific, with the critical events leading to inhibition of DNA synthesis occurring during the G_1 interval. Another possibility is an effect mediated by the immune system. It has been suggested (Roberts et al. 1979) that leukocyte interferon type I is primarily elaborated by the macrophages in the buffy coat of blood, and this may be one of their antitumor activities, as interferon can render macrophages tumoricidal. Interferon can also enhance lymphocyte cytotoxicity and the activity of natural killer cells. It also has an effect on the surface membranes of tumor cells, reducing their tumorigenicity.

The problem of increasing the availability of interferon is being attacked in a multitude of ways. The National Institutes of Health (NIH) had given support to research for about 15 years through the National Institute of Allergy and Infectious Diseases (NIAID) (Friedman 1978), but in relatively small (less than one million dollars a year) amounts. This year NIAID is increasing its allocation to $3.59 million. Since the heavy investment by ACS, there has been increased congressional pressure for NCI to support this field generously. Accordingly, it has earmarked $13.5 million for this type of research and has contracted with the New York Blood Center and with Warner Lambert Laboratories for more leukocyte interferon. It has negotiated with Flow Laboratories for fibroblast interferon, and with the Wellcome Foundation laboratories for lymphoblastoid interferon. All this activity (and money) did not go unnoticed by industry. The three current producers of interferon in the United States, Calbiochem in La Jolla, Calif., Biotechnology in West Hartford, Conn., and HEM Research Inc. in Rockville, Md., are increasing their capacity. A number of companies are investing in plants or converting existing facilities to interferon production, including G. D. Searle and Co., Chicago; Abbott Laboratories, Chicago; Merck Sharpe & Dohme, West Point, Pa.; Revlon Health Care Group (U.S. Vitamin), Tuckahoe, N.Y.; and Life Sciences, Inc., St. Petersburg, Fla. The estimated combined investment may exceed $150 million.

An exciting potential source of interferon is from bacterial genetic engineering. Nagata and co-workers (1980) have reported the synthesis in *E. coli* of a polypeptide with human leukocyte interferon activity. So far, only part of the interferon 180-amino acid—polypeptide chain has been sequenced, but it is anticipated that it will be fully characterized in a year. Meanwhile, Biogen, a Swiss pharmaceutical firm, announced that it had successfully produced a material similar to human leukocyte interferon using recombinant DNA techniques. Several other laboratories are approaching the problem in a similar manner.

As an alternative to the continuous use of exogenous interferon, interferon inducers are being actively explored. The early attempts to use poly-I:C led to unacceptable toxicity and little or no efficacy. Two new efforts using less toxic poly-ICLC were presented recently (Kerr et al. 1980; Voakes et al. 1980). Interferon production was elicited in all patients who received one milligram or more per square meter of body surface, but high fever and shaking chills were more than some patients were willing to accept as side effects. Investigators are exploring ways to reduce toxicity while retaining the interferon-inducing properties of poly-ICLC.

While new sources of higher-activity interferon are being explored, the ACS is continuing with its pilot study of four cancers: breast, non-Hodgkin's lymphoma, multiple myeloma, and melanoma. Although the number of patients who can be included in the trials is limited to about 150 because of an average cost of $30,000 per patient for the interferon alone, outside referrals are being accepted to the extent that they meet the specifications of the protocol and the availability of the interferon.

Participating institutions are as follows (lead institution named first):

Breast:

M. D. Anderson Hospital and Tumor Institute, Houston, Tex.

Mt. Sinai Medical Center, New York City

University of Wisconsin Center for Health Sciences, Madison, Wisc.

Roswell Park Memorial Institute, Buffalo, N.Y.

Non-Hodgkin's lymphoma:

Stanford University Medical Center, Palo Alto, Calif.

M. D. Anderson Hospital and Tumor Institute, Houston, Tex.

Memorial Sloan—Kettering Institute for Cancer Research, New York City

Multiple myeloma:

Columbia University College of Physicians and Surgeons, New York City

M. D. Anderson Hospital and Tumor Institute, Houston, Tex.

Johns Hopkins Oncology Center, Baltimore, Md.

Melanoma:

Memorial Sloan—Kettering Institute for Cancer Research, New York City

Yale University School of Medicine, New Haven, Conn.

U.C.L.A. Medical Center, Los Angeles, Calif.

The principal investigators are:

M. D. Anderson—Dr. Jordan Gutterman

Columbia—Dr. Elliot F. Osserman

Johns Hopkins—Dr. Albert H. Owens, Jr.

Memorial Sloan—Kettering—Dr. Herbert Oettgen

Mt. Sinai—Dr. James F. Holland

Roswell Park—Dr. Thomas L. Dao

Stanford—Dr. Thomas C. Merigan, Jr.

U.C.L.A.—Dr. Donald L. Morton

Wisconsin—Dr. Ernest C. Borden

Yale—Dr. Joseph R. Bertino

We can now answer our original questions. We devoted a whole chapter to interferon because it is potentially the most exciting new agent for the treatment of virus infections and some cancers. It is not just another drug, but the first of a class of biologic modifiers that may be important in future therapy. Its study has been scientific, systematic, and controlled. Its distribution has not been exploited for private gain, and its publicity in the lay press has been commensurate with its news value.

References

Ahstrom, L. et al. Interferon in acute leukemia in children. *Lancet* 1:166–167, 1974.

Blomgren, H. et al. Interferon therapy in Hodgkin's disease. *Acta Med. Scand.* 199:527–532, 1976.

Borden, E. et al. Interferon in recurrent breast carcinoma: preliminary report of the American Cancer Society clinical trials program. *Proc. Am. Assoc. Cancer Res.* 21:187, 1980.

Cheeseman, S. H. et al. Controlled clinical trial of prophylactic human leukocyte interferon in renal transplantation. *N. Engl. J. Med.* 300:1345–1349, 1979.

Dunnick, J. K., and Galasso, G. J. Clinical trials with exogenous interferon: summary of a meeting. *J. Infect. Dis.* 139:109–123, 1979.

Friedman, R. M. Interferon and cancer treatment. *CA* 28:278–283, 1978.

Gresser, I., ed. *Interferon.* New York: Academic Press, 1980.

Gutterman, J. et al. Leukocyte interferon (IF)-induced tumor regression in patients (PTS) with breast cancer and B cell neoplasms. *Proc. Am. Assoc. Cancer Res.* 20:167, 1979.

Hill, N. O. et al. Human leukocyte interferon responsiveness of acute leukemia. *J. Clin. Hematol. Oncol.* 9:137–149, 1979.

Hill, N. O. et al. Phase I human leukocyte interferon trials in leukemia and cancer. *Proc. Am. Soc. Clin. Oncol.* 21:361, 1980.

Horoszewicz, J. S. et al. Human fibroblast interferon in human neoplasia: clinical and laboratory study. *Cancer Treat. Rep.* 11:1899–1906, 1978.

Isaacs, A., and Lindenmann, J. Virus interference. I. The interferon. *Proc. R. Soc. Lond.* B 147:258–267, 1957.

Kerr, D. et al. Phase I trial of poly ICLC in advanced cancer. *Proc. Am. Assoc. Cancer Res.* 21:178, 1980.

Krim, M. Interferon as an antiviral and anticancer agent. *Memorial Sloan–Kettering Cancer Center Clin. Bull.* 5:34–36, 1975.

Krim, M. Toward tumor therapy with interferons. I. Interferons: production and properties. *Blood* 55:711–721, 1980a.

Krim, M. Toward tumor therapy with interferons. II. Interferons: in vivo effects. *Blood* 55:875–884, 1980b.

Krim, M. et al., eds. *Report of the Second International Workshop on Interferons.* New York: Rockefeller University Press, 1980.

Krown, S. E. et al. Phase II trial of human leukocyte interferon (IF) in non-small cell lung cancer (NSCLC). *Proc. Am. Assoc. Cancer Res.* 21:179, 1980.

McPherson, T. A., and Tan, Y. H. Phase I study of human fibroblast interferon (FI) in human malignancy. *Proc. Am. Soc. Clin. Oncol.* 20:378, 1979.

Mellstedt, H. et al. Interferon therapy in myelomatosis. *Lancet* 1:245–247, 1979.

Merigan, T. C. et al. Human leukocyte interferon for the treatment of herpes zoster in patients with cancer. *N. Engl. J. Med.* 298:981–987, 1978a.

Merigan, T. C. et al. Preliminary observations on the effect of human leukocyte interferon in non-Hodgkin's lymphoma. *N. Engl. J. Med.* 299:1449–1453, 1978b.

Nagata, S. et al. Synthesis in *E. coli* of a polypeptide with human leukocyte interferon activity. *Nature* 284:316–320, 1980.

Nemoto, T. et al. Human interferons and intralesional therapy of melanoma and breast carcinoma. *Proc. Am. Assoc. Cancer Res.* 20:246, 1979.

Osserman, E. F. et al. Preliminary results of the American Cancer Society (ACS)-sponsored trial of human leukocyte interferon (IF) in multiple myeloma (MM). *Proc. Am. Assoc. Cancer Res.* 21:161, 1980.

Priestman, R. J. Interferon: an anticancer agent? *Cancer Treat. Rev.* 6:223–237, 1979.

Roberts, N. J., Jr. et al. Virus-induced interferon production by human macrophages. *J. Immunol.* 123:365–369, 1979.

Stewart, W. E., II. *The interferon system.* New York: Springer-Verlag, 1979.

Stewart, W. E., II., ed. *Interferons and their actions.* Cleveland: Chemical Rubber Co., 1977.

Strander, H. Interferons: antineoplastic drugs? *Blut* 35:277–288, 1977.

Toufexis, A., and Jucius, A. Interferon, the big IF in cancer. *Time* 115:60–66, 1980.

Voakes, J. et al. Poly (ICLC) as an interferon inducer in refractory multiple myeloma. *Proc. Am. Assoc. Cancer Res.* 21:187, 1980.

Vyas, G. N.; Cohen, S. N.; and Schmidt, R., eds. *Clinical trials with interferons as antivirals.* Philadelphia: Franklin Institute, 1978.

part three

General Principles of Treatment

seventeen

General Principles of Radiation Therapy

ARTHUR H. KNOWLTON

Therapeutic radiology, or as it is commonly called, radiation therapy, dates back approximately to 1900 when the first patient with malignant disease was cured with this modality. Greater understanding of the biology of cancer together with technologic advances led to the development of separate training programs in therapeutic radiology in 1969. Until that time, the specialty had always been a branch of general radiology. Today, the field combines technical and medical experts employing extremely sophisticated equipment to cure and palliate cancer (figs. 17.1 – 17.3).

Approximately one-half of all patients with cancer will at some time during the course of treatment for their malignancy receive radiation therapy. The quality of care is extremely important, and efforts are constantly made to upgrade this modality to enhance overall outcome. Some examples of tumors that can be radically treated with radiation are carcinoma of the head and neck region especially those of the larynx, malignancies of the skin, cervix, bladder, and prostate, as well as Hodgkin's disease and seminomas. When used alone for these cancers it is extremely important that careful treatment planning be undertaken so as to encompass all the tumor in the irradiated field and avoid a geographic miss, which, of course, would lead to recurrence. At the same time, the volume under treatment must be as small as possible so that injury to normal tissue remains minimal.

Physical Basis

The amount of radiation delivered to a patient is measured in units referred to as rad (radiation-absorbed dose). The rad is an indication of how much energy has been absorbed in the body and corresponds to 100 erg/gm. All matter is composed of atoms that have a central positively charged nucleus, and circulating peripheral electrons with a negative charge. Electrons move in orbit about the nucleus in a fashion similar to the movement of earth around the sun. X-rays are produced when a substance of high atomic number is bombarded by electrons generated by a hot filament and accelerated across the x-ray tube by high voltage, resulting in great velocity. The electrons move across the vacuum tube and crash into a target, which results in x-rays. Radiation machines are labeled according to the voltage that accelerates the electrons. Thus there is a 250,000-volt machine (also referred to as a 250-KV or an orthovoltage unit). This machine produces 250,000 volts across the tube, accelerating the electrons. Once the energy imparted to the electron is above 600,000 volts the machines are referred to as supervoltage units, an example of which is a 4-million-volt linear accelerator (4 meV). These high-speed electrons hit a target and interact with the metal of the target to produce x-rays (photons) that pass out through the tube. The patient is placed a few feet from the machine (tube) and the x-rays pass into the patient where they interact with the patient's tissue, depositing their energy as they do so.

Most treatments in modern radiotherapy are delivered from a supervoltage unit. The unit most widely used today in the United States is a cobalt machine that produces a beam of photons similar to that of a linear accelerator, but these gamma rays emanate from a small lead-filled steel container near the center of the unit that contains a radioactive substance. The main advantage of the cobalt machine is its non-complex nature that results in very few breakdowns. Disadvantages are its slower treatment times, the necessity to replace the radioactive source every five years, and most importantly, the lack of sharpness of the edge of the beam, which makes it difficult to treat tumors near critical organs.

Biological Basis

Photons enter the patient and traverse normal tissue as well as the tumor. In their path, they eject electrons from atoms or molecules, resulting in charged particles. Since the body is composed mostly of water, many of the excited atoms and molecules are those of hydrogen and oxygen. These particles cause biologic damage, usually to DNA, which may result in cell death. These charged particles generally will cause a sublethal event within the cell, and it is the accumulation of these events that eventually leads to cell death. The cell may continue to function while lethally injured, and its death does not actually take place until it divides.

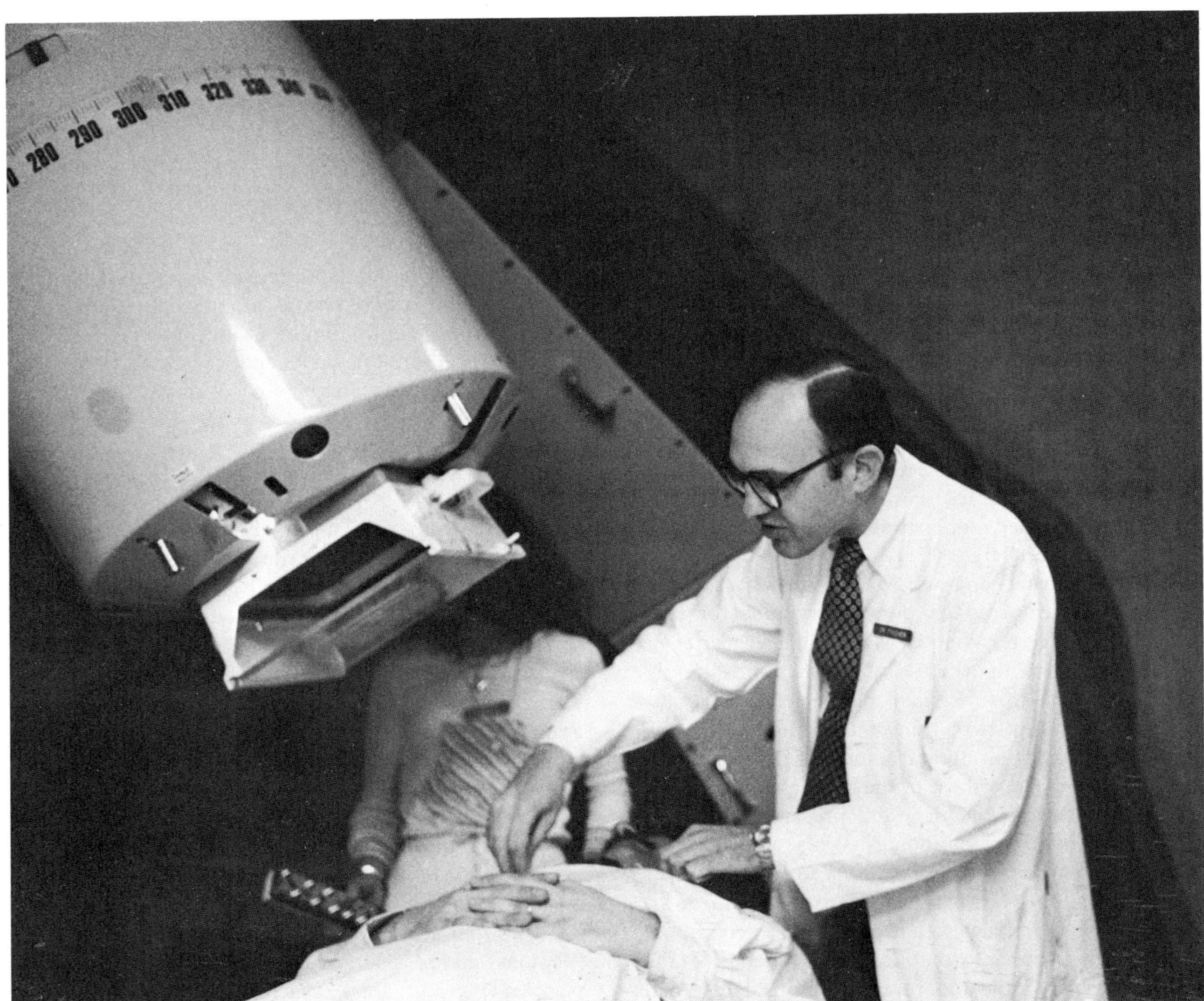

Fig. 17.1. *The Sagittaire. A linear accelerator used in the treatment of cancer. This machine produces an x-ray beam of 25 million electron volts and an electron beam of various energies to a maximum of 32 million volts. The electron capability allows the physician to treat cancers in the head and neck region with an adequate dose of radiation while avoiding overtreatment of critical normal organs. (Courtesy of Yale Comprehensive Cancer Center, New Haven, Conn.)*

At the end of a long course of successful radiation therapy that will result in a tumor cure, all the cells are dead; however, the tumor may look on x-ray and feel to palpation exactly as it did before radiation therapy was started. For a tumor to shrink the cells must divide, which will lead to their death and eventual disintegration. It is for these reasons that rapidly dividing tumors will disappear more quickly than slowly dividing tumors that may take quite some time to change in bulk. In clinical medicine this is important if one is attempting to decide whether or not radiation has actually failed. For example, a large prostate tumor may take many months to disappear, and a positive biopsy may be obtained as late as one or two years following radiation therapy although the patient will be cured of this tumor. Often, the bulk never completely disappears and is replaced by stromal reactions such as fibrosis. There is a lack of correlation between curability and the disappearance of a tumor, and thus it is a mistake to interrupt treatment part way through a course of radiation therapy in favor of another modality because the neoplasm has not shrunk.

Cellular Basis

The sensitivity of cells to radiation depends on many factors, three of which are the position of the cell in its cycle, the oxygen concentration within the cell during radiation, and the type of cell involved. Cells of different animals are more sensitive in different phases of the cell cycle, although in general, they are most sensitive in the resting phase between synthesis and mitosis.

The effect of radiation therapy is enhanced in the presence of oxygen, and the biologic effect is greater in the oxygenated than the hypoxic state. The ratio of sensitivity of these two states is referred to as the oxygen-enhancement ratio, and varies from 2 to 3 when photons are employed. This means that a well-oxygenated tumor is considerably easier to cure and thus more sensitive than a tumor with a hypoxic compartment. It is felt that radiation therapy may fail in the treatment of large tumors because of their hypoxic aspects. The oxygen does not diffuse across the tissue for such a great distance and thus cells far from blood vessels are short of oxygen and more resistant to radiation.

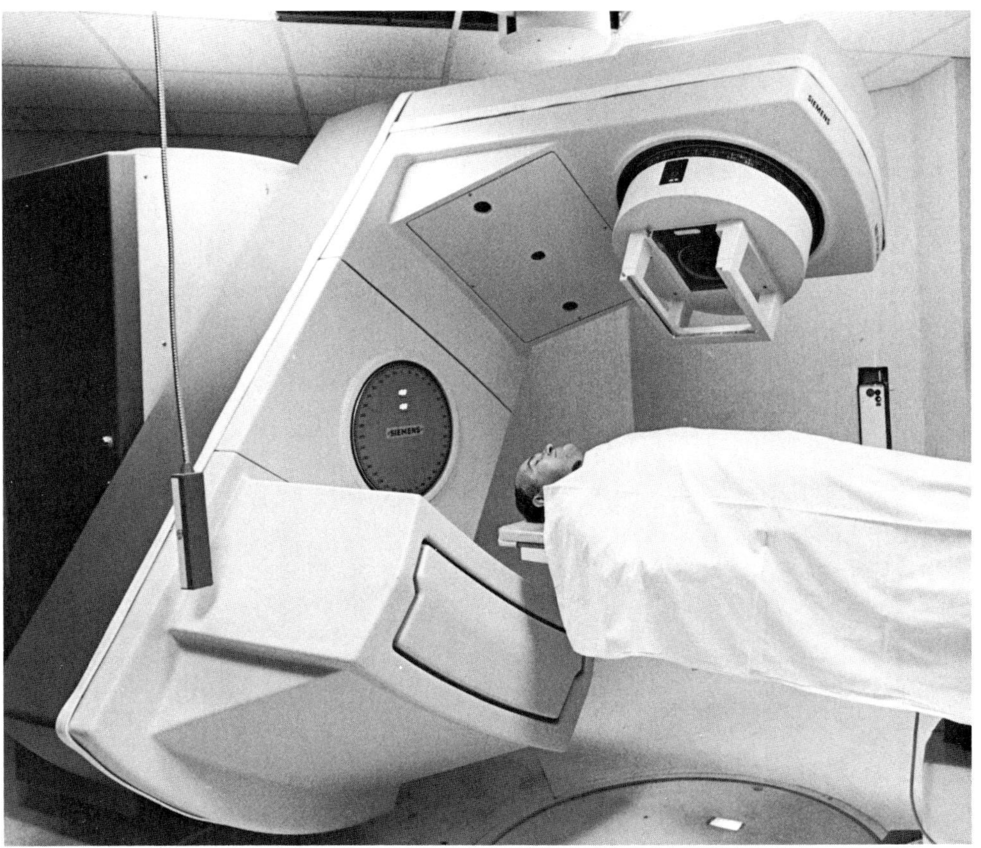

Fig. 17.2. *The Mevatron 12. A linear accelerator producing a photon beam of 10 million electron volts. The machine is shown treating a patient in a fixed position. (Courtesy of Ovid Gallo, Hospital of St. Raphael, New Haven, Conn.)*

Attempts have been made to convert hypoxic areas of tumors into well-oxygenated ones by having the patient treated in a sealed hyperbaric chamber. Some research centers are attempting to bombard tumors with high-energy heavy particles that may destroy oxygenated and hypoxic cells equally well. Because of this sensitivity of well-oxygenated cells it seems reasonable to make sure patients are not anemic during radiation therapy; generally it is best to keep the hematocrit above 30%.

Cells themselves have inherent sensitivity to radiation, perhaps related to their ability to repair sublethal radiation damage. For example, lymphocytes and seminoma cells are exquisitely sensitive, while epithelial cells and sarcoma cells are less sensitive.

Therapeutic Strategy

It is possible to cure almost every tumor in vitro with enough radiation, thus one may ask why we do not cure all tumors in patients. The tolerance of the body's normal tissues limits the amount of radiation that may be delivered to the tumor. A tumor that is very large and hypoxic may require more radiation to control than the local part of the body can withstand without serious injury. Split-course treatment is often employed in patients with large bulky tumors. This means the patient is given approximately 60% of the overall amount of treatment, and then a two- to three-week rest is followed by the last 40%. Hopefully, the first course of treatment will cause the tumor to shrink and the hypoxic cells may actually then be closer to blood vessels, become reoxygenated, and develop increased sensitivity.

Improving the oxygen status of the tumor improves the therapeutic ratio without causing increased damage to normal tissues, which are always well oxygenated. Normal cells are as sensitive to radiation as tumor cells; however, radiation may cure a tumor and yet preserve normal cell function. Although both normal and tumor cells receive multiple sublethal injuries, there is a slight increase in the ability of normal cells to repair this damage, and thus by slow daily fraction the accumulation of damage is greatest within the tumor. Also, tumors that are actively growing have more cells in a

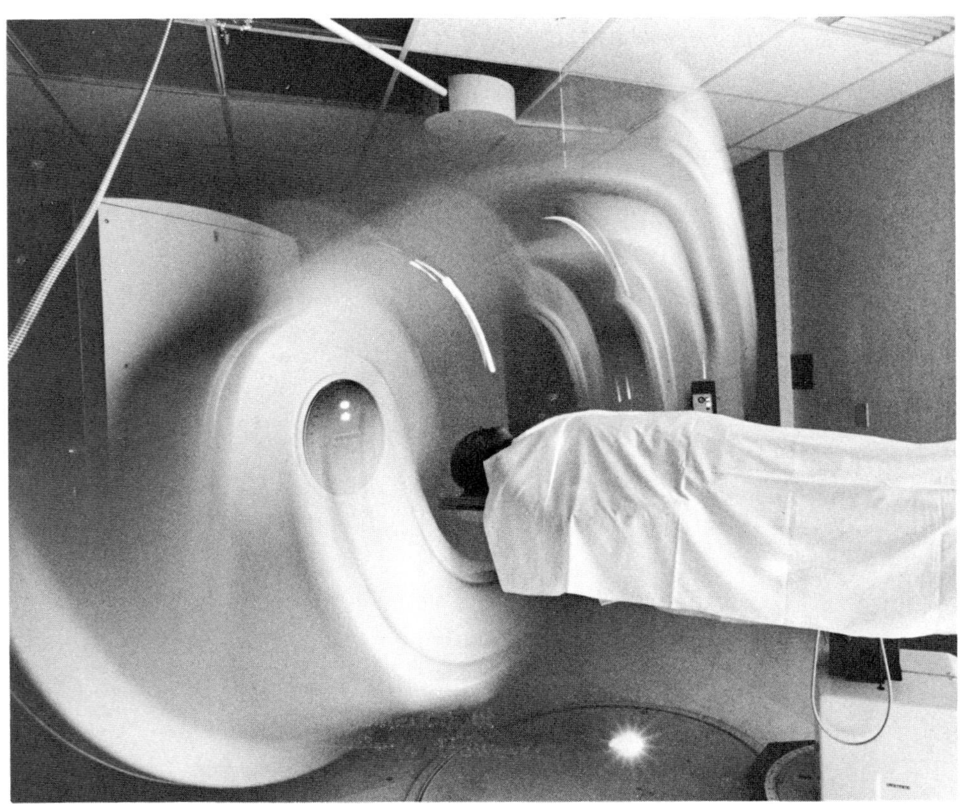

Fig. 17.3. *The Mevatron 12. A linear acelerator which also produces an electron beam of varying energies to a maximum of 12 million volts. The machine pictured is carrying out rotational treatment. The photon beam is actually directed at the patient's cancer while the machine rotates through 360 degrees. (Courtesy of Ovid Gallo, Hospital of St. Raphael, New Haven, Conn.)*

sensitive phase of the mitotic cycle, and a slight differential is accomplished here. Normal cells have a great potential for regeneration and may quickly divide and repair damage in a stressful situation such as that experienced with radiation. The bone marrow stem cells and cells of the gastrointestinal tract, oral mucosa, and skin can actively regenerate and quickly divide to fill in for their dead counterparts.

Tumor Histology, Site, and Size

Because many other diseases often mask a malignancy, one should always have a histologic diagnosis before undertaking a course of radiation therapy. Exceptions to this should be rare, but may include tumors along the base of the brain and brain stem where the pursuit of tissue for histology may jeopardize a patient's life. Cell type can be most important and will eventually determine the amount of radiation necessary and its effectiveness. In some instances, it is often best to start a course of radiation therapy without histologic diagnosis because of the acute condition of the patient, but when the situation improves one should be obtained. An example of this is the superior vena cava syndrome caused by a tumor in the midchest region. An immediate course of radiation therapy should be started but as soon as the syndrome has been relieved, histologic diagnosis should be established and radiation therapy completed.

Aside from the nature of the tumor, the amount of radiation is also determined by its site of origin and size. For example, a small early tumor of the head and neck region is very amenable to cure with primary radiation therapy, whereas the locally advanced tumor might be better eradicated with a surgical approach and postoperative external radiation.

Problems of Dosimetry

In attempting radical treatment the general approach is to treat the primary tumor and the surrounding areas where local spread is likely to have occurred. In a prostate or bladder tumor it is the usual practice to treat the entire pelvis to approximately 4000 to 5000 rad (the amount of radiation needed to eradicate subclinical disease) and then to reduce the treatment volume to the primary tumor. The biologic effect of a course of therapy depends on the amount of radiation delivered each day, the number of treatments per week, and the overall treatment time. For radical radiation of an epidermoid carcinoma of the head and neck region, many radiotherapy departments will treat at 200 rad a day, five days a week, to a total dose of approximately 6000 to 7000 rad. This will take 30 to 35 treatments. Some institutions obtain the same biologic effect using 10 to 12 treatments delivered five days a week at 400 rad each, for a total dose of 4000 to 4800 rad. It is extremely difficult to compare the biologic effectiveness of the two schedules, and thus a total dose of 6000 rad delivered at 200 rad per day, five days a week for six weeks will have a considerably different effect than 6000 rad given in four treatments of 1500 rad each twice a week.

One attempt to compare different treatment schedules has been the nominal standard dose (NSD) derived by Ellis, which combines the number of fractionations, total dose, and overall treatment time to arrive at a single number. The unit of the NSD is the ret, which is an abbreviation for rad-equivalent therapeutic. There is great debate whether or not the Ellis formula is of value on a practical, clinical basis. In general, it has not proved to be so.

Combined Modality Therapy

Radiation therapy may be given in a curative or radical approach as well as a palliative one. We should, however, be guided by the patient in our decision to administer radiation, and not just by the disease. For an elderly, frail, weak person, a prolonged course of therapy may not be wise.

When used as curative treatment, radiation therapy is often undertaken in conjunction with chemotherapy and surgery, as modalities used in combination are often considerably more effective than when used individually.

Radiation in combination with surgery either preoperatively or postoperatively is undertaken in the treatment of tumors of the brain, head and neck area, lung, rectum, bladder, uterus, breast, ovary, and some soft tissue sarcomas and pediatric tumors. Preoperative therapy has been used for many years in several different types of cancer to achieve a better cure rate. It is most useful preoperatively when the initial tumor is large and resectability is borderline. Radiation will reduce the size of the tumor and often convert it to a resectable one. Radiation is employed postoperatively when there is a question of tumor left behind or in diseases that are known to have a high local recurrence rate, such as advanced disease of the head and neck. Although surgery may be employed to save a radiation failure, it is generally rare for radiation to salvage a surgical failure.

Perhaps the greatest advances made over the past few years have been in radiation therapy combined with chemotherapy. Diseases treated by single modalities in the past are now frequently treated by combination, for example, advanced head and neck tumors, and cancer of the brain, breast, lung (especially the small cell variety), gastrointestinal tract, and lymphomas and Hodgkin's disease. Research continues very actively to develop better treatment using combination therapy.

Palliative Therapy

Palliative radiation is intended to relieve a patient's symptoms, not to prolong life although this often results. On occasion, palliative therapy may be carried out to prevent an impending problem even at a time when the patient may be asymptomatic.

Symptoms that respond well to radiation are headache, nausea, and vomiting due to brain metastasis, difficulty in swallowing, pain, bleeding, pulmonary infections and atelectasis from stenotic lesions of the bronchus, and ulcerative skin problems with their unpleasant odor and associated drainage. Large bulky masses causing venous and lymphatic obstruction may be reduced in size with relief of associated edema. Bleeding, which may take the form of hemoptysis, hematemesis, hematuria, and melena, may also be treated effectively with radiation therapy when they are caused by malignancy. Almost all of these symptoms can be quickly and easily relieved with a short intensive course.

Keen clinical judgment is required for the application of palliative therapy as the end point is immediate relief of symptoms, with as little distress as possible from acute radiation reactions to the patient. More recently there has been the use of half-body radiation to palliate pain from widespread metastatic disease. Although the toxic effect initially was radiation pneumonitis, with reduction of the dose to approximately 600 to 700 rad this distressing side effect has been eliminated. A relatively safe single treatment is given that results in partial pain relief in over 80% of patients, and complete relief in over 40%. This occurs usually very dramatically and within the first three to four days after therapy.

Side Effects

During the course of radiation, which may take several weeks, the patient may experience acute side effects. Following completion of treatment as the months and years go on, more chronic side effects may show up, as can radiation complications. The acute side effects during treatment are both systemic and local. Loss of appetite, fatigue, nausea and vomiting, and occasionally, reduction in platelet and leukocyte counts constitute the usual systemic side effects. Acute skin effects are erythema or a dry desquamation. In treatment of the head and neck and chest areas the patient may experience a dry mouth, loss of taste, difficulty swallowing, and esophagitis. Abdominal and pelvic treatment often causes diarrhea and crampy abdominal pain. These symptoms rapidly clear on completion of therapy.

Over time, some chronic effects are noted such as continuation of dry mouth, loss of taste, perhaps some mild atrophy of the skin, and occasional subcutaneous fibrosis. These are radiation reactions and are not considered radiation complications. In a very few cases, long-term complications will arise. This is injury to an organ that is not the usual side effect of radiation and is considered rare. A radiation complication does not mean that therapy was delivered incorrectly, because everybody who undergoes treatment is at a small risk for a long-term complication or serious injury. These most often occur in patients receiving radical and curative treatment where a high dose of radiation is given or a very large tumor volume is treated. Such injuries may be stenosis or necrosis of the gastrointestinal tract, especially in the pelvic area following treatment for carcinoma of the cervix. In patients with head and neck tumors an occasional osteoradionecrosis of the mandible is noted. The most dreaded complication, and thus one that physicians try to avoid most, is radiation myelopathy. This may lead to complete paralysis. Brain necrosis also occurs very rarely.

As the dose is increased, not only is the effect on the tumor increased but so is the possibility of a complication. Thus the radiotherapist will attempt to achieve maximum antitumor activity yet at the same time subjecting the patient to a minimal chance for a complication. For instance, most patients undergoing curative treatment are at 3% risk for an injury. By increasing the dosage one may increase the risk from 3% to 50% or 60% and yet only increase the chance of curing the patient from 4% to 5%. A radiation therapy physician whose patients develop few complications and no serious injuries may in general be giving patients an insufficient dose to affect the tumor; as a result, although the complication rate is low, the cure rate remains very low as well.

Radiotherapy may also cause anorexia during the actual time of treatment, which may lead to loss of weight. Good nutritional care during treatment may offset this, and a dietitian skilled in these problems should be a member of the health care team. Patients will experience inability to eat, difficulty swallowing, sore mouth, nausea and vomiting, and diarrhea. Food absorption by the gastrointestinal tract can also be altered. The patient must be encouraged to eat a high-protein high-calorie diet, most often by frequent small feedings. Local anesthetics and baking soda rinses are often used to relieve pain in the mouth or throat and thus improve oral intake. Occasionally, a patient with extreme weight loss may be hospitalized for hyperalimentation. For those undergoing abdominal radiation, a low-residue diet, prochlorperazine, and diphenoxylate (Lomotil) are among the various modalities used to prevent the common side effects of nausea, vomiting, and diarrhea.

Future Progress

Continued progress takes place daily in radiotherapy through research and clinical trials. Better tumor definition than ever before is now available through use of a CAT scanner, leading to more precise delivery of the radiation therapy, and avoidance both of normal tissues and geographic miss of the tumor. Linear accelerators have the ability to deliver radiation doses very accurately and precisely. Particle irradiation with its increased oxygen-enhancement ratio is being carried out in a few institutions on a trial basis. Research continues to arrive at an agent that will sensitize hypoxic cells to radiation therapy. New treatment schedules are attempting to carry out the best time-dose relationship to achieve better tumor control and less normal tissue reaction. Hyperthermia in combination with radiation therapy is starting to show some positive results. Combined treatment with chemotherapy and surgery is being exploited with greater benefits. Although progress is slow it is nevertheless steady. Today over 40% of the patients with malignant diseases are cured completely of their tumor, whereas in the not too distant past only 25% were cured.

References

Fletcher, G. *Textbook of radiotherapy.* Philadelphia: Lea & Febiger, 1980.

Moss, W. T.; Brand, W. N.; and Battifora, H. *Radiation oncology, rationale, technique, results,* 4th edition. St. Louis: C. V. Mosby, 1973.

Murphy, W. *Radiation therapy.* Philadelphia: W. B. Saunders, 1967.

Paterson, R. *The treatment of malignant disease by radiotherapy.* Baltimore: Williams & Wilkins, 1963.

Steinfeld, A. D. Radiation oncology. *Am. Fam. Prac.* 21:131–138, 1980.

eighteen

Blood Component Therapy

JOSEPH R. BOVE

The modern management of malignant disease, especially when aggressive chemotherapy or radiotherapy is used, cannot be undertaken successfully without the skillful use of blood component therapy. No other group of patients is more demanding of blood bank resources or requires more judicious use of blood products than do these patients. Every clinician who is responsible for the treatment of patients with cancer must have a deep knowledge of the available blood products, their appropriate use, and their potential for complications. This chapter does not deal with blood derivatives such as normal serum albumin, plasma protein fraction, or antihemophiliac factor, but discusses only those components that are prepared from single donations or by cytapheresis and, in general, are processed in the blood bank or transfusion service. These include red cell products intended to correct the signs and symptoms of anemia, fresh frozen plasma for treatment of coagulation abnormalities, platelets to control or prevent bleeding in patients with severe thrombocytopenia, and granulocytes that are useful in some patients with granulocytopenia and infection.

Red Cell Products

Red cell products are indicated to correct or improve the signs and symptoms of anemia when these are sufficient to interfere significantly with the patient's well-being. They are also used to replace significant blood loss that may occur during major surgery. Finally, red cell products may be indicated to forestall the development of cardiac complications of anemia.

Currently available red blood cell products are as follows:

- Whole blood
- Red blood cells
- Leukocyte-poor red blood cells
- Washed red blood cells
- Thawed deglycerolized red blood cells*
- Red blood cell components

Whole Blood

Whole blood is usually collected in citrate-phosphate-dextrose (CPD), an anticoagulant-preservative solution. Each unit of whole blood contains 63 ml of this solution and 450 plus or minus 45 ml of donor blood. It is well to remember that over 10% of the contents of a bag of so-called whole blood represents the CPD solution, not donor blood. With this anticoagulant, blood can be stored for up to 21 days. Although modest changes such as a rise in plasma potassium, a fall in red cell 2,3-DPG (diphosphoglucose), and some loss of red cell viability occur during storage, there is no evidence that fresh blood is beneficial or necessary in the management of any patients. Even massive transfusion with

*Usually, but improperly, called frozen red blood cells.

stored blood is well tolerated, although in some cases additional therapy with platelets or fresh frozen plasma may be indicated. Fresh blood is no longer available, and clinicians should replace requests for it with requests for whatever components are required to treat specific lesions.

Whole blood is the component of choice when treating patients who require simultaneous restoration of volume and oxygen-carrying capacity. In this author's opinion it should be used in acute bleeding, hypovolemic shock, and for most patients who require transfusion during major surgery.

Red Blood Cells

Red blood cells, also known as packed cells, are prepared by removing most of the plasma from a unit of whole blood. Usually this is done at the collecting center as part of its blood component program. Understandably, centers are anxious to obtain maximum yields of plasma or platelets, and to do so often remove enough plasma to leave the red blood cell preparation with a hematocrit value between 75% and 85% and a total volume of about 200 ml. While these red blood cells have the same storage characteristics as the whole blood from which they were harvested, the high hematocrit value makes the product difficult to infuse. Up to 100 ml of normal saline solution can, and usually should, be added before infusion to improve the flow characteristics.

The average red blood cell transfusion should take less than two hours; only patients who have compromised cardiovascular dynamics benefit from a slower infusion. Even in these patients the transfusion time should not be unduly prolonged; four hours is adequate for all but the most unusual cases. When any blood component, including red blood cells, is allowed to hang for a longer period, the risk of infection or thermal damage to the product is increased.

Washed Red Blood Cells

The knowledge that most febrile transfusion reactions are related to the interaction of donor white cells, particularly granulocytes, with leukocyte antibodies in the recipient (Perkins 1966) has prompted the use of various preparations of leukocyte-poor red blood cells (table 18.1). Centrifugation methods are relatively simple and are available in any blood bank or transfusion service that has a refrigerated centrifuge. The product has a very high hematocrit and about 100 ml of saline must be added so that the transfusion will flow properly. In addition, the red cell loss is rather high, especially considering the relatively poor efficiency of white cell removal.

Table 18.1. *Available Preparations of Leukocyte-Poor Red Blood Cells*

Preparation	*RBC Loss %*	*WBC Remaining %*
Centrifugation	20–40	15–25
Nylon filtration	12	35
Dextran sedimentation	9	7
Washing	13	7
Deglycerolization of frozen RBC	10–30	3–9

One particularly effective way to prepare leukocyte-poor red cells is by washing (Buchholz, Charette, and Bove 1978). In areas where the appropriate equipment is available—and this should include nearly all centers treating cancer patients—washed red cells can be prepared safely in about 15 minutes. The usual unit has about 175 ml of red cells suspended in normal saline. At least 85% to 90% of the original white cells has been removed, and the product can be transfused with a much diminished incidence of febrile transfusion reactions. Since equipment, solutions, and technical time required increase cost, we cannot advocate routine use of washed red cells for patients with cancer.

These cells are, however, indicated in patients who have had two or more febrile transfusion reactions. In addition, they may properly be used for all outpatient transfusions. The rationale is that the extra difficulty attending outpatient transfusions, for example, the need for the patient to arrive early for compatibility testing, the need to travel to and from the hospital, the desire to leave promptly, and the difficulty of providing a second unit of blood should there be a reaction, make it worthwhile to spend the extra money to ensure, if at all possible, that the transfusion will not have to be stopped because of a reaction.

Finally, patients with typing or cross-matching problems are reasonable candidates for washed red cells, as it is important to know that a reaction, should one occur, is almost surely not from granulocytes.

Frozen and Thawed Deglycerolized Red Blood Cells

Current technology allows the frozen storage of red cells for at least five years, although federal regulations permit routine storage for only three. The freezing process requires the addition of a cryoprotective agent, usually glycerol, which is removed by multiple washes after thawing. Clearly, the correct name of the product is thawed deglycerolized red blood cells, but in common use they are referred to as frozen red cells.

Deglycerolized red blood cells have all the advantages of washed red blood cells, in fact, they have even fewer remaining leukocytes and can be used to prevent febrile reactions in those few patients who react to other forms of leukocyte-poor transfusions. The prime indication for frozen storage of red blood cells is to maintain an inventory of rare blood types (Chaplin et al. 1974), and they best meet transfusion needs for patients with unusual antibodies or mixtures of several antibodies. In treating such patients the clinician and blood bank should maintain close communication, since frozen red blood cells must be discarded 24 hours after deglycerolization. The cost of this product is usually three to four times that of regular blood cells, and the loss of a rare donor unit is particularly distressing, hence every effort must be made to ensure the product's optimum use.

There is evidence that the product is not entirely hepatitis-free (Haugen 1979); however, it seems reasonable to assume that the risk is lower. While some institutions favor the widespread use of frozen blood, I cannot accept this because of the high cost. There is no doubt that the deglycerolized red blood cells are safe, efficacious, and well-tolerated, nor is there any doubt that they are the product of choice in selected situations. Unfortunately, the high cost and the 24-hour post-thaw expiration time make it unreasonable to use them when less costly products are nearly as effective.

Fresh Frozen Plasma

The use of fresh frozen plasma has increased dramatically without a clear-cut understanding of exactly why (fig. 18.1). Fresh frozen plasma is prepared within four hours of blood collection by removing about 175 to 225 ml of plasma (with CPD solution) from a donation of whole blood. The material is immediately frozen and is a good source of all known coagulation factors including V and VIII, both of which are labile.

There are few indications for fresh frozen plasma therapy in cancer, although it may be of some value as an adjunct in the treatment of bleeding associated with disseminated intravascular coagulation (DIC). Here, of course, the major effort must be dedicated to correction of the cause; component therapy with fresh frozen plasma or platelets or both is useful, if at all, only as a temporary measure. Fresh frozen plasma is also a good source of immunoglobulins but is almost never needed for this indication in cancer patients. Plasma or blood volume expansion can be accomplished with plasma, but albumin or plasma protein fraction, which have no hepatitis risk, is preferred.

Platelets

It is difficult to overestimate the importance of platelet therapy in the management of patients with cancer. Thrombocytopenia, whether from the disease or from chemotherapy-induced marrow failure, is a major and life-threatening complication. The widespread availability of platelet transfusion has led to a situation in which bleeding is no longer the leading cause of death in malignant disease. Almost no patient can be treated adequately with modern chemotherapy without developing thrombocytopenia, and some require several, if not more, platelet transfusions.

There is abundant evidence that the probability of abnormal bleeding increases as the platelet count falls; however, many additional factors are equally important:

Platelet count:
- below 10,000/mm^3—high risk
- 10,000 to 75,000/mm^3—moderate risk
- above 70,000/mm^3—low risk

Age of circulating platelets—young platelets function better

Rapidity of onset

Vascular integrity

Steroid therapy

Associated problems such as aspirin, coagulation factor deficiencies, and so forth

For example, it is well known that patients in whom thrombocytopenia develops slowly or those with chronic idiopathic thrombocytopenic purpura (especially during treatment with adrenal steroids) often show remarkably little evidence of bleeding despite low platelet counts. In general, patients with platelet counts above 75,000 to 80,000/mm^3 have little risk; those whose counts are below 10,000/mm^3 have high risk; those with counts between 10,000 and 80,000/mm^3 are at intermediate risk. When there is evidence of widespread purpuric bleeding in the thrombocytopenic patient, platelet therapy is clearly warranted.

A decision to use prophylactic treatment is far more difficult. Platelet therapy is expensive and carries with it the risk of hepatitis and alloimmunization; hence it is prudent to withhold prophylactic treatment unless the count is below 10,000 to 20,000/mm^3 (Schiffer,

Aisner, and Wiernick 1978). Patients with counts that are low but above 20,000/mm^3 are, of course, at risk, but in most cases the risk is acceptable when viewed in light of potential complications, the difficulty in obtaining adequate supplies of platelets, and the cost. In particular one needs to remember that sooner or later persistent platelet therapy will lead to development of antibody and a refractory state. It is important to delay the onset of refractoriness as long as possible, and one practical way to do this is by using as few platelet transfusions as possible.

The usual preparation is harvested from a regular blood donation and contains about 5.5×10^{10} platelets. These are suspended in 30 to 70 ml of plasma. Since the average platelet transfusion in an adult is 10 units, the patient also receives the equivalent of 2 or 3 units of fresh plasma. It is reasonable to expect the recipient's platelet count to rise by 7000 to 10,000/mm^3/M^2 of body surface area for each unit of platelets transfused. Failure of the expected rise is evidence that (1) platelet preparation or storage has been inadequate, (2) the patient is refractory for some reason (fever, sepsis, splenomegaly, etc.), or (3) the platelets are incompatible. In that regard platelets probably do possess ABO antigens, but it is difficult to be sure that these are really part of the platelet membrane structure rather than passively adsorbed from plasma. In either case it is unimportant, since ABO blood group compatibility is not essential for adequate platelet recovery or function. It is, in fact, more important to avoid administering large quantities of ABO-incompatible plasma to the recipient, as this may lead to a positive direct Coombs' test and hemolytic anemia.

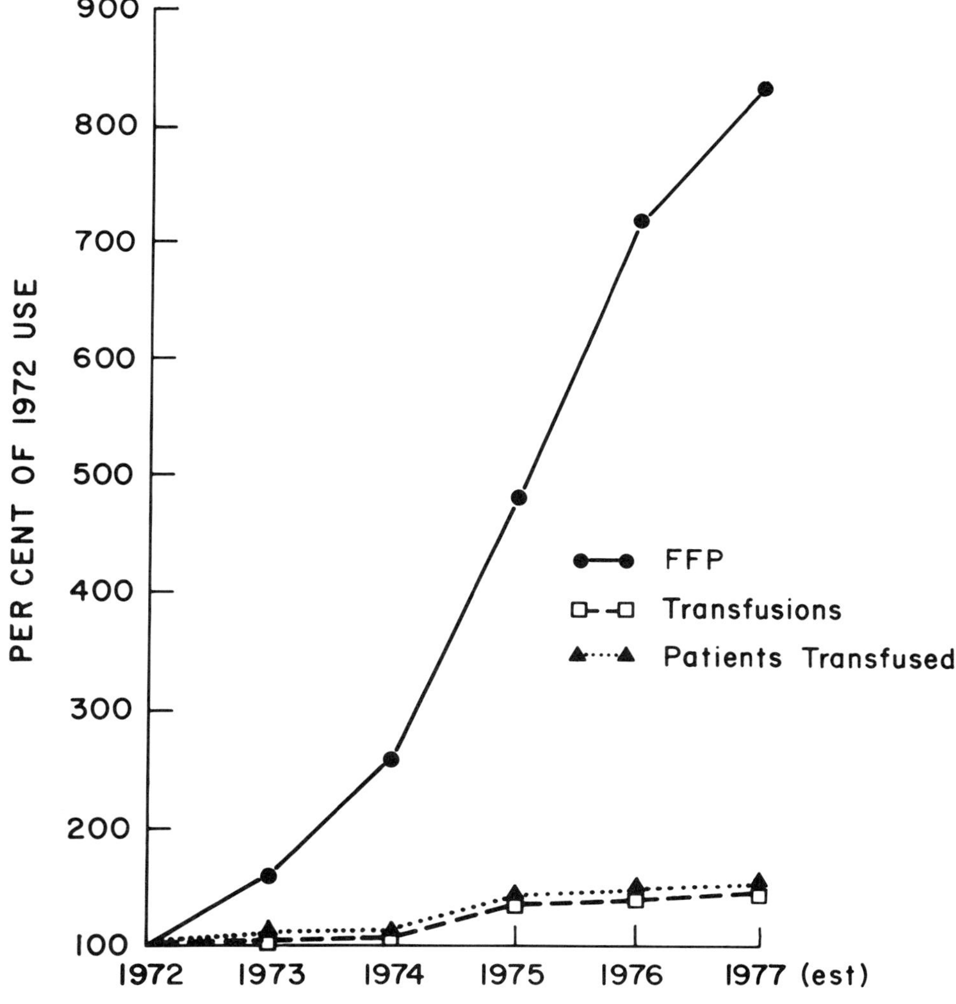

Fig. 18.1. *Use of fresh frozen plasma at Yale–New Haven Hospital, 1972–1977 (Bove 1978).*

Platelet Refractoriness

The failure of the platelet count to rise appropriately after transfusion is most likely a sign that a refractory state has developed. It is then necessary to determine the cause rather than to order larger doses or HLA-matched platelets. First, it is important to be sure that platelet preparation, transportation, and storage are proper. Usually, they are prepared in large blood centers and are used by patients throughout a blood service area. Difficulties with preparation or storage should, therefore, be obvious in more than one hospital or in several patients. If this is not the case, and it usually is not, one needs to evaluate the patient for causes of refractoriness.

While many clinicians think first of platelet antibody, the problem often lies elsewhere. Daly and coworkers (1980) presented evidence that *in some patients* it is possible to differentiate between refractoriness caused by antibody and that from other causes by comparing the postinfusion counts immediately after transfusion with those taken about 24 hours later. In the case of platelet antibody or splenomegaly neither count shows the expected increment, while in refractoriness from other causes such as fever or sepsis, the early count taken 10 minutes after infusion rises appropriately, but platelets are rapidly destroyed or removed so that 24-hour counts are disappointingly low.

There is evidence that in some patients with demonstrable antibody, HLA-matched platelets show improved or normal recovery and survival (Yankee, Grument, and Rogentine 1969). This, however, is not always the case and even the best-matched platelets, at times, seem ineffective. Furthermore, Duquesnoy and associates (1977) have shown that platelets mismatched for cross-reacting antigens may show surprisingly good survival. Finally, there have been many attempts to apply multiple serologic approaches to platelet crossmatching, all with limited success at best. Clearly, the state of the art as regards serology and compatibility is far from that associated with red blood cell transfusions. One reasonable approach is to try HLA-compatible transfusion only after refractoriness has been established and other causes clearly excluded. At that point single-donor platelets from a compatible donor—a family member is usually the best choice—should be given, and recovery, survival, and clinical effect carefully followed. If the results are satisfactory, a trial of HLA-matched single-donor platelets collected by pheresis is probably worthwhile.

Some clinicians are anxious to use single-donor platelets for transfusion in all patients, reasoning that exposure to fewer donor antigens will delay the onset of the refractory state or pose a lower hepatitis risk. Neither proposition has been proved, and the cost and difficulties associated with obtaining the single-donor product should limit their use to situations in which their benefit is clearly shown. While our program is willing to provide single-donor platelets that are not HLA-matched for refractory patients without demonstrable HLA antibody, we do so reluctantly since evidence of their effectiveness is absent.

Granulocyte Transfusions

Modern methods of granulocyte collection have opened a whole new avenue of treatment for patients with granulocytopenia. For the first time, granulocyte replacement therapy is practical and clinicians can think about the possibility of adequate support for patients in whom temporary bone marrow failure or ablation has occurred. The availability of several automated cell separators, together with evidence that these can be used safely to remove large quantities of granulocytes from normal donors, has overnight transferred granulocyte transfusion from an experimental to an almost routine procedure. The development of regional blood centers allows clinicians in all hospitals access to granulocytes, where formerly their use had been restricted to major teaching hospitals. Unfortunately, our clinical intensity has advanced beyond properly controlled studies so that we do not yet know how best to use this new and potentially valuable therapeutic tool.

There seems to be adequate evidence that granulocyte transfusion can improve rates of recovery in patients with granulocytopenia and documented infection (Graw et al. 1972). Some studies suggest, however, that this effect is seen only if eventual bone marrow recovery ensues (Buchholz, Blumberg, and Bove 1979). There is considerably less evidence about the potential efficacy of transfusions in patients with granulocytopenia and fever but without documented infection. The optimum dose is unknown nor do we really know how often or for how long the transfusions should be given. The difficult area of cost-effectiveness is only now being investigated (Rosenshein et al. 1980), and as yet we know almost nothing about the long-term effect of the collection procedure on healthy donors. Despite all these reservations, granulocyte transfusions are widely used and are, without doubt, of some value.

Granulocyte Collection

In most blood centers granulocytes are collected by hemapheresis, a procedure in which a normal donor is connected to a machine in which leukocytes, platelets, and plasma are separated by centrifugation. The leukocytes (predominately granulocytes) can be harvested with or without platelets while the red blood cells and plasma are returned to the donor. The usual run takes two to three hours, during which time about 0.8 to 2.5×10^{10} cells are collected. To induce a leukocytosis the donor is given steroids before pheresis, and a rouleaux-inducing agent, almost always hydroxyethyl starch, is added to the separation system. Much of this hydroxyethyl starch is infused into the donor during reinfusion of the plasma. While no toxicity is currently obvious, the long-term effect is unknown.

Other collection systems such as sedimentation and pooling the buffy layer from multiple units of blood, or reversible adhesion of granulocytes to nylon filters, are also used, but less frequently.

The final product as collected by pheresis contains about 0.8 to 2.5×10^{10} white blood cells, 4 to 7×10^{11} platelets, and 30 to 50 ml of red blood cells sufficient to require cross-matching before use. The total volume is about 300 to 500 ml and the product contains a considerable amount of hydroxyethyl starch.

Donor reactions are usually mild although, as stated before, the long-term effects of hydroxyethyl starch infusion are unknown.

Indications for Granulocyte Transfusion

There is almost universal agreement that these transfusions are indicated for patients who have granulocyte counts below 300/mm^3, evidence of bone marrow aplasia, documented infection, and a failure to respond to 48 hours of treatment with appropriate antibiotics. Evidence is lacking that granulocytes are also of value when these rather stringent criteria are liberalized. For example, there is often pressure on the part of clinicians to provide transfusions when febrile granulocytopenic patients with no obvious site of infection do not respond to antibiotics. The argument, and it is reasonable, is that these patients are infected and that granulocytes are essential. Unfortunately, there are no data to support this view, and some evidence suggests that granulocyte transfusions do not help (Lowenthal et al. 1975). Nonetheless, it is almost impossible to continue treating such patients without succumbing to the rational desire to "try everything, including white cells." Similar reasoning often is applied to desperately ill patients with fever and granulocytopenia, with or without documented infection. Here again, the pressure is to do everything possible to prevent what appears to be imminent death. What little evidence there is suggests that many of these patients respond dramatically to appropriate therapy including antibiotics and do not require granulocyte transfusion. In the absence of a controlled experimental protocol or an extremely unusual circumstance, the following indications seem reasonable, and all should be present before considering granulocytes:

- Peripheral neutropenia of less than 300 to 500/mm^3
- Myeloid hypoplasia
- Clinical evidence of infection without response to 24 to 48 hours of appropriate antibiotic therapy
- A reasonable expectation that recovery or remission is possible

Granulocyte Transfusion

Transfusions can be prepared with or without platelets. The regional blood center should be informed which product is required so as to make optimum use of available donor resources.

Granulocytes are stored at 4° C and, in general, are out of date 24 hours after collection. Here again, there are few data about optimum practice, and as yet no federal regulations.

Granulocytes need not be ABO- or HLA-compatible, but the red blood cells in the unit should in general be compatible with the recipient. In addition, compatibility between donor plasma and recipient red blood cells is important to avoid transfusion reactions, a positive direct Coombs' test, and at times, hemolytic anemia.

About 10% of patients who receive granulocyte transfusions will have reactions with chills and/or fever. These can be severe. Premedication with antihistamines, antipyretics, or steroids is probably appropriate, although again, there is no controlled study showing that such measures are either necessary or beneficial. Slow infusion so that the transfusion takes two to three hours seems wise. In the event of a reaction it is appropriate to discontinue the infusion for about 30 minutes, treat with antihistamines if these had not been given, and restart the transfusion at a somewhat slower rate. Reactions are more common with cells collected by filtration leukapheresis. If this technique has been used, use of cells collected by intermittent flow centrifugation may be better tolerated.

Autologous Frozen Blood Components

One of the most recent developments in the use of component therapy in cancer relates to the use of frozen autologous platelets. (This chapter will not discuss frozen autologous bone marrow that has been used for experimental marrow repopulation after intensive therapy.) These can be collected by pheresis from patients in remission, stored frozen, and then reinfused to treat thrombocytopenia. Such therapy avoids entirely the risks of incompatibility, alloimmunization, or hepatitis and may be the next dramatic step forward. This procedure is at present experimental. Data suggest that these platelets can be used in the supportive care of patients, but that further improvements are necessary (Schiffer et al. 1976).

Summary

Modern cancer therapy depends to a large extent on the intelligent use of blood components. Although all indications are not yet fully established there is little doubt that red blood cells, platelets, and granulocytes have an important role to play. Their judicious use is important to provide the best possible treatment to the patient and to make optimum use of a scarce resource.

References

Bove, J. Which is the factual basis in theory and clinical practice, for the use of fresh frozen plasma? (International Forum) *Vox Sang.* 35:426–435, 1978.

Buchholz, D. H.; Blumberg, N.; and Bove, J. R. Long-term granulocyte transfusions in patients with malignant neoplasms. *Arch. Intern. Med.* 139:317–320, 1979.

Buchholz, D. H.; Charette, J. R.; and Bove, J. R. Preparation of leukocyte-poor red blood cells using the IBM 2991 blood cell processor. *Transfusion* 18:653–662, 1978.

Chaplin, H., Jr. et al. Current status of red-cell preservation and availability in relation to the developing national blood policy. *N. Engl. J. Med.* 291:68–74, 1974.

Daly, P. A. et al. Platelet transfusion therapy. One-hour posttransfusion increments are available in predicting the need for HLA-matched preparations. *JAMA* 243:435–438, 1980.

Duquesnoy, R. J. et al. Successful transfusion of platelets "mismatched" for HLA antigens to alloimmunized thrombocytopenic patients. *Am. J. Hematol.* 2: 219–226, 1977.

Graw, R. G. et al. Normal granulocyte transfusion therapy: treatment of septicemia due to gram-negative bacteria. *N. Engl. J. Med.* 287:367–371, 1972.

Haugen, R. H. Hepatitis after the transfusion of frozen red cells and washed red cells. *N. Engl. J. Med.* 301:393–395, 1979.

Lowenthal, R. M. et al. Granulocyte transfusions in treatment of infections in patients with acute leukemia and aplastic anemia. *Lancet* 1:353–358, 1975.

Perkins, H. A. et al. Nonhemolytic febrile transfusion reactions: quantitative effects of blood components with emphasis on isoantigenic incompatibility of leukocytes. *Vox Sang.* 11:578–600, 1966.

Rosenshein, M. S. et al. The cost effectiveness of therapeutic and prophylactic leukocyte transfusion. *N. Engl. J. Med.* 302:1058–1062, 1980.

Schiffer, C. A. et al. Frozen autologous platelets in the supportive care of patients with leukemia. *Transfusion* 16:321–329, 1976.

Schiffer, C. A.; Aisner, J.; and Wiernick, P. H. Platelet transfusion therapy for patients with leukemia. In *The blood platelet in transfusion therapy,* eds. T. J. Greenwalt and G. A. Jamieson. New York: Alan R. Liss, 1978, pp. 267–279.

Yankee, R. A.; Grument, F. C.; and Rogentine, G. N. Platelet transfusion therapy: the selection of compatible platelet donors for refractory patients by lymphocyte HL-A typing. *N. Engl. J. Med.* 281:1208–1212, 1969.

nineteen

Pain Management

DAVID S. FISCHER

Probably the most frightening aspect of cancer to most people is not the potential for dying as much as the stereotyped anticipation of prolonged and persistent pain. While it is true that only half of all patients with cancer have no significant pain (Twycross 1975), the other half have varying degrees ranging from mild discomfort to the excruciating pain of expanding tumors in bones, visceral organs, nerve plexuses, and so on. While we cannot yet cure most patients with advanced metastatic cancer, we do have the ability to control their pain. It is an abdication of responsibility and trust if the physician does not provide adequate palliation of pain.

Types of Pain

Pain is an initially somatic event that is perceived by the peripheral sensory nervous system and transmitted to the thalamus where it is further processed and ultimately relayed to the cortex where it is interpreted.

Acute pain is usually sudden in origin and may last from a few seconds to several days or weeks. It is generally associated with an identifiable event, but not always. It may be protective and prevent further injury. It may be distressing in terms of discomfort, like a fractured finger. It may be ominous and life-threatening like the constricting substernal pain of evolving myocardial infarction. It can usually be relieved with reasonable or standard doses of analgesics, and it gradually subsides and disappears with healing or recovery. Its chief characteristic is that it is temporally limited.

Chronic pain is most often gradual in onset and gradually increases in intensity up to a plateau around which it waxes and wanes. It may be non–life-threatening as in chronic back strain or nonprogressive arthritis, or it may be terrifying and life-threatening as in cancer. It is the latter type that this discussion concerns.

The perception of pain is entirely subjective and we have no scientifically objective methods for measuring it. It is as severe as the patient tells us it is. Perception of pain will be modified by acculturation, prior experience, the situational context, and whether the patient is frightened or reassured. The behavior of the patient's medical attendants can enhance or reduce pain. Chronic cancer pain may be a purely destructive factor that interferes with nutrition and concentration. It may increase anxiety, depression, sleeplessness, and irritability, and ultimately lead to psychological and physical deterioration.

Character and Distribution

Patients with cancer frequently have a low threshold for pain, partly because of the life-threatening context, and partly because its persistence wears out mental and physical reserves. The pain may be severe and yet dull, and frequently the patient has difficulty describing its location with precision (Perret 1967). Malignancies of the female genital tract, the lower colon, and the rectum frequently involve the lumbosacral plexus and the pain may follow a dermatomal pattern. In the upper gastrointestinal tract, pain is often vague and may be referred to the thoracolumbar region of the spine. Invasion of the brachial plexus by cancer of the breast or lung is usually very severe and may be referred to the entire upper extremity. Constant, sharp, severe pain is associated with invasion or compression of sensory nerves and is seen when tumor spreads to the epidural space of the spine, the base of the skull, or deep in the face. Paresthesias or hypesthesias usually follow.

Techniques of Pain Control

The best way to relieve pain is to eliminate or ameliorate its cause. Thus if pain is due to obstruction and dilation by tumor of a hollow viscus, decompression may give relief at least temporarily. If it is from a tumor compressing or infiltrating a neural structure, a bone, or a viscus, frequently radiation therapy will shrink the tumor and provide relief. In the case of intracranial neoplasms, associated edema may exacerbate pain so much that the use of steroids to reduce swelling may lead to prompt and dramatic relief of headache and associated symptoms long enough for other techniques to be employed to provide more long-lasting control.

Non-narcotic Analgesics

While attempts are being made to remove the cause of pain, or when the cause cannot be advantageously modified, analgesics should be used to raise the pain threshold and make the patient more comfortable (table 19.1).

Non-narcotic analgesics are familiar to all and frequently self-administered in our society (Moertel 1974). The ubiquitous aspirin is so common that most people forget that it was originally Bayer's trade name for their brand of acetylsalicylic acid. It is an effective analgesic in the usual adult dose of 650 mg (2 tablets) for minor to moderate pain, and is the standard against which all the non-narcotic analgesics must be compared (table 19.1). It can be given every four hours to most individuals, but in some it causes gastrointestinal irritation and occult bleeding, and on occasion, gross hemorrhage. In addition, a single dose of aspirin interferes with platelet adhesiveness for several days and can cause a prolonged bleeding time. It also prolongs the prothrombin time in patients on warfarin sodium (Coumadin) or dicumerol. I tend to use it infrequently because of its potential for side effects, especially in thrombocytopenic patients.

Acetaminophen (Tylenol, Datril, Tempra, Nebs) has become our non-narcotic analgesic of choice because of its efficacy and relative lack of side effects. It is available in standard tablets of 325 mg and extra-strength capsules of 500 mg. It has also been compounded with codeine (Tylenol with codeine, Capital with codeine), with oxycodone (Percoset, Tylox), and with propoxyphene (Darvocet). Many of our patients find these combination products useful and prefer them in some instances to narcotics that we generally regard as stronger. Some, however, object to drugs containing either aspirin or acetaminophen because they cause perspiration. Since narcotics act centrally and the non-narcotic analgesics act peripherally, using them in combination is rational and results in enhanced analgesia.

In spite of some reports of controlled studies (Moertel et al. 1972) suggesting a lack of efficacy of propoxyphene (Darvon), many of our patients report very satisfying results with it and prefer it to narcotics. There is a low but definite risk of addiction with chronic usage, but it has minimal side effects. Abuse of the agent has been reported and it has been associated with some suicides and some tragedies when mixed with alcohol or other psychotropic drugs (Barclay 1979; Ballin 1979). Accordingly, some consumer activist groups have petitioned to change the drug from narcotic control class IV to more rigidly monitored class II, or to have it removed from the market altogether. I find a definite but limited role for propoxyphene in my management of chronic cancer pain.

A recently marketed non-narcotic analgesic, zomepirac sodium (Zomax), seems to be promising as a potent nonaddicting oral agent. It is a prostaglandin synthetase inhibitor that is structurally and pharmacologically unrelated to drugs that possess narcotic agonist or antagonist properties. In early studies, 100 mg of zomepirac gave as good results as 200 mg, and had analgesic activity equivalent to or better than aspirin, 650 mg; codeine phosphate, 60 mg; and intramuscular morphine sulfate, 8 mg. When compared to aspirin in clinically equivalent doses, it produced less fecal blood loss and its dose-related effects on platelet function were of shorter duration (Forrest 1980). The drug is a nonsteroidal antiinflammatory agent with antipyretic properties. Onset of action is significant in 30 minutes and reaches a maximum in 1 to 2 hours with a duration of 4 to 6 hours. The primary route of excretion of the drug and its metabolites is in the urine. It does not bind warfarin or affect the prothrombin time. The most frequent adverse effects are nausea, gastrointestinal dis-

Table 19.1. *Approximate Equivalent Analgesic Dose*

Drug	*Brand Name*	*Oral Dose (mg)*	*Antiinflammatory*	*Addiction Liability*	*Significant Adverse Effects*
Aspirin	(The standard of comparison)	650	Yes	None	GI, platelet effect, coagulation
Acetaminophen	Tylenol, Datril, Tempra, Nebs	650	No	None	Liver
Pentazocine	Talwin	30	No	Moderate	CNS
Codeine		32	No	Moderate	Constipation
Meperidine	Demerol	50	No	High	CNS
Propoxyphene-HCl Propoxyphene napsylate	Darvon Darvon-N	65 100	No	Low	CNS
Indomethacin	Indocin	25	Yes	None	GI, CNS
Ibuprofen	Motrin	400	Yes	None	GI
Zomepirac	Zomax	100	Yes	None	GI, nausea

tress, dizziness, insomnia, edema, and rash. Antacids do not affect bioavailability or analgesic potency. The drug is marketed in 100-mg tablets.

Recently, several nonsteroidal antiinflammatory agents have been shown to have analgesic properties (Brodie 1974). I have used them only when inflammation was one of the components of the pain constellation, and hence have no experience with more general usage.

Narcotic Analgesics

The use of morphine (or opium) began before recorded history and today we still find morphine one of the most efficacious drugs available. It predictably relieves severe pain in most patients if an adequate dose is used. To my personal knowledge, none of the morphine derivates or synthetic narcotics has demonstrated superiority. For a time, diamorphine (heroin) was used in England (Twycross and Wald 1976), and claims of its superiority have stimulated attempts to legislate its use in the United States. Ironically, now that the movement for its legalization has gathered momentum, many of our British colleagues have discovered its lack of superiority and ceased using it. The famous Brompton cocktail (Mount, Ajemian, and Scott 1976) containing diamorphine, chloroform, cocaine, and ethanol was first used at the Brompton Chest Hospital in London. It was later popularized in the United States and Canada by Dr. Cecily Saunders (1967) after its use at St. Christopher's Hospice in London. After careful study, however, that institution was returned to the use of morphine solution with a phenothiazine to control nausea. We have been similarly inclined.

Currently, we favor the scheduled use of morphine for the control of chronic severe cancer pain (Lewis 1979). We have watched patients receive narcotic analgesics on a demand basis and have seen them go through torture until relief is finally obtained. Regrettably, many young house officers make the well-meaning mistake of ordering inadequate analgesia with the erroneous assumption that they are protecting the patient from the horrors of addiction (Marks and Sacher 1973). The tragedy is then compounded too often by the well-meaning but inexperienced nurse who tries further to reduce addiction potential by stalling delivery of the narcotic while the patient suffers unbelievably (McCaffrey and Hart 1976). One of the problems here is disbelief on the part of the healthy young professional, who has probably never experienced chronic or severe pain, that the cancer patient is suffering *real* pain. Instead, personal exposure has often been to a generation of young people with a high addiction rate, where malingering to get a narcotic is not a rare phenomenon. The two divergent experiences must be placed in their separate contexts. We have rarely seen a cancer patient whose addiction could not be easily alleviated by eradicating the pain. In fact, Porter and Jick (1980) reviewed 11,882 patients who received at least one narcotic and found only four cases of reasonably well-documented addiction in patients who had no history of prior addiction, and the addiction was considered major in only one case.

To control intractable severe cancer pain, I favor an oral solution of morphine sulphate, 2 mg/ml in a cherry syrup vehicle given every four hours *around the clock*. My aim is to prevent pain by anticipating its occurrence and thus to decrease apprehension. With adequate treatment, the required analgesic dose frequently may be reduced and the patient kept pain-free, without sedation or euphoria and with a normal affect and unclouded sensorium. Doses of 5 to 20 mg are usually adequate to start, with escalation of the amount as needed, usually to 30 mg and rarely more than 60 mg every four hours. To avoid the complication of nausea, an antiemetic is given with or one-half hour before the analgesic. We have found oral solutions, tablets, or capsules well-tolerated, and use prochlorperazine (Compazine), triethylperazine (Torecan), trimethobenzamide (Tigan), or promethazine (Phenergan) in the doses in the chart in chapter 31. The phenothiazines may exaggerate the sedative effects of morphine.

Tolerance and dependence are traditionally associated with chronic narcotic usage. Interestingly, once an adequate pain control regimen is established in the patient with cancer, tolerance to opiate analgesics is generally not observed. Increased dose requirements under these circumstances usually indicate a change in the patient's condition. Sudden withdrawal can precipitate the abstinence syndrome with its serious sequelae. Thus if the patient becomes unable to take the analgesic by mouth, we give it rectally or parenterally. If the patient enters a state of unresponsiveness or coma, we continue the analgesic in attenuated dose to prevent dysphoria, which may be unpleasant, and the withdrawal syndrome, which may be more life-threatening than the slight respiratory depression induced by small narcotic dosages. The emphasis throughout is on keeping the patient essentially pain-free.

In a variety of circumstances, other narcotic analgesics are useful (Catalano 1975; Shimm et al. 1979) (table 19.2). Meperidine (Demerol) and anileridine (Leritine) cause little biliary or ureteral spasm and are less constipating than most of the other narcotics. Unfortunately, meperidine is very poorly absorbed orally so that very high doses in the range of 300 mg are needed for adequate analgesia and such high doses are rarely ordered or given. Instead, meperidine, 50 mg is usually ordered and is no more analgesic than the aspirin or acetaminophen, 650 mg dosage.

Methadone (Dolophine) has the advantage of good oral absorption. At one time I favored it because of its relative lack of euphoriant effect and its long serum half-life. We have since realized that the drug may cause dysphoria in some patients. For the cancer patient with chronic pain, anxiety, and depression, the euphoria of morphine and some of the other narcotics is desirable. Recently, Ettinger, Vitale, and Trump (1979) have pointed out that the manufacturer's recommended dose of methadone for oral or parenteral administration in adults is 2.5 to 10 mg every three to four hours while the average plasma half-life is 25 hours (range 13 to 47 hours). With repeated use, the monoexponential plasma half-life is about 22.4 hours, but the analgesia lasts only three to five hours. Thus the potential for drug accumulation is high and patients may develop lethargy or coma from the methadone. The authors present three such instances in their paper and I had three similar occurrences in my practice before I drastically restricted our use of the drug.

For the patient who needs a narcotic analgesic by the rectal route, I have used two excellent preparations, oxymorphone (Numorphan) and hydromorphone (Dilaudid). These are well absorbed, may be given in the presence of nausea or vomiting, and do not require a health professional to administer them. Hydromorphone has a shorter duration of action than oxymorphone and is also available for oral and parenteral use.

For longer duration of action with the choice of oral and parenteral routes, levorphanol (Levodromoran) has become popular. It is as potent as morphine, but acts for six to eight hours. Thus it should not be given more often than every six hours to avoid accumulation with lethargy and somnolence. We have found good patient acceptance in general, especially of the oral tablet.

In recent years, there has been a fad with analgesics based on scanty literature or advice from drug detail people. This usually consists of giving a relatively weak analgesic like meperidine with a supposed potentiator like promethazine or hydroxyzine. These agents do not enhance the analgesia to the best of our knowledge (Rogers 1977). What they do is to sedate the patient, and somnolent people rarely complain. There are occasions where this somnolence is desirable, but in general, especially during the day, I prefer to see my patients alert and pain-free.

Table 19.2. *Strong Analgesics: Approximate Equivalent Analgesic Dose*

Drug	*Brand Name*	*Parenteral Dose (mg)*	*Oral Dose (mg)*	*Onset Peak Effect (min)*	*Duration of Analgesic Action (hrs)*	*Serum Half-life (hrs)*	*Abuse Potential*	*Respiratory Depression*	*Effect on Cardiac Work*	*Comment*
Morphine	—	10	30	30–60	4–5	2.6	high	high	decrease	standard of comparison
Meperidine	Demerol	75	300	30–50	2–3	3.2	high	high	decrease	short duration poor oral absorption
Methadone	Dolophine	10	20	30–60	3–6	22.4	high	high	decrease	long serum half-life good oral absorption
Oxycodone	Percodan (with aspirin) Percocet and Tylox (with acetaminophen)	—	10	15–30	3–4	?	high	high	—	avoid Percodan in thrombocytopenic patients
Hydromorphone	Dilaudid	1.5	4	15–30	3–4	?	high	high	decrease	short duration of action
Oxymorphone	Numorphan	1.5	(rectal) 5	15–30	3–6	?	moderate	moderate	—	excellent rectal absorption
Anileridine	Leritine	30	50	30–50	2–3	?	moderate	moderate	—	good oral absorption
Pentazocine	Talwin	60	100	20	3–4	2	moderate	slight	increase	CNS toxicity
Codeine	—	120	200	30–60	2–4	—	low	slight	—	only for mild pain
Levorphanol	Levodromoran	2	4	60–90	6–8	—	high	high	—	long duration of action
Butorphanol	Stadol	2	—	30	3–4	—	low	limited	increase	only available by injection
Nalbuphine	Nubain	10	—	15	3–6	5	low	limited	decrease	only available by injection
Propoxyphene	Darvon	—	240	30–60	2–4	6–12	low	low	—	only for mild pain

Most patients taking narcotic analgesics develop some degree of constipation if not given a regimen to prevent it. Liberal use of stool softeners and laxatives of all kinds are indicated. I have seen several cases of pseudoobstruction that required hospitalization because the patients ignored the need for bowel regulation.

Agonists-Antagonists

This is a new group of analgesics designed to provide the benefits of morphine without some of its adverse effects. The first agent marketed, pentazocine (Talwin), is available orally and parenterally (Payne 1973). It has a relative potency equivalent to that of codeine, but less of an abuse potential. Its side effects are similar to those of the other narcotics at equianalgesic doses. Dysphorias characterized by hallucinations and bizarre thoughts can occur in a substantial number of patients, particularly the elderly. This has seriously limited its acceptability. It is important not to start pentazocine in a narcotic-dependent patient, as its narcotic antagonist activity could precipitate the acute narcotic withdrawal syndrome.

Two newer agonist-antagonist analgesics are now available, nalbuphine (Nubain) and butorphanol (Stadol) (Vandam 1980). So far, both are available only for parenteral use. They are equipotent to morphine, and have a similar duration of action but a lower abuse potential. They both cause about as much respiratory depression as morphine with initial dosage, but are said to have a ceiling effect with increasing dosage. It remains to be seen how advantageous this will be in pathophysiologic states. Nalbuphine is said to decrease the workload of the heart while pentazocine and butorphanol may increase this and thereby aggravate myocardial ischemic states. The studies available so far are preliminary observations and more extensive experience is needed before clinicians are in a position to use these new agents with any degree of confidence. These drugs should not be used in a patient who is narcotic-dependent lest the abstinence syndrome occur.

Opiate Withdrawal

It is occasionally necessary to withdraw a dependent individual from the opiates. This has always been difficult and is sometimes painful for the patient. In the past, simple discontinuance was tried and the patient went "cold turkey." Early attempts at hastening withdrawal with narcotic antagonists such as nalorphine (Nalline) and levallorphan (Lorfan) were complicated and dangerous. Naloxone (Narcan) proved to be safe and effective for reversing acute narcotic overdosages, but provoked the abstinence syndrome in chronically dependent individuals. Preliminary studies indicate that the antihypertensive clonidine (Catapres) may be useful in acute opiate withdrawal (Gold et al. 1980). It can, however, cause hypotension and must be monitored.

Other Modalities

It is obvious that control of pain has not been solved by the narcotic analgesics in spite of our better understanding of their use. Attempts at superior control are being explored with hypnosis, acupuncture, biofeedback, and transcutaneous electrical stimulators. Each of these modalities is in a state of research development. Surgical approaches have been used with variable degrees of success and could occupy a volume of their own. Two major approaches predominate—nerve blocks and neurosurgical interruption of pain pathways.

The nerve blocks have generally been performed with tetracaine, lidocaine, dibucaine, absolute ethyl alcohol, and phenol. Successful blocks have been performed on the trigeminal nerve, Gasserian ganglion, ophthalmic nerve, maxillary nerve, mandibular nerve, glossopharyngeal nerve, vagus nerve, cervical sympathetic chain, lumbar sympathetic, celiac plexus, and splanchnic nerve. In addition, selective blocks of spinal areas may be performed as epidural, intrathecal, nerve root, paravertebral, and caudal blocks.

Neurosurgical procedures may include cranial nerve sections, sympathectomy, splanchnicectomy, posterior rhizotomy (intradural section of the sensory root of the nerve), dorsal ganglionectomy, commissural myelotomy (section of the anterior pain fibers of the cord at the decussation), cordotomy (section of the spinothalamic tract in the spinal cord), thalamotomies (lesions produced stereotactically in the thalamus), and unilateral prefrontal lobotomy. Each of these procedures has advantages and side effects and should only be considered with a neurosurgeon experienced in this area.

A Last Word

In considering the ingenuity of the human mind to solve difficult problems, we can all learn from the personal approach of great teachers and physicians. When Dr. Maurice B. Strauss was dying from inoperable esophageal cancer, he chose to spend his last days at home. He medicated himself with oral morphine on a regular four-hour schedule and remained mentally alert and productive. To maintain his caloric intake and sooth his painful esophagus, he sipped a liquid diet of gin, orange juice, and eggs. The account of this is given by

Hollander and Williams (1975) and appropriately ends with two quotations: "It is as much the business of a physician to alleviate pain, and to smooth the avenues of death, when unavoidable, as to cure diseases"; and, "There is a dignity in dying that doctors should not dare to deny."

References

Ballin, J. C. Propoxyphene: is it a hazard to health? *JAMA* 241:1618, 1979.

Barclay, W. R. Propoxyphene. *JAMA* 241:1689, 1979.

Brodie, G. N. Indomethacin and bone pain. *Lancet* 2:1160, 1975.

Catalano, R. B. The medical approach to management of pain caused by cancer. *Semin. Oncol.* 2:379–392, 1975.

Ettinger, D. S.; Vitale, P. J.; and Trump, D. L. Important clinical pharmacologic considerations in the use of methadone in cancer patients. *Cancer Treat. Rep.* 63:457–459, 1979.

Forrest, W. H., Jr. Orally administered zomepirac and parenterally administered morphine. *JAMA* 244:2298–2302, 1980.

Gold, M. S. et al. Opiate withdrawal using clonidine. *JAMA* 243:343–346, 1980.

Hollander, W., and Williams, T. F. Dr. Strauss' last teaching session. *Arch. Intern. Med.* 135:1391–1392, 1975.

Lewis, B. J. The use of opiate analgesics in cancer patients. *Cancer Treat. Rep.* 63:341–342, 1979.

Marks, R. M., and Sacher, E. J. Undertreatment of medical inpatients with narcotic analgesics. *Ann. Intern. Med.* 78:173–181, 1973.

McCaffery, M., and Hart, L. L. Undertreatment of acute pain with narcotics. *Am. J. Nurs.* 76:1586–1591, 1976.

Moertel, C. G. Relief of pain by oral medications. *JAMA* 229:55–59, 1974.

Moertel, C. G. et al. A comprehensive evaluation of marketed analgesic drugs. *N. Engl. J. Med.* 256:813–815, 1972.

Mount, B. M.; Ajemian, I.; and Scott, J. Use of the Brompton mixture in treating the chronic pain of malignant disease. *Can. Med. Assoc. J.* 115:122–124, 1976.

Payne, J. J. Focus on pentazocine. *Drugs* 5:1–96, 1973.

Perret, G. Management of pain in the patient with cancer. In *Palliative care of the cancer patient,* ed. R. C. Hickey. Boston: Little, Brown & Co., 1967, pp. 361–373.

Porter, J., and Jick, H. Addiction rare in patients treated with narcotics. *N. Engl. J. Med.* 302:123, 1980.

Rogers, A. Drugs for pain. In *Second National Conference on Cancer Nursing.* New York: American Cancer Society, 1977, pp. 39–43.

Saunders, C. *The management of terminal illness.* London: Hospital Medical Publishers, 1967.

Shimm, D. S. et al. Medical management of chronic cancer pain. *JAMA* 241:2408–2412, 1979.

Twycross, R. G. Diseases of the central nervous system. *Br. Med. J.* 4:212–214, 1975.

Twycross, R. G., and Wald, S. J. Long-term use of diamorphine in advanced cancer. In *Advances in pain research and therapy,* eds. J. J. Bonica and D. Albe-Fessard. New York: Raven Press, 1976, pp. 653–661.

Vandam, L. D. Drug therapy: butorphanol. *N. Engl. J. Med.* 302:381–383, 1980.

twenty

Treatment of Infection in the Compromised Host

RAUL E. ISTURIZ
WILLIAM H. GREENE

The extraordinary progress that has been made in the field of cancer medicine over the past several decades has permitted the physician to modify favorably the natural history of many oncologic disorders. Hence increasing numbers of patients are benefiting from better diagnostic capabilities, intensive radiotherapy, improved surgical techniques, combination chemotherapy, immunotherapy, and bone marrow transplantation (Gale 1979). These measures, as well as the host defects that the neoplasms themselves impose on patients, are associated with infectious complications. Therefore advances in the treatment of cancer have also depended on the progress made in the prevention, diagnosis, and management of infection (Greene 1977; Levine et al. 1974).

This chapter deals with the major advances made in this field over the past half-decade, using as a background occasional reference to older studies. It should serve as a guide to physicians in family practice, internists, surgeons, and pediatricians who have been encountering increasing numbers of patients with cancer who have a predisposition to infection.

Factors Responsible for Infection

A careful consideration of the specific host-immune defenses that are impaired and thus render the patient compromised will usually define the most likely sites and organisms of infection, and therefore lead to a logical individualized approach to diagnosis and treatment. In addition, knowledge of the predominant flora and their antibiotic susceptibilities in the patient's hospital environment is likely to provide helpful clues as to the new organisms the patient might acquire while hospitalized and the appropriate therapy should infection occur.

Four major categories of immune impairment are observed in cancer patients: (1) deficiencies in the components of the inflammatory response, particularly neutrophil numbers and function; (2) defects in humoral immune mechanisms, for example, complement and immunoglobulins; (3) depression of cellular immune mechanisms (anergy); and (4) transgressions of anatomic and functional boundaries (mucocutaneous ulcerations, organ obstruction) (Greene 1977) (table 20.1). The inflammatory response is most commonly impaired by the presence or induction of granulocytopenia and by therapy with high doses of corticosteroids that impair neutrophil chemotaxis. Occasionally, neutrophil dysfunction is seen among patients with acute leukemia, or as a consequence of appropriate therapy (Levine et al. 1974; Pickering et al. 1978) and can be present at a time when neutrophil counts and morphology are normal. Neutropenia remains the most important factor responsible for increased susceptibility to infection with hematologic malignancy and probably among cancer patients in general (Bodey et al. 1966; Gurwith et al. 1978a, 1978b). The incidence and severity of infection have been shown to be inversely proportional to the absolute granulocyte count, and directly

Table 20.1. *Impaired Host Resistance and Infection*

Defect	*Disease*	*Therapy Causing Similar Defect*	*Infections*
Breakdown of organ structure, e.g., ulceration, obstruction, altered normal flora	Solid tumors Malnutrition	Invasive medical procedures Antineoplastic chemotherapy, e.g., 5-FU, Mtx Radiation therapy Surgery Broad-spectrum antibiotics	Local—mixed, aerobic—anaerobic *Candida*
Impaired phagocyte function, e.g., granulopenia, phagocyte mobilization	Acute leukemia	Alkylating agents Antimetabolites Corticosteroids	Local and disseminated, *S. aureus,* Gram-negative aerobes, fungi
Reduced antibody levels	Multiple myeloma Chronic lymphocytic leukemia	—	Encapsulated bacteria, *P. carinii*
Impaired cell-mediated immunity	Hodgkin's disease Malnutrition	Corticosteroids Antineoplastic chemotherapy	Intracellular organisms, TB, fungi, protozoa, viruses

proportional to the rate of fall and to the duration of granulopenia. Furthermore, a favorable response of infection to antibiotics can be correlated with a concurrent rise in the number of circulating neutrophils (Love et al. 1980). The organisms often involved in infections that develop in the setting of neutropenia are the aerobic, enteric Gram-negative bacilli (especially *Escherichia coli, Klebsiella,* and *Pseudomonas*), *Staphylococcus aureus,* and the visceral opportunistic fungi (*Candida, Aspergillus, Torulopsis,* and *Mucor*) (Feld and Bodey 1977; Levine et al. 1974; Singer et al. 1977), although the latter are also associated with coexisting factors such as prolonged broad-spectrum antibiotic therapy.

Humoral immune dysfunction, leading to decreased circulating immunoglobulins or decreased reticuloendothelial clearance, is common post-splenectomy and in patients with chronic lymphocytic leukemia (CLL), lymphosarcoma, and in some patients with multiple myeloma (Levine et al. 1974). These patients tend to have infections with organisms that have antiphagocytic capsules, such as *Streptococcus pneumoniae* and *Hemophilus influenzae,* which require serum-opsonizing factors for efficient phagocytosis. Aggressive chemotherapy and radiation also impair humoral defense, and have been felt to magnify the risk of post-splenectomy sepsis in patients with Hodgkin's disease (Weitzman and Aisenberg 1977; Weitzman et al. 1977).

Thymus-derived lymphocytes in conjunction with mononuclear phagocytes are largely responsible for protection against intracellular organisms such as bacteria (*Salmonella, Listeria, Mycobacteria,* and *Nocardia*), fungi (*Cryptococcus* and others), protozoa (*Toxoplasma, Pneumocystis*) and viruses, especially the herpesviruses (varicella-zoster, cytomegalovirus, herpes simplex), and rubeola. Abnormal cellular immunity (anergy) with a predisposition to infection by these organisms is expected in lymphomas such as Hodgkin's disease, in the untreated state, or as a consequence of aggressive antineoplastic therapy, as in the induction of remission in acute leukemia or following bone marrow engraftment (Greene 1977; Kaplan et al. 1974; Levine et al. 1974; Mazur and Dolin 1978; Reboul et al. 1978; Winston et al. 1979; Young et al. 1979).

Finally, and perhaps most important, cutaneous and mucosal barriers are violated in multiple ways as a result of the disease itself (obstruction secondary to tumor, central nervous system disease with impaired mental state, and aspiration), iatrogenically (intravenous needles, intravenous and urethral catheters, invasive procedures), or in the functional sense, such as changes in the normal flora induced by debility or antibiotics, with resultant prolonged colonization with potentially pathogenic organisms (Green 1977; Freeman and McGowan 1978). As examples, the association of *S. bovis* bacteremia with carcinoma of the colon (Klein et

Table 20.2. *Changes in Spectrum of Infection in Granulopenic Cancer Patients*

I. Sites of infection have remained the same:

Site	*Percent of All Recognized Sites*
Oral cavity	19
Lung and bronchi	19
Skin and soft tissue	14
Urinary tract	11
Anorectum	9
Primary bacteremia	7

II. But organisms have changed—despite considerable inter-hospital variation, in general:

Class of Organism	*Decreasing*	*Increasing*	*New*
Bacteria	*P. aeruginosa*	*S. aureus*	Legionnaire's bacillus
		E. coli	Pittsburgh pneumonia agent
		Klebsiella	*S. bovis*
Fungi	—	*Candida* sp.	—
		Aspergillus sp.	
		?*Torulopsis glabrata*	
Viruses	—	Varicella-zoster	Non-A, non-B hepatitis
		Cytomegalovirus	
		Herpes simplex	
Other	*P. carinii*	—	*Strongyloides stercoralis*
	M. tuberculosis		

SOURCE: Part I EORTC 1978.

al. 1979), of *Candida* fungemia and hyperalimentation (Plouffe et al. 1977; Montgomerie and Edwards 1978), and of intraarterial catheters for cancer chemotherapy and the recently described septic endarteritis (Maki et al. 1979), are infectious diseases, some of medical "progress" which can be ascribed to changes in the functional or anatomic barriers to infection posed by normal organ structure.

Finally, many cancer patients have the added burden, at some point in the course of the disease, of associated malnutrition. This factor, which has received greatest attention in the surgical literature and in developing nations, synergizes with other defects, especially in mucocutaneous and cell-mediated defenses, in leading to infection (Greene 1977).

Etiology of Infections

Bacteria continue to be the most common group of agents responsible for infection in patients with cancer. Aerobic Gram-negative bacilli, usually *E. coli, Klebsiella, Pseudomonas aeruginosa,* or *Serratia,* are the most prevalent, followed by *S. aureus,* and other Gram-positive cocci; fungi, viruses, and protozoa are less common.

Although individual variations in the frequency of isolation of different pathogens is the rule in different centers, four recent trends have been evident (table 20.2): (1) the resurgence of *S. aureus* (and other Gram-positive organisms) as a major pathogen (EORTC 1978; Pearson et al. 1977; Pizzo et al. 1978) after its marked diminution in the 1960s, perhaps related in some instances to the use of indwelling Broviac or Hickman catheters and other intravenous lines; (2) the decline in mortality due to *Pseudomonas* sepsis, probably caused by (a) prompt and more adequate therapy with newer semisynthetic penicillins (carbenicillin and ticarcillin) used in combination with an aminoglycoside (gentamicin, tobramycin, amikacin), and (b) a true decrease in the incidence of *Pseudomonas* sepsis, with a concomitant increase in *E. coli* and *Klebsiella* infections; (3) the unwelcome appearance of Gram-negative (Meyer et al. 1976) and Gram-positive organisms (Jacobs et al. 1978; Lewis and Altemeier 1978) resistant to multiple antibiotics. Although not yet widespread, these bacteria represent not only potential threats to the lives of severely immunosuppressed cancer patients but to the adequacy of present antimicrobial therapy among more "normal" hosts; (4) the recognition of new organisms and infectious diseases that must be added to the differential diagnosis of cancer patients with fever, particularly if accompanied by a pulmonary infiltrate. Pneumonia caused by *Legionella pneumophila* has been recognized in patients with cancer (Gump et al. 1979), and its clinical presence does not permit its certain distinction from other pulmonary infections. As a result, and because of the severity of the untreated disease, early diagnosis, at times requiring invasive procedures and special microbiology, may be required. Further, these difficulties have often prompted the empiric use of parenteral erythromycin among such patients (Gump et al. 1979; Lewis et al. 1978).

Another distinct organism, the Pittsburgh pneumonia agent (now classed in the *Legionella* genus) has been described from two institutions as an opportunistic pulmonary pathogen in immunosuppressed patients, particularly after renal transplant and high-dose corticosteroids, but has also been seen in patients with cancer (Myerowitz et al. 1979; Rogers et al. 1979). This Gram-negative, weakly acid-fast bacterium is distinct from *Legionella pneumophila* but also appears to be susceptible to erythromycin, rifampin, and cotrimoxazole (trimethoprim-sulfamethoxazole). An indirect fluorescent antibody technique is useful to demonstrate seroconversion. Three other new organisms are worth mentioning; although rare, they have all been reported in cancer patients. One, a slowly growing Gram-negative rod recovered from the blood of patients with histories of dog bites, has been seen in patients with fever and cellulitis, although endocarditis and meningitis have been reported (Butler et al. 1977). The organism is sensitive in vitro to conventional and newer penicillins and cephalosporins, but resistant to aminoglycosides. The second is a bacterium that, although different in some respects, resembles *L. pneumophila* in growth characteristics and pathogenicity (Isenberg 1979; Thomason 1979). Finally, the JK group of *Corynebacteria* have increasingly been reported as causes of sepsis in patients with cancer, especially those with indwelling intravenous catheters. The significance of these new organisms and their impact on the overall issue of care of the cancer patient are yet to be fully determined.

Clinical Syndromes and Diagnosis of Infection

A detailed description of the infectious syndromes of patients with varied oncologic disorders is beyond the space limitations of this chapter. Therefore this section deals with the most common and serious clinical setting in this field, granulocytopenia (less than 1000 PMNs/mm^3) and infection. We will also mention briefly certain aspects of infection in other, nongranulocytopenic hosts.

Generalized Infection

Bacteremia is usually secondary to a localized source, and of course, the organisms recovered from the blood may serve as a clue to their origin. For example, the association of *Pseudomonas aeruginosa* bacteremia with perirectal infection is well described. Other common sources in the patient with granulocytopenia include the oropharynx (Greenberg and Cohen 1977), lungs and bronchi (Matthay and Greene 1980), urinary tract, and skin. In only about 5% to 10% of all infections (although as much as 25% of all bacteremias) (EORTC 1978) is the source of bacteremia not found. Therefore persistence in the search for a primary site is likely to be revealing. Surveillance cultures of throat, axilla, and stool will assist in identifying the colonizing organisms. Because infection often involves such organisms, the results of these cultures may be useful when an antibiotic choice must be made, especially among those patients colonized with organisms that are unusual in type or in antibiotic susceptibility.

The clinical picture initially consisting of fever and sometimes rigors, is specific neither for the site of origin nor for any particular group of organisms. Indeed, in the neutropenic patient, the absence of most signs and symptoms in a given area does not eliminate the possibility of infection in that site. Severe granulocytopenia (less than 100/mm^3) is associated with a marked diminution of signs such as exudate, abscess formation, and ulceration, and the physician must rely on "softer" symptoms such as pain, and signs such as erythema and tenderness, to diagnose and follow infection (Sickles et al. 1975). Although almost any organism can be responsible for generalized infection (Guerrant et al. 1978; Lehman et al. 1977; Pearson et al. 1977), *E. coli, Pseudomonas, Klebsiella,* and *S. aureus* are the most common; polymicrobial bacteremia is not rare.

Generalized nonbacterial infection, when it occurs, is most often caused by opportunistic fungal pathogens and is being recognized more frequently (up to 30% of fatal infections in acute leukemia and lymphoma, but far less often in patients with solid tumors). This is particularly true among patients with prolonged granulocytopenia, long courses of broad-spectrum antibacterials, and indwelling vascular catheters (Levine et al. 1974; Montgomerie and Edwards 1978; Plouffe et al. 1977; Singer et al. 1977; Winston et al. 1979), especially those delivering hyperalimentation. *Candida* and *Aspergillus* are by far the most common fungal offenders among acute leukemic patients, while *Cryptococcus* is prominent among patients with lymphoma and those receiving steroids. Although many other organisms are potential pathogens in this setting, apart from some epidemic situations, the frequency with which one encounters infection with *Nocardia, Toxoplasma gondii,* and *Strongyloides* remains quite low. Thus from the point of view of diagnosis, major attention must focus on bacterial and fungal infections.

Although it is nonspecific, fever is one of the most reliable signs of infection and in the neutropenic patient should originate an intensive search for other diagnostic clues. The characteristic ecthyma gangrenosum should always suggest *Pseudomonas* (or rarely, *Aeromonas*) sepsis; endophthalmitis should suggest fungemia. Early biopsy of a new skin lesion may provide the only clue to disseminated *Candida, Aspergillus,* or *Nocardia* infection; the importance of assessing skin lesions histologically rather than just clinically cannot be over emphasized. The importance of immediate and appropriate cultures and strains and frequent routine chest x-rays should be obvious. Indeed, apart from fever, the chest x-ray is the single best clue to pneumonia. Further diagnostic procedures such as computed tomographic scanning, ultrasound, ordinary radionuclide scanning, gallium scanning, or the infusion of indium^{111} labeled autologous leukocytes for localization of abscess may be employed if the clinical condition in less critically ill patients permits the movement and delay inherent in such procedures.

Pneumonia

Pneumonia is one of the most commonly documented localized infections among granulocytopenic patients (Matthay and Greene 1980), and is the localized infection with the highest associated mortality. Clearance of viable organisms (commonly, Gram-negative rods) that colonize the upper airway and reach the alveoli is severely impaired by debility, neutropenia, and cytotoxic therapy (Goldstein et al. 1974; Pennington 1977; Pennington and Ehrie 1978) and allows establishment and propagation of parenchymal infection.

Approximately the same range of organisms is seen as in generalized infection, but some less common pathogens deserve mention. Among them the tubercle bacillus (Kaplan et al. 1974), when present, is most commonly found in patients with Hodgkin's disease, chronic lymphocytic leukemia, bronchogenic and gastric carcinoma, and multiple myeloma. Atypical mycobacteria, often disseminated, also occur with an unusually high incidence in cancer patients (Bodey 1975). *Nocardia* infections also occur more frequently in patients with neoplasia, especially those with hematologic malignancies and those receiving corticosteroid therapy (Young et al. 1979). Available sulfonamides have accounted for the decreased mortality from nocardiosis and continue to be the treatment of choice for this disease. Two protozoa, *Pneumocystis carinii* and *Toxoplasma gondii,* also cause pulmonary infection in cancer patients (Hughes 1977; Matthay and Greene 1980). Indeed, up to 45% of cases of interstitial pneumonia in some patients with cancer (especially children with acute lymphocytic leukemia) have been due to the former. Clinical diagnosis is difficult. Profound hypoxemia, interstitial-to-alveolar infiltrates, and absence of response to antimicrobials may suggest the diagnosis in the appropriate clinical setting, which often includes steroid administration. Trimethoprim-sulfamethoxazole is as effective as and much less toxic than the prior and alternative therapy, pentamidine, and is the treatment of choice (Wormser and Keusch 1979). Moreover, one excellent study has shown its efficacy in prevention of *P. carinii* infections in children with neoplasia (Hughes et al. 1977), and this has become standard practice where pneumocystosis has been common. Toxoplasmosis causes pneumonia, but also a mononucleosis-like syndrome, chorioretinitis, and disseminated infection characterized by cerebral and (heart) muscle involvement. Treatment is pyrimethamine and sulfa drugs (Krick and Remington 1978). Severe viral pulmonary infections are common among transplant recipients but less so among cancer patients. In both groups the major viruses are the herpesviruses, especially cytomegalovirus (CMV) (Abdallah et al. 1976; Meyers et al. 1975), herpes simplex and varicella-zoster virus (Mazur and Dolin 1978; Reboul et al. 1978), and measles.

Perhaps of greatest importance in the management of pulmonary infections is the realization that neither the clinical presentation nor the appearance on chest radiograph is specific. Further, infection may disseminate and be rapidly fatal from the time of or shortly after presentation. Thus repeated chest x-rays and a stepwise, often invasive, evaluation is necessary to establish an early and specific diagnosis and to arrive at specific therapeutic decisions (Matthay et al. 1977; Matthay and Greene 1980). It is essential that the clinician undertake further diagnostic maneuvers, including transbronchoscopic biopsy or open lung biopsy, if initial assumptions about and therapy of a pneumonia of unknown etiology do not result in prompt improvement.

Perirectal Infections

Anorectal lesions are easy to overlook especially in granulocytopenic patients (Sickles et al. 1975). They are common in acute monocytic or myelomonocytic leukemia, but they also occur in other diseases associated with leukopenia. Pain on defecation and erythema or tenderness on gentle palpation of the region should suggest the diagnosis. In addition to antibiotics, including anti-pseudomonal therapy, a reduction in volume of stool, softening of stools, and the institution of sitz baths are important therapeutic measures.

Oral Infections and Pharyngitis

The oral bacterial flora are a potential and common source of infection, and a possible threat to the favorable outcome of antineoplastic therapy in immunosuppressed patients (Greenberg and Cohen 1977). It becomes of particular importance among those patients with oral neoplastic lesions (for example, head and neck cancer, gingival hypertrophy in monocytic leukemia) or those receiving ulcerogenic antineoplastic therapy, for example, methotrexate or daunorubicin. In addition, candidal infection (thrush) is perhaps the most common oral infection, causing local discomfort, and perhaps progressing to esophagitis or dissemination. The use of oral nystatin for prevention is of uncertain value (Pizzuto et al. 1978). Bacterial pharyngitis is frequent following chemotherapy and, unlike the intact host, is a significant source of bacteremia in the granulopenic patient.

Esophagitis

Retrosternal pain and dysphagia should suggest esophagitis and prompt a barium swallow and possibly esophagoscopy, which can be useful in making a positive diagnosis of candidal esophagitis, or to recognize other etiologic agents such as herpes simplex (Lightdale et al. 1977) or tumor invasion.

Skin

The skin may be the source of infection, or a manifestation of dissemination from another source as previously noted. Indeed a recent study suggests that scalp vein needles and intravascular catheters may be two of the primary sources of Gram-positive coccal infection in the granulopenic host. In the setting of a fever of unknown origins (FUO) and granulopenia, the appearance of a skin lesion is a mandate for biopsy.

Central Nervous System (CNS) Infection

These infections are common in patients with lymphoma, leukemia, and head and spine tumors, and those undergoing CNS surgery. Bacterial infection (*Listeria monocytogenes, S. aureus,* and Gram-negative rods) closely followed by fungal infection (*Aspergillus, Candida, Mucor, Cryptococcus*) predominate (Chernick et al. 1977). Dysfunction of the CNS in an immunosuppressed cancer patient should prompt a diagnostic lumbar puncture and extensive CSF evaluation if risk of cerebral herniation is minimal or if bacterial meningitis is suspected. Early recognition of CNS infection and aggressive therapy appear to increase survival.

Urinary Tract Infection (UTI)

Urinary infections are common but are predictable in that they are usually the consequence of instrumentation or of factors predisposing to obstruction (catheter, tumor, etc.). Etiologic agents correlate with the aerobic stool flora, especially *E. coli.* The decreased inflammatory response of granulocytopenia limits symptoms and makes less likely the visualization of white blood cells in urinary specimens. The physician must therefore rely on findings of bacteria in the unspun urine specimen or a positive culture to make the diagnosis. If diagnosis is prompt the outcome in UTIs is usually favorable even in the granulopenic host.

Hepatitis

Hepatic dysfunction during induction of acute leukemia may be secondary to drug therapy, may be a consequence of bacterial sepsis (for which evaluation should be carried out), or may reflect viral hepatitis usually secondary to blood product transfusion. Non-A–non-B hepatitis (NANB) is presently the most frequent form of viral hepatitis. Diagnosis is sustained on the basis of clinical features plus elimination of other likely causes. It is possible that accurate markers for NANB hepatitis may become available in the next year or two, contributing greatly not only to diagnosis but also prophylaxis.

Therapy of Infection

From the preceding discussion it should be clear that the cancer patient, and especially the patient with granulocytopenia, is particularly susceptible to infection, and that infection when it occurs is frequently severe. This section attempts to provide some guidelines for therapy of presumed or established infection in the neutropenic patient.

Empiric, Broad-Spectrum Antimicrobial Therapy Initiated at the Onset of Fever

Rationale (Greene 1977):

1. About 70% of all febrile episodes in the granulocytopenic patient are caused by bacterial infection.
2. Mortality in untreated bacterial sepsis in these patients is high, up to 50% in the first 48 to 72 hours.
3. Other than fever, symptoms and physical (as well as radiologic) findings of infection are often minimal at first examination.

The implications of these data are that fever in the granulopenic patient is most likely an indication of true infection, of which most will be bacterial. Furthermore, the absence of confirmatory findings on physical examination does not reliably exclude infection. Finally, to withhold antibacterial therapy in these patients until cultures or examination document infection means running a considerable risk that a patient will die or be irretrievably ill before such therapy begins. In short, fever in a granulopenic patient in whom there is clinical suspicion of infection warrants a prompt diagnostic work-up and initiation of broad-spectrum antibiotics.

Drugs

Several recent studies have described improved cure rates of neutropenic patients with infection (Bodey et al. 1978b; Love et al. 1979). The information provided from some of these studies (Bodey et al. 1978a, 1979; EORTC 1978; Feld et al. 1979; Gurwith et al. 1978a, 1978b; Keating et al. 1979; Lau et al. 1977) will be summarized below, but in choosing a particular agent the physician must be aware of the particular locally important pathogenic isolates as well as the local patterns of antibiotic resistance. The following guidelines can be used as background:

1. Aminoglycosides alone are inadequate therapy for *Pseudomonas* infections in granulocytopenic patients, although it has been suggested that their efficacy is substantially improved when they are given by continuous infusion. Cell-wall-active agents, notably carbenicillin (or ticarcillin), are preferable.

2. Combination therapy with two agents to which the pathogen is susceptible is better than administration of a single antibiotic, especially if in vitro synergy is demonstrated by the combination against the infecting organism (Anderson et al. 1978; Andriole 1971; Lau et al. 1977; Love et al. 1980).

3. The combination of cephalothin plus an aminoglycoside is probably more nephrotoxic than either agent used alone (EORTC 1978), particularly in the elderly. This potentiation of nephrotoxicity may not hold true for newer cephalosporins such as cefamandole and cefoxitin, although conclusive data are lacking. The issue of comparative nephrotoxicity of tobramycin and gentamicin will not be discussed any further than to note that the recent study by Smith and co-workers (1980) does not, to these writers, appear to be definitive.

4. The addition of a third (or more) antibiotic does not seem to result in improved efficacy and may produce increased toxicity and an increased theoretical risk of superinfection.

5. Gentamicin (and other newer aminoglycosides) is adequate initial coverage for *S. aureus* (EORTC 1978), and carbenicillin (or ticarcillin) in full dosages is adequate therapy for most instances of anaerobic sepsis.

It is ironic and disappointing that despite a decade of studies, many comparative and controlled, the regimen of carbenicillin and gentamicin (or equivalent) described by Schimpff (1977) has not been improved on. Thus a satisfactory current choice for initial empiric antibiotic therapy at most institutions would be the combination of carbenicillin (or ticarcillin) plus an aminoglycoside. Gentamicin is generally chosen when *P. aeruginosa* is not highly suspected and, of course, in hospitals where isolation of gentamicin-resistant Gram-negative bacteria is not substantial. (In the former, tobramycin may be preferable and in the latter amikacin may be required). Because most infections are caused by the organisms colonizing, a reasonable although expensive aid to antibiotic choice is to obtain serial surveillance cultures (throat, axilla, and stool) to follow flora and their antibiotic susceptibility patterns. After initiation of antibiotics their subsequent manipulation will depend on full daily reevaluations, and may be guided by bacterial isolation and by clinical response. A simplified guide to such adjustments is shown in figure 20.1, but a full explanation is beyond the scope of this paper (Greene 1977). The question of discontinuing antibiotics in persisting granulopenia is controversial and no certain guidelines can be offered. Nevertheless, it is the authors' preference to minimize the duration of antibiotics because of the high rate of superinfection

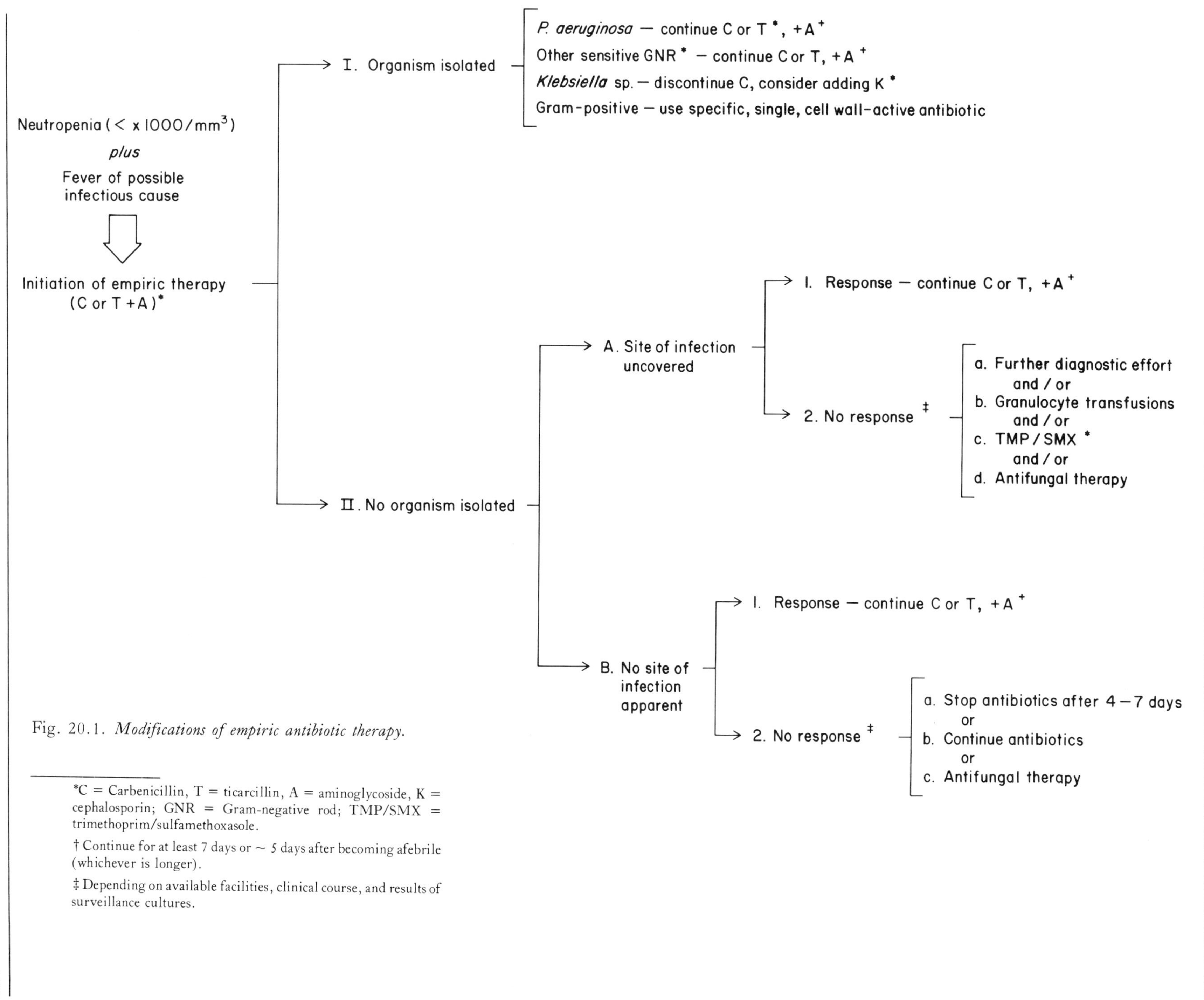
Neutropenia (< x 1000/mm³)
plus
Fever of possible infectious cause
Initiation of empiric therapy (C or T + A)*
I. Organism isolated
P. aeruginosa — continue C or T*, + A†
Other sensitive GNR* — continue C or T, + A†
Klebsiella sp. — discontinue C, consider adding K*
Gram-positive — use specific, single, cell wall-active antibiotic
II. No organism isolated
A. Site of infection uncovered
1. Response — continue C or T, + A†
2. No response ‡
a. Further diagnostic effort
and / or
b. Granulocyte transfusions
and / or
c. TMP / SMX *
and / or
d. Antifungal therapy
B. No site of infection apparent
1. Response — continue C or T, + A†
2. No response ‡
a. Stop antibiotics after 4 – 7 days
or
b. Continue antibiotics
or
c. Antifungal therapy

Fig. 20.1. *Modifications of empiric antibiotic therapy.*

*C = Carbenicillin, T = ticarcillin, A = aminoglycoside, K = cephalosporin; GNR = Gram-negative rod; TMP/SMX = trimethoprim/sulfamethoxasole.

† Continue for at least 7 days or ~ 5 days after becoming afebrile (whichever is longer).

‡ Depending on available facilities, clinical course, and results of surveillance cultures.

associated with prolonged antibiotic therapy (EORTC 1978).

Granulocyte Transfusions

Therapeutic granulocyte transfusions are probably of value if reasonable criteria based on recent trials (Alavi et al. 1977; Herzig et al. 1977) are developed and used. Although further ongoing research is expected to identify specific subsets of patients deriving maximum benefit from these transfusions, it is useful to recognize those who are less likely to respond to antibiotics alone and may thus require additional measures. This would include patients with Gram-negative bacteremia, pneumonia, and those likely to have persistent rather than transient granulocytopenia (Alavi et al. 1977; Schiffer 1977). Nevertheless, as recently noted (Love et al. 1980), most granulopenic patients with infection, even those with bacteremia, will improve with antibiotics alone. Further, febrile granulopenic patients without definite signs and symptoms (i.e., those with "possible" infection) have a very high response rate (more than 80% to 90%) to antibiotics alone. Thus the initiation of polymorphonuclear cell (PMN) transfusions in all febrile granulopenic patients would waste a limited resource and expose them to the potential toxicities, including CMV infection, alloimmunization, pulmonary reactions, and the formidable constitutional reactions. It seems judicious therefore to use PMN transfusions when the patient:

1. Is granulopenic (less than $500/mm^3$)
2. Has a documented site and/or organism causing the infection
3. Has failed to respond to appropriate antiinfective therapy after 48 to 72 hours

When granulocyte transfusions are given, they should be continued throughout the entire course of treatment (Aisner et al. 1978; Schiffer 1977) either until antibiotics are discontinued or the patient is no longer granulopenic.

Fungal Infections

The increasing frequency of visceral fungal infections (Edwards et al. 1978; Krick and Remington 1976; Wingard et al. 1979; Young et al. 1974) and their poor outcome with standard treatment have raised the question of empiric initiation of antifungal therapy. Survival from invasive disease has been associated with early diagnosis and therapy (Aisner et al. 1977; Pennington 1976), usually as a result of aggressive diagnostic approaches. Since (1) fungal infections are uncommon as compared to bacterial infections, and (2) effective therapy has significant toxicity, the empiric use of antifungal therapy should be reserved for consideration in patients who have a new fever after a prolonged course of antibacterials and granulocytopenia, or in whom other epidemiologic or serologic evidence of fungal colonization and possibly invasion is present. Patients who would not tolerate invasive diagnostic procedures are also candidates for empiric therapy (e.g., intravenous amphotericin-B). Treatment for established fungal infection has been recently reviewed (Medoff and Kobayashi 1980). Novel forms of therapy, among these miconazole and ketoconazole, and synergistic combinations of agents (Beggs et al. 1976; Kitahara et al. 1976; Medoff and Kobayashi 1980) have not received adequate clinical trials to be certain of their value. Some seem promising on the basis of in vitro and animal experiments and may be essayed in the desperate clinical situation. Finally, granulocyte transfusions have been used. Several reports have suggested they are beneficial in patients with host-defense abnormalities as well as fungal infections (Gesovich et al. 1975; Lowenthal et al. 1975).

Prevention of Infections

Prevention is, of course, the best way of dealing with disease. Development of a program to prevent infection depends on knowledge of predisposing factors as mentioned above. Such programs should include a review of the risk of infection for specific diseases and their therapy, and a detailed analysis of those infections that are occurring within the given institution. Several other factors merit further discussion.

Improve Host Defenses

Vaccination

The recent licensure of a polyvalent pneumococcal vaccine has led to its recommendation for high-risk patients (Pneumococcal vaccine 1978). Although patients with Hodgkin's disease have shown impaired antibody responses particularly shortly after treatment (Minor et al. 1979; Siber 1978), the excellent risk/benefit ratio should encourage its use. Similarly, killed influenza vaccine should be given to patients with cancer prior to or between chemotherapy courses (Ortbals et al. 1977). Equally important is the avoidance of live virus vaccines, such as polio or measles.

Prophylactic Granulocyte Transfusions

These have been noted to be protective in one study of patients receiving bone marrow transplants (Clift et al. 1978). Further evaluation by another group has led to the discontinuation of the protocol due to an unacceptably high incidence of severe CMV infections (Winston et al. 1980) felt to be secondary to transmission by way of the transfused PMNs. Further studies are under way and may help decide their true value.

Lithium Carbonate

The agent has been used to offset the neutropenia associated with malignant disease (Stein et al. 1977; Lyman et al. 1980). Neutrophils obtained from patients taking the medication function normally (Cohen et al. 1979), but the side effects of lithium and the uncertainties of benefit argue against its routine use at present.

Other accepted approaches include zoster-immune globulin following varicella exposure in immunosuppressed children with a negative history of varicella, and immune serum globulin following measles exposure in nonimmunized children. When corticosteroids must be given, an alternate-day regimen should be used if possible.

Reduce Invasive Procedures

Large intravenous catheters and urinary catheters should be avoided unless absolutely necessary. Intravenous catheters when used and scalp vein needles should be changed every 48 hours. The increasing use of long-term indwelling subcutaneously tunneled subclavian catheters (Hickman or Broviac) can only be viewed with alarm in the context of the severely immunosuppressed patient, unless carefully controlled studies establish their safety.

Decrease Acquisition of Potential Pathogens

Hospitalization should be avoided when possible, and patients in hospital should be discharged without undue delay. Those who need hospitalization should be placed in single-bed rooms if possible. Hygiene should be stressed for ward personnel, especially effective hand-washing, but so-called protective or reverse isolation does not seem superior to standard ward care (Nauseef and Maki 1979) based on limited clinical data. Modified reverse isolation (gloves and masks) is neither onerous nor expensive and is probably worth continuing. Laminar airflow rooms and "sterile diets" will substantially reduce the acquisition of new organisms, and their use in association with oral nonabsorbable antibiotics will clearly decrease the frequency of infection. These remain experimental measures, and are both cumbersome and expensive (Greene 1977).

Suppress Organisms Already Colonizing

The use of expensive and often unpalatable oral nonabsorbable antibiotics will suppress the gut flora and as noted, can be effective in reducing infection (Greene 1977). Recent studies have shown that oral trimethoprim-sulfamethoxazole (T/S), clearly efficacious in chemoprophylaxis for *Pneumocystis carinii* pneumonitis (Hughes et al. 1977), can be effective as prophylaxis of bacterial infection in hospitalized granulocytopenic patients (Gurwith et al. 1979; Hughes et al. 1977). Further studies are in progress, at least one of which has reportedly been negative. Nevertheless, this remains an exciting prospect and many oncologists have adopted use of T/S routinely.

Future Directions

Although great progress has been made, infection continues to be a leading cause of mortality among patients with cancer. The attention of the medical community continues to be focused on means to prevent or better treat infection in these compromised patients. New bacterial and viral vaccines and immune sera have been prepared, and clinical trials are currently under way (Pennington 1978; Sabin 1977; Wolf and McCuthan 1979). Newer aminoglycosides (Yap and Bodey 1979) are still under evaluation, as are innovative (third generation) cephalosporins that have an extended spectrum including resistant *Enterobacteriaceae, Pseudomonas aeruginosa* (Wise and Rollason 1978), and *Bacteroides fragilis*. Even more exciting are novel approaches to the possible prevention and therapy of severe local or disseminated viral infections, especially those caused by the herpesviruses, herpes simplex, cytomegalovirus, and varicella-zoster virus using biologic and chemical products such as human leukocyte interferon, adenine arabinoside, and acyclovir (Hirsch and Swartz 1980).

Despite all the potential improvements to come, there *have* been previous clinical trials in which infectious morbidity has been markedly reduced and mortality eliminated in patients with severe host compromise and malignancy. Limitation of application of these seemingly effective measures (laminar airflow rooms, oral nonabsorbable antibiotics) has come from their effort and cost, and the lack of resultant improvement in remission and survival (Greene 1977). The ultimate challenge for cancer care in the 1980s lies in finding those means of preventing infectious mortality that are cost-effective and in discovering modes of tumor therapy that will improve the remission rate among patients no longer dying from infection, and be cancer-specific, causing little or no suppression of host immune defenses.

References

Abdallah, P. S. et al. Diagnosis of cytomegalovirus pneumonia in compromised hosts. *Am. J. Med.* 61:326–332, 1976.

Aisner, J. et al. Treatment of invasive aspergillosis: relation of early diagnosis and treatment to response. *Ann. Intern. Med.* 86:539–543, 1977.

Aisner, J. et al. Granulocyte transfusions: evaluation of factors influencing result and a comparison of filtration and intermittent centrifugation leukapheresis. *Br. J. Haematol.* 38:121–129, 1978.

Alavi, J. B. et al. A randomized clinical trial of granulocyte transfusions for infection in acute leukemia. *N. Engl. J. Med.* 296:706–711, 1977.

Anderson, E. T. et al. Antimicrobial synergism in the therapy of gram-negative rod bacteremia. *Chemotherapy* 24:45–54, 1978.

Andriole, V. T. Synergy of carbenicillin and gentamicin in experimental infection with *Pseudomonas*. *J. Infect. Dis.* 124 (suppl.):46–55, 1971.

Beggs, W. H. et al. Synergistic action of amphotericin B and rifampin against *Candida* species. *J. Infect. Dis.* 133:206–209, 1976.

Bodey, G. P. Infections in cancer patients. *Cancer Treat. Rev.* 2:89–128, 1975.

Bodey, G. P. et al. Quantitative relationships between circulating leucocytes and infection in patients with acute leukemia. *Ann. Intern. Med.* 64:328–340, 1966.

Bodey, G. P. et al. Carbenicillin plus cefamandole in the treatment of infections in patients with cancer. *J. Infect. Dis.* 137:139–143, 1978a.

Bodey, G. P. et al. Fever and infection in leukemic patients. *Cancer* 41:1610–1627, 1978b.

Bodey, G. P. et al. A randomized study of carbenicillin plus cefamandole in the treatment of febrile episodes in cancer patients. *Am. J. Med.* 67:608–616, 1979.

Butler, T. B. et al. Unidentified gram-negative rod infection. A new disease of man. *Ann. Intern. Med.* 86:1–5, 1977.

Chernick, N. L. et al. Central nervous system infections in patients with cancer. *Cancer* 40:268–274, 1977.

Clift, R. A. et al. Granulocyte transfusion for the prevention of infection in patients receiving bone marrow transplants. *N. Engl. J. Med.* 298:1052–1057, 1978.

Cohen, M. S. et al. Granulocyte function during lithium therapy. *Blood* 53:913–915, 1979.

Edwards, J. E. Severe candidal infections. *Ann. Intern. Med.* 89:91–106, 1978.

EORTC. Three antibiotic regimens in the treatment of infection in febrile granulocytopenic patients with cancer. *J. Infect. Dis.* 137:14–29, 1978.

Feld, R. et al. Empiric therapy for infections in granulocytopenic cancer patients. *Arch. Intern. Med.* 139:310–314, 1979.

Feld, R., and Bodey, G. P. Infections in patients with malignant lymphoma treated with combination chemotherapy. *Cancer* 39:1018–1025, 1977.

Freeman, J., and McGowan, J. E. Risk factors for nosocomial infection. *J. Infect. Dis.* 138:811–819, 1978.

Gale, R. P. Advances in the therapy of acute myelogenous leukemia. *N. Engl. J. Med.* 300:1189–1190, 1979.

Gesovich, F. G. et al. Successful control of systemic *Aspergillus niger* infection in two patients with acute leukemia. *Cancer* 36:2271–2276, 1975.

Goldstein, E. et al. Pulmonary alveolar macrophage: defender against bacterial infection in the lung. *J. Clin. Invest.* 54:519–528, 1974.

Greenberg, M. S., and Cohen, G. Oral infection in immunosuppressed renal transplant patients. *Oral Surg.* 43:879–885, 1977.

Greene, W. H. Supportive care in the cancer patient. In *Cancer: a comprehensive treatise,* vol. 5, ed. F. Becker. New York: Plenum Press, 1977, pp. 238–270.

Guerrant, R. L. et al. Campylobacteriosis in man. *Am. J. Med.* 65:584–592, 1978.

Gump, D. W. et al. Legionnaires' disease in patients with associated serious disease. *Ann. Intern. Med.* 90:538–542, 1979.

Gurwith, M. J. et al. Granulocytopenia in hospitalized patients. I. *Am. J. Med.* 64:121–126, 1978a.

Gurwith, M. J. et al. Granulocytopenia in hospitalized patients. II. *Am. J. Med.* 64:127–132, 1978b.

Gurwith, M. J. et al. A prospective controlled investigation of prophylactic trimethoprim/sulfamethoxazole in hospitalized granulocytopenic patients. *Am. J. Med.* 66:248–256, 1979.

Herzig, R. H. et al. Successful granulocyte transfusion therapy for gram-negative septicemia. *N. Engl. J. Med.* 296:701–705, 1977.

Hirsch, M. S., and Swartz, M. N. Antiviral agents. *N. Engl. J. Med.* 203:903–907, 949–953, 1980.

Hughes, W. T. Pneumocystis carinii pneumonia. *N. Engl. J. Med.* 297:1381–1383, 1977.

Hughes, W. T. et al. Successful chemoprophylaxis for Pneumocystis carinii pneumonitis. *N. Engl. J. Med.* 297:1419–1426, 1977.

Isenberg, H. D. *Legionella,* WIGA, et cetera: pathogens? Editorial. *Ann. Intern. Med.* 91:785–786, 1979.

Jacobs, M. R. et al. Emergence of multiply resistant pneumococci. *N. Engl. J. Med.* 299:735–740, 1978.

Kaplan, M. H. et al. Tuberculosis complicating neoplastic disease. *Cancer* 33:850–858, 1974.

Keating, M. C. et al. A randomized comparative trial of three aminoglycosides. *Medicine* 58:159–170, 1979.

Kitahara, M. et al. Activity of amphotericin B, 5-fluorocytosine and rifampin against six clinical isolates of *Aspergillus. Antimicrob. Agents Chemother.* 9:915–919, 1976.

Klein, R. S. et al. *Streptococcus bovis* septicemia and carcinoma of the colon. *Ann. Intern. Med.* 91:560–562, 1979.

Krick, J. A., and Remington, J. S. Opportunistic invasive fungal infection in patients with leukemia and lymphoma. *Clin. Haematol.* 5:149–310, 1976.

Krick, J. A., and Remington, J. S. Toxoplasmosis in the adult—an overview. *N. Engl. J. Med.* 298:550–553, 1978.

Lau, W. K. et al. Comparative efficacy and toxicity of amikacin/carbenicillin versus gentamicin/carbenicillin in leucopenic patients. *Am. J. Med.* 62:959–966, 1977.

Lehman, T. J. A. et al. *Clostridium septicum* infection in childhood leukemia. *Cancer* 40:950–953, 1977.

Levine, A. S. et al. Hematologic malignancies and other marrow failure states: progress in the management of complicating infections. *Semin. Hematol.* 11:141–202, 1974.

Lewis, S. A., and Altemeier, W. A. Emergence of clinical isolates of *Staphylococcus aureus* resistant to gentamicin and correlates of resistance with bacteriophage type. *J. Infect. Dis.* 137:314–317, 1978.

Lewis, V. J. et al. In vivo susceptibility of the legionnaires' disease bacterium to ten antimicrobial agents. *Antimicrob. Agents Chemother.* 13:419–422, 1978.

Lightdale, C. J. et al. Herpetic esophagitis in patients with cancer: ante-mortem diagnosis by brush biopsy cytology. *Cancer* 39:223–226, 1977.

Love, L. J. et al. Randomized trial of empiric antibiotic therapy with ticarcillin in combination with gentamicin, amikacin, or netilmicin in febrile patients with granulocytopenia and fever. *Am. J. Med.* 66:603–610, 1979.

Love, L. J. et al. Improved prognosis for granulocytopenic patients with gram-negative bacteremia. *Am. J. Med.* 68:643–648, 1980.

Lowenthal, R. H. et al. Granulocyte transfusions in treatment of infections in patients with acute leukemia and aplastic anemia. *Lancet* 1:353–358, 1975.

Lyman, G. H. et al. The use of lithium carbonate to reduce infection and leukopenia during systemic chemotherapy. *N. Engl. J. Med.* 302:257–260, 1980.

Maki, D. G. et al. Septic endarteritis due to intraarterial catheters for cancer chemotherapy. *Cancer* 44: 1228–1240, 1979.

Matthay, R. A. et al. Diagnostic fiberoptic bronchoscopy in the immunocompromised host with pulmonary infiltrates. *Thorax* 32:539–545, 1977.

Matthay, R. A., and Greene, W. H. Pulmonary infections in the immunocompromised patient. *Med. Clin. North Am.* 64:529–551, 1980.

Mazur, M. H., and Dolin, R. Herpes zoster at the NIH: a 20-year experience. *Am. J. Med.* 65:738–744, 1978.

Medoff, G., and Kobayashi, G. Strategies in the treatment of systemic fungal infections. *N. Engl. J. Med.* 302:145–155, 1980.

Meyer, R. D. et al. Gentamicin-resistant *Pseudomonas aeruginosa* and *Serratia marcescens* in a general hospital. *Lancet* 1:580–583, 1976.

Meyers, J. D. et al. Cytomegalovirus pneumonia after human marrow transplantation. *Ann. Intern. Med.* 82:181–188, 1975.

Minor, D. R. et al. Response of patients with Hodgkin's disease to pneumococcal vaccine. *Ann. Intern. Med.* 90:887–892, 1979.

Montgomerie, J. Z., and Edwards, J. E. Association of infection due to *Candida albicans* with intravenous hyperalimentation. *J. Infect. Dis.* 137:197–201, 1978.

Myerowitz, R. L. et al. Opportunistic lung infection due to the "Pittsburgh pneumonia agent." *N. Engl. J. Med.* 301:953–958, 1979.

Nauseef, W. M., and Maki, D. G. A study of conventional isolation in granulocytopenic patients. Proceedings of the 19th Interscience Conference on Antimicrobial Agents and Chemotherapy, 1979, Boston.

Ortbals, D. W. et al. Influenza immunization of adult patients with malignant disease. *Ann. Intern. Med.* 87:552–557, 1977.

Pearson, T. A. et al. *Corynebacterium* sepsis in oncology patients. *JAMA* 238:1737–1740, 1977.

Pennington, J. E. Successful treatment of *Aspergillus* pneumonia in hematologic neoplasia. *N. Engl. J. Med.* 295:426–427, 1976.

Pennington, J. E. Bronchoalveolar cell response to bacterial challenge in immunosuppressed lung. *Am. Rev. Respir. Dis.* 116:885–889, 1977.

Pennington, J. E. Infection in the compromised host. Recent advances and future directions. In *Seminars in infectious diseases,* eds. L. Weinstein and B. Fields. New York: Stratton Intercontinental, 1978, pp. 142–168.

Pennington, J. E., and Ehrie, M. G. Pathogenesis of *Pseudomonas aeruginosa* pneumonia during immunosuppression. *J. Infect. Dis.* 137:764–774, 1978.

Pickering, L. K. et al. Effect of chemotherapeutic agents on metabolic and bactericidal activity of polymorphonuclear leucocytes. *Cancer* 42:1741–1746, 1978.

Pizzo, P. A. et al. Increasing incidence of gram-positive sepsis in cancer patients. *Med. Pediatr. Oncol.* 5:241–244, 1978.

Pizzuto, J. et al. Nystatin prophylaxis in leukemia and lymphoma. *N. Engl. J. Med.* 299:661–662, 1978.

Plouffe, J. F. et al. Nosocomial outbreak of *Candida parapsilosis* fungemia related to intravenous infusions. *Arch. Intern. Med.* 137:1686–1689, 1977.

Pneumococcal vaccine. *Medical Letter* 20:13–14, 1978.

Reboul, F. et al. Herpes zoster and varicella infections in children with Hodgkin's disease. *Cancer* 41:95–99, 1978.

Rogers, B. H. et al. Opportunistic penumonia. *N. Engl. J. Med.* 301:959–961, 1979.

Sabin, A. B. Varicella-zoster virus vaccine. *JAMA* 238:1731–1733, 1977.

Schiffer, C. A. Granulocyte transfusion therapy. *Med. Clin. North Am.* 61:1119–1131, 1977.

Schimpff, S. C. Therapy of infection in patients with granulocytopenia. *Med. Clin. North Am.* 61:1101–1118, 1977.

Siber, G. R. Impaired antibody response to pneumococcal vaccine after treatment for Hodgkin's disease. *N. Engl. J. Med.* 299:442–448, 1978.

Sickles, E. A. et al. Clinical presentation of infection in granulocytopenic patients. *Arch. Intern. Med.* 135:715–719, 1975.

Singer, C. et al. Bacteremia and fungemia complicating neoplastic disease. *Am. J. Med.* 62:731–742, 1977.

Smith, C. R. et al. Double-blind comparison of the nephrotoxicity and auditory toxicity of gentamicin and tobramycin. *N. Engl. J. Med.* 302:1106–1109, 1980.

Stein, R. S. et al. Lithium carbonate attenuation of chemotherapy-induced leukopenia. *N. Engl. J. Med.* 297:430–431, 1977.

Thomason, B. M. et al. A *Legionella*-like bacterium related to WIGA in a fatal case of pneumonia. *Ann. Intern. Med.* 91:673–676, 1979.

Weitzman, S. A. et al. Impaired humoral immunity in treated Hodgkin's disease. *N. Engl. J. Med.* 297: 245–248, 1977.

Weitzman, S. A., and Aisenberg, A. C. Fulminant sepsis after the successful treatment of Hodgkin's disease. *Am. J. Med.* 62:47–50, 1977.

Wingard, J. R. et al. *Candida tropicalis:* a major pathogen in immunocompromised patients. *Ann. Intern. Med.* 91:539–543, 1979.

Winston, D. J. et al. Infectious complications of human bone marrow transplantation. *Medicine* 58:1–31, 1979.

Winston, D. J. et al. Prophylactic granulocyte transfusions during human bone marrow transplantation. *Am. J. Med.* 68:893–897, 1980.

Wise, R., and Rollason, T. HR756, a highly active cephalosporin. Comparison with cefazolin and carbenicillin. *Antimicrob. Agents Chemother.* 14:807–811, 1978.

Wolf, J. L., and McCuthan, J. A. Prophylactic antibody to core lipopolysaccharide in neutropenic patients. Proceedings of the 19th Interscience Conference on Antimicrobial Agents and Chemotherapy, 1979, Boston.

Wormser, G. P., and Keusch, G. T. Trimethoprim-sulfamethoxazole in the United States. *Ann. Intern. Med.* 91:420–429, 1979.

Yap, B-S., and Bodey, G. P. Netilmicin in the treatment of infections in patients with cancer. *Arch. Intern. Med.* 139:1259–1262, 1979.

Young, L. S. et al. *Nocardia asteroides* infection complicating neoplastic disease. *Am. J. Med.* 50:356–367, 1979.

Young, R. C. et al. Fungemia with compromised host resistance. *Ann. Intern. Med.* 80:605–612, 1974.

part four

Chemotherapy

twenty-one

Chemotherapy: An Introduction

DAVID S. FISCHER

To give some perspective on a time scale of when the major drugs became available for clinical trials, table 21.1 presents them in order of their use, with a tumor type in which each has demonstrated some efficacy.

Tumors that grew progressively were described in papyruses 3600 years ago in ancient Egypt (Kardinal and Yarbro 1979). General therapy was with surgical incision and cauterization, and superficial skin lesions were treated with caustic arsenic pastes. Use of arsenic pastes continued into this century. In fact, the first specific anticancer drug was potassium arsenite, introduced by Lissauer in 1865 against chronic leukemia and regarded as standard therapy early in this century (Osler 1909). As Fowler's solution, its use was still enthusiastically being reported 66 years later for treatment of chronic myelogenous leukemia by Forkner and Scott (1931). Although many other agents were tried, none achieved this degree of acceptance. On the contrary, a general attitude developed that cancer could be treated only by surgery and radiation, and drugs had no role in therapy.

The nihilistic attitude about anticancer drugs persisted until the mid-1930s when Prontosil, sulfonilamide, and penicillin were shown to be effective antibacterial agents. This reexcited interest in the search for antitumor agents, and set the stage for further research. Burchenal (1977) regards this change in attitude as a decisive turning point. He lists the five phases of the history of cancer chemotherapy as follows:

1. Realization that the chemotherapy of cancer might be possible (1935–1945)
2. Discovery and evaluation of new antitumor agents (1945–present)
3. Development of sanctuary therapy with intrathecal methotrexate or craniospinal irradiation or both (1957–1965)
4. Development of intensive intermittent combination therapy (1960–present)
5. Development of combined modality (adjuvant) therapy (early era 1955–1971, current era 1971–present)

Some of the high points of those phases can shed light on our current practices. Bibliographic citations may be found in reviews by Burchenal (1977) and Zubrod (1979).

In the period of reawakening interest in the drug therapy of cancer, natural agents such as hormones were evaluated and found to be active. Huggins and Hodges (1941) demonstrated the salutary effects of estrogens and castration in the treatment of disseminated prostatic cancer, while in 1896, Beatson observed that oophorectomy was beneficial for the premenopausal patient with breast cancer. A large and often controversial literature compared the relative benefits of androgens and estrogens in perimenopausal and postmenopausal patients. Cortisone was shown to produce regressions in mouse lymphosarcomas, and the drug and its derivates were later used in combinations for treatment of human leukemias, lymphomas, and carcinomas.

Table 21.1. *Introduction of Major Anticancer Agents*

Year	*Agent*	*Major Indication*
1600 BC	Arsenic paste	Skin tumors
1865 AD	Potassium arsenite	Chronic leukemia
1895	Oophorectomy	Breast
1939	Androgens	Breast
1941	Estrogens	Prostate
1942	Mechlorethamine	Hodgkin's disease
1948	Methotrexate	Acute leukemia
1949	Steroids	Lymphomas
1951	6-Mercaptopurine	Acute leukemia
1952	Chlorambucil	Chronic leukemia
1953	Triethylenethio-phosphoramide	Ovary
1954	Dactinomycin	Wilms' tumor
1955	Busulfan	Chronic leukemia
1956	Mitomycin	Stomach
1957	5-Fluorouracil	Colon
1958	Cyclophosphamide	Lymphomas
1959	Mitotane	Adrenal
1960	Vinblastine	Hodgkin's disease
	Vincristine	Lymphomas
1961	Methyl-GAG	Leukemia
	Carmustine	Brain tumors
1962	Hydroxyurea	Chronic leukemia
	Melphalan	Myeloma
1963	Lomustine	Brain tumors
	Procarbazine	Hodgkin's disease
	Cytarabine	Acute leukemia
1964	Daunorubicin	Acute leukemia
1966	L-Asparaginase	Acute leukemia
1967	Dacarbazine	Melanoma
1968	Doxorubicin	Breast
1969	Tamoxifen	Breast
1970	Bleomycin	Testicle
1971	Cisplatin	Testicle
1977	Interferon	Breast

During the early years of World War II, the U.S. Chemical Warfare Service demonstrated in experimental animals the same toxic effects of nitrogen mustard on bone marrow and lymphoid tissues that had been noted in World War I victims of sulfur mustard gas. Discovery of the antitumor activity of nitrogen mustard (mechlorethamine) was made at Yale by Gilman, Goodman, Philips, Dougherty, and Allen in their work with animals (Gilman 1963). The first patient was treated by Lindskog at the New Haven Hospital in December 1942. The patient had a far-advanced lymphosarcoma resistant to radiation and had a dramatic, albeit transient, response to the drug. In a sense this was the beginning of the modern chemotherapy era, and gave impetus to studies of the pharmacology, kinetics, and chemistry of alkylating agents.

In a relatively short period of time many alkylating agents were synthesized and tested, but only a few had much clinical success and even fewer are used today. Of these, both chlorambucil and busulfan were developed and used for chronic lymphocytic and chronic myelocytic leukemia respectively at the Chester Beatty Institute in London, where melphalan was also synthesized. In Germany, cyclophosphamide was synthesized based on the idea that tumor cells contained phosphatases and phosphoramidases that would convert this inactive compound into the active cytotoxic agent in the tumor cell, with lethal local consequences and without adverse effects on normal cells. This attempt at selective toxicity was admirable but unfortunately was not realized, as normal liver microsomes metabolize the drug to its active state.

Numerous other alkylating agents are used less frequently. The Memorial Sloan–Kettering group (Burchenal et al. 1950) studied triethylenemelamine (TEM), triethylenephosphoramide (TEPA), and triethylenethiophosphoramide (thiotepa), but only the last is used clinically now. A Hungarian group introduced and studied dibromomannitol (Eckhardt et al. 1963) and dibromodulcitol (Sellei et al. 1969), but both remain experimental in this country. Dacarbazine was developed as an intermediate in the synthesis of purine analogues, but its mechanism of action is thought to be akin to that of the alkylating agents with which it is frequently grouped.

An astute follow-up was made by Rosenberg, Van Camp, and Krigas (1965) of a serendipitous observation of bacteria clumping in an electrical field with platinum electrodes. This led to study of the composition of the solution that surprisingly contained platinum, and development of cisplatin as a major new chemotherapeutic agent (Rosenberg et al. 1969) with curative potential in testicular and ovarian neoplasms. Although its mechanism of action is still under investigation, it seems to bind to DNA and causes cross-linkages similar to those of alkylating agents, and is therefore tentatively grouped with them.

The nitrosoureas were initially synthesized and studied at the Southern Research Institute (Skipper et al. 1961), and two of them, carmustine (BCNU) and lomustine (CCNU) have been marketed. At least three others—semustine (methyl-CCNU), streptozocin (Zanosar), and chlorozotocin—are in active stages of clinical evaluation. These drugs act by alkylation and carbamoylation, and probably other mechanisms not fully understood. They are usually grouped with the alkylating agents but are sufficiently unique that we treat them as a subgroup.

The interest in antibacterial chemotherapy and its mechanisms of action had direct consequences for antitumor drug development. Shortly after sulfonilamide was found to be an antimetabolite of paraaminobenzoic acid, an essential growth factor for streptococci, the group at Lederle Laboratories (Seeger et al. 1947) synthesized antimetabolites of folic acid—first aminopterin and later amethopterin, better known as methotrexate. These antifolates were shown by Farber (1948) and the group at Children's Hospital of Boston to be palliative in acute lymphoblastic leukemia of children. This observation gave tremendous impetus to further studies of anticancer drugs in leukemia and other childhood tumors, and to the search for other antimetabolites. The Burroughs Wellcome group led by Hitchings and Elion (1954) studied the antimetabolites of purines and pyrimidines and developed many agents, the most significant ones being antipurines. The first, 6-mercaptopurine (6-MP), was found to be effective in acute lymphocytic, acute myelocytic, and chronic myelocytic leukemias, while 6-thioguanine (6-TG) has been used primarily in acute myelogenous leukemia. As a byproduct of these studies, azathioprine (Imuran) was developed as an effective immunosuppressive agent (Hitchings and Elion 1963; Rosman and Bertino 1973), and allopurinol (Zyloprim) as a xanthine oxidase inhibitor useful in the prevention and treatment of gout (Klinenberg, Goldfinger, and Seegmiller 1965) and of the hyperuricemia caused by the destruction of tumors by cytotoxic drugs. Interestingly, allopurinol blocks the degradation of 6-MP to thiouric acid (Elion et al. 1963) so that the 6-MP must be reduced about 40% from the usual dose when allopurinol is given. Since 6-TG is not so affected, it is used in its usual dose.

The first major antipyrimidine that saw widespread use was 5-fluorouracil, synthesized by Heidelberger at the McArdle Institute in Wisconsin (Heidelberger, Chanduri, and Dannenberg 1957). It was adopted for the treatment of gastrointestinal tumors by Ansfield and Curreri (1963) and was later incorporated into combinations. Other fluorinated, brominated, and iodinated pyrimidines were developed but never played a major role in anticancer therapy, although iododeoxyuridine, synthesized by Prusoff (1963) at Yale has been a major topical antiviral agent in the treatment of herpetic keratitis (Kaufman 1961).

In addition to halogenating the pyrimidine, one can make antimetabolites by altering the ring by substituting a nitrogen for a carbon, as was done to make 5-azacytidine by a Czechoslovakian group (Piskala and Sorm 1964). It is also possible to substitute arabinose for ribose, as the Upjohn Company laboratories did in synthesizing cytarabine (cytosine arabinoside). This compound has been a major component of all effective modern combinations for treatment of acute nonlymphocytic leukemia and is being evaluated in combination therapy of lymphomas and as a synchronizing agent for other therapeutic approaches.

The search for antibacterial drugs, particularly for antituberculous agents, led to isolation of the actinomycetes (Waksman and Woodruff 1940). After neglect for some years because of a low order of activity against tuberculosis, they were reevaluated and found to be effective antineoplastic agents. Dactinomycin (actinomycin D) has been curative alone and in combination with other drugs in gestational trophoblastic disease, and in Wilms' tumor when combined with surgery and radiation. It is also used in a multitude of combinations for childhood solid tumors, testicular carcinoma, and some adult sarcomas. Its effectiveness encouraged exploration of other possible antibiotics with gratifying results, as bleomycin and mitomycin were developed in Japan and daunorubicin and doxorubicin in Italy.

Research into new agents to treat diabetes mellitus prompted exploration of folk myths about the activity of the periwinkle plant *Vinca rosea* (Linn.) in producing hypoglycemia. Instead, investigators at the Collip Laboratories in Canada (Beer 1955) and the Eli Lilly laboratories in the United States (Johnson, Wright, and Svoboda 1959) found that their extracts produced leukopenia. They joined forces and found antitumor activity in their extracts. The most important isolates were vinblastine, which is active in testicular, breast, and choriocarcinoma, and in lymphomas; and vincristine, which is relatively bone marrow-sparing and active in lymphomas and sarcomas, breast cancer, and small cell carcinoma of the lung. Since these two drugs were marketed, three additional plant extracts have been undergoing clinical investigation: etoposide (VP-16-213), teniposide (VM-26), and vindesine (Eldisine). Much of the perspective and data for the appropriate use of these drugs has been developed by the clinical trials program of the National Cancer Institute (DeVita et al. 1979).

Numerous additional effective antineoplastic drugs are available for use alone or in combination, and will be mentioned with their drug group or in a subsequent chapter on miscellaneous antitumor agents. The hypersensitivity reactions to these drugs have recently been reviewed (Weiss and Bruno 1981). There is an extensive literature on their toxicity (Ghione 1978; Ignoffo and Friedman 1980; USP 1980; Sartorelli and Johns 1975; Schilsky et al. 1980; Weiss, Walker, and Wiernik 1974; Weiss and Muggia 1980).

General Principles

In approaching a clinical situation for cancer chemotherapy it is important to be certain of the precise histologic diagnosis and the extent (stage) of disease. With this information plus an appreciation of the patient's overall health status and the available therapeutic armamentarium (at this time), a decision can be made whether to aim for cure, prolongation of survival, for palliation, or whether to give only supportive care. When the goal is cure, a considerably greater degree of toxicity may be acceptable than for prolongation of survival, and relatively little toxicity is tolerable if palliation is the best that can be expected.

Cell Kinetics

To cure cancer it is necessary in one way or another to kill every last cancer cell in the body. In 1937, Furth and Kahn showed that a single leukemic cell injected into a mouse would produce a lethal leukemia. This was confirmed by Skipper and associates (1964) in a series of pioneering studies that laid the groundwork for laboratory screening of new antitumor agents on a rational basis. Among other things, it was shown that tumor cell kill by cytotoxic drugs is by first order (or pseudo-first order) kinetics. A given dose of a cytotoxic drug will kill the same fraction (not the same number) of widely different sizes of tumor cell populations so long as they are similarly exposed, and both the growth fraction and the ratio of drug-sensitive to drug-resistant cells in the different-sized populations are the same. Thus if a given drug has a 99.9% cell kill, it will dissolve a 100-gm tumor (10^{11} cells = 100,000,000,000 = 100 billion cells) to a 0.1-gm tumor mass; although too small to detect (10^8 cells = 100,000,000 = 100 million cells) and an apparent clinical remission, the tumor will soon regrow to lethal size. If a second independently active drug has the same cell kill, the tumor burden may be reduced from 10^8 to 10^5 (100,000 cells), a level that is regarded by some immunologists as being controllable by the body's immune response so that there is a potential for cure.

To plan therapy further, an understanding of the cell cycle and its relation to anticancer drugs is important (Chabner et al. 1975; Shackney 1976). Following division (mitosis = M), the proliferating cell goes into a state called G_1 ("gap") for a variable period of time (in humans, about 9 to 25 hours) and then into a synthetic (S) phase of DNA replication during which it is very vulnerable to anything that interferes with normal DNA synthesis. Finally, the cell enters G_2 phase before its next mitosis. Cells that are not in a proliferative state remain in G_1 for prolonged periods; this has been called G_0, a phase during which the cell is not vulnerable to any cycle-specific agents but is still susceptible to cycle-nonspecific agents.

Bruce, Meeker, and Valeriote (1966) attempted to place the scheduling of anticancer agents on a more scientific basis according to their different effects on normal and malignant cell lines. The spleen colony assay was used to measure colony-forming units (CFU) from a rapidly proliferating lymphoma (LCFU) and normal hematopoietic stem cells (NCFU) as representatives of malignant and normal cell populations respectively. Drugs were classified into three groups:

I. Cycle-nonspecific agents affecting resting NCFU and proliferating LCFU equally. Dose-survival curves for both cell lines were exponential. Mechlorethamine is the prototype of this group, and behaves like irradiation.

II. Phase-specific agents generated dose-survival curves for both groups that reached plateau levels. The sensitive cells were assumed to be those proliferating cells in a specific phase of the cycle, since nonproliferating cells would not be sensitive to single applications of such drugs. Representative examples include cytarabine, hydroxyurea, vinblastine, vincristine, bleomycin, methotrexate, and asparaginase. Skipper has called this group "cell cycle stage-specific."

III. Cycle-specific agents produced exponential dose-survival curves for both, but the curve for LCFU (rapidly proliferating cells) was steeper than for NCFU, suggesting proliferation-dependent sensitivity. Examples of this group include 5-fluorouracil, dacarbazine, cyclophosphamide, dactinomycin, and mitomycin. Skipper called this group "cell cycle stage-nonspecific.")

It should be added that there is still considerable disagreement in the literature as to which drugs are phase-specific and which are cycle-specific; reputable investigators have reached varying conclusions (Hill and Baserga 1975). A tentative formulation is proposed in figure 21.1.

Some guidelines have been suggested (Valeriote and Edelstein 1977) from the foregoing studies: (1) chemotherapy should be started early when the tumor burden is small; (2) phase-specific agents should be administered in fractionated schedules or infusions unless they have long half-lives; (3) cycle-specific agents should be administered as single large doses in intermittent schedules; (4) treatment should be repeated for a number of cycles if tumor cell populations are greater than 10^4, and the greater the initial tumor burden the longer the treatment necessary; (5) courses should be spaced widely enough to allow recovery of normal tissues, a minimum of two weeks; (6) if acute toxicity is dose-limiting the drug should be given over a few days; (7) since drug resistance can arise after a few courses and some tumors do not respond to single-agent chemotherapy, combination chemotherapy should be considered for many or most tumors, and to exploit synchronization (manipulation of a cell population so that an increased proportion is in a drug-sensitive phase of the cycle) and recruitment techniques (increasing the fraction of proliferating cells). In addition, drugs may be selected for combination chemotherapy based on their differing modes of action. Some of the major drugs and their mechanisms of action are illustrated in figure 21.2.

Adjuvant Chemotherapy

Recurrent cancer and death many months or several years after apparently curative surgery (and often, postoperative radiation therapy) has made it obvious that in certain high-risk situations additional (adjuvant) therapy is indicated. What are these situations, and how does one decide when to use adjuvant therapy and with what agents? (Block and Isacoff 1977; Bagshawe 1978; DeVita 1978; Weiss and DeVita 1979).

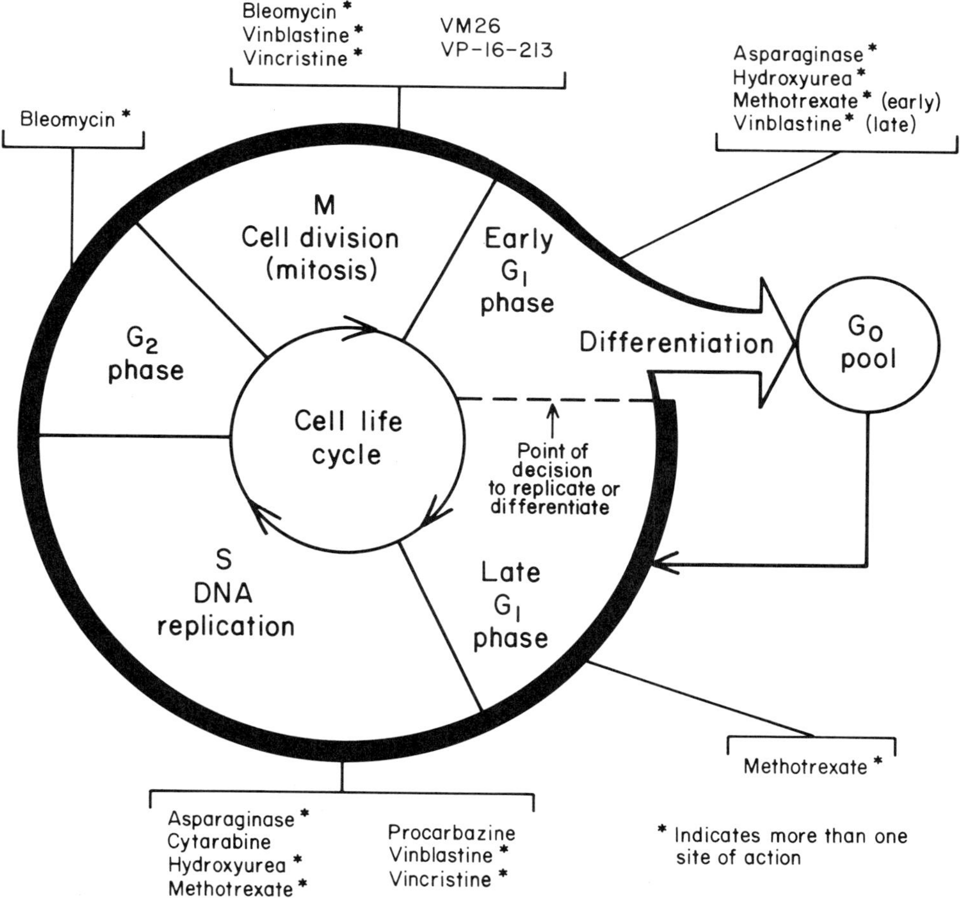

Fig. 21.1. *Action of antineoplastic agents in relation to the cell cycle. (Modified from Hill and Baserga 1975 and Adria Laboratories monograph. Reprinted by permission.)*

Tumors with a high growth fraction (GF) are at high risk for recurrence. The GF can be estimated as proliferating cells (those that are pulse-labeled with tritiated thymidine) as compared to total viable tumor cells. Typical high-GF tumors are acute leukemia, gestational trophoblastic tumors, Wilms' tumor, and some lymphomas. The great successes of adjuvant therapy have been with these. Disease recurrence in acute childhood leukemia was rapid and clinically obvious before the use of repeated cycles of adjuvant (consolidation) therapy and adjuvant treatment of potential privileged sanctuaries with intrathecal methotrexate and cranial irradiation. A similar experience with choriocarcinoma in women has been well documented (Li, Hertz, and Spencer 1956). Here chemotherapy was continued in the face of complete remission and the absence of clinical disease, and unusually high cure rates were obtained in a condition formerly almost uniformly fatal. Fortunately, the sensitive tumor marker, human chorionic gonadotropin, was available to monitor the progress of the microscopic disease. In the treatment of Wilms' tumor, addition of adjuvant chemotherapy with dactinomycin alone raised the two-year survival rate after surgery and radiation from 45% to 90% (Burgert and Glidewell 1967), and now vincristine is being added in hopes of improving those excellent results.

If these results are so good, then why not apply them to all tumors? Obviously, all tumors are not high-GF, in fact, most are not and most do not respond. To succeed, adjuvant therapy should be given: (1) immediately after the primary tumor and regional lymph nodes have been removed or ablated by surgery or radiation; (2) when clinical, laboratory, and radiologic investigations cannot rule out micrometastatic disease; (3) when historical experience indicates a high probability of ultimate relapse because of undetectable micrometastases existing before surgery or radiation; (4) when there is chemotherapy available that has demonstrated a 50% or greater response rate with acceptable toxicity in cases with measurable gross residual disease; and (5) when there can be prolonged therapy, as a single course will probably not kill all remaining cells even following debulking, when the residual tumor cells are more likely to be in a proliferative and therefore more susceptible phase.

Experiences with adjuvant therapy of breast and colon cancer and osteogenic sarcoma are detailed in the chapters devoted to those subjects. We can summarize by indicating that its efficacy in colon cancer is entirely unproved, and the early enthusiastic reports of its use in osteogenic sarcoma have been questioned by new studies and reevaluation of the old ones (Carter 1978). The

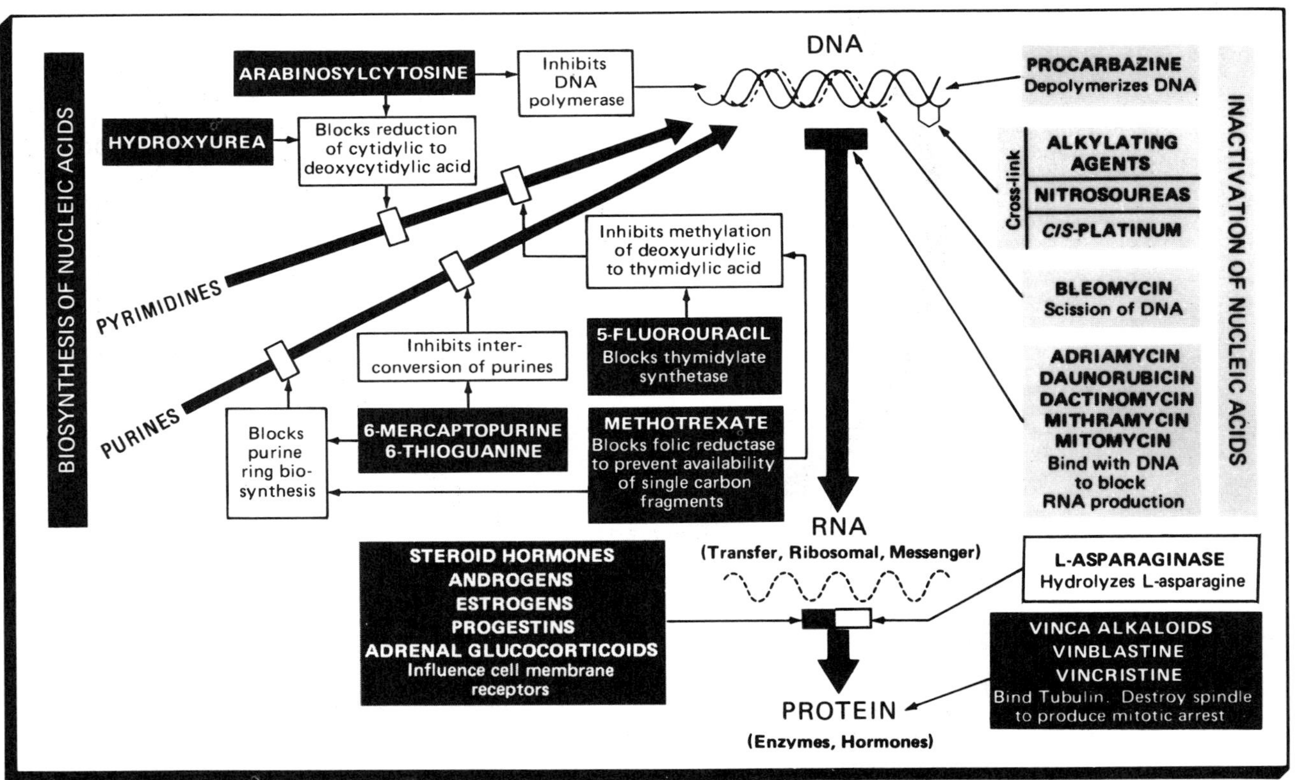

Fig. 21.2. *Mechanism of action of anticancer drugs. (Krakoff 1981. Reprinted by permission.)*

Table 21.2. *Neoplastic Diseases that Respond to Chemotherapy*

Type of Cancer	*Therapeutic Response (%)*	*Adjuvant Response*	*Survival of Responders*
	Prolonged Survival or Cure		
Gestational trophoblastic tumors	70–80	Excellent	Cured
Burkitt's tumor	50–60	Excellent	Cured
Seminoma	90–95	Excellent	50–60% cured
Embryonal cell cancer	90–95	Excellent	40–50% cured
Wilms' tumor	60–80	Excellent	Cured
Neuroblastoma	50–80	Excellent	Prolonged
Acute lymphoblastic leukemia	90	Excellent	50% cured
Lymphoma (childhood)	90	Excellent	Prolonged
Hodgkin's disease	70	Excellent	50% cured
	Palliation and Prolongation of Life		
Prostate cancer	70	Excellent	Increased
Breast cancer			
Premenopausal	60	Good (proved)	Increased
Postmenopausal	60	Fair (unproved)	Increased
Acute myelogenous leukemia	60	Fair	Slightly increased
Chronic lymphocytic leukemia	50	None	Slightly increased
Lymphoma (adult)			
Lymphocytic	60	Good (unproved)	Increased
Histiocytic	40	Fair	20% cured
Osteogenic sarcoma	20–30	Excellent	Increased
Multiple myeloma	60	Fair (unproved)	Slightly increased
Small cell carcinoma of lung	60	Good	Increased
	Palliation with Uncertain Prolongation of Life		
Chronic myelogenous leukemia	90		Probable increase
Ovarian cancer	30–50	Fair (unproved)	Probable increase
Endometrium	25	Fair (unproved)	Probable increase
Soft tissue sarcoma	30	Fair (unproved)	Probable increase
Stomach (USA)	30	Fair (unproved)	Probable increase
	Uncertain Palliation		
Lung (non-small cell)	30–40	Poor	Brief
Head and neck	20–30	Poor	Brief
Large bowel	20–30	Unproved	Slightly increased (unproved)
Pancreas	10–15	Poor–none	Brief
Liver (USA)	10–15	Poor–none	Brief
Cervix	20	Poor–none	Brief
Melanoma	20	Fair (unproved)	Brief
Adrenal cortex	20	Poor	Brief
Bladder	30	Unproved	Brief
Kidney	5–10	Unproved	Brief

Table 21.3. *Drug-Tumor Interactions*

Drug (Generic Name)	Tumor Type: Breast	Esophagus	Stomach	Pancreas	Liver	Colon-Rectum	Kidney	Bladder	Prostate	Testicle	Endometrium	Ovary	Cervix
ALKYLATING AGENTS													
Mechlorethamine	+		+						+			++	
Chlorambucil	+		+							++		++	+
Cyclophosphamide	++					+		++	++	++	++	++	++
Melphalan	++									++		++	+
Triethylene thiophosphoramide	++							++				++	
Busulfan													
Dacarbazine													
Estramustine*									++				
Estradiol mustard*	+		+			+			++				
Dibromodulcitol*	++			+			+						
Dibromomannitol*													
Cisplatin	+	+					+	++	++	++		++	+
NITROSOUREAS													
Carmustine	+		+			+							
Lomustine						++	+					+	
Semustine*			+			++							+
Streptozocin*				++									
Chlorozotocin*			+	+		+	+					+	
ANTIMETABOLITES													
Methotrexate	++					+				+		+	++
Triazinate*	+		+			+	+	+	++				
6-Mercaptopurine													
6-Thioguanine													
5-Fluorouracil	++		++	++	++	++		++	++		++	++	++
Floxuridine				+	++	+							
Ftorafur*	+	+	++			++	+		+				
Cytarabine													
5-Azacytidine*													
Hexamethylmelamine*	+					+						++	+
Hydroxyurea						+	+						

Table 21.3. *Continued*

Drug (Generic Name)	Tumor Type												
	Breast	*Esophagus*	*Stomach*	*Pancreas*	*Liver*	*Colon-Rectum*	*Kidney*	*Bladder*	*Prostate*	*Testicle*	*Endometrium*	*Ovary*	*Cervix*
ANTITUMOR ANTIBIOTICS													
Dactinomycin										++		++	
Mitomycin	++		++	++	++	++		++				+	++
Mithramycin										++			
Daunorubicin													
Doxorubicin	++		++	++	++			++	++	++	++	++	+
Bleomycin		+						+		++			++
Zinostatin*					+			+					
Streptonigrin*	+		+										+
PLANT-DERIVED ANTINEOPLASTICS													
Vinblastine	++						+	+		++			
Vincristine	++					+				+			++
Vindesine*	+						+			+			
Teniposide*	+				+		+	+				+	
Etoposide*					+			+		+			
Maytansine*	+											+	
MISCELLANEOUS ANTITUMOR													
Mitotane													
Methyl-GAG*		+	+		+	+	+	+			+		
Procarbazine													
L-Asparaginase													
Razoxane*	+					+							
Amsacrine*	++												
Metronidazole†													
Misonidazole*													
Interferon*	+												

+ = possibly active; ++ = definitely active.

*Investigational.

†Approved as anti-infective but investigational as antineoplastic.

Table 21.3. *Continued*

Drug (Generic Name)	Tumor Type: Breast	Esophagus	Stomach	Pancreas	Liver	Colon-Rectum	Kidney	Bladder	Prostate	Testicle	Endometrium	Ovary	Cervix
HORMONAL AGENTS													
Adrenal corticosteroids	++												
Androgens	++						+						
Estrogens	++								++				
Tamoxifen	++						+		+		++		
Aminoglutethimide*	++								++				
Progestins	++						+		++		++	++	

Drug (Generic Name)	Tumor Type: Acute Lymphocytic Leukemia	Chronic Lymphocytic Leukemia	Acute Non-lymphocytic Leukemia	Chronic Myelogenous Leukemia	Lymphoma	Hodgkin's Disease	Myeloma	Lung, Small Cell	Lung, Non-small Cell	Sarcoma	Melanoma	Brain	Head and Neck
ALKYLATING AGENTS													
Mechlorethamine					++	++		++	++				
Chlorambucil		++			++	++	+			+			+
Cyclophosphamide	++	++	+		++	++	++	++	++	++			++
Melphalan				++			++			+			
Triethylene thiophosphoramide					++			+	+				
Busulfan				++									
Dacarbazine					++	++				+	++		
Estramustine*													
Estradiol mustard*													
Dibromodulcitol*				++	+			+		+	+		+
Dibromomannitol*				++									
Cisplatin						+	++	+	++	+			++
NITROSOUREAS													
Carmustine					++	++	++	+	+		+	++	
Lomustine					++	++		++	++		+	++	
Semustine*								+	+		++	++	+
Streptozocin*						+							
Chlorozotocin*						+					+		

Table 21.3. *Continued*

Drug (Generic Name)	Tumor Type												
	Acute Lympho-cytic Leukemia	*Chronic Lympho-cytic Leukemia*	*Acute Non-lym-phocytic Leukemia*	*Chronic Myelo-genous Leukemia*	*Lymphoma*	*Hodgkin's Disease*	*Myeloma*	*Lung, Small Cell*	*Lung, Non-small Cell*	*Sar-coma*	*Mela-noma*	*Brain*	*Head and Neck*
ANTIMETABOLITES													
Methotrexate	++		+		++	+		++	++	+		+	++
Triazinate*								+	+			+	
6-Mercaptopurine	++		++	++	+								+
6-Thioguanine	++		++	++									
5-Fluorouracil													++
Floxuridine													+
Ftorafur*								+	+				
Cytarabine	++		++	++	++					+			+
5-Azacytidine*			++	++									
Hexamethylmelamine*					+	+		++	++				+
Hydroxyurea				++				+	+				+
ANTITUMOR ANTIBIOTICS													
Dactinomycin										++	+		
Mitomycin								+	+	+			++
Mithramycin													
Daunorubicin	++		++	++									
Doxorubicin	++		++	++	++	++	++	++	++	++			+
Bleomycin					++	++		+	+				++
Zinostatin*		+	++		+	+							
Streptonigrin*													+
PLANT-DERIVED ANTINEOPLASTICS													
Vinblastine					++	++				+			++
Vincristine	++				++	++		++	+	+	+	++	
Vindesine*	+		+		+	+		++	++		+		
Teniposide*	++		++	+	+	+		+	+			+	
Etoposide*			++		++	+		++					
Maytansine*	+				+			+	+		+		

+ = possibly active; ++ = definitely active. *Investigational.

Table 21.3. *Continued*

Drug (Generic Name)	Tumor Type: Acute Lymphocytic Leukemia	Chronic Lymphocytic Leukemia	Acute Non-lymphocytic Leukemia	Chronic Myelogenous Leukemia	Lymphoma	Hodgkin's Disease	Myeloma	Lung, Small Cell	Lung, Non-small Cell	Sarcoma	Melanoma	Brain	Head and Neck
MISCELLANEOUS ANTITUMOR													
Mitotane													
Methyl-GAG*	+		++	++				+	+		+		
Procarbazine					++	++		++	+			++	
L-Asparaginase	++												
Razoxane*			+		+			+	+				+
Amsacrine*			++	++	+	+							
Metronidazole†												++	
Misonidazole*												++	
Interferon*					+		+	+					
HORMONAL AGENTS													
Adrenal corticosteroids	++	++		++	++	++	++					++	
Androgens													
Estrogens													
Tamoxifen													
Aminoglutethimide*													
Progestins													

SOURCE: Modified from Wasserman et al. 1975 and expanded from numerous additional sources.

NOTES: The drugs listed have been found active to some degree either in the literature or in our experience. Undoubtedly many drugs have been found or will be found to be active in situations in which we have failed to indicate their usefulness either because of our ignorance of the published studies or because they have not been tested.

\+ = possibly active; ++ = definitely active.

*Investigational.

†Approved as anti-infective but investigational as antineoplastic.

proof of efficacy in breast cancer of premenopausal women seems to be confirmed by each new study (Jones and Salmon 1979); with postmenopausal women adjuvant chemotherapy remains controversial, although several studies show statistically significant benefits, including a recent report from the Milan National Cancer Institute (Bonadonna and Valagussa 1980).

A current evaluation (or educated guess) of the trends of response to curative, palliative, and adjuvant chemotherapy is given in table 21.2, based on reported results from many sources (AMA 1980; Becker 1977; Carter, Babowski, and Hellman 1977; DeVita and Schein 1973; Haskell 1980; Holland and Frei 1973; Knopf et al. 1981; Livingston and Carter 1970; Lokich 1978, 1979; Marsh 1979; National Institutes of Health 1981; Sartorelli and Creasey 1969; Sather et al. 1979). Drug—tumor interactions are shown in table 21.3.

Drug Administration

In general, current practice is to calculate dosages based on measured height and weight and then translated by calculation to body surface area (BSA). This makes it easier to work with both adults and children and to extrapolate from animal studies. Nomograms for BSA for adults and children respectively are included (figs. 21.3 and 21.4). Some early studies were conducted based on weight alone, and since no subsequent studies based on BSA are available, some of these values are still given in terms of body weight. For those individuals

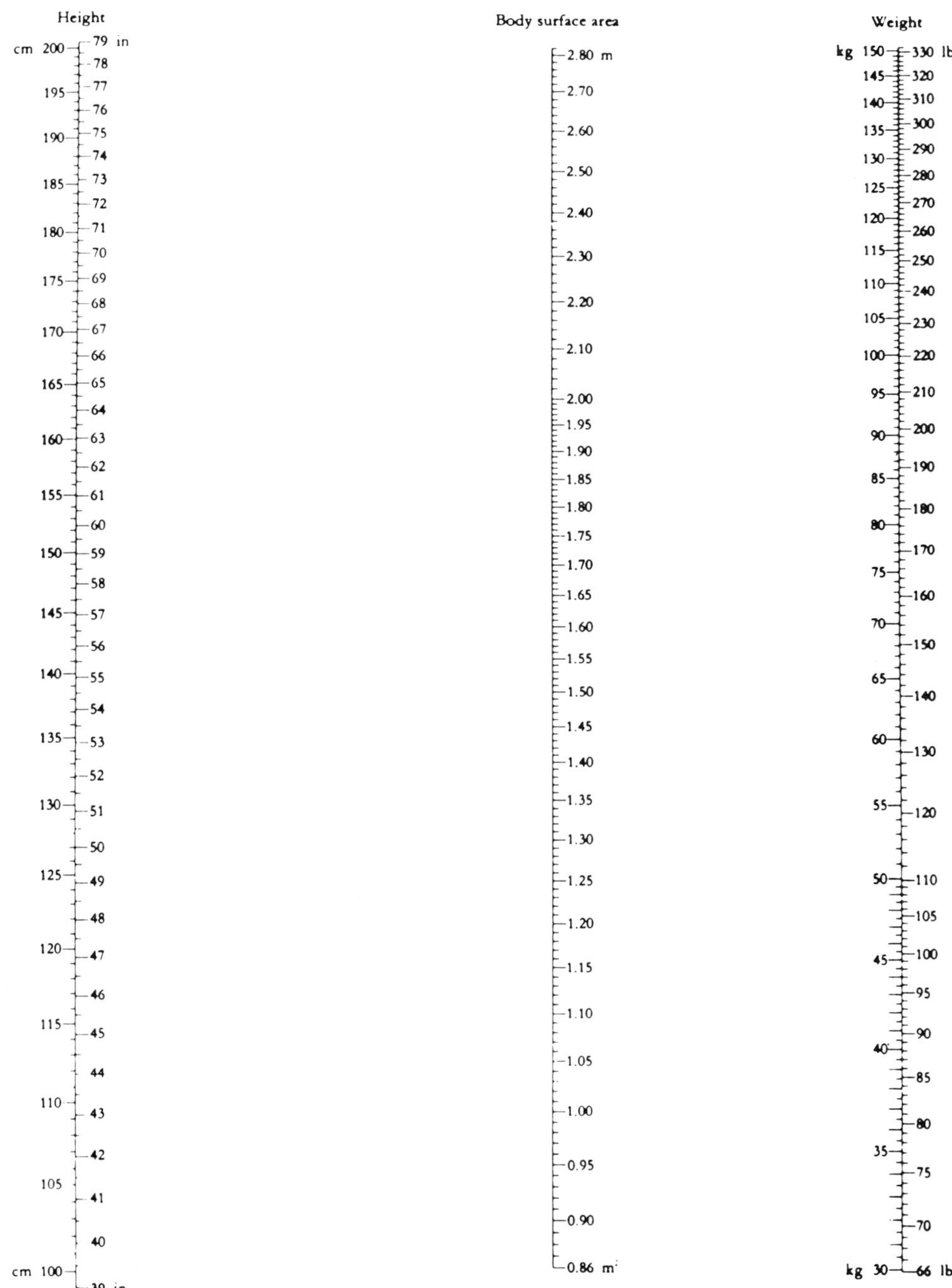

Fig. 21.3. *Nomogram for determination of body surface area of adults from height and weight. (Diem and Lentner 1962. Reprinted by permission.)*

NOTE: From the formula of DuBois and DuBois, *Arch. Intern. Med.*, 17:863, 1916: $S = W^{0.425} \times H^{0.725} \times 71.84$, or $\log S = \log W \times 0.425 + \log H \times 0.725 + 1.8564$ (S = body surface in cm^2, W = weight in kg, H = height in cm).

who are grossly obese the standard or ideal weight should be used for calculation of dosage or of BSA. A table of standard weights based on height, age, and sex is given for men and women in figure 21.5.

Chemotherapy drugs have a great potential for good or for complications. To minimize complications, careful administration procedures must be followed. Table 21.4 summarizes the guidelines we have found useful in the parenteral administration of antineoplastic drugs. Table 21.5 gives an introduction to the incompatibilities of parenteral anticancer drugs.

In the evaluation of the patient with neoplastic

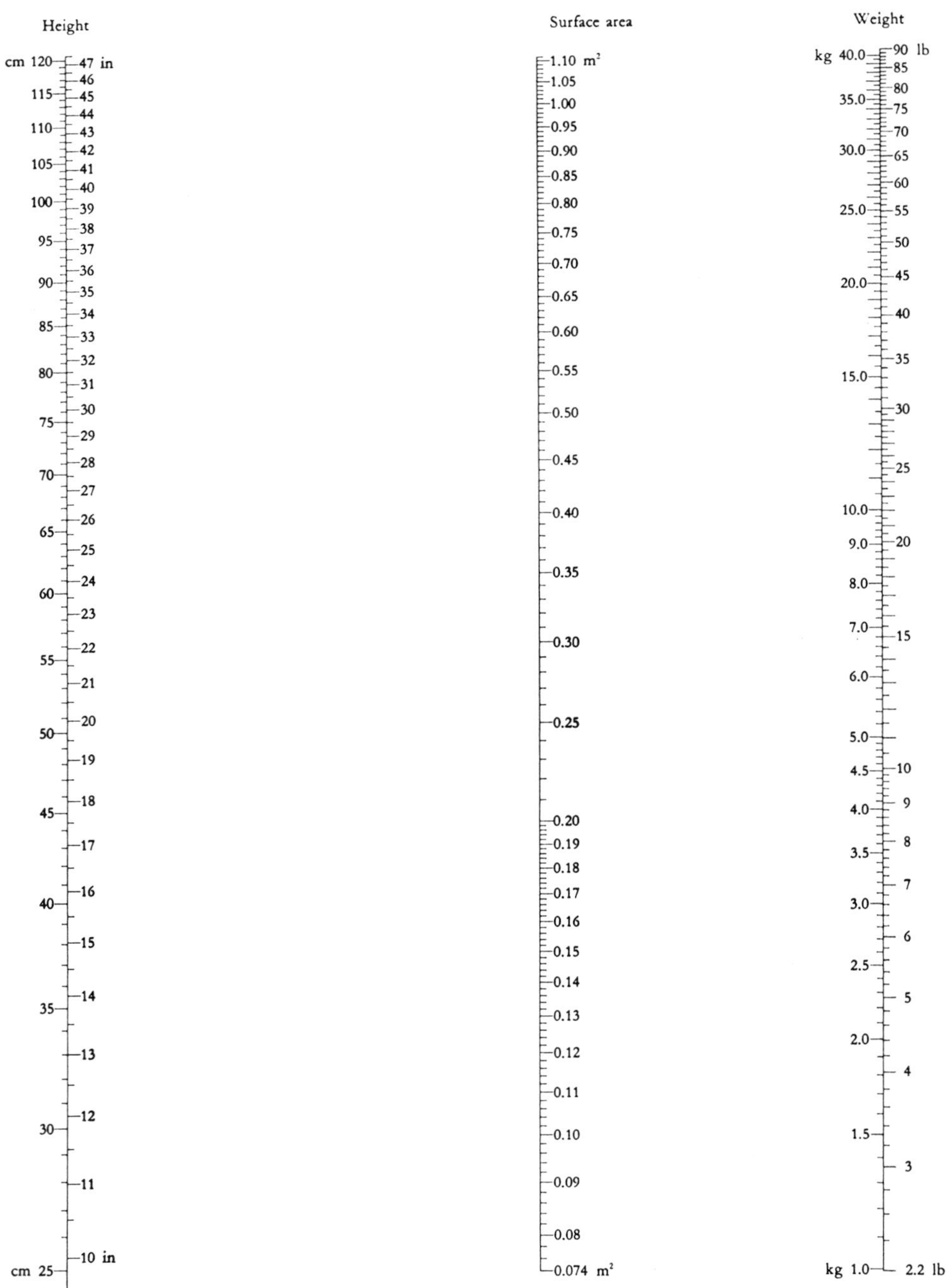

Fig. 21.4. *Nomogram for determination of body surface area of children from height and weight. (Diem and Lentner 1962. Reprinted by permission.)*

NOTE: From the formula of DuBois and DuBois, *Arch. Intern. Med.*, 17:863, 1916: $S = W^{0.425} \times H^{0.725} \times 71.84$, or $\log S = \log W \times 0.425 + \log H \times 0.725 + 1.8564$ (S = body surface in cm^2, W = weight in kg, H = height in cm).

Table 21.4. *Summary of Guidelines for Use of Parenteral Antineoplastic Drugs*

Drug	*Usual Route*	*Usual Single Dose*	*Extravasation Consequences*
ALKYLATING AGENTS			
Nitrogen mustard (Mustargen)	Push through IV drip	0.4 mg/kg	Necrosis, ulceration, skin slough
Cyclophosphamide (Cytoxan)	Direct IV push up to 750 mg, then through IV drip	20–40 mg/kg	Mild irritation
Thiotepa	IV push, IM, SC	0.2–1 mg/kg	None
Dacarbazine (DTIC)	Slow push through IV drip or volutrol	200–600 mg/m^2	Pain, ulceration, tissue necrosis
Cisplatin	IV drip with diuresis	20 mg/m^2/day to 120 mg/m^2	Local irritation
NITROSOUREAS			
Carmustine (BCNU, BiCNU)	IV drip	100–200 mg/m^2	Local necrosis, phlebitis
ANTIMETABOLITES			
Methotrexate	IV push, IM, SC	20–50 mg/m^2	None
5-Fluorouracil	IV push	500–1000 mg	Numbness, skin discoloration, tingling
Cytarabine (Ara-C, Cytosar)	IV drip, SC, IM	100 mg/m^2	None
ANTITUMOR ANTIBIOTICS			
Doxorubicin (Adriamycin)	Push through IV drip	40–75 mg/m^2	Necrosis, ulceration, tendon and skin slough
Dactinomycin (Cosmegen)	Push through IV drip	0.25–1 mg/m^2	Local pain, phlebitis, necrosis
Daunorubicin (Cerubidine)	Push through IV drip	30–60 mg/m^2	Necrosis, ulceration, tendon and skin slough
Mitomycin (Mutamycin)	Push through IV drip	2–5 mg or 10–20 mg/m^2	Local necrosis and slough
Bleomycin (Blenoxane)	IV, IM, SC	2–15 units	None
Mithramycin (Mithracin)	IV drip	1–2 mg	Local phlebitis and cellulitis
MITOTIC INHIBITORS			
Vincristine (Oncovin)	Push through IV drip	1–2 mg	Local pain, phlebitis, necrosis
Vinblastine (Velban)	Push through IV drip	7–14 mg	Local pain, phlebitis, necrosis

disease and in planning chemotherapy, a few tests will suffice in most cases. In some cases, however, a great many tests are needed and sometimes these are rare and unusual. In those instances, normal values should be obtained from the laboratory performing the determination, although sometimes these are not readily available. For convenience, we have compiled in appendix 21.1 some of the normal values that we find useful.

Finally, in discussing drug therapy with patients, it is important that they be fully informed of the nature of the drug and its side effects before they consent to therapy. To help their understanding and recall, we developed a series of cards listing general instructions to patients, and the specifics of each of the more common drugs. We give each patient the cards that pertain to his or her treatment. The text of these cards is reproduced in appendix 21.2.

Table 21.5. *Incompatibilities with Parenteral Anticancer Drugs*

Drug	*Incompatible with:*	*Reaction Noted*	*Clinical Relevance*
L-asparaginase (Elspar)	Preservative	Enzyme may be inactivated; very unstable	Diluted with normal saline; use immediately
5-Azacytidine (investigational)	Unbuffered nonphysiologic vehicles; warming above 20° C or pH > 6.5	More rapid decomposition, with half-life only 4.4 hrs in distilled water at 20° C	Mix with Ringer's lactate for maximum stability; mix fresh every 8 hrs
Bleomycin (Blenoxane)	Ascorbic acid, sulfhydryl-containing compounds, hydrogen peroxide	Not characterized	Avoid administration with ascorbic acid
Carmustine (BCNU)	Temperature greater than 27° C	Drug melts and decomposes	Keep below 27° C
Cisplatin (Platinol)	Mannitol in D5W; D5W or other solution with low sodium chloride concentration	Mannitol platinum complexes form; breakdown products form after 2 hrs admixture	Dilute in normal saline. Mannitol used sequentially and not mixed with cisplatin
Cyclophosphamide (Cytoxan)	Heating vials to 70–80° C to get solution; prolonged exposure to benzyl alcohol-preserved diluents	Accelerated decomposition	Avoid excessive heating to obtain solution; significant only after 24 hrs admixture
Cytarabine (Cytosar-U)	Fluorouracil	UV spectrum change of cytarabine	No physical alteration noted; avoid direct admixture
Dacarbazine (DTIC)	Hydrocortisone sodium succinate (solu-cortef)	Immediate pink precipitate	Mixing with hydrocortisone sodium phosphate does not do this
Dactinomycin (Cosmegen)	Preservatives in bacteriostatic diluents	Precipitation	Use sterile water, D5W, or normal saline preservative-free
Daunorubicin (Cerubidine)	Sodium heparin, dexamethasone	Immediate milky precipitate	Avoid admixture; use before or after

MEN — Age

Ft.	In.	25-29		30-34		35-39		40-44		45-49		50-54		55up	
		Lbs.	Kgs.	Lbs.	Kgs.	Lbs.	Kgs.	Lbs.	Kgs.	Lbs.	Kgs.	Lbs.	Kgs.	Lbs.	Kgs.
4	11	122	55.5	125	56.8	127	57.7	130	59.1	132	60.0	133	60.5	134	60.9
5	0	124	56.4	127	57.7	129	58.6	132	60.0	134	60.9	135	61.4	136	61.8
	1	126	57.3	129	58.6	131	59.5	134	60.9	136	61.8	137	62.3	138	62.7
	2	128	58.2	131	59.5	133	60.5	136	61.8	138	62.7	139	63.2	140	63.6
	3	131	59.5	134	60.9	136	61.8	139	63.2	141	64.1	142	64.5	143	65.0
	4	134	60.9	137	62.3	140	63.6	142	64.5	144	65.5	145	65.9	146	66.4
	5	138	62.7	141	64.1	144	65.5	146	66.4	148	67.3	149	67.7	150	68.2
	6	142	64.5	145	65.9	148	67.3	150	68.2	152	69.1	153	69.5	154	70.0
	7	146	66.4	149	67.7	152	69.1	154	70.0	156	70.9	157	71.4	158	71.8
	8	150	68.2	154	70.0	157	71.4	159	72.3	161	73.2	162	73.6	163	74.1
	9	154	70.0	158	71.8	162	73.6	164	74.6	166	75.5	167	75.9	168	76.4
	10	158	71.8	163	74.1	167	75.9	169	76.8	171	77.7	172	78.2	173	78.6
	11	163	74.1	168	76.4	172	78.2	175	79.5	177	80.5	178	80.9	179	81.4
6	0	169	76.8	174	79.1	178	80.9	181	82.3	183	83.2	184	83.6	185	84.1
	1	175	79.5	180	81.8	184	83.6	187	85.0	190	86.4	191	86.8	192	87.3
	2	181	82.3	186	84.5	191	86.8	194	88.2	197	89.5	198	90.0	199	90.5
	3	187	85.0	192	87.3	197	89.5	201	91.4	204	92.7	205	93.2	206	93.6

WOMEN — Age

Ft.	In.	25-29		30-34		35-39		40-44		45-49		50-54		55up	
		Lbs.	Kgs.	Lbs.	Kgs.	Lbs.	Kgs.	Lbs.	Kgs.	Lbs.	Kgs.	Lbs.	Kgs.	Lbs.	Kgs.
4	11	116	52.7	119	54.1	122	55.5	126	57.3	129	58.6	131	59.5	132	60.0
5	0	118	53.6	121	55.0	124	56.4	128	58.2	131	59.5	133	60.5	134	60.9
	1	120	54.5	123	55.9	126	57.3	130	59.1	133	60.5	135	61.4	137	62.3
	2	122	55.5	125	56.8	129	58.6	133	60.5	136	61.8	138	62.7	140	63.6
	3	125	56.8	128	58.2	132	60.0	136	61.8	139	63.2	141	64.1	143	65.0
	4	129	58.6	132	60.0	136	61.8	139	63.2	142	64.5	144	65.5	146	66.4
	5	132	60.0	136	61.8	140	63.6	143	65.0	146	66.4	148	67.3	150	68.2
	6	136	61.8	140	63.6	144	65.5	147	66.8	151	68.6	152	69.1	153	69.6
	7	140	63.6	144	65.5	148	67.3	151	68.6	155	70.5	157	71.4	158	71.8
	8	144	65.5	148	67.3	152	69.1	155	70.5	159	72.3	162	73.6	163	74.1
	9	148	67.3	152	69.1	156	70.9	159	72.3	163	74.1	166	75.5	167	75.9
	10	152	69.1	155	70.5	159	72.3	162	73.6	166	75.5	170	77.3	173	78.6
	11	155	70.5	158	71.8	162	73.6	166	75.5	170	77.3	174	79.1	177	80.5
6	0	159	72.3	162	73.6	165	75.0	169	76.8	173	78.6	177	80.5	182	82.7

Fig. 21.5. *Chart of standard weights.*

NOTE: Under certain circumstances such as edema, ascites, or obesity, it may be preferable to base dosage on the patient's standard (ideal) rather than actual body weight. To do this, determine the standard weight from the chart and compare this to the patient's actual weight. The lower of the two figures should be used to calculate dosage. (From *Surgical adjuvant program*, Roswell Park Memorial Institute, Buffalo, New York, 1979. Reprinted by permission of Adria Laboratories.)

Table 21.5. *Continued*

Drug	*Incompatible with:*	*Reaction Noted*	*Clinical Relevance*
Doxorubicin (Adriamycin)	Aminophylline, cephalothin sodium, dexamethasone, diazepam, fluorouracil, hydrocortisone sodium succinate, heparin sodium	Immediate precipitation or solution darkening (red to blue-purple)	Avoid admixture
Etoposide (VP16-213)	5% Dextrose solution, normal saline	Unstable precipitate; precipitates in 30 min diluted 1:20 in NS, 3 hrs at 1:50, and 6 hrs at 1:100	Use normal saline or sterile water for injection; observe time-dilution-stability relationship
5-Flourouracil (Adrucil)	Cytarabine (Cytosar-U), doxorubicin (Adriamycin), diazepam (Valium), methotrexate (Mexate)	Solution darkening or precipitation or change of UV spectrum of drugs	Avoid direct admixture
Mechlorethamine (nitrogen mustard, mustargen)	Preservative or any organic compound	Highly reactive with all but the most inert materials	Use sterile water or saline; wear gloves to mix; severe vesicant
Methotrexate (Mexate)	Cytarabine, fluorouracil	Alteration in UV spectrum	Avoid direct admixture
Mithramycin (Mithracin)	Divalent cations, Zn^{++}, Ca^{++}, Fe^{++}	Chelation	Avoid direct admixture
Mitomycin	5% Dextrose solution	Stable 3 hrs in D5W, 12 hrs in NS, and 24 hrs in sodium lactate injection	Dissolve in sterile water and dilute with NS or sodium lactate
Teniposide (VM-26)	5% Dextrose solution, normal saline	Unstable precipitate; a 1:5 to 1:20 dilution is stable 4 hrs, a 1:50 or 1:100 for 6 hrs with NS	Observe time-duration-stability relationship
Thiotepa	5% Dextrose solution, normal saline	Hypertonic solution results	Make initial solution with sterile water
Vinblastine	5% Dextrose	Unstable	Use normal saline with benzyl alcohol
Vincristine	5% Dextrose solution	Unstable	Use bacteriostatic normal saline supplied with vial

SOURCE: Modified from Dorr 1979.

References

AMA drug evaluations, 4th edition. Chicago: American Medical Association, 1980.

Ansfield, F. J., and Curreri, A. R. Further clinical comparison between 5-fluorouracil (5-FU) and 5-fluoro-2′-deoxyuridine (5-FUdR). *Cancer Chemother. Rep.* 32:101–105, 1963.

Bagshawe, K. D. Adjuvant chemotherapy. *Cancer Clin. Trials* 1:135–138, 1978.

Beatson, G. T. On the treatment of inoperable cases of carcinoma of the mamma. *Lancet* 2:104–107, 1896.

Becker, F. F., ed. *Cancer, a comprehensive treatise,* vol. 5. New York: Plenum, 1977.

Beer, C. T. The leucopenic action of extracts of *Vinca rosea. Ann. R. Br. Empire Cancer Campaign* 33:487–488, 1955.

Block, J. B., and Isacoff, W. H. Adjuvant chemotherapy in cancer. *Semin. Oncol.* 4:109–115, 1977.

Bonadonna, G., and Valagussa, P. Dose-response effect of CMF in breast cancer. *Proc. Am. Soc. Clin. Oncol.* 21:413, 1980.

Bruce, W. R.; Meeker, B. E.; and Valeriote, F. A. Comparison of the sensitivity of normal hematopoietic and transplanted lymphoma colony-forming cells to chemotherapeutic agents administered in vivo. *J. Natl. Cancer Inst.* 37:233–245, 1966.

Burchenal, J. H. The historical development of cancer chemotherapy. *Semin. Oncol.* 4:135–146, 1977.

Burchenal, J. H. et al. The action of certain ethylene amine (aziridine) derivatives on mouse leukemia. *Arch. Biochem.* 26:321–323, 1950.

Burgert, E. O., and Glidewell, O. Dactinomycin in Wilms' tumor. *JAMA* 199:464–468, 1967.

Carter, S. K. The analysis of adjuvant trials. Editorial. *Cancer Treat. Rev.* 5:1–5, 1978.

Carter, S. K.; Bakowski, M. T.; and Hellman, K. *Chemotherapy of cancer.* New York: John Wiley & Sons, 1977.

Chabner, B. A. et al. Clinical pharmacology and antineoplastic agents. *N. Engl. J. Med.* 292:1107–1113; 1159–1168, 1975.

DeVita, V. T., Jr. The evolution of therapeutic research in cancer. *N. Engl. J. Med.* 298:907–910, 1978.

DeVita, V. T., Jr. et al. The drug development and clinical trials programs of the Division of Cancer Treatment, National Cancer Institute. *Cancer Clin. Trials* 2: 195–216, 1979.

DeVita, V. T., Jr., and Schein, P. S. The use of drugs in combination for the treatment of cancer. *N. Engl. J. Med.* 288:998–1006, 1973.

Diem, K., and Lentner, C., eds. *Scientific tables,* 7th edition. Basel, Switzerland: CIBA-GEIGY, 1962.

Dorr, R. T. Incompatibilities of parenteral anticancer drugs. *Am. J. Intravenous Ther.* 6:45–46, 1979.

Eckhardt, S. et al. Effect of 1,6-dibromo-1,6-dideoxy-D-mannitol on chronic granulocytic leukemia. *Cancer Chemother. Rep.* 33:57–61, 1963.

Elion, G. B. et al. Potentiation of inhibition of drug degradation: 6-substituted purines and xanthine oxidase. *Biochem. Pharmacol.* 12:85–93, 1963.

Farber, S. et al. Temporary remissions in acute leukemia in children produced by folic acid, 4-aminopteroylglutamic acid (aminopterin). *N. Engl. J. Med.* 238: 787–793, 1948.

Forkner, C. E., and Scott, T. F. M. Arsenic as a therapeutic agent in chronic myelogenous leukemia. *JAMA* 97:3–5, 1931.

Furth, J., and Kahn, M. C. The transmission of leukemia of mice with a single cell. *Am. J. Cancer* 31:276–282, 1937.

Ghione, M. Cardiotoxic effects of antitumor agents. *Cancer Chemother. Pharmacol.* 1:25–34, 1978.

Gilman, A. The initial clinical trial of nitrogen mustard. *Am. J. Surg.* 105:574–578, 1963.

Haskell, C. M. *Cancer treatment.* Philadelphia: W. B. Saunders, 1980.

Heidelberger, C.; Chanduri, N. K.; and Dannenberg, P. Fluorinated pyrimidines, a new class of tumor-inhibitory compounds. *Nature* 179:663–669, 1957.

Hill, B. T., and Baserga, R. The cell cycle and its significance for cancer treatment. *Cancer Treat. Rev.* 2:159–175, 1975.

Hitchings, G. H., and Elion, G. B. The chemistry and biochemistry of purine analogs. *Ann. NY Acad. Sci.* 60:195–199, 1954.

Hitchings, G. H., and Elion, G. B. Chemical suppression of the immune response. *Pharmacol. Rev.* 15:365–405, 1963.

Holland, J. F., and Frei, E., III, eds. *Cancer medicine.* Philadelphia: Lea & Febiger, 1973.

Huggins, C., and Hodges, C. V. Studies on prostatic cancer. I. The effect of castration, of estrogen, and of androgen injection on serum phosphatase in metastatic carcinoma of the prostate. *Cancer Res.* 1:293–297, 1941.

Ignoffo, R. J., and Friedman, M. A. Therapy of local toxicities caused by extravasation of cancer chemotherapy drugs. *Cancer Treat. Rev.* 7:17–27, 1980.

Johnson, I. S.; Wright, H. F.; and Svoboda, G. H. Experimental basis for clinical evaluation of antitumor principles derived from *Vinca rosea* Linn. *J. Lab. Clin. Med.* 54:830, 1959.

Jones, S. E., and Salmon, S. E., eds. *Adjuvant therapy of cancer,* vol. 2. New York: Grune & Stratton, 1979.

Kardinal, C. G., and Yarbro, J. W. A conceptual history of cancer. *Semin. Oncol.* 6:396–408, 1979.

Kaufman, H. E. Clinical cure of herpes simplex keratitis by 5-iodo-2′-deoxyuridine. *Proc. Soc. Exp. Biol. Med.* 109:251–252, 1961.

Klinenberg, J. R.; Goldfinger, S. E.; and Seegmiller, J. E. The effectiveness of the xanthine oxidase inhibitor, allopurinol, in the treatment of gout. *Ann. Intern. Med.* 62:639–647, 1965.

Knobf, M. K. et al. *Cancer chemotherapy: treatment and care.* Boston: G. K. Hall & Co., 1981.

Krakoff, I. H. Cancer chemotherapeutic agents. *CA* 31:130–140, 1981.

Li, M. C.; Hertz, R.; and Spencer, D. B. Effect of methotrexate upon choriocarcinoma and chorioadenoma. *Proc. Soc. Exp. Biol. Med.* 93:361–366, 1956.

Lissauer, H. Zwei Fälle Leucaeme. *Berliner Klin. Wochnschr.* 2:403–404, 1865.

Livingston, R. B., and Carter, S. K. *Single agents in cancer chemotherapy.* New York: Plenum, 1970.

Lokich, J. J. *Primer of cancer management.* Boston: G. K. Hall & Co., 1978.

Lokich, J. J. *Clinical cancer medicine.* Boston: G. K. Hall & Co., 1980.

Marsh, J. C. Cancer chemotherapeutic agents. In *Practical drug therapy,* ed. R. I. H. Wang. Philadelphia: J. B. Lippincott, 1979.

National Institutes of Health. *Compilation of cancer therapy protocol summaries,* 5th edition. Washington, D.C.: U.S. Department of Health and Human Services, 1981.

Osler, W. *The principles and practice of medicine.* New York: Appleton, 1909.

Piskala, A., and Sorm, F. Nucleic acid components and their analogs. LI. Synthesis of 1-glycosyl derivatives of 5-azauracil and 5-azacytosine. *Co. Czech. Chem. Commun.* 29:2060–2076, 1964.

Prusoff, W. H. A review of some aspects of 5-iododeoxyturidine and azauridine. *Cancer Res.* 23: 1247–1259, 1963.

Rosenberg, B. et al. Platinum compounds: a new class of potent antitumor agents. *Nature* 222:385–386, 1969.

Rosenberg, B.; Van Camp, L.; and Krigas, T. Inhibition of cell division in *Escherichia coli* by electrolysis products from a platinum electrode. *Nature* 205:698–699, 1965.

Rosman, M., and Bertino, J. R. Azathioprine: drugs five years later. *Ann. Intern. Med.* 79:694–700, 1973.

Sartorelli, A. C., and Creasey, W. A. Cancer chemotherapy. *Ann. Rev. Pharmacol.* 9:51–72, 1969.

Sartorelli, A. C., and Johns, D. G., eds. *The handbook of experimental pharmocology.* New York:. Springer-Verlag, 1975.

Sather, M. R. et al. *Cancer chemotherapeutic agents: handbook of clinical data.* Boston: G. K. Hall & Co., 1979.

Schilsky, R. L. et al. Gonadal dysfunction in patients receiving chemotherapy for cancer. *Ann. Intern. Med.* 93:109–114, 1980.

Seeger, D. R. et al. Analogs of pteroylglutamic acid. III. 4-Amino derivatives. *J. Am. Chem. Soc.* 7:1753–1758, 1947.

Sellei, C. et al. Clinical and pharmacological experience with dibromodulcitol (NSC 104800), a new antitumor agent. *Cancer Chemother. Rep.* 53:377–384, 1969.

Shackney, S. E. Proceedings of the symposium on cell kinetics and cancer chemotherapy. *Cancer Treat. Rep.* 60:1697–2021, 1976.

Skipper, H. E. et al. Experimental evaluation of potential anticancer agents. VI. Anatomical distribution of leukemic cells and failure of chemotherapy. *Cancer Res.* 21:1154–1164, 1961.

Skipper, H. E. et al. Experimental evaluation of potential anticancer agents. XII. On the criteria and kinetics associated with "curability" of experimental leukemias. *Cancer Chemother. Rep.* 35:1–111, 1964.

United States Pharmacopoeial Convention. *USP dispensing information.* Easton, Pa.: Mack Printing Co., 1980.

Valeriote, F. A., and Edelstein, M. B. The role of cell kinetics in cancer chemotherapy. *Semin. Oncol.* 4:217–226, 1977.

Waksman, S., and Woodruff, H. B. Bacteriostatic and bacteriocidal substances produced by a soil actinomyces. *Proc. Soc. Exp. Biol. Med.* 45:609–614, 1940.

Wasserman, T. H. et al. Tabular analysis of the clinical chemotherapy of solid tumors. *Cancer Chemother. Rep.* 6:399–419, 1975.

Weiss, H. D.; Walker, M. D.; and Wiernik, P. H. Neurotoxicity of commonly used antineoplastic agents. *N. Engl. J. Med.* 291:75–81; 127–133, 1974.

Weiss, R. B., and Bruno, S. Hypersensitivity reactions to cancer chemotherapeutic agents. *Ann. Intern. Med.* 94:66–72, 1981.

Weiss, R. B., and DeVita, V. T., Jr. Multimodal primary care treatment (adjuvant chemotherapy): current results and future prospects. *Ann. Intern. Med.* 91:251–260, 1979.

Weiss, R. B., and Muggia, F. M. Cytotoxic drug-induced pulmonary disease: update 1980. *Ann. J. Med.* 68:259–266, 1980.

Zubrod, C. G. Historic milestones in curative chemotherapy. *Semin. Oncol.* 6:490–505, 1979.

Appendix 21.1. *Normal Values*

Chemistry		
Test	*Normal Range*	*Units*
Acetone, serum	None detected	
Acid phosphatase, prostatic	0–1.5	IU/L
ACTH serum (8 a.m. fasting)	20–100	pg/ml
(4 p.m.)	10–50	pg/ml
Albumin, serum	3.5–5.0	mg/dl
Albumin, urine	20–70	mg/24 hrs
Alcohol, ethyl, serum	0–50	mg/dl
Aldolase	0–6	mU/ml
Aldosterone, plasma:		
(peripheral vein)	4–30 (9 a.m. upright)	ng/dl
(adrenal vein)	200–400	ng/dl
Aldosterone, urine:		
(normal salt diet)	3–19	μg/24 hrs
(low salt diet)	20–80	μg/24 hrs
Alkaline phosphatase (adult)	10–85	IU/L
(child)	2–3 times adult values	
Alkaline phosphatase isoenzymes, serum:		
Fasting liver	0–16	% of total
Liver	60–85	% of total
Bone	0–16	% of total
Intestine	0–8	% of total
Alpha hydroxybutyric dehydrogenase	90–220	IU/L
Alpha-1 fetoprotein	Less than 25	ng/ml
Aminolevulinic acid, urine	0–0.54	mg/dl
Ammonia, blood	65–184	μg/dl
Amylase, blood	50–200	units
Amylase, urine	50–300	units/hr
Ascorbic acid	0.2–2.0	mg/dl
Bilirubin, total	0.2–1.2	mg/dl
Bilirubin, direct	0–0.3	mg/dl

Appendix 21.1. *Normal Values*, continued

Chemistry		
Test	*Normal Range*	*Units*
Bromides	None detected	
BSP (at 45 minutes)	Less than 5% retention	
BUN	7–22	mg/dl
Calcitonin	0–200	pg/ml
Calcium serum	8.5–10.5	mg/dl
Calcium urine	50–150	mg/24 hrs
Carbon dioxide	22–30	mEq/L
Carotene	50–300	mg/dl
Catecholamines, urine		
Epinephrine	0–20	μg/24 hrs
Norepinephrine	0–80	μg/24 hrs
Total, free	0–103	μg/24 hrs
Chloride, serum	98–108	mEq/L
Chloride, urine	170–254	mEq/24 hrs
Cholesterol, total	110–275	mg/dl
Cholesterol, esters	70–78	% of total
Cholinesterase	2.5–5.0	IU/ml
Compound S: (11-deoxycortisol)	30–200	ng/dl
Copper, serum	69–140	μg/dl
Copper, urine	20–50	μg/L
Cortisol, plasma (a.m.)	5–25	μg/dl
(p.m.)	Half of a.m.	
CPK isoenzymes:		
Fraction MM	98–100	% of total
Fraction MB	0–2	% of total
Fraction BB	None detected	
Creatine phosphokinase	0–80	IU/L

Appendix 21.1. *Normal Values,* continued

Chemistry		
Test	*Normal Range*	*Units*
Creatine, serum	0.2–0.9	mg/dl
Creatinine, serum	0.2–1.4	mg/dl
Creatinine, urine	0.8–2.0	gm/24 hrs
Creatinine clearance	85–125	ml/min
Dilantin, serum, therapeutic	10–20	μg/ml
D-Xylose tolerance:		
Blood (at 2 hrs)	20–52	mg/dl
Urine (at 5 hrs)	greater than 5.0	gm/5 hrs
Electrophoresis:		
Protein, serum:		
Albumin	51.6–70.2	% of total
Alpha-1	1.6–5.0	% of total
Alpha-2	5.6–11.6	% of total
Beta	7.9–15.9	% of total
Gamma	11.2–19.4	% of total
Protein, CSF:		
Prealbumin	4.0–4.3	% of total
Albumin	56.8–68.0	% of total
Alpha-1	4.1–6.5	% of total
Alpha-2	6.2–10.2	% of total
Beta	10.8–14.8	% of total
Gamma	6.7–8.9	% of total
Protein, urine:		
Albumin	Average–37.9	% of total
Alpha-1	27.3	% of total
Alpha-2	19.5	% of total
Beta	8.8	% of total
Gamma	3.3	% of total
Estradiol, 17-Beta, serum:		
Male	0.8–3.5	ng/dl
Female:		
Preovulatory	20	ng/dl
Follicular	3–10	ng/dl
Luteal	7–30	ng/dl
Estriol, urine (pregnancy):		
Week of gestation		mg/24 hrs
28		4–12
30		5–15
32		5–18
34		5–22
36		6–23
38		8–30
40		11–44

Appendix 21.1. *Normal Values*, continued

Chemistry		
Test	*Normal Range*	*Units*
Estrogens, total, serum:		
Male	60–260	pg/ml
Female:		
Days 1–10	45–200	pg/ml
Days 11–20	80–450	pg/ml
Days 21–30	140–300	pg/ml
Estrogens, total, urine, non-pregnant:		
Male	0–25	μg/24 hrs
Female:		
Proliferative	25–35	μg/24 hrs
Ovulatory	50–100	μg/24 hrs
Luteal	35–50	μg/24 hrs
Postmenopausal	0–25	μg/24 hrs
Fatty acids, free	0.45–0.90	mEq/L
Fetal hemoglobin	0–2	%
Follicle stimulating hormone, serum		
Male	5–25	mIU/ml
Female:		
Follicular	5–20	mIU/ml
Ovulatory	12–30	mIU/ml
Luteal	5–15	mIU/ml
Postmenopausal	40–200	mIU/ml
Follicle stimulating hormone, urine		
Male	5–25	IU/24 hrs
Female:		
Follicular	5–20	IU/24 hrs
Ovulatory	12–30	IU/24 hrs
Luteal	5–51	IU/24 hrs
Postmenopausal	50–100	IU/24 hrs
Gamma GTP:		
Male	6–32	mu/ml
Female	4–17	mu/ml
Glucose-6-PD	6–10	IU/gm HGB
Glucose, serum	70–105	mg/dl
Glucose, CSF	50–80% of serum glucose	
Glucose, urine	Average–0.13	gm/24 hrs
Haptoglobin	50–140	mg/dl
Hemoglobin A2	1.8–3.5	% of total
Homovanillic acid	0–15	mg/24 hrs

Appendix 21.1. *Normal Values*, continued

Chemistry		
Test	*Normal Range*	*Units*
17-Hydroxycorticosteroids, urine	5–15	mg/24 hrs
5-Hydroxy-indole acetic acid, urine	2–10	mg/24 hrs
17-Hydroxyprogesterone:		
Male:		
Adult	27–199	ng/dl
Female		
Prepuberty	3–90	ng/dl
Follicular	15–70	ng/dl
Luteal	25–290	ng/dl
Hydroxyproline, total, urine	25–75	mg/24 hrs
Iron, serum	65–175	μg/dl
Iron binding capacity	225–425	μg/dl
Ketogenic steroids, urine:		
Male	5–23	mg/24 hrs
Female	3–15	mg/24 hrs
17-Ketosteroids, urine:		
Male	5–20	mg/24 hrs
Female	3–12	mg/24 hrs
Lactic acid (fasting venous)	3.5–13.0	mg/dl
Lactic dehydrogenase (serum)	40–110	IU/L
LDH isoenzymes:		
LDH-1	21–47	% of total
LDH-2	40–53	% of total
LDH-3	10–23	% of total
LDH-4	1–5	% of total
LDH-5	0–4	% of total
Lead, blood	0–60	μg/dl
Lead, urine	0–100	μg/24 hrs
Lipase, serum	0–1.7	units
Lipids, total, serum	400–1000	mg/dl
Lithium, serum (therapeutic)	0.5–1.5	mEq/l

Appendix 21.1. *Normal Values,* continued

Chemistry		
Test	*Normal Range*	*Units*
Luteinizing hormone, urine:		
Male	5–18	IU/24 hrs
Female		
Follicular	2–25	IU/24 hrs
Ovulatory	30–95	IU/24 hrs
Luteal	2–20	IU/24 hrs
Postmenopausal	40–110	IU/24 hrs
Lysozyme (muramidase), serum	0–10	μg/ml
Magnesium, serum	1.6–2.4	mg/dl
5′Nucleotidase	0–16	IU/L
Osmolality, serum	275–295	mOsm/kg
Osmolality, urine	300–1000	mOsm/kg
Parathyroid hormone:		
Intact PTH	163–347	pg/ml
Phenobarbital, serum (therapeutic)	1.0–4.0	μg/dl
Phospholipids	150–300	mg/dl
Phosphorus, serum:		
Adult	2.5–4.5	mg/dl
Child	4.0–7.0	mg/dl
Porphyrins; urine:		
Corproporphyrin	17–100	μg/24hrs
Porphorbilinogen	None detected	
Uroporphyrin	0–10	μg/24 hrs
Potassium, serum	3.5–5.0	mEq/L
Potassium, urine	25–125	mEq/24 hrs
Pregnanediol, urine:		
Male	0.1–9.9	mg/24 hrs
Female (non-pregnant)	1.2–9.5	mg/24 hrs
Female (pregnant)	5–100	mg/24 hrs
Pregnanetriol, urine		
Male	0.4–2.4	mg/24 hrs
Female	0–1.8	mg/24 hrs

Appendix 21.1. *Normal Values,* continued

Chemistry		
Test	*Normal Range*	*Units*
Progesterone, serum:		
Male	15–150	ng/dl
Female:		
Follicular	20–150	ng/dl
Luteal	300–2400	ng/dl
Protein, total, CSF	15–40	mg/dl
Protein, total, serum	6.0–8.0	gm/dl
Protein, total, urine	0–100	mg/24 hrs
Pyruvic acid (fasting-venous)	0.2–1.0	mg/dl
Quinidine (therapeutic)	2.0–5.0	μg/ml
Salicylates (therapeutic)	8.0–12.0	mg/dl
SGOT	7–24	IU/L
SGPT	5–25	IU/L
Sodium, serum	136–145	mEq/L
Sodium, urine	50–225	mEq/24 hrs
Theophylline (therapeutic)	1.0–2.0	mg/dl
Testosterone, serum:		
Male:		
Prepuberty	20–80	ng/dl
Adult	300–1200	ng/dl
Female:		
Prepuberty	10–85	ng/dl
Transferrin	200–400	mg/dl
Triglycerides	10–190	mg/dl
Urea nitrogen (BUN)	7–22	mg/dl
Uric acid, serum	2–7	mg/dl
Vanillylmandelic acid (VMA), urine	0–7	mg/24 hrs
Vitamin A	20–60	μg/dl
Vitamin B1 (thiamine)	1.6–4.0	mg/dl

Appendix 21.1. *Normal Values,* continued

Test	Normal Range	Units
	Chemistry	
Vitamin B6 (pyridoxine)	28–87	μg/ml
Vitamin C (ascorbic acid)	0.2–2.0	mg/dl
Vitamin E	5–20	μg/ml
Zinc, serum	55–150	μg/dl
Zinc, urine	150–1300	μg/24 hrs

NOTE: In general, normal values should be specified by the laboratory performing the test. For convenience, we have compiled these normal values from three sources: Hospital of St. Raphael, *Laboratory organization, procedures and normal values,* 2nd edition, New Haven, Conn., 1979; Yale–New Haven Hospital, *Clinical laboratory manual,* New Haven Conn., 1980. Case records of the Massachusetts General Hospital, *N. Engl. J. Med.* 302:37–48, 1980.

Appendix 21.1. *Cytology Class and Interpretation*

Cytology reports will usually have a diagnostic interpretation and a class.

The following is given as a guideline for interpretation of the classes used.

Class	*General Definition*	*Relation to Malignancy*
I	Negative for tumor; this denotes absence of atypical or abnormal material	Negative
II	Atypical cytology but no evidence of malignancy	Negative
III	Atypical cytology suspicious for but not diagnostic of malignancy	Suspicious
IV	Atypical cytology strongly suggestive of malignancy	Positive
V	Atypical cytology diagnostic of malignancy	Positive

Appendix 21.1. *Cerebrospinal-Fluid Values*

Bilirubin	0
Cell count	0–5 mononuclear cells
Chloride	120–130 mEq per liter
Colloidal gold	0000000000-0001222111
Albumin	Mean 21 mg/dl Range ± 1 SD 11.4–38.4 ± 2 SD 6–71
IgG	Mean 3.4 mg/dl Range ± 1 SD 2.0–5.9 ± 2 SD 1–10
IgG/Alb Ratio	Range ± 1 SD 0.094–0.25 ± 2 SD 0.05–0.43
Glucose	50–75 mg/dl
Pressure (initial)	70–180 mm of water
Protein:	
Lumbar	15–45 mg/dl
Cisternal	15–25 mg/dl
Ventricular	5–15 mg/dl

Appendix 21.1. *Hematology*

Test	Normal Range	Units
Antithrombin III	70–130	%
Autohemolysis test	<4% in 48 hours	
Bleeding time, Ivy (lancet)	<6	min
Bleeding time, Ivy, Template	<10	min
Cerebrospinal fluid cell count	<6 lymphs	
Coagulation factor assays:		
Factor I (fibrinogen)	150–350	mg/dl
Factor II (prothrombin)	60–140	%
Factor V (proaccelerin)	60–140	%
Factor VII (proconvertin)	50–150	%
Factor VIII (antihemophilic globulin)	50–200	%
Factor IX (plasma thromboplastin component)	60–140	%
Factor X (Stuart factor)	70–130	%
Factor XI (plasma thromboplastin antecedent)	60–140	%
Factor XII (Hageman factor)	60–140	%
Factor XIII (fibrin stabilizing factor)	50–150	%
Complete blood count (CBC)		
White blood count (WBC)	4800–10,800	per μl (mm^3)
Red blood count (RBC):		
Male	$4.5-6.0 \times 10^6$	per μl (mm^3)
Female	$4.0-5.5 \times 10^6$	per μl (mm^3)
Hematocrit:		
Male	47 ± 5	%
Female	42 ± 5	%
Hemoglobin:		
Male	16 ± 2	gm/dl
Female	14 ± 2	gm/dl
RBC indices:		
Mean corpuscular volume (MCV)	82–98	fl
Mean corpuscular hemoglobin (MCH)	27–31	pg
Mean corpuscular hemoglobin conc. (MCHC)	32–36	%
Differential white cell count (absolute):		
Segmented neutrophils	1800–7000	per μl (mm^3)
Bands	0–700	per μl (mm^3)
Eosinophils	0–450	per μl (mm^3)
Basophils	0–200	per μl (mm^3)
Lymphocytes	1000–4800	per μl (mm^3)
Monocytes	0–800	per μl (mm^3)

Appendix 21.1. *Hematology*, continued

Test	*Normal Range*	*Units*
Erythrocyte sedimentation rate (Wintrobe):		
Male	0–9	mm/hr
Female	0–19	mm/hr
Euglobulin lysis time	normal >2	hr
	abnormal <1.5	hr
Ferritin	20–300	ng/ml
Fetal red blood cell stain	negative in adults	
Fibrin split products	normal <10	μg/ml
	borderline 10–40	μg/ml
	abnormal >40	μg/ml
Fibrinogen	150–350	mg/dl
Folate, RBC	>110	ng/ml
Folate, serum	>3	ng/ml
Free erythrocyte protoporphrin	5–40	μg/dl
Glucose-6 phosphate dehydrogenase	6–10	IU/gm HGB
Ham's acid hemolysis test	negative	
Heinz body stain	negative	
Hemoglobin, plasma or serum	0–4	mg/dl
Hemoglobin, urine	0	
Hemoglobin AlC (glycosylated)	5–8	%
Hemosiderin, urine	negative	
Iron, serum:		
Males	60–180	μg/dl
Females	50–170	μg/dl
Iron binding capacity (IBC)	225–425	μg/dl
LE test (lupus erythematosus)	negative	
Lee-White whole blood clotting time	<10	min
Leukocyte alkaline phosphatase	13–130	score
Lysozyme, serum	0–10	μg/ml

Appendix 21.1. *Hematology*, continued

Test	*Normal Range*	*Units*
Lysozyme, urine	0–0.5	μg/ml
Myoglobin, urine	negative	
Partial thromboplastin time (activated)	25–45	sec
Platelet adhesiveness	>70% retention	
Platelet count	150,000–350,000	per μl (mm^3)
Prothrombin time	<13	sec
Pyruvate kinase	4.5–10.5	units/10^{10} RBC
Reticulocyte count	0.5–2.0	%
Siderocyte stain	negative	
Sugar-water test	negative	
Thrombin time	20–25	sec
Vitamin B12	200–1200	pg/ml
Vitamin B12 binding capacity:	1300	pg/ml
TCII	80	%
R binders	20	%

Appendix 21.1. *Radioimmunoassays and Binding*

Test	*Normal Range*	*Units*
Aldosterone	standing 4–31	ng/dl
	recumbent 1–16	ng/dl
Beta HCG (human chorionic gonadotropin)	1st week: 10–30	mIU/ml
	2nd week: 30–100	mIU/ml
	3rd week: 100–1000	mIU/ml
	4th week: 1000–10,000	mIU/ml
	2nd–3rd month: 10,000–100,000	mIU/ml
	2nd trimester: 10,000–30,000	mIU/ml
	3rd trimester: 5000–15,000	mIU/ml
Carcinoembryonic antigen (CEA):		
Nonsmokers	<2.5	ng/ml
Smokers	<5	ng/ml
Digitoxin (therapeutic)	9–25	ng/ml
Digoxin (therapeutic):		
0.125 mg/day	0.3–0.7	ng/ml
0.25 mg/day	0.8–1.6	ng/ml
0.50 mg/day	0.9–2.4	ng/ml
Estriol	6 weeks 1.3–3.2	ng/ml
	12 weeks 1.6–4.4	ng/ml
	20 weeks 2.0–7.2	ng/ml
	25 weeks 3.5–10.0	ng/ml
	30 weeks 4.5–14.0	ng/ml
	32 weeks 5.0–16.0	ng/ml
	34 weeks 5.5–18.5	ng/ml
	36 weeks 7.0–25.0	ng/ml
	38 weeks 9.0–32.0	ng/ml
	40 weeks 10.5–34.0	ng/ml
Estrogen-binding receptors:		
Premenopausal negative	0–4	fm/mg
borderline	5–9	fm/mg
Postmenopausal negative	0–14	fm/mg
borderline	15–29	fm/mg
Ferritin	20–300	ng/ml
Free thyroxine	1.0–2.3	ng/dl
Gastrin	<190	pg/ml
Gentamycin (therapeutic)	4–12	μg/ml
Hepatitis A antibody	negative	

Appendix 21.1. *Radioimmunoassays and Binding,* continued

Test	*Normal Range*	*Units*
Hepatitis A IgM antibody	negative	
Hepatitis B surface antigen	negative	
Hepatitis B surface antibody	negative	
Hepatitis B core antigen	negative	
Hepatitis B e antigen	negative	
Hepatitis B e antibody	negative	
Human growth hormone	0–5 (adults)	ng/ml
Insulin (fasting)	5–34	μ units/ml
Progesterone binding capacity:		
Negative	0–9	fm/mg
Borderline	10–19	fm/mg
Prolactin:		
Female	6–27	ng/ml
Male	6–12	ng/ml
Renin activity, plasma:		
Supine	0.15–2.33	ng/ml/hr
Upright	1.13–3.95	ng/ml/hr
Thyroid stimulating hormone	<10	μ units/ml
Thyroxin (T_4)	4.5–11.5	μg/dl
Thyroxin binding globulin	13–20	μg/dl
Tobramycin (therapeutic)	3–10	μg/ml
Triiodothyronine (T_3)	60–190	ng/dl

Appendix 21.1. *Serology*

Test	*Normal Range*	*Units*
Alpha-1 antitrypsin	200–450	mg/dl
Anti-DNA binding capacity	<20	%
Anti-nuclear factor	<1:32	titer
Antihyaluronidase	<1:256	titer
Antimitochondrial antibody	negative	
Antiparietal cell antibody	negative	
Anti-smooth muscle antibody	negative	
Antistreptolysin O	<1:160	titer
Aspergillus antibody	<1:4	titer
Brucella antibody	<1:80	titer
Candida antibody	<1:4	titer
Carcinoembryonic antigen (CEA):		
Nonsmoker	<2.5	ng/ml
Smoker	<5	ng/ml
Cl esterase inhibitor	78–143	%
Cold agglutinins	<1:64	titer
Complement (Clq) antigen	40–150	%
Complement (C3) antigen	78–150	mg/dl
Complement (C4) antigen	20–50	mg/dl
C-reactive protein	not detected	
Cryoglobulins	absent	
Cytomegalovirus	1:4–1:32	titer
Epstein-Barr virus	<1:40	titer
Heterophile antibody (ox cell)	<1:40	titer
Heterophile antibody (sheep cell)	<1:56	titer
Herpes virus	<1:64	titer

Appendix 21.1. *Serology*, continued

Test	*Normal Range*	*Units*
Immunoglobulins, quantitative serum		
IgA	60–400	mg/dl
IgG	700–2000	mg/dl
IgM	60–250	mg/dl
IgD	<15	mg/dl
IgE	<200	IU/ml
Light chains	absent	
Latex fixation (rheumatoid factor)	<1:20	titer
Leptospira antibody	<1:80	titer
Mycoplasma antibody	<1:32	titer
Paratyphoid A and B	<1:80	titer
Rickettsial antibody (Weil-Felix)	<1:160	titer
Thyroid antibodies:		
Microsomal (hemagglutination)	absent	
Thyroglobulin (hemagglutination)	<1:250	titer
Toxoplasma	<1:256	titer
Treponemal antibody (FTA-ABS)	negative	
Tularensis	<1:80	titer
Typhoid H	<1:40	titer
Typhoid O	<1:80	titer
VDRL	negative	

SOURCES: Hospital of St. Raphael. *Laboratory organization, procedures and normal values,* Second edition. New Haven, Conn., 1979; Yale–New Haven Hospital. *Clinical laboratory manual, 1980;* Case records of the Massachusetts General Hospital. *N. Engl. J. Med.* 302:37–48, 1980.

Appendix 21.2. *Drug Information for Patients*

The following instructions and informational drug reviews were prepared by members of the nursing, pharmacy, and physician (medical-oncology) staff of Yale-New Haven Medical Center, and printed on cards. The appropriate cards are distributed to patients before they are asked to consent to chemotherapy and are retained by the patients for future reference. The more common drugs are listed alphabetically by generic name.

Chemotherapy: General Instructions

Allopurinol (Zyloprim)
L-asparaginase (Elspar)
5-Azacytidine*
Bleomycin (Blenoxane)
Busulfan (Myleran)
Carmustine (BCNU, BiCNU)
Chlorambucil (Leukeran)
Cisplatin (Platinol, cis-platinum, CDDP)
Cyclophosphamide (Cytoxan, Endoxan)
Cytarabine (Cytosar-U, Ara-C)
Dacarbazine (DTIC)
Dactinomycin (Cosmagen, actinomycin-D)
Daunorubicin (Cerubidine, daunomycin, rubidomycin)
Diethylstilbestrol (DES)
Doxorubicin (Adriamycin)
Etoposide (VP-16-213)*
5-Fluorouracil (Adrucil, Fluorouracil)
Fluoxymesterone (Halotestin)
Hexamethylmelamine*
Hydroxyurea (Hydrea)
Lomustine (CCNU, CeeNU)
Mechlorethamine (Mustargen, nitrogen mustard)
Medroxyprogesterone acetate (Provera)
Megestrol acetate (Megace)
Melphalan (Alkeran, L-PAM)
Mercaptopurine (Purinethol)
Methotrexate (Mexate)
  Leucovorin rescue
  Urine alkalinization
Mithramycin (Mithracin)
Mitomycin (Mutamycin)
Mitotane (Lysodren)
Prednisone
Procarbazine (Matulane)
Razoxin (Razoxane, ICRF-159)*
Semustine (Methyl-CCNU)*
Streptozocin (Streptozotocin)*
Tamoxifen (Nolvadex)
6-Thioguanine (Thioguanine, Tabloid)
Vinblastine (Velban)
Vincristine (Oncovin)

*Investigational.

CHEMOTHERAPY

The information on the following cards is to help you to understand your chemotherapy. You may experience some, none, or all of the side effects. Your doctor and nurses are familiar with all of these side effects and will help you to manage them should they occur.

Call ________________________ for:

- Fever higher than 101° F.
- Shaking chill.
- Unusual bleeding or bruising.
- Shortness of breath.
- Severe constipation or diarrhea.
- Vomiting that continues 72 hours after treatment.
- Painful or burning urination.
- Blood in the urine or stool.
- Soreness of the intravenous site.
- Any questions that occur.

Your chemotherapy will proceed more smoothly if you:

Eat nourishing foods and drink plenty of fluids at mealtime and between meals.

Do not take aspirin—you may take Tylenol, Datril, or Tempra if needed.

Tell your doctor all the medications you are taking.

Check with your doctor before having any dental work done.

Do not drink alcoholic beverages or do so in moderation.

NOTE: Some of the drugs may alter your sexual drive or your ability to have children. You may want to talk with your doctor about birth control and family planning before beginning chemotherapy.

Allopurinol (Zyloprim)

What It Looks Like:

Tablets:

White (100 mg).

Orange (300 mg).

How It Is Given:

Taken by mouth.

Common Side Effects:

Skin rash.

Less Common Side Effects:

Nausea and vomiting.

Diarrhea.

Loss of appetite.

This drug is not a chemotherapy drug, but it is often used in many different types of tumors to prevent uric acid from damaging the kidneys or producing gout.

L-asparaginase (Elspar)

What It Looks Like:

Clear fluid after dissolved.

How It is Given:

Injection into vein or into a muscle.

Common Side Effects:

Nausea and vomiting may occur within four to six hours after treatment.

Loss of appetite.

"Blahs" occur in most patients and generally become worse with each added dose.

Fever (100–101°F) occurs in about half of the patients receiving this drug.

Skin rash.

Sore arm muscle.

Less Common Side Effects:

Liver problems: blood counts of liver function will be done on a regular basis.

High blood sugar.

Drowsiness.

Excessive bleeding or blood clotting.

Unusual Drug Reaction:

Some patients have a severe drug reaction that consists of hives, chills, fever, facial redness, lowered blood pressure, and shortness of breath. This happens shortly after the drug is given. The doctor and nurse will be immediately available for 30 minutes after the drug is given to treat the problem if it does occur.

Call doctor if hives develop or arm soreness lasts more than one day.

5-Azacytidine*

What It Looks Like:

Clear fluid after dissolved.

How It Is Given:

Injection into vein or just below the skin.

Common Side Effects:

Symptoms of nausea and vomiting are worse for the first two days of treatment and then become less with continued treatment.

Diarrhea occurs in half of those patients receiving the drug.

Reduced blood counts occur two to two and one half weeks after treatment.

Less Common Side Effects:

Liver problems; blood counts of liver function will be done on a regular basis.

Lowered blood pressure may occur if the drug is given too rapidly. Tell the person giving the drug if you feel dizzy or lightheaded.

Fever may occur if the drug is given too rapidly. Tell the person giving the drug if you feel warm.

Temporary changes in behavior.

*This drug is investigational, which means that it can only be obtained through your oncologist.

Bleomycin (Blenoxane)

What It Looks Like:

Clear fluid after dissolved.

How It Is Given:

Injection into vein, or into muscle or under the skin.

Common Side Effects:

Fever and chills may occur 2 to 10 hours after the drug is given.

Scarring of the lungs may occur: report any problems with breathing (i.e., shortness of breath or cough) to your doctor.

Darkening, peeling, or rash on skin (especially hands).

Dark rings in the nailbeds may occur.

Pain in area where needle is inserted.

Mouth sores.

Less Common Side Effects:

Nausea and vomiting.

Tiredness or weakness.

Pain and swelling of joints.

Hair loss may occur and is not permanent.

Headache.

Busulfan (Myleran)

What It Looks Like:
White tablet (2 mg).

How It Is Given:
Taken by mouth.

Common Side Effects:
Menstrual cycle may be irregular.

Reduced blood counts particularly with long-term daily use of the tablet.

Less Common Side Effects:
Nausea and vomiting.

Diarrhea.

Darkening of skin.

Sore tongue and irritation at the corners of the mouth.

Scarring of the lungs may occur with long-term usage of the drug. Report shortness of breath, cough, and fever to your oncologist.

Larger breasts.

Carmustine (BCNU, BiCNU)

What It Looks Like:
Clear fluid after dissolved.

How It Is Given:
Injection into vein.

Common Side Effects:
There may be discomfort along vein while the drug is being given.

Nausea and vomiting generally occur two to four hours after drug is given and may last up to 24 hours.

Flushing (redness) of the face.

Fatigue, "the blahs."

Reduced blood counts usually occur three to five weeks after treatment.

Less Common Side Effects:
Hair loss may occur and is not permanent.

Mouth sores may occur.

Liver problems, blood counts of liver function will be done on a regular basis.

Chlorambucil (Leukeran)

What It Looks Like:
White tablet (2 mg).

How It Is Given:
Taken by mouth.

Common Side Effects:
Reduced blood counts.

Less Common Side Effects:
Nausea and vomiting.

Skin irritation.

Cisplatin (Platinol, cis-platinum, CDDP)

What It Looks Like:
Clear fluid after being dissolved.

How It Is Given:
Injection into vein.

Common Side Effects:
Nausea and vomiting may occur shortly after the drug is given and may last up to 24 hours.

Kidney damage may occur but is reduced by giving large amounts of fluids.

Hearing damage may occur.

Less Common Side Effects:
Reduced blood counts may occur in two to four weeks.

Numbness, tingling, and reduced feeling in fingers and toes may occur.

Very rarely, sweating, difficulty in breathing, and rapid heart beat may occur.

Cyclophosphamide (Cytoxan, Endoxan)

What It Looks Like:
Clear fluid after dissolved.

White tablet with blue specks (25 and 50 mg).

How It Is Given:
Taken by mouth or by injection into the vein.

Common Side Effects:
Nausea and vomiting usually occur about six hours after the drug is given through the vein and may last 8 to 10 hours. When the tablet is taken, nausea may occur throughout the entire day.

General thinning of hair.

Nasal stuffiness, sinus congestion, sneezing, watery eyes, and runny nose during or immediately following injection of the drug.

Reduced blood counts occur one to two weeks after treatment.

Less Common Side Effects:
Bladder irritation—may produce burning on urination or bloody urine. Adults should drink at least three quarts of fluid (whatever you prefer including water, soda, tea, coffee, milk, etc.) during the day of the injection and two days after receiving the injection of the drug. Empty your bladder frequently while taking the drug. When taking the tablet, it should be taken early enough in the day to allow for drinking large amounts of fluids and frequent emptying of the bladder. If unable to drink fluids or pass your urine, call the doctor.

Children between 2 and 12 years of age should drink two quarts of fluid, and children under two years of age should be given one quart of fluid during the day of injection.

Cytarabine (Cytosar-U, Ara-C)

What It Looks Like:

Clear fluid after dissolved.

How It Is Given:

Injection into the vein or just below the skin.

Common Side Effects:

Nausea and vomiting occur in most patients and last 8 to 12 hours after the drug is given.

Reduced blood counts occur one to two weeks after treatment.

Less Common Side Effects:

Headache.

Fever.

Redness and swelling of vein where drug is given.

Confusion, agitation, depression.

Dacarbazine (DTIC)

What It Looks Like:

Clear fluid after dissolved.

How It Is Given:

Injection into vein.

Common Side Effects:

Nausea and vomiting.

Flu-like symptoms (fever, aches, or tiredness) for one day after treatment.

Discomfort along vein while drug is being given, which may be lessened by applying ice above the place where the needle is located.

Reduced blood counts occur two to four weeks after treatment.

Less Common Side Effects:

Metal taste in the mouth.

Eye and skin may become more sensitive to the sun.

Dactinomycin (Cosmagen, actinomycin-D)

What It Looks Like:

Yellow fluid after dissolved.

How It Is Given:

Injection into vein.

Common Side Effects:

Nausea and vomiting usually occur two to five hours after drug is given and may last up to 24 hours.

Hair loss may occur a week or more after treatment and is not permanent.

Redness of skin where radiation has been given.

Mouth sores.

Reduced blood counts usually occur one to two weeks after treatment.

Less Common Side Effects:

"Blahs."

Diarrhea.

Drug can be irritating to tissue if it leaks out of the vein. Tell the person giving the drug if you feel any burning, stinging, or pain while the drug is being given. If the area of injection becomes red and swollen after the injection, notify your doctor.

Daunorubicin (Cerubidine, daunomycin, rubidomycin)

What It Looks Like:

Red fluid after dissolved.

How It Is Given:

Injection into the vein.

Common Side Effects:

Nausea and vomiting occur in about half of all patients usually within 24 hours after the drug is given.

Discolored urine (pink to red) may occur up to 48 hours after the drug is given.

Complete hair loss occurs two or more weeks after treatment begins and is not permanent.

Reduced blood counts occur one to two weeks after treatment.

Less Common Side Effects:

Mouth sores may occur.

Heart muscle damage may occur; therefore, studies are done before the drug is given and at certain times throughout treatment to assess heart function. Report any shortness of breath or ankle swelling.

The drug can be irritating to tissue if it leaks out of the vein. Tell person administering drug if you feel any burning, stinging, or pain while the drug is being given. If the area of injection becomes red and swollen after the injection, notify your doctor.

Diethylstilbestrol (DES)

What It Looks Like:

White tablet (0.1 mg, 0.25 mg, 0.5 mg, 5.0 mg)

How It Is Given:

Taken by mouth.

Common Side Effects:

Nausea and vomiting usually occur at the beginning of treatment and disappear within a few weeks.

Swelling of the legs and a possible increase in blood pressure.

Breast tenderness in females with possible worsening of cystic breast (lumps in breasts).

Larger or tender breasts may occur in males.

Increased blood calcium during the first few weeks of treatment. Report any increased thirst, drowsiness, constipation, and increased urination.

Decrease in sexual drive and voice change in males.

Less Common Side Effects:

Leakage of urine or slipping of womb in women.

Increased incidence of high blood pressure or heart disease.

Spotting between periods in women.

Effects on blood clotting.

Gallbladder disease.

Doxorubicin (Adriamycin)

What It Looks Like:

Red fluid after dissolved.

How It Is Given:

Injection into vein.

Common Side Effects:

Nausea and vomiting may occur one to three hours after the drug is given and may last up to 24 hours.

Complete hair loss generally occurs two or more weeks after treatment begins and is not permanent.

Discolored urine (pink to red) may occur up to 48 hours after the drug is given.

Reduced blood counts occur one to two weeks after treatment.

Less Common Side Effects:

Heart muscle damage may occur; therefore, studies are done before the drug is given and at certain times throughout treatment to assess heart function. Report any shortness of breath or ankle swelling.

Fatigue, weakness, the "blahs."

Mouth sores may occur.

The drug can be irritating to tissue if it leaks out of the vein. Tell the person giving the drug if you feel any burning, pain, or stinging while the drug is being given. If the area of injection becomes red and swollen after the injection, notify your doctor.

Etoposide (VP-16-213)*

What It Looks Like:

Clear fluid after dissolved.

How It Is Given:

Injection into vein.

Common Side Effects:

Nausea and vomiting immediately following treatment; usually mild.

Loss of appetite.

Hair loss may occur but is not permanent.

Reduced blood counts.

Less Common Side Effects:

Mouth sores may occur.

Diarrhea.

Special Precautions:

Some patients develop lowered blood pressure and shortness of breath when the drug is being given or shortly after. Your blood pressure will be checked while you are receiving the drug. Report any shortness of breath.

*This drug is investigational, which means that it can only be obtained through your oncologist.

5-Fluorouracil (Adrucil, Fluorouracil)

What It Looks Like:

Clear fluid.

How It Is Given:

Taken by mouth and by injection into a vein.

Common Side Effects:

Loss of appetite.

Diarrhea.

"Blahs."

Mouth sores.

Reduced blood counts occur 10 to 14 days after treatment.

Skin is sensitive to sun.

Splitting of fingernails.

Dry flaky skin.

Metal taste in mouth.

Darkening of skin especially on face and palms of hands.

Watery eyes.

Nasal dryness.

Less Common Side Effects:

Nausea and vomiting.

Hair loss occurs as thinning and loss of eyebrows.

Skin rash.

Special Precautions:

Do not stay in sun for long periods of time because your skin is more sensitive to the sun and it may burn more easily than normal.

Fluoxymesterone (Halotestin)

What It Looks Like:

Tablet:

Pink (2 mg).

Yellow (5 mg).

Green (10 mg).

How It Is Given:

Taken by mouth.

Common Side Effects:

Male features in females after using the drug for greater than three months, such as more hair on face, deeper voice, more noticeable muscles and veins, baldness, and excessive body hair.

Increased sexual drive.

Acne may develop or worsen.

Retention (holding) of body fluids.

Increased blood calcium, report any increased thirst, drowsiness, constipation, and increased urination.

Less Common Side Effects:

Nausea and vomiting.

Occasional yellow skin.

Hexamethylmelamine*

What It Looks Like:

Capsule:

White (50 mg).

Orange and white (100 mg).

How It Is Given:

Taken by mouth.

Common Side Effects:

Nausea and vomiting.

Less Common Side Effects:

Confusion, agitation, and depression.

Tingling, numbness, muscle weakness of hands, fingers, legs, and feet.

"Blahs."

Reduced blood counts.

*This drug is investigational, which means that it can only be obtained through your oncologist.

Hydroxyurea (Hydrea)

What It Looks Like:

Capsules (gray and pink 500 mg).

How It Is Given:

Taken by mouth.

Common Side Effects:

Mild to moderate nausea.

Lack of appetite.

Reduced blood counts.

Less Common Side Effects:

Diarrhea.

Hair loss.

Mouth sores.

Rash.

Lomustine (CCNU, CeeNU)

What It Looks Like:

Capsules:

Purple (10 mg).

Purple and green (40 mg).

Green (100 mg).

How It Is Given:

Taken by mouth.

Common Side Effects:

Nausea and vomiting may occur one to five hours after the drug is given.

Reduced blood counts occur four to five weeks after treatment.

Less Common Side Effects:

Mouth sores may occur.

Hair loss may occur but is not permanent.

Mechlorethamine (Mustargen, nitrogen mustard)

What It Looks Like:

Clear fluid after dissolved.

How It Is Given:

Injection into vein.

Common Side Effects:

Nausea and vomiting usually occur one-half to one hour after treatment but may occur up to eight hours later and last 24 to 48 hours.

Redness and swelling of vein; may be painful. Can apply warm soaks.

Vein turns brown color and may remain that way.

Menstrual cycle may be irregular.

Impaired sperm production.

Reduced blood counts occur one to two weeks after treatment.

Less Common Side Effects:

Skin rash.

The drug can be irritating to tissue if it leaks out of vein. Tell person administering drug if you feel any burning, stinging, or pain while the drug is being given. If the area of injection becomes red and swollen after the injection, notify your oncologist.

Medroxyprogesterone acetate (Provera)

What It Looks Like:
Small white tablets (10 mg).
White fluid.

How It Is Given:
Taken by mouth.
Injection into muscle.

Common Side Effects:
Nausea.
Skin rash.
Swelling (or puffiness) of the legs.

Megestrol acetate (Megace)

What It Looks Like:
Light blue scored tablets (20 mg, 40 mg).

How It Is Given:
Taken by mouth.

Common Side Effects:
Fluid retention.

Less Common Side Effects:
Can cause fetal damage in first trimester, hence contraindicated in early pregnancy.

Melphalan (Alkeran, L-PAM)

What It Looks Like:
White tablet (2 mg).

How It Is Given:
Taken by mouth.

Common Side Effects:
Reduced blood counts may occur three to five weeks after treatment.

Less Common Side Effects:
Nausea and vomiting may occur after use of high doses.
Menstrual cycle may become irregular.

Mercaptopurine (Purinethol)

What It Looks Like:
White tablets (50 mg).

How It Is Given:
Taken by mouth.

Common Side Effects:
Nausea is occasional and mild.
Reduced blood counts.

Less Common Side Effects:
Mouth sores may occur.
Diarrhea.
Fever.
Skin rash.

Methotrexate (Mexate)

What It Looks Like:

Yellow fluid after dissolved.

Yellow tablet (2.5 mg).

How It Is Given:

Taken by mouth or injection into a vein or muscle.

Common Side Effects:

Hair loss—thinning rather than complete loss.

Mouth sores.

Diarrhea.

"Blahs."

Reduced blood counts occur one to two weeks after treatment.

Less Common Side Effects:

Lung changes—report any cough, shortness of breath, or fever to your doctor. This will disappear when the drug is no longer taken.

Kidney problems—blood and urine counts of kidney function will be on a regular basis.

Liver problems—Blood counts of liver function will be done on a regular basis.

Nausea and vomiting.

Back pain while the drug is being given.

Special Precautions:

Report mouth sores to your physician immediately.

Do not take aspirin or anything containing aspirin (Percodan, Empirin) within 72 hours after receiving the drug without checking with your doctor.

Leucovorin rescue*

What It Looks Like:

Yellow fluid.

Small white pills (5 mg).

How It Is Given:

Taken by mouth.

This is a drug that will stop the action of the methotrexate. You *must* begin taking this at a time prescribed by your doctor. It is extremely important that you take your leucovorin rescue (pills or fluid) at the correct time and for the number of doses prescribed by the doctor.

Should you forget to take the medicine or not be able to keep it in your stomach, you should report this to your doctor. The leucovorin rescue will be absorbed if it remains in your stomach for 30 minutes. If you vomit after 30 minutes have gone by, it is not necessary to repeat the leucovorin rescue.

*The tablets are investigational, which means they can only be obtained through your oncologist.

Urine alkalinization

You should have already collected your urine for at least one 24-hour period. This is to determine your kidney function.

At ________ p.m. the evening before your treatment, you will begin taking the number of bicarbonate pills that your doctor has prescribed every three hours. You will continue doing this until you are treated. You should also begin at this time to drink large amounts of fluid by mouth.

After you have been treated with methotrexate, you will continue your bicarbonate pills every four hours for a total of 48 hours after you are given the methotrexate.

Throughout this entire time (about 72 hours), you will have to test the pH of your urine and record the results.

If at any time during this 72 hours, your urine pH is less than 7, you should immediately take three extra bicarbonate pills and test your urine one-half hour later.

If your urine pH continues to be less than 7 or you are unable to take the pills, you should call your oncologist.

Mithramycin (Mithracin)

What It Looks Like:
Pale yellow fluid after dissolved.

How It Is Given:
Injection into vein.

Common Side Effects:
Nausea and vomiting occur within six hours after treatment and last 12 to 24 hours.

Loss of appetite.

Weakness, drowsiness.

Headache.

Interference with clotting of blood—watch for and report new or unusual bleeding (nose, gums), bruising, facial redness.

The drug can be irritating to tissue if it leaks out of the vein. Tell the person giving the drug if you feel any burning, stinging, or pain while the drug is being given. If the area of injection becomes red and swollen after the injection, notify your doctor.

Less Common Side Effects:
Mouth sores.

Diarrhea.

Possible liver and kidney problems—blood counts of liver and kidney function will be done on a regular basis.

Decreased calcium, which may lead to muscle stiffness or twitching. If this occurs, call your doctor. In some cases when the calcium is abnormally high, the doctor may use this drug to reduce the calcium.

Mitomycin (Mutamycin)

What It Looks Like:
Purple fluid after dissolved.

How It Is Given:
Injection into vein.

Common Side Effects:
Mild to moderate nausea and vomiting usually occur one to two hours after treatment and may last up to 24 hours.

"Blahs."

Hair loss may occur and is not permanent.

Reduced blood counts occur four to five weeks after treatment and may last two to three weeks.

Less Common Side Effects:
Mouth sores may occur.

Diarrhea.

Fever.

The drug can be irritating to tissue if it leaks out of vein. Tell person administering drug if you feel burning, stinging, or pain while the drug is being given. If the area of injection becomes red and swollen after the injection, notify your oncologist.

Mitotane (Lysodren)

What It Looks Like:
Tablet (500 mg).

How It Is Given:
Taken by mouth.

Common Side Effects:
Nausea and vomiting occur in some patients.

Loss of appetite.

Less Common Side Effects:
Diarrhea.

Fatigue and sleepiness.

Dizziness.

Lightheadedness.

Skin irritation.

Prednisone

What It Looks Like:
Tablet (5 mg, 10 mg, 20 mg, 50 mg).

How It Is Given:
Taken by mouth.

Common Side Effects:
Stomach upset occurs in most patients. This can often be helped by taking the pill with an antacid, milk, and/or meals.

Acne of the face, neck, and upper chest may develop or worsen.

High blood sugar.

A feeling of well-being while taking the drug.

Difficulty in falling asleep.

Increased appetite and weight gain.

Less Common Side Effects:
Stomach ulcers: old one may become active again or a new one may develop.

More likely to get infections.

Increased blood pressure.

Nervousness, depression (small percentage of patients have this side effect).

With long-term use, a round face, increasing thickness of the back of the neck, abdominal obesity, cataracts, loss of muscle mass, more facial and body hair, and weak bones may occur.

Patients taking prednisone for long periods of time should not stop taking the drug suddenly without talking to their doctor. Prednisone is available in many different strength tablets. Check your dose carefully.

Call oncologist for fever over 101° F while taking prednisone or in children with fever over 102° F within six months after taking prednisone.

Procarbazine (Matulane)

What It Looks Like:
Yellow capsule.

How It Is Given:
Taken by mouth.

Common Side Effects:
Nausea and vomiting.

Drowsiness, weakness, fatigue.

Confusion, restlessness.

Reduced blood counts occur two to three weeks after treatment.

Special Precautions:
Do not drink alcohol, beer, or wine.

Do not eat yogurt, Brewer's yeast, cheese, bananas, chicken livers, pickled herring.

These alcoholic beverages and foods may cause unpleasant side effects (vomiting, abdominal cramps) if taken while on this medicine.

Since this drug may make you drowsy, other drugs that may make you sleepy (sleeping pills, pain medications, or tranquilizers) should be avoided if at all possible.

Razoxin (Razoxane, ICRF-159)*

What It Looks Like:
White Tablets (50 and 500 mg).

How It Is Given:
Taken by mouth.

Common Side Effects:
Nausea and vomiting, which are usually mild.

Diarrhea.

Hair loss may occur and is not permanent.

Reduced blood counts.

Less Common Side Effects:
Flu-like condition consisting of chills, muscle aches, and crusty eyes.

Skin rash.

*This drug is investigational, which means it can only be obtained through your oncologist.

Semustine (Methyl-CCNU)*

What It Looks Like:
Solid white capsule (10 mg).

Brown capsule (40 mg).

Brown and black capsule (100 mg).

How It Is Given:
Taken by mouth.

Common Side Effects:
Nausea and vomiting occur one to five hours after treatment.

Less Common Side Effects:
Kidney damage may occur.

Reduced blood counts occur four to six weeks after treatment.

*This drug is investigational, which means it can only be obtained through your oncologist.

Streptozocin (Streptozotocin)*

What It Looks Like:
Clear fluid after dissolved.

How It Is Given:
Injection into vein.

Common Side Effects:
Nausea and vomiting usually occur one to four hours after treatment and may last up to 24 hours.

Diarrhea may occur.

Kidney problems—blood and urine counts of kidney function will be done on a regular basis.

Less Common Side Effects:
Low blood sugar, which may make you feel dizzy, nervous, shaky, or have headaches.

Redness or swelling in area where needle is inserted.

The drug can be irritating to tissue if it leaks out of vein. Tell the person administering the drug if you feel burning, stinging, or pain while the drug is being given. If the area of injection becomes red and swollen after the injection, notify your doctor.

*This drug is investigational, which means it can only be obtained through your oncologist.

Tamoxifen (Nolvadex)

What It Looks Like:
Tablet (10 mg).

How It Is Given:
Taken by mouth.

Common Side Effects:
Hot flashes.

Menstrual cycle may be irregular.

Bone or tumor pain (during the first several weeks of treatment).

Bleeding or discharge from the vagina.

Less Common Side Effects:
Nausea and vomiting.

Changes in vision may occur.

Reduced blood count.

Hair loss may occur and is not permanent.

Dizziness.

6-Thioguanine (Thioguanine, Tabloid)

What It Looks Like:
Green tablet (40 mg).

How It Is Given:
Taken by mouth.

Common Side Effects:
Occasional nausea.

Reduced blood counts.

Vinblastine (Velban)

What It Looks Like:
Clear fluid after dissolved.

How It Is Given:
Injection into vein.

Common Side Effects:
Reduced blood counts occur one week after treatment.

Less Common Side Effects:
Constipation.

Nausea and vomiting.

Headache.

Tingling, numbness, or muscle weakness of hands or feet.

Depression.

Loss of appetite.

Fatigue.

Acne.

Drug can be irritating to tissues if it leaks out of the vein. Tell the person administering the drug if you feel burning, stinging, or pain while the drug is being given. If the area of injection becomes red and swollen after the injection, notify your oncologist.

Vincristine (Oncovin)

What It Looks Like:
Clear fluid after dissolved.

How It Is Given:
Injection into vein.

Common Side Effects:
Hair loss may occur and is not permanent.

Numbness and tingling of fingers and toes. After prolonged use you may find it difficult to button your clothes or tie your shoes.

Constipation.

Weakness or cramps in legs.

Less Common Side Effects:
Jaw pain.

Metal taste in the mouth.

The drug can be irritating to tissue if it leaks out of vein. Tell person administering drug if you feel any burning, stinging, or pain while the drug is being given. If the area of injection becomes red and swollen after injection, notify your oncologist.

twenty-two

Alkylating Agents

DAVID S. FISCHER

Alkylating agents are highly reactive compounds that can covalently attach electrophilic (positively charged) alkyl groups to nucleophilic (negatively charged) cellular substances. The most significant biologic targets are the nucleic acids of DNA, especially the 7-nitrogen position of guanine, which is strongly nucleophilic; its alkylation may lead to chain fragmentation, miscoding, and depurination. Polyfunctional alkylating agents may cause cross-linking of two nucleic acid chains, intrachain linkages, or the linking of a nucleic acid to a protein. Any one of these events would prevent separation of the strands of DNA, with failure of replication and resultant cell injury or death. Monofunctional alkylating agents may simply attach to a DNA strand and cause base-pair miscoding and lead to mutagenic and carcinogenic cell damage that may be propagated as an inherited mutation. The DNA synthesis is inhibited more than RNA synthesis. Other systems inhibited in order of decreasing effect include protein synthesis, energy-generating pathways, active transport pathways, and glycolytic pathways (Ochoa 1969; Warwick 1963; Wheeler 1962; Whitelock 1958).

Resistance to alkylating agents can be explained by cell lines with increased capacity to repair altered nucleic acids. There is much cross-resistance in the effect of different alkylating agents on the same cell line. This is probably because some, like mechlorethamine, melphalan, and chlorambucil, form identical ethylenimonium ions as their active alkyl group. Cyclophosphamide and to a lesser extent nitrosoureas do not follow this pattern and are frequently not cross-reactive. Most of these drugs are cleared from the plasma in minutes and inactivated. Urinary excretion products are usually inactive although the metabolites of cyclophosphamide can be very irritating to the bladder mucosa (Johnson and Meadows 1971). Hemolytic anemia (especially with cyclophosphamide) and skin pigmentation (especially with busulfan) can occur with any of these agents.

With reference to the cell cycle, alkylating agents appear to be most effective against cells in the M or G_1 phase, but nonproliferating cells in G_0 may be affected also. Graphs of cell survival after administration of alkylating agents demonstrate exponentially decreasing curves corresponding to groups I or III of Bruce, the cycle-nonspecific or the cycle-specific agents. There is some confusion in the literature (Hill and Baserga 1975) with regard to whether most alkylating agents are cycle-nonspecific (Bruce I), like mechlorethamine, and work at all phases including G_0, or whether most of the other alkylating agents do not affect G_0 and are cycle-specific (Bruce III) but not phase-specific (Bruce II). Inhibition of mitosis and synthesis of RNA and protein can lead to cell injury or death. These agents can be used for tumors with a small growth fraction and can be combined with antimetabolites that are usually considered group II of Bruce, the phase-specific agents. The survival curve after a phase-specific agent usually reaches a plateau up to a threshold regardless of the dose given. Thus when given in a combined protocol alkylating agents are frequently given first to reduce the total population; antimetabolites are given when the residual cell population is more likely to be in a proliferative

Table 22.1. *Alkylating Agents*

Generic Name	*Trade or Common Name*	*Major Route(s)*	*Frequent Dose*	*Major Indication(s)*	*Major Toxicities*
Mechlorethamine	Mustargen, (HN2, nitrogen mustard)	IV	8–16 mg/m^2	Lymphoma; lung cancer	Marrow, G.I. vesicant
Chlorambucil	Leukeran	p.o.	10–16 mg/day × 5 days	Lymphoma, CLL	Marrow, G.I.
Cyclophosphamide	Cytoxan, Endoxan	p.o.	60–120 mg/m^2/day	Lymphoma, breast, myeloma	Marrow, G.I., bladder, alopecia
		IV	500–1500 mg/m^2		
Melphalan	Alkeran (L-PAM)	p.o.	6 mg/m^2/day	Myeloma, ovary	Marrow
Triethylenethio-phosphoramide	Thiotepa	IV, IM, SC	40 mg/m^2	Ovary	Marrow
		Intravesical	60 mg total	Bladder	
Busulfan	Myleran	p.o.	4–8 mg/m^2 × 2–3 wks	CML	Marrow
Dacarbazine	DTIC-Dome	p.o.	250 mg/m^2/day × 5 days	Melanoma	G.I.
Estramustine*	Estracyt	p.o.	400–800 mg/m^2	Prostate	G.I.
Estradiol mustard*		p.o.	40–80 mg/m^2 × 14 days	Breast	Marrow, G.I.
Dibromodulcitol*	Mitolactol	p.o.	100 mg/m^2/day	Breast, CML	Marrow
Dibromomannitol*	(Myelobromal, mitobronitol)	p.o.	250 mg/day	CML	Marrow
Cisplatin	Platinol	IV	50–120 mg/m^2	Ovary, testicle, lung	Marrow, renal, auditory

*Investigational.

phase and hence more susceptible to phase-specific agents such as the antimetabolites.

Although more than 700 alkylating agents have been synthesized, only 10 are widely used, with many additional ones in active experimental programs (table 22.1). We will consider (1) nitrogen mustards—mechlorethamine (Mustargen), chlorambucil (Leukeran), cyclophosphamide (Cytoxan), and melphalan (Alkeran); (2) ethyleneimine—triethylenethiophosphoramide (thiotepa); (3) alkyl sulfonate—busulfan (Myleran); (4) triazene—dacarbazine (DTIC-Dome); (5) experimental agents—estramustine phosphate (Estracyt); estradiol mustard; dibromodulcitol (Mitolactol); and dibromomannitol (Myelobromol); (6) nitrosoureas released for commercial distribution—carmustine (BiCNU, BCNU) and lomustine (CeeNU, CCNU); (7) experimental nitrosoureas—semustine (methyl-CCNU); streptozocin (Zanosar, streptozotocin); and chlorozotocin (DCNU); (8) heavy metal—cisplatin (Platinol, cis-diamminedichloroplatinum). The nitrosoureas are grouped together with their references in chapter 23.

Mechlorethamine

Mechlorethamine (nitrogen mustard, HN2, Mustargen) is a bifunctional alkylating agent developed during World War II (fig. 22.1). The designation HN2 was its secret code name and has no chemical significance (Gilman 1963; Goodman et al. 1946; Rhoads 1946). It was the first of the modern antineoplastic drugs and is therefore the oldest of these agents still in use (Lynch et al. 1918; Krumbhaar and Krumbhaar 1919). Since it is unstable in solution, it must be carefully and freshly prepared to avoid splashing onto the skin or into the eyes. It is highly vesicant and therefore is injected through the tubing of a rapidly running intravenous that has been placed in a good vein several minutes earlier to permit observation of its free flow and absence of infiltration. The drug should be injected within 10 to 15 minutes of reconstitution to obtain its full effect (Hunt and Philips 1949). It can also be administered into the pleural cavity (and occasionally the pericardial cavity) and is sometimes given intraarterially (Lathrop and Frates 1980). It should not be put into the peritoneal cavity as it may cause adhesions with resulting bowel obstruction.

Mechlorethamine is used systemically, primarily in the MOPP (mechlorethamine, Oncovin, procarbazine, and prednisone) combination program in Hodgkin's disease or in the non-Hodgkin's lymphomas and lung cancer. It has been used topically in treatment of mycosis fungoides with controversial results (Van Scott and Winters 1970). It is given intrapleurally for hydrothorax due to lymphomas, carcinoma of the breast or lung, and so forth, and is partially absorbed with the consequence of a variable degree of myelosuppression.

Side effects most frequently include nausea and vomiting (which are centrally mediated probably by the chemoreceptor trigger zone, and can be ameliorated with an antiemetic and a short-acting hypnotic or sedative), anorexia, weakness, and diarrhea. A more serious toxic effect is bone marrow depression, with lymphopenia developing within 24 hours and the nadir of granulocytopenia and thrombocytopenia in 7 to 21 days. Recovery is usual by the fourth week, with rebound hyperplasia frequently seen in the fifth to seventh week (Zubrod et al. 1960). Other toxic effects include alopecia, skin eruptions, vertigo, jaundice, menstrual irregularities, impaired spermatogenesis, and potential sterility. Thrombosis and thrombophlebitis may result from direct contact of the drug with the intima of the vessel, especially if the intravenous infusion is not rapid enough to dilute the drug promptly. Extravasation of drug into the subcutaneous tissue can cause severe brawny induration with slough of the overlying tissues, necessitating later surgical debridement and grafting. For extravasation, the specific antidote is isotonic sterile sodium thiosulfate (1/6 molar) solution, which should be infiltrated into the area immediately to neutralize the mechlorethamine (Ignoffo and Friedman 1980). Cold compresses should be applied intermittently for 6 to 12 hours.

Dosage depends on protocol use. In the MOPP combination regimen it is given as 6 mg/m^2 on days 1 and 8 of a 28-day cycle. As a single agent in lung cancer it is given intravenously in a dose of 10 to 16 mg/m^2; when given intrapleurally for effusion the usual dose is 0.2 to 0.4 mg/kg (equivalent to 8 to 16 mg/m^2). It is available as Mustargen (Merck Sharp & Dohme) powder, 10 mg per vial with sodium chloride and is reconstituted with sterile water for immediate administration.

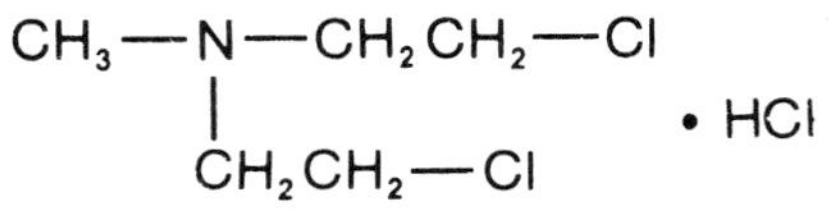

$$CH_3-N(-CH_2CH_2-Cl)-CH_2CH_2-Cl \cdot HCl$$

Fig. 22.1. *Mechlorethamine, NSC 762*

Chlorambucil

Chlorambucil (Leukeran, NSC 3088) is an aminophenylbutyric acid derivative of mechlorethamine (fig. 22.2). It is the slowest acting of the standard derivatives with a latent period of about two weeks. It is given orally since it is well absorbed from the gastrointestinal tract,

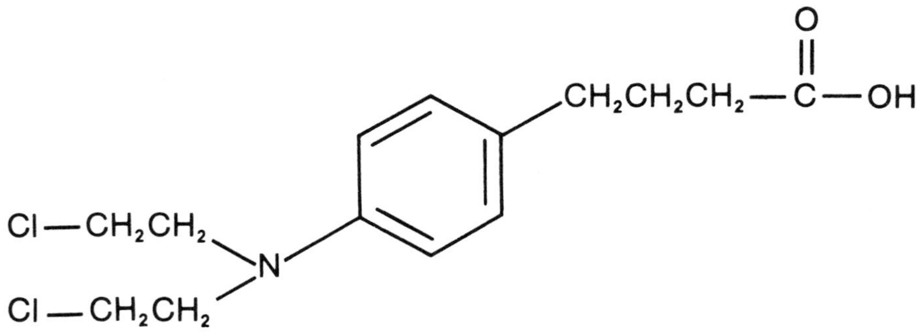

$$(Cl-CH_2CH_2)_2N-C_6H_4-CH_2CH_2CH_2-C(=O)-OH$$

Fig. 22.2. *Chlorambucil, NSC 3088*

but its further metabolism has not been clarified (Alberts et al. 1979b; McLean et al. 1979). It suppresses lymphoid tissues proportionally more than myeloid cells and has found its greatest use in treatment of chronic lymphocytic leukemia and lymphomas (Rundles et al. 1959; Galton et al. 1961; Kaung et al. 1964). At one time it was widely used in the therapy of advanced ovarian carcinoma but has been superceded by newer agents and combinations. It is probably still the drug of choice in Waldenström's macroglobulinemia, and finds occasional application in breast carcinoma, multiple myeloma, polycythemia vera, agnogenic myeloid metaplasia, mycosis fungoides, testicular carcinoma, primary thrombocythemia, and choriocarcinoma (Miller, Diamond, and Craver 1950; Moore et al. 1968). It has also been used in nonmalignant disorders such as vasculitis, hemolytic anemia, cold agglutinin diseases, lupus erythematosis, and nephritis (Snaith et al. 1973). Chlorambucil has been used in the treatment of nodular lymphocytic and well-differentiated diffuse lymphocytic lymphomas, either alone in a dose of 12 to 16 mg/m^2 for five days every four weeks, or as continuous therapy of 4 to 8 mg/m^2 per day for the first week and then a lower maintenance dose adjusted to the peripheral blood and bone marrow response. I have used chlorambucil in a variety of combination programs to replace oral cyclophosphamide when a patient developed hemorrhagic cystitis from that drug or refused therapy entirely because of anticipated hair loss. In those situations, I use 2 mg chlorambucil for each 50 mg of oral cyclophosphamide intended. The substitution for intravenous drug is more difficult.

Acute toxicity includes nausea and vomiting with high dosage. Most patients are able to tolerate up to four tablets at a time before breakfast and after supper without ill effects. If higher dosages are used, then schedules of medication three or four times a day are necessary; at very high doses an antiemetic may be required. Liver toxicity is rare. Hematologic toxicity is the major problem and is usually mild to moderate, with myelosuppression developing by the third week and continuing for 7 to 10 days before bone marrow recovery. Patients with damaged marrow from previous radiation, chemotherapy, or infiltration with neoplastic cells will have delayed and incomplete recovery. Because they are at higher risk, an attenuated dose may be used with more frequent monitoring of white cell and platelet counts.

Patients with a high lymphoid burden may respond dramatically to effective chemotherapy or radiation therapy with lysis of many cells and excretion of large amounts of nucleic acids. To avoid a high concentration of uric acid, which could precipitate an attack of gout or an obstructive uropathy, a xanthine oxidase inhibitor such as allopurinol, 300 mg/day, is given prophylactically until the lymphoid tumor burden is greatly reduced.

Amenorrhea, cessation of menstruation, oligospermia, and even sterility can occur from therapeutic doses of chlorambucil. Alopecia and dermatitis are rare. Second malignancies have been reported, especially acute myelogenous leukemia.

Two popular dosage regimens are:

1. 0.1 to 0.2 mg/kg daily for two or three weeks, with subsequent doses based on platelet and white cell counts
2. A five-day regimen of 10 to 16 mg/m^2 per day repeated in four weeks (occasionally three weeks if the nadir has passed with good recovery)

The drug is available as Leukeran (Burroughs Wellcome) in 2-mg tablets and is stable at room temperature.

Cyclophosphamide

Cyclophosphamide (Cytoxan, Endoxan, NSC 26271) is available in both oral and intravenous forms. It is the most widely used alkylating agent at present because it is relatively platelet-sparing, the parenteral preparation is not vesicant, and it has a broad spectrum of activity against a variety of tumors (Gershwin, Groetzl, and Steinberg 1974) (fig. 22.3). In addition, it appears not to be fully cross-reactive with the other nitrogen mustard derivatives, and responses have been documented after demonstrated resistance to mechlorethamine and melphalan. It has also been used effectively in disorders that do not ordinarily respond to alkylating agents, for example, acute lymphoblastic leukemia in children and adult acute non-lymphocytic leukemia (Hoogstraten et al. 1960).

In its administered form cyclophosphamide is inactive, but is converted to the active phosphoramide mustard by liver microsomal oxidase systems and liver

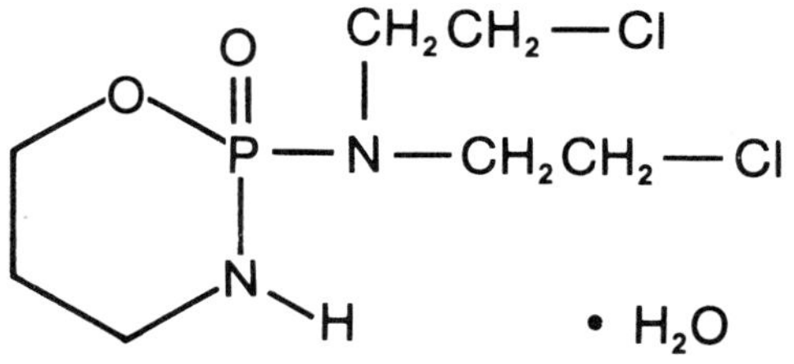

Fig. 22.3. *Cyclophosphamide, NSC 26271*

and plasma phosphamidases. The enzyme systems may be stimulated by inducing agents such as phenobarbital or inhibited by drugs such as corticosteroids and sex hormones. Metabolism occurs in the liver by the aldehyde oxidase system, resulting in products that are relatively inactive as systemic cytotoxic agents. In concentrated form in the urinary bladder, however, it can result in frequent hemorrhagic cystitis, less often in fibrosis and telangiectasia, and very rarely in carcinoma of the bladder (Johnson and Meadows 1971). About 5% of an intravenous dose of cyclophosphamide is excreted unchanged in the urine, but its relation to bladder toxicity is unclear. Following intravenous administration, peak plasma levels of the cytotoxic metabolite are achieved in two to three hours. The plasma half-life of the parent compound is from two to nine hours and 70% to 80% is still present at eight hours (Cox, Farmer, and Jarman 1976; Torkelson et al. 1974).

Cyclophosphamide as a single agent remains the drug of choice for Burkitt's lymphoma at present and achieves a cure in approximately 50% of cases (Ziegler 1972). It has been used as the alkylating agent of preference in the nodular non-Hodgkin's lymphomas, either alone or combined with vincristine and prednisone, and by either modality has resulted in complete remission in over 50% of patients (Bagley et al. 1972). In the diffuse histiocytic lymphomas it has been used in several combinations that have included procarbazine, vincristine, prednisone, bleomycin, doxorubicin, and lomustine. With these, complete remissions have resulted in approximately 45% of cases and long-term survival (apparent cures) in about 20% of cases (Schein et al. 1976). It is also active in chronic lymphocytic leukemia, small cell undifferentiated carcinoma of the lung, and adenocarcinoma of the ovary. In multiple myeloma it is particularly useful in thrombocytopenic patients because of its relative platelet-sparing effect, and has also induced responses alone or in combination in melphalan failures (Bergsagel, Cowan, and Hasselback 1972).

In childhood neoplasms, cyclophosphamide combinations have been variably successful in rhabdomyosarcoma, neuroblastoma, retinoblastoma, and Ewing's sarcoma, both in active and in adjuvant therapy. In cancer of the breast in women, cyclophosphamide is widely used in combination with methotrexate and 5-fluorouracil and often with other drugs, especially doxorubicin, vincristine, and prednisone. Although cyclophosphamide has been used in treatment of carcinomas of the gastrointestinal tract and cervix, melanoma, squamous cell carcinoma of the head and neck, non-small cell cancer of the lung, and adenoid cystic carcinoma of the salivary glands, its efficacy in these neoplasms remains to be demonstrated by future research (Wall and Conrad 1961).

The major toxic effect of this drug is bone marrow depression with leukopenia. The white cell nadir occurs at about two weeks after a single dose, and recovery is usually noted within 17 to 28 days. Mild to moderate leukopenia in the range of 3000 to 4000 white cells per mm^3 is common and safe, but severe and prolonged leukopenia exposes the patient to the danger of infection and should be avoided if possible. Anemia is common but rarely a problem. Thrombocytopenia is less common and less severe than with most other alkylating agents.

With large intravenous doses, nausea and vomiting are common and usually occur 3 to 6 hours later and may last from 3 to 24 hours. Oral cyclophosphamide frequently causes anorexia and nausea at usual doses and vomiting at higher doses. Antiemetics are helpful in controlling these symptoms.

Hair loss is very common and is not prevented by scalp tourniquets or ice packs. It is seen in about one-third of patients taking oral doses and 75% to 90% of those receiving intravenous medication. It usually begins three weeks after initiation of therapy and is reversible, with new hair developing at the cessation of therapy and frequently, in spite of continued therapy. The new hair may be of a different color or texture, and the patient should be advised of these possibilities before treatment starts. Other toxicities include amenorrhea, depression of sperm count, and less frequently, pulmonary interstitial fibrosis (Spector, Zimbler, and Ross 1979), cardiomyopathy (Mills and Roberts 1979), acute water intoxication (DeFronzo et al. 1973) due to the syndrome of inappropriate antidiuretic hormone (SIADH) secretion, nasal stuffiness, sneezing, rhinorrhea, dermatitis, dizziness, facial flushing, sweating, and at least one patient has had anaphylaxis or acute hemolytic anemia. Second malignancies are being reported with most alkylating agents and radiation after prolonged exposure (Kyle, Pierre, and Bayrd 1975). The most common is acute myelogenous leukemia that generally has been quite resistant to therapy (Karchmer et al. 1974). Cyclophosphamide can cause carcinoma of the bladder (Wall and Clausen 1975).

Dosage regimens vary, and for use in combinations the section on combination therapy or the original protocol report should be consulted. In single-agent therapy intravenous dosages range from 500 to 1500 mg/m^2 every three to four weeks, while oral daily doses range from 60 to 120 mg/m^2, and are adjusted according to the bone marrow response.

The drug is available as Cytoxan (Mead Johnson) in the United States, and as Endoxan overseas. Oral tablets are available in 25-mg and 50-mg sizes, and for intravenous use a lyophilized powder is supplied in sterile vials of 100, 200, and 500 mg to be reconstituted with sterile water on the day of use, although they can be stored refrigerated for six days. An oral suspension can be prepared from the sterile powder but this substantially increases the expense.

Melphalan

Melphalan (Alkeran, L-phenylalanine mustard, L-PAM, L-sarcolysin, NSC 8806) is the phenylalanine derivative of mechlorethamine (fig. 22.4). Its general mode of action is similar to that of chlorambucil and mechlorethamine. Following oral administration peak blood levels are seen at two hours. Between 20% and 50% of the label of ^{14}C-melphalan is recovered in the feces in six days, and 30% in the urine over nine days (Alberts et al. 1979a). In contrast, following intravenous administration melphalan is distributed in the total body water and disappears with a biphasic half-life of 67 minutes and 160 hours. This long terminal plasma half-life of nearly seven days may help explain the prolonged action of the drug. Up to 65% of label is recovered in the urine over seven days, and a negligible amount in the feces after intravenous injection (Tattersall et al. 1978; Brox, Birkett, and Belch 1979). Drug metabolism is not extensive, and the majority of the label recovered from the plasma in 5 minutes and from the urine in 40 minutes of intravenous administration cochromatographed with melphalan, suggesting that it is not degraded significantly to metabolites. One can also conclude that absorption following oral ingestion is erratic and incomplete. Hence fixed oral doses are unreliable, and the clinician must gauge the dose by the hematologic response (Tattersall et al. 1978). In contrast to the other mechlorethamine derivatives, the granulocyte and platelet response to melphalan is more like that to carmustine and gamma irradiation. The counts fall to a nadir on days 8 to 10, then plateau or recover slightly through day 25, and have a second nadir about day 27 to 32 before recovering between days 42 and 50. Many clinicians give melphalan every six or seven weeks when using intermittent oral therapy to avoid severe cumulative bone marrow suppression.

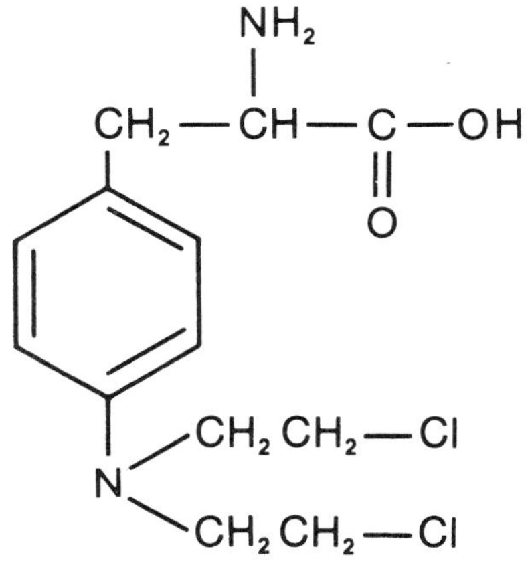

Fig. 22.4. *Melphalan, NSC 8806*

Melphalan is now the most frequently used drug for the treatment of multiple myeloma (McArthur et al. 1970; Brook et al. 1973). Used alone or in combination with prednisone (Costa et al. 1973), it has led to a significant prolongation of survival, decrease in bone pain (Rodriguez et al. 1972) and anemia, a reduction in the quantity of abnormal protein in the serum and/or urine, amelioration of renal function and hypercalcemia, and a decrease in the number of plasma cells and blasts in the bone marrow. Recently it has been incorporated into combination chemotherapy regimens in an attempt to improve the therapeutic index. Preliminary reports of four-drug (Presant and Klahr 1978) and five-drug regimens (Lee et al. 1974) claim a significant increase in the rate of complete remission and duration of survival compared to controls treated with melphalan and prednisone (Case, Lee, and Clarkson 1977).

For many years melphalan has been the standard single-agent treatment for adenocarcinomas of the ovary, and it remains the base against which newer combination regimens must be compared (Young et al. 1978; Park et al. 1980). It has also been used as a single agent in active and adjuvant therapy of breast carcinoma (Fisher et al. 1975) but is less effective than the combination regimens to which it has been compared. It is currently being studied in combination with 5-fluorouracil in an adjuvant protocol with breast cancer (Fisher et al. 1977). It has been used occasionally in treatment of chronic myelocytic leukemia, polycythemia vera, and seminoma.

Toxicity is primarily hematologic, with dose-related depression of the white cell, red cell, and platelet counts with a slower recovery than is seen with mechlorethamine, chlorambucil, and cyclophosphamide. It has been recommended that intermittent therapy be given no more often than every four to six weeks (Alexanian et al. 1968). Nausea and vomiting are mild with the usual doses but may be severe with high-dose therapy. Pulmonary fibrosis, amenorrhea, and oligospermia have been noted.

Although second malignancies occur with most of the alkylating agents, more have been reported with melphalan than with any of the others so far (Kyle,

Pierre, and Bayrd 1975). This may be related to the large numbers of patients with multiple myeloma and ovarian carcinoma treated over a long period of time; it may reflect to some extent the low-dose chronic regimens popular at one time; it may be a result of the increased survival of these patients; or it may be something peculiar to melphalan. Whatever it is, these patients usually develop acute myelogenous leukemia and their response to therapy is poor compared to patients in a cohort with apparently de novo disease (Karchmer et al. 1974).

Dosage regimens (George et al. 1972) include:

1. 0.25 mg/kg for 4 consecutive days every 6 weeks
2. 0.1 to 0.15 mg/kg daily for 2 or 3 weeks, then up to 2 to 4 mg daily following a rest period of 2 to 4 weeks (the dosage is then adjusted to keep the white cell count in the range of 3500 and the platelet count around 100,000)
3. 6 mg/m^2 daily for 5 days every 6 weeks

The drug is available commercially as Alkeran (Burroughs Wellcome) in 2-mg tablets. It has also been used experimentally for intraarterial perfusion of locally or regionally confined melanoma (Stehlin 1969), and for this purpose is available to registered investigators from the Division of Cancer Therapy, National Cancer Institute (NCI) in 100-mg vials. It is ironic that this is its only use in melanoma now in spite of the fact that melphalan was originally developed as the phenylalanine derivative of nitrogen mustard with the idea that it would be metabolized to tyrosine, a precursor of melanin, and would be specific for that neoplasm.

Triethylenethiophosphoramide

Triethylenethiophosphoramide (Thiotepa, NSC 6396) is an ethyleneimine derivative (fig. 22.5), the only trifunctional alkylating agent still commercially available. Its mechanism of action is similar to that of the other alkylating agents although it is not a nitrogen mustard derivative. It is incompletely absorbed from the gastrointestinal tract and is variably absorbed from serous membranes and the bladder (Jones and Swinney 1961). Most of the drug is excreted in the urine as metabolites in one to two days.

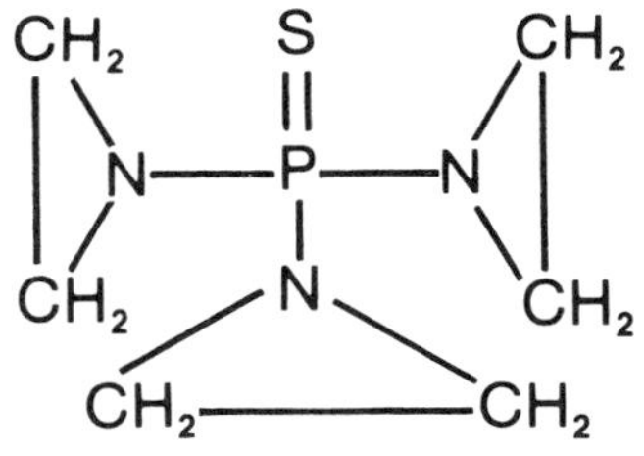

Thiotepa was once widely used intravenously, intramuscularly, or subcutaneously for the treatment of ovarian carcinoma, lymphoma, and breast, prostate, and lung cancer (Moore 1958; Ultman et al. 1957; Bateman 1955; Levine 1960; Weyrauch and Nesbet 1959; Noer et al. 1962; Bateman and Carleton 1956; Bateman and Winship 1956). Currently, it finds its major application in the treatment of serous effusions (pleural, pericardial, and peritoneal) (Groesbeck and Cudmore 1962) and superficial papillary carcinomas of the bladder (Murphy and Soloway 1980; Veenema et al. 1962).

Toxicity is mainly hematologic, with depression of the white cell and platelet counts in 7 to 18 days. Nadir cell counts are usually seen in about 15 days, but may remain depressed up to 30 days. The drug is not vesicant so its action on serous surfaces is cytotoxic rather than sclerosing. Nausea and vomiting occur occasionally and are dose-dependent. Headaches and fever are occasional but not dose-related. Late second malignancies have been reported after prolonged use (Kardinal and Donegan 1980).

For bladder instillation the sterile lyophilized powder is diluted to 1 mg/ml, and 60 ml is used once a week. For systemic administration or intracavitary instillation, 45 to 60 mg is used in adults or children over 12 years of age.

The drug is available as Thiotepa (Lederle) in 15-mg vials as a lyophilized powder to be kept refrigerated until reconstituted with 1.5 ml of sterile water for injection. The reconstituted solution is stable for five days at 4° C.

Fig. 22.5. *Triethylenethiophosphoramide, NSC 6396*

Busulfan

Busulfan (Myleran, NSC 750) is an alkyl sulfonate (fig. 22.6). Although it does not resemble the mustard-derived alkylating agents structurally, it behaves in the same way and its mechanism of action is the same. It seems to affect granulocytes and platelets more than lymphocytes and red cells and is therefore used primarily in the treatment of chronic granulocytic leukemia (CGL) (Galton 1953; Huguley 1963; Haut et al. 1961; Schilling and Meyer 1956; Unugur, Schulman, and Dameshek 1957; Schullenberger 1962). It is not effective in acute leukemia or in the blast crisis of CGL. It is also used in primary thrombocythemia, polycythemia vera, and agnogenic myeloid metaplasia with high white cell and/or platelet counts. Some patients with myeloid metaplasia are particularly sensitive to the drug and have a precipitous fall in those counts resulting in leukopenia, thrombocytopenia, and anemia, which may not respond to discontinuation. Hence therapy in this condition should be cautious and gradual, and counts should be monitored frequently.

Busulfan is well absorbed orally and is largely metabolized to compounds not yet identified, but 10% to 50% is excreted in the urine in 24 hours (Vodopick et al. 1969). Reduction in white cell counts usually begins after 10 days of therapy and continues for 2 weeks after the drug is stopped.

Toxicity is primarily hematologic and dose-related, but occasionally thrombocytopenia is idiosyncratic and the drug has to be discontinued. With high initial white cell counts and a good response, large amounts of nucleic acids may be liberated with the danger of hyperuricemia and resultant renal tubular problems. To avoid this, allopurinol and vigorous hydration should be employed at the initiation of therapy and maintained until the white count is reduced adequately. Prolonged therapy may result in hyperpigmentation alone or as part of an addisonian-like wasting syndrome that can include hypotension, fatigue, nausea, vomiting, and weight loss (Feingold and Koss 1969). There is usually no objective evidence of adrenal hypofunction, and use of corticosteroids does not prevent or reverse it. Busulfan may also cause late complications such as ovarian fibrosis, amenorrhea, testicular atrophy, aspermia, gynecomastia, endocardial fibrosis (Weinberger et al. 1975), and cataracts. One of the most feared toxicities is irreversible pulmonary fibrosis, the so-called busulfan lung (Oliner et al. 1961). It is manifested by cough, low-grade fever, and dyspnea that may progress to pulmonary insufficiency and death.

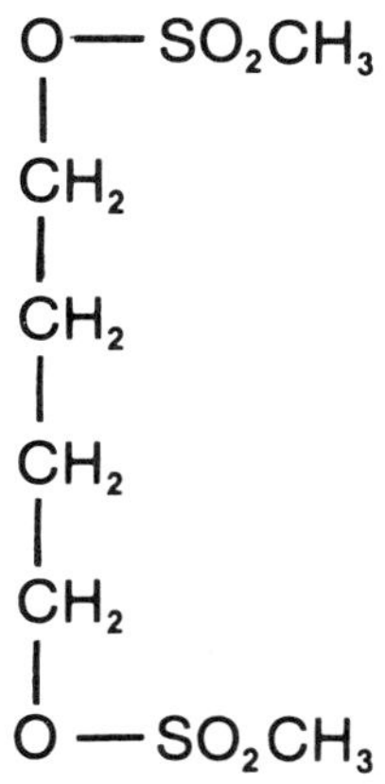

$$\begin{array}{l} O-SO_2CH_3 \\ | \\ CH_2 \\ | \\ CH_2 \\ | \\ CH_2 \\ | \\ CH_2 \\ | \\ O-SO_2CH_3 \end{array}$$

Fig. 22.6. *Busulfan, NSC 750*

Therapy is usually initiated with a loading dose of 4 to 8 mg/m^2 per day for two or three weeks or until the white cell count begins to fall. Then intermittent or continuous therapy can be used. With continuous therapy, the aim is to keep the white cell count in the range of 10,000 to 20,000 per mm^3. With intermittent therapy, the aim is to reduce the count to about 10,000 per mm^3, then discontinue therapy until it increases to 50,000 per mm^3, and begin another course.

The drug is available as Myleran (Burroughs Wellcome) in 2-mg tablets.

Dacarbazine

Dacarbazine (DTIC-Dome, dimethyltriazenoimidazole carboxamide, NSC 45388), a triazine derivative (fig. 22.7), is a synthetic analogue of the naturally occurring intermediate 5-aminoimidazole 4-carboxamide (AIC). Dacarbazine was synthesized with the intention of developing a purine antimetabolite, but it appears to act primarily as an alkylating agent. It shows cross-resistance with other alkylating agents. The drug is inactive and has to be metabolized (presumably in the liver) to a methylcarbonium ion that interacts with DNA, and to a residual diazo-molecule capable of reacting with both RNA and DNA.

The drug is erratic in its oral absorption and is used primarily intravenously but occasionally intra-arterially. Following administration there is a biphasic half-life of 19 minutes and of 5 hours. Forty percent of the unchanged drug is excreted in the urine in six hours. In addition to the liver, the kidney apparently is involved in drug metabolism.

Dacarbazine is the most commonly used single agent for the treatment of disseminated melanoma, with a response rate in a large number of trials fairly consistently in the 20% to 30% range (Carter 1976). So far, no other agent has a better response rate. Responses

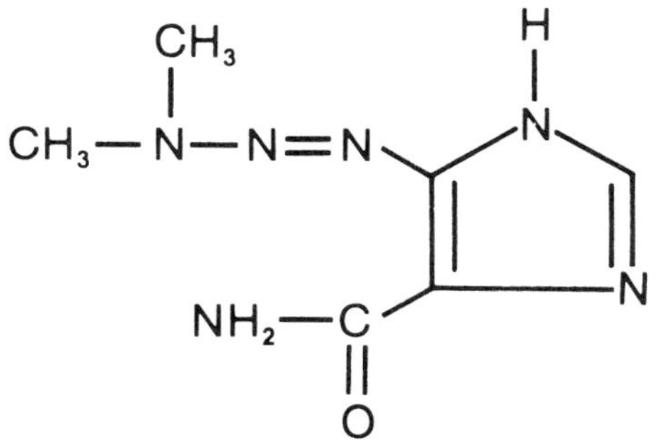

CH$_3$ | CH$_3$—N—N=N— (imidazole ring with N–H, N; NH$_2$—C(=O)—)

Fig. 22.7. *Dacarbazine, NSC 45388*

average six months and are most frequently seen in women with soft tissue, nodal, and skin involvement who have not been previously treated with drugs (Comis 1976; Burke et al. 1971; Luce et al. 1970). It is also being used in combination with BCG, transfer factor, and melphalan (Schwartz et al. 1980).

In combination with doxorubicin, bleomycin, and vinblastine, dacarbazine has been used (ABVD) in the treatment of advanced Hodgkin's disease refractory to the MOPP combination (Bonadonna et al. 1975). In patients with a presumed poor prognosis the two combinations have been alternated as primary therapy in hopes of achieving a prolonged complete remission and cure. In a variety of soft tissue sarcomas dacarbazine has been used with doxorubicin (Gottlieb et al. 1975). Whether dacarbazine contributes to the response rate of about 20% remains to be seen. Kaposi's sarcoma appears to be especially responsive to the combination (Bhasin et al. 1980).

Acute toxicity is manifested by severe nausea and vomiting that occur within 1 to 3 hours of administration and may persist for 12 hours, and are only partially ameliorated by antiemetics the first day of a multiple-day course. By the third day the same dose produces much less nausea and vomiting, but an influenza-like syndrome may develop with nasal stuffiness, rhinorrhea, facial flushing, myalgias, fever, and malaise. Myelosuppression with leukopenia and thrombocytopenia is frequent but usually mild. Liver enzymes are transiently elevated. Hepatic veno-occlusive disease secondary to dacarbazine has been reported (Asbury et al. 1980).

The drug is usually given by intravenous infusion over 20 to 40 minutes because severe pain develops at the site of infusion, even with a perfect IV, if the rate is too rapid. A cold pack placed over the vein may reduce the discomfort. Caution must be exercised to avoid extravasation into the tissues as this results in prolonged pain and may lead to ulceration and sloughing of skin. Intraarterial infusion for local or regional tumor, particularly melanoma, has been reported experimentally (Einhorn et al. 1973; Jönsson et al. 1980).

Dosage regimens include:

1. IV, 2 to 4.5 mg/kg daily for 10 days and repeated after 28 days
2. IV, 250 mg/m^2 daily for 5 days every 3 weeks
3. Single large doses of 650 to 1450 mg/m^2 every 4 to 6 weeks

For dosage in combination regimens, see the section on combinations or the original publications.

The drug is available as DTIC-Dome (Dome) as a sterile lyophilized powder in vials of 100 and 200 mg, which are reconstituted with 9.9 ml or 19.7 ml respectively of sterile water to achieve a concentration of 10 mg/ml. The unopened vials should be refrigerated until used. The reconstituted solution may be stored in the dark for 8 hours at 20° C, or 72 hours at 4° C if necessary, without significant loss of potency.

Estramustine Phosphate (Investigational)

Estramustine phosphate (Estracyt, Emcyt, NSC 89199) is the 3,17-diester of the steroidal hormone estradiol with an alkylating nitrogen mustard moiety (fig. 22.8). It is thought that the compound localizes in the prostate because of its steroidal nature and exerts an alkylating action there (Von Hoff et al. 1977). The disodium salt is well absorbed orally and is metabolized in the liver.

The drug was originally used by European investigators as an intravenous preparation for advanced carcinoma of the prostate, and was found to be clinically effective although there was a high incidence of regional toxicity. In this country there are ongoing active investigational, individual, and cooperative studies of the oral preparation in advanced hormonally resistant carcinoma of the prostate (Fossa and Miller 1976; Mittelman et al. 1975). Objective responses have generally been confined to regression of soft tissue or prostatic masses, and return of elevated acid and alkaline phosphate values to normal (Nilsson and Jonsson 1976). No significant or consistent improvement in osteoblastic lesions was noted (Nilsson and Jonsson 1975). Subjective improvement consisted of decrease or disappearance of pain, increased appetite with measured weight gain, and improved performance status (Murphy et al. 1977). Results were the same when 5-fluorouracil was used in combination (Kennealey et al. 1978).

Toxicity consists primarily of nausea and vomiting at high doses, and can be ameliorated with antiemetics in some and dose reduction in others. Diarrhea, impotence, and fluid retention are occasionally seen; gynecomastia is rare. Most significantly, myelosuppression either does not occur or is mild.

The drug is available to approved NCI investigators as Emcyt (Roche) by application to the Division of Cancer Therapy. It is supplied in 140-mg capsules that should be refrigerated. The usual daily dose is 400 to 800 mg/m^2 orally in three divided doses.

Estradiol Mustard (Investigational)

Estradiol mustard (NSC 112259) is the 3,17-diester of the steroidal hormone estradiol with the alkylating agent chlorphenacyl (fig. 22.9). Thus it should be readily distinguished from estramustine phosphate (with which it has been confused) by the presence of phenyl groups at the 3 and 17 positions linked to a nitrogen mustard moiety at both ends of the compound. The rationale for its use is that the steroid moiety will target the molecule to receptors in tumor cells and then the alkylating agent will act on these cells (Vollmer et al. 1970). A possible role for estrogen-binding protein in mediating its activity has been suggested (Everson et al. 1974).

The drug has been tested in a large number of animal tumor systems with varying but many favorable responses (Wall et al. 1969). Clinical trials are in an early stage, but a few responses or stabilizations of disease have been reported in breast cancer and gastrointestinal tumors, with relief of pain and some transient tumor regressions (Schapira et al. 1978). Toxicity consists of mild to moderate hematologic depression of platelet and white cell counts and mild gastrointestinal side effects including anorexia, nausea, and vomiting.

Dosage is still being worked out, but schedules of 40 to 80 mg/m^2 daily for 14 days of each 28-day course seem tolerable (Schapira et al. 1978). Intermittent schedules of 160 mg/m^2 led to severe or life-threatening hemorrhage and had to be abandoned. The drug needs further testing in hormonally dependent or responsive tumors.

Estradiol mustard is available to registered investigators through the Division of Cancer Treatment, NCI. It is supplied as 5- and 50-mg tablets in amber-colored bottles and may be stored at room temperature away from light.

Dibromodulcitol (Investigational)

Dibromodulcitol (D-galactitol, mitolactol, NSC 104800) is an alpha-, omega-substituted hexitol (fig. 22.10). Its mechanism of action is thought to be that of a bifunctional alkylating agent based on cross-resistance studies. While generally regarded as an alkylating agent, however, its actions cannot all be explained by this mechanism (Handelsman, Carter, and Slavik 1974). In vivo, the major conversion product is to the diepoxide (Institoris et al. 1967), dianhydrogalactitol (NSC 132313), which is apparently more active as an an-

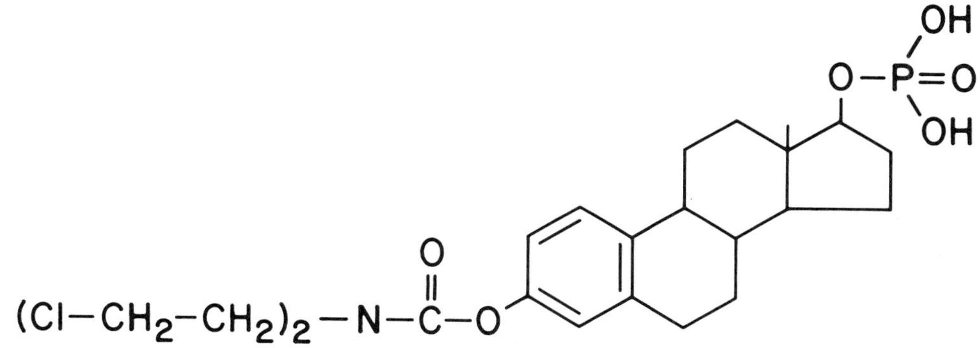

$(Cl-CH_2-CH_2)_2-N-C(=O)-O-$ [steroid] $-O-P(=O)(OH)_2$

Fig. 22.8. *Estramustine phosphate, NSC 89199*

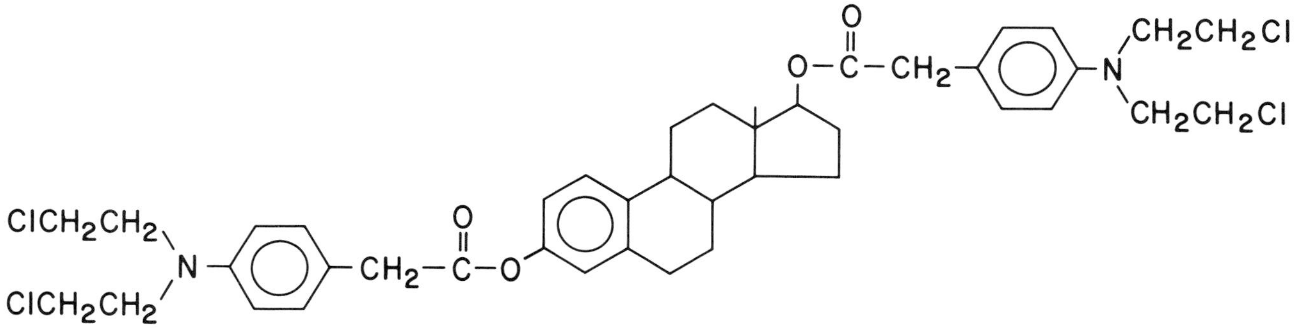

$(ClCH_2CH_2)_2N-C_6H_4-CH_2-C(=O)-O-$ [steroid] $-O-C(=O)-CH_2-C_6H_4-N(CH_2CH_2Cl)_2$

Fig. 22.9. *Estradiol mustard (phenestradiol), NSC 112259*

titumor agent and is being investigated independently (Mischler et al. 1979). These compounds inhibit synthesis of DNA more than RNA, and cause interstrand DNA links.

Dibromodulcitol is rapidly absorbed on oral administration and is detectable in the blood in 15 minutes; peak plasma levels are reached in 1 hour. The compound is sufficiently lipid-soluble that it crosses cell membranes and enters serous cavities and the central nervous system. Maximum concentrations in spinal, pleural, and ascitic fluid are achieved in five hours, and maximum levels are equal to half the maximum serum levels. Distribution in normal and tumor tissues is about the same.

Renal excretion is the major route of elimination, but much of the drug is metabolized in the liver and undergoes an enterohepatic circulation. The plasma half-life is 8 hours for ^{14}C-labeled drug, and it is essentially undetectable at 48 hours unless there is ascites that retards elimination.

The drug has shown clinical activity in breast (Andrews et al. 1971; Van Amburg et al. 1979) and head and neck carcinoma (Sellei et al. 1969), melanoma (Bellet et al. 1978), and lymphoma. In chronic myelogenous leukemia an overall 85% response rate has been reported, which included many patients who failed with busulfan (Sellei et al. 1969). In polycythemia vera a 60% response rate was observed, but the results were not as good as with the isomer dibromomannitol (Nagy, Lehi, and Petranyi 1975). In combination with doxorubicin, dibromodulcitol produced a 46% remission rate in women with previously treated metastatic breast carcinoma, with a median remission duration of five months (Tormey et al. 1975). With the addition of the antiestrogen tamoxifen, the response rate rose to 64% and the duration of remission was increased twofold to threefold (Tormey et al. 1977).

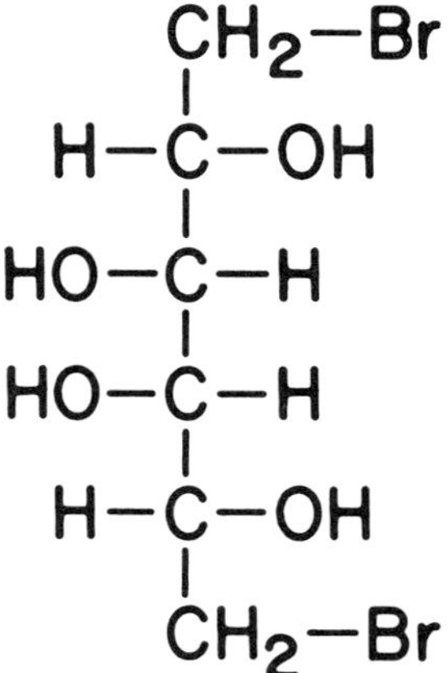

Fig. 22.10. *Dibromodulcitol, NSC 104800*

In childhood acute lymphocytic leukemia in remission, dibromodulcitol maintenance chemotherapy resulted in only 1 of 23 patients developing CNS recurrence, compared to 9 of 17 on cyclophosphamide concurrently (Sitarz et al. 1974). Studies of the drug in therapy of brain tumors, lung cancer, and breast cancer are in progress (Andrews et al. 1974; Mischler et al. 1979).

Dose-limiting toxicity is myelosuppression especially of the granulocytes, and is dose-related. Synergism with cyclophosphamide, 5-fluorouracil, doxorubicin, and carmustine seems to occur. Minor toxicity includes anorexia, nausea, vomiting, diarrhea, dyspnea, abnormal liver function tests, skin pigmentation, pruritus, vertigo, alopecia, dysuria, allergic reactions, local tumor pain, and hemorrhage.

Effective oral dosage regimens include:

1. 2.5 to 3.5 mg/kg daily for 5 to 7 weeks
2. 4 to 5 mg/kg daily for 10 to 20 days repeated monthly
3. 100 mg/m^2 daily with adjustments determined by blood counts
4. 400 mg/m^2 every week

With all schedules, frequent monitoring of hematologic, hepatic, and renal function is indicated. The drug is supplied to registered investigators by the Division of Cancer Treatment as mitolactol in 50-mg and 100-mg tablets that are stable in the unopened bottle for two years at room temperature.

Dibromomannitol (Investigational)

Dibromomannitol (mitobronital, myelobromol, NSC 94100) is an alpha-, omega-substituted hexitol and isomer of dibromodulcitol (fig. 22.11). Although its structure is very similar to dibromodulcitol's, that compound is active against L 1210 leukemia in animals and dibromomannitol is not (Livingston et al. 1968). It is generally agreed that dibromomannitol behaves as a bifunctional alkylating agent in many respects, but there are some features of its behavior that suggest mechanisms more commonly associated with an antimetabolite. One group of investigators concluded that the compound may represent a transitional form between alkylating agents and antimetabolites (Livingston et al. 1968). Absorption is rapid after oral administration. Excretion is primarily renal but the drug is also metabolized in the liver.

Dibromomannitol is an agent of proved clinical usefulness in the treatment of chronic myelocytic leukemia (Tura et al. 1973; Eckhardt et al. 1963; Tomov et al. 1976; Canellos et al. 1975). In clinical trials, 80% of previously untreated patients went into remission (Casazza, Cahn, and Carbone 1967), and 67% of those previously treated with busulfan or radiation went into complete remission. With intermittent therapy, average duration of remission was 20.2 months and with continuous therapy it was 26.5 months. Although 40% of those who were treated in blast crisis of CML responded, those remissions were short-lived (Eckhardt 1967). Dibromomannitol appears to be at least as effective as busulfan in the treatment of CML, and better than 6-mercaptopurine, hydroxyurea, and demecolcin (NSC 3096). Perhaps its greatest virtue is that it appears to be effective in most cases that are busulfan-resistant (Bohnel and Stacher 1967). On the other hand, cases that are resistant to dibromomannitol do not respond to busulfan (Eckhardt 1967).

In the treatment of polycythemia vera, responses to dibromomannitol have been almost uniformly good even after ^{32}P failure.

Toxicity has been mainly hematologic and is dose-related, with leukopenia and thrombocytopenia being somewhat prolonged when excessive dosage was given (Elson, Jarman, and Ross 1968). Nausea and vomiting are rare. Liver toxicity has not been reported.

The drug is still available from the Division of Cancer Treatment (DCT) to investigators who already have patients on therapy with this agent. The DCT is not planning to supply the drug for new investigations. Tablets are available in 50- and 100-mg sizes, and the usual dose is 250 mg daily.

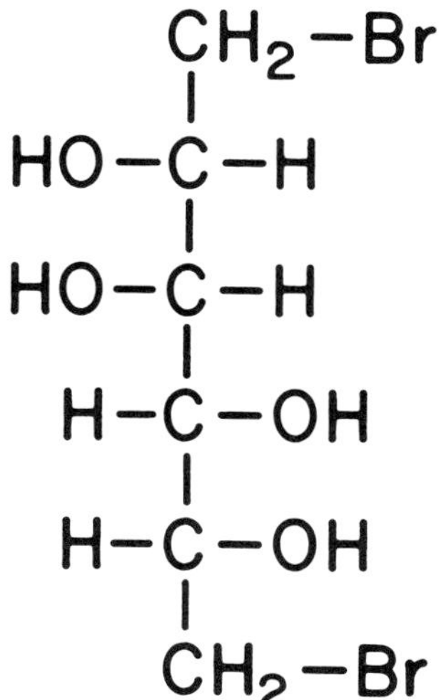

Fig. 22.11. *Dibromomannitol, NSC 94100*

Cisplatin

Cisplatin (Platinol, cis-dichlorodiammineplatinum II, DDP, CDDP, NSC 119875) is a heavy metal complex with a central atom of platinum complexed to two chloride atoms and two ammonia molecules in the cis-position (fig. 22.12). It behaves like a bifunctional alkylating agent and produces interstrand and intrastrand cross-linkages in DNA. It was developed for antitumor therapy after a chance observation that bacteria in an electrical field with platinum electrodes tended to aggregate and failed to reproduce, although they continued to grow (Rosenberg, Van Camp, and Krigas 1965). Investigation of the growth medium revealed the presence of cisplatin as the active inhibitory compound and led to studies of it in tumor cells in cell culture, then in animals, and finally in humans (Prestayko et al. 1979).

Following intravenous administration the drug is rapidly distributed in the tissues, especially the liver, kidney, ovary, uterus, skin, and bone. There is no apparent increased concentration in the tumor. Plasma levels decline in a biphasic manner, with a distribution phase half-life of minutes and an elimination phase half-life of days. Urinary excretion is extensive on the first day, with recovery of 70% to 90% of the administered dose. Cisplatin is excreted more rapidly from well-hydrated individuals.

Cisplatin has been approved for use in testicular and ovarian carcinomas where it has been most effective. Currently, combination chemotherapy for nonseminomatous testicular carcinoma consisting of cisplatin, bleomycin, and vinblastine (Einhorn and Donahue 1977) with or without doxorubicin, cyclophosphamide, and chlorambucil, has raised the response rate to over 80% and the cure rate to 60% (Anderson, Javadpour, and Zwelling 1979). In ovarian carcinoma, the best responses so far have been from combinations of cisplatin and doxorubicin with or without cyclophosphamide. So far, significant responses in better than 40% of

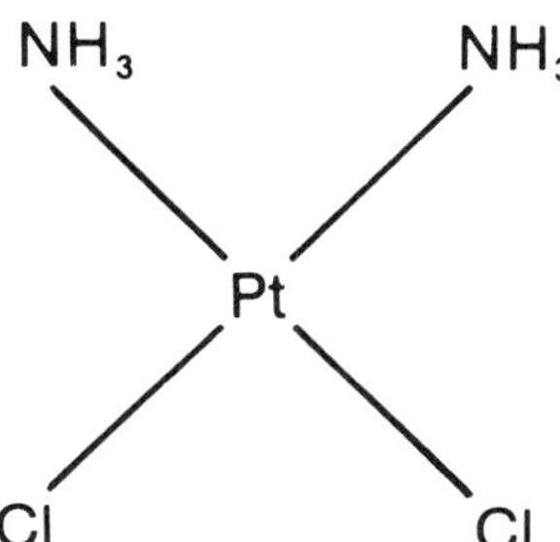

Fig. 22.12. *Cisplatin, NSC 119875*

patients have been documented by several groups using one of the cisplatin regimens (Bruckner et al. 1978; Thigpen et al. 1979).

At present, studies are under way to evaluate the role of cisplatin in head and neck, lung, breast, and renal cell carcinoma, Hodgkin's disease and non-Hodgkin's lymphoma, sarcomas, bladder, esophageal, cervical, and prostatic cancer (Prestayko, Crooke, and Carter 1979; Yagoda et al. 1978; Gutierrez and Crooke 1979; Rozencweig et al. 1977).

The major toxicity is renal and auditory. The former is irreversible renal tubular necrosis (Dentino et al. 1978). It is best avoided by adequate hydration so that the patient voids at least 100 to 200 ml each hour for several hours after the drug is administered. Mannitol, 12.5 to 37.5 gm may be given intravenously just before the cisplatin, with a strong diuretic such as furosemide to enhance diuresis (Hayes et al. 1977). Prior to administration, blood urea nitrogen (BUN), creatinine, and creatinine clearance should be checked, and the drug withheld if any of these values is seriously impaired. Nephrotoxicity is dose-related and cumulative, and on occasion has been fatal (Vogl, Zaravinos, and Kaplan 1980).

Ototoxicity may be manifested by high-frequency hearing loss and tinnitus in one-third of patients treated. It may be unilateral or bilateral, and worsens with continued treatment. So far there is no good way to prevent this except by reducing the dose, with risk of diminished tumor response.

Other major dose-related toxicities are nausea and vomiting. These occur in almost all patients and can be so severe and prolonged that the drug sometimes must be discontinued. Vomiting may begin 1 to 4 hours after treatment and last up to 24 hours. Nausea may persist for a week.

Myelosuppression is not usually severe at the low doses used in some patients, but at high doses it may occur in one-fourth to one-third of patients treated. Nadir counts are usually seen between two and four weeks, with recovery by the fifth or sixth week.

Peripheral neuropathy is not common, but when it occurs it is usually not easily reversible. Loss of taste and onset of seizures have been reported. Electrolyte imbalances are a common complication of the diuresis. Anaphylactoid reactions have occurred in patients receiving a second or subsequent dose.

A number of dosage schedules have been used:

1. 50 to 120 mg/m^2 once every 3 or 4 weeks
2. 15 to 20 mg/m^2 daily for 5 days, and repeat every 4 weeks
3. As part of a multidrug protocol. (Consult chapter 29 or the original description in the literature.)

The drug should be given after pretreatment hydration of 1 to 2 liters and then administered with mannitol to enhance diuresis.

Cisplatin is supplied as Platinol (Bristol) in vials of 10 and 50 mg of a lyophilized powder that need not be refrigerated. The reconstituted solution is stable at room temperature for 20 hours and should not be refrigerated lest it precipitate.

References

Alberts, D. S. et al. Oral melphalan kinetics. *Clin. Pharmacol. Ther.* 26:737–745, 1979a.

Alberts, D. S. et al. Pharmacokinetics and metabolism of chlorambucil in man: a preliminary report. *Cancer Treat. Rev.* 6(suppl.):9–18, 1979b.

Alexanian, R. et al. Melphalan therapy for plasma cell myeloma. *Blood* 31:1–10, 1968.

Anderson, T.; Javadpour, N.; and Zwelling, L., eds. Proceedings of the National Cancer Institute conference on cis-platinum and testicular cancer. *Cancer Treat. Rep.* 63:1431–1699, 1979.

Andrews, N. C. et al. Phase I study of dibromodulcitol (NSC 104800). *Cancer Chemother. Rep.* 55:61–65, 1971.

Andrews, N. C. et al. Phase II study of dibromodulcitol (NSC 104800). *Cancer Chemother. Rep.* 58:653–660, 1974.

Asbury, R. F. et al. Hepatic veno-occlusive disease due to DTIC. *Cancer* 45:2670–2674, 1980.

Bagley, C. M. et al. Advanced lymphosarcoma: intensive cyclical combination chemotherapy with cyclophosphamide, vincristine, and prednisone. *Ann. Intern. Med.* 76:227–234, 1972.

Bateman, J. C. Chemotherapy of solid tumors with triethylenethiophosphoramide. *N. Engl. J. Med.* 252: 879–887, 1955.

Bateman, J. C., and Carleton, H. N. Palliation of mammary carcinoma with phosphoramide drugs. *JAMA* 162:701–706, 1956.

Bateman, J. C., and Winship, T. Palliation of ovarian carcinoma with phosphoramide drugs. *Surg. Gynecol. Obstet.* 102:347–354, 1956.

Bellet, R. E. et al. Positive phase II trial of dibromodulcitol in patients with metastatic melanoma refractory to DTIC and a nitrosourea. *Cancer Treat. Rep.* 62:2095–2099, 1978.

Bergsagel, D. E.; Cowan, D. H.; and Hasselback, R. Plasma cell myeloma: response of melphalan-resistant patients to high-dose intermittent cyclophosphamide. *Can. Med. Assoc. J.* 107:851–855, 1972.

Bhasin, R. et al. Kaposi's sarcoma (KS): a review of 49 patients. *Proc. Am. Assoc. Cancer Res.* 21:157, 1980.

Bohnel, J., and Stacher, A. The effect of a new cytostatic (myelobromol) in chronic myeloid leukemia. *Wien. Med. Wochenschr.* 117:535–538, 1967.

Bonadonna, G. et al. Combination chemotherapy of Hodgkin's disease with Adriamycin, bleomycin, vinblastine, and imidazole carboxamide (ABVD) vs. MOPP. *Cancer* 36:252–259, 1975.

Brook, J. et al. Long-term low-dose melphalan treatment of multiple myeloma. *Arch. Intern. Med.* 131:545–548, 1973.

Brox, L.; Birkett, L.; and Belch, A. Pharmacology of intravenous melphalan in patients with multiple myeloma. *Cancer Treat. Rev.* 6(suppl.):27–32, 1979.

Bruckner, H. W. et al. Adriamycin and cis-dichlorodiammineplatinum (II) after failure of initial chemotherapy. *Cancer Treat. Rep.* 62:1021–1023, 1978.

Burke, P. J. et al. Imidazole carboximide therapy in advanced malignant melanoma. *Cancer* 27:744–750, 1971.

Canellos, G. P. et al. Dibromomannitol in the treatment of chronic granulocytic leukemia: a prospective randomized comparison with busulfan. *Blood* 45:197–203, 1975.

Carter, S. K. Proceedings of the sixth new drug seminar: DTIC. *Cancer Treat. Rep.* 60:123–214, 1976.

Casazza, A. R.; Cahn, E. L.; and Carbone, P. P. Preliminary studies with dibromomannitol (NSC 94100) in patients with chronic myelogenous leukemia. *Cancer Chemother. Rep.* 51:91–97, 1967.

Case, D.; Lee, B. J. III; and Clarkson, B. D. Improved survival times in multiple myeloma treated with melphalan, prednisone, cyclophosphamide, vincristine, and BCNU: M-2 protocol. *Am. J. Med.* 63:897–903, 1977.

Comis, R. L. DTIC (NSC 45388) in malignant melanoma: a perspective. *Cancer Treat. Rep.* 60:165–176, 1976.

Costa, G. et al. Melphalan and prednisone: an effective combination for the treatment of multiple myeloma. *Am. J. Med.* 54:589–599, 1973.

Cox, P. J.; Farmer, P. B.; and Jarman, M. Proceedings of the symposium on the metabolism and mechanism of action of cyclophosphamide. *Cancer Treat. Rep.* 60:299–525, 1976.

DeFronzo, R. A. et al. Water intoxication in man after cyclophosphamide therapy. *Ann. Intern. Med.* 78:861–869, 1973.

Dentino, M. et al. Long-term effect of cis-diamminedichloride platinum (CDDP) on renal function and structure in man. *Cancer* 41:1274–1281, 1978.

Eckhardt, S. Chronic myelogenous leukemia and its treatment with dibromomannitol. In *Fifth International Congress of Chemotherapy,* vol. 3, Vienna, Austria, 1967, pp. 259–264.

Eckhardt, S. et al. Effect of 1,6-dibromo-1,6-dideoxy-D-mannitol on chronic granulocytic leukemia. *Cancer Chemother. Rep.* 33:57–61, 1963.

Einhorn, L. H. et al. Intra-arterial infusion therapy with 5-(3,3-dimethyl-1-triazeno) imidazole-4-carboxamide (NSC 45388) for malignant melanoma. *Cancer* 32:749–752, 1973.

Einhorn, L. H., and Donahue, J. P. Cis-diamminedichloroplatinum, vinblastine, and bleomycin combination chemotherapy in disseminated testicular cancer. *Ann. Intern. Med.* 87:293–298, 1977.

Elson, L. A.; Jarman, M.; and Ross, W. C. J. Toxicity, haematologic effects, and antitumor activity of epoxides derived from disubstituted hexitols. Mode of action of mannitol, Myleran, and dibromomannitol. *Eur. J. Cancer* 4:617–625, 1968.

Everson, R. B. et al. Estradiol mustard (NSC 112259) and phenesterin (NSC 116785): possible mediation of action by estrogen-binding protein. *Cancer Chemother. Rep.* 58:353–359, 1974.

Feingold, M. L., and Koss, L. G. Effects of long-term administration of busulfan. *Arch. Intern. Med.* 124:66–71, 1969.

Fisher, B. et al. L-phenylalanine mustard(L-PAM) in the management of primary breast cancer: a report of early findings. *N. Engl. J. Med.* 292:117–122, 1975.

Fisher, B. et al. L-phenylalanine mustard (L-PAM) in the management of primary breast cancer. *Cancer* 39: 2883–2903, 1977.

Fossa, S. D., and Miller, A. Treatment of advanced carcinoma of the prostate with estramustine phosphate. *J. Urol.* 115:406–408, 1976.

Galton, D. A. G. Myleran in chronic myeloid leukemia. *Lancet* 1:208–213, 1953.

Galton, D. A. G. et al. The use of chlorambucil and steroids in the treatment of chronic lymphocytic leukemia. *Br. J. Haematol.* 7:73–98, 1961.

George, R. P. et al. Multiple myeloma—intermittent combination chemotherapy compared to continuous therapy. *Cancer* 29:1665–1670, 1972.

Gershwin, M. E.; Goetzl, E. J.; and Steinberg, A. D. Cyclophosphamide: use in practice. *Ann. Intern. Med.* 80:531–540, 1974.

Gilman, A. The initial clinical trial of nitrogen mustard. *Am. J. Surg.* 105:574–578, 1963.

Goodman, L. S. et al. Nitrogen mustard therapy. *JAMA* 132:126–132, 1946.

Gottlieb, J. A. et al. Adriamycin (NSC 123127) used alone and in combination for soft tissue and bone sarcomas. Part III. *Cancer Chemother. Rep.* 6:271–282, 1975.

Groesbeck, H. P., and Cudmore, J. J. P. Intracavitary thiotepa for malignant effusions. *Am. Surg.* 28:90–95, 1962.

Gutierrez, M. L., and Crooke, S. T. Pediatric cancer chemotherapy: an updated review. I. Cis-diamminedichloroplatinum (cisplatin), VM-26 (teniposide), VP-16 (etoposide), mitomycin C. *Cancer Treat. Rev.* 6:153–164, 1979.

Handelsman, H.; Carter, S. K.; and Slavik, M. *Dibromodulcitol, NSC 104800.* Clinical brochure. Bethesda, Md.: National Cancer Institute, 1974.

Haut, A. et al. Busulfan in the treatment of chronic myelocytic leukemia. The effect of long-term intermittent therapy. *Blood* 17:1–19, 1961.

Hayes, D. M. et al. High-dose cis-platinumdiamminedichloride: amelioration of renal toxicity by mannitol diuresis. *Cancer* 39:1372–1381, 1977.

Hill, B. T., and Baserga, R. The cell cycle and its significance for cancer treatment. *Cancer Treat. Rev.* 2:159–175, 1975.

Hoogstraten, B. et al. Cyclophosphamide (Cytoxan) in acute leukemia, preliminary report. *Cancer Chemother. Rep.* 8:120–135, 1960.

Huguley, C. M., Jr. Comparison of 6-mercaptopurine and busulfan in chronic granulocytic leukemia. *Blood* 21:89–100, 1963.

Hunt, C. C., and Philips, F. S. Acute pharmacology of methyl-bis(2-chloroethyl) amine (HN_2). *J. Pharmacol. Exp. Ther.* 95:131–144, 1949.

Ignoffo, R. J., and Friedman, M. A. Therapy of local toxicities caused by extravasation of cancer chemotherapeutic drugs. *Cancer Treat. Rev.* 7:17–27, 1980.

Institoris, L. et al. Metabolic pathway of cytostatic dibromohexitols. *Cancer Chemother. Rep.* 51:261–270, 1967.

Johnson, W. W., and Meadows, D. C. Urinary bladder fibrosis and telangiectasia associated with long-term cyclophosphamide therapy. *N. Engl. J. Med.* 284:290–294, 1971.

Jones, H. C., and Swinney, J. Thiotepa in the treatment of tumors of the bladder. *Lancet* 2:615–618, 1961.

Jönsson, P-E. et al. Treatment of malignant melanoma with dacarbazine (DTIC-Dome) with special reference to urinary excretion of 5-S-cysteinyldopa. *Cancer* 45:245–248, 1980.

Karchmer, R. K. et al. Alkylating agents as leukemogens in multiple myeloma. *Cancer* 33:1103–1107, 1974.

Kardinal, C. G., and Donegan, W. L. Second cancers after prolonged adjuvant thiotepa for operable carcinoma of the breast. *Cancer* 45:2042–2046, 1980.

Kaung, D. et al. Treatment of chronic lymphocytic leukemia with chlorambucil and cyclophosphamide. *Cancer Chemother. Rep.* 39:41–45, 1964.

Kennealey, G. T. et al. Treatment of advanced carcinoma of the prostate with estramustine and 5-fluorouracil. *Am. Soc. Clin. Oncol.* 19:394, 1978.

Krumbhaar, E. B., and Krumbhaar, H. D. The blood and bone marrow in yellow cross gas (mustard gas) poisoning; changes produced in the bone marrow of fatal cases. *J. Med. Res.* 40:497–507, 1919.

Kyle, R. A.; Pierre, R. V.; and Bayrd, E. D. Multiple myeloma and acute leukemia associated with alkylating agents. *Arch. Intern. Med.* 135:185–192, 1975.

Lathrop, J. C., and Frates, R. E. Arterial infusion of nitrogen mustard in the treatment of intractable pelvic pain of malignant origin. *Cancer* 45:432–438, 1980.

Lee, B. J. et al. Combination chemotherapy of multiple myeloma with Alkeran, Cytoxan, vincristine, prednisone, and BCNU. *Cancer* 33:533–538, 1974.

Levine, B. The effect of triethylenethiophosphoramide in the treatment of incurable neoplastic disease. *J. Chron. Dis.* 12:258–264, 1960.

Livingston, R. B. et al. *Dibromomannitol, NSC 94100.* Clinical brochure. Bethesda, Md.: National Cancer Institute, 1968.

Luce, J. K. et al. Clinical trials with the antitumor agent 5(3,3-dimethyl-triazeno) imidazole-4-carboximide (NSC 45388). Part I. *Cancer Chemother. Rep.* 54: 119–124, 1970.

Lynch, V. et al. On dichloroethylsulphide (mustard gas). I. The systemic effects and mechanism of action. *J. Pharmacol. Exp. Ther.* 12:265–290, 1918.

McArthur, J. R. et al. Melphalan and myeloma. *Ann. Intern. Med.* 72:665–670, 1970.

McLean, A. et al. Pharmacokinetics and metabolism of chlorambucil in patients with malignant disease. *Cancer Treat. Rev.* 6(suppl.):33–42, 1979.

Miller, D. G.; Diamond, H. D.; and Craver, L. F. The clinical use of chlorambucil. A critical study. *N. Engl. J. Med.* 261:525–528, 1950.

Mills, B. A., and Roberts, R. W. Cyclophosphamide-induced cardiomyopathy. *Cancer* 43:2223–2226, 1979.

Mischler, N. E. et al. Dibromodulcitol. *Cancer Treat. Rev.* 6:191–204, 1979.

Mittelman, A. et al. Oral estramustine phosphate (NSC 89199) in the treatment of advanced (stage D) carcinoma of the prostate. *Cancer Chemother. Rep.* 59:219–223, 1975.

Moore, G. E. Clinical experience with triethylenethiophosphoramide, with special reference to carcinoma of the breast. *Ann. NY Acad. Sci.* 68:1074–1080, 1958.

Moore, G. E. et al. Effects of chlorambucil in 374 patients with advanced cancers. *Cancer Chemother. Rep.* 52:661–666, 1968.

Murphy, G. P. et al. A comparison of estramustine phosphate and streptozotocin in patients with advanced prostatic carcinoma who have had extensive radiation. *J. Urol.* 118:288–291, 1977.

Murphy, W. M., and Soloway, M. S. The effect of thiotepa on developing and established mammalian bladder tumors. *Cancer* 45:870–875, 1980.

Nagy, G.; Lehi, M.; and Petranyi, G. Cytostatic treatment of polycythaemia rubra vera. Comparison of the effects of some cytostatics in 100 patients in a period of 5 years. *Hematologia* (Budapest) 9:283–286, 1975.

Nilsson, T., and Jonsson, G. Clinical results with estramustine phosphate: a comparison of intravenous and oral preparations. *Cancer Chemother. Rep.* 59:229–232, 1975.

Nilsson, T., and Jonsson, G. Primary treatment of prostatic carcinoma with estramustine phosphate: preliminary report. *J. Urol.* 115:168–169, 1976.

Noer, R. J. et al. Surgical adjuvant chemotherapy breast group: effectiveness of thiotepa as adjuvant to radical mastectomy for breast cancer. A preliminary report. *Cancer Chemother. Rep.* 16:137–140, 1962.

Ochoa, M. Alkylating agents in clinical cancer chemotherapy. *Ann. NY Acad. Sci.* 163:921–930, 1969.

Oliner, H. et al. Interstitial pulmonary fibrosis following busulfan therapy. *Am. J. Med.* 31:134–139, 1961.

Park, R. C. et al. Treatment of women with disseminated or recurrent advanced ovarian cancer with melphalan alone in combination with 5-fluorouracil and dactinomycin or with the combination of Cytoxan, 5-flourouracil, and dactinomycin. *Cancer* 45: 2529–2542, 1980.

Presant, C. A., and Klahr, C. Adriamycin, 1,3-bis(2-chloroethyl)-1-nitrosourea (BCNU, NSC 409962), cyclophosphamide plus prednisone (ABC-P) in melphalan-resistant multiple myeloma. *Cancer* 42:1222–1227, 1978.

Prestayko, A. W. et al. Cisplatin (cis-diammine-dichloroplatinum II). *Cancer Treat. Rev.* 6:17–39, 1979.

Prestayko, A. W.; Crooke, S. T.; and Carter, S. K., eds. *Cisplatin: current status and new developments.* New York: Academic Press, 1979.

Rhoads, C. P. Nitrogen mustards in treatment of neoplastic disease. Official statement. *JAMA* 131:656–658, 1946.

Rodriguez, L. H. et al. Bone healing in multiple myeloma with melphalan chemotherapy. *Ann. Intern. Med.* 76:551–556, 1972.

Rosenberg, B.; Van Camp, L.; and Krigas, T. Inhibition of cell division in *Escherichia coli* by electrolysis products from a platinum electrode. *Nature* 205:698–699, 1965.

Rozencweig, M. et al. Cis-diamminedichloroplatinum II, a new anticancer drug. *Ann. Intern. Med.* 86:803–812, 1977.

Rundles, R. W. et al. Comparison of chlorambucil and Myleran in chronic lymphocytic and granulocytic leukemia. *Am. J. Med.* 27:424–432, 1959.

Schapira, D. et al. A phase II study of estradiol mustard (NSC 112259) by the Eastern Cooperative Oncology Group. *Cancer Clin. Trials* 1:5–8, 1978.

Schein, P. S. et al. Bleomycin, adriamycin, cyclophosphamide, vincristine, and prednisone (BACOP) combination chemotherapy in the treatment of advanced diffuse histiocytic lymphoma. *Ann. Intern. Med.* 85:417–422, 1976.

Schilling, R. F., and Meyer, O. O. Treatment of chronic granulocytic leukemia with 1,4 dimethanesulfonoxybutane (Myleran). *N. Engl. J. Med.* 254:986–989, 1956.

Schwartz, M. D. et al. Chemoimmunotherapy of disseminated malignant melanoma with DTIC-BCG, transfer factor plus melphalan. *Cancer* 45:2506–2515, 1980.

Sellei, C. et al. Clinical and pharmacological experience with dibromodulcitol (NSC 104800), a new antitumor agent. *Cancer Chemother. Rep.* 53:377–384, 1969.

Shullenberger, C. C. Evaluation of the comparative effectiveness of Myleran and 6-MP in the management of patients with chronic myelocytic leukemia. *Cancer Chemother. Rep.* 16:203–207, 1962.

Sitarz, A. L. et al. Incidence of CNS leukemia in children with ALL or AUL receiving cytoxan or dibromodulcitol for remission maintenance. *Proc. Am. Assoc. Cancer Res.* 15:48, 1974.

Snaith, M. L. et al. Treatment of patients with systemic lupus erythematosus including nephritis with chlorambucil. *Br. Med. J.* 2:197–201, 1973.

Spector, J. I.; Zimbler, H.; and Ross, J. S. Early-onset cyclophosphamide-induced interstitial pneumonitis. *JAMA* 242:2852–2854, 1979.

Stehlin, J. S. Hyperthermic perfusion with chemotherapy for cancers of the extremities. *Surg. Gynecol. Obstet.* 129:305–308, 1969.

Tattersall, M. H. N. et al. Pharmaco-kinetics of melphalan following oral or intravenous administration in patients with malignant disease. *Eur. J. Cancer* 14:507–513, 1978.

Thigpen, T. et al. Cis-dichlorodiammine platinum (II) in the management of gynecologic malignancies: phase II trials by the Gynecologic Oncology Group. *Cancer Treat. Rep.* 63:1549–1555, 1979.

Tomov, C. et al. Treatment of chronic myelocytic leukemia with dibromomannitol (myelobromol). *Ther. Hung.* 24:56–59, 1976.

Torkelson, A. R. et al. The metabolic fate of cyclophosphamide. *Drug Metab. Rev.* 3:131–165, 1974.

Tormey, D. C. et al. Adriamycin and dibromodulcitol in metastatic breast cancer. *Proc. Am. Assoc. Cancer Res.* 16:129, 1975.

Tormey, D. C. et al. Evaluation of Adriamycin and dibromodulcitol in metastatic breast carcinoma. *Cancer Res.* 37:529–534, 1977.

Tura, S. et al. Report of the Dibromomannitol Cooperative Study Group: survival of chronic myeloid leukemia patients treated by dibromomannitol. *Eur. J. Cancer* 9:583–589, 1973.

Ultmann, J. E. et al. Triethylenethiophosphoramide (thiotepa) in the treatment of neoplastic disease. *Cancer* 10:902–911, 1957.

Unugur, A.; Schulman, E.; and Dameshek, W. Treatment of chronic granulocytic leukemia with Myleran. *N. Engl. J. Med.* 256:727–734, 1957.

Van Amburg, A. L., III. et al. Phase I-II study of hexamethylmelamine plus dibromodulcitol in refractory carcinoma of the breast. *Cancer Treat. Rep.* 63:141–142, 1979.

Van Scott, E., and Winters, O. Responses of mycosis fungoides to intensive external treatment with nitrogen mustard. *Arch. Derm.* 102:507–514, 1970.

Veenema, R. J. et al. Bladder carcinoma treated by direct instillation of thiotepa. *J. Urol.* 88:60–63, 1962.

Vodopick, H. et al. Metabolic fate of tritiated busulfan in man. *J. Lab. Clin. Med.* 73:266–276, 1969.

Vogl, S. E.; Zaravinos, T.; and Kaplan, B. H. Toxicity of cis-diamminedichloroplatinum II given in a two-hour outpatient regimen of diuresis and hydration. *Cancer* 45:11–15, 1980.

Vollmer, E. P. et al. *Estradiol mustard, NSC 112259.* Clinical brochure. Bethesda, Md.: National Cancer Institute, 1970.

Von Hoff, D. D. et al. Estramustine phosphate: a specific chemotherapy agent? *J. Urol.* 117:464–466, 1977.

Wall, M. E. et al. The effect of some steroidal alkylating agents on experimental animal mammary tumor and leukemia systems. *J. Med. Chem.* 12:810–818, 1969.

Wall, R. L., and Conrad, F. G. Cyclophosphamide therapy. *Arch. Intern. Med.* 108:456–482, 1961.

Wall, R. L., and Clausen, K. P. Carcinoma of the urinary bladder in patients receiving cyclophosphamide. *N. Engl. J. Med.* 293:271–273, 1975.

Warwick, G. P. The mechanism of action of alkylating agents. *Cancer Res.* 23:1315–1333, 1963.

Weinberger, A. et al. Endocardial fibrosis following busulfan treatment. *JAMA* 231:495, 1975.

Weyrauch, H. M., and Nesbet, J. D. Use of triethylenethiophosphoramide (thiotepa) in the treatment of advanced carcinoma of the prostate. *J. Urol.* 81:185–193, 1959.

Wheeler, G. P. Studies related to the mechanisms of action of cyctotoxic alkylating agents: a review. *Cancer Res.* 22:651–688, 1962.

Whitelock, O. V. S. Comparative clinical and biological effects of alkylating agents. *Ann. NY Acad. Sci.* 68:657–1266, 1958.

Yagoda, A. et al. Diamminedichloride platinum and cyclophosphamide in the treatment of advanced urothelial cancer. *Cancer* 41:2121–2130, 1978.

Young, R. C. et al. Advanced ovarian adenocarcinoma. A prospective clinical trial of melphalan (L-PAM) versus combination therapy. *N. Engl. J. Med.* 299:1261–1266, 1978.

Ziegler, J. L. Chemotherapy of Burkitt's lymphoma. *Cancer* 30:1534–1540, 1972.

Zubrod, C. G., et al. Appraisal of methods for the study of chemotherapy in man: comparative therapeutic trials of nitrogen mustard and triethylenethiophosphoramide. *J. Chron. Dis.* 11:7–33, 1960.

twenty-three

Nitrosoureas

DAVID S. FISCHER

Nitrosoureas represent both a valuable addition to our chemotherapy arsenal and an instructive lesson in drug development (Schepartz 1976). In 1959, 1-methyl-1-nitroso-3-nitroguanidine (MNNG, NSC 9369) was found in screening trials to prolong the life span of mice given intraperitoneal inoculations of L 1210 leukemia cells. Although MNNG had a brief and unproductive clinical trial, its efficacy in animal studies stimulated the search for structurally related compounds; and activity was demonstrated with 1-methyl-1-nitrosourea, MNU (NSC 23909). Systematic variations of this molecule were synthesized and tested, primarily at the Southern Research Institute, and the twenty-third analogue screened was 1,3-bis(2-chloroethyl)-2-nitrosourea (BCNU, NSC 409962), now known as carmustine. By 1962, this had sufficient animal tumor activity to merit clinical trials. These were so encouraging that further synthetic work was pursued and led to eventual clinical trials in 1969 of 1-2(chloroethyl)-3-cyclohexyl-1-nitrosourea (CCNU, NSC 79037), now known as lomustine, and in 1971 of its methyl derivative, methyl-CCNU (NSC 95441), now known as semustine. Carmustine and lomustine were marketed in 1977, and semustine remains investigational at this writing.

The mechanism of action of the nitrosoureas is still being investigated (Wheeler 1974). They behave in part as alkylating agents with which they have in common a chloroethyl arm linked to a nitrosourea. Carmustine has two such active arms and can act as a bifunctional alkylating agent, while lomustine and semustine have only one and are monofunctional. The nitrosoureas can alkylate DNA and prevent its repair, and inhibit the synthesis and alter the structure of RNA. They can also cause carbamoylation of DNA synthetic enzymes and other proteins. It is thought that lomustine and semustine are more active in this respect than carmustine.

There is some discrepancy in the literature as to whether the nitrosoureas behave as Bruce group I (cycle-nonspecific) or group III (cycle-specific), but it is agreed that they are not group II (phase-specific). There is a somewhat greater degree of cell kill in the M phase and G_1/S phase boundary of the cell cycle (Bono 1976).

Pharmacokinetic studies in animals indicate that the nitrosoureas are very rapidly degraded, with little or no intact drug detectable in blood, urine, or spinal fluid (Prestayko et al. 1981). The two oral agents are rapidly absorbed and reach a peak plasma level in one to six hours, depending on which part of the molecule is labeled and studied (Sponzo, DeVita, and Oliverio 1973). Their plasma half-lives are biphasic. Lomustine has a 5-hour first phase and greater than 27-hour second phase; semustine has a 24-hour first phase and a 72-hour second phase. Urinary excretion of ^{14}C-labeled semustine is about 60% in 48 hours, and of lomustine 56% to 72% depending on the location of the label. The prolonged plasma levels suggest a degree of enterohepatic recirculation of the degradation products of these drugs. Part of their metabolism occurs in the hepatic microsomal system.

The unique characteristic of the nitrosoureas is their lipid-solubility. This accounts for their rapid entry

Table 23.1. *Nitrosoureas*

Generic Name	*Trade or Common Name*	*Major Route(s)*	*Frequent Dose*	*Major Indication(s)*	*Major Toxicities*
Carmustine	BiCNU (BCNU)	IV	200 mg/m^2	Brain, lymphoma, myeloma	Marrow, G.I.
Lomustine	CeeNu (CCNU)	p.o.	130 mg/m^2	Brain, lung	Marrow, G.I.
Semustine*	(Methyl-CCNU)	p.o.	200 mg/m^2	G.I.	Marrow, G.I., renal
Streptozocin*	Zanosar	IV	1.0 to 1.5 gm/m^2/week	Carcinoid, pancreas	Renal, G.I.
Chlorozotocin*	(DCNU)	IV	120 to 175 mg/m^2	G.I.	Marrow, renal

*Investigational.

into the cerebrospinal fluid (CSF), which occurs in 30 to 60 minutes and closely parallels changes in plasma levels. Absolute levels of carmustine in the CSF are 15% to 30% of the simultaneous plasma levels of the radio-labeled degradation products of the parent compound. Lomustine and semustine are more lipid-soluble than carmustine and hence achieve higher CSF levels.

In addition to the three mentioned, two additional nitrosoureas are available for investigation: streptozocin (NSC 85998), also known as streptozotocin and Zanosar; and chlorozotocin (NSC 178248), also known as DCNU for 2-deoxy-D-glucopyrano-(2-chloroethyl)-3-nitrosourea.

The various nitrosoureas (table 23.1) have found different clinical uses that are best described in discussion of the individual drugs. The uses have ranged from treatment of primary and metastatic brain tumors (Levin and Wilson 1976) to Hodgkin's disease and other lymphomas (Prestayko et al. 1981), and have included multiple myeloma (Salmon 1976), melanoma, lung, ovary and kidney carcinomas, and gastrointestinal tumors as diverse as colon, stomach, pancreas, carcinoid, and insulinomas. The precise role and choice of drug are evolving (Carter 1976; Katz and Glick 1979).

The most common and serious toxicity is hematologic; it is frequently delayed and eventually cumulative. Thrombocytopenia is usually the most hazardous problem, with the platelet nadir at four to five weeks and the lowest leukocyte counts at four to six weeks. With continued use of these drugs alone or in combination, prolonged marrow depression may occur with incomplete recovery, especially in patients previously treated with radiation or chemotherapy. There is some evidence that early multipotential hematopoietic stem cells are profoundly influenced by these agents even when the cells are not rapidly proliferating. Streptozocin and chlorozotocin are less toxic to marrow.

Nausea and vomiting are usual after administration of nitrosoureas and are incompletely ameliorated by antiemetics. Nausea may occur within a few minutes after intravenous administration and usually two to four hours after the oral agents, and may persist for 6 to 24 hours. It is centrally mediated, and hence the oral drugs should not be repeated unless vomiting is so prompt that the drug (capsule) can be seen in the vomitus. Hepatic and renal toxicity may occur occasionally with elevation of liver enzymes and BUN, but these are rarely serious problems.

Pulmonary toxicity with interstitial fibrosis progressing to a fatal outcome has been reported in many cases with carmustine and in a few instances with semustine. No cases associated with lomustine or chlorozotocin had been reported by mid-1979 when the subject was reviewed in a report from the Cancer Therapy Evaluation Program of the NCI (Weiss and Muggia 1980). Patients at particular hazard were those who had had prior pulmonary radiation therapy, who had received or were simultaneously receiving bleomycin, busulfan, mitomycin, or cyclophosphamide, or were receiving respiratory therapy with high concentrations of inspired oxygen.

Less serious and less common side effects include alopecia, stomatitis, diarrhea, anorezia, dizziness, gynecomastia, and conjunctival flushing. Local phlebitis may occur with the intravenous preparations. A very few cases of acute non-lymphocytic leukemia have been reported in patients treated with nitrosoureas (Cohen, Wiernik, and Walker 1976). It is not yet clear whether this is a coincidental finding or a direct association. The latter would not be surprising in view of the known association of leukemia with the other alkylating agents, especially those with chlorethyl groups such as mechlorethamine, melphalan, chlorambucil, and cyclophosphamide.

Carmustine

Carmustine (BiCNU, BCNU, NSC 409962) was the first nitrosourea used clinically (fig. 23.1). Its mechanism of action by alkylation and carbamoylation has been described. Although the drug is rapidly absorbed orally, clinical trials with this form have not produced satisfactory results to date, and it is commercially available only for intravenous use (Carter et al. 1972).

After intravenous administration of ^{14}C-labeled carmustine, the intact drug is detectable for less than 15 minutes according to some studies, and almost not at all as reported in others. The plasma half-life of some radioactive fragments is 67 hours. The label is detectable in the CSF almost immediately and at one hour the amount is almost equal to that in the plasma. Plasma levels decline thereafter but significant levels remain in the CSF for nine hours. Small amounts appear in the urine at 30 minutes, and 70% of the label is excreted in the urine in 96 hours. About 10% is eliminated in 24 hours as respiratory carbon dioxide and less than 1% appears in the feces. It is presumed that the remainder is metabolized. The highest specific activity has been found in the spleen, liver, and ovary.

Carmustine has been used alone or in combination with radiation therapy in the treatment of a variety of primary brain tumors after noncurative resections (Walker and Hurwitz 1970). There is a continuing disagreement about whether to give carmustine with radiation immediately after palliative resection of glioblastoma multiforme or to wait until the tumor recurs before initiating chemotherapy. Controlled studies have demonstrated an overall response rate of 47%, with an average duration of response between three and six months. In most studies the drug has been used as a single agent, but there is an increasing number of reports of combination chemotherapy with vincristine, methotrexate, procarbazine, and/or dexamethasone (Levin et al. 1976). There are some claims of better results with the combinations. In a four-arm prospective postsurgical randomized study with median survival as the measure of response, carmustine plus radiation therapy was superior to radiation alone, carmustine alone, and surgery alone, with efficacy in that order (Solero et al. 1979).

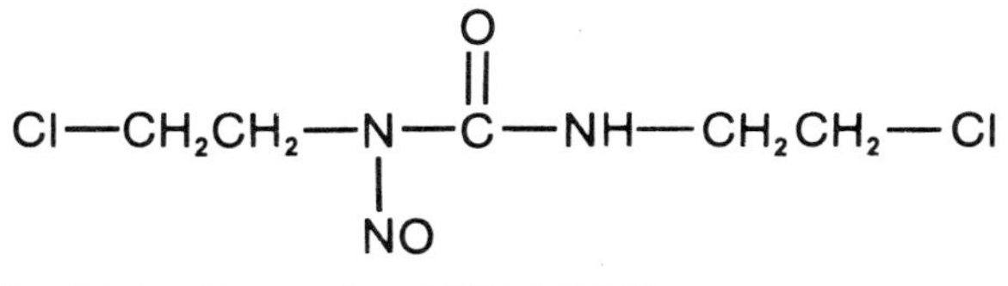

$$
\begin{array}{c}
\qquad\qquad\qquad\quad O \\
\qquad\qquad\qquad\quad \| \\
Cl{-}CH_2CH_2{-}N{-}C{-}NH{-}CH_2CH_2{-}Cl \\
\qquad\qquad\quad | \\
\qquad\qquad\quad NO
\end{array}
$$

Fig. 23.1. *Carmustine, NSC 409962*

In the treatment of multiple myeloma, carmustine has demonstrated good responses alone but better responses combined with prednisone or in a five-drug regimen that adds cyclophosphamide, melphalan, and vincristine (Case, Lee, and Clarkson 1977). These and other combinations are still being evaluated.

Studies of carmustine in Hodgkin's disease indicate a response rate of 40% to 50% as a single agent (Marsh, DeConti, and Hubbard 1971) and 70% to 90% in combinations with other active agents. In the non-Hodgkin's lymphomas, single-agent activity has been in the range of 33% and a four-drug combination produced a 50% complete remission rate and 75% overall remission rate. Studies of responses in various lung cancers are in an early stage (Katz and Glick 1979).

Toxicity is mainly hematopoietic and delayed. The platelet nadir is at 25 to 30 days and does not recover for an additional 8 to 10 days. The leukocyte nadir is seen at 30 to 35 days and recovers 10 to 12 days later. In some cases recovery is much slower.

Gastrointestinal side effects are dose-related and include nausea and vomiting, which begin two hours after the drug is administered and seldom last beyond six hours. Antiemetics can ameliorate the problem.

Rapid intravenous infusion is often associated with intense flushing of the skin, suffusion of the conjunctiva, and burning at the site of infusion. These can all be decreased by slowing the rate of infusion; the pain may be lessened with ice packs placed over the vein. When multiple drugs are used carmustine should be administered last unless one of the other drugs is a vesicant, in which case the agent should be given last.

In 1976, the first case of interstitial fibrosis caused by carmustine was reported, and since then there have been more than a dozen additional reports of patients who received only carmustine (Durant et al. 1979; Melato and Tuveri 1980). They experienced progressive dyspnea, nonproductive cough, and tachypnea, and on examination had rales and decreased breath sounds. Pulmonary function studies showed hypoxemia and ventilation-perfusion defects. The patients had generally been taking the drug for six months or more and had received a cumulative dose of 580 mg/m^2 to 2100 mg/m^2. The incidence of pulmonary fibrosis was higher in patients who had been taking bleomycin or cyclophosphamide, or had chest irradiation or higher concentrations of inspired oxygen.

Other side effects include elevation of hepatic function tests, transient elevation of the BUN, dizziness, ataxia, and brown discoloration of the skin.

Recommended dosage is 200 mg/m^2 as a single dose every six weeks, or divided into consecutive daily injections of 100 mg/m^2 on two successive days. The drug is available as BiCNU (Bristol) in ampules of 100 mg that are usually shipped by the distributor packed in dry ice and should be refrigerated from time of receipt until reconstituted for use. The package contains 3 ml of absolute ethanol with which to dissolve the lyophilized powder, which is then further diluted with 27 ml of sterile water so that each milliliter of solution contains 3.3 mg of carmustine in 10% ethanol, with a pH of 5.6 to 6.0. This can be further diluted with normal saline or 5% dextrose in water and given by IV drip over 30 to 120 minutes. Since no preservative is included, any drug not used in that period of time should be discarded.

Lomustine

Lomustine (CeeNu, CCNU, NSC 79037) was synthesized and investigated as part of a systematic study of nitrosourea derivatives (fig. 23.2). It differs from carmustine in having a cyclohexyl group instead of a second chloroethyl group. As a result of this, lomustine is more lipid-soluble and has had higher activity in advanced Lewis lung tumors and murine glioma tumor models. It is rapidly absorbed orally in a predictable pattern, and because of its high lipid-solubility and lack of ionization at physiologic pH it readily crosses the blood-brain barrier.

Several mechanisms of action have been suggested. It can cause alkylation by the formation of diazoalkanes and/or 2-chloroethylamine. It can interfere selectively with the use of histidine in one carbon metabolism and can decrease DNA nucleotidyltransferase activity. It can modify proteins mainly by cyclohexylcarbamoylation of lysine residues. The rather complex mechanism of action is not fully understood but it involves modification of proteins on one hand, and inhibition of both DNA and RNA on the other.

Like carmustine, unmodified lomustine is detectable in the plasma for less than 15 minutes, if at all. Its products have been labeled with ^{14}C at different positions in the molecule (choroethyl, carbonyl, and cyclohexyl) and give slightly different plasma half-lives, patterns of excretion, and transit into the CSF. In general, absorption after oral administration occurs in 1 to 4 hours, 50% of the radioactive label is excreted in 12 hours in the urine, and essentially all is excreted in 48 to 72 hours. The labeled activity rapidly enters the CSF and its concentration is almost equal to that of the plasma in an hour; its disappearance from the CSF is much slower than it is from the plasma.

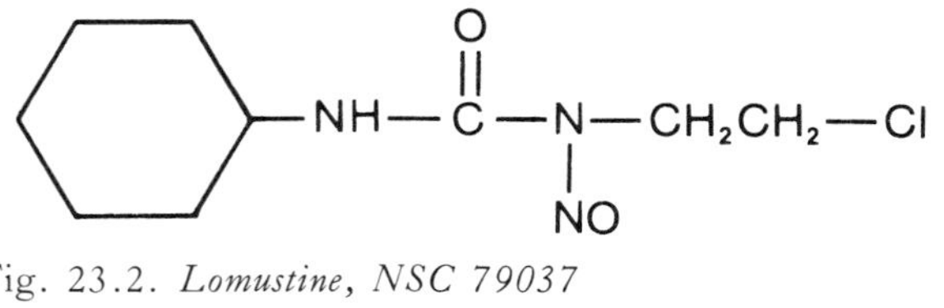

Fig. 23.2. *Lomustine, NSC 79037*

Lomustine has been shown in several studies to be slightly more effective than carmustine in therapy of glioblastoma multiforme (Solero et al. 1979; Wasserman, Slavik, and Carter 1975). In a European Organization for Research in Treatment of Cancer (EORTC) brain tumor group study, it was shown that lomustine prolongs total survival time, produces objective remissions in about 30% of cases, and that in patients with a tumor-free interval it should be administered after relapse (Hildebrand et al. 1978). In another study, there was a 41% overall response rate. In a randomized trial with radiation and surgery, it appeared to improve the quality and duration of survival (Cianfriglia et al. 1980).

In the treatment of patients with Hodgkin's disease who failed primary therapy, one report showed a 47% response rate with lomustine alone (Wasserman, Slavik, and Carter 1974). In general, the drug has been used in combination chemotherapy with response rates ranging from 50% to 85%, with satisfactory durations of remission and survivals that compare with the best of the other regimens that omit nitrosoureas.

Some activity for lomustine has been reported in lung cancer, melanoma, ovarian cancer, and non-Hodgkin's lymphomas (Reynolds et al. 1978). A few responses of renal cell carcinoma, a notoriously unresponsive tumor, have been reported with lomustine alone or combined with vinblastine. Responses in a small series of colon cancer to lomustine as a single agent range from 7% to 18% (Carter 1979). Studies in combination with 5-fluorouracil have recently been initiated (Katz and Glick 1979).

Toxicity is primarily myelosuppression after a latent period (Hoogstraten et al. 1973). After the usual recommended oral dosage of 130 mg/m^2 every six weeks, a nadir for thrombocytopenia was noted on days 26 to 34 with a duration of 6 to 10 days, and leukopenia with a nadir on days 41 to 46 with a duration of 9 to 14 days. Hence some clinicians prefer to give the drug at eight-week intervals. Anemia and renal, hepatic, and pulmonary toxicity have not been problems.

Nausea and vomiting occur 4 to 6 hours after a dose and rarely persist to 24 hours. The effect is centrally mediated and can be ameliorated with antiemetics.

The drug is available as CeeNU (Bristol) in capsules of 100 mg, 40 mg, and 10 mg, which are stable for two years at room temperature in well-closed containers. A dose reduction schedule is available to compensate for leukopenia and/or thrombocytopenia.

Semustine (Investigational)

Semustine (Methyl-CCNU, NSC 95441) has not been marketed yet (July 1, 1981) (fig. 23.3). Its mechanism of action and absorption are similar to those of lomustine. The plasma half-life is biphasic, with the first phase 24 hours and the second 72 hours. Equilibration of the portion between the CSF and plasma occurs in about one hour, and concentration in the CSF falls off more slowly than that in plasma.

Although semustine has some demonstrated activity in sarcoma (Rivkin et al. 1980), lung (Richards et al. 1973; Takita et al. 1973) melanoma, lymphoma, (Tranum et al. 1975) and brain tumors, its most exciting role has been in the treatment of gastrointestinal tumors (Wasserman, Slavik, and Carter 1974a, 1974b; Young et al. 1973).

Following reports from the University of Pretoria (Falkson and Falkson 1976) and the Mayo Clinic (Moertel et al. 1971) of responses in advanced colon cancer of 37% and 43% respectively using combination therapy of semustine, 5-fluorouracil, and vincristine, there was wide hope that a significant breakthrough had been made in the management of this common tumor. Unfortunately, it proved not to be the case. In a large Eastern Cooperative Oncology (ECOG) study, this same combination gave a 12% response rate, and when the Mayo Clinic repeated its own study the result was a 19% response rate, essentially the same as for 5-fluorouracil alone (Katz and Glick 1979). There was no survival advantage for the combination. Semustine is now being investigated in combination with 5-fluorouracil for gastric cancer.

Toxicity of semustine is essentially the same as with lomustine except for the recent report of chronic renal failure (Harmon et al. 1979). Usual dosage is 200 to 225 mg/m^2 every six weeks. The drug is available to registered investigators as semustine (methyl-CCNU, NSC 95441) from the Division of Cancer Treatment in 100-mg, 50-mg, and 10-mg capsules.

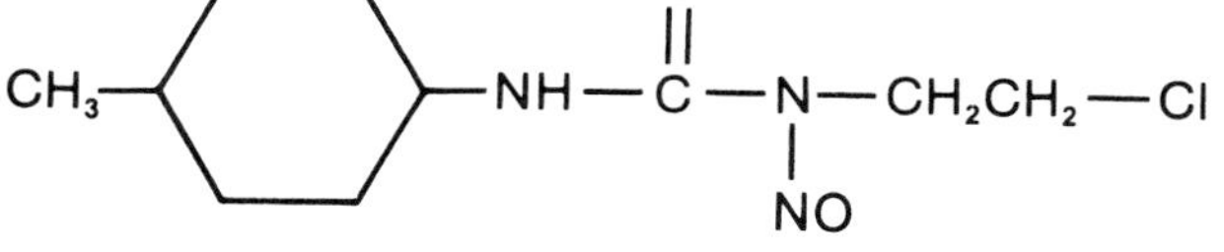

CH_3—C$_6$H$_{10}$—NH—C(=O)—N(NO)—CH_2CH_2—Cl

Fig. 23.3. *Semustine, NSC 95441*

Streptozocin (Investigational)

Streptozocin (Streptozotocin, Zanosar, NSC 85998) is 1-methyl nitrosourea glucosamine, an antibiotic derived originally from *Streptomyces acromogenes,* but now synthesized (fig. 23.4). The primary mode of action is inhibition of DNA synthesis but it affects all stages of the cell cycle. In addition, biochemical studies indicate inhibitory effects on pyridine nucleotides and enzymes involved in gluconeogenesis (Handelsman et al. 1974).

The drug is not significantly absorbed from the gastrointestinal tract and must be given intravenously. Following a dose the drug rapidly disappears from the plasma (in 15 minutes or less) and 10% to 20% appears in the urine, mostly in the first hour (Seibert et al. 1979).

The drug is a specific beta cell toxin and therefore useful in the treatment of islet cell carcinomas of the pancreas (Taylor et al. 1970). It has been active in 64% of functional tumors (mostly insulin-secreting, but some producing gastrin, glucagon, or ACTH). Responses included a lowering of serum insulin, decreased gastric acidity, or a return to normoglycemia. The response rate in nonfunctioning tumors has been about 50%. Still, most patients with these tumors eventually died.

In malignant carcinoid a 40% response rate is obtained, but so far the duration of response has been brief with single-agent therapy (Schein et al. 1973). Combinations of streptozocin, doxorubicin, 5-fluorouracil, and mitomycin look very promising but remain investigational. They are also being tried in adenocarcinoma of the pancreas, a tumor that has generally been unresponsive to all agents, and in gastric (Moertel et al. 1971) and lung cancer (Mauer, Weiss, and Aisner 1979).

Streptozocin has been used in combination chemotherapy of colorectal carcinoma with semustine, vincristine, and 5-fluorouracil (Kemeny et al. 1980), and in Hodgkin's disease in combination with bleomycin, vinblastine, and doxorubicin. Results have been positive but far from dramatic in both situations.

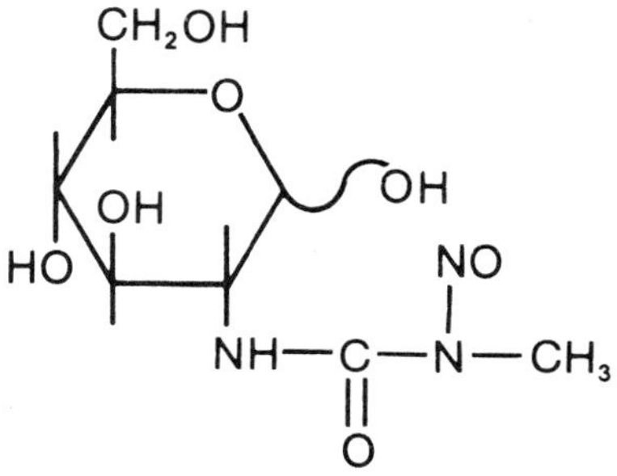

CH_2OH / O / OH / OH / HO / NO / NH—C(=O)—N(NO)—CH_3

Fig. 23.4. *Streptozocin, NSC 85998*

Toxicity is primarily renal (Sadoff 1970) and gastrointestinal (Stolinsky et al. 1972). Within two to four hours nausea and vomiting occur in virtually all patients, and antiemetics are only partially effective. Nephrotoxicity and cytoproliferative side effects occur together with azotemia in a small number of patients, but can progress to a fatal outcome (Myerowitz, Sartiano, and Cavallo 1976). Mild proteinuria is one of the first signs of toxicity, as is a rising BUN. Renal tubular acidosis, proximal tubular damage, and anuria are all potential dangers, but generally renal toxicity is reversible if the drug is stopped in time, and if patients with prior renal disease are not given the drug.

Myelosuppression is rare compared to that with other nitrosoureas, but can occur. If streptozocin is used with a strong myelosuppressive drug, the danger of synergism with profound marrow toxicity remains. Transient elevations of liver enzymes are frequently seen but their significance is not clear.

Hyperinsulinism may be caused by streptozocin, but in general this has not happened often (Broder and Carter 1973). At one time nicotinamide was used to block this problem, but it is not effective and is rarely used today.

Dosage depends on the protocol being used. Common regimens as a single agent include:

1. 1 to 1.5 gm/m^2 once a week for four weeks and continued if effective
2. 0.5 to 1.6 gm/m^2 five times a week every two or three weeks

The drug is available as streptozocin (Streptozotocin, Zanosar) to registered investigators from the Division of Cancer Therapy, which obtains it from Upjohn Company. It is distributed in vials of 2 gm and 100 mg, lyophilized to be reconstituted with bacteriostatic water and then diluted in sterile isotonic saline for intravenous administration. Vials are stored unopened and refrigerated. The reconstituted solution is stable between 4° C and 20° C for 48 hours.

Chlorozotocin (Investigational)

Chlorozotocin (DCNU, NSC 178248) is a 2-chloroethyl analogue of the glucose-substituted N-methyl-N-nitrosourea antibiotic streptozocin (fig. 23.5). It was deliberately synthesized to develop a nitrosourea with minimal myelosuppression, presumably caused by the sugar group, and still retain the antitumor activity (Schein et al. 1976). Chlorozotocin has retained the alkylating activity and inhibits tumor DNA, but it has little carbamoylating activity.

The drug is water-soluble and is degraded in part in the liver. There is some enterohepatic recirculation. Significant amounts of drug are excreted in the urine (Plowman 1978).

Experience with this drug is limited and phase II studies are just beginning (Kovach et al. 1979; Gralla et al. 1979). Some activity has been noted in colon, renal, pancreatic, ovarian, and gastric carcinomas, and in Hodgkin's disease and melanoma. No dramatic results have been reported, but some transient tumor shrinkage has been observed (Prestayko et al. 1981).

Toxicity is hematologic, albeit less than that seen with carmustine, lomustine, and semustine. Thrombocytopenia is frequent and dose-limiting. Leukopenia is less severe. Platelet nadir counts occur between four and five weeks with recovery a week or two later. Leukocyte nadir counts occur between five and six weeks and recover in a week, but they are usually mild unless another cytotoxic drug is used simultaneously (Anderson, McMenamin, and Schein 1975).

Elevations of BUN and creatinine occur infrequently (Kovach et al. 1979), but patients who already have azotemia should not receive chlorozotocin. If the BUN rises to 30 mg/dl, or the creatinine to 1.5 mg/dl during therapy with this drug, it should be discontinued. When recovery from nephrotoxicity occurs, it can be readministered at 60% of the previously calculated dose. The usual dose is 120 to 175 mg/m^2 intravenously every six weeks. The greater amount may cause severe and frequently prolonged nausea and vomiting, but these are usually partially ameliorated with antiemetics.

The drug is available as chlorozotocin to registered investigators from the Division of Cancer Treatment in 50-mg vials. The lyophilized powder is dissolved with sterile water or saline without preservative immediately before administration. The drug is some-

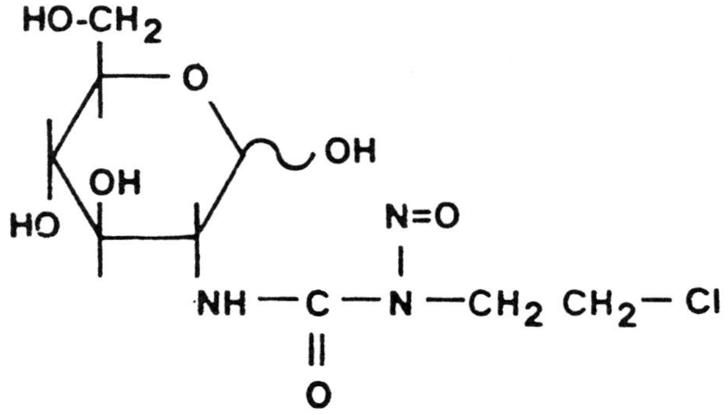

Fig. 23.5. *Chlorozotocin, NSC 178248*

what light-sensitive and therefore is packaged in amber vials. It should be stored at 2° C to 8° C. It is stable in aqueous solution at pH 4 for at least three hours. It is hoped that this drug will give better antitumor responses with less toxicity.

References

Anderson, T.; McMenamin, M.; and Schein, P. S. Chlorozotocin, [3-(2-chloroethyl)3-nitrosoureido], D-glucopyranose, an antitumor agent with modified bone marrow toxicity. *Cancer Res.* 35:761–765, 1975.

Bono, V. H., Jr. Review of mechanism of action studies of the nitrosoureas. *Cancer Treat. Rep.* 60:699–702, 1976.

Broder, L. E., and Carter, S. K. Pancreatic islet cell carcinoma: II, results in therapy with streptozotocin in 52 patients. *Ann. Intern. Med.* 79:108–118, 1973.

Carter, S. K., ed. Proceedings of the seventh new drug seminar: nitrosoureas. *Cancer Treat. Rep.* 60:645–811, 1976.

Carter, S. K. et al. 1,3-bis(2-chloroethyl)-1-nitrosourea (BCNU) and other nitrosoureas in cancer treatment: a review. *Adv. Cancer Res.* 16:273–332, 1972.

Case, D.; Lee, B. J., III; and Clarkson, B. D. Improved survival times in multiple myeloma treated with melphalan, prednisone, cyclophosphamide, vincristine, and BCNU: M-2 protocol. *Am. J. Med.* 63:897–903, 1977.

Cianfriglia, F. et al. CCNU chemotherapy of hemispheric supratentorial glioblastoma multiforme. *Cancer* 45:1289–1299, 1980.

Cohen, R. J.; Wiernik, P. H.; and Walker, M. D. Acute non-lymphocytic leukemia associated with nitrosourea chemotherapy: report of two cases. *Cancer Treat. Rep.* 60:1257–1261, 1976.

Durant, J. R. et al. Pulmonary toxicity associated with bis-chloroethylnitrosourea (BCNU). *Ann. Intern. Med.* 90:191–194, 1979.

Falkson, G., and Falkson, H. C. Fluorouracil, methyl-CCNU, and vincristine in cancer of the colon. *Cancer* 38:1468–1470, 1976.

Gralla, R. J. et al. Phase I trial of chlorozotocin. *Cancer Treat. Rep.* 63:17–20, 1979.

Handlesman, H. et al. *Streptozotocin NSC 85998.* Clinical brochure. Bethesda, Md.: National Cancer Institute, 1974.

Harmon, W. E. et al. Chronic renal failure in children treated with methyl-CCNU. *N. Engl. J. Med.* 300:1200–1203, 1979.

Hildebrand, J. et al. Effect of CCNU on survival rate of objective remission and duration of free interval in patients with malignant brain glioma—final evaluation of EORTC brain tumor group. *Eur. J. Cancer* 14:851–856, 1978.

Hoogstraten, B. et al. CCNU in the treatment of cancer. *Cancer* 32:38–43, 1973.

Katz, M. E., and Glick, J. H. Nitrosoureas: a reappraisal of clinical trials. *Cancer Clin. Trials* 2:297–316, 1979.

Kemeny, M. et al. Therapy for metastatic colorectal carcinoma with combination of methyl-CCNU, 5-fluorouracil, vincristine, and streptozotocin, (MOF-Strep.). *Cancer* 45:876–881, 1980.

Kovach, J. S. et al. A phase I study of chlorozotocin (NSC 178248). *Cancer* 43:2189–2196, 1979.

Levin, V. A., and Wilson, C. B. Nitrosourea chemotherapy for primary malignant gliomas. *Cancer Treat. Rep.* 60:710–722, 1976.

Levin, V. A., and Wilson, C. B. Nitrosourea chemotherapy for primary malignant gliomas. *Cancer Treat. Rep.* 60:710–722, 1976.

Marsh, J. C.; DeConti, R. C.; and Hubbard, S. P. Treatment of Hodgkin's disease and other cancers with BCNU (NSC 409962). *Cancer Chemother. Rep.* 55:599–606, 1971.

Mauer, L. H.; Weiss, R. B.; and Aisner, J. Streptozotocin: an inactive agent in small cell carcinoma. *Cancer Clin. Trials* 2:59–62, 1979.

Melato, M., and Tuveri, G. Pulmonary fibrosis following low-dose 1,3-bis(2-chloroethyl)-1-nitrosourea (BCNU) therapy. *Cancer* 45:1311–1314, 1980.

Moertel, C. G. Natural history of gastrointestinal cancer. In *Advanced gastrointestinal cancer clinical management and chemotherapy,* eds. C. G. Moertel and R. J. Reitemeier. New York: Harper & Row, 1969, pp. 3–14.

Moertel, C. G. et al. Phase II study of streptozotocin (NSC 85998) in the treatment of advanced gastrointestinal carcinoma. *Cancer Chemother. Rep.* 55:303–307, 1971.

Myerowitz, R. L.; Sartiano, G. P.; and Cavallo, T. Nephrotoxic and cytoproliferative effects of streptozotocin. *Cancer* 38:1550–1555, 1976.

Plowman, J. Disposition of chlorozotocin in rats and dogs. *Cancer Treat. Rep.* 62:31–44, 1978.

Prestayko, A. W. et al. *Nitrosoureas: current status and new developments.* New York: Academic Press, 1981.

Reynolds, R. D. et al. CCNU (NSC 79037): experience and review. *Cancer Clin. Trials* 1:43–48, 1978.

Richards, R. et al. Study of methyl-CCNU in the treatment of lung cancer. *Cancer Chemother. Rep.* 57:419–422, 1973.

Rivkin, S. E. et al. Methyl-CCNU and Adriamycin for patients with metastatic sarcomas. *Cancer* 46:446–451, 1980.

Sadoff, L. Nephrotoxicity of streptozotocin (NSC 85998). *Cancer Chemother. Rep.* 54:457–459, 1970.

Salmon, S. E. Nitrosoureas in multiple myeloma. *Cancer Treat. Rep.* 60:789–794, 1976.

Schein, P. et al. Streptozotocin for malignant insulinomas and carcinoid tumor. *Arch. Intern. Med.* 132:555–561, 1973.

Schein, P. S. et al. Pharmacology of chlorozotocin (NSC 178248), a new nitrosourea antitumor agent. *Cancer Treat. Rep.* 60:801–805, 1976.

Schepartz, S. Early history and development of the nitrosoureas. *Cancer Treat. Rep.* 60:647–649, 1976.

Seibert, K. et al. Continuous streptozotocin infusion: a phase I study. *Cancer Treat. Rep.* 63:2035–2037, 1979.

Solero, C. L. et al. Controlled study with BCNU vs. CCNU as adjuvant chemotherapy following surgery plus radiotherapy for glioblastoma multiforme. *Cancer Clin. Trials* 2:43–48, 1979.

Sponzo, R. W.; DeVita, V. T.; and Oliverio, V. T. Physiologic disposition of CCNU and methyl-CCNU in man. *Cancer* 31:1154–1159, 1973.

Stolinsky, D. C. et al. Streptozotocin in the treatment of cancer: phase II study. *Cancer* 30:61–67, 1972.

Takita, H. et al. Phase II study of the effect of methyl-CCNU on bronchogenic carcinoma. *Cancer Chemother. Rep.* 4(3):257–259, 1973.

Taylor, S. G. et al. Streptozotocin therapy for metastatic insulinoma. *Arch. Intern. Med.* 126:654–657, 1970.

Tranum, B. L. et al. A phase II study of methyl-CCNU in the treatment of solid tumors and lymphomas: a Southwest Oncology Group study. *Cancer.* 35: 1148–1153, 1975.

Walker, M. D., and Hurwitz, B. S. BCNU in the treatment of malignant brain tumor, a preliminary report. *Cancer Chemother. Rep.* 54:263–271, 1970.

Wasserman, T. H.; Slavik, M.; and Carter, S. K. Methyl-CCNU in clinical cancer therapy. *Cancer Treat. Rev.* 1:251–269, 1974a.

Wasserman, T. H.; Slavik, M.; and Carter, S. K. Review of CCNU in clinical cancer therapy. *Cancer Treat. Rev.* 1:131–151, 1974b.

Wasserman, T. H.; Slavik, M.; and Carter, S. K. Clinical comparison of the nitrosoureas. *Cancer* 36:1258–1268, 1975.

Weiss, R. B., and Muggia, F. M. Cytotoxic drug-induced pulmonary disease. Update 1980. *Am. J. Med.* 68:259–266, 1980.

Wheeler, G. P. Mechanism of action of nitrosoureas. In *Antineoplastic and immunosuppressive agents, handbook of experimental pharmacology,* vol. 38, part 2, eds. A. C. Sartorelli and D. G. Johns. New York: Springer-Verlag, 1974, pp. 65–84.

Young, R. C. et al. Initial clinical trials with methyl-CCNU 1-(2-chloroethyl)3-(4-methylcyclohexyl)-1-nitrosourea. *Cancer* 31:1164–1169, 1973.

twenty-four

Antimetabolites

DAVID S. FISCHER

In many ways, especially to those who are biochemically and pharmacologically minded, the antimetabolites are the most interesting antineoplastic agents because they were developed by design and not by serendipity (Welch 1965). With the effective use of sulfonamides in the 1930s, interest in drug therapy of disease was reawakened. In the 1940s, the mechanism of action of the antibacterial sulfonamides was shown to be as antagonists of the use of paraaminobenzoic acid in the biosynthesis of compounds related to folic (pteroylglutamic) acid (Woods 1940). Many microorganisms are dependent on coenzymes related to tetrahydrofolic acid, but are unable to use exogenous folic acid as a precursor of these coenzymes. The dependence of these microorganisms on the internal biosynthesis de novo of dihydrofolic acid, using either endogenously or exogenously formed paraaminobenzoic acid, affords an opportunity for selective interference with the use of a substance that is critical to the reproduction of bacteria, whereas it is of no significance to the life of the mammalian cell that uses exogenous folic acid to make its essential coenzymes (Bertino and Johns 1967).

The presence of an exploitable qualitative difference between the metabolic pathways of bacteria and mammalian cells gave tremendous impetus to the concept of competitive antagonism between enzyme substrates and their analogues. Not only was the development of new and potentially useful drugs given a more rational basis, but through logical syntheses of new competitive antagonists of other metabolites (Oliverio and Zubrod 1965), tools of much value were provided for the study of the mechanisms of a variety of important metabolic reactions. With an understanding of some of these metabolic pathways, scientists were prepared to look for ways to exploit *qualitative* biochemical differences between normal and neoplastic mammalian cells (Chabner, Myers, and Oliverio 1977). Alas, few have been found. The only one of clinical significance so far relates to asparaginase, which is discussed in chapter 27.

If *qualitative* differences between normal and neoplastic mammalian cells could not be readily elucidated, then *quantitative* differences had to be exploited. When the observation was made by Heinle and Welch (1948) and by Farber (1949) that folic acid accelerated the leukemic process, the call went out to develop folic acid antagonists. Chemists at Lederle Laboratories produced a series of such agents, and aminopterin (4-aminopteroylglutamic acid) (Seeger, Smith, and Hultquist 1947) was first used in 1947 with some temporary regressions in acute childhood lymphoblastic leukemia. In 1949, amethopterin (4-amino-N^{10}-methylpteroylglutamic acid), now called methotrexate, was developed (Seeger et al. 1949) and quickly replaced aminopterin because of its better therapeutic index. Promising results were reported in leukemia from several institutions in the ensuing years (Huennekens et al. 1963). Then came the exciting report of the cure of a solid tumor, choriocarcinoma, by methotrexate (Li, Hertz, and Spencer 1956). There was now a strong impetus to the study and development of antineoplastic drugs, and of antimetabolites in particular.

Table 24.1. *Antimetabolites*

Generic Name	*Trade or Common Name*	*Major Route(s)*	*Frequent Dose*	*Major Indication(s)*	*Major Toxicities*
Methotrexate	Methotrexate, Mexate	IV, SC	30–40 mg/m^2	Head and neck, ALL, breast, choriocarcinoma, osteosarcoma	Marrow, G.I., hepatic, pulmonary
		p.o.	5–15 mg/day		
Triazinate*	Baker's antifol	IV	250 mg/m^2 × 3 days	Breast, G.I.	Pulmonary, neurologic
6-Mercaptopurine	Purinethol	p.o.	100 mg/m^2/day	AML, ALL, CLL	Marrow
6-Thioguanine	Tabloid	p.o.	100 mg/m^2 b.i.d.	AML	Marrow
5-Fluorouracil	Fluorouracil, Adrucil	IV	400–600 mg/m^2	G.I., breast	Marrow, G.I., CNS
Floxuridine	FUDR	IV, IA	16–24 mg/m^2	Hepatic	Marrow, G.I.
Ftorafur*	Tegafur	IV	2400 mg/m^2	G.I., breast	Marrow, G.I.
Cytarabine	Cytosar-U	IV, SC	100 mg/m^2	AML, lymphoma	Marrow, G.I.
5-Azacytidine*	—	IV, SC	250–300 mg/m^2 × 5 days	AML	Marrow, G.I.
Hexamethyl-melamine*	—	p.o.	480 mg/m^2/day × 21 days	Ovary	Neurologic, G.I., marrow
Hydroxyurea	Hydrea	p.o.	1–2 gm/m^2	CML	Marrow

*Investigational.

With the growing knowledge of the structure of DNA and RNA from the ribose and deoxyribose sugars of purines and pyrimidines, it was natural to look for antimetabolites of these structures. A large number of such compounds have been synthesized and tested, but only a very few have reached or remained in clinical use (table 24.1). Of those still used, the purine antagonists 6-mercaptopurine and 6-thioguanine were developed by Hitchings and Elion (1954) and have found their major use in treatment of acute and chronic leukemias. The fluorinated pyrimidines were first synthesized (Heidelberger et al. 1957) and tested (Curreri et al. 1958) at the University of Wisconsin. They have been employed principally against adenocarcinomas of the gastrointestinal tract and breast. Brominated and iodinated pyrimidines have not been useful in antineoplastic therapy, although iododeoxyuridine has been useful in antiviral ophthalmic therapy (Prusoff, Bakhle, and Sekely 1965; Kaufman 1965), and it and iododeoxycytidine have been shown to inhibit development of polyoma virus-induced tumors in animals (Fischer et al. 1965; Fischer, Black, and Welch 1965). Pyrimidine nucleosides are also immunosuppressive agents (Fischer, Cassidy, and Welch 1966).

A significant contribution to the clinical armamentarium for leukemia and lymphoma was the synthesis of the arabinoside of cytosine (Carter and Livingston 1969; Ellison et al. 1968). This left the basic pyrimidine molecule intact but used an isomer of ribose as the sugar moiety, so as to interfere with DNA synthesis. This compound is known generically as cytarabine but is also referred to in common usage as Ara-C. It has become the cornerstone of most current regimens for acute myelocytic and monocytic leukemia. When these regimens fail, a noncross-reactive cytidine antimetabolite, 5-azacytidine, has been used in a number of investigational studies with some success (Saiki et al. 1978; Vogler, Miller, and Keller 1976). The drug has a nitrogen substituted for the carbon in the 5 position and acts against RNA, DNA, and protein synthesis, probably in that order.

An interesting investigational drug that resembles an alkylating agent structurally, but not mechanistically, is hexamethylmelamine. At the present time (Legha,

Slavik, and Carter 1976), it appears to function as a pyrimidine antimetabolite with demonstrated inhibition of RNA and DNA synthesis. Its precise classification and mode of action remain for future studies to elucidate. Hydroxyurea is also regarded by some authorities as an antimetabolite because of its mechanism of action (Belt et al. 1980).

Methotrexate

Methotrexate (amethopterin, Methotrexate, Mexate, NSC 740) (fig 24.1) was introduced for the treatment of acute childhood lymphocytic leukemia in 1949 by Farber and has since been used for several other malignancies. It has been studied extensively and used by many investigators in a variety of schedules and combinations (Porter and Wiltshaw 1962; Djerassi 1975; Shapiro, Young, and Mehta 1975; DeConti 1976).

Methotrexate is a 2,4-diamino folate antagonist. It competitively binds to dihydrofolate reductase, the enzyme that reduces folic acid to tetrahydrofolic acid, which is important in the metabolic transfer of one carbon units in a variety of biochemical reactions. These include the biosynthesis of thymidylic acid (the nucleoside specific to DNA) and inosinic acid, the precursor of adenine and guanine nucleotides in de novo purine biosynthesis. Methotrexate is cell cycle phase-specific for the S phase, with arrest of cells at the G_1/S interphase of the cell cycle. The major factors that determine cytotoxicity are duration of exposure and drug concentration. There has been a great deal of interest in drug concentration and attempts to increase it (Djerassi 1975), but insufficient emphasis is given to the vital importance of duration of exposure of the cell to the free drug. There is rapid reversal of the inhibition of DNA synthesis when levels of free intracellular drug fall, as only a small fraction of dihydrofolate reductase is required to maintain reduced folate pools at levels adequate to sustain DNA synthesis. Other important factors in determining cytotoxicity are the rate of transport of the drug into the cell; the level of folate cofactors in the cell; the presence of substrates, such as thymidine, in alternate pathways of DNA synthesis; and the proportion of cells proliferating in the cell cycle. The specific antidote is leucovorin (5-formyltetrahydrofolic acid, folinic acid, citrovorum factor), which is able to bypass the block in the reduction of dihydrofolate to tetrahydrofolate caused by methotrexate (Bleyer 1977). Leucovorin has been given systemically with high doses of methotrexate to prevent otherwise lethal toxicity. The use of other substances such as thymidine or 5-methyltetrahydrofolate as differential protectors of normal cells from antifolate toxicity is under investigation (Bertino 1977).

Drug absorption orally is complete at low doses (less than 30 mg/m^2) but is erratic at high doses, suggesting an intestinal absorption saturation mechanism. In addition, the gastrointestinal epithelium is even more sensitive to methotrexate than bone marrow, and high doses have led to denudation of the intestinal mucosa with bleeding and infection, and an occasional lethal outcome with very high doses (Von Hoff et al. 1977). Following intravenous administration, three phases of plasma clearance have been observed with half-lives of 0.75, 3.5, and 10.4 hours (Bleyer 1978). There is probably extensive enterohepatic circulation and some bacterial metabolism. The third phase of plasma disappearance is of particular importance in determining bone marrow toxicity in humans. About one-half to three-quarters of the drug is bound to albumin, and low doses are actively transported into cells. In the case of methotrexate resistance, decreased transport ability is thought to be one mechanism. Another is an increase in dihydrofolate reductase activity after therapy. A possible third mechanism is the presence of dihydrofolate reductase with an altered affinity for the inhibitor.

Excretion of methotrexate is largely through the kidney, and as much as 55% to 88% is reported to appear in unchanged form in the urine in 24 hours (*Physicians' Desk Reference* 1981). It is felt that this initial

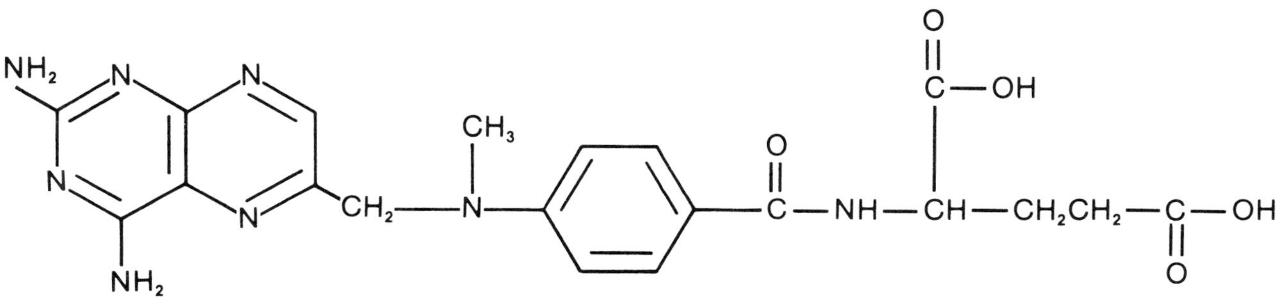

Fig. 24.1. *Methotrexate, NSC 740*

excretion represents primarily "surplus" drug that is not bound to tissue dihydrofolate reductase. There is a detectable urinary excretion rate of 1% to 2% of the retained dose for several weeks after a single dose, suggesting a slow release from tissue dihydrofolate reductase and from intestinal absorption from enterohepatic recirculation. Small amounts of drug undergo metabolism with the 7-hydroxy derivative as the probable metabolite. About 1% to 2% of the drug is detectable in the stool after an intravenous dose, probably from enterohepatic circulation (Bleyer 1977). Drug also enters cerebro-spinal fluid (Shapiro, Young, and Mehta, 1975) and ascites and pleural fluids.

Methotrexate was initially used as a single agent in treatment of acute childhood leukemia with significant responses but no cures (Farber 1949). It is now used in this leukemia as a key component of an oral or parenteral maintenance regimen after other agents have induced a remission. With this combination chemotherapy, once remission has been achieved, cranial irradiation and intrathecal methotrexate are used to prevent recurrence from so-called sanctuary sites. Unfortunately, methotrexate does not achieve high levels in the testes, which are now recognized as another sanctuary site. Survival with no evidence of disease at five years is achieved in approximately 50% of cases, and it is believed that most of these are cures (George et al. 1979).

In choriocarcinoma in women, methotrexate alone or in combination has produced cures in more than 75% of cases if treated within four months of onset (Lewis 1972). The presence of HCG as a sensitive tumor marker to help direct duration and intensity of therapy has been pivotal in this success. It has also been suggested that the tumor may be recognized in part as foreign by the body's immunologic system, as the genetic makeup of the tumor is 50% from the father (Lewis 1972). With those antigens being foreign, the small residual tumor population after chemotherapy may be cleared by the immunologic system.

Methotrexate has been effective in head and neck cancer, Burkitt's lymphoma, mycosis fungoides, carcinoma of the cervix, and in combination chemotherapy of embryonal rhabdomyosarcoma, breast, testis, lung, and ovarian carcinoma. A major use has been in the treatment of dermatoses, especially psoriasis (Weinstein 1977).

In osteogenic sarcoma, high-dose methotrexate with leucovorin rescue has been reported to be effective, both in active therapy and as adjuvant therapy after surgery (Jaffe et al. 1973). This has raised a number of questions. The early reports of success were based on comparisons with historical controls (Muggia and Louie 1978). More recent studies suggest that modern therapy with surgery alone, low-dose methotrexate, or other drugs is as effective as high-dose methotrexate and better than historical controls (Edmonson et al. 1980). Further studies will be necessary to resolve this.

High-dose methotrexate with leucovorin rescue (HDMTX-LCV) has been reported as highly effective in several individual institutional studies of head and neck cancer, non-Hodgkin's lymphoma, small cell lung cancer, breast cancer, and osteogenic sarcoma (Frei et al. 1980; Ervin and Canellos 1980). In the only cooperative prospective randomized trial in which HDMTX-LCV and conventional-dose methotrexate were compared (in head and neck cancer), there was no difference in response or survival, but among the responders, survival was greatest with standard-dose methotrexate (DeConti 1976; DeConti and Schoenfeld 1981). The criticism of that study has been that the high dose (240 mg/m^2) was not high enough. Now doses of 3 to 7.5 g/m^2 are being routinely used (Frei et al. 1980) in some studies. At this level an average individual whose size is 1.7 m^2 would receive 12,750 mg every week. At an average wholesale cost of $24 per 100 mg, this drug alone would cost $3060 per week or $159,120 per year, not to mention the cost of leucovorin, blood cell counts, creatinine clearance studies, plasma methotrexate levels, and some hospitalization for management of toxic reactions. Although these studies have in general been conducted by experienced investigators at university medical centers, there have been reports of significant numbers of drug deaths and probably larger numbers have gone unreported (Von Hoff et al. 1977). Obviously, this is not a technique to be undertaken except as part of a controlled clinical trial by those experienced in the area, and with the clinical facilities and backup of a first-class university research laboratory. An NCI group (Catane et al. 1978) pointed out that HDMTX-LCV is not a conventional treatment, and that in 1977 it cost the NCI over one million dollars just for the drug; in those days, much lower doses were called high-dose. Except in special circumstances, it is unlikely that third party payers will honor bills for this kind of therapy, and very few individuals can afford to bear such an expense themselves.

The toxicities of conventional-dose methotrexate include both gastrointestinal reactions and bone marrow suppression. Nausea and vomiting are frequent but mild. Diarrhea and stomatitis are common and are indications to discontinue therapy until they clear. Hemorrhagic enteritis and intestinal perforation can occur if therapy is continued after these early toxic signs. Toxicity can be reduced with proper attention to plasma pharmacokinetics (Stoller et al. 1977).

Myelosuppression is very common and dose-limiting. A severe leukopenia and thrombocytopenia may occur in six to nine days and can be life-threatening.

Megaloblastic anemia occurs almost routinely, as one would expect, but rarely causes significant problems. Hepatic damage has been reported and is usually evidenced by abnormal liver function tests that revert to normal when the drug is stopped (Djerassi et al. 1967); however, some patients have progressed to cirrhosis with its consequences (Dahl, Gregory, and Scheuer 1971). Anaphylactoid reactions have also been reported (Goldberg et al. 1978).

Acute reversible allergic pneumonitis that is not dose-related can occur with methotrexate (Sostman et al. 1978). It is characterized by fever, cough, shortness of breath, peripheral eosinophilia, and patchy pulmonary infiltrates. It seems to occur more commonly with intermittent therapy. A more serious complication is interstitial pneumonitis which may be fatal; interestingly, this has been seen with intrathecal as well as oral and parenteral methotrexate. In these cases, steroids should be given a therapeutic trial. To prevent this toxicity (and others), systemic leucovorin is frequently given concomitantly with intrathecal or intraarterial therapy (Shapiro, Mehta, and Hutchison 1977).

Because methotrexate is excreted primarily by the kidneys, any renal impairment poses a serious hazard to its use. The BUN and creatinine should be routinely checked before and intermittently in the course of therapy. If anything more than a usual dosage level is planned, a creatinine clearance should be obtained. When using HDMTX-LCV adequate hydration is essential, and alkalinization of the urine with sodium bicarbonate and/or acetazolamide is desirable, as the drug is more soluble at alkaline pH (Pitman and Frei 1977). Crystallization of drug in the renal tubules and renal tubular necrosis have been reported, with usually serious or fatal consequences.

Alopecia, dermatitis, vasculitis, and occasional osteoporosis have been reported with methotrexate. Headache, fever, and severe neurologic toxicity (including paraplegia and brain atrophy) have been seen on occasion following intrathecal administration of the drug (Gagliano and Costanzi 1976). Methotrexate has been used as an abortifacient and should not be administered during the first trimester of pregnancy. No late second malignancies have been attributed to this drug.

Interactions with other drugs are common. Since there is binding to serum albumin, other agents that bind may displace it and raise the level of free methotrexate. These include aspirin, sulfa drugs, chloral hydrate, chloramphenicol, phenytoin (Dilantin), and tetracycline. Vincristine augments the cellular uptake of methotrexate. Cytarabine and hydroxyurea may prevent progression of cells into the S phase and thereby diminish the effect of methotrexate when it is given later. The inhibition of protein synthesis by L-asparaginase may have a similar effect, and this enzyme has been deliberately used in some experimental protocols to terminate the cytotoxic action of methotrexate. It would seem that leucovorin could do that more safely and at a lower cost. Methotrexate given a few hours before 5-fluorouracil increases the incorporation of the fluoropyrimidine in target cells and thereby enhances cytotoxicity.

The routes of administration are oral, subcutaneous, intramuscular, intravenous, intraarterial, intralesional, intrathecal, and intracavitary. The oral dose seldom exceeds 30 mg/day, and subcutaneous (SC) and intramuscular (IM) doses are usually 50 mg or less. When given intravenously the suggested schedule is:

5 to 149 mg	— slow IV push
150 to 500 mg	— IV drip over 20 minutes
Over 500 mg	— IV infusion as specified in experimental protocol

The usual dose for patients with normal renal function is 30 to 40 mg/m^2 IV, SC, or IM weekly. The intrathecal dose is 8 to 12 mg/m^2 and should be given only with preservative-free methotrexate prepared freshly from the lyophilized powder.

The drug is supplied as Methotrexate (Lederle) in 2.5-mg tablets and as the sodium salt in 2-ml vials containing either 2.5 mg total dose or 50 mg total dose (25 mg/ml) with preservative, and as a lyophilized powder in 20-mg, 50-mg, and 100-mg vials preservative-free, and as constituted preservative-free solutions of 50 mg, 100 mg, and 200 mg. It is also supplied as Mexate (Bristol) in 50-mg, 100-mg, and 250-mg vials as a lyophilized powder. The investigational preparation in 500-mg and 1000-mg vials of lyophilized powder formerly distributed by the NCI is no longer available.

Storage is at room temperature. Reconstituted drug without preservative should be used the day it is prepared for intrathecal administration. For intravenous use, it is stable for a week but should be used earlier because of the danger of microbial contamination.

Folinic acid (citrovorum factor) is commercially available as Leucovorin Calcium Injection (Lederle), a liquid in ampules of 3 mg/ml, and as a cryodessicated powder in vials of 50 mg. Folinic acid, 5-mg tablets are still investigational and must be obtained from NCI as calcium leucovorin (NSC 3590).

Triazinate (Investigational)

Triazinate (Baker's antifol, TZT, NSC 139105) is a triazine folate antagonist that causes inhibition of DNA synthesis by a potent reversible inhibition of the enzyme dihydrofolate reductase (fig. 24.2). It should be noted that there are two distinct types of inhibitors of dihydrofolate reductase. The first is the aminofols as represented by aminopterin and methotrexate. These are classical antimetabolites with a close structural resemblance to the substrate, that is, folic acid. The second type includes diaminopyrimidines such as pyrimethamine (Daraprim) and trimethoprim, and various quinazoline derivatives. Because they have gross structural differences from the substrate they are called nonclassical antimetabolites. Therefore, TZT is a nonclassical antimetabolite designed as an analogue of pyrimethamine (Skeel et al. 1973; Legha and Slavik 1975).

Triazinate is poorly absorbed when administered by mouth. After intravenous injection the serum half-life is 1.2 to 4 hours. Measurable levels of drug are present in the serum 24 hours after injection. Cumulative urinary excretion varies between 15% and 60% of the injected dose at 12 hours, and there is still some drug excretion at 24 and 48 hours. Levels in CSF are 1% to 5% of the serum level, but levels in the brain may be very high following brain surgery. The drug is metabolized by the liver and some is excreted through the bile (Cashmore et al. 1975).

In phase I and II studies responses have been reported in small numbers of cases with cancer of the stomach, breast, lung, bladder, colon, kidney, and brain (Rodrigues et al. 1976; McCreary et al. 1977). Further investigations are in progress.

Dose-limiting toxicity has been neurologic and respiratory. Diplopia, lightheadedness, and other visual disturbances have occurred and seem to be dose- and rate-related. Acute respiratory distress with difficulty breathing may occur and is frightening to the patient and to the medical staff. To minimize toxicity, the drug should be given by slow intravenous infusion over at least one hour. The patient should be kept in bed in an area where there is good observation by nurses and physicians. If visual or respiratory disturbances occur the drug should be discontinued.

Myelosuppression occurs in about 20% of cases with leukopenia and thrombocytopenia, but beyond a certain threshold this is not dose-related. Mild nausea and vomiting can be controlled with antiemetics. Dermatitis, stomatitis, diarrhea, somnolence, and skin pigmentation are fairly common. The diarrhea and stomatitis are indications to discontinue the drug temporarily before gastrointestinal bleeding occurs. In the presence of liver impairment the dose should be reduced substantially.

Dosage on the M. D. Anderson Hospital schedule (Rodriguez, Richman, and Benjamin 1977) is 250 mg/m^2 IV administered daily for three consecutive days every two or three weeks with moderate myelosuppression and nadirs on or about the ninth day. The Yale schedule is 500 mg/m^2 IV weekly, resulting in minimal myelosuppression but with the worrisome neurologic and pulmonary symptoms mentioned (Skeel et al. 1976).

The drug is available as Baker's antifol from the Division of Cancer Treatment in 10-ml vials containing 100 mg of a lyophilized white cake, or in 20-ml vials containing 250 mg/vial of the material. The dry unopened vials may be stored at room temperature for two years or more, but once reconstituted the drug should be used within eight hours. The excess should be discarded because the preparation has no preservative and is susceptible to microbial contamination.

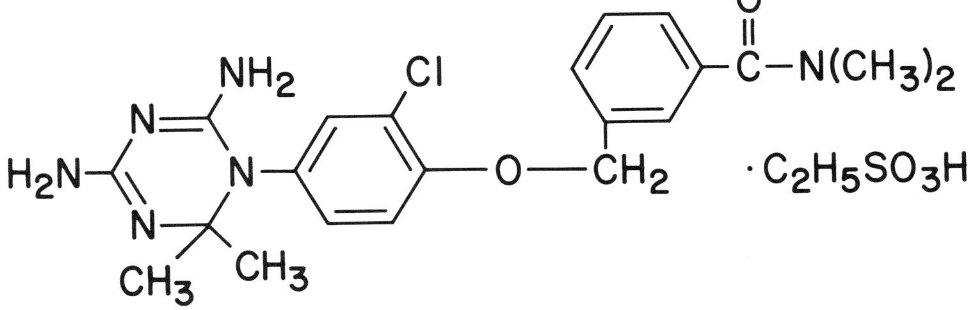

Fig. 24.2. *Triazinate, NSC 139105*

6-Mercaptopurine

6-Mercaptopurine (Purinethol, 6-MP, NSC 755) (fig. 24.3) is the thio-analogue of the naturally occurring purine hypoxanthine, a precursor of adenine and guanine in the de novo synthetic pathway. It also inhibits the biosynthesis of purines from small molecule precursors such as glycine, formate, and phosphate by inhibiting the conversion of phosphoribosylpyrophosphate to phosphoribosylamine, a pseudofeedback inhibition by thioinosinic acid, one of the products of 6-MP. The drug is cell cycle phase-specific with inhibition of synthesis of DNA and RNA. It is apparently not incorporated into DNA. The drug is also an immunosuppressant (Brockman 1963; Patterson and Tidd 1975).

About half of an oral dose is absorbed and maximal plasma levels are achieved in 2 hours, with a serum half-life after intravenous administration of about 90 minutes. Plasma protein binding occurs to the extent of 20%. The drug is metabolized in the liver and kidney by the enzyme xanthine oxidase to thioxanthine and thiouric acid. The enzyme is blocked by allopurinol, and 6-MP may achieve toxic levels unless dosage is reduced about 60% to 75% when allopurinol is used. The kidney excretes some unchanged drug and some metabolites. About 50% of an oral dose is recovered in the urine in 24 hours. It is usually cleared from the plasma by eight hours (Loo et al. 1968; Elion 1967).

Although the drug was originally used for the treatment of acute lymphoblastic and myeloblastic leukemia as a single agent (Moore et al. 1968; Rhoads 1954), it has been supplanted by other drugs, especially cytarabine. It has achieved good responses in combination therapy with cytarabine, or with vincristine, methotrexate, and prednisone (Henderson and Serpick 1967). Currently, it is more often used in maintenance therapy of acute lymphoblastic leukemia (Frei and Sallan 1978) and in some cases of chronic myelocytic leukemia. It has been used experimentally in choriocarcinoma, lymphocytic lymphoma, the blast crisis of chronic myelocytic leukemia, and as an immunosuppressive agent (Patterson and Tidd 1975).

Toxicity is primarily bone marrow depression. Leukocyte and platelet counts begin to fall in five or six days and may continue to go down for several additional days. Hence the drug should be discontinued until the counts start to rise again. In patients with renal impairment it is best to start with smaller than usual doses to avoid a cumulative effect from slower elimination of the drug.

Other toxic manifestations include nausea, vomiting, anorexia, stomatitis, rash, weight loss, drug fever, hyperuricemia, and diarrhea. Jaundice has been observed in a few instances, suggesting liver damage or biliary stasis. The drug should not be given to patients with liver disease or in the first trimester of pregnancy.

The usual single-agent initial dosage is 100 mg/m^2 daily, with adjustments based on white cell and platelet counts and disease response. In combination therapy, dosage is determined from the protocol. The drug is available as Purinethol (Burroughs Wellcome) in 50-mg scored tablets in bottles of 25 and 250. An investigational preparation of 500 mg per vial for intravenous injection is available to registered investigators from the Division of Cancer Treatment.

6-Thioguanine

6-Thioguanine (thioguanine, Tabloid, 6-TG, 2-amino-6-mercaptopurine, NSC 752) is an analogue of guanine in which a single oxygen atom is replaced by a sulfur atom (fig. 24.4). It acts by substituting for guanine and producing functionally altered polynucleotides. Unlike 6-MP, which it resembles, 6-TG is incorporated into DNA, which is thought to be its major mode of cytotoxic action (Nelson et al. 1975; LePage and Whitecar 1971). To a lesser extent, it is incorporated into RNA, and interferes with de novo purine biosynthesis by feedback inhibition.

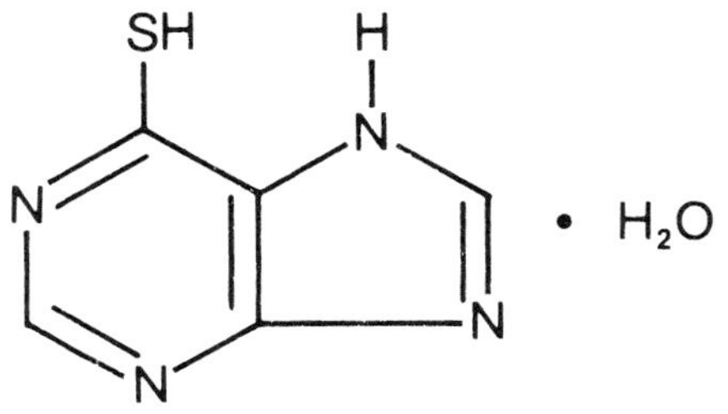

SH H N N N N • H_2O

Fig. 24.3. *6-Mercaptopurine, NSC 755*

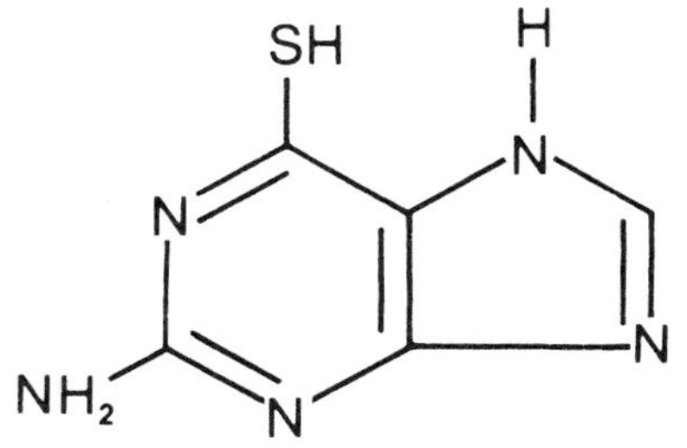

SH H N N N NH_2 N

Fig. 24.4. *6-Thioguanine, NSC 752*

The drug is partially absorbed from the gastrointestinal tract with a short plasma half-life; the significance of this is questionable, as the drug enters anabolic and catabolic pathways rapidly. About 20% to 25% of the drug is excreted in the urine. The remainder is metabolized to inactive compounds by methylation and deamination. The deamination by guanase results in thioxanthine, some of which is excreted in the urine and some of which is oxidized by xanthine oxidase to thiouric acid, which is excreted in the urine. Although allopurinol inhibits the action of xanthine oxidase, it has no effect on the antitumor activity or toxicity of 6-TG, since deamination to thioxanthine renders the 6-TG inactive (Grindey 1979).

The major use of 6-TG has been in the treatment of acute non-lymphocytic leukemia in combination with cytarabine (Gee, Yu, and Clarkson 1969), with or without the addition of daunorubicin (Gale 1979; Wiernik et al. 1976) or doxorubicin. It has been used experimentally in chronic myelocytic leukemia alone early in the disease and in combination in the blast crisis. It is being investigated as an immunosuppressive agent (Patterson and Tidd 1975).

Major toxicity has been myelosuppression manifested by leukopenia, thrombocytopenia, and to a lesser extent, anemia. Depression of blood cell counts begins five or six days after initiation of daily therapy in most cases, but occasionally can take three or four weeks. Counts usually begin to recover a week after the drug is discontinued, and therapy may be resumed when they rise to a reasonable level. Nausea, vomiting, and anorexia are common and usually dose-related, but milder than with 6-MP possibly because guanase is present in high concentrations in the gastrointestinal tract. The drug should be used in reduced initial dosage in the presence of liver or kidney impairment.

Dosage is usually 100 mg/m^2 twice a day in combination with cytarabine until the desired effect is produced or toxicity supervenes. The drug is available as Tabloid (Burroughs Wellcome) in 40-mg scored tablets in bottles of 25. An investigational parenteral preparation is available to registered investigators from the NCI as a lyophilized power in 75-mg vials.

5-Fluorouracil

5-Fluorouracil (Fluorouracil, Adrucil, 5-FU, NSC 19893) is a fluorinated pyrimidine (fig. 24.5). It was designed to be an antimetabolite of uracil, the pyrimidine unique to RNA, but the molecular size of the fluorine atom approaches that of a methyl group, which is the substituent in the 5 position of thymine, the pyrimidine unique to DNA. Although 5-FU can be phosphorylated to 5-FU ribonucleotides and incorporated into RNA, it can also be converted to fluorouracil-deoxyriboside (FUdR) and thereby act as an inhibitor of thymidylate synthetase, the crucial enzyme that promotes methylation of deoxyuridylate to thymidine. This block appears to be its major focus of action, as little if any is incorporated into DNA (Heidelberger and Ansfield 1963). While 5-FU has been shown to act in all phases of the cell cycle except G_0, its major loci of activity are in S and G_1 phases.

Oral administration of 5-FU as a tablet led to fairly poor absorption in most individuals (Bruckner and Creasey 1974), and was never approved. Oral absorption of the intravenous liquid preparation is good in the majority of individuals but poor in a substantial minority. Thus unless the clinician has a laboratory equipped to measure blood or urine levels, the drug is best not given orally because of this erratic pattern of absorption. Indeed, after a brief period of popularity, this route of administration has been abandoned by most major centers (Cohen et al. 1974). The claim that oral 5-FU yields high levels and hence better responses with liver lesions has been withdrawn by its original proponent after additional study in a larger number of cases.

Following intravenous administration the plasma half-life is about 20 minutes, and half of the drug (and its metabolites) is excreted in the urine in 9 hours and about 85% in 24 hours in patients with normal renal function (Sitar et al. 1977). Degradation occurs primarily in the liver, proceeding through dihydrofluorouracil to ring cleavage, so that little unchanged drug is excreted in the urine. Dosage must be reduced in patients with either hepatic or renal impairment to avoid toxicity (Myers et al. 1976).

The drug has been used extensively in treatment of colorectal carcinoma with about a 20% response rate in several large series when used alone or in various com-

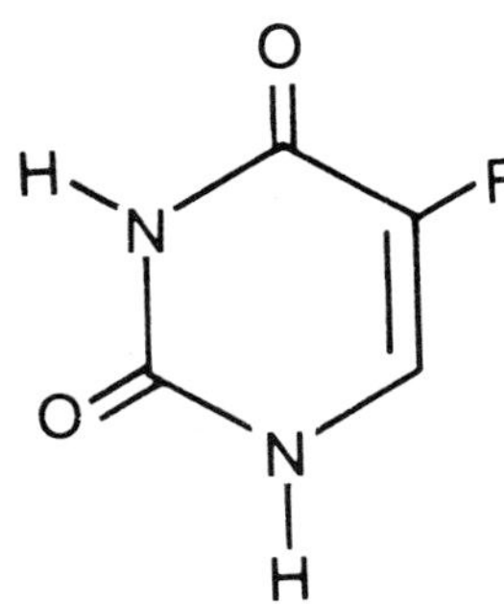

Fig. 24.5. *5-Fluorouracil, NSC 19893*

binations (Carter 1970). It has been used alone or with other drugs and/or radiation for treatment of gastric and pancreatic adenocarcinoma with a degree of efficacy the extent of which remains controversial (Ansfield et al. 1962). Nonetheless, it is the agent against which all others must be compared in therapy of gastrointestinal adenocarcinomas.

The role of 5-FU is well established in breast cancer where it is used in combination with methotrexate and cyclophosphamide (CMF) to achieve an approximate 50% remission rate (Canellos et al. 1976). In adjuvant therapy of the breast, CMF plus vincristine and prednisone has been highly effective in both premenopausal and postmenopausal women, while CMF has been clearly effective in premenopausal women but less convincingly so in the postmenopausal group who apparently tend to get much less than the protocol dose. In the subgroup of postmenopausal women who did receive 85% or more of the intended CMF dose, response was statistically significantly better than in the control group (Bonadonna and Valagussa 1980). Adjuvant therapy of colon carcinoma with 5-FU is controversial (Higgins et al. 1978).

Other tumors that respond in varying degree to 5-FU alone or in combination include ovarian, bladder, hepatoma, prostatic, and biliary adenocarcinomas, head and neck tumors, adenoid cystic and uterine cervix carcinoma, and topically, some skin cancers. The use of intraarterial and intracavitary 5-FU is discussed in chapter 30.

Major toxicity is primarily gastrointestinal and myelosuppressive. Anorexia, nausea, and vomiting are common and indicate the need to reduce the dosage and perhaps try antiemetics. Stomatitis and diarrhea are more ominous and dictate the interruption of therapy until they resolve. Persistence of treatment in spite of these signs can lead to hemorrhage and sloughing of the gastrointestinal mucosa. Leukopenia is the major dose-limiting side effect, with the nadir being reached in 7 to 14 days after the first dose and recovery occurring in the following week. Thrombocytopenia is usually less prominent and the nadir is seen between 7 and 17 days.

Other toxicity includes cerebellar ataxia, which usually resolves when the drug is discontinued but may be persistent and troublesome. Alopecia is seen more commonly with five-day courses of therapy than with single weekly doses and may include loss of eyebrows and eyelashes. A maculopapular rash occurs occasionally on the extremities and trunk and usually disappears spontaneously with steroid or antihistamine therapy. Ridging and cracking of the nails is more common than the few reports would indicate. Occasionally, loss of nails occurs. Increased lacrimation is a rare problem.

Photosensitivity can be a serious problem in the summer or in sunny climates. Increased skin pigmentation, erythema, and even bullous formation may occur with exposure to sunlight. Patients should be warned to use sun screens or to avoid unnecessary exposure. Hyperpigmentation at the site of injection or as a general phenomenon is occasionally seen.

A wide variety of dosage schedules have been used. The most popular has been 12 mg/kg daily for five days with a maximum of 800 mg on any one day, and then 6 mg/kg every other day for two to four doses if toxicity does not occur sooner. Some advocate repeating this type of course every 28 days, while others allow recovery from toxicity and give weekly doses of 12 to 15 mg/kg with a maximum single dose of 1000 mg (Horton et al. 1970). The drug is given by intravenous push directly into the vein. At one time, prolonged IV infusions were popular because larger doses could be given with little or no toxicity, but resulted in little or no antitumor efficacy.

The drug is available in 500-mg ampules as Fluorouracil (Roche) or Adrucil (Adria). The solution may discolor slightly during storage, but potency and safety are not adversely affected. In the rare instance when the drug is used in an IV drip, it may be added to either 5% dextrose in water or normal saline. Ampules should be stored at room temperature away from light. If they are exposed to cold the drug may precipitate. It can be put back into solution by heating to 140° F (60° C) in a water bath and then allowing it to cool to room temperature before use. A topical preparation, Efudex (Roche), is available for treatment of actinic keratoses and superficial basal cell carcinomas. It is supplied in 2% and 5% solutions in 10-ml containers and as a 5% cream in 25-g containers.

Floxuridine

Floxuridine (FUDR, 5-FUdR, 5-fluor-2′-deoxyuridine, NSC 27640) is the deoxyriboside of 5-FU (fig. 24.6). It is four orders of magnitude more potent than 5-FU in inhibiting the action of thymidylate synthetase (Papac and Calabresi 1966). Unfortunately, the increased activity is approximately equal in tumor cells and normal cells, so there is no therapeutic advantage in routine intravenous use. When 5-FUdR is given rapidly by intravenous route, it is broken down to 5-FU and urea and its effects and toxicity are the same as those of 5-FU. When 5-FUdR is given by slow continuous intraarterial infusion, it is anabolized to 5-FUdR-monophosphate, which inhibits thymidine synthetase and thus DNA synthesis. Accordingly, the drug has been released exclusively for intraarterial slow continuous infusion.

It is administered into the hepatic artery when primary or metastatic tumor is confined to the liver. It has also been used with some benefit in external carotid artery infusion for head and neck tumors, and for pelvic tumors by hypogastric artery infusion (see chapter 30).

Toxicity is similar to that seen with 5-FU, except that mucositis may be more severe with external carotid artery infusion. Abnormalities of liver function tests are common with intrahepatic artery infusion and must be monitored carefully to reduce or discontinue therapy when significant abnormalities occur.

The drug is usually given by an infusion pump at a rate of 0.1 to 0.6 mg/kg continuously over a 24-hour period. For hepatic artery infusions 0.4 to 0.6 mg/kg/day is used. The drug is available as FUDR (Roche) as a lyophilized powder in 500-mg vials of 5 ml to be reconstituted with sterile water as needed. The solution is stable for two weeks refrigerated.

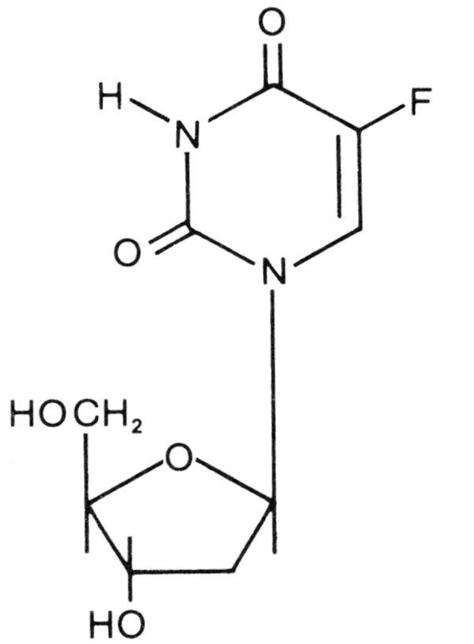

O
H
N
F
O
N
$HOCH_2$
O
HO

Fig. 24.6. *Floxuridine, NSC 27640*

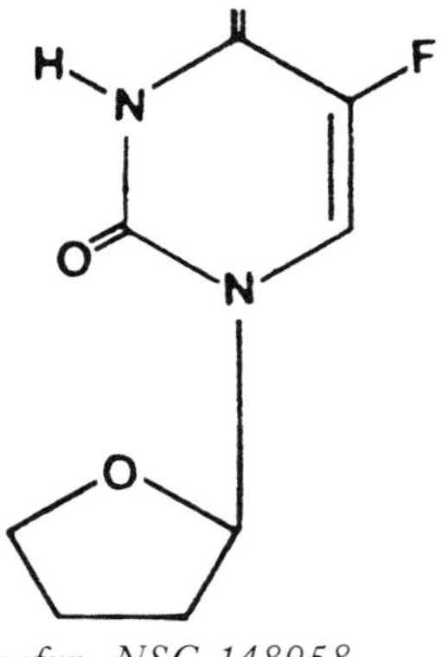

O
H
N
F
O
N
O

Fig. 24.7. *Ftorafur, NSC 148958*

Ftorafur (Investigational)

Ftorafur (Tegafur, 5-fluoro-1-tetrahydro-2-furyluracil, NSC 148958, N′[2′-furanidyl]5-fluorouracil) (fig. 24.7) is a pyrimidine antimetabolite first synthesized in the Soviet Union in 1966 as part of a detailed program for the synthesis of fluorinated nucleosides (Smart et al. 1975). The rationale was that modification of a known active pyrimidine antimetabolite, 5-fluoro-2′-deoxyuridine (5-FUdR), on a carbohydrate moiety might result in significant biochemical and pharmacodynamic differences in both antitumor activity and toxicity.

Although ftorafur may be viewed as a 5-FU derivative, it is actually a representative of a new class of compounds named furanidylpyrimidines, and has many pharmacologic and biochemical properties and clinical effects essentially different from those of 5-FU. The drug is classified as a heterocyclic compound, and is structurally similar to 5-FUdR (Handelsman and Slavik 1974).

Ftorafur acts as a weak inhibitor of thymidine synthetase and hence DNA. It also weakly inhibits RNA pyrimidine synthesis, but is neither a substrate nor an inhibitor of pyrimidine nucleoside phosphorylases.

When 4 to 5 gm/m^2 of ^{14}C-labeled drug is given by intravenous infusion over 1 to 2 hours, the plasma disappearance is biphasic with a mean terminal $t_{1/2}$ of 16.8 hours. A significant metabolite is 5-FU, which persists in the plasma for up to 96 hours after drug administration. The 24-hour cumulative urinary excretion of ^{14}C-labeled ftorafur is 15% to 30% of the administered dose. In addition to 5-FU, the urine contains ftorafur, 5-FUdR, 5-FUdR-5′-monophosphate, and 5-fluorouridine. Metabolism is primarily in the liver, and because it is slow the effect of ftorafur is essentially that of low-dose continuous infusion of 5-FU (Hall et al. 1976).

Clinical responses have been obtained in carcinomas of the stomach, colon, rectum, genitourinary tract, breast, lung, and esophagus (Buroker et al. 1977; Hall, Valdivieso, and Benjamin 1977). It has been claimed that the response rate in rectal carcinoma to ftorafur is three times that of 5-FU. Clinical investigation of this drug is continuing.

Dose-limiting toxicity is neurologic. Hallucinations, headache, and anxiety occur at 4 gm/m^2, and at 5 gm/m^2 there is frequently ataxia, lethargy, confusion, and dizziness. The lethargy is most common and usually begins one hour after infusion. If the infusion is too rapid, flushing, apprehension, dizziness, orthostatic hypotension, and chest tightness may occur. The drug should be stopped and additional normal saline given to raise the blood pressure back to pretreatment level.

Other toxicity includes moderate nausea and vomiting that are dose-related. Diarrhea, stomatitis, and liver toxicity occur occasionally. Myelosuppression is surprisingly uncommon and when it occurs is usually mild.

The dose of ftorafur in clinical trials in the Soviet Union was generally 15 mg/kg by intravenous infusion every 12 hours to a total dose of 30 to 40 gm (Handelsman and Slavik 1974). The Japanese clinical trials were less extensive.

In the United States, an early phase I study using 80 mg/kg/day IV resulted in leukopenia, diarrhea, and two drug-related deaths. Hence the recommended dose has been 60 mg/kg/day IV in normal saline over 30 to 45 minutes for a total dose of 30 to 40 gm (Smart et al. 1975). A dose of 3, 4, or 5 gm/m^2 IV in 100 ml 5% dextrose in water or normal saline infused over 15 minutes to 2 hours has been given every two to three weeks in controlled clinical trials and resulted in the toxicity described (Hall, Valdivieso, and Benjamin 1977).

The drug is available from the NCI in 500-mg vials of lyophilized powder that can be reconstituted with 9.7 ml sterile water to make a solution of 50 mg/ml. The drug is chemically stable for 96 hours or more at room or refrigerated temperatures, but since it has no preservative added the unused solution should be discarded after 8 hours because of the danger of microbial contamination.

Cytarabine

Cytarabine (Cytosar-U, cytosine arabinoside, Ara-C, arabinosylcytosine, NSC 63878) is a synthetic pyrimidine nucleoside that differs from its natural analogue cytidine in having the pentose sugar arabinose instead of its isomer, ribose (fig. 24.8). Its primary action is to inhibit DNA synthesis in the S phase of the cell cycle. Originally, it was thought that the primary drug action was inhibition of the conversion of cytidine to deoxycytidine, thereby resulting in a block of DNA synthesis. The fact that deoxycytidine reverses the cytotoxic effects of cytarabine supports this suggested mechanism of action, but it is no longer thought to be the major effect. It is now believed that the primary mode of action involves phosphorylation to cytarabine triphosphate by a series of nucleotide kinases, and then the triphosphate of cytarabine competes with the other trinucleotides for DNA polymerase, and this leads to decreased DNA synthesis. The drug can be incorporated into RNA and DNA (Cohen 1977).

Oral absorption is incomplete and deamination occurs in the gastrointestinal tract so that less than 20% reaches the circulation unchanged. Hence the oral route is not clinically useful, and the preferred routes are intravenous or subcutaneous. After intravenous administration there is a biphasic plasma half-life with an initial phase of 10 to 15 minutes and a second phase of 2 to 3 hours. The drug is rapidly deaminated to inactive uracil arabinoside, primarily in the liver. Only 4% to 10% of the drug is excreted unchanged in the urine, but 85% of the metabolites (mainly uracil arabinoside) are recovered in 24 hours in the urine (Ho and Frei 1971).

Because most of the unchanged drug is not found in the circulation after 20 minutes, to obtain prolonged plasma levels and thus expose as many cells in the S phase as possible, continuous intravenous infusion or frequent subcutaneous injection is necessary. Occasionally, tetrahydrouridine is administered to block the deaminase and thereby "protect" the cytarabine.

Although cytarabine crosses into the cerebrospinal fluid (CSF) when given by constant infusion, CSF concentration rarely exceeds 40%, or at the most 50%, of the simultaneous plasma concentration. Hence direct intrathecal administration has become popular. Since there is little or no deaminase in the CSF, the half-life there varies from 2 to 11 hours, and most of the drug there remains unchanged (Wang and Pratt 1970).

The major use of cytarabine has been in the treatment of acute non-lymphoblastic leukemia (which usually is abbreviated ANLL and includes acute myelogenous, myelomonocytic, monocytic, and erythroid leukemia). The use of cytarabine has changed the response picture from a 10% or 15% response rate for 3 or 4 months, to a 45% to 85% response rate in various

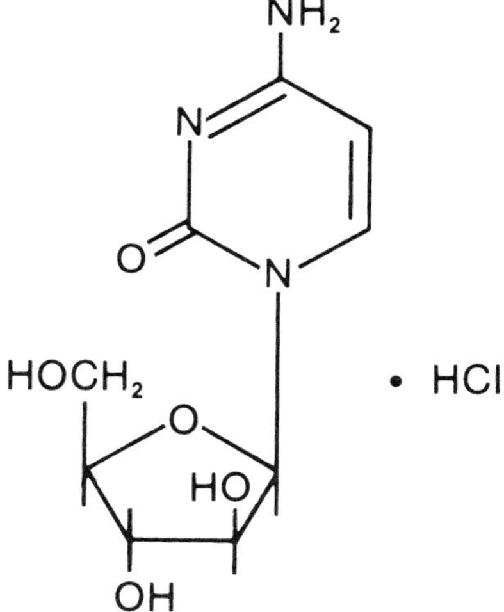

Fig. 24.8. *Cytarabine, NSC 63878*

combination regimens with remissions lasting for 8 to 12 months on the average (Kremer 1975; Southwest Oncology group 1974; Skeel et al. 1980). Combination therapy began with cytarabine infusions of 5 to 10 days and oral 6-thioguanine given every 12 hours for as many days. Either or both drugs were then used in many different schedules to maintain the remission induced by vigorous initial therapy.

The anthracycline antibiotics daunorubicin and doxorubicin have greatly enhanced the rate and duration of cytarabine responses. Active clinical trials are evaluating different schedules of these drug combinations in regard to selection of optimal doses and durations of administration (Gale 1979). We are currently trying an induction regimen that uses cytarabine, daunorubicin, and 6-thioguanine, and then has a separate maintenance schedule. Like most groups, we seem to be more successful in inducing remissions than in maintaining them.

Other indications for cytarabine have included head and neck cancers and some sarcomas. In diffuse histiocytic lymphoma, a combination regimen using cyclophosphamide, vincristine, cytarabine, and methotrexate with leucovorin rescue was pioneered at Yale (Cadman et al. 1977) and further developed at the University of Chicago (Sweet et al. 1980). This seems to produce excellent results in about 50% of cases. Sometimes doxorubicin is added to the regimen. Cytarabine has also demonstrated immunosuppression (Mitchell et al. 1969).

Meningeal leukemia and carcinomatous meningitis have been treated with intrathecal cytarabine either as an alternative to methotrexate or after failure of that drug (Wang and Pratt 1970).

The major toxicity is bone marrow depression, which is more directly related to duration of exposure than to dose. Severe myelosuppression with neutropenia and thrombocytopenia can occur. Megaloblastic changes are common, especially in red cell precursors, as the drug inhibits DNA synthesis. Drug effect can be seen for five to seven days after its discontinuation, and recovery of white cell and platelet counts may take two to three weeks and occasionally longer.

Other toxicities include severe nausea, vomiting, and stomatitis which may be dose-limiting. Less common are thrombophlebitis, fever, hepatic dysfunction, headache, and dizziness if intravenous infusion is too rapid. Cases of paraparesis have been reported after intrathecal use (Breuer et al. 1977), and this route should be used only when indications for it are strong, and even then with great caution. For good or for ill, the drug is a potent immunosuppressant.

A variety of regimens have been used and new ones are being evaluated (Skeel et al. 1980). The most popular pulse therapy has been cytarabine, 100 mg/m^2 every 12 hours by IV or SC injection for seven days, combined with 6-thioguanine or daunorubicin or both (Gale 1979; Yates et al. 1973). Another approach is continuous infusion of cytarabine, 100 mg/m^2 daily for seven days and concomitant use of 6-thioguanine, daunorubicin, or doxorubicin. The intrathecal dose ranges from 10 to 30 mg/m^2 and may be given once, twice, or three times a week.

The drug is available as Cytosar-U (Upjohn) in 100-mg and 500-mg freeze-dried vials that are reconstituted with bacteriostatic water for injection when intended for IV or SC administration. For intrathecal use, preservative-free diluent is essential. The unopened vials are stable at room temperature for long periods and are dated. The reconstituted solution is stable at room temperature for 48 hours, and for 7 days in the refrigerator. Crystallization occasionally occurs in highly concentrated solutions in the refrigerator.

5-Azacytidine (Investigational)

5-Azacytidine (NSC 102816) is an antimetabolite analogue of cytadine synthesized in Czechoslovakia with a nitrogen in place of a carbon in the 5 position of the ring (fig. 24.9). It is phosphorylated by uridine-cytidine kinase, and as the triphosphate is incorporated into RNA and DNA, where it miscodes and interrupts the translation of nucleic acid sequences into significant protein. It also inhibits de novo pyrimidine synthesis by

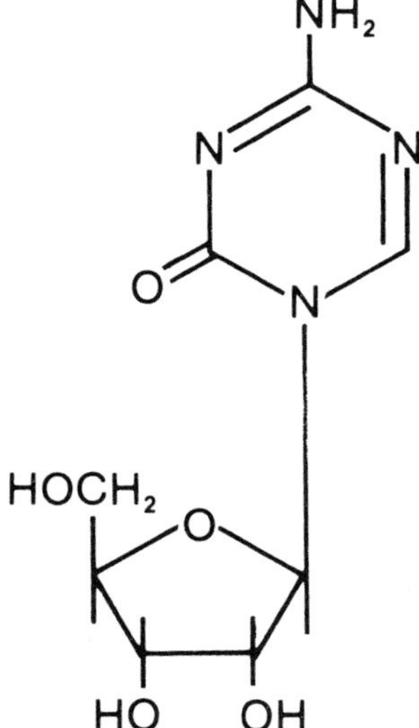

Fig. 24.9. *5-Azacytidine, NSC 102816*

inhibiting orotidylic acid decarboxylase. It acts in the S phase of the cell cycle and is phase-spcific. It is not cross-reactive with cytarabine, and its cytotoxicity can be prevented by cytidine that competes for uridine kinase (Von Hoff, Handelsman, and Slavik 1975).

The drug is usually given intravenously but may also be administered subcutaneously. It is relatively unstable in solution and undergoes rapid hydrolysis in neutral and basic media. The radioactively labeled drug has a plasma half-life of three and a half hours. About 90% of the radioactivity appears in the urine in 24 hours and accounts in part for the rapid plasma clearance. The other explanation is relatively rapid deamination by cytidine deaminase in the liver to 5-azauridine, which is extremely unstable and undergoes spontaneous ring cleavage. Studies show that 5-azacytidine concentrates to some extent in the lymphatic organs and very little enters the CSF.

The major indication for the drug so far has been in acute myelogenous leukemia (AML) refractory to other drugs and combinations. Given as a single agent, the response rate is about 20% to 36% but remissions are brief (Von Hoff, Slavik, and Muggia 1976). Investigations have been initiated to include the drug in first-line combination chemotherapy of AML (Cassileth et al. 1979). The drug is also being tried in melanoma, and breast, ovary, and colon carcinoma, lymphoma, and mesothelioma (Weiss et al. 1977). Experience so far is very limited.

The major toxicity is bone marrow hypoplasia with inhibition of all elements, whereas in AML the desired effect is inhibition of the leukocyte line. The range of the leukocyte nadir is 18 to 30 days with a mean of 25 days in patients with solid tumors (nonhematologic). Recovery usually occurs in 7 to 21 days. For patients with AML on a 5-day schedule of intravenous therapy the nadir is usually 14 to 17 days. Thrombocytopenia of less than 100,000 has been reported in 17% of patients with a nadir of 13 to 21 days, and it may last for 2 weeks (Von Hoff, Slavik, and Muggia 1976).

Gastrointestinal toxicity can be severe with nausea and vomiting in 75% of patients and usually occurring one to three hours after intravenous injection. Antiemetics are occasionally helpful and appear to give best results when begun a day or two before chemotherapy, and continued throughout the course. Vomiting can become so severe that some patients choose to stop therapy. Although diarrhea occurs in half the cases, it is not dose-limiting but should be watched carefully.

Abnormal liver function tests occur in 7% of patients and hepatic coma in 0.5% (Von Hoff, Slavik, and Muggia 1976). A strange neurologic syndrome with lethargy, myalgia, and coma has been described. Fever may occur in 6% of patients and begins one to four hours after the drug is given. A pruritic skin rash has been seen, and occasionally, phlebitis and stomatitis. Hypotension occurs if intravenous drug is given too rapidly.

The drug is available as a lyophilized 100-mg vial of azacytidine. It is reconstituted with 19.9 ml of sterile water and can then be further diluted in Ringer's lactate solution, which provides the best pH and stability. The solution should be used in 30 minutes for maximum potency but is often given over 4 hours with a sacrifice of potency. Usual dose is a course of 250 to 300 mg/m^2 per day IV for five days every two to three weeks, depending on recovery blood counts.

Hexamethylmelamine (Investigational)

Hexamethylmelamine (HMM, NSC 13875) is a synthetic chemical whose structure resembles that of triethylene melamine (TEM), an alkylating agent (fig. 24.10). Studies in humans and in animals suggest that the small structural difference leads to different activities and probably different mechanisms. Triethylene melamine reacts positively with 4-(nitrobenzyl) pyridine (NBP) in the classical in vitro alkylating function test, while HMM does not. Hexamethylmelamine has been implicated in nucleic acid metabolism and inhibits incorporation of thymidine and uridine into DNA and RNA. Prolonged exposure of cells to the drug also inhibits protein synthesis, but the clinical significance of this is uncertain (Legha et al. 1974).

The drug is well absorbed orally and the peak plasma level is reached in one hour. The plasma half-life of radioactive drug or metabolites is 3 hours with

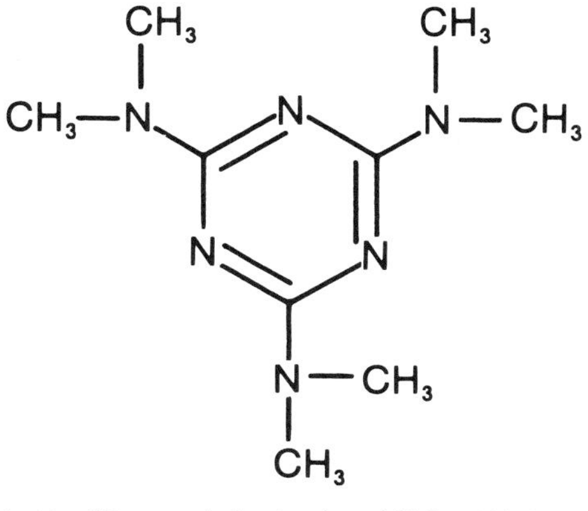

Fig. 24.10. *Hexamethylmelamine, NSC 13875*

measurable levels still detectable at 24 hours. About 60% of the metabolites is excreted in the urine in 24 hours, another 25% in the second 24 hours, and 5% more during the third day. Some of the methyl groups are oxidized to CO_2 and the melamines are excreted in the urine. The N-demethylation occurs primarily in the liver (I ouis et al. 1967; Legha, Slavik, and Carter 1976).

The major use of the drug at present is in therapy of ovarian carcinoma, alone or in combination (Smith and Rutledge 1975). A popular combination known as hexa-CAF is made up of HMM, cyclophosphamide, amethopterin (methotrexate), and 5-FU, and has resulted in some of the best response rates reported in ovarian carcinoma (Young et al. 1978). Activity has been reported in cervical carcinoma and in head and neck tumors (Blum et al. 1973; Legha et al. 1974). In small cell undifferentiated carcinoma of the lung, an approximate 30% response rate has been noted (Wilson et al. 1969). In adenocarcinoma of the breast, the response rate has been 30%, with half being partial responses (PR) (Denefrio and Vogel 1978). In lymphoma of both the Hodgkin's and non-Hodgkin's varieties, responses of 25% to 40% are seen (Borden et al. 1977; Wampler et al. 1972).

The major dose-limiting toxicity is gastrointestinal (Bergevin, Tormey, and Blom 1973). It manifests as anorexia, nausea, vomiting, abdominal cramps, and diarrhea. It occurs in 40% to 70% of patients and can be ameliorated by dividing the dose into four portions, and giving one portion about two hours after each meal and at bedtime. Antiemetics are quite helpful, and symptoms cease soon after the drug is discontinued. Toxicity is dose-related; 10% of patients are unable to tolerate the drug and discontinue its use.

Hematologic toxicity occurs in 20% to 40% of patients with standard-dose therapy, and is mild and tolerable. The onset of leukopenia and thrombocytopenia is usually at the end of the first week of therapy, reaches a nadir in three to four weeks, and returns to normal by the sixth week. The incidence of leukopenia and thrombocytopenia is about the same, but the former is usually more severe.

Central nervous system (CNS) toxicity is seen in 10% to 20% of patients. It is manifested by confusion, agitation, and depression. Some have hallucinations and petit mal spells, and rarely, ataxia and parkinsonian-like symptoms. These are all reversible when the drug is stopped.

Peripheral neuropathy manifests as paresthesias, hypesthesia, impaired sense of touch, vibration, and position sensation.

As a single agent, low-dose, medium-dose, and high-dose schedules have been used. The low-dose schedule employed 4 mg/kg/day for 42 days; the medium-dose schedule used 8 mg/kg/day for 42 days, or in some studies for 90 days (Bergevin, Tormey, and Blom 1973). The high-dose schedule was 12 mg/kg/day for 21 days repeated at four weekly intervals. The low-dose schedule resulted in more toxicity but better responses. The high-dose schedule is more commonly used (Legha, Slavik, and Carter 1976). For combination usage, see chapter 29 or original protocols.

The drug is available to registered investigators as hexamethylmelamine in capsules of 50 mg and 100 mg from the Division of Cancer Treatment.

Hydroxyurea

Hydroxyurea (Hydrea, NSC 32065) is a simple molecule (fig. 24.11) that directly inhibits DNA synthesis by inhibiting ribonucleoside diphosphate reductase, an enzyme that catalyzes the conversion of ribonucleotides to deoxyribonucleotides, a crucial step in the biosynthesis of DNA. Hydroxyurea is an S-phase-specific agent that behaves in some respects as an antimetabolite (Belt et al. 1980; Yarbro 1968).

After oral administration the drug is rapidly absorbed from the gastrointestinal tract, and peak plasma level is achieved in two hours. The half-life is three to four hours and plasma levels decline rapidly; there is no cumulative effect with repeated administration. About 50% of an oral dose is metabolized in the liver to CO_2 and urea. The other 50% is excreted in the urine, with 80% of the radioactive label recovered in 12 hours.

Although hydroxyurea was originally marketed with treatment of melanoma in mind, it has had limited value in this tumor (Nathanson and Hall 1967). It has been used for renal cell carcinoma with marginal results. Its major application has been in management of chronic myelogenous leukemia (CML) refractory to busulfan (Schullenberger 1964). As we have acquired more experience with it, hydroxyurea has become the drug of choice in CML (Kennedy 1972; Spiers 1979). It is more difficult to use than busulfan, as the white blood cell counts bounce up and down and must be monitored often for frequent dose adjustments. I have been particularly pleased with the prompt fall in high

$$NH_2-\overset{\displaystyle O}{\overset{\|}{C}}-NH-OH$$

Fig. 24.11. *Hydroxyurea, NSC 32065*

white cell counts in contrast to the much slower response with busulfan. Several patients have survived for long periods of time while taking this drug. I have also used it in combination with vincristine and prednisone to induce remissions in the acute blastic phase of CML in four patients, with one patient having been induced into remissions on three separate occasions. The remissions are, unfortunately, usually brief and we need to concentrate more on maintaining them.

I have also used hydroxyurea to reduce the very high white cell counts in several patients with newly diagnosed AML in preference to treating them with a cell separator. Although brief, the responses were usually good and allowed us to begin the more definitive therapy without danger of leukostasis in cerebral vessels. Hydroxyurea has also been effective in the hypereosinophilic syndrome (Parrillo, Fauci, and Wolff 1978) and in some solid tumors (Ariel 1970; Lerner, Beckloff, and Godwin 1969; Thurman et al. 1963).

Primary toxicity is myelosuppression, which is also the desired action. Leukopenia is more common than thrombocytopenia. Anemia is also common, and at one time the drug was used for treatment of polycythemia.

Anorexia occurs frequently, but nausea, vomiting, stomatitis, and mucosal ulcerations are all rare. Occasional skin rash is seen. High doses can cause drowsiness. Renal impairment with elevated BUN is a rare side effect.

Usual single-agent doses are 1000 to 2000 mg/m^2/day in two or more divided doses, with subsequent adjustments based on blood cell counts. The same initial dose is used with prednisone and vincristine. When used in other combinations, the original protocol should be consulted.

Hydroxyurea is available as Hydrea (Squibb) in capsules of 500 mg each. An experimental preparation for injection is available from the Division of Cancer Treatment in 2-gm vials.

References

Ansfield, F. J. et al. Five years' clinical experience with 5-fluorouracil. *JAMA* 181:295–299, 1962.

Ariel, I. M. Therapeutic effects of hydroxyurea: experience with 118 patients with inoperable solid tumors. *Cancer* 25:705–714, 1970.

Belt, R. J. et al. Studies of hydroxyurea administered by continuous infusion. *Cancer* 46:455–462, 1980.

Bergevin, P. R.; Tormey, D. C.; and Blom, J. Clinical evaluation of hexamethylmelamine (NSC 13875). *Cancer Chemother. Rep.* 57:51–58, 1973.

Bertino, J. R. "Rescue" techniques in cancer chemotherapy. *Semin. Oncol.* 4:203–216, 1977.

Bertino, J. R., and Johns, D. G. Folate antagonists. *Ann. Rev. Med.* 18:27–34, 1967.

Bleyer, W. A. Methotrexate: clinical pharmacology, current status, and therapeutic guidelines. *Cancer Treat. Rev.* 4:87–102, 1977.

Bleyer, W. A. The clinical pharmacology of methotrexate. New applications of an old drug. *Cancer* 41:36–51, 1978.

Blum, R. H. et al. Hexamethylmelamine—a new drug with activity in solid tumors. *Eur. J. Cancer* 9:195–202, 1973.

Bonadonna, G., and Valagussa, P. Dose-response effect of CMF in breast cancer. *Proc. Am. Soc. Clin. Oncol.* 21:413, 1980.

Borden, E. C. et al. Hexamethylmelamine treatment of sarcomas and lymphomas. *Med. Pediatr. Oncol.* 3:401–406, 1977.

Breuer, A. C. et al. Paraparesis following intrathecal cytosine arabinoside. *Cancer* 40:2817–2822, 1977.

Brockman, R. W. Biochemical aspects of mercaptopurine inhibition and resistance. *Cancer Res.* 23:1191–1201, 1963.

Bruckner, H. W., and Creasey, W. A. The administration of 5-fluorouracil by mouth. *Cancer* 33:14–18, 1974.

Buroker, T. et al. Phase II clinical trial of ftorafur in 5-fluorouracil—refractory colorectal carcinoma. *Cancer Treat. Rep.* 61:1579–1580, 1977.

Cadman, E. et al. Combination chemotherapy for diffuse histiocytic lymphoma that includes antimetabolites. *Cancer Treat. Rep.* 61:1109–1116, 1977.

Canellos, G. P. et al. Combination chemotherapy for advanced breast cancer: response and effect on survival. *Ann. Intern. Med.* 84:389–392, 1976.

Carter, S. K. ed. *Proceedings of the chemotherapy conference on the chemotherapy of solid tumors. An appraisal of 5-fluorouracil and BCNU.* Bethesda, Md.: National Cancer Institute, 1970.

Carter, S. K., and Livingston, R. B., eds. *Proceedings of the chemotherapy conference on Ara-C: development and application.* Bethesda, Md.: National Cancer Institute, 1969.

Cashmore, A. R. et al. Pharmacology of a new triazine antifolate in mice, rats, dogs, and monkeys. *Cancer Res.* 35:17–22, 1975.

Cassileth, P. A. et al. Feasibility and efficacy of 5-azacytidine used early in the therapy of adult acute nonlymphocytic leukemia: an ECOG pilot study. *Cancer Clin. Trials* 2:339–344, 1979.

Catane, R. et al. High-dose methotrexate, not a conventional treatment. *Cancer Treat. Rep.* 62:178–180, 1978.

Chabner, B. A.; Myers, C. E.; and Oliverio, V. T. Clinical pharmacology of anticancer drugs. *Semin. Oncol.* 4:165–191, 1977.

Cohen, J. L. et al. Clinical pharmacology of oral and intravenous 5-fluorouracil (NSC 19893). *Cancer Chemother. Rep.* 58:723–731, 1974.

Cohen, S. The mechanisms of lethal action of arabinosyl cytosine (Ara-C) and arabinosyl adenines (Ara-A). *Cancer* 40:509–518, 1977.

Curreri, A. R. et al. Clinical studies with 5-fluorouracil. *Cancer Res.* 18:478–484, 1958.

Dahl, M. G. C.; Gregory, M. M.; and Scheuer, P. J. Liver damage due to methotrexate in patients with psoriasis. *Br. Med. J.* 1:625–630, 1971.

DeConti, R. C. Phase III comparison of methotrexate with leucovorin vs. a combination of methotrexate plus leucovorin, cyclophosphamide, and cytosine arabinoside in head and neck cancer. *Proc. Am. Soc. Clin. Oncol.* 17:248, 1976.

DeConti, R. C., and Schoenfeld, D. A randomized prospective comparison of intermittent methotrexate, methotrexate with leucovorin, and a methotrexate combination in head and neck cancer. *Cancer* 48:1061–1072, 1981.

Denefrio, J. M., and Vogel, C. L. Phase II study of hexamethylmelamine in women with advanced breast cancer refractory to standard cytotoxic therapy. *Cancer Treat. Rep.* 62:173–175, 1978.

Djerassi, I. High-dose methotrexate and citrovorum factor rescue: background and rationale. *Cancer Chemother. Rep.* 6:3–6, 1975.

Djerassi, I. et al. Continuous infusion of methotrexate in children with acute leukemia. *Cancer* 20:233–242, 1967.

Edmonson, J. H. et al. Post-surgical treatment of primary osteosarcoma of bone—comparison of high dose methotrexate vs. observation: preliminary report. *Proc. Am. Soc. Clin. Oncol.* 21:476, 1980.

Elion, G. B. Biochemistry and pharmacology of purine analogues. *Fed. Proc.* 26:898–904, 1967.

Ellison, R. R. et al. Arabinosyl cytosine: a useful agent in the treatment of acute leukemia in adults. *Blood* 32:507–523, 1968.

Ervin, T., and Canellos, G. P. Successful treatment of recurrent primary central nervous system lymphoma with high-dose methotrexate. *Cancer* 45:1556–1557, 1980.

Farber, S. H. Some observations on the effect of folic acid antagonists on acute leukemia and other forms of incurable cancer. *Blood* 4:160–167, 1949.

Fischer, D. S. et al. Inhibition of tumor virus production by halogenated deoxyribonucleosides. *Ann. NY Acad. Sci.* 130:213–216, 1965.

Fischer, D. S.; Black, F. L.; and Welch, A. D. Inhibition by nucleoside analogues of tumor formation. *Nature* 206:839–840, 1965.

Fischer, D. S.; Cassidy, E. P.; and Welch, A. D. Immunosuppression by pyrimidine nucleoside analogues. *Biochem. Pharmacol.* 15:1013–1022, 1966.

Frei, E., III et al. High-dose methotrexate with leucovorin rescue. *Am. J. Med.* 68:370–376, 1980.

Frei, E., III, and Sallan, S. E. Acute lymphoblastic leukemia; treatment. *Cancer* 42:828–838, 1978.

Gagliano, R. G., and Costanzi, J. J. Paraplegia following intrathecal methotrexate. *Cancer* 37:1663–1668, 1976.

Gale, R. P. Advances in the treatment of acute myelogenous leukemia. *N. Engl. J. Med.* 300:1189–1199, 1979.

Gee, T. S.; Yu, K. P.; and Clarkson, B. D. Treatment of adult acute leukemia with arabinosyl cytosine and thioguanine. *Cancer* 23:1019–1032, 1969.

George, S. L. et al. A reappraisal of the results of stopping therapy in childhood leukemia. *N. Engl. J. Med.* 300:269–273, 1979.

Goldberg, N. H. et al. Anaphylactoid-type reactions in two patients receiving high-dose intravenous methotrexate. *Cancer* 41:52–55, 1978.

Grindey, G. B. Clinical pharmacology of the 6-thiopurines. *Cancer Treat. Rev.* 6(suppl.):19–25, 1979.

Hall, S. W. et al. Pharmacokinetics and metabolism of ftorafur in man. *Proc. Am. Assoc. Cancer Res.* 17:128, 1976.

Hall, S. W.; Valdivieso, M.; and Benjamin, R. S. Intermittent high single-dose ftorafur. *Cancer Treat. Rep.* 61:1495–1498, 1977.

Handelsman, H., and Slavik, M. *Ftorafur (FT-207), NSC 148958.* Clinical brochure. Bethesda, Md.: National Cancer Institute, 1974.

Heidelberger, C. et al. Fluorinated pyrimidines, a new class of tumor-inhibitory compounds. *Nature* 179:663–666, 1957.

Heidelberger, C., and Ansfield, F. J. Experimental and clinical use of fluorinated pyrimidines in cancer chemotherapy. *Cancer Res.* 23:1226–1243, 1963.

Heinle, R. W., and Welch, A. D. Experiments with pteroylglutamine acid and pteroylglutamic acid deficiency in human leukemia (abstr.) *J. Clin. Invest.* 27:539, 1948.

Henderson, E. S., and Serpick, A. The effect of combination drug therapy and prophylactic antibiotic treatment in adult acute leukemia. *Clin. Res.* 15:336, 1967.

Higgins, G. E., Jr. et al. The case for adjuvant 5-fluorouracil in colorectal carcinoma. *Cancer Chemother. Trials* 1:35–41, 1978.

Hitchings, G. H., and Elion, G. B. The chemistry and biochemistry of purine analogues. *Ann. NY Acad. Sci.* 60:195–199, 1954.

Ho, D. H. W., and Frei, E., III. Clinical pharmacology of 1-B-D-arabinofuranosyl cytosine (Ara-C). *Clin. Pharmacol. Ther.* 12:944–954, 1971.

Horton, J. et al. 5-Fluorouracil in cancer: an improved regimen. *Ann. Intern. Med.* 73:897–900, 1970.

Huennekens, F. M. et al Antimetabolites in the chemotherapy of leukemia. *Exp. Cell Res.* 19(suppl.): 441–461, 1963.

Jaffe, N. et al. Favorable responses of metastatic osteogenic sarcoma to pulse high-dose methotrexate with citrovorum rescue and radiation therapy. *Cancer* 31: 1367–1373, 1973.

Kaufman, H. E. In vivo studies with antiviral agents. *Ann. NY Acad. Sci.* 130:168–180, 1965.

Kennedy, B. J. Hydroxyurea therapy in chronic myelogenous leukemia. *Cancer* 29:1052–1056, 1972.

Kremer, W. B. Cytarabine. *Ann. Intern. Med.* 82:684–688, 1975.

Legha, S. S. et al. *Hexamethylmelamine (NSC 13875).* Clinical brochure. Bethesda, Md.: National Cancer Institute, 1974.

Legha, S. S., and Slavik, M. *Baker's antifol (NSC 139105).* Clinical brochure. Bethesda, Md.: National Cancer Institute, 1975.

Legha, S. S.; Slavik, M.; and Carter, S. K. Hexamethylmelamine: an evaluation of its role in the therapy of cancer. *Cancer* 38:27–35, 1976.

LePage, G. A., and Whitecar, J. P., Jr. Pharmacology of 6-thioguanine in man. *Cancer Res.* 31:1627–1631, 1971.

Lerner, H. J.; Beckloff, G. L.; and Godwin, M. C. Hydroxyurea (NSC 32065) intermittent therapy in malignant diseases. *Cancer Chemother. Rep.* 53: 385–395, 1969.

Lewis, J. L., Jr. Chemotherapy of gestational choriocarcinoma. *Cancer* 30:1517–1521, 1972.

Li, M. C.; Hertz, R.; and Spencer, D. B. Effect of methotrexate upon choriocarcinoma and chorioadenoma. *Proc. Soc. Exp. Biol. Med.* 93:361–366, 1956.

Loo, T. L. et al. Clinical pharmacologic observations on 6-mercaptopurine and 6-methylmercaptopurine riboside. *Clin. Pharmacol. Ther.* 9:180–194, 1968.

Louis, J. et al. The clinical pharmacology of hexamethylmelamine: a phase I study. *Clin. Pharmacol. Ther.* 8:55–64, 1967.

McCreary, R. H. et al. A phase II study of triazinate (NSC 139105) in advanced colorectal carcinoma. *Cancer* 40:9–13, 1977.

Mitchell, M. S. et al. Immunosuppressive effects of cytosine arabinoside and methotrexate in man. *Ann. Intern. Med.* 70:535–547, 1969.

Moore, G. E. et al. Effects of 6-mercaptopurine (NSC 755) in 290 patients with advanced cancer. *Cancer Chemother. Rep.* 52:655–660, 1968.

Muggia, F. M., and Louie, A. C. Five years of adjuvant treatment of osteosarcoma: more questions than answers. *Cancer Treat. Rep.* 62:301–305, 1978.

Myers, C. E. et al. Pharmacokinetics of the fluoropyrimidines: implications for their clinical use. *Cancer Treat. Rev.* 3:175–183, 1976.

Nathanson, L., and Hall, T. Phase II study of hydroxyurea (NSC 32065) in malignant melanoma. *Cancer Chemother. Rep.* 51:503–505, 1967.

Nelson, J. A. et al. Mechanism of action of 6-thioguanine, 6-mercaptopurine, and 8-azaguanine. *Cancer Res.* 35:2872–2878, 1975.

Oliverio, V. T., and Zubrod, C. G. Clinical pharmacology of the effective antitumor drugs. *Ann. Rev. Pharmacol.* 5:335–356, 1965.

Papac, R. J., and Calabresi, P. Infusion of floxuridine in the treatment of solid tumors. *JAMA* 197:237–241, 1966.

Parrillo, J. E.; Fauci, A. S.; and Wolff, S. M. Therapy of the hypereosinophilic syndrome. *Ann. Intern. Med.* 89:167–172, 1978.

Patterson, A. R. P., and Tidd, D. M. 6-Thiopurines. In *Antineoplastic and immunosuppressive agents. Handbook of experimental pharmacology,* vol. 38, part II, eds. A. C. Sartorelli and D. G. Johns. Berlin: Springer-Verlag, 1975.

Physicians' desk reference, 35th edition. Oradell, N.J.: Medical Economics Co., 1981, p. 1007.

Pitman, S .W., and Frei, E., III. Weekly methotrexate-calcium leucovorin rescue: effect of alkalinization on nephrotoxicity; pharmacokinetics in the CNS; and use in non-Hodgkin's lymphoma. *Cancer Treat. Rep.* 61:695–701, 1977.

Porter, R., and Wiltshaw, E. *Methotrexate in the treatment of cancer.* Bristol: John Wright & Sons, 1962.

Prusoff, W. H.; Bakhle, Y. S.; and Sekely, L. Cellular and antiviral effects of halogenated deoxyribonucleosides. *Ann. NY Acad. Sci.* 130:135–150, 1965.

Rhoads, C. P., ed. Conference on 6-mercaptopurine. *Ann. NY Acad. Sci.* 60:183–508, 1954.

Rodriguez, V. et al. Phase I studies with Baker's antifol (BAF) (NSC 139105). *Cancer* 38:690–694, 1976.

Rodriguez, V.; Richman, S.; and Benjamin, R. Phase II study with Baker's antifol in solid tumors. *Cancer Res.* 37:980–983, 1977.

Saiki, J. K. et al. 5-Azacytidine in acute leukemia. *Cancer* 42:2111–2114, 1978.

Seeger, D. R. et al. Analogs of pteroylglutamic acid. III. 4-amino derivatives. *J. Am. Chem. Soc.* 71:1753–1758, 1949.

Seeger, D. R.; Smith, J. M., Jr.; and Hultquist, M. E. Antagonist for pteroylglutamic acid. *J. Am. Chem. Soc.* 69:2567–2569, 1947.

Shapiro, W. R.; Mehta, B. M.; and Hutchison, D. J., eds. Proceedings of the workshop on antimetabolites and the central nervous system. *Cancer Treat. Rep.* 61:505–757, 1977.

Shapiro, W. R.; Young, D. F.; and Mehta, B. M. Methotrexate: distribution in cerebrospinal fluid after intravenous, ventricular, and lumbar injections. *N. Engl. J. Med.* 293:161–166, 1975.

Shullenberger, C. Phase II studies of hydroxyurea in adults: leukemia. *Cancer Chemother. Rep.* 40:49–50, 1964.

Sitar, D. S. et al. Disposition of 5-fluorouracil after intravenous bolus doses of a commercial formulation to cancer patients. *Cancer Res.* 37:3981–3984, 1977.

Skeel, R. T. et al. The basis for the disparate sensitivity of L 1210 leukemia and Walker 256 carcinoma to a new triazine folate antagonist. *Cancer Res.* 33:2972–2976, 1973.

Skeel, R. T. et al. Clinical and pharmacological evaluation of triazinate in humans. *Cancer Res.* 36:48–54, 1976.

Skeel, R. T. et al. Cyclophosphamide, cytosine arabinoside, and methotrexate versus cytosine arabinoside and thioguanine for acute non-lymphocytic leukemia in adults. *Cancer* 45:224–231, 1980.

Smart, C. et al. Phase I study of ftorafur, an analogue of 5-fluorouracil. *Cancer* 36:103–106, 1975.

Smith, J. P., and Rutledge, F. N. Random study of hexamethylmelamine, 5-fluorouracil, and melphalan in the treatment of advanced carcinoma of the ovary. *Natl. Cancer Inst. Monogr.* 42:169–172, 1975.

Sostman, H. D. et al. Methotrexate-induced pneumonitis. *Medicine* 55:67–84, 1978.

Southwest Oncology Group. Cytarabine for acute leukemia in adults; effects of schedule on the therapeutic response. *Arch. Intern. Med.* 133:251–259, 1974.

Spiers, A. S. D. Chronic granulocytic leukemia: practical aspects of diagnosis and management. *Am. Soc. Hemat. Educ. Program* 22:21–26, 1979.

Stoller, R. G. et al. Use of plasma pharmacokinetics to predict and prevent methotrexate toxicity. *N. Engl. J. Med.* 297:630–634, 1977.

Sweet, D. L. et al. Cyclophosphamide, vincristine, methotrexate with leucovorin rescue, and cytarabine (COMLA) combination sequential chemotherapy for advanced diffuse histiocytic lymphoma. *Ann. Intern. Med.* 92:785–790, 1980.

Thurman, W. et al. A phase I study of hydroxyurea. *Cancer Chemother. Rep.* 29:103–107, 1963.

Vogler, W.; Miller, D. S.; and Keller, J. W. 5-Azacytidine (NSC 102816): a new drug for treatment of myeloblastic leukemia. *Blood* 48:331–337, 1976.

Von Hoff, D. D. et al. Incidence of drug-related deaths secondary to high-dose methotrexate and citrovorum factor administration. *Cancer Treat. Rep.* 61:745–748, 1977.

Von Hoff, D. D.; Handelsman, H.; and Slavik, M. *5-Azacytidine (NSC 102816).* Clinical brochure. Bethesda, Md.: National Cancer Institute, 1975.

Von Hoff, D. D.; Slavik, M.; and Muggia, F. M. 5-Azacytidine. *Ann. Intern. Med.* 85:237–245, 1976.

Wampler, G. L. et al. Hexamethylmelamine (NSC 13875) in the treatment of advanced cancer. *Cancer Chemother. Rep.* 56:505–514, 1972.

Wang, J. J., and Pratt, C. B. Intrathecal arabinosyl cytosine in meningeal leukemia. *Cancer* 25:531–534, 1970.

Weinstein, G. D. Drugs five years later: methotrexate. *Ann. Intern. Med.* 86:199–204, 1977.

Weiss, A. J. et al. Phase II study of azacytidine in solid tumors. *Cancer Treat. Rep.* 61:55–58, 1977.

Welch, A. D. Some mechanisms involved in selective chemotherapy. *Ann. NY Acad. Sci.* 123:19–41, 1965.

Wiernik, P. H. et al. Randomized clinical comparison of daunorubicin (NSC 82151) alone with a combination of daunorubicin, cytosine arabinoside (NSC 63878), 6-thioguanine (NSC 752), and pyrimethamine (NSC 3061) for the treatment of acute nonlymphocytic leukemia. *Cancer Treat. Rep.* 60:41–53, 1976.

Wilson, W. L. et al. Phase II study of hexamethylmelamine (NSC 13875). *Cancer* 23:132–136, 1969.

Wilson, W. L., and de la Garza, J. G. Phase I study of hexamethylmelamine (NSC 13875). *Cancer Chemother. Rep.* 48:49–52, 1965.

Woods, D. D. The relation of p-aminobenzoic acid to the mechanism of action of sulfanilamide. *Br. J. Exp. Pathol.* 21:74–90, 1940.

Yarbro, J. W. Further studies on the mechanisms of action of hydroxyurea. *Cancer Res.* 28:1082–1087, 1968.

Yates, J. W. et al. Cytosine arabinoside (NSC 63878) and daunorubicin (NSC 82151) therapy in acute nonlymphocytic leukemia. *Cancer Chemother. Rep.* 57:485–488, 1973.

Young, R. C. et al. Advanced ovarian adenocarcinoma: a prospective clinical trial of melphalan (L-PAM) versus combination chemotherapy. *N. Engl. J. Med.* 299:1261–1266, 1978.

twenty-five

Antitumor Antibiotics

DAVID S. FISCHER

The antitumor antibiotics are a heterogeneous group whose common denominator is their microbial origin and an ability to inhibit the growth of animal tumor cells. Many hundreds have been isolated, purified, and tested, but only six are marketed. At present, many are being actively investigated, but only two in this stage of development merit discussion at this time. The mechanisms of action are diverse, ranging from those of alkylating agents to antimetabolites, from S–phase-specific agents to noncycle-specific agents.

The first antibiotic shown to be a useful anticancer agent was actinomycin D, now generically dactinomycin. It was isolated from *Streptomyces parvullus* by Waksman and Woodruff (1940) as part of a systematic search for antituberculous agents. Because it was not active against tuberculosis, it was neglected for almost a decade before it was "rediscovered" as an antitumor agent. When that did happen, it served as an example for the subsequent development of additional antitumor antibiotics (Waksman 1960). In addition, the elucidation of its mechanism of action, inhibition of DNA-directed RNA synthesis, served as a key to unlock many of the secrets of molecular biology.

It is interesting that only two of the six antitumor antibiotics commercially available—dactinomycin and mithramycin—were isolated and developed in the United States. Daunorubicin and doxorubicin come from Italy and mitomycin and bleomycin from Japan (as does zinostatin).

An additional antitumor antibiotic, streptozocin, remains investigational but promising. We have already discussed it with the nitrosoureas because its behavior and mechanism of action follow the pattern of those agents.

Dactinomycin

Dactinomycin (actinomycin D, Cosmegen, NSC 3053) was the first antitumor antibiotic (fig. 25.1). It inhibits both DNA-dependent (so-called messenger) RNA polymerase and DNA-dependent DNA polymerase. In addition, it apparently binds to the guanine moieties of DNA, and thus further inhibits RNA and DNA synthesis, and hormonal pathways (Samuels 1964).

The drug is poorly absorbed after oral administration and is therefore given intravenously. It is cleared from the plasma rapidly, and very little is detected there two minutes after injection. About 50% to 90% is excreted unchanged in the bile and 10% to 20% in the urine. There is little metabolism of the drug, and it does not cross the blood-brain barrier.

The drug has a wide spectrum of usefulness. In childhood Wilms' tumor the addition of dactinomycin to surgery and radiation has more than doubled response and long-term survival rates (Farber et al. 1960) to the point that we can predict a very respectable number of cures with these combined modalities (Meienhofer and Frei 1974). Alone and in combination it has proved curative in a large majority of cases of gestational trophoblastic neoplasms, and has been used both in methotrexate failures and also as a first-line drug (Goldstein, Winig, and Shirley 1972; Osathanondh, Goldstein, and Pastorfide 1975). For a time, it was the key in a three-drug combination for testicular carcinoma (Li, Whitmore, and Golbey 1960). It has since been preempted by more active drugs, although it is still used in the highly successful VAB III and VAB IV regimens of the Memorial Sloan–Kettering Medical Center (Golbey, Reynolds, and Vurgrin 1979). It is also used in combination chemotherapy of childhood rhabdomyosarcoma, neuroblastoma, and retinoblastoma (Wilbur et al. 1975). In adults, it has demonstrated some efficacy in combination therapy of Ewing's, Kaposi's, and other soft tissue sarcomas (Gottlieb et al. 1975; Jaffe et al. 1976). It is being tried in melanoma.

Dactinomycin appears to be synergistic with radiation, probably because of interference by the drug with the repair of DNA damage induced by radiation (Pearson et al. 1978). While this may be helpful in some instances, it poses problems of serious toxicity for combined modality therapy and for anamnestic toxicity, and requires some dosage reduction. Other major toxicity is hematologic and gastrointestinal. Bone marrow depression occurs two to seven days after completion of therapy. Thrombocytopenia is often seen two to four days after treatment, and leukopenia is noted perhaps a day later. The latter tends to be more severe, is dose-limiting, and may last for two weeks. Anorexia, nausea, and vomiting usually occur within a few hours after injection and may be very severe (Philips et al. 1960). Antiemetics often ameliorate the vomiting, but with some patients it is so violent that they discontinue therapy with this drug. Other problems include stomatitis, cheilitis, glossitis, proctitis, diarrhea, and occasional alopecia and acne. Cutaneous erythema, desquamation, and hyperpigmentation are seen especially in previously irradiated areas.

Dactinomycin is an irritant and therefore should be administered through a rapidly running IV. The drug is available as Cosmegen (Merck Sharp & Dohme) in 0.5-mg vials of a yellow lyophilized powder that is reconstituted with 1.1 ml of sterile water without preservative (any other solvent may cause precipitation). For combination therapy, the original protocol should be consulted. For single-agent use the common dosage is 0.3 to 0.5 mg/m^2 IV for five consecutive days once a month, or 0.5 mg/m^2 IV weekly. Additional drug may be given if there is no toxicity, which is rare. If there is hepatic (or a question of renal) impairment, the dosage should be reduced. No more than 2 mg can be given as a single bolus dose because of severe nausea and vomiting. Children are sometimes given daily doses for 10 to 14 days. Although the reconstituted drug is stable for a week, any unused amounts should be discarded after one day because it lacks preservative and may undergo bacterial contamination.

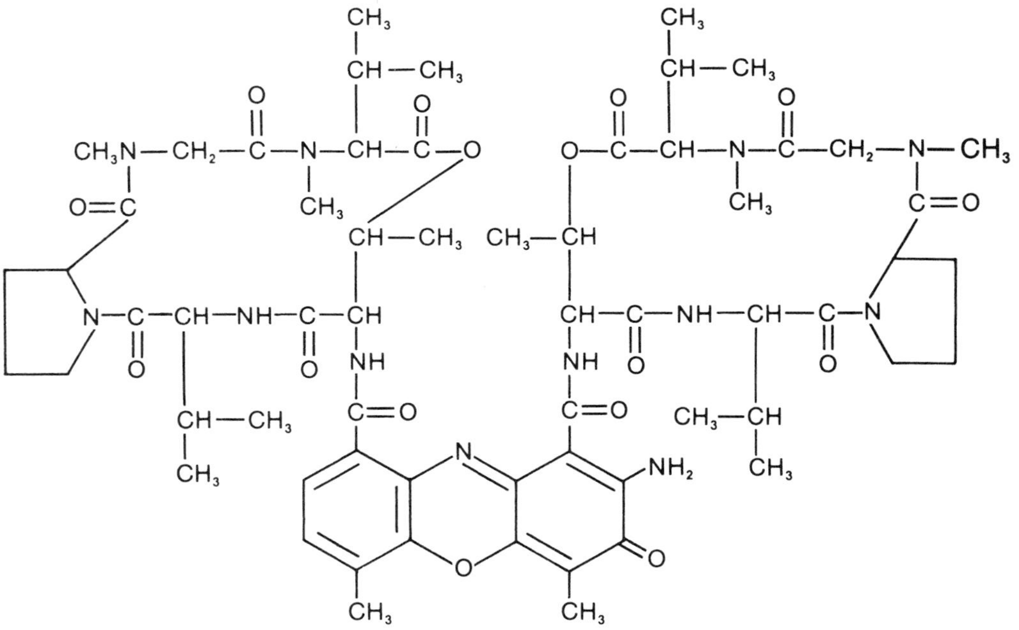

Fig. 25.1. *Dactinomycin, NSC 3053*

Mitomycin

Mitomycin (Mutamycin, mitomycin C, NSC 26980) is an antibiotic isolated in Japan in 1956 from *Streptomyces caespitosus* (Carter and Crooke 1979) as blue-violet crystals (fig. 25.2). Actually, what we generically call mitomycin is really mitomycin C, as two structurally related compounds were isolated earlier and called mitomycin A and B respectively. They are more toxic, however, and were never developed for human use. The N-methyl homologue of mitomycin C was discovered in 1960 by a group at the Upjohn Company and called porfiromycin. It was less toxic and underwent phase I clinical trials, but proved to be less effective than mitomycin C, and was not marketed. Although the Japanese had reported good results with mitomycin C and were using it extensively in clinical practice by 1960 (Carter 1968), an American study in 1959 was disappointing. The drug was neglected for another decade in this country when it was finally introduced clinically by Bristol Laboratories in 1974 (Crooke and Bradner 1976b).

Mitomycin is activated in vivo by intracellular reductases and then functions as a potent alkylating agent and induces interstrand and intrastrand cross-links in DNA in relation to guanine and cytosine. In addition, it has been shown to degrade DNA, to inhibit DNA synthesis, and to prevent the unwinding of the DNA double helix. It is most effective during the late G_1 and S phases of the cell cycle.

After oral administration mitomycin is absorbed erratically. It is reported to be absorbed after intrapleural and intraperitoneal administration, but not after intravesical instillation. After intravenous injection the drug is cleared rapidly from the blood with half-life values ranging from 9 to 17 minutes. About 10% is recovered in the urine in 24 hours after usual doses.

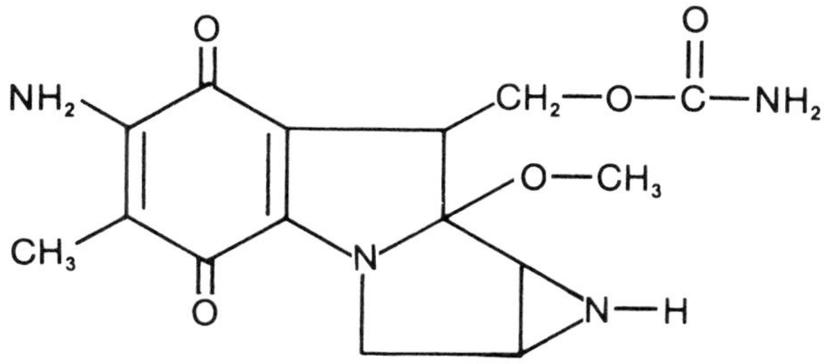

Fig. 25.2. *Mitomycin, NSC 26980*

Most of the drug is metabolized in the liver. Few additional pharmacokinetic data are available.

As a single agent, mitomycin is effective against adenocarcinoma of the stomach, biliary tree, liver, colon, pancreas, ovary, and breast, squamous cell carcinoma of the cervix, lung, head, and neck, and melanoma. Intravesically administered mitomycin is reported to be highly effective against superficial transitional cell carcinomas of the bladder. Complete response rates in phase I and II evaluations appeared to be dose-related (Carter and Crooke 1979). Doses of 25 mg instilled intravesically every week for eight weeks resulted in a complete remission rate of 67% with no absorption, no systemic toxicities, and no significant local toxicities (Crooke, Johnson, and Bracken 1978). Pediatric indications for mitomycin were recently reviewed (Gutierrez and Crooke 1979).

Combination chemotherapy is undergoing active investigation with encouraging results in breast, gastrointestinal, and uterine cervix tumors using MA (mitomycin-Adriamycin), FAM (5-fluorouracil, Adriamycin, and mitomycin), MOB (mitomycin, Oncovin, and bleomycin), and VAM (vinblastine, Adriamycin and mitomycin).

The principal dose-limiting toxicity of mitomycin is delayed cumulative myelosuppresion. The nadirs of leukopenia and thrombocytopenia are typically reached more than 28 days after a single dose. Toxicity is so cumulative that in many regimens an automatic dose reduction is employed after two full doses. Leukopenia persists for one or two weeks and thrombocytopenia for two or three weeks. The blood count recovers in most patients within eight weeks; however, in about 25% of patients it never returns to normal levels. Cumulative toxicity is seen with each subsequent course. A microangiopathic hemolytic anemia has been noted in patients treated with mitomycin and 5-FU and is probably the result of mitomycin (Gulati et al. 1980).

Other toxicity includes malaise, anorexia, nausea, and vomiting in almost all patients. The nausea and vomiting usually begin one to two hours after treatment; vomiting may persist for three to four hours, with nausea sometimes lasting two or three days. Antiemetics are often helpful, and attention to adequate hydration is important. An unusual but well-documented toxicity is a form of glomerular sclerosis that may occur after several months of therapy in about 2% of patients (Liu et al. 1971). It does not appear to be dose-related and is manifested by a rising level of BUN and serum creatinine. Rare abnormalities in liver function tests have been noted. Cardiac toxicity with doxorubicin may be synergistic (Buzdar et al. 1978).

An originally rare toxicity but one that is being recognized with increasing frequency is interstitial pneumonitis and alveolitis (Buzdar et al. 1980; Orwell, Kiessling, and Patterson 1978). The 15 patients reviewed recently (Weiss and Muggia 1980) all had symptoms of progressive dyspnea and nonproductive cough. Pulmonary function studies showed hypoxia and diffusion abnormalities. Seven patients had some improvement during steroid therapy but five died of pulmonary insufficiency. These patients should not be exposed to inspired oxygen concentration greater than 50% unless absolutely necessary, because it appears to exert a synergistic toxicity.

Minor toxicities include rash, stomatitis, fever, drowsiness, diarrhea, and alopecia. Extravasation may lead to cellulitis, ulceration, and sloughing of the involved tissue.

Dosage has varied widely (Carter and Crooke 1979). Early schedules called for 2 mg/m^2 daily for five days, followed by a drug-free interval of two days, and then 2 mg/m^2 daily for five more days (total dose 20 mg/m^2 over 12 days). An alternate schedule is 10 to 20 mg/m^2 every six to eight weeks. Doses greater than 20 mg/m^2 are more toxic but no more effective. Subsequent doses should not be given until the white blood cell count has returned to 3000 and the platelet count to 75,000. The dose of mitomycin must be reduced appropriately, and the protocol in the original or follow-up publications should be consulted before using this potent and dangerous drug in combination chemotherapy.

The drug is available as Mutamycin (Bristol) as a lyophilized blue-violet powder in 5-mg and 20-mg vials. It is reconstituted with sterile water for injection and administered through a rapidly running IV of 5% dextrose in water or normal saline. As a powder, it is stable for two years at room temperature. Reconstituted it is stable for 7 days at room temperature and 14 days in the refrigerator.

Mithramycin

Mithramycin (Mithracin, NSC 24559) is a yellow crystalline antibiotic produced by *Streptomyces plicatus* (fig. 25.3). It is interesting that it was active against only one of the animal tumors used for screening and was almost discarded without clinical trials (Carter and Friedman 1970). It is structurally closely related to chromomycin A_3 discovered in Japan, and olivomycin discovered in the Soviet Union, with minor differences in the structure of the sugar components (Legha, Slavik, and Carter 1975). The mechanism of action of mithramycin has not been precisely defined but is believed to involve initial binding to divalent magnesium ions, resulting in a complex with the capacity to bind to the guanine residues of DNA in such a manner as to obstruct the function of RNA polymerase in the minor groove of the DNA helix. It is cell cycle-specific for the S phase. The effect on calcium is thought to be due to a direct effect on osteoclasts, thereby blocking bone resorption and possibly also blocking parathyroid hormone production, leading to a fall in plasma calcium.

Mithramycin is minimally active orally and is given intravenously. About 25% of the radioactively-labeled drug is excreted in the urine in 2 hours and 40% in 15 hours. Levels in the CSF approach those of the plasma in four to six hours. Little more is known about its pharmacokinetics.

The major antineoplastic indication at present is in the treatment of embryonal cell carcinoma of the testis (Kennedy 1970b), and even there the drug has been supplanted by superior agents given in combination. There have been some indications of activity in glioblastoma multiforme, but they have not been explored very extensively.

Most of the mithramycin used at this time is for treatment of the hypercalcemia of malignancy (Mazzaferri, O'Dorisio, and LoBuglio 1978), for which it is usually quite effective as a single 900-μg/m^2 dose. It has also been used in the treatment of Paget's disease of

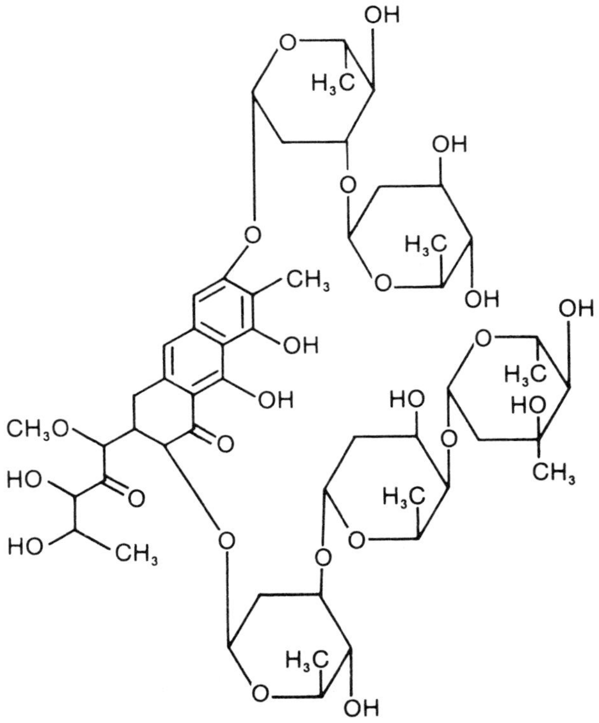

Fig. 25.3. *Mithramycin, NSC 24559*

bone to diminish the elevated osteoclast activity, particularly in symptomatic cases refractory to other treatment modalities (Lebbin, Ryan, and Schwartz 1974; Ryan 1977).

Toxicity is to a considerable extent dose-related. In early studies (Kennedy 1970a) the drug was given in a daily schedule for 10 days, and hemorrhagic diathesis was common. Epistaxis was frequently the first sign, but hematemesis could be first. Although a low platelet count was frequently noted, abnormalities of plasma protein coagulation factors caused by liver impairment were the major signs. Modification of the treatment schedule to every other day has greatly diminished the incidence of coagulation problems. Still, when using the drug as an anticancer agent, careful monitoring of platelet count, prothrombin time, and partial thromboplastin time (PTT) is necessary. In addition to thrombocytopenia, which may be rapid in onset (Ahr et al. 1978), leukopenia is also seen but much less frequently.

Anorexia, nausea, and vomiting are quite common and begin 1 or 2 hours after therapy and may persist for 12 to 24 hours. Antiemetics may help if given before the drug and repeated at intervals. Gastrointestinal toxicity is decreased by infusing the drug over four to six hours as recommended in the product brochure. Most clinicians at our hospital give it over 15 to 60 minutes to minimize the potential for drug infiltration, which can lead to local tissue irritation and cellulitis.

Hepatic and renal toxicity are fairly common and one should watch for a rise in SGOT, lactic dehydrogenase, and BUN. The drug is contraindicated in patients with underlying significant hepatic or renal disease, as it then may lead to severe impairment of production of coagulation in proteins with clinical bleeding. Azotemia is also an occasional complication.

Other side effects include facial flushing (an indication to discontinue the drug), stomatitis, headache, fever, depression, drowsiness, diarrhea, confusion, rash, pigmentation, epistaxis, and delirium.

Dosage is critical to minimize toxicity. For testicular embryonal carcinoma, 0.025 to 0.050 mg/kg is given intravenously on alternate days for three to eight doses unless toxicity develops sooner. For treatment of hypercalcemia, 0.015 to 0.025 mg/kg is used as a single dose in 100 to 150 ml of 5% dextrose in water over 15 to 60 minutes in a good vein. Response may take 24 to 48 hours, and therapy should not be repeated before this.

The drug is available as Mithracin (Pfizer) in 2.5-mg vials as a lyophilized powder that is reconstituted with 4.9 ml sterile water for injection. Unused reconstituted drug should be discarded.

Daunorubicin

Daunorubicin (Cerubidine, daunomycin, rubidomycin, NSC 82151) is an antitumor antibiotic isolated in Italy from *Streptomyces peucetius* (fig. 25.4). The red crystalline powder is an anthracycline glycoside that forms a stable complex with DNA by intercalation between base pairs and inhibits RNA synthesis by template disordering and steric obstruction (Livingston and Carter 1970). It is cell cycle specific.

Oral absorption is poor and usually leads to breakdown of the compound. After intravenous injection it is cleared rapidly from the plasma with a half-life of 45 minutes. It is metabolized in the liver but also has some enterohepatic circulation, as it is excreted in the bile and has a second plasma peak. The cumulative five-day urine excretion is only about 20%. It does not cross the blood-brain barrier.

Although daunorubicin has been used experimentally with some response in acute lymphocytic leukemia, neuroblastoma, and non-Hodgkin's lymphoma, its only currently recommended use is in the treatment of adult acute non-lymphocytic leukemia (ANLL—myelogenous, monocytic, and erythroid) (Boiron et al. 1969; Cassileth and Katz 1977; Gale 1979). In this disease it has achieved complete remission rates of 40% to 50% used alone, and 53% to 65% when combined with cytarabine. In a three-drug combination with cytarabine and 6-thioguanine, a 79% complete remission rate was achieved (Gale and Cline 1977; Wiernik et al. 1976). It should be clear that therapy is pushed to almost total aplasia of the bone marrow, so this is a "brinksmanship" type of treatment. Thus it can only be done in a hospital with facilities for platelet and leukocyte transfusion, multiple-drug antibiotic therapy, and reverse isolation to carry the patient through the hazard-

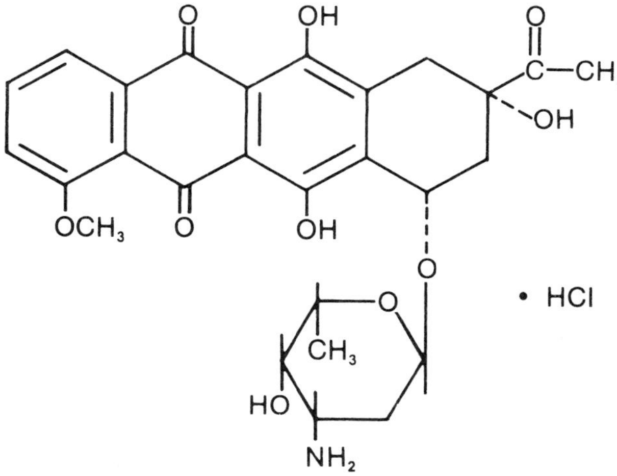

O OH O C—CH_3 OH OCH_3 O OH O O • HCl CH_3 HO NH_2

Fig. 25.4. *Daunorubicin, NSC 82151*

ous period of thrombocytopenia and neutropenia. Even in expert hands, these inductions have an incidence of drug-related mortality that can be minimized with careful supervision by an experienced oncology team. In childhood acute lymphocytic leukemia, daunorubicin has been used with prednisone (Holten et al. 1969) and more recently with both prednisone and vincristine.

The two major dose-limiting toxicities are myelosuppression and cardiotoxicity. Leukopenia is more severe than thrombocytopenia, but both are predictably very severe and may last several weeks until partial or complete remission is achieved, if it occurs. Therapy should be performed cautiously if at all in patients with marrow damage from any cause, but especially from prior radiation therapy or cytotoxic chemotherapy.

Cardiotoxicity is a clear danger in patients with preexisting heart disease, prior doxorubicin therapy, or radiation therapy to the heart. At total cumulative doses of less than 550 mg/m^2 acute congestive heart failure is seldom encountered, but rare instances of pericarditis-myocarditis, not dose-related, have been reported (Von Hoff et al. 1977). As the cumulative dose increases above 550 mg/m^2 the incidence of drug-induced congestive heart failure increases proportionally. It has been recommended that patients who have had radiation therapy that included part or all of the heart not exceed 400 mg/m^2 cumulative dose. Although there is no reliable method for predicting acute congestive heart failure, warning signs help to recognize patients at greatest risk. We have found two tests to be particularly useful. On the standard electrocardiogram (EKG) a decrease equal to or greater than 30% in limb lead QRS voltage has been associated with a significant risk of drug-associated cardiomyopathy. We do an EKG before each course of therapy. We have also been impressed with the value of measuring the left ventricular ejection fraction (LVEF) as described by Alexander and associates (1979) either before or after the first course and again at any time there is doubt about the safety of another dose, usually as one approaches the previously enumerated limiting dosages. The LVEF is much simpler and less traumatic than the left ventricular myocardial biopsies advocated by some, and at least as reliable. It helps in estimating the risk-benefit ratio of therapy. Studies of vitamin E, an antioxidant, to diminish cardiac toxicity are in progress now.

Since the drug is largely metabolized in the liver, hepatic function should be checked before administration. If the serum bilirubin is greater than 1.2 mg/dl the dose should be reduced by 50%, and if greater than 3.0 mg/dl the dose should be reduced by 75% or omitted. Renal function should also be checked because there is some renal excretion. Patients should be warned that their urine may be red for one or two days as the drug is excreted.

Nausea and vomiting are common but usually mild. Alopecia occurs in about 80% of patients with sudden onset in three or four weeks. We have attempted to reduce its severity by applying a scalp tourniquet and an ice pack while the drug is being injected and for a few minutes afterward, with variable success. The hair ultimately grows back but is sometimes a different color or consistency. Febrile reactions may occur. Stomatitis typically begins as a burning sensation with erythema of the oral mucosa leading to ulceration in two or three days.

Extravasation can cause local tissue necrosis that initially may or may not be painful. Later, swelling and erythema become prominent, and if the dose was large, skin sloughing may occur with necrosis of underlying muscles and tendons. Eventually, plastic surgery may be necessary to preserve limb function. The entire situation is best avoided by giving the drug only through a rapidly running intravenous in a good vein under careful supervision. Veins in the extremities with poor venous or lymphatic drainage should be avoided. If infiltration occurs or is suspected, infusion should be stopped and the area infiltrated with 5 ml of 8.4% sodium bicarbonate followed by 4 mg of dexamethasone. Early plastic surgery consultation is recommended, as an extravasation ulcer can progress for weeks. Early wide excision of all inflamed, involved tissue should be considered.

Usual single-agent dosage is 30 to 60 mg/m^2 daily for three consecutive days every three to six weeks. When used in combination with cytarabine with or without 6-thioguanine, the doses are modified according to the protocol being used.

The drug is available as Cerubidine (Ives) in 20-mg vials of lyophilized powder that should be reconstituted with 10 ml of sterile water for injection. Reconstituted material not used within six hours should be discarded.

Doxorubicin

Doxorubicin (Adriamycin, 14-Hydroxydaunorubicin, NSC 123127) is an antitumor antibiotic isolated in Italy from *Streptomyces peucetius*, variant *caesius* (fig. 25.5). The red crystalline powder is an anthracycline glycoside that differs from daunorubicin only by the presence of a hydroxyl group in the carbon-14 position. Its mechanism of action is essentially the same—formation of stable complexes with DNA by intercalation between base pairs, and inhibition of RNA synthesis by template disordering and steric obstruction. It does not inhibit single-stranded DNA. Chromosome breaks and gaps have been found, and scission of strands of DNA by the drug has been noted. It appears to be cell cycle-specific. In spite of its near identical structure and mechanism of action, doxorubicin has one of the broadest ranges of activity compared to the narrow spectrum of daunorubicin.

Oral absorption is poor. When the drug is given intravenously it (or its fluorescent metabolites) has a plasma half-life of about one to one and a half hours and a secondary phase of 14 to 20 hours. Urinary excretion ranges from 3% to 40% (mean 12%) in the first 72 hours. Metabolism is primarily in the liver, and about 40% of the drug can be recovered in the bile or feces in a week (Lee et al. 1980). Hence hepatic impairment can potentially lead to slower metabolism and a build-up of high blood levels if caution is not used to decrease the dose substantially. As a guide, we tend to reduce the dose by 50% if the serum bilirubin exceeds 1.2 mg/dl and, by 75% if greater than 3 mg/dl, if we give it at all. The drug does not cross the blood-brain barrier. Intra-arterial use of the drug is being evaluated (Shah, Baker, and Vaitkevicius 1977).

The indications for doxorubicin are as great as or greater than those for any other single chemotherapeutic antineoplastic agent (Blum and Carter 1974). It is the single best drug for carcinoma of the breast, and has been used alone (Creech, Catalano, and Shah 1980) and in combinations that may include 5-FU, cyclophosphamide, methotrexate, vincristine, vinblastine, mitomycin, dibromodulcitol, and/or a nitrosourea. Response rates in previously untreated disease usually exceed 50% (Hoogstraten and George 1974), and even after prior chemotherapy failures thay range from 18% to 52%.

In Hodgkin's disease, doxorubicin (Adriamycin) has been used in a four-drug regimen with bleomycin, vinblastine, and dacarbazine (ABVD) as an alternate noncross-reactive therapy for MOPP failures (Bonadonna et al. 1975). In poor-risk patients, we and others have been alternating MOPP with ABVD on a monthly basis in hopes of achieving a cure with tolerable therapy. In non-Hodgkin's lymphoma, especially of the large cell variety (formerly histiocytic), good responses have been obtained with combinations where doxorubicin (Adriamycin) is combined with bleomycin, cyclophosphamide, vincristine (Oncovin), and prednisone (BACOP) (Schein et al. 1976); with bleomycin, lomustine (CCNU), and vincristine (Oncovin) as BACO (Davis et al. 1977); or cyclophosphamide, hydroxydaunorubicin, vincristine (Oncovin), and prednisone as CHOP (McKelvey et al. 1976). It is probably the most active agent for thyroid carcinoma (Gottlieb and Hill 1975). In soft tissue sarcomas it is the cornerstone of most current combination regimens (Gottlieb et al. 1975). It has found an important place in regimens for lung cancer of all varieties, and even for mesothelioma. In urothelial cancers it has demonstrated some efficacy in bladder, prostate, and nonseminoma testicular cancers. It has been used in therapy of malignant salivary gland tumors, Ewing's sarcoma, neuroblastoma, and gastric, pancreatic, and ovarian carcinomas (Bachur, Benjamin, and Hall 1975).

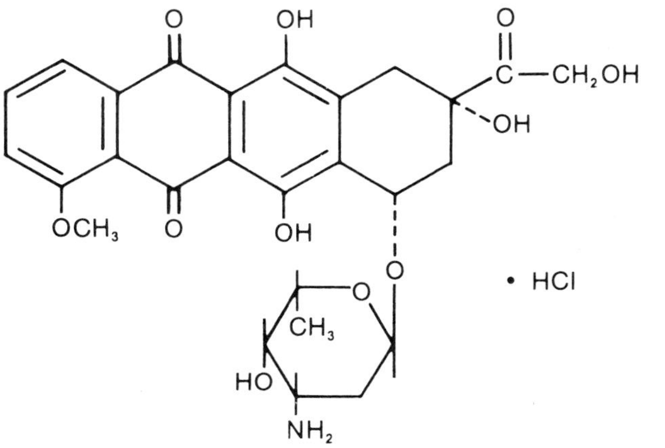

Hematologic neoplasms have been good responders. Although there is a general feeling that daunorubicin is superior to doxorubicin in acute leukemias of both the lymphocytic and non-lymphocytic types (Gale 1979), "head-to-head" comparison is only in progress now. In multiple myeloma doxorubicin is used in second-line therapy after primary drug failure (Presant and Klahr 1978).

Toxicity is severe (Praga et al. 1979) and in general is parallel or identical to that of daunorubicin (Gilladoga et al. 1976); the section on toxicity for that drug should be consulted. At one time the recommended maximum cumulative dose for patients who had previous radiotherapy to the heart or cyclophosphamide therapy was 450 mg/m^2 (Bachur, Benjamin, and Hall 1975). This has since been revised down to 400 mg/m^2 by the manufacturer to the same dose level as daunorubicin. The total cumulative dose for patients without antecedent heart disease and the two therapies just mentioned remains 550 mg/m^2 (Myers and McGuire 1978). In predicting cardiomyopathy, the manufacturer now raises doubts about the value of the reduction of voltage in the QRS EKG lead, the systolic time interval, and echocardiography (Lenaz and Page 1976). They grant that radionuclide angiography (Alexander et al. 1979) appears promising but awaits confirmation. They also caution that serious arrhythmias can occur with doxorubicin, including ventricular tachycardia or fib-

Fig. 25.5. *Doxorubicin, NSC 123127*

rillation, which can be fatal. The physician in charge of administration of this drug should be prepared to deal with arrhythmias, congestive heart failure, and hypotension (Von Hoff et al. 1979). Results of tests of vitamin E to decrease myocardial toxicity are eagerly awaited.

The manufacturer has recently paid more attention to the serious and increasingly common problem of extravasation which can produce ulceration and can damage skin, subcutaneous tissue and even tendons, nerves, and joints. Extravasation can occur with or without accompanying pain. If there is any suggestion that it has occurred, even if blood can still be aspirated, the injection should be stopped and a new intravenous site used. Veins in the extremities with poor venous or lymphatic drainage should be avoided since there is an increased chance for doxorubicin to leak along the side of the needle.

Several methods have been described for immediate treatment of the site of extravasation (Reilly, Neifeld, and Rosenberg 1977; Ignoffo and Friedman 1980). Infiltration with a corticosteroid followed by flooding with normal saline has been suggested. Although still to be confirmed, the method of Zweig and Kabakow (1978) appears effective if given early after the infiltration. It consists of infiltrating the area with 5 ml of 8.4% sodium bicarbonate followed by 4 mg of dexamethasone. Careful, frequent examination of any suspected extravasation, with a plastic surgery consultation, is recommended, as an ulcer can progress for weeks. Early wide excision of all inflamed, involved tissue should be considered.

A wide variety of dosage schedules have been tried for different indications (Blum and Carter 1974). As a single agent, the most widely used range is from 60 to 75 mg/m^2 every three weeks as a single IV push. Other schedules include 30 mg/m^2 on two or three consecutive days and repeated every three or four weeks. Still another option is 15 mg/m^2 every week, a schedule that has gained popularity recently because of reports of decreased cardiac toxicity. The objection is that each additional intravenous injection poses the danger of another chance for extravasation and its dire consequences.

Combination therapy has become increasingly popular, and doxorubicin has been used in a great many combinations (Bachur, Benjamin, and Hall 1975). For those dosages, consult chapter 29 on combination chemotherapy or the original publication.

The drug is available as Adriamycin (Adria) as a lyophilized powder in 10- and 50-mg vials. The recommendation for the use of bacteriostatic saline to reconstitute has been dropped, and the preferred agent is sterile water without preservative. The drug is more rapidly soluble in water than saline and is stable in the refrigerator for 48 hours. In view of the lack of bacteriostatic agent, however, the danger of microbial contamination is high after eight hours. The patient should be warned about the possibility of red urine for two days, which poses no danger.

Bleomycin

Bleomycin (Blenoxane, NSC 125066) is a group of 13 antitumor glycopeptides with the A_2 peptide representing more than 50% of the mixture (fig. 25.6). It is extracted from a strain of *Streptomyces verticillus*. The discovery of bleomycin and identification of its clinical activity are credited to Drs. Hamao Umezawa and Tokuji Ichikawa respectively (Rosenbaum and Carter 1970). Bleomycin binds to DNA, leading to single-strand breaks and double-stranded scissions (Crooke and Bradner 1976a). Cells are most sensitive during the G_2 and M phases of the cell cycle.

The drug is not orally active presumably because the peptide is hydrolyzed and digested before it can be absorbed. The intravenous drug is rapidly distributed throughout the body with highest concentrations in the skin, kidneys, lungs, and lymph nodes (Broughton et al. 1977). It is rapidly inactivated in all tissues except skin and lung, possibly explaining selective toxicity in those locations. Between 20% and 40% is excreted in the urine in 24 hours, and urinary concentration may exceed the relatively high plasma concentration. The drug tends to accumulate in some tumor tissues; bleomycin labeled with ^{99m}Tc has been relatively reliable as a marker in large, superficial tumors of the head and neck and lung, lymphomas, testicular tumors, brain tumors, and thyroid and breast cancer.

Bleomycin has been most successful in treatment of testicular tumors, lymphomas, uterine cervix carcinoma (Krakoff et al. 1977), and head and neck squamous cell carcinomas (Mosher, DeConti, and Bertino 1972). It has been used as a sclerosing agent in malignant hydrothorax and hydroperitoneum (Paladine et al. 1976), but more experience is needed. Intravesical therapy has been employed in recurrent superficial bladder tumors. Systemically, the drug is rarely used alone. Since it has little significant myelosuppressive activity it lends itself particularly well to combination chemotherapy with other agents that do.

Bleomycin has been particularly useful in a variety of regimens for treatment of testicular neoplasms (Golbey et al. 1979). Early experience was confined to embryonal cell carcinoma, but has since been broadened to several other histologic types. The drug is used in conjunction with vinblastine and cisplatin most of the time (Bosl et al. 1980), and frequently with cyclophosphamide, dactinomycin, chlorambucil, and doxorubicin (Golbey et al. 1979). Response rates of 60% to 80% are achieved in disease that is confined locally, and lesser responses in more widespread disease (Bennet and Reich 1979), including extragonadal germ cell tumors (Feun, Samson, and Stephens 1980).

In Hodgkin's disease, it has been incorporated in the noncross-resistant ABVD regimen, including doxorubicin (Adriamycin), bleomycin, vincristine, and dacarbazine for MOPP failures (Bonadonna et al. 1975). In cases with poor prognosis, ABVD and MOPP are alternated as primary therapy. In the non-Hodgkin's lymphomas bleomycin has been combined with doxorubicin (Adriamycin), cyclophosphamide, vincristine (Oncovin), and prednisone (BACOP) to produce response rates over 50% (Schein et al. 1976). It has also been used with doxorubicin (Adriamycin), lomustine (CCNU), mechlorethamine (nitrogen mustard) and vincristine (Oncovin) in the BACON regimen (Soper and Gott 1974), or with cyclophosphamide, doxorubicin (hydroxydaunorubicin), vincristine (Oncovin), and prednisone (CHOP-bleo).

In cervical carcinoma bleomycin has been used in combination with methotrexate or in combination with mitomycin and vincristine (Carter, Crooke, and Umezawa 1978). In head and neck tumors it has recently been combined with methotrexate and cisplatin (Caradonna et al. 1979).

The major life-threatening toxicity is pulmonary (Iacovino et al. 1976). Bleomycin is known to produce pulmonary pneumonitis (Holoye et al. 1978) and fibrosis in 10% to 40% of patients treated (Weiss and Muggia 1980). The incidence of this complication increases with cumulative dose; most clinicians watch for this very carefully after a total dose of 150 units, and stop therapy at 400 units. I generally stop therapy at 300 units and note an increasing trend among my colleagues to do the same. Toxicity is enhanced when radiation is used simultaneously or even sequentially (Carter, Crooke, and Umezawa 1978). Recently, it has been suggested that high oxygen concentrations in the inspired air often potentiate bleomycin fibrosis or pneumonitis (Weiss and Muggia 1980). To monitor for this toxicity, there has been a tendency to follow patients with pulmonary function tests, especially forced vital capacity and diffusing capacity for carbon monoxide; however, it has been suggested that these tests may be ineffective and potentially misleading (Lewis and Izbicki 1980). It must be remembered that complications can occur after very few doses and have been reported after as little as 75 units or less. Clinical examination may give the first clue to toxicity as one hears rales, rhonchi, and occasionally, a pleural friction rub. Later, x-ray changes develop. Pathologically, the lesions are most frequently seen in the lower lobes and consist of a

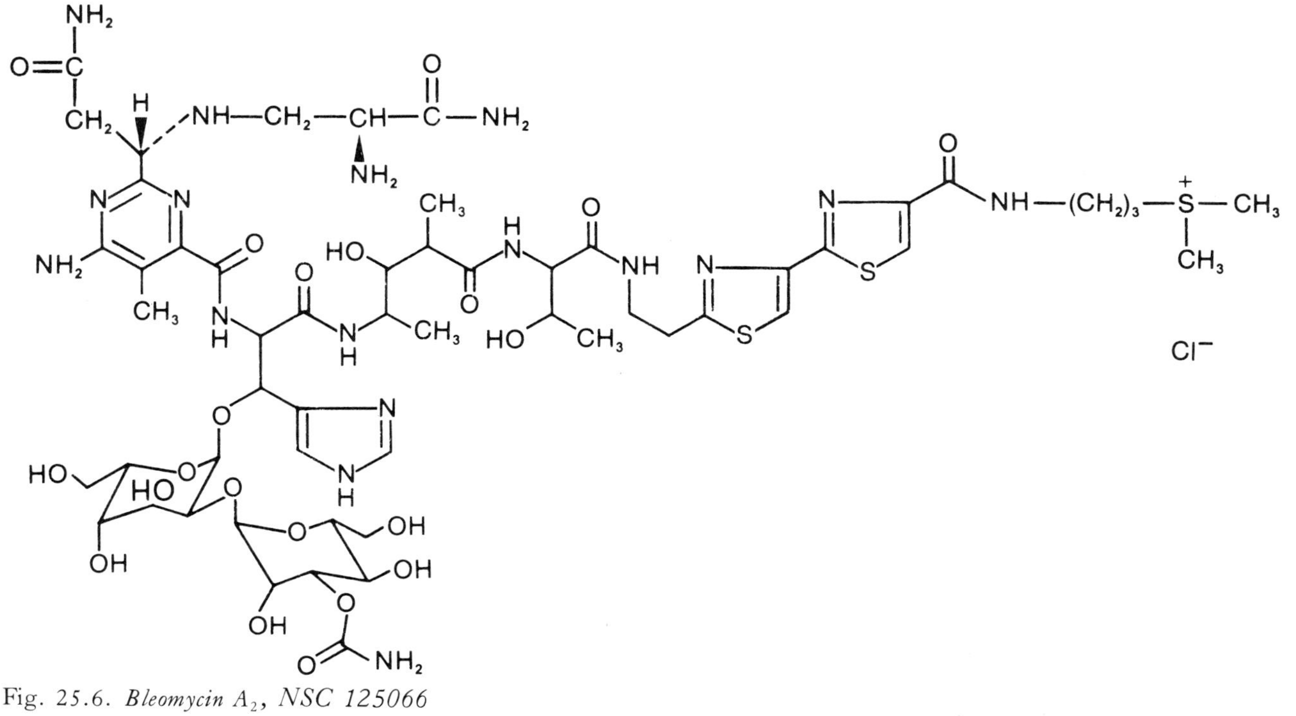

Fig. 25.6. *Bleomycin A_2, NSC 125066*

fibrinous exudate, atypical proliferation of alveolar cells, hyaline membranes, interstitial and intraalveolar fibrosis, and squamous metaplasia of the distal air spaces. Older patients are at greater risk than younger patients. The side effects may not show up for 10 to 12 weeks.

About 60% of patients have a febrile response (103° to 105° F) usually occurring 4 to 10 hours after drug administration; it may last for 48 hours. Rarely, in a patient with lymphoma the first dose of bleomycin may cause a fever to 106° to 107°, with hypotension, anaphylaxis, and death. I have seen three such reactions, but fortunately they did not end fatally. Most of us avoid this problem by giving bleomycin first as a test dose of 1 unit intravenously after premedication with oral acetaminophen and diphenhydramine, and observing for one hour before giving the remainder of the dose. Generally, patients receiving bleomycin are instructed to take acetaminophen and diphenhydramine every four hours for two or three doses after the drug is given.

About 50% of patients develop skin hyperpigmentation and hyperkeratosis on the palms and fingers. Skin tenderness and peeling, urticaria, pruritus, and rash occur in about 5%. Although these reactions can be so severe that the drug must be discontinued, they are rarely prolonged and cease soon after therapy is stopped.

Myelosuppression is rare. Nausea, vomiting, alopecia, lethargy, headache, joint swelling and pain, and a bad taste in the mouth have all been reported but are usually not dose-limiting.

The drug may be given subcutaneously (SC), intramuscularly (IM), IV, or intraarterially. When given SC or IM there may be local burning or pain at the injection site. Intravenous drug is given at the rate of 1 unit/min. Usual dosage is 10 to 20 units/m^2 once or twice a week. For protocols, see chapter 29 on combination chemotherapy or the original publication.

The drug was originally marketed as Blenoxane (Bristol) as a lyophilized powder in glass ampules of 15 units. It is now available as a lyophilized powder in vials of 15 units intended for single use. The drug, however, is chemically stable after reconstitution, and if sterility can be insured, may be used up to two weeks if kept at room temperature and up to four weeks if refrigerated. To prepare for injection of the entire 15 units, sterile normal saline is added as follows:

SC	0.5 ml
IM	1.5 ml
IV	5 ml (without preservative) to achieve a concentration of 3 units/ml

For the test dose, about 0.33 ml is given IV and washed in well. If there is no adverse reaction the rest of the dose is given. If small doses are to be given (for example two units or five units), then dilute to 5 ml with extreme care to maintain sterility and withdraw the necessary dose and save the remainder for use within two to four weeks depending on storage conditions.

Zinostatin (Investigational)

Zinostatin (Neocarzinostatin, NSC 157365) is a protein antibiotic first isolated and purified from *Streptomyces carzinostaticus,* variant *F47* by Ishida in Japan in 1965 (Legha et al. 1976). It is an acidic protein macromolecule with a molecular weight of 10,700. It is a single polypeptide chain of 109 amino acids cross-linked by two disulfide bridges. The amino acid sequence of zinostatin is shown in figure 25.7 (Meienhofer et al. 1972). It is stable in water but not in most organic solvents. It is sensitive to ultraviolet light and should be protected from it.

The mechanism of action appears to be selective inhibition of DNA synthesis with strand scission. In addition, it may exert a toxic effect on the cell by binding to receptors on the cell membrane. Activity seems to be predominantly in the G_2 phase of the cell cycle (Issell et al. 1979).

Oral administration is ineffective, as presumably the protein is digested. Following intravenous administration there is a biphasic plasma half-life of 3 to 9 minutes and 25 to 231 minutes. The longer elimination phase half-lives were found in patients with impaired creatinine clearances. Intact drug is excreted rapidly in the urine by glomerular filtration. There is no significant accumulation in pleural or peritoneal effusions, and bile excretion has not been demonstrated.

Although some activity has occurred in a few cases of hepatoma and other gastrointestinal cancers and bladder cancer (Natale et al. 1980; Sakamato et al. 1978), the major encouraging activity has been in acute leukemia (Griffin et al. 1978, 1979). In 58 patients who had failed on prior chemotherapy, there were four complete remissions. Among 18 previously untreated patients there were seven complete remissions (39%). Most responses were seen in acute myelomonocytic and monocytic leukemia. The effect was more pronounced on peripheral blood than marrow, suggesting that the drug is unlikely to be useful as a single agent but might be better in combination therapy of these diseases (Van Echo and Wiernik 1978).

As might be expected, myelosuppression is the dose-limiting toxicity in most studies, especially those using continuous infusion schedules (McKelvey et al. 1979). The white cell count usually starts to drop in 5 to

10 days and then recovers rapidly. About 30% of cases have prolonged leukopenia lasting more than four weeks. Thrombocytopenia is less common but recovery is a little later, usually about 20 days after treatment.

Another potential use-limiting toxicity is severe chills and fever sometimes associated with rigors. Onset is usually in one or two hours after administration. Since the drug is a foreign protein, it can be immunogenic. If a rash occurs, as it occasionally does, the drug should be discontinued to avoid hypotension and possible anaphylaxis. Nausea is common, usually without vomiting but with moderately severe anorexia. Mucositis is seen only with continuous infusion therapy. If the drug extravasates, it is very irritating. Slight hepatic toxicity has been noted, usually manifested by elevations of serum transaminase and only rarely by elevation of bilirubin and alkaline phosphatase.

Pulmonary toxicity has been reported (Weiss and Muggia 1980). In addition to the histologic changes of interstitial pneumonitis and fibrosis, there was also evidence of endothelial edema and endothelial cell hypertrophy of pulmonary vessels. It is thought that this may be due to an allergic reaction.

The drug is only given intravenously because the IM and SC routes are associated with local necrosis. Two types of IV schedules have been used, continuous and intermittent (McKelvey et al. 1979), the former allowing higher doses resulting in the same toxicity. In solid tumors, the drug is given continuously in doses of 3000 to 4500 units/m^2, or intermittently over 30 minutes in doses of 2250 to 3600 units/m^2 for five consecutive days. In acute leukemia higher doses are tolerated, and 6500 to 12,000 units/m^2 are given continuously, or 3000 to 6750 units/m^2 are given intermittently for five days. The drug is available as an experimental preparation in ampules of 2000 units/2 ml from the Division of Cancer Treatment, to registered investigators.

Streptonigrin (Investigational)

Streptonigrin (NSC 45383, Nigrin, bruneomycin, rufocromonycin) is an antitumor antibiotic isolated from *Streptomyces flocculus* (fig. 25.8). Like mitomycin and dactinomycin, it has an aminoquinone moiety. It is thought that these drugs may act in part by producing superoxide and hydroxyl radicals that cause single-stranded DNA breaks. Superoxide radicals also interfere with cell respiratory mechanisms. Thus streptonigrin may interfere with both cellular replicative and metabolic mechanisms. It appears to be cell cycle-nonspecific.

The drug is well absorbed orally but can also be given intravenously and intraarterially. Little is known about its metabolism or excretion.

It has been used primarily in treatment of lymphomas, Hodgkin's disease, and chronic lymphocytic leukemia. Response rates of 30% to 35% have been reported (Kaung et al. 1969b). In direct comparisons with chlorambucil it appears to possess equal efficacy but

H–Ala–Ala–Pro–Thr–Ala–Thr–Val–Thr–Pro–Ser–Ser–Gly–Leu–Ser–Asp–
5 10 15

Gly–Thr–Val–Val–Lys–Val–Ala–Gly–Ala–Gly–Leu–Gln–Ala–Gly–Thr–
20 25 30

Ala–Tyr–Asp–Val–Gly–Gln–Cys–Ala–Ser–Val–Asn–Thr–Gly–Val–Leu–
35 40 45

Trp–Asn–Ser–Val–Thr–Ala–Ala–Gly–Ser–Ala–Cys–Asn–Pro–Ala–Asn–
50 55 60

Phe–Ser–Leu–Thr–Val–Arg–Arg–Ser–Phe–Glu–Gly–Phe–Leu–Phe–Asp–
65 70 75

Gly–Thr–Arg–Trp–Gly–Thr–Val–Asp–Cys–Thr–Thr–Ala–Ala–Cys–Gln–
80 85 90

Val–Gly–Leu–Ser–Asp–Ala–Ala–Gly–Asp–Gly–Glu–Pro–Gly–Val–Ala–
95 100 105

Ile–Ser–Phe–Asn–OH.

Fig. 25.7. *Amino acid sequence of zinostatin, 157365*

Table 25.1. *Antitumor Antibiotics*

Generic Name	*Trade or Common Name*	*Major Route(s)*	*Frequent Dose*	*Major Indication(s)*	*Major Toxicities*
Dactinomycin	Cosmegen (Actinomycin D)	IV	0.3 to 0.5 mg/m^2 × 5 days	Wilms' tumor, sarcomas	Marrow, G.I., vesicant
Mitomycin	Mutamycin	IV, intravesical	10 to 20 mg/m^2	G.I., breast, bladder	Marrow, G.I., pulmonary, renal
Mithramycin	Mithracin	IV	0.9 mg/m^2	Testicular	Hemorrhagic, marrow, G.I.
Daunorubicin	Cerubidine (Daunomycin)	IV	30 to 60 mg/m^2 × 3 days	AML	Marrow, cardiac, vesicant, alopecia
Doxorubicin	Adriamycin	IV	60 to 75 mg/m^2	Lymphoma, G.I., sarcomas, breast	Marrow, cardiac, vesicant, alopecia
Bleomycin	Blenoxane	IV, SC	10 to 20 units/m^2	Lymphoma, head and neck, testicular	Pulmonary, cutaneous
Zinostatin*	(Neocarzinostatin)	IV	3000 to 6750 units/m^2 × 5 days	AML	Marrow, G.I., fever
Streptonigrin*	Nigrin (Bruneomycin, rufocromonycin)	IV p.o.	0.2 to 0.28 mg/m^2/day for 5 days 1.0 mg/m^2	Lymphoma, CLL	Marrow, G.I.

*Investigational

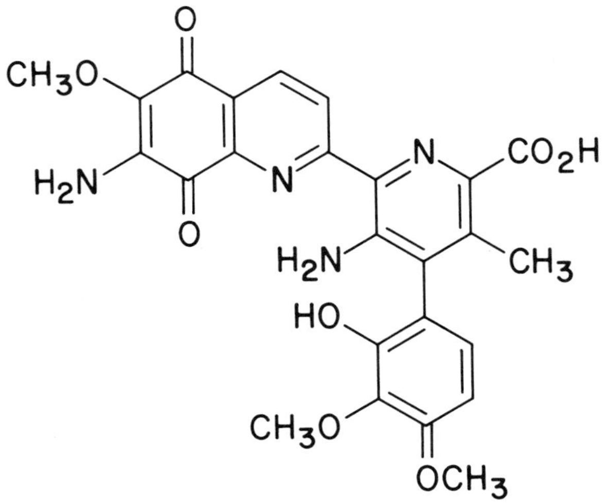

Fig. 25.8. *Streptonigrin, NSC 45383*

more gastrointestinal toxicity (Kaung et al. 1969a). It has been combined with vincristine and prednisone, and the combination gives better responses in histiocytic lymphoma than streptonigrin does alone (Silver, Lauper, and Jarowski 1977). It has also been tried in squamous cell carcinoma of the head and neck, cervical carcinoma, and adenocarcinoma of the breast, but those studies are preliminary and the numbers have been small (Livingston and Carter 1970).

The major dose-limiting toxicity is myelosuppression, which may be prolonged. Onset of leukopenia is usual in three weeks, reaching a nadir after four weeks. Thrombocytopenia also occurs over a similar time course. Anemia may be severe and require transfusions. Hematologic problems have been a major cause of abandoning therapy with this drug.

Nausea and vomiting are frequent and may be prolonged, leading to patient drop-out from the therapy program. Antiemetics should be tried. Stomatitis and diarrhea are less frequent.

Low-grade fever occurs in about one-third of the

patients treated with intravenous drug. If extravasation occurs, local skin necrosis with ulceration may eventuate. Alopecia is rare. Toxic psychosis and flapping tremor have been noted.

The drug is investigational and is available from the Division of Cancer Treatment in 0.2-mg capsules for oral use, and 0.5-mg vials for injection with diluent.

Dosage schedules are still being evaluated. One popular oral dose is 1 mg/m^2 each week for four to six weeks (Silver, Lauper, and Jarowski 1977). An alternative is 0.004 mg/kg/day for four to six weeks. The capsules are usually given over a period of 30 minutes at bedtime with antiemetics to minimize nausea and vomiting. The intravenous preparation is reconstituted by adding 2.5 ml of diluent (10% dimethyl sulfoxide, 10% ethanol, 2.2% 0.05 M citric acid, and 77.8% 0.1 M disodium phosphate) to the 0.5-ml vial. This is then infused with 5% dextrose in water taking care to protect it from light, as photodegradation occurs. For continuous or prolonged infusion, the bottle containing the streptonigrin should have an opaque cover.

A summary of guidelines for the use of the most frequently employed chemotherapeutic agents discussed thus far is shown in table 25.1.

References

Ahr, D. J. et al. Acquired platelet dysfunction following mithramycin therapy. *Cancer* 41:448–454, 1978.

Alexander, J. et al. Serial assessment of doxorubicin cardiotoxicity with quantitative radionuclide angiocardiography. *N. Engl. J. Med.* 300:278–283, 1979.

Bachur, N. R.; Benjamin, R. S.; and Hall, T. C., eds. Proceedings of the fifth new drug seminar on Adriamycin. *Cancer Chemother. Rep.* 6:83–419, 1975.

Bennet, J. M., and Reich, S. D. Drugs five years later: bleomycin. *Ann. Intern. Med.* 90:945–948, 1979.

Blum, R. H., and Carter, S. K. Adriamycin. *Ann. Intern. Med.* 80:249–259, 1974.

Boiron, M. et al. Daunorubicin in the treatment of acute myelocytic leukemia. *Lancet* 1:330–333, 1969.

Bonadonna, G. et al. Combination chemotherapy of Hodgkin's disease with Adriamycin, bleomycin, vinblastine, and imidazole carboxamide (ABVD) vs. MOPP. *Cancer* 36:252–259, 1975.

Bosl, G. J. et al. Vinblastine, bleomycin, and cis-diamminedichloroplatinum in the treatment of advanced testicular carcinoma. *Am. J. Med.* 68:492–496, 1980.

Broughton, A. et al. Clinical pharmacology of bleomycin following intravenous infusion as determined by radioimmunoassay. *Cancer* 40:2772–2778, 1977.

Buzdar, A. U. et al. Adriamycin and mitomycin C: possible synergistic cardiotoxicity. *Cancer Treat. Rep.* 62: 1005–1008, 1978.

Buzdar, A. U. et al. Pulmonary toxicity of mitomycin. *Cancer* 45:236–244, 1980.

Caradonna, R. et al. Methotrexate, bleomycin, and high-dose cis-dichlorodiammineplatinum (II) in the treatment of advanced epidermoid carcinoma of the head and neck. *Cancer Treat. Rep.* 63:489–491, 1979.

Carter, S. K. Mitomycin C (NSC 26980). Clinical brochure. *Cancer Chemother. Rep.* 1:99–114, 1968.

Carter, S. K., and Crooke, S. T. *Mitomycin C: current status and new developments.* New York: Academic Press, 1979.

Carter, S. K.; Crooke, S. T.; and Umezawa, H., eds. *Bleomycin: current status and new developments.* New York: Academic Press, 1978.

Carter, S. K., and Friedman, M. A., eds. *Proceedings of the chemotherapy conference on mithramycin (Mithracin): development and application.* Bethesda, Md.: National Cancer Institute, 1970, pp. 1–77.

Cassileth, P. A., and Katz, M. E. Chemotherapy for adult acute non-lymphocytic leukemia with daunorubicin and cytosine arabinoside. *Cancer Treat. Rep.* 61:1441–1445, 1977.

Creech, R. H.; Catalano, R. B.; and Shah, M. K. An effective low-dose Adriamycin regimen as secondary chemotherapy for metastatic breast cancer patients. *Cancer* 46:433–437, 1980.

Crooke, S. T., and Bradner, W. T. Bleomycin, a review. *J. Med.* 7:333–428, 1976a.

Crooke, S. T., and Bradner, W. T. Mitomycin C: a review. *Cancer Treat. Rev.* 3:121–139, 1976b.

Crooke, S. T.; Johnson, D. E.; and Bracken, R. B. A phase I–II study of mitomycin C (MMC) topical therapy in early transitional cell carcinoma of the bladder—a preliminary report. *Proc. Am. Soc. Clin. Oncol.* 19:321, 1978.

Davis, L. K. et al. Bleomycin, Adriamycin, CCNU, and Oncovin combination chemotherapy (BACO) in advanced and recurrent lymphomas. *Proc. Am. Soc. Clin. Oncol.* 18:273, 1977.

Farber, S. H. et al. Clinical studies of actinomycin D with special reference to Wilms' tumor in children. *Ann. NY Acad. Sci.* 89:421–425, 1960.

Feun, L. G.; Samson, M. K.; and Stephens, R. L. Vinblastine (VLB), bleomycin (BLEO), cis-diamminedichloroplatinum (DDP) in disseminated extragonadal germ cell tumors. *Cancer* 45:2543–2549, 1980.

Gale, R. P. Advances in the treatment of acute myelogenous leukemia. *N. Engl. J. Med.* 300:1189–1199, 1979.

Gale, R. P., and Cline, M. J. High remission induction rate in acute myeloid leukemia. *Lancet* 1:497–499, 1977.

Gilladoga, A. C. et al. The cardiotoxicity of Adriamycin and daunorubicin in children. *Cancer* 37:1070–1078, 1976.

Golbey, R. B. et al. Chemotherapy of metastatic germ cell tumors. *Semin. Oncol.* 6:82–86, 1979.

Golbey, R. B.; Reynolds, T. F.; and Vugrin, D. Chemotherapy of metastatic germ cell tumors. *Semin. Oncol.* 6:82–86, 1979.

Goldstein, D. P.; Winig, P.; and Shirley, R. L. Actino D as initial therapy of gestational trophoblastic disease. *Obstet. Gynecol.* 39:341–345, 1972.

Gottlieb, J. A. et al. Adriamycin used alone and in combination for soft tissue and bony sarcomas. *Cancer Chemother. Rep.* 6:271–282, 1975.

Gottlieb, J. A., and Hill, C. S., Jr. Adriamycin (NSC-123127) therapy in thyroid carcinoma. *Cancer Chemother. Rep.* 6:283–296, 1975.

Griffin, T. W. et al. Phase I and preliminary phase II study of neocarzinostatin. *Cancer Treat. Rep.* 62:2019–2025, 1978.

Griffin, T. W. et al. Treatment of acute non-lymphocytic leukemia with neocarzinostatin. *Cancer Treat. Rep.* 63:1853–1856, 1979.

Gulati, S. C. et al. Microangiopathic hemolytic anemia observed after treatment of epidermal carcinoma with mitomycin C and 5-fluorouracil. *Cancer* 45:2252–2257, 1980.

Gutierrez, M. L., and Crooke, S. T. Pediatric cancer chemotherapy: an updated review. I. Cis-diamminedichloroplatinum (cisplatin), VM-26 (teniposide), VP-16 (etoposide), mitomycin C. *Cancer Treat. Rev.* 6:153–164, 1979.

Holoye, P. Y. et al. Bleomycin hypersensitivity pneumonitis. *Ann. Intern. Med.* 88:47–49, 1978.

Holten, C. P. et al. Clinical study of daunomycin and prednisone for induction of remission in children with advanced leukemia. *N. Engl. J. Med.* 280:171–174, 1969.

Hoogstraten, B., and George, S. Adriamycin and combination chemotherapy in breast cancer. *Proc Am. Assoc. Cancer Res.* 15:60, 1974.

Iacovino, J. R. et al. Fatal pulmonary reaction from low doses of bleomycin. *JAMA* 235:1253–1255, 1976.

Ignoffo, R. J., and Friedman, M. A. Therapy of local toxicities caused by extravasation of cancer chemotherapeutic drugs. *Cancer Treat. Rev.* 7:17–27, 1980.

Issell, B. F. et al. Zinostatin (neocarzinostatin). *Cancer Treat. Rev.* 6:239–249, 1979.

Jaffe, N. et al. Improved outlook for Ewing's sarcoma with combination chemotherapy (vincristine, actinomycin D, and cyclophosphamide) and radiation therapy. *Cancer* 38:1925–1930, 1976.

Kaung, D. T. et al. Comparison of chlorambucil and streptonigrin (NSC 45383) in the treatment of chronic lymphocytic leukemia. *Cancer* 23:597–600, 1969a.

Kaung, D. T. et al. Comparison of chlorambucil and streptonigrin (NSC 45383) in the treatment of malignant lymphomas. *Cancer* 23:1280–1283, 1969b.

Kennedy, B. J. Metabolic and toxic effects of mithramycin. *Am. J. Med.* 49:494–503, 1970a.

Kennedy, B. J. Mithramycin therapy in advanced testicular neoplasms. *Cancer* 26:755–766, 1970b.

Krakoff, I. H. et al. Clinical pharmacology and therapeutic studies of bleomycin given by continuous infusion. *Cancer* 40:2027–2037, 1977.

Lebbin, D.; Ryan, W. G.; and Schwartz, T. B. Outpatient treatment of Paget's disease of bone with mithramycin. *Ann. Intern. Med.* 81:635–637, 1974.

Lee, Y. T. N. et al. Distribution of Adriamycin in cancer patients. *Cancer* 45:2231–2239, 1980.

Legha, S. S. et al. Neocarzinostatin (NSC 157365): a new cancerostatic compound. *Oncology* 33:265–270, 1976.

Legha, S. S.; Slavik, M.; and Carter, S. K. *Chromomycin A3*–NSC 58514 (Toyomycin). Clinical brochure. Bethesda, Md.: National Cancer Institute, 1975.

Lenaz, L., and Page, J. A. Cardiotoxicity of Adriamycin and related anthracyclines. *Cancer Treat. Rev.* 3:111–120, 1976.

Lewis, B. M., and Izbicki, R. Routine pulmonary function tests during bleomycin therapy. *JAMA* 243:347–351, 1980.

Li, M. C.; Whitmore, W. F., Jr.; and Golbey, R. B. Effects of combined drug therapy in metastatic cancer of testis. *JAMA* 174:1291–1299, 1960.

Liu, K. et al. Renal toxicity in man treated with mitomycin C. *Cancer* 28:1314–1320, 1971.

Livingston, R. B., and Carter, S. K. Daunomycin (NSC 82151). *Chemotherapy Fact Sheet.* Bethesda, Md.: National Cancer Institute, 1970a.

Livingston, R. B., and Carter, S. K. *Single agents in cancer chemotherapy.* New York: IFI/Plenum, 1970b.

Mazzaferri, E. L.; O'Dorisio, T. M.; and LoBuglio, A. F. Treatment of hypercalcemia associated with malignancy. *Semin. Oncol.* 5:141–153, 1978.

McKelvey, E. M. et al. Hydroxydaunomycin (Adriamycin) combination chemotherapy in malignant lymphoma. *Cancer* 38:1484–1493, 1976.

McKelvey, E. M. et al. Neocarzinostatin: a phase I clinical trial with five-day intermittent and continuous infusions. *Cancer* 44:1182–1188, 1979.

Meienhofer, J. et al. Primary structure of neocarzinostatin, an antitumor protein. *Science* 178:875–876, 1972.

Meienhofer, J., and Frei, E., III, eds. Selman A. Waksman conference on actinomycins. Their potential for cancer chemotherapy. *Cancer Chemother. Rep.* 58:1–121, 1974.

Mosher, M. B.; DeConti, R. C.; and Bertino, J. R. Bleomycin therapy in advanced Hodgkin's disease and epidermoid cancer. *Cancer* 30:56–60, 1972.

Myers, C. E., and McGuire, W. P. Proceedings of the conference on noninvasive and invasive prospective monitoring for anthracycline cardiotoxicity. *Cancer Treat. Rep.* 62:855–892, 1978.

Natale, R. B. et al. Phase II trial of neocarzinostatin in patients with bladder and prostatic cancer. *Cancer* 45:2836–2842, 1980.

Orwell, E. S.; Kiessling, P. J.; and Patterson, J. R. Interstitial pneumonia from mitomycin. *Ann. Intern. Med.* 89:352–355, 1978.

Osathanondh, R.; Goldstein, D. P.; and Pastorfide, G. B. Actinomycin D as the primary agent for gestational trophoblastic disease. *Cancer* 36:863–866, 1975.

Paladine, W. et al. Intracavitary bleomycin in the management of malignant effusions. *Cancer* 38:1903–1908, 1976.

Pearson, D. et al. The interaction of actinomycin D and radiation. *Int. J. Radiat. Oncol. Biol. Phys.* 4:71–73, 1978.

Philips, F. S. et al. The toxicity of actinomycin D. *Ann. NY Acad. Sci.* 89:348–360, 1960.

Praga, C. et al. Adriamycin cardiotoxicity: a survey of 1273 patients. *Cancer Treat. Rep.* 63:827–834, 1979.

Presant, C. A., and Klahr, C. Adriamycin, 1,3-bis(2-chloroethyl)-1-nitrosourea (BCNU NSC 409962), cyclophosphamide plus prednisone (ABC-P) in melphalan resistant multiple myeloma. *Cancer* 42:1222–1227, 1978.

Reilly, J. J.; Neifeld, J. P.; and Rosenberg, S. A. Clinical course and management of accidental Adriamycin extravasation. *Cancer* 40:2053–2056, 1977.

Rosenbaum, C., and Carter, S. K. *Bleomycin.* (NSC 125066 "Bleo" BLM). Clinical brochure. Bethesda, Md.: National Cancer Institute, 1970.

Ryan, W. G. Treatment of Paget's disease of bone with mithramycin. *Clin. Orthop.* 127:106–110, 1977.

Sakamato, S. et al. Effects of systemic administration of neocarzinostatin, a new protein antibiotic on human bladder cancer. *Cancer Treat. Rep.* 62:453–454, 1978.

Samuels, L. D. Actinomycin and its effects: influence on an effector pathway for hormonal control. *N. Engl. J. Med.* 271:1252–1258, 1301–1308, 1964.

Schein, P. S. et al. Bleomycin, Adriamycin, cyclophosphamide, vincristine, and prednisone (BACOP) combination chemotherapy. *Ann. Intern. Med.* 85:417–422, 1976.

Shah, P.; Baker, L. H.; and Vaitkevicius, V. K. Preliminary experiences with intra-arterial Adriamycin. *Cancer Treat. Rep.* 61:1565–1567, 1977.

Silver, R. T.; Lauper, R. D.; and Jarowski, C. I. *A synopsis of cancer chemotherapy.* New York: Dun-Donnelley, 1977.

Soper, W. T., and Gott, A. B., eds. *New drug seminar on bleomycin.* Bethesda, Md.: National Cancer Institute, 1974.

Van Echo, D. A., and Wiernik, P. H. Phase I study of neocarzinostatin in patients with acute leukemia. *Cancer Treat. Rep.* 62:1363–1365, 1978.

Von Hoff, D. D. et al. Daunomycin-induced cardiotoxicity in children and adults. *Am. J. Med.* 62:200–208, 1977.

Von Hoff, D. D. et al. Risk factors for doxorubicin-induced congestive heart failure. *Ann. Intern. Med.* 91:710–717, 1979.

Waksman, S. A., ed. The actinomyces and their importance in the treatment of tumors in animals and man. *Ann. NY Acad. Sci.* 89:283–486, 1960.

Waksman, S. A., and Woodruff, H. B. Bacteriostatic and bacterial substances produced by a soil actinomyces. *Proc. Soc. Exp. Biol. Med.* 45:609–614, 1940.

Weiss, R. B., and Muggia, F. M. Cytotoxic drug-induced pulmonary disease: update 1980. *Am. J. Med.* 68:259–266, 1980.

Wiernik, P. H. et al. Randomized clinical comparison of daunorubicin alone and the combination of daunorubicin, cytosine arabinoside, 6-thioguanine and pyrimethamine for the treatment of acute nonlymphocytic leukemia. *Cancer Treat. Rep.* 60:41–53, 1976.

Wilbur, J. R. et al. Chemotherapy of sarcomas. *Cancer* 36:765–769, 1975.

Yagoda, A. et al. Bleomycin, an antitumor antibiotic. *Ann. Intern. Med.* 77:861–870, 1972.

Young, C. W. Actinomycin and antitumor antibiotics. *Am. J. Clin. Pathol.* 52:130–137, 1969.

Zweig, J. I. et al. Rational effective medical treatment of skin ulcers due to Adriamycin. *Cancer Treat. Rep.* 63:2101–2103, 1979.

Zweig, J. I., and Kabakow, B. An apparently effective countermeasure for doxorubicin extravasation. *JAMA* 239:2116, 1978.

twenty-six

Plant-Derived Antineoplastic Drugs

DAVID S. FISCHER

For centuries people have derived some of their medicinals from plants. The poppy, which provides the opium family of narcotic analgesics, was known to humans before history was recorded. Two centuries ago Withering (1785) learned from an old woman of Shropshire of the value of the foxglove leaf in treating "dropsy" and set out the guidelines for the use of digitalis that we follow, in general, to this day. Podophyllin was used as a cancer remedy by the Penobscot Indians of Maine and by private practioners treating cancer in the United States before 1897 (Carter and Livingston 1976). A half century ago, western physicians learned about the use of *Rauwolfia serpentina* which practitioners in India had been using for two millennia (Sen and Bose 1931). Even a century ago the average pharmacy in this country carried primarily plant-derived materials such as rhubarb, castor oil, alcohol, olive oil, and paregoric; the list is too long to enumerate further here.

There are thousands of complex molecules synthesized by plants of both higher and lower orders that are not known to biochemists. Some of these are highly toxic and could become hazardous to the environment, but they do not accumulate because microbes use and degrade them. Interestingly, it is the toxic plants that have most often been found to yield materials worthy of being studied and developed into drugs. For a long time, folklore was the only guide to selection and testing of the most promising of the 230,000 plants available.

In 1937, the National Cancer Institute (NCI) was established, and one of its early activities was a study of plant extracts carried out under the direction of Dr. M. J. Shear (Perdue and Hartwell 1976). Working in that program, Hartwell (1976) isolated podophyllotoxin from podophyllin. From that early start, two investigational antineoplastic agents have been derived from the podophyllotoxin: etoposide and teniposide. Both appear to be very active agents and are discussed for use in cancer chemotherapy. Podophyllin had been used for years as a topical cytotoxic agent in treatment of condylomata acuminata.

A more systematic approach to screening drugs began with the establishment of the Cancer Chemotherapy National Service Center in the NCI in 1955 (Zubrod et al. 1966). By 1961, systematic screening of plant extracts was initiated; in the next 15 years, 25,000 species of higher plants were screened. Materials were sent to the contract facility at Madison, Wisconsin where extracts were prepared and concentrated. They were then sent out to be tested both in vitro and in vivo (Schepartz 1976). If the compound showed activity in one of these experimental systems, it was sent out for large-batch chemical isolation and further study. The better compounds were isolated and purified, and when possible, characterized. So far the only compound derived directly from that screening is maytansine, an ansa macrolide, a class of compounds that includes the antibiotics rifamycin and streptovaricin (Perdue and Hartwell 1976). Now that the program is well established, it is anticipated that new and useful compounds will be developed more frequently.

Table 26.1. *Plant-Derived Antineoplastic Drugs*

Generic Name	*Trade or Common Name*	*Major Route(s)*	*Frequent Dose*	*Major Indication(s)*	*Major Toxicities*
Vinblastine	Velban	IV	6 mg/m^2	Lymphoma, testicular	Marrow, G.I. neurologic
Vincristine	Oncovin	IV	1.4 mg/m^2	Lung, sarcoma, lymphoma	Neurologic, alopecia
Vindesine*	Eldisine	IV	3 to 4 mg/m^2	Lung, lymphoma, breast	Marrow, alopecia, neurologic
Teniposide*	(VM-26)	IV	100 mg/m^2	Lymphoma, ALL, brain	Marrow, alopecia
Etoposide*	(VP-16-213); Vepesid	IV	45 to 100 mg/m^2 × 5 days	Lung, lymphoma, AML	Marrow, alopecia, bronchospasm
Maytansine*		IV	0.7 to 1.25 mg/m^2	ALL, lymphoma	G.I., neurologic

*Investigational.

The most useful plant alkaloids were developed through investigation of folk tales, and their result had nothing to do with the original reason for the search. There had been folk use of the periwinkle *Catharanthus roseus* G. Don (*Vinca rosea* Linn.) as a remedy for diabetes. Studies were initiated independently by the Eli Lilly and Company research laboratories (Johnson et al. 1960; Johnson et al. 1963) and the Collip Laboratories at the University of Western Ontario (Noble, Beer, and Cutts 1958). It was found that extracts of the plant produced peripheral granulocytopenia and bone marrow depression in rats. Tests were then performed in rodents with transplanted tumors, and increased survival was documented. About 60 alkaloids were isolated and tested, and eventually vinblastine and vincristine proved to be sufficiently active that they were approved for marketing (Neuss et al. 1964). An additional derivative, vindesine (desacetyl vinblastine amide sulfate) is now being evaluated in phase I and II studies. It is interesting that although the only difference between vinblastine and vincristine is a methyl group or a formyl group respectively on the indole nitrogen of the vindoline moiety, significant differences have been observed in the spectrum of toxicity and antitumor activity, and there is a remarkable lack of cross-resistance.

Plant products that were tested but no longer used in chemotherapy include colchicine and demecolcin, alkaloids that are mitotic inhibitors. The plant-derived drugs in current use are listed in table 26.1.

Vinblastine

Vinblastine (Velban, NSC 49842) is the sulfate salt of a dimeric alkaloid derived from the periwinkle plant, *Vinca rosea* Linn., a species of myrtle (fig. 26.1). It binds to microtubules, thereby impairing formation of a functional mitotic spindle and arresting cell division in metaphase. In the absence of an intact mitotic spindle the chromosomes may disperse throughout the cytoplasm or appear as clusters, ultimately leading to cellular death. The drug can bind to other types of microtubules as well, and affect the function of phagocytes and neurons. In addition, inhibition of uridine transport and of RNA

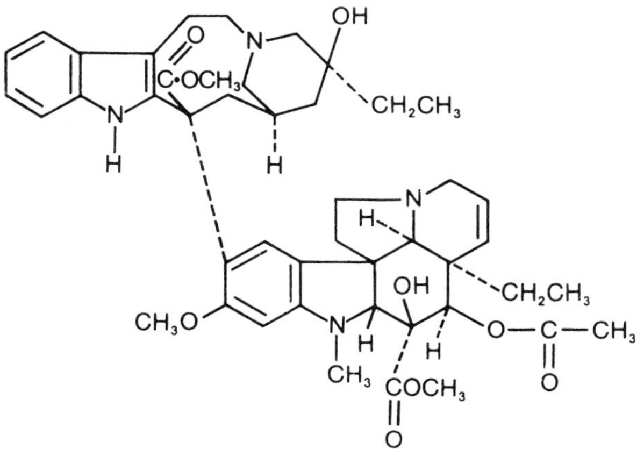

Fig. 26.1. *Vinblastine, NSC 49842*

and DNA synthesis has been reported. The uptake of glutamic acid is inhibited and there is some suppression of protein synthesis. The drug is cell cycle phase-specific with metaphase arrest in the M phase (Chabner, Myers, and Oliverio 1977).

Although vinblastine is absorbed orally and has been used in tablet form, absorption was erratic. This route has been abandoned, and only intravenous use is approved. Following administration, clearance from the blood of drug-derived tritiated thymidine on the 4-acetyl group is biphasic with initial and terminal half-lives of about 4.5 minutes and 190 minutes respectively (Beer, Wilson, and Bell 1964). Binding of the drug is strongest to plasma, platelets, red blood cells, and leukocytes in that order. The drug is extensively metabolized by the liver and excreted in the bile. A major metabolite is desacetyl vinblastine, which is biologically active. About 20% of the drug or its metabolite appears in the urine by three days, and 25% to 45% in the stool. The remainder is presumably bound to tissues and indeed, some is slowly released later. It does not penetrate the blood-brain barrier.

Although vinblastine is the single most active agent for the treatment of Hodgkin's disease and has kept patients in remission for more than a year, it is seldom of ever curative as a single agent. Hence it should generally be used in combinations. The British use it in a four-drug combination designated MVPP (mechlorethamine, vinblastine, procarbazine, and prednisone) for the treatment of Hodgkin's disease (Nicholson et al. 1970), and we have used it in a five-drug combination, MVVPP, adding vincristine to the regimen. It has been used in a three-drug regimen with lomustine and doxorubicin (Rosenberg and Kaplan 1973) as an alternative to or for failures from MOPP; in Italy it is used in a noncross-reactive combination designated ABVD (Adriamycin, bleomycin, vinblastine, and dacarbazine) (Bonadonna et al. 1975). For poor-risk patients, MOPP and ABVD are frequently alternated. These various combinations produce remissions in the range of 40% to 80% and cures in about 40% to 50% of cases (Coltman 1979). It is also used in the therapy of non-Hodgkin's lymphoma, albeit less frequently.

In the management of testicular carcinoma, especially embryonal cell carcinoma, vinblastine has been combined with bleomycin and has produced striking responses and some cures. Combined with cisplatin and bleomycin, the response rate has been 70% complete remission and 30% partial, with about a 50% cure rate (Bosl et al. 1980; Feun, Samson, and Stephens 1980). More extensive combinations (VAB III and IV at Memorial Sloan-Kettering Cancer Center) give comparable results.

Vinblastine has efficacy alone or more often in combination in breast cancer, renal cell carcinoma (Amiel et al. 1979), neuroblastoma, Kaposi's sarcoma (Klein et al. 1980), head and neck cancer (Brown et al. 1980), and choriocarcinoma (Hertz et al. 1960).

Dose-limiting toxicity is hematologic, primarily leukopenia with a nadir of 4 to 10 days, and recovery one to two weeks later. Thrombocytopenia is usually worse in patients who have had previous radiation or chemotherapy. Anemia is rarely a result of this drug.

Nausea, vomiting, and anorexia are common but seldom lead to discontinuance of therapy. Antiemetics are helpful. Diarrhea and stomatitis are encountered but are not common. At high doses, constipation and paralytic ileus may occur. This can be avoided by use of laxatives in a preventive modality.

Neurotoxicity is not as severe as it is with vincristine, but it can be a problem. Patients complain of numbness, paresthesias, headaches, malaise, and severe jaw and face pain. The paresthesias may occur within a few hours of drug administration and last for hours or days. Loss of deep tendon reflexes, mental depression, peripheral neuropathy, urinary retention, and constipation may be noted. Alopecia and rash occur infrequently. The drug is teratogenic and should not be used in early pregnancy.

As a single agent, the usual dose is 6 mg/m^2 every week. Since it is a potent irritant and can cause severe pain and necrosis if extravasation occurs, we give the drug into the side-arm of a rapidly running IV. In the MVPP regimen for Hodgkin's disease, the dose of vinblastine is 6 mg/m^2 days 1 and 8. In the most popular regimen for testicular carcinoma, the original dose was 0.2 mg/kg on each of two consecutive days (Einhorn, Furnas, and Powell 1976), but this was found to be too toxic and was modified to 0.3 mg/kg once a course (Einhorn and Donahue 1979). For other regimens, see chapter 29 on combination therapy or the original publication or protocol.

The drug is available as Velban (Lilly) in lyophilized vials of 10 mg. It is reconstituted with 10 ml bactericidal sterile normal saline. The unopened vial should be refrigerated until reconstituted. The solution is stable for about 30 days when refrigerated.

Vincristine

Vincristine (Oncovin, NSC 67574) is the sulfate salt of a dimeric alkaloid derived from the periwinkle plant, *Vinca rosea* Linn. (fig. 26.2). It is cell cycle phase-specific and blocks mitosis with metaphase arrest in the M phase, apparently because of binding to microtubules (Sullivan 1968).

Absorption from the gastrointestinal tract of tablets is erratic and incomplete. Following an intravenous dose of tritiated vincristine, disappearance of the radioactively labeled drug is biphasic, with half-lives of 5 minutes and 191 minutes respectively. Over a three-day period, about 70% is excreted in the feces and 15% in the urine. The gastrointestinal tract excretion is derived primarily from biliary sources with enterohepatic circulation. Relatively little of the drug is metabolized, and the rate of excretion varies with the dose administered (Owellen et al. 1977). There is some evidence that levels in the brain continue to increase for 24 hours, which is interesting in view of its known neurotoxicity. Our understanding of vincristine's mode of neurotoxicity remains rudimentary, however.

As a single agent, vincristine has few indications (Costa et al. 1962). It has been used in the treatment of some refractory cases of idiopathic thrombocytopenic purpura with success (Ahn et al. 1974) while vinblastine has been used bound to platelets (Ahn et al. 1978). It has been used alone in attempts at remission induction in acute lymphoblastic leukemia (Haggard et al. 1968; Howard 1967; Heyn et al. 1966) with 41% complete and 73% total response rates. In combination chemotherapy, however, it has been highly successful in a multitude of tumors.

Combined with prednisone (Hardisty, McElwain, and Darby 1969), it induces complete remissions in 80% (Smithson, Gilchrist, and Burgert 1980) of children with acute lymphoblastic leukemia, and is probably even more effective in combination with daunorubicin. When vincristine, prednisone, and L-asparaginase are used together, incidence of remission remains the same, but duration is significantly prolonged.

In the treatment of Hodgkin's disease, vincristine (Oncovin) is part of the MOPP (mechlorethamine, Oncovin, procarbazine, prednisone) regimen (DeVita, Serpick, and Carbone 1970), which is fairly standard and yields 80% remissions and about 50% cures (Coltman 1979). In the non-Hodgkin's lymphomas it has been part of the CVP (cyclophosphamide, vincristine, prednisone) regimen (Bagley et al. 1972) for nodular lymphocytic lymphomas, and COPP (cyclophosphamide, Oncovin, procarbazine, prednisone) regimen (DeVita et al. 1975) and BACOP (bleomycin, Adriamycin, cyclophosphamide, Oncovin, prednisone) regimen (Schein et al. 1976) for diffuse histiocytic lymphomas.

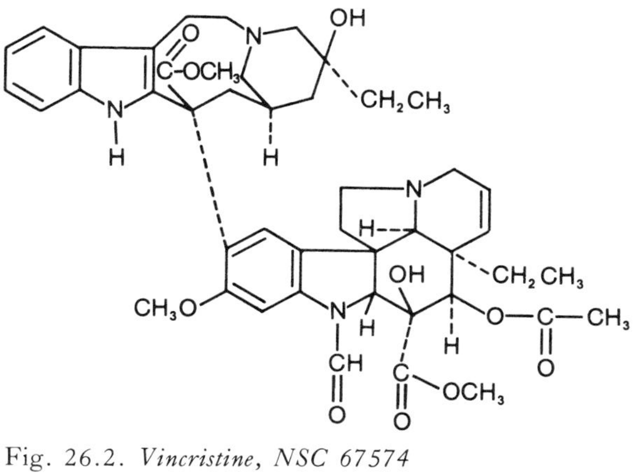

Fig. 26.2. *Vincristine, NSC 67574*

In breast cancer, vincristine is an integral part of the original five-drug regimen (5-FU, methotrexate, cyclophosphamide, prednisone, and vincristine) introduced in 1969 by Cooper. No one has reported better adjuvant results (Cooper, Holland, and Glidewell 1979). Although there has been some question as to the single-drug activity of vincristine in this disease, it has been used in combination with doxorubicin (Adriamycin) in the AV regimen, which has been relatively successful for CMF (cyclophosphamide, methotrexate, 5-fluorouracil) failures (Bonadonna et al. 1974).

Vincristine has been used extensively in several effective combinations for small cell carcinoma of the lung (Livingston et al. 1978) and is being evaluated in non-small cell lung cancer. It has been an integral part of the VAC (vincristine, actinomycin D, cyclophosphamide) regimen for childhood rhabdomyosarcoma, retinoblastoma, and other soft tissue sarcomas (Wilbur et al. 1975). It has been a part of effective combination chemotherapies for Wilms' tumor, Ewing's sarcoma, and neuroblastoma (James et al. 1965; Finkelstein et al. 1974). It has been used in combination chemotherapy for several other tumors where its efficacy has not been established, for example, melanoma, testicle, colon, (Moertel et al. 1975), and brain (Gutin et al. 1975).

In marked contrast to vinblastine, there is relatively minor bone marrow toxicity associated with vincristine. This has been one of the major reasons for its wide use in combination with myelosuppressive agents. Its dose-limiting toxicity is neurologic (Rosenthal and Kaufman 1974). This is manifested by paresthesias, loss of deep tendon reflexes, peripheral neuropathy (fig. 26.3), foot drop, constipation, abdominal pain, hoarseness, ptosis, and double vision, any of which can be so troublesome as to cause the patient to abandon therapy. Paralytic ileus is less common but very frightening because it mimics intestinal obstruction in a patient possibly susceptible to that complication. Laxatives should be used prophylactically, and bowel function should be followed carefully, with the patient instructed to report apparent constipation promptly. While many of the neurologic side effects are ultimately reversible, recovery is frequently slow and incomplete. Loss of the Achilles' tendon reflex and fine finger movements and development of numbness are early warning signs to decrease or discontinue the drug.

Alopecia occurs in at least half of patients and is reversible (Simister 1966). It is one of the most disagreeable side effects from the patient's perspective, however, and has caused many to avoid or discontinue therapy. Since vincristine binds to tissues rapidly (biphasic plasma half-life with first peak at five minutes), alopecia can be greatly reduced by decreasing circulation to the scalp with a tourniquet applied 5 minutes before and maintained for 15 to 20 minutes after the drug is administered (O'Brien et al. 1970).

Other toxicities may include seizures, lethargy, and coma. A syndrome of inappropriate antidiuretic hormone secretion with hyponatremia and high urinary sodium concentration has been associated with vincristine and is thought to result from a direct effect on the hypothalamus (Stuart et al. 1975). It can be treated with fluid restriction.

The usual dose of vincristine alone or in combination is 1.4 mg/m^2, but not to exceed 2 mg per dose on any one day. In the treatment of the blast crisis of chronic myelogenous leukemia with prednisone and vincristine, the authors recommend 2 mg/m^2 with no limitation of dose other than toxicity (Canellos et al. 1971). In general, it is felt that the therapeutic effect is not dose-related, and significantly greater toxic reactions without increased benefit occur with larger doses.

Vincristine is a local irritant, and extravasation causes severe cellulitis and phlebitis. Hence the drug should be administered through a running intravenous infusion or injected with particular care to prevent extravasation. Liver impairment increases the drug's toxicity, so doses should be decreased in those with liver disease. Elderly individuals tolerate the drug less well than young people, and experience more frequent and more severe toxicity.

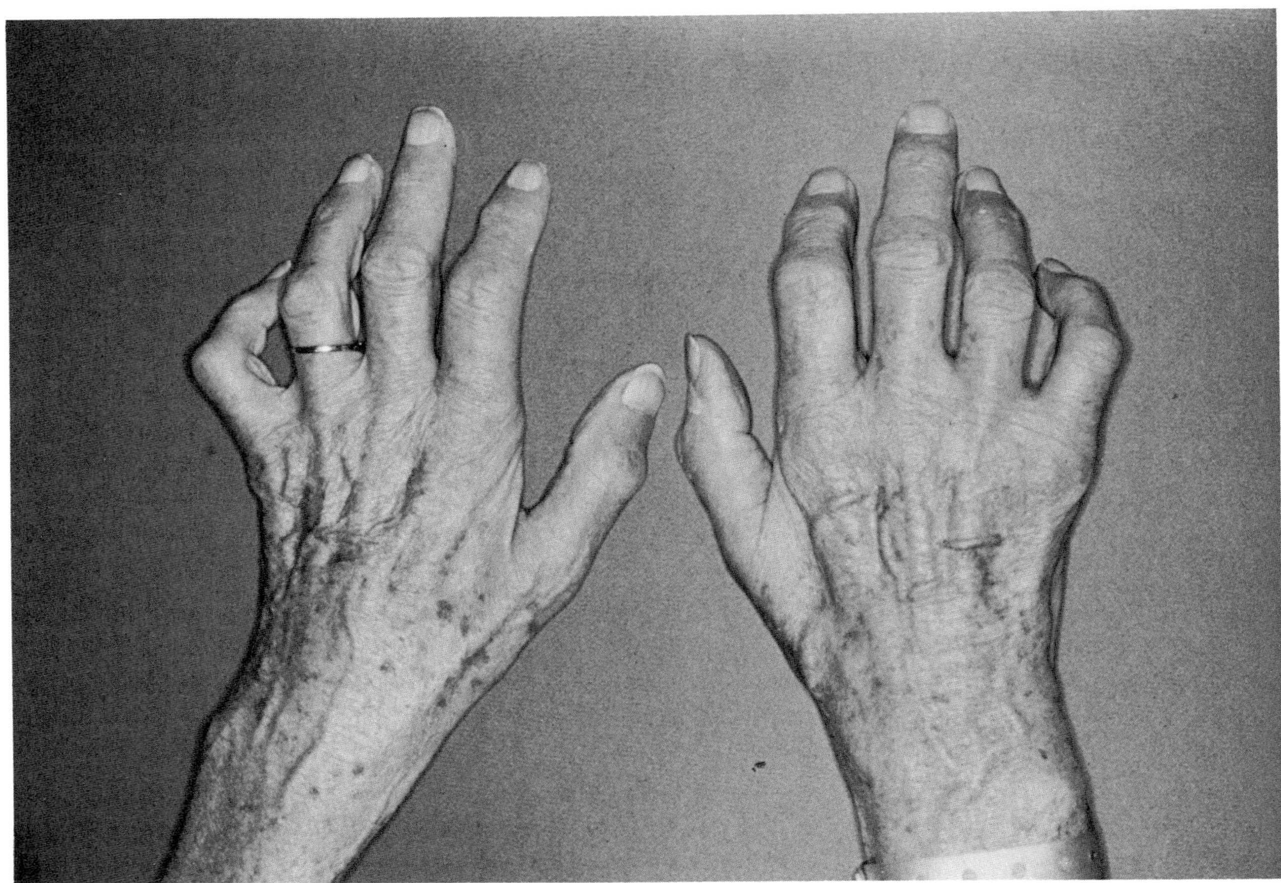

Fig. 26.3. *Severe vincristine neuropathy complicating underlying arthritis. Patient essentially lost use of both hands after excessive and prolonged use of vincristine.*

The drug is available as Oncovin (Lilly) as a lyophilized powder in 1- and 5-mg vials that come as a duo-pack with a bacteriostatic diluent with 10 and 50 mg of lactose respectively. The vials should be refrigerated until used. The reconstituted product is stable for up to 14 days when refrigerated. Having seen both physicians and nurses administer 5 mg or 10 mg when 1 or 2 mg was intended (the vials are the same size and shape), I have not permitted the 5-mg vial to be stocked in my office, and the Pharmacy and Therapeutics Committee of Yale–New Haven Hospital has removed the 5-mg vial from the formulary and hence from the pharmacy.

Vindesine (Investigational)

Vindesine (Eldisine, Lilly compound 99094, desacetyl vinblastine amide sulfate, NSC 24567) is derived from vinblastine by chemical modification (fig. 26.4). The primary amide at position 3 replaces the carboxy methyl ester, and an alcohol at position 4 replaces the acetyl group. Its mode of action appears to be the same as that of vinblastine—binding to microtubules with inhibition of the formation of the mitotic spindle resulting in metaphase arrest. The drug is cell cycle phase-specific for the M phase. There is some suggestion that it may also serve to inhibit RNA and DNA synthesis, but that remains to be demonstrated.

Oral absorption is erratic and unsatisfactory. Following rapid intravenous injection the plasma decay is

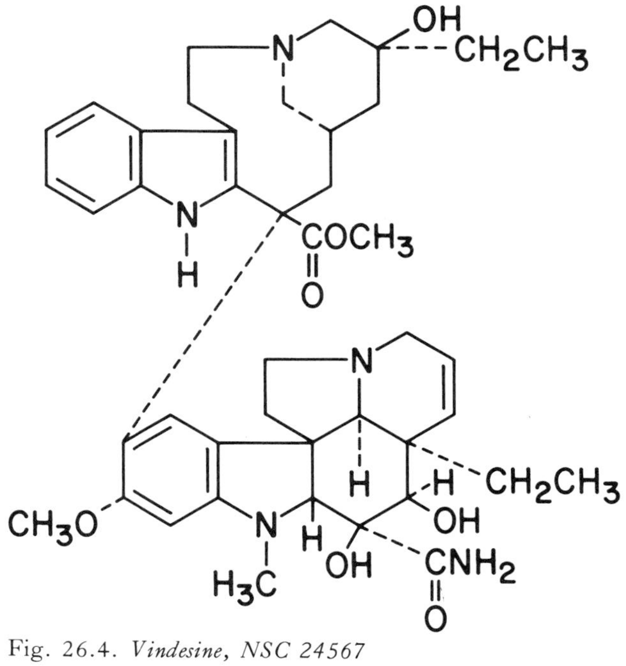

Fig. 26.4. *Vindesine, NSC 24567*

triphasic. The initial half-life is 2 minutes, secondary half-life is 1 hour, and tertiary half-life is 24 hours (Nelson, Dyke, and Root 1980; Dyke and Nelson 1977). Urinary excretion is minor with only 6% recovered in three days. The major excretory pathway is through the bile. The large volume of distribution and long elimination half-life suggest that extensive but reversible tissue binding is primarily responsible for the rapid clearance of vindesine from plasma. Just as the body clearance of vindesine is intermediate between that of vinblastine and vincristine, so is its dose and its toxicity per unit weight intermediate.

Preliminary reports of phase I and II trials suggest clinical activity in the treatment of melanoma (Smith et al. 1978), lung cancer (Gralla et al. 1979), acute leukemias (Mathé et al. 1978), testicular carcinoma (Currie et al. 1978), Hodgkin's disease, non-Hodgkin's lymphoma, colon cancer (Carroll, Gralla, and Kemeny 1979; Bedikian et al. 1980), nephroblastoma, histiocytosis X, and breast cancer. The response rate in one report with 21 evaluable patients with breast carcinoma was 29%, with two patients achieving complete remission (CR), four a partial remission (PR), and five others obtaining a measurable response (Smith et al. 1978). Responses were seen most often in soft tissue, nodal, and pulmonary metastases. Two of 12 evaluable patients with melanoma (16%) achieved a PR and a third achieved a measurable response.

Dose-limiting toxicity is myelosuppression with leukopenia in about half the cases. It is usually mild and transient and not associated with severe infections. The nadir is seen at 4 to 10 days, with recovery one or two weeks later. Thrombocytopenia is mild and never dangerous except with severe overdosage or in patients heavily pretreated with radiation or other cytotoxic agents. Neurotoxicity occurs in about 40% and most commonly starts with peripheral paresthesias. Constipation to a disturbing degree is seen in about 20% of patients and requires use of laxatives and stool softeners. Neurotoxicity may be dose-limiting in a few patients (Young et al. 1978; Ohnuma, Greenspan, and Holland 1980).

Alopecia occurs in about half the patients, and with its rapid binding to tissues can be treated with a head band with the same guidelines as described for vincristine. A potentially serious problem with vindesine is the frequency of inapparent infiltrations associated with its administration (Dorr and Jones 1979). The group at the University of Arizona found that when using their standard intravenous push technique with thin 21- to 25-gauge steel butterfly sets, they had 8 significant local reactions to the drug in 34 separate injections. In only one patient was infiltration noted at the time of the injection by the highly skilled oncology nurses administering them. By contrast, these same individuals administered 1126 other chemotherapy injections with only 1 infiltration. It would appear that vindesine should be administered by the technique I have advocated for vinblastine and vincristine, that is, injection through the side arm of a rapidly running intravenous. Other minor toxicities include nausea and vomiting, fatigue, malaise, rash, photophobia, stomatitis, pyrexia, anorexia, and diarrhea.

Dosage schedules are still being evaluated. At present, the most popular is 3 to 4 mg/m^2 IV every 7 to 14 days. An alternative for hospitalized patients is 1 to 1.3 mg/m^2/day for five to seven days every three or four weeks as tolerated. Because of kinetic considerations, a twice-weekly schedule of 1.5 to 2 mg/m^2 per dose has been advocated, but little experience with it has accumulated so far.

The drug is available as Eldisine (Lilly) to investigators by application to the Eli Lilly and Company research laboratories. It is supplied as a lyophilized powder in 10-mg vials to be reconstituted with 10 ml of bacteriostatic normal saline. Combination therapy is in an early investigative phase, and those dosages need much more study. An early response to vindesine plus cisplatin in lung cancer has been reported, and is quite exciting (Casper, Gralla, and Golbey 1979; Itri et al. 1981).

Teniposide (Investigational)

Teniposide (VM-26, 4′-demethyl-epidophyllotoxin-B-D-thenylidene glucoside, NSC 122819) is a semisynthetic derivative of podophyllotoxin, a natural product of the mayapple or American mandrake plant *(Podophyllum peltatum)* (fig. 26.5). The drug was synthesized by Sandoz Pharmaceuticals. It is highly water-insoluble and requires a lipid solvent for intravenous administration. The mode of action is at least twofold: immediate metaphase arrest of dividing cells, and subsequent prevention of cells from entering mitosis. Protein and RNA synthesis are not affected. Tritiated thymidine incorporation is inhibited, suggesting inhibition of DNA synthesis. Alterations of the microtubules have not been demonstrated. Finally, the drug inhibits mitochondrial electron transport in the respiratory chain at the NADH dehydrogenase level, and this inhibition could prevent formation of the energy necessary in the premitotic period (Strauss, Goldsmith, and Slavik 1975). The drug is cell cycle phase-specific primarily for the M phase. It is not cross-reactive with the *Vinca* alkaloids or their derivatives.

After intravenous infusion a triexponential decay curve is seen, with the half-life of the terminal phase varying from 11 to 38 hours (Rosencweig et al. 1977). At three days, 44% of the drug is recovered in the urine with 9% as unchanged drug and 35% as metabolites. Cerebrospinal fluid levels are less than 1% of plasma concentrations in spite of the lipid-solubility of the drug. This value increased to 27% in a patient who had undergone previous brain surgery and radiotherapy. Recovery in the feces is 0% to 10%. The drug is strongly protein-bound.

Antitumor responses have been seen in brain tumors, neuroblastoma, Hodgkin's disease, non-Hodgkin's lymphoma, bladder, lung, breast (Spremulli et al. 1980), ovary, and kidney cancer, blast crisis of chronic myelogenous leukemia, acute lymphocytic (Rivera et al. 1980) and non-lymphocytic leukemia, hepatoma, and melanoma (Bellet et al. 1978).

The most promising results so far have been in intracranial tumors with 12 PRs in 23 patients (52%), and in 20 cases of ovarian carcinoma, with 1 CR and 7 PRs for a 40% response rate (Radice, Bunn, and Ihde 1979). Bladder tumors have been treated both topically and systemically. Of 142 cases treated systemically, there were 14 CRs and 32 PRs, yielding a response rate of 32% (Radice, Bunn, and Ihde 1979). The results in lymphoma are equally encouraging. In diffuse histiocytic lymphoma there were 30 PRs in 71 cases (42%), in lymphocytic lymphoma 22 PRs in 48 cases (45%), and

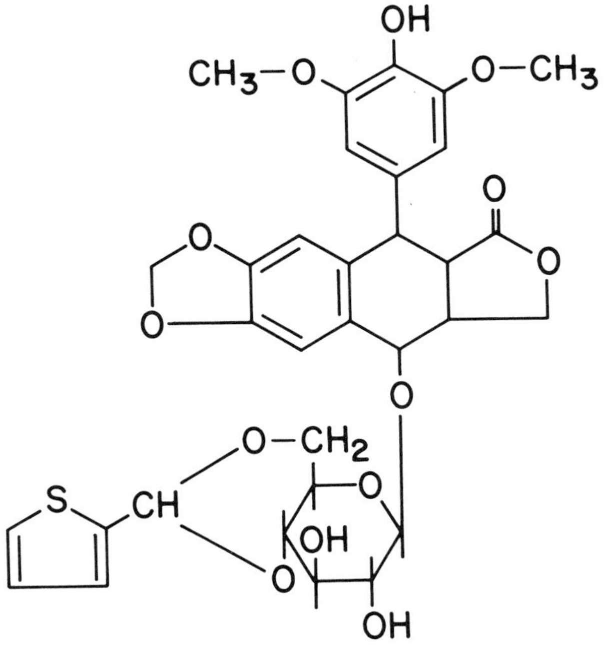

Fig. 26.5. *Teniposide, NSC 122819*

in Hodgkin's disease 3 CRs and 30 PRs in 92 cases (36%) (Radice, Bunn, and Ihde 1979). Clearly, the drug is not active enough in lymphomas for single-agent use, but it looks promising as a component of new combinations. In a French study teniposide plus lomustine was used in 57 patients with renal cell carcinoma with proved metastases, and resulted in 2 CRs and 5 PRs (Amiel et al. 1979).

The major dose-limiting toxicity is hematologic. Leukopenia is most severe, with 20% of patients having a nadir of $1000/mm^3$ or less, usually reached in 10 to 14 days and with recovery by day 16 to 21. The thrombocytopenia was mild and occurred in 16% of patients. No cumulative toxicity has been noted.

Gastrointestinal toxicity includes nausea, vomiting, diarrhea, anorexia, and stomatitis, but these are generally mild and infrequent. Alopecia has been seen in 27% of cases and there is no experience yet with scalp tourniquets to reduce its incidence. Recovery is nearly universal following cessation of therapy. Other toxicities include fever, mild elevation of liver function tests, phlebitis, palpitations, and mild peripheral neuropathy.

Dosages are still being worked out, but a great many have been or are being tried. The more popular are $100 mg/m^2$/week IV for six to eight weeks and then reevaluate. Some investigators increase the dosage to $130 mg/m^2$ without toxicity. Administration twice a week is thought by some to give better responses; so $50 mg/m^2$ on that schedule is being given for four weeks before reevaluation (Gutierrez and Crooke 1979; Rosencweig et al. 1977). In the French study with lomustine, the dose of teniposide was 50 mg/day for two days (Amiel et al. 1979).

The drug is available as teniposide from the Division of Cancer Treatment for clinical trials. It is supplied to NCI by Bristol Laboratories in 50-mg ampules each containing 5 ml. They should be stored at room temperature and protected from the light. Although the compound is basically unstable, it has been skillfully formulated to remain chemically stable for four years at room temperature. Each 5-ml ampule contains teniposide, 50 mg; benzyl alcohol, 150 mg; N'N-dimethylacetamide, 300 mg; polyethoxylated castor oil, purified, 2.5 gm; maleic acid q.s. pH 5.1; absolute alcohol q.s. 4.75 gm. For reconstitution, the ampule must be diluted with 5 volumes, and preferably 10 to 20 volumes, of normal saline or 5% dextrose in water before administration by IV infusion. Solutions that show evidence of a precipitate should be discarded. A slight opalescence is caused by surfactant in the preparation. This preparation is physically stable for four hours, and six hours if diluted to 50 or 100 volumes. It should be given by slow IV infusion.

Etoposide (Investigational)

Etoposide (VP-16-213, Vepesid, 4′-demethylepipodophyllotoxin-B-D-ethylidene glucoside, NSC 141540) is a semisynthetic derivative of podophyllotoxin, a natural product of the mayapple or American mandrake plant *(Podophyllum peltatum)* (fig. 26.6). The drug was synthesized and studied at Sandoz Pharmaceuticals (Handelsman, Goldsmith, and Slavik 1974) and is being developed now at Bristol Laboratories (Issell and Crooke 1979). It is water-insoluble and requires a lipid solvent for intravenous administration. An oral formulation has been made available by Sandoz Laboratories (Basel, Switzerland) but has not yet been approved for clinical trials in the United States (Nissen et al. 1976; Falkson et al. 1975).

The mechanism of action is thought to be arrest of mitosis at metaphase and prevention of cells from entering mitosis possibly by inhibition of DNA synthesis. There may be an effect on RNA and protein synthesis but no binding to microtubules. It is not cross-reactive with *Vinca* alkaloids. It appears to act on proliferating cells and is cell cycle phase-specific, with the G_2 and S phases more sensitive than G_1 (Drewinko and Barlogie 1976).

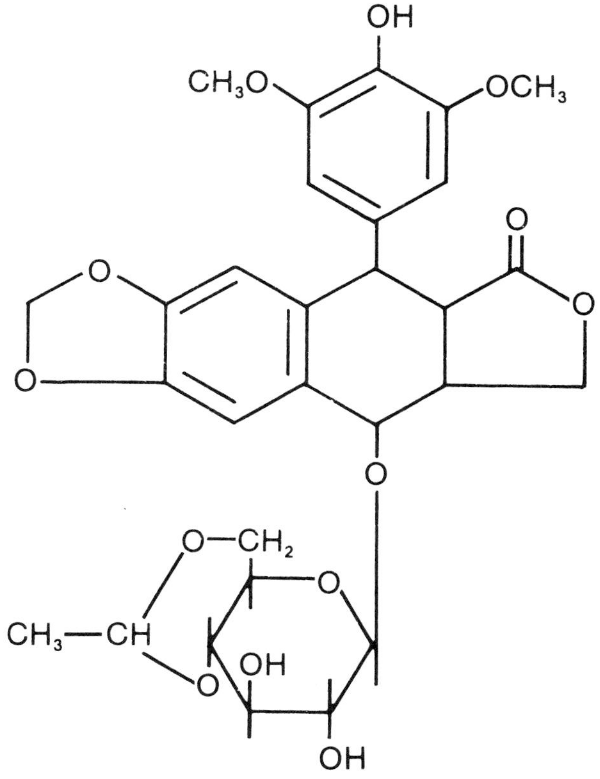

OH

CH_3O OCH_3

O

O O

O

O

O—CH_2

O

CH_3—CH

OH

O

OH

Fig. 26.6. *Etoposide, NSC 141540*

The drug is protein-bound and is evenly distributed throughout the body, except for the brain from which it appears to be excluded. Following intravenous infusion, it has a biexponential decay curve with a terminal half-life of 11.5 hours. After 72 hours, 44% of the drug is excreted in the urine with only 33% as metabolites. Plasma clearance is three times greater than with teniposide, renal clearance is nearly six times greater, accounting for equitoxic weekly doses of etoposide (290 mg/m^2) being three times larger than of teniposide (100 mg/m^2). There is a substantial enterohepatic circulation with variable bile excretion. Cerebrospinal fluid concentration is 1% of the plasma concentration (Issell and Crooke 1979; Allen and Creaven 1975). There are fewer published studies on the pharmacokinetics of orally administered etoposide. In an early phase I trial with the oral lipophil capsule, there were no dose-dependent hematologic toxic effects over a dose range of 120 to 300 mg/m^2 (Nissen et al. 1976). Subsequent studies with samples of tritiated drug showed erratic absorption of this formulation. Two newer formulations, the "drinking ampule" and a hydrophilic soft gelatin capsule, appear to give consistent gastrointestinal absorption of 47% to 50% in studies of the tritiated drug. These oral formulations exhibited dose-dependent toxic effects in phase I studies and cause less gastrointestinal toxicity than the initial capsule (Lau et al. 1979). Although only one study has compared the oral versus the intravenous route for tumor response (Cavalli et al. 1978), preliminary cumulative data in small cell carcinoma of the lung suggest equipotent antitumor activity.

The best tumor responses with etoposide have been in small cell carcinoma of the lung (SCCL), lymphoma (Ambruso et al. 1980), and acute nonlymphocytic leukemia (ANLL) (Issell and Crooke 1979). Cumulative figures from phase I and II studies in SCCL using different doses and schedules show an objective response rate of 44% in 201 patients, with 14 CRs and 74 PRs. Many of these patients received less than optimal doses, and the majority were heavily pretreated and had failed first-line drugs (Radice, Bunn, and Ihde 1979). Data from different institutions are remarkably similar, with objective response rates in phase II trials of 25% to 50%. Oral administration appears to give equivalent if not superior response rates compared to intravenous administration (Cavalli et al. 1978). At present there are many combination chemotherapy trials in progress, and preliminary reports suggest an even higher response rate than in monotherapy trials (Valdivieso et al. 1979; Dhafir et al. 1981). Experience with non-SCCL is limited, but a few responses have been reported and further studies seem indicated.

It is difficult to compare adequately the reports of etoposide therapy in lymphoma with our more standard drugs, because a large percentage of etoposide use was reported from Europe (Radice, Bunn, and Ihde 1979) and was not classified according to the Rappaport guidelines for non-Hodgkin's lymphomas. If we lump together the responses in reticulum cell sarcoma and diffuse histiocytic lymphoma, we find a 32% response rate with 1 CR and 35 PRs in 111 cases. In lymphosarcoma, there were 5 PRs in 22 cases (23%), and in unspecified lymphomas there were 14 PRs in 52 cases (27%). The drug seems promising for future trials of combination chemotherapy.

In acute leukemias, responses are highly specific for cell type. In 158 cases of ANLL there were 19 CRs and 19 PRs for a total objective response rate of 24%. For acute myelomonocytic leukemia the response rate was up to 41% with 10 CRs and 4 PRs in 34 cases. The response rate in acute lymphocytic leukemia was a disappointing 7% (Radice, Bunn, and Ihde 1979). Other tumors that have shown some response include mycosis fungoides, hepatoma, rhabdomyosarcoma, testicular tumors, and uterine, prostate, and bladder carcinomas (Nissen et al. 1980).

The dose-limiting toxicity is leukopenia, which occurred in 43% of patients with about 10% having a nadir less than 1000/mm^3. Thrombocytopenia was noted in 14% of patients and was rarely severe. The white blood cell nadir was reached in 10 to 14 days with recovery by day 16 to 21 (Radice, Bunn, and Ihde 1979). No cumulative toxicity has been noted.

Gastrointestinal toxicity occurred in 15% of patients receiving intravenous treatment and in 55% of those given oral drug. Stomatitis was also noted in 23% of patients treated orally and only 5% receiving intravenous therapy. There was no significant difference in other toxicities between the two routes of administration (Radice, Bunn, and Ihde 1979). Alopecia occurs commonly but recovers with cessation of the drug, and frequently with continued therapy. Bronchospasm with wheezing is a relatively unique problem associated with intravenous administration, and usually responds satisfactorily to cessation of infusion and administration of antihistamines such as diphenhydramine. Fever, chills, and hypotension have also been associated with intravenous therapy. Hypotension occurred most often with a rapid infusion of etoposide and responded to slowing or stopping the infusions.

The drug is available as etoposide to registered investigators from the Division of Cancer Treatment, which obtains it from Bristol Laboratories. Only the injectable preparation is available in the United States at this time although oral etoposide is available in Europe (Brunner et al. 1976; Lau et al. 1979). It is hoped that an oral preparation will be available soon here.

The injectable etoposide is supplied in a 100-mg ampule with citric acid, anhydrous, 10 mg; benzyl alcohol, 150 mg; polysorbate 80, purified, 400 mg; polyethylene glycol 300, 3.25 gm; and absolute alcohol q.s. 5.12 gm. The drug is prepared as a solution in 5-ml ampules, with 10 in a box. The solution in each ampule must be diluted with 20 to 50 volumes of sterile normal saline before administration by slow IV infusion. In time, solutions tend to show a precipitate, depending on concentration. A 1:20 solution shows precipitate in 30 minutes, 1:50 in 3 hours, and 1:100 in 6 hours. Solutions with precipitate should be discarded. Five percent dextrose should not be used as a vehicle as it causes instability. Unopened ampules are stable at room temperature for one to five years.

Maytansine (Investigational)

Maytansine (NSC 153858) is a naturally occurring ansa macrolide with antitumor activity (Division of Cancer Treatment 1975) first isolated from the East African shrub *Maytenus serrata* (formerly known as *Maytenus ovatus*), and later from the wood and bark of *Maytenus buchananii* (fig. 26.7). It is a member of a class of compounds usually isolated from microorganisms such as the antibiotics rifamycin and streptovaricin. Its mechanism of action appears to be interference with tubulin polymerization in the mitotic spindle, leading to metaphase arrest. More generally it interferes with microtubule formation in many organs (Issell and Crooke 1978). It inhibits incorporation of tritiated thymidine into DNA and thereby inhibits DNA synthesis. It is cell cycle phase-specific primarily in the M and S phases.

As an antimitotic agent, maytansine is about 100 times more potent than vincristine on sea urchin eggs and 20 times more potent in Chinese hamster ovary-K cells in tissue cultures (Issell and Crooke 1978). Blood levels of maytansine are so low that so far no satisfactory method has been developed for measuring the concentration present in human blood and tissues following dosage in the clinical range. Thus there are no pharmacokinetic data available at present. It is hoped that when a microbiologic source becomes available so that the supply problem is relieved, there will also be enough to develop immunoassay procedures for measuring blood levels.

Antitumor activity has been noted in phase I studies. In four patients with acute lymphoblastic leukemia there was one CR and three PRs. In lymphoma there was one CR and three patients who had been treated previously and failed with vincristine

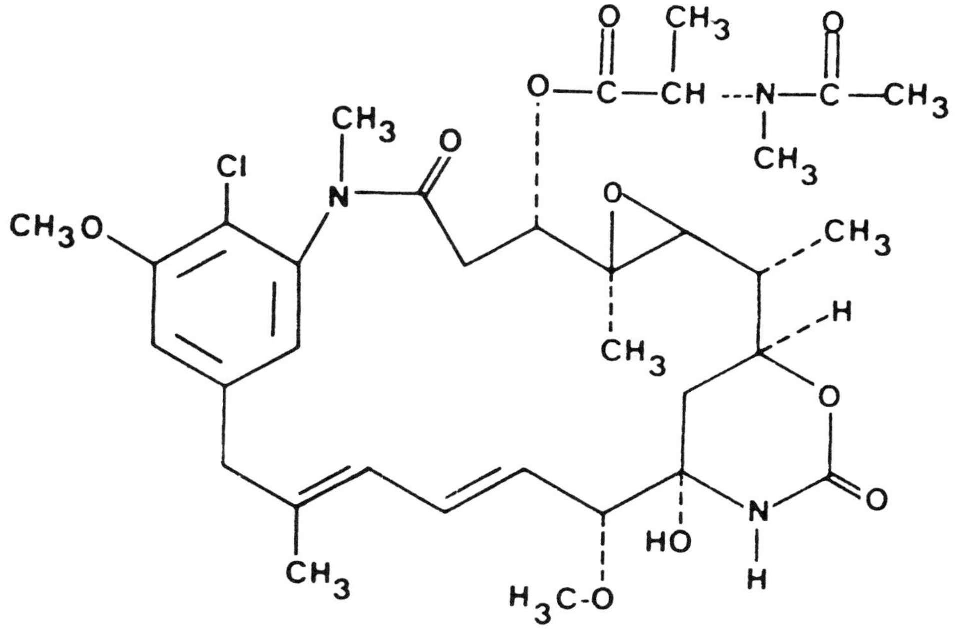

Fig. 26.7. *Maytansine, NSC 153858*

(Chabner et al. 1978). Occasional responses have been reported in thymoma, ovarian carcinoma, melanoma, and breast and lung cancer.

Dose-limiting toxicities are nausea, vomiting, and early diarrhea often followed by late constipation (Blum and Kahlert 1978; Eagan et al. 1978). These all seem to be dose-related and become more severe at higher drug levels. Other incapacitating toxicities also considered to be dose-limiting were caused by the effect of maytansine on the central nervous system (Blum et al. 1978). These included weakness, lethargy, dysphoria, and insomnia. Peripheral neuropathy was reported with jaw pain, paresthesias, and severe myalgias. Loss of deep tendon reflexes and marked prolongation of nerve conduction times are seen (Chahinian et al. 1979). Transient abnormal liver function tests occur frequently (Franklin et al. 1980), but serious hepatotoxicity has only been reported in patients with prior liver impairment (Cabanillas et al. 1978). Myelosuppression is mild and infrequent, occurring primarily in patients with liver impairment. Neurologic toxicity is cumulative and only slowly reversible.

Local phlebitis can be troublesome but is usually ameliorated by diluting the drug in a larger volume of fluid (250 to 500 ml). Paravenous infiltration leads to cellulitis and potentially this could go on to a slough. To minimize this, the drug should be administered through the tubing or three-way stopcock of a rapidly running intravenous, or at a predetermined rate in a monitored infusion.

Dosage is still being evaluated but the recommended weekly schedule is 0.07 to 1.25 mg/m^2 by IV bolus for six doses, at which point cumulative toxicity becomes a problem. The maximum tolerated dose (MTD) was 2 mg/m^2 repeated at 21-day intervals. Using a three-day schedule, the MTD was 1.8 to 2.1 mg total for the three days, or 0.6 to 0.7 mg per day for each of the three days.

The drug is available as maytansine from the Division of Cancer Treatment only to cooperative study groups and comprehensive cancer center directors. It is supplied for injection in 0.25 mg vials with mannitol, 100 mg, as a white lyophilized powder in 10-ml vials. It is reconstituted with 5 ml of sterile normal saline or water for injection to make a solution containing 0.05 mg/ml maytansine. For infusion, this is diluted further to at least 0.01/mg/ml with 5 volumes 5% dextrose in saline. The intact vials are stable for two years under refrigeration. Reconstituted solution is chemically stable for four days, but the unused portion should be discarded after eight hours because of danger of microbial contamination.

References

Ahn, Y. S. et al. Vincristine therapy of idiopathic and secondary thrombocytopenias. *N. Engl. J. Med.* 291:376–380, 1974.

Ahn, Y. S. et al. The treatment of idiopathic thrombocytopenia with vinblastine-loaded platelets. *N. Engl. J. Med.* 298:1101–1107, 1978.

Allen, L. M., and Creaven, P. J. Comparison of the human pharmacokinetics of VM-26 and VP-16, two antineoplastic epidophyllotoxin glucopyranoside derivatives. *Eur. J. Cancer* 11:69–70, 1975.

Ambruso, D. R. et al. Successful treatment of lymphohistiocytic reticulosis with phagocytosis with epipodophyllotoxin VP-16-213. *Cancer* 45:2516–2520, 1980.

Amiel, J. L. et al. Cancer of the kidney: chemotherapy trial in 97 patients. *Nouv. Presse Med.* 8:2335–2337, 1979.

Bagley, C. M., Jr. et al. Advanced lymphosarcoma: intensive cyclical combination chemotherapy with cyclophosphamide, vincristine, and prednisone. *Ann. Intern. Med.* 76:227–234, 1972.

Bedikian, A. Y. et al. Evaluation of vindesine and MER in colorectal cancer. *Cancer* 46:463–467, 1980.

Beer, C. T.; Wilson, M. L.; and Bell, J. A preliminary investigation of the fate of tritiated vinblastine in rats. *Can. J. Physiol. Pharmacol.* 42:368–373, 1964.

Bellet, R. E. et al. Phase II trial of VM-26 in patients with metastatic malignant melanoma. *Cancer Treat. Rep.* 62:445–447, 1978.

Blum, R. H. et al. A therapeutic trial of maytansine. *Cancer Clin. Trials* 1:113–118, 1978.

Blum, R. H., and Kahlert, T. Maytansine: a phase I study of an ansa macrolide with antitumor activity. *Cancer Treat. Rep.* 62:435–438, 1978.

Bonadonna, G. et al. Controlled study with multiple drug combination in advanced breast cancer. *Proc. Am. Soc. Clin. Oncol.* 15:176, 1974.

Bonadonna, G. et al. Combination chemotherapy of Hodgkin's disease with Adriamycin, bleomycin, vinblastine, and imidazole carboxamide (ABVD) vs. MOPP. *Cancer* 36:252–259, 1975.

Bosl, G. J. et al. Vinblastine, bleomycin, and Cis-diamminedichloroplatinum in the treatment of advanced testicular carcinoma. *Am. J. Med.* 68:492–496, 1980.

Brown, A. W. et al. Combination chemotherapy with vinblastine, bleomycin, and Cis-diamminedichloroplatinum (II) in squamous cell carcinoma of the head and neck. *Cancer* 45:2830–2835, 1980.

Brunner, K. W. et al. Comparison of the biologic activity of VP-16-213 given IV and orally in capsules or drink ampules. *Cancer Treat. Rep.* 60:1377–1379, 1976.

Cabanillas, F. et al. Phase I study of maytansine using a 3-day schedule. *Cancer Treat. Rep.* 62:425–428, 1978.

Canellos, G. P. et al. Hematologic and cytogenetic remission of blastic transformation in chronic granulocytic leukemia. *Blood* 38:671–679, 1971.

Carroll, D. S.; Gralla, R. J.; and Kemeny, N. E. Phase II evaluation of vindesine in patients with advanced colorectal carcinoma. *Cancer Treat. Rep.* 63:2097–2098, 1979.

Carter, S. K., and Livingston, R. B. Plant products in cancer chemotherapy. *Cancer Treat. Rep.* 60:1141–1156, 1976.

Casper, E. S.; Gralla, R. J.; and Golbey, R. B. Vindesine (DVA) and Cis-dichlorodiammineplatinum II (DDP) combination chemotherapy in non-small cell lung cancer (NSCLC). *Proc. Am. Soc. Clin. Oncol.* 20:337, 1979.

Cavalli, F. et al. VP-16-213 monotherapy for remission induction of small cell lung cancer: a randomized trial using three dosage schedules. *Cancer Treat. Rep.* 62:473–475, 1978.

Chabner, B. A. et al. Initial clinical trials of maytansine, an antitumor plant alkaloid. *Cancer Treat. Rep.* 62:429–433, 1978.

Chabner, B. A.; Myers, C. E.; and Oliverio, V. T. Clinical pharmacology of anticancer drugs. *Semin. Oncol.* 4:165–191, 1977.

Chahinian, A. P. et al. Phase I study of weekly maytansine given by IV bolus or 24-hour infusion. *Cancer Treat. Rep.* 63:1953–1960, 1979.

Coltman, C. A., Jr. Chemotherapy of advanced Hodgkin's disease. *Semin. Oncol.* 6:87–93, 1979.

Cooper, R. G. Combination chemotherapy in hormone-resistant breast cancer. *Proc. Am. Assoc. Cancer Res.* 10:15, 1969.

Cooper, R. G.; Holland, J. F.; and Glidewell, O. Adjuvant chemotherapy of breast cancer. *Cancer* 44:793–798, 1979.

Costa, G. et al. Initial clinical studies with vincristine. *Cancer Chemother. Rep.* 24:39–44, 1962.

Currie, V. E. et al. Phase I trial of vindesine in patients with advanced cancer. *Cancer Treat. Rep.* 62:1333–1336, 1978.

DeVita, V. T., Jr. et al. Advanced diffuse histiocytic lymphoma, a potentially curable disease. *Lancet* 1:248–250, 1975.

DeVita, V. T., Jr.; Serpick, A. A.; and Carbone, P. P. Combination chemotherapy in the treatment of advanced Hodgkin's disease. *Ann. Intern. Med.* 73:881–895, 1970.

Dhafir, R. A. et al. The effect of etoposide (VP-16), used alone or in combination, on the survival of patients (Pts) with refractory testicular cancer (RTC). *Proc. Am. Soc. Clin. Oncol.* 21:464, 1981.

Division of Cancer Treatment. *Maytansine, NSC 153858.* Clinical brochure. Bethesda, Md.: National Cancer Institute, 1975.

Dorr, R. T., and Jones, S. E. Inapparent infiltrations associated with vindesine administration. *Med. Pediatr. Oncol.* 6:285–288, 1979.

Drewinko, B., and Barlogie, B. Survival and cycle-progression delay of human lymphoma cells in vitro exposed to VP-16-213. *Cancer Treat. Rep.* 60:1295–1306, 1976.

Dyke, R. W., and Nelson, R. L. Phase I anti-cancer agents. Vindesine (desacetyl vinblastine amide sulfate). *Cancer Treat. Rev.* 4:135–142, 1977.

Eagan, R. T. et al. Phase II evaluation of maytansine in patients with metastatic lung cancer. *Cancer Treat. Rep.* 62:1577–1579, 1978.

Einhorn, L. H.; and Donahue, J. P. Combination chemotherapy in disseminated testicular cancer: the Indiana University experience. *Semin. Oncol.* 6:87–93, 1979.

Einhorn, L. H.; Furnas, B. E.; and Powell, N. Combination chemotherapy of disseminated testicular carcinoma with cis-platinum diammine dichloride (CPDD), vinblastine (VBL), and bleomycin (BLEO). *Proc. Am. Soc. Clin. Oncol.* 17:240, 1976.

Falkson, G. et al. A clinical trial of the oral form of 4′-demethyl-epidophyllotoxin-B-D-ethylidene glucoside (NSC 141540) VP-16-213. *Cancer* 35:1141–1144, 1975.

Feun, L. G.; Samson, M. K.; and Stephens, R. L. Vinblastine (VLB), bleomycin (Bleo), Cis-diamminedichloroplatinum (DDP) in disseminated extragonadal germ cell tumors. *Cancer* 45:2543–2549, 1980.

Finkelstein, J. Z. et al. Combination chemotherapy for metastatic neuroblastoma. *Proc. Am. Assoc. Cancer Res.* 15:44, 1974.

Franklin, R. et al. A phase I-II study of maytansine utilizing a weekly schedule. *Cancer* 46:1104–1108, 1980.

Gralla, R. J. et al. Phase II evaluation of vindesine in patients with non-small cell carcinoma of the lung. *Cancer Treat. Rep.* 63:1343–1346, 1979.

Gutierrez, M. L., and Crooke, S. T. Pediatric cancer chemotherapy: an updated review. I. Cis-diamminedichloroplatinum (cisplatin), VM-26 (teniposide), VP-16 (etoposide), mitomycin C. *Cancer Treat. Rep.* 6:153–164, 1979.

Gutin, P. H. et al. Phase II study of procarbazine, CCNU, and vincristine combination chemotherapy in the treatment of malignant brain tumors. *Cancer* 35:1398–1404, 1975.

Haggard, M. E. et al. Vincristine in acute leukemia of childhood. *Cancer* 22:438–444, 1968.

Handelsman, H.; Goldsmith, M. A.; and Slavik, M. *4'-demethyl-epidophyllotoxin-B-D-ethylidene glucoside (NSC 141540), VP-16-213*. Bethesda, Md.: National Cancer Institute, 1974.

Hardisty, R. M.; McElwain, R. J.; and Darby, C. W. Vincristine and prednisone for the induction of remissions in acute leukemia of childhood. *Br. Med. J.* 2:662–665, 1969.

Hartwell, J. L. Types of anticancer agents isolated from plants. *Cancer Treat. Rep.* 60:1031–1067, 1976.

Hertz, R. et al. Effect of vincaleukoblastine on metastatic choriocarcinoma and related trophoblastic tumors in women. *Cancer Res.* 20:1050–1058, 1960.

Heyn, R. M. et al. Vincristine in the treatment of acute leukemia in children. *Pediatrics* 38:82–91, 1966.

Howard, J. P. Response of acute leukemia in children to repeated courses of vincristine. *Cancer Chemother. Rep.* 51:465–469, 1967.

Issell, B. F., and Crooke, S. T. Maytansine. *Cancer Treat. Rev.* 5:199–208, 1978.

Issell, B. F., and Crooke, S. T. Etoposide (VP-16-213). *Cancer Treat. Rev.* 6:107–124, 1979.

Itri, L. M. et al. Vindesine with cisplatin in non-small cell lung cancer (NSCLC): the influence on survival and the effect of adding conventional agents. *Proc. Am. Soc. Clin. Oncol.* 22:521, 1981.

James, D. H. et al. Combination chemotherapy for childhood neuroblastoma. *JAMA* 194:123–126, 1965.

Johnson, I. S. et al. Antitumor principles derived from *Vinca rosea* Linn. I. Vincaleukoblastine and leurosine. *Cancer Res.* 20:1016–1022, 1960.

Johnson, I. S. et al. The *Vinca* alkaloids: a new class of oncolytic agents. *Cancer Res.* 23:1390–1427, 1963.

Klein, E. et al. Treatment of Kaposi's sarcoma with vinblastine. *Cancer* 45:427–431, 1980.

Lau, M. E. et al. Phase I trial of a new form of an oral administration of VP-16-213. *Cancer Treat. Rep.* 63:485–487, 1979.

Livingston, R. B. et al. Small cell carcinoma of the lung: combined chemotherapy and radiation. *Ann. Intern. Med.* 88:194–199, 1978.

Mathé, G. et al. Phase II clinical trial with vindesine for remission induction in acute leukemia, blastic crisis of chronic myeloid leukemia, lymphosarcoma, and Hodgkin's disease: absence of cross-resistance with vincristine. *Cancer Treat. Rep.* 62:805–809, 1978.

Moertel, C. G. et al. Brief communication: therapy of advanced colorectal cancer with a combination of 5-fluorouracil, methyl-1-3-cis(2-chloroethyl)-1-nitrosourea and vincristine. *J. Natl. Cancer Inst.* 54:69–71, 1975.

Nelson, R. L.; Dyke, R. W.; and Root, M. A. Comparative pharmacokinetics of vindesine, vincristine, and vinblastine in patients with cancer. *Cancer Treat. Rev.* 7(suppl.):17–24, 1980.

Neuss, N. et al. The *Vinca* alkaloids. *Adv. Chemother.* 1:133–174, 1964.

Nicholson, W. M. et al. Combination chemotherapy in generalized Hodgkin's disease. *Br. Med. J.* 3:7–10, 1970.

Nissen, N. I. et al. Phase I clinical trial of an oral solution of VP-16-213. *Cancer Treat. Rep.* 60:943–945, 1976.

Nissen, N. I. et al. Clinical trial of VP-16-213 (NSC 141540) IV twice weekly in advanced neoplastic disease. *Cancer* 45:232–235, 1980.

Noble, R. L.; Beer, C. T.; and Cutts, J. H. Role of chance observations in chemotherapy: *Vinca Rosea*. *Ann. N.Y. Acad. Sci.* 76:882–894, 1958.

O'Brien, R. et al. Scalp tourniquet to lessen alopecia after vincristine. Letter to the editor. *N. Engl. J. Med.* 283:1469, 1970.

Ohnuma, T.; Greenspan, E. M.; and Holland, J. F. Initial clinical study with vindesine: tolerance to weekly IV bolus and 24-hour infusion. *Cancer Treat. Rep.* 64:25–30, 1980.

Owellen, R. J. et al. Pharmacokinetics of vindesine and vincristine in humans. *Cancer Res.* 37:2603–2607, 1977.

Perdue, R. E., and Hartwell, J. L., eds. Proceedings of the sixteenth Annual Meeting of the Society for Economic Botany: plants and cancer. *Cancer Treat. Rep.* 60:973–1214, 1976.

Radice, P. A.; Bunn, P. A., Jr.; and Ihde, D. C. Therapeutic trials with VP-16-213 and VM-26: active agents in small cell lung cancer, non-Hodgkin's lymphomas, and other malignancies. *Cancer Treat. Rep.* 63:1231–1239, 1979.

Rivera, G. et al. Combined VM-26 and cytosine arabinoside in treatment of refractory childhood lymphocytic leukemia. *Cancer* 45:1284–1288, 1980.

Rosenberg, S. A., and Kaplan, H. A. CCNU, Adriamycin, and vinblastine (CAV) combination chemotherapy for advanced Hodgkin's disease. *Cancer* 35:55–63, 1973.

Rosenthal, S., and Kaufman, S. Vincristine neurotoxicity. *Ann. Intern. Med.* 80:733–737, 1974.

Rozencweig, M. et al. VM-26 and VP-16-213: a comparative analysis. *Cancer* 40:334–342, 1977.

Schein, P. S. et al. Bleomycin, Adrianycin, cyclophosphamide, vincristine, and prednisone (BACOP) combination chemotherapy. *Ann. Intern. Med.* 85:417–422, 1976.

Schepartz, S. A. History of the National Cancer Institute and the plant screening program. *Cancer Treat. Rep.* 60:975–977, 1976.

Sen, G., and Bose, K. C. *Rauwolfia serpentina,* a new Indian drug for insanity and high blood pressure. *Indian Med. Wld.* 2:194–201, 1931.

Simister, J. M. Alopecia and cytotoxic drugs. *Br. Med. J.* 2:1138, 1966.

Smith, I. E. et al. Vindesine: phase I study in the treatment of breast cancer, malignant melanoma, and other tumors. *Cancer Treat. Rep.* 62:1427–1433, 1978.

Smithson, W. A.; Gilchrist, G. S.; and Burgert, E. O., Jr. Childhood acute lymphocytic leukemia. *CA* 30:158–181, 1980.

Spremulli, E. et al. Phase II study of VM-26 in adult malignancies. *Cancer Treat. Rep.* 64:147–149, 1980.

Strauss, G. M.; Goldsmith, M. A.; and Slavik, M. *4′-demethylepidophyllotoxin-B-D-thenylidene glucoside (NSC 122819), VM-26.* Clinical brochure. Bethesda, Md.: National Cancer Institute, 1975.

Stuart, M. J. et al. Syndrome of recurrent increased secretion of antidiuretic hormone following multiple doses of vincristine. *Blood* 45:315–320, 1975.

Sullivan, M. P. Symposium on vincristine. *Cancer Chemother. Rep.* 52:453–535, 1968.

Valdivieso, M. et al. Intensive induction chemotherapy (IIC) of small cell lung cancer (SCLC) with ECHO: E = epipodophyllotoxin VP-16, C = Cytoxan, H = hydroxydaunorubicin, O = Oncovin. *Proc. Am. Soc. Clin. Oncol.* 20:383, 1979.

Wilbur, J. R. et al. Chemotherapy of sarcomas. *Cancer* 36:765–769, 1975.

Withering, W. *An account of the fox-glove and some of its medical uses.* Birmingham: Swinney, 1785.

Young, C. W. et al. Early phase II evaluation of vindesine in patients with advanced cancer. Proceedings of the Tenth International Congress of Chemotherapy, Zurich, 1977. In *Current Chemotherapy,* vol. 2, eds. W. Siegenthaler and R. Luthy. Washington, D.C.: American Society of Microbiology, 1978, pp. 1330–1331.

Zubrod, C. G. et al. The chemotherapy program of the National Cancer Institute: history, analysis, and plans. *Cancer Chemother. Rep.* 50:349–540, 1966.

twenty-seven

Miscellaneous Antineoplastic Drugs

DAVID S. FISCHER

This group represents drugs that did not readily fit into the earlier chapters based on classification by mechanism of action or origin. It includes three drugs of restricted indication already marketed, three investigational agents, and two radiosensitizers, one marketed for other indications and one investigational (table 27.1). At least 10 additional investigational drugs could have been included, but those that seemed most likely to be approved for commercial distribution were selected.

Mitotane has been used for two decades for palliation of the rare metastatic adrenal cortical carcinoma (Gutierrez and Crooke 1980). It has no other indications. At about the same time, methyl-GAG was investigated as a drug for acute leukemia (Livingston et al. 1968). Although it had well-documented efficacy, its toxicity was unacceptable in the dosage schedule then used and the drug was abandoned. After a period of neglect, it is now being reevaluated with new schedules that are less toxic in both solid tumors (Hart et al. 1980; Killen et al. 1980) and acute leukemias of the non-lymphocytic type (Levi and Wiernik 1975).

Procarbazine is a methylhydrazine derivative used primarily in the treatment of lymphomas (Carter 1970). It has achieved its greatest fame as a component of the MOPP regimen (mechlorethamine, Oncovin, prednisone, and procarbazine). Initially, methotrexate was used instead of procarbazine. The combination MOPP has revolutionized the treatment of stage III and stage IV Hodgkin's disease by producing complete remissions (CR) in up to 80% and cures in 68% of those achieving CR (DeVita et al. 1980).

L-asparaginase is an enzyme that hydrolyzes the amino acid asparagine, which is required for many tumor cells but is synthesized by normal cells. Thus it is the first anticancer agent that has a qualitatively different effect on neoplastic as compared to normal cells, rather than simply a quantitative advantage. Although the drug is only useful clinically in acute lymphoblastic leukemia, its significance is enormous as biochemical proof that qualitative differences can be found between normal and neoplastic animal cells and not simply between plant (bacteria) and animal (human) cells (Capizzi, Bertino, and Handschumacher 1970).

An investigational drug that seemed to show great promise in acute non-lymphocytic leukemias, amsacrine is an acridine dye derivative that acts to inhibit DNA synthesis and transcription by intercalation between base pairs in a manner reminiscent of the anthracycline antibiotics—daunorubicin and doxorubicin. Not surprisingly then, after being initially judged relatively nontoxic, amsacrine has recently been found to be cardiotoxic (Marsoni 1980). The extent of this and its implications for future therapy are still being investigated.

The response to radiation therapy is usually cell cycle-nonspecific with all cells affected regardless of their proliferative status. Interestingly, cells that are hypoxic are resistant to radiation destruction by a dose factor of nearly 3. This resistance is believed to be a major determinant in the failure of radiation therapy to

Table 27.1. *Miscellaneous Antitumor Drugs*

Generic Name	*Trade or Common Name*	*Major Route(s)*	*Frequent Dose*	*Major Indication(s)*	*Major Toxicities*
Mitotane	Lysodren (o, p'-DDD)	p.o.	9–10 gm/day	Adrenal cortical	G.I., neuromuscular, cutaneous
Methyl-GAG*	—	IV	500 mg/m^2	Bladder, G.I.	Mucositis, marrow
Procarbazine	Matulane	p.o.	100 mg/m^2 × 14 days	Lymphoma	Marrow, G.I., neurologic MAO inhibitor
L-asparaginase	Elspar	IV	4000–400,000 IU/m^2	ALL	Neurologic, hepatic, allergic
Razoxane*	(ICRF-159, Razoxin)	p.o.	800–1200 mg/m^2 × 4 days	G.I., ALL	Marrow
Amsacrine*	(m-AMSA)	IV	75–90 mg/m^2 × 7 days	AML	Marrow, G.I., cardiac
Metronidazole†	Flagyl	p.o., IV	2.5 gm/m^2 × 2–6 weeks	Glioblastoma	G.I.
Misonidazole*	(RO-07-582)	p.o., IV	Under study	Under study	G.I., neurologic

*Investigational.

†Approved as anti-infective but investigational as antineoplastic.

cure some tumors. To enhance radiation responses, several approaches have been used. Treatment in hyperbaric chambers is difficult, expensive, and of marginal efficacy. Use of heavy nuclear particle beams such as neutrons or negative π (pi) mesons is being evaluated at present, but it is very expensive and the equipment is very scarce. A more popular and affordable approach is to use chemical agents that selectively increase the radiosensitivity of hypoxic cells without affecting the radiation sensitivity of well-oxygenated cells of most normal tissues. These are called radiosensitizers or hypoxic-cell radiosensitizers. Many agents have been investigated for this type of action. One of the more popular ones was 5-bromouracil-2′-deoxyriboside, which was incorporated into and damaged the DNA of dividing cells when exposed to radiation (Hodnett 1963). A new investigational antineoplastic agent, razoxane (ICRF-159) is not only efficacious as a tumor cell inhibitor, but appears to improve response in hypoxic cells by increasing the vascular supply and by enhancing capillary growth. The drug has had marginal success in acute leukemia and several solid tumors (Wasserman et al. 1973). Data are still preliminary, but evaluation as a hypoxic-cell sensitizer is proceeding concomitant to study of the neoplastic cell response and separate from surgery or radiation (Kanazir 1969).

Still another group of hypoxic-cell sensitizers is the oxygen-mimetic drugs, especially those with affinity for electrons. At the present time, those of greatest clinical interest are the nitroimidazoles, some of which have low toxicity, distribute freely in tissues, and have a long metabolic half-life (Fowler, Adams, and Denekamp 1976). Preliminary trials have been carried out with metronidazole, a commercially available antitrichomonal marketed for many years as Flagyl, and a 2-nitro-imidazole, misonidazole, an investigational preparation that appears to be more effective. Unlike razoxane, which has independent cellular toxicity against cancer cells, metronidazole and misonidazole are not in themselves antitumor agents, but only behave so by enhancing radiation response. It is felt that these may achieve considerable importance in the future, and the question has even been raised as to whether they may play a role in selective chemotherapy of the hypoxic cell (Kelly, Hannam, and Giles 1979).

Mitotane

Mitotane (Lysodren, o,p′-DDD, NSC 38721) (fig. 27.1) is the ortho, para prime isomer of the insecticide dichlorodiphenyl-dichloroethane, a close relative of the better known insecticide DDT (dichloro-diphenyl-trichloroethane). It was introduced into clinical medicine following the observation that DDD caused severe atrophy of the adrenal cortex in dogs. It exerts a direct cytotoxic effect on the mitochondria of the adrenal cortical cells, producing focal degeneration of the fascicular and reticular zones (Broder and Carter 1970). The exact biochemical mechanism of action is unknown.

Following oral administration, absorption is about 40%, and maximum plasma concentration is reached in three to five hours. Equilibrium between plasma and tissue drug levels is achieved in 12 hours, with 20% to 30% of the administered drug stored in the tissues and about 10% metabolized and excreted in the urine (Moy 1961). The liver and kidney are primary metabolic sites. The highest tissue concentrations are found in the adipose tissue, but this lipid-soluble drug is also detected in the brain, adrenals, liver, bile, and serum with *no* preferential accumulation in the adrenals (Gutierrez and Crooke 1980).

The only clinical indication for mitotane is in therapy of patients with inoperable, residual, or recurrent adrenal cortical carcinoma (Bergenstal et al. 1960). In more than 70% of patients it results in a decrease of more than 30% in urinary steroid excretion from the increased pretreatment levels (Gallagher et al. 1962). Response with regression in measurable disease has been reported in 34% to 61% of cases (Hutter and Kayhoe 1966; Lubitz, Freeman, and Okun 1973). A small number of patients with measurable tumor regression did not have elevated pretreatment steroid levels, suggesting that the drug is effective in both functioning and nonfunctioning adrenal cortical carcinoma. Comparison with historical controls suggests that survival is increased with mitotane therapy (Montgomery and Welbourn 1965; Molnar, Mattox, and Bahn 1963). The drug should not be used in treatment of obesity (Danowski et al. 1964).

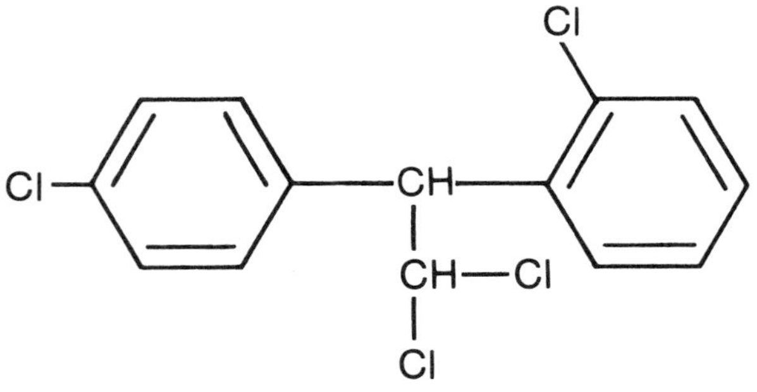

The major toxic effects are gastrointestinal, neuromuscular, and dermatologic. Anorexia, nausea, vomiting, and/or diarrhea occur in about 80% of cases and are the most common reasons for patients discontinuing the drug. Antiemetics may be helpful, and in severe reactions dose reduction or suspension is necessary. Central nervous system depression manifested by lethargy and somnolence occurs in one-third of cases, and dizziness, vertigo, headache, muscle tremors, confusion, and/or weakness occur in an additional one-sixth of patients. Thus half of all those treated experience some neuromuscular side effects.

Skin rash occurs in about 15% of cases, does not appear to be dose-related, and frequently disappears with continuance of the drug. Less common toxicities include visual blurring, diplopia, lens opacification, retinopathy, hematuria, albuminuria, hemorrhagic cystitis, flushing, hypertension, or orthostatic hypotension.

The recommended dosage of mitotane is 9 to 10 gm per day in three or four divided doses. Tolerance has varied widely, and some patients can only tolerate 2 gm per day, while others have been reported to tolerate 16 gm per day without ill effects. Treatment should be initiated in the hospital or other professionally monitored environment until a stable dosage is achieved. Response may require three months and may be manifested only by maintenance of clinical status or slowing of growth of metastatic lesions. Treatment is usually continued for many months, sometimes more than a year. Exogenous steroids may have to be administered if adrenal cortical insufficiency develops, or in situations of added stress such as trauma, infection, or hypotension.

The drug is available as Lysodren (Bristol) in 500-mg scored white tablets in bottles of 100.

Cl CH CH—Cl Cl Cl

Fig. 27.1. *Mitotane (o,p′-DDD), NSC 38721*

Methyl-GAG (Investigational)

Methyl-GAG (methyl-glyoxal-bis-guanylhydrazone, MGBG, methyl-G, NSC 32946) is a synthetic chemical compound chosen for clinical trials in humans because of its activity in L 1210 mouse leukemia and other animal tumor systems (fig. 27.2). It is believed to inhibit 5′-adenosyl-methionine-decarboxylase, thereby inhibiting production of spermidine from putrescine. It inhibits DNA and RNA presumably by complexing with the nucleic acids. It also acts as a mitochondrial poison and inhibits cellular respiration.

Oral administration leads to gastrointestinal upset and poor absorption. Following brief intravenous infusion, the drug has a triphasic plasma half-life of 18 minutes, 3 hours, and 100 hours. The drug appears to undergo very little metabolism and has a biphasic urine excretion with 25% excreted in the first 24 hours and the remainder slowly excreted over 3 weeks. Little is detectable in CSF, but ascites fluid levels sometimes exceed plasma levels.

In its initial trials, methyl-GAG was administered intravenously on a daily schedule for the treatment of acute non-lymphocytic leukemia (ANLL) (Levin et al. 1965). Although it had objectively demonstrable efficacy, associated toxicity was so severe that the drug was withdrawn from clinical trials for many years. The most common side effect was diffuse mucositis involving the oropharynx, larynx, vagina, rectum, and presumably the entire gastrointestinal tract, associated with anorexia, abdominal pain, and diarrhea (Mihich et al. 1962). Progressive unexplained weight loss persisted for several weeks and was frequently accompanied by oral and esophageal moniliasis. Hypoglycemia was also a common side effect, and several deaths from drug toxicity were noted.

After several years of neglect, interest in clinical trials of methyl-GAG has revived. Using weekly or biweekly schedules of 500 mg/m^2 intravenously over 30 minutes (Knight et al. 1979a), responses have been seen in transitional cell carcinoma of the bladder, adenocarcinoma of the colon esophageal, gastric, renal cell, lung and endometrial carcinoma, melanoma, hepatoma, and ANLL (Knight et al. 1979b).

Dosage schedules are still being worked out. Below 500 mg/m^2 weekly no significant toxicity was noted (Knight et al. 1979a). Toxicity did occur at that dosage and consisted of mucositis (usually beginning on day 5 to 14), generalized malaise, and fatigue. As the dose was slowly escalated, toxicity became more severe and was dose-limiting at 850 mg/m^2. Dysesthesias were common; myelosuppression, nausea, and vomiting were less common; and fever, arrhythmia, and hypoglycemia were rare at 500 mg/m^2. For ANLL doses are being tested in the range of 100 mg/m^2/day for five days and if toxicity is acceptable, then 150 to 200 mg/m^2/day to toxicity or response. Very preliminary observations have caused investigators to suggest that continuous infusions will reduce toxicity and improve the therapeutic index (Hart et al. 1980). An intramuscular route has been effective for maintenance therapy in some cases (Shnider et al. 1974).

The drug is available from the Division of Cancer Treatment in 1-gm vials for reconstitution with 30 ml normal saline, but it will go into solution with 10 ml. Intravenous infusion should be done cautiously because extravasation may lead to cellulitis. Systemic toxicity may be increased by concurrent 5-azacytidine. The dry powder is stable for six years at room temperature and the reconstituted liquid for 20 days at 22° C.

Procarbazine

Procarbazine (Matulane, NSC 77213) is one of a group of methylhydrazine derivatives originally synthesized and evaluated for monoamine oxidase inhibitory activity (fig. 27.3). It was also shown to be effective in inhibiting the growth of several rodent tumors and was then introduced into clinical trials (Carter 1970). Its precise mechanism of action is unknown, but it is thought to be

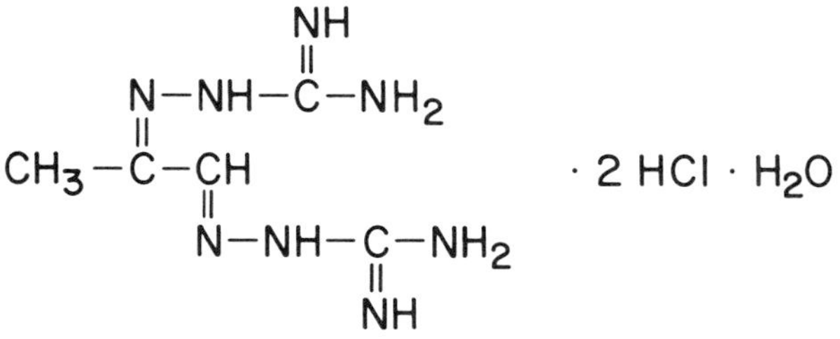

Fig. 27.2. *Methyl-GAG, NSC 32946*

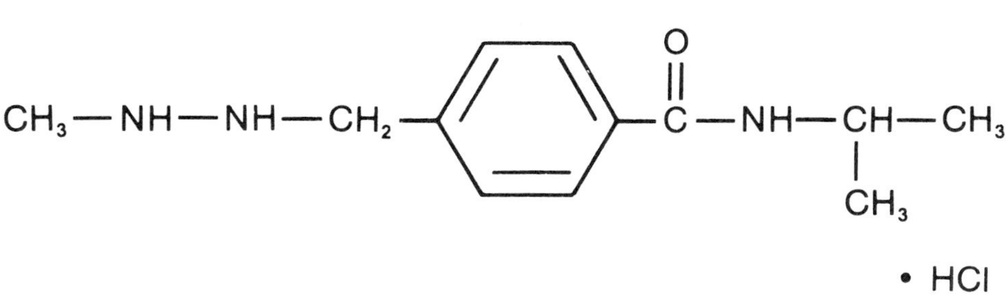

Fig. 27.3. *Procarbazine, NSC 77213*

converted to a biologically active metabolite to exert its carcinostatic effect. It degrades DNA in vitro without significantly disrupting its double helical structure, possibly due to the effect of the hydroxyl radicals. Methylation of nucleic acids by the N-methyl group of procarbazine may also play a role, particularly in the 1 position of adenine. Although procarbazine is not cross-resistant with alkylating agents, patients rapidly develop resistance to the drug when it is used alone. It is cell cycle S phase-specific.

The drug is readily absorbed from the gastrointestinal tract and easily crosses the blood-brain barrier so CSF and plasma levels are soon in equilibrium. The plasma half-life in humans is about 10 minutes. Metabolism to the azo derivative occurs primarily in the liver and kidney. About 70% of the carbonyl-^{14}C-procarbazine is excreted in human urine as the acid during the first 24 hours. Approximately 30% of the N-methyl group appears in respiratory CO_2.

The primary role of procarbazine has been as a replacement for methotrexate used in conjunction with mechlorethamine, vincristine (Oncovin), and prednisone in the MOPP or MVPP treatment of stage III or IV Hodgkin's disease (DeVita et al. 1970; Nicholson et al. 1970), or with cyclophosphamide, vincristine, and prednisone in the treatment of non-Hodgkin's lymphoma with C-MOPP (DeVita et al. 1975). In these instances, it is part of a potentially curable regimen (Spivack 1974). It has been used with responses but no cures in primary and metastatic brain tumors, bronchogenic carcinoma, melanoma, bladder, ovarian, and testicular carcinoma, and neuroblastoma (Jellife and Marks 1965; Carter 1970; Martz et al. 1963).

Primary toxic manifestations are myelosuppression and gastrointestinal disturbances. Leukopenia and thrombocytopenia are usually dose-limiting and their onset may be delayed for several weeks after the start of treatment. Anemia may result from a direct effect on the marrow or from hemolysis. Nausea and vomiting occur frequently and may be dose-limiting, but tolerance can develop with use. Non-phenothiazine antiemetics may be helpful. Stomatitis, dysphagia, and diarrhea are less common. Lethargy, depression, drowsiness, hyperexcitability, ataxia, psychosis, and nystagmus have been noted. Less common are myalgia, arthralgia, dermatitis, pruritus, hyperpigmentation, and alopecia (Brunner and Young 1965).

Central nervous system depressants may be enhanced by procarbazine, and a disulfiram-like reaction may occur when alcohol and procarbazine are used concomitantly. Because procarbazine inhibits monoamine oxidase, tricyclic antidepressants, phenothiazines, sympathomimetics, and foods with a high tyramine content should be avoided. This includes, but is not limited to, strong cheeses, wine, beer, yogurt, brewer's yeast, bananas, chicken livers, and pickled herring. Disregard of this caution may lead to hypertensive crisis, intracranial hemorrhage, manic reactions, and headache (Mann and Hutchison 1967). The drug is also immunosuppressive, teratogenic, and carcinogenic (Kelly et al. 1964), so it is best avoided in pregnancy.

The usual dosage is 50 to 200 mg/day orally for three to four weeks, and should be reduced in patients with hepatic, renal, or bone marrow impairment. As a component of the MOPP and C-MOPP regimens, 100 mg/m^2 is given daily for 14 days every 4 weeks, but for only 10 days in the COPP regimen.

The drug is available as Matulane (Roche) in 50-mg capsules that are stable at room temperature.

L-asparaginase

L-asparaginase (Elspar, NSC 109229) is an enzyme of unknown structure produced by *Escherichia coli*, which exerts antitumor activity through catalyzing the hydrolysis of asparagine in tumor cells incapable of synthesizing sufficient L-asparaginase for their own needs. This mechanism is unique in at least two respects: (1) it is extracellular in its locus of action, and the drug does not get into the cell but hydrolyzes the L-asparagine before it reaches the dependent tumor cell; and (2) it exploits a qualitative difference between normal cells and some cancer cells, namely the inability of the latter to synthesize sufficient L-asparagine and the ability of the former to do so. All the other antineoplastic agents so far available depend on quantitative differences in the response between normal and cancer cells.

In addition to its hydrolytic effect on L-asparagine, the drug has resulted in measurable inhibition of asparagine synthetase in tumor cells. The asparagine-depleting action interferes with tumor cell protein synthesis and thereby leads to enzyme depletion and ultimately to inhibition of DNA and RNA synthesis. It probably is cell cycle phase-specific for the postmitotic G_1 phase (Ohnuma et al. 1970).

Following intravenous administration, the plasma half-life is about 15 to 30 hours (Livingston and Carter 1969). The drug is a foreign protein and elicits antibody in spite of the patient's state of relative immunosuppression due to the underlying disease. Hypersensitivity reactions ranging from urticaria to anaphylactic shock occur in approximately 10% of patients during the initial course, and more frequently with each subsequent administration. Allergic reactions are not completely predictable on the basis of an intradermal test. In a series of 562 patients reported by Jones and co-workers (1977), there were six anaphylactic deaths due to L-asparaginase.

At present, the only indication for this agent is as a component of a combination regimen to induce remission in acute childhood lymphocytic leukemia (Leventhal and Henderson 1970; Sutow et al. 1971). It should not be used for maintenance. Although a few responses were noted in acute myelogenous leukemia and in non-Hodgkin's lymphoma when the drug was being evaluated (Clarkson et al. 1970), both of these disorders can be treated far more effectively with other agents without the addition of L-asparaginase. There are, however, reports of its use in combination with daunorubicin, especially in T cell lymphomas (Bodey et al. 1974).

For a drug that exerts a qualitatively different effect on normal and tumor cells and has no bone marrow or gastrointestinal mucosal toxicity, L-asparaginase has a multitude of other toxicities. Neurotoxic reactions are common, ranging from decreased level of consciousness to coma. Seizures or focal neurologic signs are rare. Since the drug does not cross the blood-brain barrier, toxicity may be related to the sudden release of ammonia from asparagine. Malaise is common and usually worsens with each successive dose. Fever of at least 1° C occurs in more than half the patients. Hepatotoxicity with abnormal liver function tests occurs in 50% to 75% of patients. Low serum albumin and hypocholesterolemia, as well as other clotting factors including V, VII, VIII, and IX, may be decreased. If reduction of platelets occurs, one should suspect a disseminated intravascular coagulation and check for fibrin split products.

Less common side effects include hyperglycemia (leading to nonketotic hyperosmolar coma that requires insulin therapy), pancreatitis, azotemia, and weight loss (most patients average a 6% loss of body weight). Nausea and vomiting are seen in about half the patients.

The most worrisome side effect is a syndrome consisting of rapid onset of urticaria, chills, fever, flushing, fall in blood pressure, and dyspnea. If untreated or inadequately treated this can progress to death, and has done so in several cases. Therefore the drug should be administered to patients only in a hospital setting under the supervision of a physician who is qualified by training and experience to administer cancer chemotherapeutic agents. In addition, there should be available an experienced nurse, a running intravenous, oxygen, suction, a syringe filled with epinephrine, 1:1000, and vials of diphenhydramine, 50 mg and hydrocortisone, 100 mg. The nurse-physician team must be prepared to treat anaphylaxis at each administration of the drug, and the incidence increases with each successive dose. In choosing treatment for induction in the child with acute lymphocytic leukemia, the physician must weigh carefully the possibility of achieving therapeutic benefits versus the risk of toxicity.

Usual dosages range from 1000 to 10,000 IU/kg given daily, triweekly, or weekly for 10 to 28 days. Regimens of this type have induced 33% to 66% remissions in acute lymphocytic leukemia and 12% in acute myelocytic leukemia. In general, if L-asparaginase is used as a single agent remissions are of short duration. Although combination with vincristine and prednisone does not produce a higher remission rate than vincristine and prednisone alone, the median duration of remission with the three drugs appears to be significantly prolonged (Jones et al. 1977). L-asparaginase should always be given after the vincristine, never before or simultaneously with it. L-asparaginase has also been used to potentiate the effect of methotrexate (Capizzi et al. 1971).

L-asparaginase of *E. coli* derivation is available as Elspar (Merck Sharpe & Dohme) as a lyophilized powder in vials of 10,000 IU and 50,000 IU in 10-ml containers. They are reconstituted with 5 or 10 ml respectively of sterile normal saline. An investigational preparation of L-asparaginase derived from *Erwinia carotovora* (NSC 106977) is available from NCI in 10,000-IU vials to be reconstituted with 2 ml sterile normal saline. Either preparation should be injected into the tubing of a running infusion of 5% dextrose in water or normal saline over a period of at least 30 minutes, or given intramuscularly.

Razoxane (Investigational)

Razoxane (ICRF-159, Razoxin, NSC 129943) (fig. 27.4) belongs to a family of bis-dioxopiperazines, the parent compound being ethylenediamine tetraacetic acid (EDTA), a powerful chelating agent. Razoxane is less polar than EDTA and therefore is able to penetrate cells. It was shown to be tumor-inhibitory in several murine tumor systems (Wasserman et al. 1973), and appears to block the entrance of proliferating cells into mitosis when given during the premitotic and early mitotic

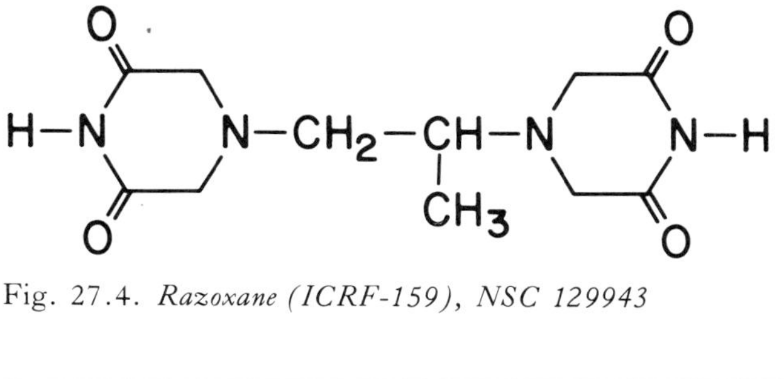

Fig. 27.4. *Razoxane (ICRF-159), NSC 129943*

(G_2/M) phases of cell growth. It also tends to normalize tumor vasculature somewhat so that there is a decreased incidence of metastases.

Absorption is better with multiple small doses rather than a single large dose. Following an oral dose of 3 gm/m^2, the peak plasma level was noted at two hours and the plasma half-life was three and one half hours. Drug was detectable in the plasma at 12 hours but not at 24 hours. Initially, the major urinary excretion product is razoxane, but at 72 hours more metabolite is excreted. Apparently the urinary and plasma metabolite are the same, but the biologic activity of the metabolite is unknown.

Phase II investigations are still in progress, but some activity has been demonstrated in colon carcinoma (Bellet et al. 1976; Marciniak et al. 1975), head and neck tumors, osteosarcoma, lung cancer, carcinoma of the breast, lymphoma, and acute leukemias (Bellet et al. 1973; Bakowski 1976). In a group of children with acute lymphocytic leukemia who had failed most of the available drugs, there were two complete and seven partial remissions lasting from one to six months.

Razoxane is also being evaluated as a radiosensitizer. Factors that suggest potential activity in this role include: (1) its normalization of tumor blood vessels which may decrease tumor hypoxia and increase sensitivity to radiation; (2) it potentiates radiomimetic alkylating agents; (3) it acts at the G_2/M phase of the cell cycle, a point at which cells are particularly sensitive to radiation. In two clinical trials, radiation plus razoxane gave better results than historical controls in the treatment of soft tissue and osteosarcomas. In a study of 16 patients with bronchogenic carcinoma, 6 were given radiation therapy alone, 10 were given razoxane plus radiation, and 8 stayed on maintenance razoxane (Bakowski 1976). The mean survival time of these 8 patients was 11.4 months compared to 8.3 months in those treated with radiation alone. Use of the drug in combination is in an early stage (Paul, Catalano, and Engstrom 1978).

Another interesting property of razoxane in animal studies has been its ability to decrease the toxicity of daunorubicin, and to act synergistically with daunorubicin, doxorubicin, cisplatin, cytarabine, cyclophosphamide, 5-fluorouracil, and hexamethylmelamine (Bakowski 1976).

The dose-limiting toxicity is hematologic, with leukopenia being quite marked. Thrombocytopenia and anemia are usually mild. The nadir of the leukopenia is usually 12 days, and blood counts return to normal 8 days later. Thrombocytopenia is usually mild and occurs in about 20% of patients. Nausea and vomiting occur in about 40% but are usually mild and respond to antiemetics (Wasserman et al. 1973). Diarrhea and alopecia are experienced by about 10% of patients. No significant renal, hepatic, or pulmonary toxicity has been reported so far.

When used as a single agent, the usual dose has been 20 to 30 mg/kg daily by mouth for four consecutive days. When used as a radiation sensitizer, the dose has been 125 mg/day. Other schedules being tried include:

1. 850 mg/m^2 by mouth in divided doses for three consecutive days repeated every four weeks
2. 1 to 2 gm/m^2 once weekly by mouth in three divided doses
3. 300 mg/m^2 by mouth daily

For doses in combination therapy, see the published protocol.

The drug is available in 50-mg and 500-mg scored tablets from the Division of Cancer Treatment to registered investigators. It may be stored at room temperature.

Amsacrine (Investigational)

Amsacrine (m-AMSA, acridinyl anisidine, 4′-(9-acridinylamino)methanesulfon-m-anisidine, NSC 249992) is an acridine dye derivative that inhibits DNA synthesis and transcription by intercalation and external binding to DNA (fig. 27.5). It is also an inhibitor of DNA synthetase. At nonphysiologic concentrations, inhibition of DNA polymerase is observed as well (Cain and Atwell 1974). Cycling cells are two to four times more sensitive to the drug's cytotoxic effects than resting cells, with a transitory accumulation of cells in S phase followed by an arrest in G_2 phase.

When administered intravenously, the drug is distributed to all tissues except the central nervous system. It is rapidly metabolized to a thioether of acridine and glutathione in the liver and excreted principally

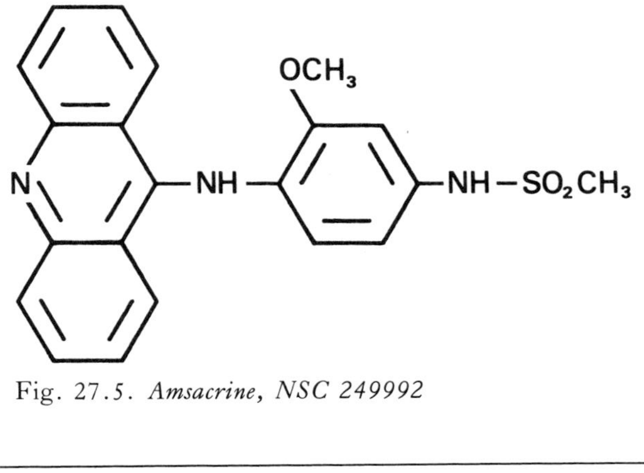

Fig. 27.5. *Amsacrine, NSC 249992*

through the biliary system. Hepatic dysfunction prolongs biliary excretion, and dose reduction is recommended when this is significant. Urinary excretion plays a secondary but significant role, and impaired renal function prolongs clearance from the blood. The importance of renal excretion increases proportionately when there is hepatic dysfunction. Much or most of the drug is degraded before excretion.

The most exciting role for amsacrine appears to be in the treatment of acute leukemia, especially the acute non-lymphocytic leukemias (Legha et al. 1980; Weiss, Charles, and Macdonald 1980). In early phase I and II studies there were 17 complete remissions in 81 patients (Weiss, Charles, and Macdonald 1980), with a smaller number of patients achieving lesser responses. Some of those who responded had previously failed regimens that included doxorubicin. Subsequently, a large phase II study in a single institution reported on 62 adults with previously treated acute leukemia who were treated with a total intravenous dose of 150 to 1320 mg/m^2 over 3 to 14 days (Legha et al. 1980). Of the 56 evaluable patients, 13 achieved a complete remission and 6 had partial remission. Best results occurred at a dose level of 75 to 90 mg/m^2 for seven days, which resulted in 9 complete remissions in 30 patients. Of 38 patients with acute myeloblastic leukemia, 11 achieved complete remission, and 3 of 13 with lymphoblastic disease had a partial remission.

Five of 38 patients with breast cancer treated with either 40 mg/m^2/day for three days, or 100 mg/m^2 as a single dose, both every three weeks, have had partial remissions (Weiss, Charles, and Macdonald 1980). Antitumor responses with amsacrine have occurred in previously treated patients with melanoma, which is unusual but encouraging, and suggests the need for testing it as a first-line drug (Legha et al. 1978). Hepatomas have also regressed with systemic therapy, but no intraarterial hepatic infusions have been tried yet. A few objective responses have been seen in heavily pretreated patients with Hodgkin's disease and non-Hodgkin's lymphoma (Goldsmith et al. 1980). So far, trials of amsacrine in colon and non-small cell carcinoma of lung have shown no responses.

Published toxicity is primarily hematologic. Leukopenia is the dose-limiting toxicity (Issell 1980). Nadir counts occur between 7 and 14 days and recovery is usually seen by day 24. Thrombocytopenia is usually mild except in patients with prior radiation to major marrow-bearing sites, in which case it may be severe (VonHoff et al. 1978; Legha et al. 1979).

Pain on infusion occurs when the drug is not adequately diluted. When given in 500 ml 5% dextrose in water immediate pain is uncommon, but late phlebitis may be a problem. The drug is a potent tissue irritant, so care must be exercised to avoid extravasation that may lead to tissue necrosis, slough, and pain. Phlebitis may occur in spite of perfect technique, and cold packs and corticosteroid creams have been used for symptomatic relief. In such instances, future drug administration should use a larger volume of diluent.

The frequency and severity of nausea and vomiting depend on dose and rate of administration, but is rarely a limiting factor. Premedication with antiemetics is frequently effective. Stomatitis is usually mild to moderate. During early testing, very high doses caused seizures in several patients. Post infusion headache and dizziness were reported with some frequency but usually disappeared within two hours. Abnormal liver function tests have occurred with frequency and severity depending on dosage. This was not entirely unexpected, since animal studies showed frequent hepatic damage. Because it is primarily excreted by the liver, patients with prior hepatic dysfunction are poor risks for this drug.

Published studies had indicated that at very high repetitive doses for acute leukemia, several patients developed ventricular fibrillation. On July 29, 1980, the NCI sent an urgent update letter (Marsoni 1980) to all investigators indicating a recent report of four cases of serious cardiac abnormalities associated with amsacrine. This brought to eight the number of documented cases with acute arrhythmia during or immediately after infusion. Four patients had ventricular fibrillation, one had supraventricular tachycardia, and three had reported cardiac arrest. Of these eight patients, five were pretreated with one or more anthracyclines, and four had low potassium values. In one patient, death was directly attributed to the arrhythmia. Five other patients died, but probably as a result of complications of their disease. To put this in perspective, there were at least 1500 patients already treated with amsacrine by the time of the update letter. Whether cardiac monitoring during administration, with appropriate antiarrhythmic agents and resuscitative equipment available, will become an official NCI recommendation remains to be seen. Probably, after further study guidelines will be issued. At present, we monitor all patients and have standby resuscitative equipment.

Dosage is still being worked out. For solid tumors, 40 mg/m^2/day for three days every three weeks was found to produce severe leukopenia, especially in patients with breast cancer. A tolerable and efficacious dosage seems to be 30 mg/m^2/day for three days every three weeks. Single doses of 90 to 120 mg/m^2 IV every 28 days have also been used. For acute leukemia, dosages of 50 to 90 mg/m^2/day for three days have been tried, but response rates were low. The current favored dosage is 90 mg/m^2/day for 5 to 10 days depending on response. The daily dose of amsacrine is mixed in 500 ml 5% dextrose in water and given intravenously over 60 to 90 minutes. It must *not* be put in saline because the chloride is less soluble than the lactate, and it may precipitate. The solution should not be refrigerated or it may precipitate.

Amsacrine is available from the Division of Cancer Treatment to registered investigators. It is supplied in a duo-pack containing two sterile liquids that must be aseptically combined prior to use, forming what will be termed the "combined solution." Each 2-ml flint ampule contains 1.5 ml of 50-mg/ml solution of amsacrine (total 75 mg) in anhydrous N,N-dimethylacetamide (DMA). Each 20-ml amber vial contains 13.5 ml of 0.0353 M L-lactic acid diluent.

Aseptically add 1.5 ml of amsacrine to 13.5 ml L-lactic acid diluent to produce an orange-red solution containing 5 mg/ml of amsacrine. The combined solution is physically and chemically stable for at least 48 hours at room temperature (22° to 25° C) under ambient lighting, but since it does not contain antibacterial agents it should be used within eight hours and the residual discarded. The unopened drug and diluent are stable for at least four years at room or refrigerator temperature. A new 20-mg/ml vial containing 1 ml is being added to available formulations.

Metronidazole

Metronidazole (Flagyl, NSC 69587) is a systemic trichomonad and amebicide (fig. 27.6). It is a 5-nitroimidazole and is relatively well tolerated in the clinical doses needed for treating trichomonal and amebic infections. Experience with the very high doses required for radiosensitization is limited (Fowler, Adams, and Denekamp 1976). Patients seem to tolerate 300 mg/kg (10 to 15 gm) in a single dose. Limiting toxicity is nausea.

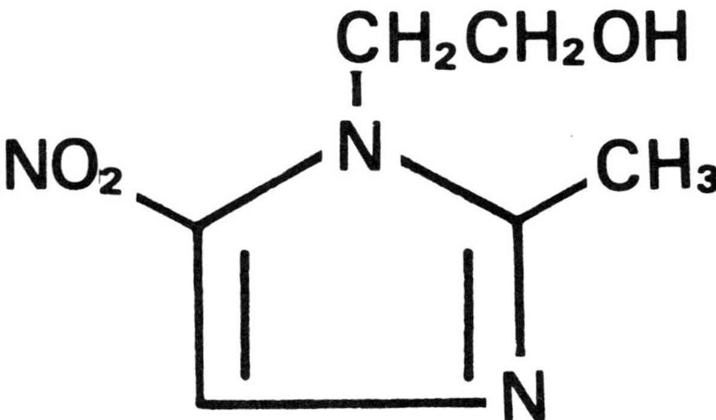

Fig. 27.6. *Metronidazole, NSC 69587*

Following oral administration peak concentration is achieved (200 mg/ml) in one-half to six hours. Mean plasma half-life is 7.9±1.4 hours. The peak plasma level is lower and occurs later if food is taken shortly before the drug. Serum concentrations fall to 25% of peak levels in 24 hours and to less than 10% after 48 hours. There is good CSF penetration (75% to 90%). Liver function tests and blood counts show no abnormalities. Five percent to 20% is excreted in the urine unchanged. Metabolism is in the liver by hydroxylation of the 2-methyl group and oxidation of the 1-hydroxyethyl group.

In one clinical trial with glioblastoma, 31 patients were randomized into two groups two weeks after surgery. Both groups received a total tumor dose of 3000 rad in nine fractions, given three times a week in an overall time of 18 days. Fifteen patients received radiation treatment alone and 16 received 6 gm/m^2 of metronidazole in divided doses. Half of the patients treated with metronidazole returned home self-sufficient. Of those receiving radiation alone, 6 out of 15 were discharged home. The difference in survival between the two groups shows a significant difference, $P \sim 0.02$ (Urtasun 1976). Ultimately patients in both groups succumbed, but in the treated group there was a delay of mortality of four and one-half months before 50% of patients died.

The logical explanation for improved survival of patients taking metronidazole is that tumor regrowth is delayed by killing more of the radioresistant hypoxic cells (Workman 1980). The demonstration of a significant difference in survival time undoubtedly indicates a beneficial effect of the radiosensitizer. Whether this holds up in future trials is yet to be determined. A role for metronidazole as a cytocidal agent with other chemotherapy drugs is being evaluated (Kelly, Hannam, and Giles 1979).

Dose-limiting toxicity is nausea and vomiting. Other adverse effects are headache, anorexia, grand mal seizures, diarrhea, abdominal cramping and constipation, and a sharp and unpleasant metallic taste (Thomas et al. 1980). Occasionally, stomatitis and leukopenia have occurred. Dosage is usually 2.5 gm/m^2 (3 to 4 gm per dose) orally over two to six weeks. The drug is available as Flagyl (Searle) in 250-mg tablets. An investigational intravenous preparation is in development. Caution must be exercised in selection of patients at present because metronidazole is carcinogenic in mice and possibly rats. It is also mutagenic to some bacteria in concentrations reached in human therapy, and this often predicts carcinogenesis. No carcinogenesis has been shown in hamsters or in humans.

Misonidazole (Investigational)

Misonidazole (RO-07-582, NSC 261037) is a 2-nitroimidazole that is being studied as a hypoxic-cell radiosensitizer of greater potency (fig. 27.7). There is also early evidence to suggest that it may have a similar role in hyperthermia and with selected chemotherapy drugs (Stratford et al. 1980).

Absorption is good following oral administration, and maximum serum concentration is reached in two to four hours. Serum half-life is 9.8 to 17.5 hours. The serum concentration at four hours rises linearly with dose and is disproportionately high after large amounts, suggesting saturation of the metabolic enzyme systems or the saturation of tissue depots. Metabolism is in the liver by O-demethylation. Excretion in the urine is 5% to 20%. Penetration into CSF is excellent and approaches plasma levels.

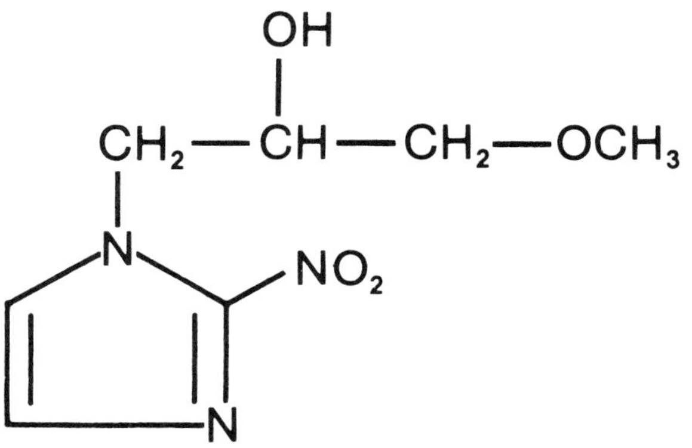

OH

$CH_2—CH—CH_2—OCH_3$

N

NO_2

N

Fig. 27.7. *Misonidazole, NSC 261037*

Tumor response to radiation plus misonidazole is spotty (Fu et al. 1980; Arcangeli et al. 1980). There have been responses in squamous cell carcinoma of the cervix, sarcoma, and skin tumors. Several additional tumors have shown less quantifiable responses. Much of the data have been reported orally and are not yet published.

Toxicity always includes nausea and vomiting. The latter is severe in patients given 10 gm/day, and antiemetics diminish it. Dose-limiting toxicity is peripheral neuropathy, a problem that arises from continued use and the high plasma levels required for hypoxic-cell radiosensitization.

The drug is available from the Division of Cancer Treatment to registered investigators. It is supplied in opaque off-white capsules of 100 mg and 500 mg with 50 to the bottle, and stored at room temperature. In addition, a parenteral preparation is supplied as 500 mg of a light yellow lyophilized powder in 30-ml amber vials. After reconstitution, it is chemically stable for 14 days at room temperature and unaffected by exposure to light. Since there is no antibacterial preservative, however, it is suggested that reconstituted unused solution be discarded after eight hours.

References

Arcangeli, G. et al. Multiple daily fractionation (MDF) radiotherapy in association with hyperthermia and/or misonidazole: experimental and clinical results. *Cancer* 45:2707–2711, 1980.

Bakowski, M. T. ICRF 159, (±) 1,2-di(3,5-dioxopiperazin-1-yl) propane, NSC 129943; razoxane. *Cancer Treat. Rev.* 3:95–107, 1976.

Bellet, R. E. et al. Phase II study of ICRF-159 in solid tumors. *Cancer Chemother. Rep.* 57:185–189, 1973.

Bellet, R. E. et al. Phase II study of ICRF-159 in patients with metastatic colorectal cancer previously exposed to systemic chemotherapy. *Cancer Treat. Rep.* 60:1395–1397, 1976.

Bergenstal, D. M. et al. Chemotherapy of adrenocortical cancer with o,p′-DDD. *Ann. Intern. Med.* 53:672–682, 1960.

Bodey, G. P. et al. Therapy of adult acute leukemia with daunorubicin and L-asparaginase. *Cancer* 33:626–630, 1974.

Broder, L. E., and Carter, S. K., eds. *Proceedings of chemotherapy conference on ortho para′ DDD.* Bethesda, Md.: National Cancer Institute, 1970.

Brunner, K. W., and Young, C. W. A methylhydrazine derivative in Hodgkin's disease and other malignant neoplasms. Therapeutic and toxic effects studied in 51 patients. *Ann. Intern. Med.* 63:69–86, 1965.

Cain, B. F., and Atwell, G. J. The experimental antitumor properties of three congeners of the acridylmethansulphonanilide (AMSA) series. *Eur. J. Cancer* 10:539–549, 1974.

Capizzi, R. L. et al. L-asparaginase: clinical, biochemical, pharmacological and immunological studies. *Ann. Intern. Med.* 74:893–901, 1971.

Capizzi, R. L.; Bertino, J. R.; and Handschumacher, R. E. L-asparaginase. *Ann. Rev. Med.* 21:433–444, 1970.

Carter, S. K., ed. *Proceedings of the chemotherapy conference on procarbazine (matulane: NSC 77213): development and applications*. Bethesda, Md.: National Cancer Institute, 1970.

Clarkson, B. et al. Clinical results of treatment with *E. coli* L-asparaginase in adults with leukemia, lymphoma and solid tumors. *Cancer* 25:279–305, 1970.

Danowski, T. S. et al. O,p′ DDD therapy in Cushing's syndrome and in obesity with cushingoid changes. *Am. J. Med.* 37:235–250, 1964.

DeVita, V. T., Jr. et al. Combination chemotherapy in the treatment of advanced Hodgkin's disease. *Ann. Intern. Med.* 73:881–895, 1970.

DeVita, V. T., Jr. et al. Advanced diffuse histiocytic lymphoma, a potentially curable disease. *Lancet* 1:248–250, 1975.

DeVita, V. T., Jr. et al. Curability of advanced Hodgkin's disease with chemotherapy. *Ann. Intern. Med.* 92:587–595, 1980.

Fowler, J. F.; Adams, G. E.; and Denekamp, J. Radiosensitizers of hypoxic cells in solid tumors. *Cancer Treat. Rev.* 3:227–256, 1976.

Fu, K. K. et al. The effects of misonidazole during continuous low-dose rate irradiation. *Cancer Clin. Trials* 3:257–265, 1980.

Gallagher, T. F. et al. The effect of ortho para′ DDD on steroid hormone metabolites in adrenal cortical carcinoma. *Metabolism* 11:1155–1161, 1962.

Goldsmith, M. A. et al. Phase I study of m-AMSA in patients with solid tumors and leukemias. *Cancer Clin. Trials* 3:197–202, 1980.

Gutierrez, M. L., and Crooke, S. T. Mitotane (o,p′-DDD). *Cancer Treat. Rev.* 7:49–55, 1980.

Hart, R. D. et al. Clinical and pharmacologic studies with weekly and biweekly methyl-glyoxal-bis-guanylhydrazone (methyl-G). *Proc. Am. Assoc. Cancer Res.* 21:181, 1980.

Hodnett, E. M. Drugs used with radiation in the treatment of cancer. *Cancer Chemother. Rep.* 32:55–65, 1963.

Hutter, A., and Kayhoe, D. Adrenal cortical carcinoma, results of treatment with o,p′ DDD in 138 patients. *Am. J. Med.* 41:581–592, 1966.

Issell, B. F. Amsacrine (AMSA). *Cancer Treat. Rev.* 7:73–83, 1980.

Jellife, A. M., and Marks, J., eds. *Symposium on natulan*. London: John Wright & Sons, 1965.

Jones, B. et al. Optimal use of L-asparaginase in acute lymphocytic leukemia. *Med. Pediatr. Oncol.* 3: 387–400, 1977.

Kanazir, D. T. Radiation-induced alteration in DNA. *Progr. Nucl. Acid Res.* 9:117–122, 1969.

Kelly, J. P.; Hannam, T. W.; and Giles, G. R. The cytocidal action of metronidazole in combination with other antineoplastic agents. *Cancer Treat. Rev.* 6(suppl.):53–61, 1979.

Kelly, M. G. et al. Carcinogenic activity of a new antitumor agent, N-isopropyl-α-(2-methylhydrazino)-p-toluamide hydrochloride (NSC 77213). *Cancer Chemother. Rep.* 39:77–80, 1964.

Killen, J. et al. Methyl-glyoxal-bis-guanylhydrazone (NSC 32946) (methyl-G): phase II experience and clinical pharmacology. *Proc. Am. Soc. Clin. Oncol.* 21:368, 1980.

Knight, W. A., III et al. Phase I-II trial of methyl-GAG: a Southwest Oncology Group pilot study. *Cancer Treat. Rep.* 63:1933–1937, 1979a.

Knight, W. A., III et al. Methyl-glyoxal bis-guanylhydrazone (methyl-GAG, MGBG) in advanced human malignancy. *Proc. Am. Soc. Clin. Oncol.* 20: 319, 1979b.

Legha, S. S. et al. Phase I clinical investigation of 4′-(9-acridinylamino methansulfon-m-anisidide (NSC 249992), a new acridine derivative. *Cancer Res.* 38: 3712–3716, 1978.

Legha, S. S. et al. 4′-(acridinylamino) methanesulfon-m-anisidide (AMSA) in metastatic breast cancer. *Cancer Treat. Rep.* 63:1961–1964, 1979.

Legha, S. S. et al. 4′(9-acridinylamino) methanesulfon-m-anisidide (AMSA): a new drug effective in the treatment of adult acute leukemia. *Ann. Intern. Med.* 93:17–20, 1980.

Leventhal, B. G., and Henderson, E. S. Therapy of acute leukemia with drug combinations which include asparaginase. *Cancer* 25:825–829, 1970.

Levi, J. A., and Wiernik, P. H. Combination therapy with 5-azacytidine and methyl-GAG in previously treated patients with acute non-lymphocytic leukemia. *Cancer Chemother. Rep.* 59:1043–1045, 1975.

Levin, R. H. et al. Treatment of acute leukemia with methylglyoxal-bis-guanylhydrazone (methyl-GAG). *Clin. Pharmacol. Ther.* 6:31–42, 1965.

Livingston, R. B. et al. *Methyl-GAG, NSC 32946*. Clinical brochure. Bethesda, Md.: National Cancer Institute, 1968.

Livingston, R. B., and Carter, S. K. *L-asparaginase, NSC 109229*. Clinical brochure. Bethesda, Md.: National Cancer Institute, 1969.

Lubitz, J. A.; Freeman, L.; and Okun, R. Mitotane use in inoperable adrenal cortical carcinoma. *JAMA* 223:1109–1112, 1973.

Mann, A. M., and Hutchison, J. L. Manic reaction associated with procarbazine hydrochloride therapy of Hodgkin's disease. *Can. Med. Assoc. J.* 97:1350–1353, 1967.

Marciniak, T. A. et al. Phase II study of ICRF-159 in advanced colorectal cancer. *Cancer Chemother. Rep.* 59:761–763, 1975.

Marsoni, S. Urgent NCI update on m-AMSA cardiotoxicity. National Cancer Institute (letter), July 29, 1980.

Martz, G. et al. Preliminary clinical results with a new antitumor agent Ro 4-6467 (NSC 77213). *Cancer Chemother. Rep.* 33:5–14, 1963.

Mihich, E. et al. Pharmacology of methylglyoxal-bis (guanylhydrazone) (CH_3-G). Toxic and pathologic effects. *Cancer Res.* 22:962–972, 1962.

Molnar, G. D.; Mattox, V. R.; and Bahn, R. C. Clinical and therapeutic observations in adrenal cancer. A report on 7 patients treated with o,p′ DDD. *Cancer* 16:259–268, 1963.

Montgomery, D. A. D., and Welbourn, R. B. Adrenocortical carcinoma treated with o,p′ DDD. *Br. Med. J.* 1:1356–1358, 1965.

Moy, R. H. Studies on the pharmacology of o,p′ DDD in man. *J. Lab. Clin. Med.* 58:296–304, 1961.

Nicholson, W. M. et al. Combination chemotherapy in generalized Hodgkin's disease. *Br. Med. J.* 3:7–10, 1970.

Ohnuma, T. et al. Biochemical and pharmacological studies with asparaginase in man. *Cancer Res.* 30:2297–2305, 1970.

Paul, A. R.; Catalano, R. B.; and Engstrom, P. F. Phase I trial of ICRF-159 in combination with 1,3 bis-(2-chloroethyl)-1-nitrosourea (MeCCNU). *Cancer Clin. Trials* 1:99–102, 1978.

Shnider, B. I. et al. Effectiveness of methyl-GAG (NSC 32946) administered intramuscularly. *Cancer Chemother. Rep.* 58:689–695, 1974.

Spivack, S. D. Procarbazine. Drugs five years later. *Ann. Intern. Med.* 81:795–800, 1974.

Stratford, I. J. et al. The interaction of misonidazole with radiation, chemotherapeutic agents or heat. *Cancer Clin. Trials* 3:231–236, 1980.

Sutow, W. W. et al. L-asparaginase therapy in children with advanced leukemia. *Cancer* 28:819–824, 1971.

Thomas, G. M. et al. A toxicity study of daily dose metronidazole with pelvic irradiation. *Cancer Clin. Trials* 3:223–230, 1980.

Urtasun, R. C. Radiation and high-dose metronidazole in supratentorial glioblastomas. *N. Engl. J. Med.* 294:1364–1367, 1976.

VonHoff, D. D. et al. Phase I study of methanesulphonamide, N-[4-(9-acridinyl amino)-3-methoxyphenyl] using a single-dose schedule. *Cancer Treat. Rep.* 62:1421–1426, 1978.

Wasserman, T. et al. *±1,2-di(3,5-dioxopiperazin-1-yl) propane, ICRF-159, NSC 129943.* Clinical brochure. Bethesda, Md.: National Cancer Institute, 1973.

Weiss, R. B.; Charles, L. M.; and Macdonald, J. S. M-AMSA: an exciting new drug in the National Cancer Institute Drug Development Program. *Cancer Clin. Trials* 3:203–210, 1980.

Workman, P. Pharmacokinetics of hypoxic-cell radiosensitizers. *Cancer Clin. Trials* 3:237–251, 1980.

twenty-eight

Hormones and Cancer Therapy

DAVID S. FISCHER

Palliation of cancer by methods of endocrine manipulation still practiced, antedates the use of modern cytotoxic chemotherapy.

During the last century it was noted that the ovaries influenced mammary physiology in animals and humans. Accordingly, in 1896 Beatson removed the ovaries in women with breast cancer and reported striking palliation in a few cases. In the next 10 years English surgeons did about 100 such cases with temporary improvement in about one-third of their patients (Lett 1905), but the operation lost favor for the next four decades. In the 1920s, radiation oophorectomy was introduced with favorable reports of response in about one-third of cases.

Bilateral orchiectomy for advanced disseminated prostatic cancer was first used in 1941 by Huggins, Stevens, and Hodges and continues to be central to current management. Bilateral total adrenalectomy for prostatic carcinoma was first employed in 1945 by Huggins and Scott, but was complicated by the fact that corticosteroid replacement therapy did not become available until a few years later. In 1951, Huggins and Bergenstal described adrenalectomy for metastatic breast carcinoma. The theoretical basis for the surgery was belief in the common embryologic origin of the gonads and the adrenals, and the assumption that these are the only structures having the capacity to synthesize endogenous steroid hormones. In various series, reports of objective responses varied somewhat, but grouped at about one-third (Fracchia, Randall, and Farrow 1970). Later, when hypophysectomy became popular for breast cancer and large series were reported, the response rate, particularly in postmenopausal women, was very close to that of the other ablative procedures (Miller 1970).

Although the hormones and their antagonists play a role in many areas of modern medicine, the discussion here is confined largely to their role in cancer. Figure 28.1 shows molecular structures of several principal steroid hormones. Figure 28.2 shows several fluorinated steroids.

With the development of the adrenocorticosteroids in the late 1940s and early 1950s, replacement therapy became available to provide maintenance for patients subjected to ablative surgery (Huggins and Bergenstal 1951). As more potent preparations were created by chemists through manipulation of the basic molecules, it soon became possible to explore the effects of pharmacologic doses instead of physiologic doses. It was noted that in high doses, corticosteroids caused temporary shrinkage of some breast tumors, lymphomas, and Hodgkin's disease. In combination therapy with cytotoxic drugs, the responses were often striking, and in the MOPP program for Hodgkin's disease they could be curative (DeVita et al. 1980). Corticosteroids were also found to be effective in temporarily reducing edema around some tumors.

Androgens have been used since 1939 in the palliation of breast cancer. Figure 28.3 shows the molecular structure of the major androgens used in cancer therapy. Objective and subjective responses have been reported for many years, with an approximate 20% regression rate (Goldenberg 1964; Kennedy and Nathanson 1953).

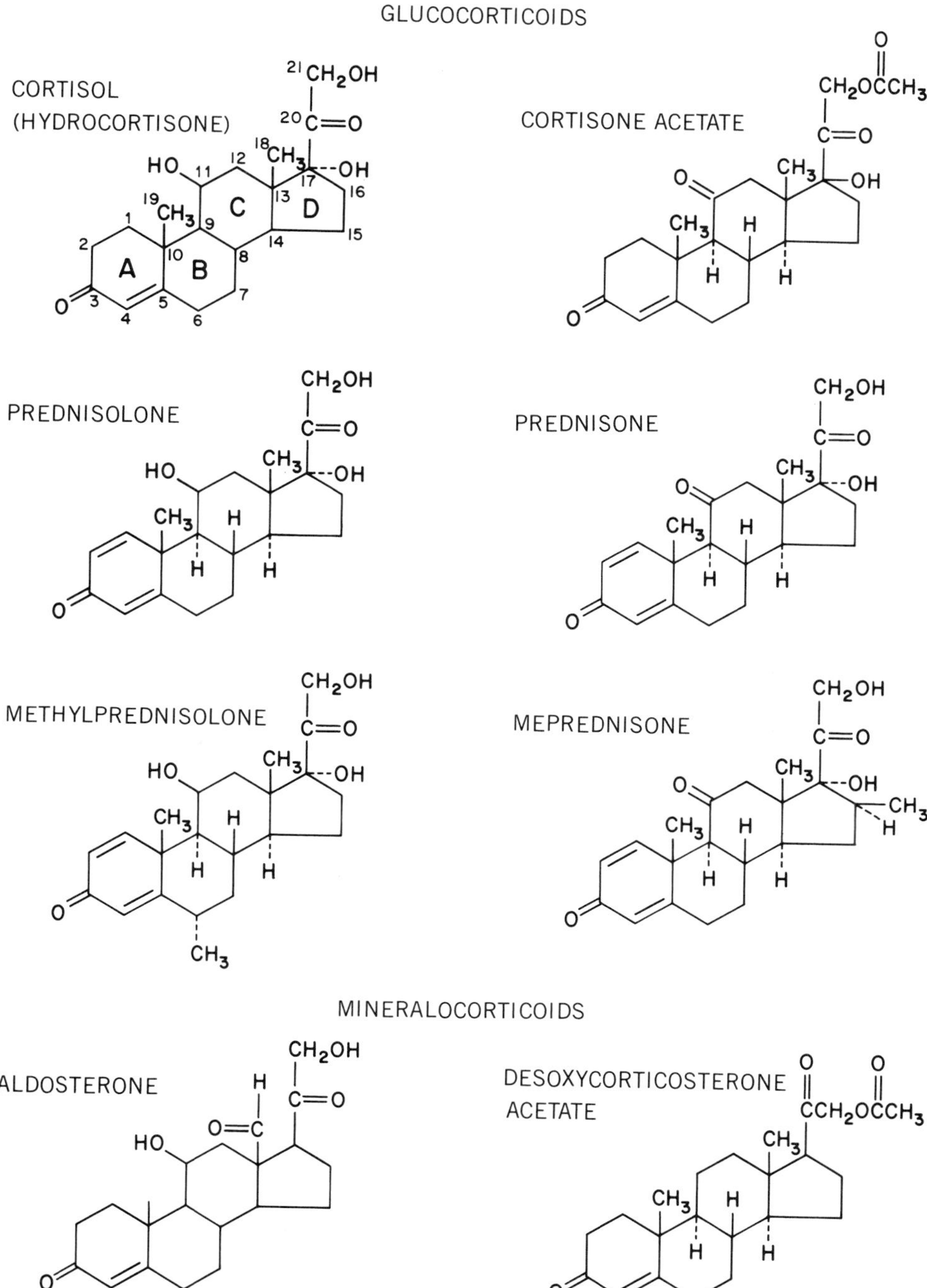

Fig. 28.1. *Cortisol (hydrocortisone) is the basic glucocorticoid of the body. Its basic structure is numbered in standard fashion. Prednisolone is the delta-1 (Δ^1) derivative, having lost a hydrogen in the one position and acquired a double bond in the 1-2 position. Prednisone is the Δ^1 derivative of cortisone. Each of the Δ^1 derivatives has its methyl derivative, which has slightly greater potency.*

Aldosterone is the physiologic mineralocorticoid of the body. Desoxycorticosterone acetate was the first mineralocorticoid available as a drug.

The masculinizing side effects are so troublesome to many women, however, that androgens have frequently been abandoned even when relieving pain. Their anabolic effects are desirable in patients who are frequently in negative nitrogen balance. To use the beneficial anabolic effects and avoid unpleasant masculinization, chemical modifications of the basic molecules have been attempted, with the development of a group of anabolic steroids that are less virilizing. Although not used directly as antitumor agents, they play a significant role in anticancer management and are worthy of a brief discussion and listing. Figure 28.4 shows the molecular structure of the major anabolic steroids.

Estrogens have been employed in the management of disseminated prostatic cancer and produce 75% to 85% subjective response (Nesbit and Baum 1950; Herbst 1941). It is impossible at this time to find reliable data on objective response rates. Recent studies suggest that the formerly high doses predisposed to an increased incidence of cardiac morbidity and mortality, and much lower doses are now used (Bailar, Byar, and VA Cooperative Group 1970; Scott, Menon, and Walsh 1980).

While one would expect estrogens to be valuable in prostatic cancer based on physiologic considerations, their value in breast cancer would not seem to be so obvious. Nonetheless, well documented large studies indicated a 20% to 40% objective response rate to estrogen therapy in patients with breast cancer who are more than four years beyond the natural menopause (Haagen-

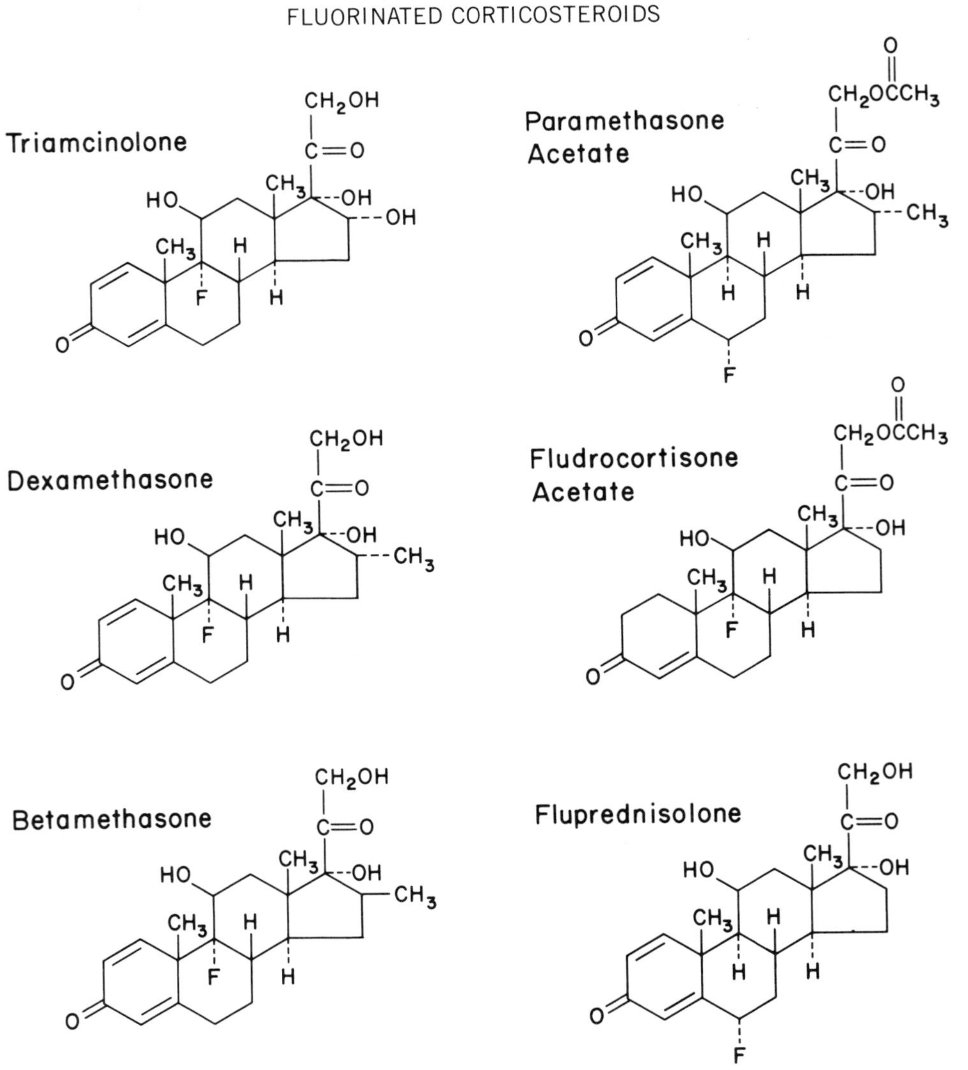

FLUORINATED CORTICOSTEROIDS

Triamcinolone

Paramethasone Acetate

Dexamethasone

Fludrocortisone Acetate

Betamethasone

Fluprednisolone

Fig. 28.2. *These synthetic fluorinated corticosteroids are very potent. Fludrocortisone has primarily mineralocorticoid properties while the others have almost exclusively glucocorticoid effects.*

sen 1971; Nathanson 1947). The molecular structures of the major estrogens used as antineoplastic drugs are shown in figure 28.5.

With development of knowledge of estrogen-binding receptors (EBR), it is estimated that when given some form of endocrine therapy, 55% to 65% of patients with EBR positivity will obtain objective tumor regression, as opposed to 0% to 11% of the EBR-negative group (Legha, Davis, and Muggia 1978). One of the newest such therapies is the nonsteroidal antiestrogen tamoxifen, recently made available in this country. So far it has had minimal side effects and a better than 50% response rate in EBR-positive patients (Heusen 1976; Mouridsen et al. 1978; Tagnon 1977). Although it is still in clinical trials, aminoglutethimide, an adrenal-blocking agent, has produced 25% to 38% objective responses in patients with metastatic breast cancer (Ciba-Geigy Co. 1976; Wells et al. 1978).

The progestins have been demonstrated to be effective in one-third or more cases of endometrial carcinoma (Kelly and Baker 1961). They are also being evaluated for efficacy in breast (Bloom et al. 1980) and renal cell carcinoma (Bloom 1973). The molecular structure of some of those used in cancer therapy is shown in figure 28.6.

Adrenal Corticosteroids

These compounds are produced by the adrenal cortex and then isolated from it. Now, most of these drugs are synthesized and many have been chemically modified to analogues that are more potent or more selective for a particular property.

Both the natural and synthetic corticosteroids can be divided into the glucocorticoids and the mineralocorticoids (Thorn et al. 1953). In physiologic amounts, the glucocorticoids are carbohydrate-storing, protein-catabolic, and corticotropin-suppressive. In pharmacologic doses they are immunosuppressive, an-

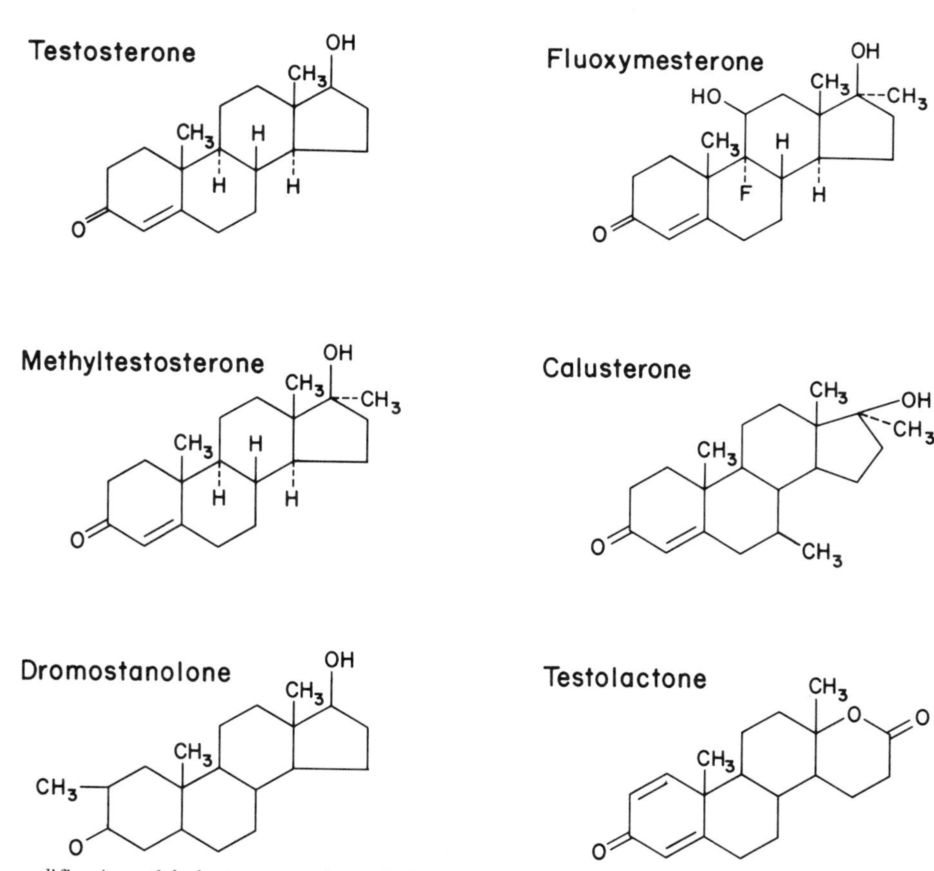

Fig. 28.3. *Most of the androgens are modifications of the basic four-ring structure of testosterone (including calusterone, which looks slightly different by virtue of the way in which its D ring is drawn). Testolactone is different as can be seen from the lactone ring structure and is a quasi-male hormone with minimal hormonal effects and some limited activity in breast cancer.*

tiinflammatory, lympholytic, and tend to reduce hypercalcemia secondary to malignancy and central nervous system edema secondary to metastasis.

The mineralocorticoids have primarily sodium-retaining and potassium-excreting effects and are used in physiologic amounts for replacement therapy. Occasionally they are used in orthostatic hypotension to increase extracellular fluid volume. In humans, aldosterone is physiologically the most important mineralocorticoid, but desoxycorticosterone acetate (DOCA) was the first corticosteroid synthesized (1937) and used clinically (Forsham and Thorn 1955). Although DOCA is secreted in the same amount as aldosterone, it is only 3% to 5% as potent on an equimolar basis. Since aldosterone is not commercially available, and as DOCA is only available for intramuscular injection or subcutaneous pellet implantation, the major oral clinically therapeutic mineralocorticoid is fludrocortisone. This is a fluorinated derivative of hydrocortisone and is the only oral mineralocorticoid sold. It is available as Florinef acetate (Squibb) in 0.1-mg tablets. The usual replacement dose for adrenal insufficiency is 0.05 to 2.0 mg daily, and it

ANABOLIC STEROIDS

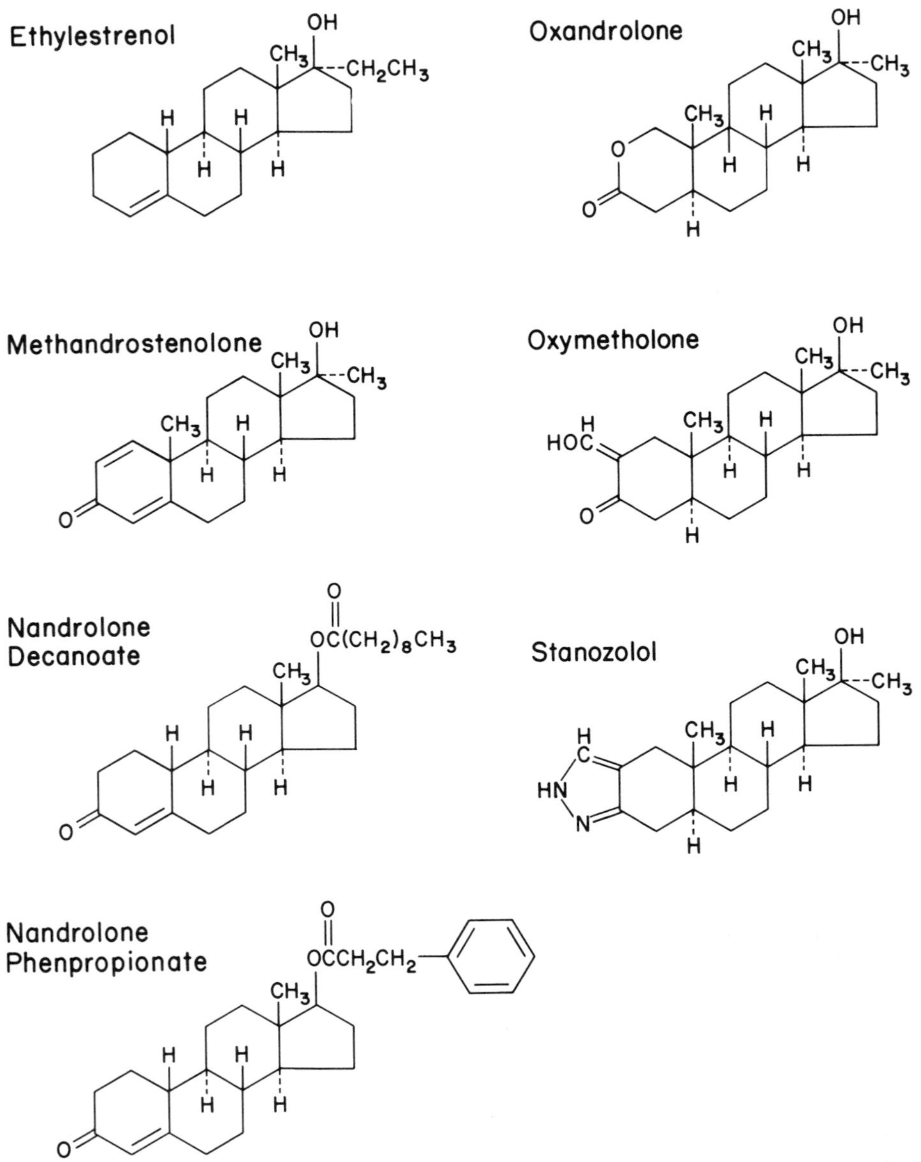

Ethylestrenol

Oxandrolone

Methandrostenolone

Oxymetholone

Nandrolone Decanoate

Stanozolol

Nandrolone Phenpropionate

Fig. 28.4. *Reference to the formula of testosterone in figure 28.3 will make it clear that all these drugs are modifications of the basic testosterone four-ring structure with additional side-chains.*

should be given with a glucocorticoid after bilateral adrenalectomy. Table 28.1 lists the trade and generic names of the corticosteroids and their usual doses.

Each day the normal adrenal cortex ordinarily secretes 15 to 25 mg (12 to 15 mg/m^2) of hydrocortisone and 1.5 to 4 mg corticosterone, the major natural glucocorticoids. Under situations of stress this can increase as much as tenfold. The adrenal cortex also secretes androgens, principally dehydroepiandrosterone (DHEA) and smaller amounts of androstenedione and testosterone. It secretes physiologically insignificant amounts of estrogens, but androstenedione can be converted to estrogen both by the ovary and peripherally, principally in the adipose tissues. Hydrocortisone exerts a negative feedback on the pituitary secretion of adrenocorticotropin (ACTH), which regulates both hydrocortisone and androgen secretion from the adrenal cortex.

Corticosteroids are transported in the blood reversibly bound to albumin or corticosteroid-binding globulin (CBG). Hydrocortisone is about 90% bound and dexamethasone is entirely unbound; it is the unbound hormone that is active. This decreased binding, as well as slower metabolic degradation (primarily in the liver), explain the greater potency and longer duration of action of the synthetic as compared to the physiologic hormones, and the need to reduce dosage in cases of liver impairment.

The mechanism of action of steroids is thought to be primarily their effect on protein synthesis. The

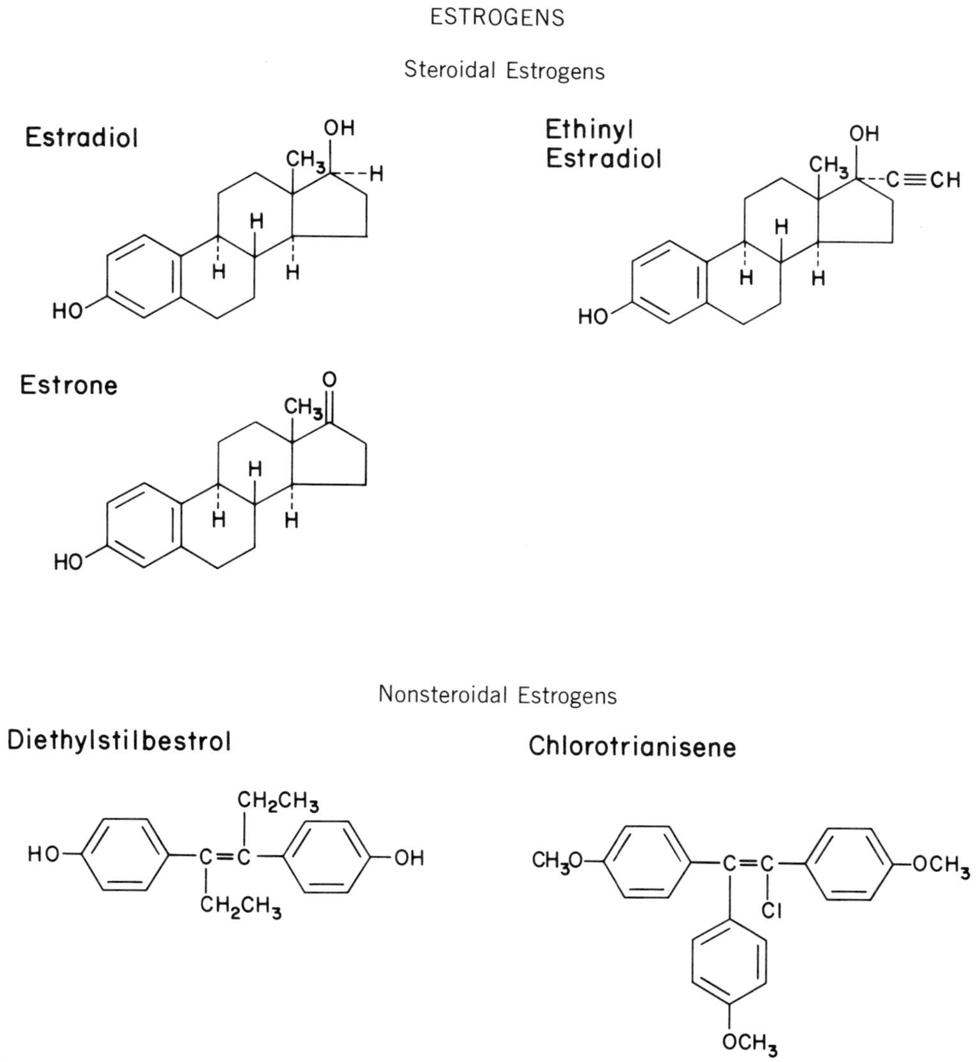

ESTROGENS

Steroidal Estrogens

Estradiol

Ethinyl Estradiol

Estrone

Nonsteroidal Estrogens

Diethylstilbestrol

Chlorotrianisene

Fig. 28.5. *The resemblance of the ring structure of the steroidal estrogens to that of testosterone (fig. 28.3) with just a different double bond structure in the A ring is striking. Metabolic interconversions have been suggested. Both diethylstilbestrol and chlorotrianisene have totally different structures but have potent estrogenic properties.*

steroid molecule enters the cell and forms complexes in the cytoplasm with specific receptors in target cells. These steroid-receptor complexes enter the nucleus where the transcription of a messenger RNA is influenced. This results in a degree of control of the nature and rate of protein, and particularly enzyme, synthesis.

By mechanisms not yet well defined, glucocorticoids increase hemoglobin, erythrocyte, and total leukocyte counts and polymorphonuclear leukocyte counts, but cause lysis of eosinophils, lymphocytes, basophils, and monocytes. In pharmacologic doses these properties can be maximized, resulting in the desired reduction of an immunologic effect, and in helping to lyse lymphoid cells in leukemias and lymphomas. In acute childhood lymphocytic leukemia the combination of prednisone and vincristine is successful in inducing remission in 80% to 90% of children so afflicted (Necheles 1979). In chronic lymphocytic leukemia of adults, the combination of prednisone and chlorambucil achieves a therapeutic response in about 50% of cases (Han et al. 1973). In multiple myeloma, the combination of prednisone plus melphalan is claimed to induce remissions in 55% of patients, compared to 23% treated with melphalan alone (Costa et al. 1973). In the MOPP regimen for Hodgkin's disease, prednisone, 40 mg/m^2, is given on days 1 to 14 during the first and fourth course of therapy. In the CVP regimen for non-Hodgkin's lymphomas, prednisone, 100 mg/m^2, is given for five days every three weeks. In the original Cooper regimen for breast cancer (Cooper 1969), prednisone is one of the five drugs. In the treatment of the blast crisis of chronic myelocytic leukemia, transient remissions have been induced in 30% of patients with prednisone plus vincristine (Canellos et al. 1971). In breast cancer, 48% of 31 patients had an objective response to prednisone (Lemon 1959).

In addition to their use in direct chemotherapy of tumors, corticosteroids have reduced the hypercalcemia associated with breast cancer, lymphoma, and multiple myeloma, possibly because in these tumors prednisone has an antineoplastic effect. It is less successful with hypercalcemia of other etiologies. In tumors of the brain or spinal cord, corticosteroids frequently reduce associated edema, thereby relieving pain and improving cerebral function and nerve conduction for a time. This allows other treatment modalities to be employed that get slower responses, but hopefully of greater duration.

Additional potential therapeutic effects include a reduction in bleeding in patients with thrombocytopenia either by strengthening capillaries or raising the platelet count. Corticosteroids may reduce autoimmune hemolysis and raise the white cell count transiently to help patients over the nadir of a chemotherapy treatment. It may produce nonspecific symptomatic im-

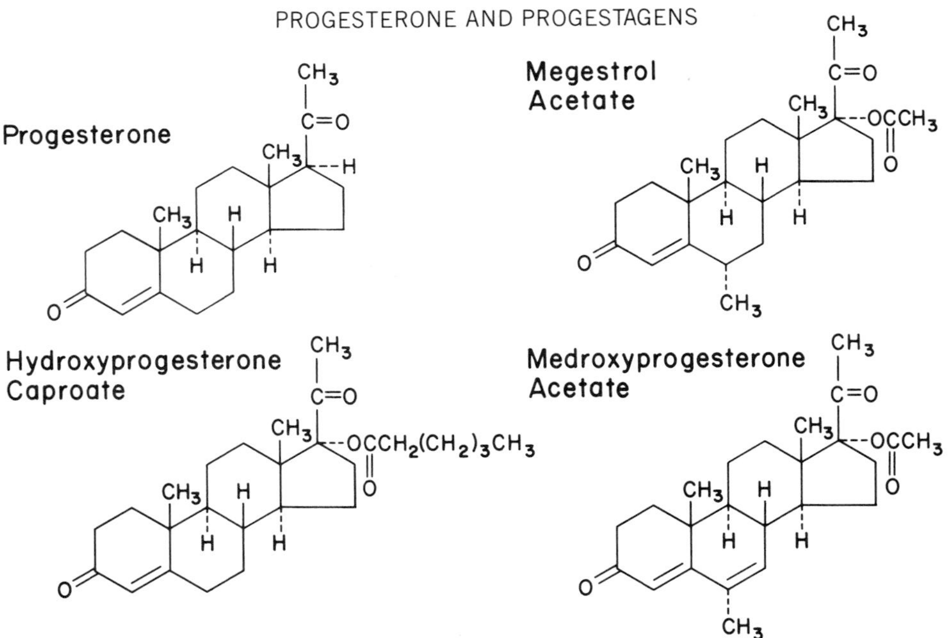

Fig. 28.6. *The progestagens are all derivatives of progesterone, which differs from testosterone primarily in having an oxygen at C-2 and an acetyl group at C-17. It differs from cortisol (hydrocortisone) which has the hydroxy group at C-11 and the glycolic (hydroxyacetic) group at C-17. Megestrol acetate is available in oral form whereas the others are injectable preparations.*

Table 28.1. *Corticosteroids*

Generic Name	*Brand Name*	*Usual Dose in Cancer Therapy*
Betamethasone	Celestone	1.2–7.2 mg/m^2/day
Cortisone	Cortone	50–300 mg/m^2/day
Dexamethasone	Decadron Hexadrol	1.5–9.0 mg/m^2/day
Hydrocortisone	Hydrocortone	50–300 mg/m^2/day
Hydrocortisone sodium phosphate	Hydrocortone phosphate	IV 100–300 mg/m^2
Hydrocortisone sodium succinate	Solucortef	IV 100–300 mg/m^2
Meprednisone	Betapar	8–48 mg/m^2/day
Methylprednisolone	Medrol	8–48 mg/m^2/day
Methylprednisolone sodium succinate	Solu-Medrol	IV 8–48 mg/m^2
Paramethasone	Haldrone, Stemex	5–30 mg/m^2/day
Prednisolone	Delta-Cortef	10–60 mg/m^2/day
Prednisolone sodium phosphate	Hydeltrasol	IV 10–60 mg/m^2
Prednisolone sodium succinate	Meticortelone Soluble	IV 10–60 mg/m^2
Prednisone	Delta-Dome, Deltasone, Meticorten	10–60 mg/m^2/day
Triamcinolone	Aristocort, Kenacort	8–48 mg/m^2/day

provement by an antiinflammatory effect, and reduce fever, sweating, and pain and restore appetite, strength, and a feeling of well-being.

Adverse reactions should be expected and evaluated in estimating the relative benefit to side effect ratio, that is, the therapeutic index. Most of these unwanted effects are extensions of the physiologic or pharmacologic actions of the drugs and are dose- and time-related. These values can sometimes be manipulated to reduce toxicity, and sometimes other drugs or maneuvers are desirable to cut down the unwanted action or ameliorate its effect.

In children, long-term, daily divided doses of glucocorticoid therapy can lead to growth suppression. To avoid this, alternate-day therapy with intermediate-acting glucocorticoids (prednisone, prednisolone, or methylprednisolone) have been used in many situations. When the entire therapeutic dose is given once every 48 hours in the morning, the diurnal pattern of the adrenal cortex is not suppressed very much and growth is not inhibited. This therapy seems to work well in asthma, lupus erythematosus, nephrotic syndrome, and uveitis, but not in arthritis or ulcerative colitis. In those situations, a single daily dose has been employed. The efficacy of alternate-day therapy is still being evaluated (Harter, Reddy, and Thorn 1963; Breitenfield et al. 1980) in hematologic and oncologic disorders, but many clinicians have empirically found single daily doses as effective as divided daily doses while awaiting controlled clinical trials. Research in relation to hormones and cancer remains active (Iacobelli, Nehci, and Ranelletti 1979).

Infection is a major threat to the patient with neoplastic disease who may have immunosuppression from the disease or malnutrition. Glucocorticoids further impair host defenses and increase susceptibility to or reactivation of tuberculosis, fungal infections, pneumocystis, and bacterial and viral infections. They also tend to mask the signs and symptoms of infection so that it is often detected in a more advanced stage.

Carbohydrate and lipid metabolism is deranged by glucocorticoids so that latent diabetes is frequently unmasked. The patients usually do not become ketotic and can be managed with diet or oral hypoglycemic agents; insulin is sometimes required. Gastric mucosal defenses are impaired by glucocorticoids, and acid and pepsinogen secretions are increased in some patients. Although a review by Conn and Blitzer (1976) questioned their role in producing or reactivating peptic ulcers with perforation or bleeding, a majority of clinicians still have patients take antacids and sometimes antisecretory agents when using high-dose glucocorticoids.

Mental and emotional changes are seen with high doses of these agents. Sometimes the euphoria produced is desirable in a depressed patient with advanced malignancy. The potential for undesirable effects is great, however, and includes nervousness, hyperkinesia, irritability, insomnia, and psychoses. Although frank psychoses are fortunately uncommon, they can be devastating and include manic-depressive, paranoid, and acute toxic psychoses.

Electrolyte imbalance with retention of sodium and water and depletion of potassium is less frequent now that synthetic glucocorticoids with less mineralocorticoid activity have replaced hydrocortisone for most indications. Since the intermediate-acting agents do re-

Table 28.2. *Adrenal Corticosteroids Compared to Hydrocortisone*

Generic Name	*Brand Name(s)*	*Glucocorticoid Potency*	*Mineralocorticoid Potency*	*Equivalent Dose*
Hydrocortisone (cortisol)	Many	1.0	1.0	20 mg
Cortisone	Cortone	0.8	0.8	25 mg
Prednisone	Many	4	0.8	5 mg
Prednisolone	Many	4	0.8	5 mg
Meprednisone	Betapar	5	0	4 mg
Methylprednisone	Medrol	5	0	4 mg
Triamcinolone	Kenacort, Aristocort	5	0	4 mg
Paramethasone	Haldrone	10	0	2 mg
Fluprednisolone	Alphadrol	10	0	1.5 mg
Desoxycorticosterone*	Many	0	10	1.5 mg
Fludrocortisone*	Florinef	12	125	0.1 mg
Dexamethasone	Decadron, Hexadrol	30	0	0.75 mg
Betamethasone	Celestone	30	0	0.6 mg
Aldosterone*	—	0.3	3000	—
Corticosterone*	—	0.3	15	—

*Only used for mineralocorticoid effect.

tain some mineralocorticoid effect and are widely used because of their economy and other desirable properties, edema and hypokalemia may occur and require therapy. Edema may be treated with diuretics, including potassium-sparing agents such as triamterene (Dyrenium) or spironolactone (Aldactone), when necessary, but spironolactone has been associated with breast cancer in animals. Potassium replacement is indicated for hypokalemia lest that condition lead to cardiac arrhythmias, weakness, fatigue, or paralysis. As glucocorticoids are catabolic and cause protein breakdown, negative nitrogen balance may result. A high protein diet and anabolic steroids are frequently helpful.

Long-term glucocorticoids can lead to Cushing's syndrome with cataracts, glaucoma, truncal obesity, acne, osteoporosis, swollen facies, atrophy of the skin, hirsutism, and development of striae. Weakness in the proximal musculature of the upper and lower extremities can occur with any glucocorticoid, but seems to have a higher incidence with 9-alpha-fluorinated steroids such as triamcinolone and dexamethasone (Drachman 1980).

Relative potency and equivalent dosages of the major corticosteroids are compared to hydrocortisone in table 28.2. We have tended to use prednisone for most purposes; it is used in large amounts and is available in several dosage sizes as a generic drug from multiple manufacturers, and therefore is quite economical. It is metabolized in the liver to an active form. Neurosurgeons frequently use dexamethasone to reduce cerebral edema as it has no mineralocorticoid properties. For replacement therapy where relatively low doses are indicated, as with aminoglutethimide therapy, hydrocortisone seems to be the drug of choice. Specific dosages must be selected based on the agent being used, the protocol being followed, or the particular condition being treated. Formulations and dose forms are described in *AMA drug evaluations, Physicians desk reference, United States pharmacopeia dispensing information,* and *The American hospital formulary service.*

Androgens

Androgens are virilizing hormones secreted by the testis, adrenal, and ovary. Normal adult men produce 2.5 to 10 mg of testosterone daily and lesser amounts of 4-androstenedione and dehydroepiandrosterone. About 99% of circulating testosterone, the most active androgen, is bound to sex hormone-binding globulin

(SHBG), and the free hormone is the biologically active material. It is metabolized primarily in the liver and excreted in the urine as metabolites. Like other hormones, it has a secretory diurnal variation. The synthetic derivatives, especially those alkylated in the 17-alpha position (methyltestosterone and fluoxymesterone), are orally active, metabolized more slowly by the liver, and are potentially hepatotoxic, occasionally causing jaundice that clears when the drug is discontinued.

There are three major indications for androgens in cancer therapy: (1) for the palliation of breast cancer in selected patients; (2) to stimulate erythropoiesis in patients with anemia caused by renal disease, aplasia, chronic inflammation or infection, and the vague entity of neoplastic suppression; and (3) to stimulate positive nitrogen balance as part of a general anabolic effect. Items 2 and 3 are in general served by a group of androgens chemically modified to decrease their virilizing properties and preserve their anabolic activity. They are discussed as a group in the next section, Anabolic Steroids.

Relatively large doses of androgens have produced objective regression in women with metastatic carcinoma of the breast. Responses have been seen most often with soft tissue, nodal, and osseous metastases and rarely with visceral spread, except possibly pulmonary metastases. The incidence of response overall is about 20%, but is higher in women beyond the menopause; the further removed from the menopause, the greater the response. Other factors that predict for success are a long relapse-free interval and positive estrogen-binding receptors. The synthetic analogues are at least as effective as testosterone and probably more effective. In addition, they are less virilizing and have therefore been used in preference to testosterone. Androgens in general are being used less often because of their adverse effects and the availability of a relatively nontoxic alternative in the antiestrogen tamoxifen. Androgen therapy has been added to chemotherapy in acute myelogenous leukemia (Hollard et al. 1980).

The major adverse effect that is unacceptable to most women is physiologic and pharmacologic virilization. This is manifested by hirsutism with increased facial and body hair, deepening of the voice, acne, clitoral enlargement, increased libido, alopecia, and erythrocythemia. Accordingly, many women with breast cancer either refuse to start androgens or discontinue them even when deriving obvious palliation from them. Other side effects include fluid retention, occasional cholestatic jaundice with the 17-alpha oral agents, and possibly, an increased tendency to hypercalcemia, although the evidence for a causal connection with this condition is not yet convincing.

Table 28.3. *Androgens*

Generic Name	*Brand Name*	*Usual Dose in Cancer Therapy*
Calusterone	Methosarb	50–75 mg q.i.d., p.o.
Dromostanolone proprionate	Drolban	100 mg IM 3 ×/wk
Fluoxymesterone	Halotestin, Ora-Testryl	20–30 mg/day, p.o.
Methyltestosterone	Metandren, Oreton Methyl, Testred	50–200 mg/day, p.o.
Testolactone	Teslac	250 mg q.i.d., p.o. or 100 mg IM 3 ×/wk
Testosterone cypionate	Depo-testosterone, T-Ionate-PA	200–400 mg IM q 2–4 wks
Testosterone enanthate	Delatestryl	200–400 mg IM q 2–4 wks
Testosterone propionate	Neo-Hombreol	50–100 mg IM 3 ×/wk
	Oreton Propionate	10 mg/day boccal

The available preparations with their brand and generic names and usual dosages are shown in table 28.3.

Anabolic Steroids

These are basically androgens that have been modified to maintain their anabolic properties while minimizing their virilizing potential. When given to patients who can and will ingest an adequate diet, they contribute to a positive nitrogen balance and thereby help the cachectic patient achieve a condition where a salutary response to surgery, radiation, or chemotherapy is more likely.

In aplastic or other aregenerative anemias, high doses (100 mg/day) of oxymethalone orally or of the injectable nandrolone preparations have led to erythropoietic responses with a rise in red cell mass. No convincing rise in white cells or platelets has been noted. Since oxymethalone has been implicated in causing neoplasms of the liver, it is rarely used now.

All the oral anabolic steroids are 17-alpha–alkylated; accordingly there is a potential for cholestatic

Table 28.4. *Anabolic Steroids*

Generic Name	*Brand Name*	*Usual Dose in Adults*
Ethylestrenol	Maxibolin	8–16 mg/day p.o.
Methandrostenolone	Dianabol	2.5–5 mg/day p.o.
Nandrolone decanoate	Deca-durabolin	50–100 mg IM q 3–4 wks
Nandrolone phenpropionate	Durabolin, Nandrolin	25–50 mg IM weekly
Oxandrolone	Anavar	2.5–10 mg/day p.o.
Oxymetholone	Adroyd, Anadrol	5–10 mg/day p.o.; 50–100 mg/day p.o. for erythropoiesis
Stanozolol	Winstrol	6 mg/day p.o.

jaundice with any of them. Nandrolone is not alkylated at the 17-alpha position and is rarely associated with jaundice. Other adverse effects are the tendency to fluid retention and a greatly diminished but not absent capacity for virilization.

The available preparations with their generic and brand names and usual dosages are given in table 28.4.

Estrogens

The estrogens are a group of compounds that produce feminization. The estrogenic steroids are produced primarily by the ovary, but small amounts are produced by the adrenal, the testis, and adipose tissue. Estradiol is the major estrogenic steroid produced in the premenopausal nonpregnant woman. About 100 to 600 μg is secreted daily by the ovary, where androstenedione is converted to testosterone, which in turn is demethylated and aromatized to estrogen. Androstenedione may also be converted to estrone and then to estradiol, and these two compounds may be metabolized peripherally to estriol. The major conversion of androstenedione to estrone occurs in adipose tissue and accounts for 25% of the estrone produced, the remainder coming from the ovary (Segaloff 1963).

In addition to the steroidal estrogens, there is a group of synthetic compounds that are nonsteroidal but have feminizing properties. These include diethylstilbestrol, the first to be synthesized, a stilbene in chemical structure. Further modifications in structure yielded other nonsteroidal compounds including hexestrol, dienestrol, methallenestril, and chlorotrianisene. Estradiol is about 80% bound to SHBG and only the free compound is metabolically active. In general, the synthetic nonsteroidal estrogens are not SHBG-bound.

The estrogens stimulate development of the breast and uterus, linear growth of the skeleton, female distribution of body hair, sodium and water retention, skin elasticity, a weak anabolic effect, and the female distribution of adipose tissue. They play a role in the regulation of puberty and the menstrual cycle and in the negative feedback to inhibit pituitary follicle-stimulating hormone (FSH), and luteinizing hormone (LH).

The mechanism of action of estrogens appears to be an increase in the cellular synthesis of DNA and RNA. The hormone penetrates the cell wall and in the cytoplasm binds to estrogen-binding receptors (EBR). These complexes then migrate to the nucleus and are transferred to the ribosomes where enzymes and other proteins are synthesized that carry out the specific cellular function of the hormone. Recent studies have correlated the presence of EBR in primary or metastatic breast cancers with responsiveness to ablative and additive hormonal manipulations (Jensen 1975).

The major indications for estrogens in cancer therapy are in the management of metastatic prostatic cancer and in metastatic breast cancer in postmenopausal women (Haddow et al. 1944). The response rate increases with greater remoteness from the natural menopause. Additive estrogen therapy results in a remission rate of 31% to 37% overall and 55% to 65% in those with positive estrogen receptors in the group more than five years postmenopausal (Fischer, Katz, and Wiggans 1978; McGuire et al. 1977; Kennedy 1974). Patients who are EBR-positive have a predictably higher response rate, but the response may not be apparent for several weeks or months. Median remission duration is 15 months but can be several years. When relapse occurs, a second remission is occasionally achieved by estrogen withdrawal. The standard drug has generally been diethylstilbestrol (DES) because it is economical and effective. Unfortunately, it may produce nausea and vomiting in effective doses, so many clinicians prefer conjugated estrogens in spite of their greater expense. Objective response may be demonstrated by shrinkage in tumor mass, a fall in carcinoembryonic antigen (CEA) level, and x-ray evidence of bone improvement.

Metastatic prostatic carcinoma frequently responds to oral or parenteral estrogens. In general, orchiectomy is preferred as the first endocrine manipulation, but many men object to this. The response rate for orchiectomy and estrogens is about the same. There

Table 28.5. *Estrogens*

Generic Name	*Brand Name*	*Dosage in Breast Cancer*	*Dosage in Prostate Cancer*
Chlorotrianisene	TACE	—	12–25 mg/day p.o.
Conjugated estrogens	Premarin	10 mg t.i.d., p.o	1.25–2.5 mg/day, p.o.
Diethylstilbestrol	Many	5 mg t.i.d., p.o.	1–3 mg/day p.o.
Diethylstilbestrol diphosphate	Stilphostrol	—	50 mg. t.i.d., p.o. IV (see text)
Esterified estrogens	Many	10 mg t.i.d., p.o.	1.25–2.5 mg t.i.d., p.o.
Ethinyl estradiol	Estinyl, Feminone	1 mg. t.i.d., p.o.	0.15–2.0 mg/day p.o.

appears to be no advantage to doing both simultaneously. Following relapse from the first procedure, the remission rate by the second hormonal maneuver is of a low order statistically (Brendler 1969; DeWys 1976), but secondary responses have been documented.

Curiously, patients who have failed oral DES or chlorotrianisene after a response frequently obtain at least a subjective response (pain relief) from intravenous DES diphosphate. The method of administration is somewhat complicated and is therefore described here. On the first day, 500 mg DES diphosphate in 300 ml 5% dextrose solution is administered at the rate of 20 to 30 drops per minute for 15 minutes. The flow rate is then increased to permit completion of the dose in one hour. The dosage is then increased to 1000 mg a day for five or more days as needed to relieve bone pain. Maintenance therapy may be 250 to 500 mg in 300 ml solution of 5% dextrose, administered once or twice a week at the same flow rate as during induction. Alternatively, maintenance can be oral DES diphosphate tablets, 50 mg three times a day, and gradually increased to as much as 200 mg three times a day as needed and as tolerated. Pruritus and burning pain in the anogenital region or at metastatic sites is occasionally noted and usually responds to antihistamines.

The side effects of estrogens are numerous and can be severe. There may be a tendency to stimulate thrombosis with resulting thrombophlebitis, pulmonary embolism, or cerebrovascular accident. Nausea and vomiting may be severe at the higher doses. Edema is frequent, and in men has been associated with an increased incidence of cardiovascular death when the standard 15 mg/day or 5 mg/day DES regimens were used (Bailar, Byar, and VA Cooperative Group 1970; Byar 1973). Since DES oral dosage for prostatic carcinoma has been reduced to 1 to 3 mg/day, this has not been a problem. In men, breast swelling and tenderness can be very disturbing, but low-dose irradiation of the nipples before initiation of estrogen therapy can usually avoid this problem.

Changes in vaginal bleeding pattern with spotting, breakthrough bleeding, prolonged bleeding, or cessation of menstrual periods can be confusing to both patient and physician. Pigmentation of nipples and areolae occurs in almost all patients, but painful breast swelling in women is fortunately uncommon. Changes in libido may be disturbing, with a decrease in men and an increase in women. Hypercalcemia is a potentially fatal complication, but its direct relationship to hormonal therapy has been suggested, not proved. Nonetheless, if hypercalcemia occurs, hormones should be discontinued and appropriate antihypercalcemic measures begun, such as diuresis, phosphates, calcitonin, corticosteroids, or mithramycin if necessary. A syndrome of vaginal adenomatosis sometimes progressing to cancer has been described in offspring of women who received estrogens during pregnancy (Ulfelder 1980).

Less common side effects include cholestatic jaundice, urinary incontinence, exacerbation of bone pain, depression, headache, anorexia, and skin rash. In women, estrogen may cause changes in mammographic patterns (Bland et al. 1980).

In selecting a drug, we have tended to favor DES initially. For breast cancer, we begin with 5 mg daily for a few days, and if tolerated, raise the dose to 5 mg twice a day and evaluate side effects for a few days. If this is tolerated, we go to 5 mg three times a day. If it is not tolerated, we use conjugated estrogens, 10 mg/day, or give the dose at bedtime. In men, 1 to 3 mg of DES is well tolerated. Urologists tend to use chlorotrianisene, but we have avoided this drug because it is stored in the adipose tissue and causes sodium and fluid retention with resulting cardiovascular problems.

The available preparations with their generic and brand names and usual dosages are shown in table 28.5.

Antiestrogens

The antiestrogens are a group of synthetic compounds, not necessarily steroidal, that are able to decrease the specific uptake of estrogens in vitro and in vivo by various target organs in rats and in humans. More specifically, it is thought that the antiestrogens block the binding of estradiol to cytoplasmic estrogen-binding receptors by competitively binding themselves. It has been further suggested that the antiestrogen is unable to maintain elevated receptor concentrations in the cytoplasm. Probably the antiestrogen-receptor complex migrates to the nucleus where it exerts an estrogenic stimulus, possibly a mechanism of the so-called "flare," but then the cell is receptor depleted, which prevents further estrogenic action (Plotkin et al. 1978). When estradiol combines with receptor and migrates to the nucleus it stimulates more receptor formation.

Other physiologic effects of antiestrogens include inhibition of prolactin secretion and, to a lesser extent, of LH, FSH, estradiol, and progesterone. Most authors believe that the action of antiestrogens is on the cancer tissue itself and not through action on prolactin (Heel et al. 1978).

The majority of early studies of antiestrogens were performed in Europe and included clomiphen, nafoxidin, MER-25, and tamoxifen (Tagnon 1977; Heusen 1976; Proceedings 1976). So far, only tamoxifen has been approved for use in the United States, and we will confine our discussion to that drug. In a way, it is a medical attempt at producing an ovariectomy result (Nissen-Meyer 1964).

Tamoxifen

Tamoxifen (Nolvadex, ICI 46474, NSC 180973) is the nonsteroidal transisomer of a triphenylethylene derivative (fig. 28.7). It was developed by Imperial Chemical Industries in England, and the earliest studies were reported by Cole, Jones, and Todd in 1971. It became clinically available in Great Britain in 1973. Clinical studies in the United States began in 1974 under the sponsorship of Stuart Pharmaceuticals (Proceedings 1976; Lippman 1980), and the drug became available for general use in 1978.

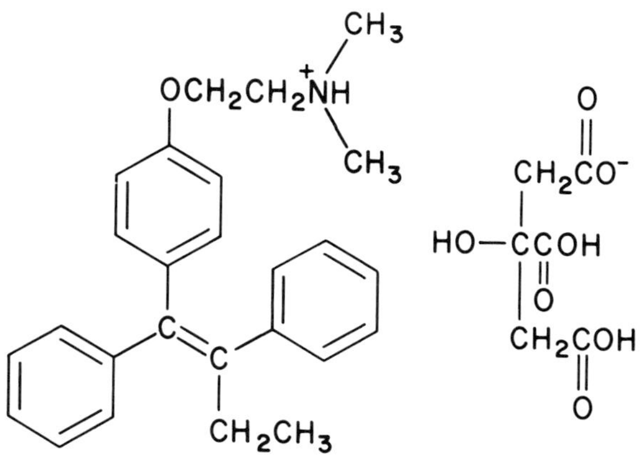

Fig. 28.7. *Tamoxifen, NSC 180973*

The mechanism of action is similar to the other antiestrogens, with tamoxifen competitively binding to the estrogen-binding receptor (EBR) and then failing to stimulate further EBR formation. Following the migration of tamoxifen-EBR complex to the nucleus, DNA synthesis decreases, shifting the equilibrium between cell death and cell renewal in the tumor in favor of cell death.

After oral ingestion, maximum plasma levels of drug appear in several hours. There is a greater concentration of uptake in ovaries and uterus than in other tissues. Metabolism is primarily in the liver by hydroxylation. The monohydroxylated metabolite is more active than tamoxifen itself, but the dihydroxylate metabolite is only weakly active. There is enterohepatic circulation with major ultimate excretion through the bile into the stools. Elimination half-life has been about seven days in the small number of patients studied so far.

The major indication for the drug has been in treatment of postmenopausal women with recurrent or metastatic breast carcinoma that is EBR-positive (Wiggans et al. 1979; Kiang and Kennedy 1977). Responses have been better in women more than five years postmenopausal as compared to those less than five years postmenopausal (Heel et al. 1978). Relatively few premenopausal patients have been treated because tissue and animal studies show that estradiol can reverse the tamoxifen effect, and the premenopausal patient should have ample estradiol. Nonetheless, a few premenopausal (Manni et al. 1979) and a few EBR-negative patients have been reported to respond, particularly if they had previous response to hormone therapy. Hence a mechanism of prolactin inhibition has been postulated as a major pathway in such instances.

Combining tamoxifen with cytotoxic chemotherapy regimens concurrently or sequentially has yielded mixed reports. Most groups indicated an increased response rate in patients known to be EBR-positive (Manni, Trujillo, and Pearson 1980) or more than five years postmenopausal, but there have been a few studies that showed no enhancement of the combination as compared to either modality alone (Glick et al. 1980). These problems continue under active study. Postmenopausal patients who have failed combination chemotherapy have frequently responded to tamoxifen if they were EBR-positive, particularly if they had soft tissue involvement (Legha et al. 1979). Patients with osseous and visceral metastases do not respond as well. Tamoxifen has been compared to fluoxymesterone in an open, randomized, cross-over trial. Overall remission in the first course of treatment was 30% with tamoxifen and 19% with fluoxymesterone (Westerberg 1980). In a comparison with hypophysectomy, tamoxifen gave approximately equivalent responses (Kiang et al. 1980).

Side effects have been gratifyingly mild and uncommon. Less than 3% of postmenopausal women have discontinued therapy because of adverse reactions, in contrast to the large numbers who abandon androgen and estrogen therapy because of toxicity. The most common side effects are caused by the drug's antiestrogenic actions and include hot flushes (10% to 20%), and less frequently pruritus vulvae and vaginal bleeding or discharge. Nausea and vomiting occur in about 10% of patients with tamoxifen and in about 5% with a placebo. Transient thrombocytopenia, mild leukopenia, and anemia have occurred on rare occasions but were not dose-limiting (Legha and Carter 1976). Pulmonary emboli have been reported in a few patients receiving tamoxifen, but a causal relationship has not been established (Lerner et al. 1976). A small number of patients develop bone pain or increased soft tissue swelling when therapy is started, the so-called flare, but this usually subsides promptly with a response to the drug in the majority of cases (Plotkin et al. 1978). In fact, a flare almost predicts a response.

The recommended starting dosage of tamoxifen is 10 mg twice daily. If a response does not occur in a month, this is increased to 20 mg twice daily. Higher doses than that do not seem to increase the response rate, although amounts up to 100 mg per day have been given without significant side effects, except possibly retinopathy (Kaiser-Kupser and Lippman 1978) and corneal changes.

Tamoxifen is available as Nolvadex (Stuart) in 10-mg tablets in bottles of 60. It is stable at room temperature.

Aminoglutethimide (Investigational)

Aminoglutethimide (Cytadren, BA 16038, Elipten) (fig. 28.8) is a derivative of the hypnotic glutethimide. It was originally introduced in 1958 as an anticonvulsant. The development of adrenal insufficiency in an epileptic child being treated with aminoglutethimide stimulated investigation of the drug in adrenal hyperfunction syndromes.

Its mechanism of action appears to be blockage of estrogen biosynthesis at two separate sites: (1) the adrenal cortex, and (2) extraglandular tissue. In the adrenal it interrupts the conversion of cholesterol to pregnenolone and subsequently reduces production of the major estrogen precursor androstenedione, as well as glucocorticoids and mineralocorticoids. In peripheral tissues, aminoglutethimide blocks the formation of estrogens by inhibiting the aromatizing enzymes responsible for conversion of androstenedione to estrone. Histologically, the adrenal cortex shows cellular hypertrophy, cytoplasmic vacuolization, and excessive accumulation of lipid. In rats, aminoglutethimide has an antithyroid action similar to that of propylthiouracil, with diminished uptake of radioactive iodine and an intrathyroidal block in the formation of triiodothyronine and thyroxine, resulting in the accumulation of monoiodotyrosine.

The drug is well absorbed after oral administration, with onset of action in several hours. Pharmacokinetic studies are still in progress in humans, but metabolism is believed to be by hydroxylation in the liver. There is enterohepatic circulation, so major excretion appears to be in the feces.

So-called medical adrenalectomy is attempted by giving aminoglutethimide with a glucocorticoid (Sanford et al. 1976; Santen, Lipton, and Kendall 1974). Originally, dexamethasone was used but it does not prevent the reflex ACTH rise and its metabolism is accelerated by the action of the aminoglutethimide on the liver's inducible enzymes. Substituting hydrocortisone gives a much more predictable result. The combination of these two drugs effectively blocks adrenal function in patients with breast cancer and produces an objective response rate of about 38% (Santen et al. 1977). Compared to surgical hypophysectomy or adrenalectomy (Newsome et al. 1977), the response rate is about the same but the side effects are considerably less with aminoglutethimide-hydrocortisone compared to either surgical procedure (Harvey et al. 1979). Best results are obtained in patients with positive estrogen-binding receptors (Lawrence et al. 1980).

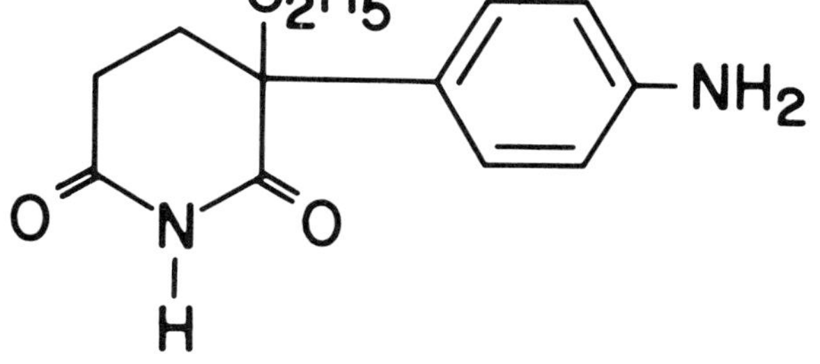

C_2H_5 NH_2 O N O H

Fig. 28.8. *Aminoglutethimide, BA 16038*

Table 28.6. *Progesterones*

Generic Name	*Brand Name*	*Usual Dose in Cancer Therapy*
Hydroxyprogesterone caproate	Delalutin	1 gm 2 × weekly IM
Medroxyprogesterone acetate	Depo-Provera	Initially, 400–1000 mg IM weekly, then 400 mg monthly
Megestrol acetate	Megace	Breast: 40 mg q.i.d., p.o. Endometrium: 40–80 mg q.i.d., p.o.

In metastatic carcinoma of the prostate, therapy with aminoglutethimide and a glucocorticoid has resulted in a 30% response rate in a small series, with diminution of pain and fall in the acid phosphatase (Sanford et al. 1976). Further studies in this area are indicated. Aminoglutethimide has also been used in adrenocortical carcinoma to ameliorate the symptoms of Cushing's syndrome caused by high steroid levels.

Adverse effects have been noted in about 50% of patients but they are usually not dose-limiting. The most common reaction is a morbilliform rash that usually appears within the first week of treatment and disappears in five to eight days (Santen et al. 1977). Lethargy, ataxia, and dizziness have been reported but usually subside spontaneously. Anorexia, gastric discomfort, periorbital edema, nausea, vomiting, and nystagmus are occasionally seen. Adrenal insufficiency with hyponatremia and facial fullness are to be expected. Idiosyncratic bone marrow suppression with leukopenia, agranulocytosis, and pancytopenia occurs rarely. A few instances of thyroid enlargement and mild hypothyroidism have been reported in children treated for longer than six months. Masculinization, hirsutism, and sexual precocity have been reported in prepubertal and adolescent patients, but very few if any of them would be candidates for therapy.

Dosage of aminoglutethimide is 1000 mg per day usually divided into 250 mg four times a day, with hydrocortisone, 10 mg four times a day, or total 40 mg per day. Earlier literature (Griffith et al. 1973) and company brochures suggested use of dexamethasone but the dose had to be monitored and changed frequently, whereas the hydrocortisone dose is stable (Santen et al. 1977). Doses as high as 1500 mg to 2500 mg aminoglutethimide have been used.

Aminoglutethimide remains an investigational drug but may be obtained as Elipten or Cytadren (BA 16038) from CIBA-GEIGY for clinical investigation on a protocol with the patient fully informed and signing a consent form. FDA approval and marketing is expected soon.

Progestins

Progesterone is produced primarily by the corpus luteum of the ovary after each ovulation, and to a lesser extent by the adrenal cortex. Preovulatory production is about 3 mg per day, while luteal phase secretion is 20 to 30 mg per day. During pregnancy very large amounts are produced by the placenta.

Progesterone is bound largely to corticosteroid-binding globulin (CBG), which also binds hydrocortisone. It is the free hormone that is active. The anticancer progestins are all chemical derivatives of 17-alpha-hydroxyprogesterone.

The mechanism of action of progestins is primarily to increase the synthesis of RNA by means of interaction with DNA. Larger doses inhibit the release of luteinizing hormone (LH) from the anterior pituitary. Relatively small doses cause an increase in cervical mucus viscosity.

Only megestrol of the anticancer agents is significantly absorbed from the gastrointestinal tract. Medroxyprogesterone acetate (Provera) is also available orally but only in 10-mg tablets, and the dose for cancer is 160 to 320 mg/day. Hence an injectable preparation is used. Metabolism is primarily hepatic, and excretion is primarily renal.

The major indication for progestins is in the treatment of endometrial adenocarcinoma (Piver et al. 1980). It seems to have the best efficacy in patients whose tumors are well differentiated. Tumor shrinkage has been objectively demonstrated in some cases, and roughly one-third of patients derive significant benefit (Kelly and Baker 1961). Responses in breast cancer are beginning to accumulate, but it remains third- or fourth-line therapy (Kennedy 1974) and frequently fails because it is used in late stages of the disease when tumor burden is heavy. Anecdotal responses in prostatic and renal carcinoma have been reported, but for these diseases they are almost all experimental.

Hydroxyprogesterone caproate (Delalutin) comes as 125 mg/ml and 250 mg/ml in oil for deep intramuscular injection. The usual initial dosage is 1000 mg twice a week, and is later tapered. Medroxyprogesterone acetate (Depo-Provera) is given intramuscularly every week as an aqueous suspension, starting with 1000 mg initially, and later 400 mg per week. It comes in vials of 100 mg/ml in 5-ml size, and as 400 mg/ml in 1-, 2.5-, and 10-ml sizes. The only oral progestin used widely for cancer is megestrol (Megace). It comes in 20-mg and 40-mg tablets. Divided doses of 160 mg/day are used for breast carcinoma, but for endometrial and renal cell carcinoma 320 mg/day in four doses of 80 mg each is preferred.

Side effects of progestins are relatively mild. As would be expected, there are changes in the vaginal bleeding pattern, including irregular cycle time, spotting, breakthrough bleeding, and amenorrhea. Less frequent are headaches, loss of coordination, skin rash, and jaundice. An association with thrombophlebitis and thrombosis or embolization has been suggested but not proved.

The generic and trade names and usual dosages of the anticancer progestins are recapitulated in table 28.6.

References

AMA drug evaluations, 4th edition. Chicago: American Medical Association, 1980.

American Society of Hospital Pharmacists. *The American hospital formulary service.* Washington, D.C.: ASHP, 1980.

Bailar, J. C., III; Byar, D. P.; and the VA Cooperative Urological Research Group. Estrogen treatment for cancer of the prostate; early results with three doses of diethylstilbestrol and placebo. *Cancer* 26:257–261, 1970.

Beatson, G. T. On the treatment of inoperable cases of carcinoma of the mamma; suggestions for a new method of treatment. *Lancet* 2:104–107; 162–165, 1896.

Bland, K. I. et al. The effects of exogenous estrogen replacement therapy of the breast: breast cancer risk and mammographic parenchymal patterns. *Cancer* 45: 3027–3033, 1980.

Bloom, H. J. G. Hormone-induced and spontaneous regression of metastatic renal cancer. *Cancer* 32: 1066–1071, 1973.

Bloom, N. B. et al. The role of progesterone receptors in the management of advanced breast cancer. *Cancer* 45:2992–2997, 1980.

Breitenfield, R. V. et al. Stability of renal transplant function with alternate day corticosteroid therapy. *JAMA* 244:151–156, 1980.

Brendler, H. Therapy with orchiectomy or estrogens or both. *JAMA* 210:1074–1075, 1969.

Byar, D. P. The Veteran's Administration's Cooperative Urological Research Group's studies of cancer of the prostate. *Cancer* 32:1126–1130, 1973.

Canellos, G. P. et al. Hematologic and cytogenetic remission of blast transformation in chronic granulocytic leukemia. *Blood* 38:671–679, 1971.

CIBA-GEIGY Company. *Orientation data: Cytadren (BA 16038), aminoglutethimide.* Summit, N.J.: CIBA-GEIGY, 1976.

Cole, M. P.; Jones, C. T. A.; and Todd, I. D. H. A new anti-oestrogenic agent in late breast cancer. An early clinical appraisal of ICI 46474. *Br. J. Cancer* 25:270–275, 1971.

Conn, H. O., and Blitzer, B. L. Nonassociation of adrenocorticoid therapy and peptic ulcer. *N. Engl. J. Med.* 294:473–479, 1976.

Cooper, R. G. Combination chemotherapy in hormone resistant breast cancer. *Proc. Am. Assoc. Cancer Res.* 10:15, 1969.

Costa, C. et al. Melphalan and prednisone: an effective combination for the treatment of multiple myeloma. *Am. J. Med.* 54:589–599, 1973.

DeVita, V. T., Jr. et al. Curability of advanced Hodgkin's disease with chemotherapy. *Ann. Intern. Med.* 92:587–595, 1980.

DeWys, W. D. Perspectives and overview. *Semin. Oncol.* 3:189–192, 1976.

Drachman, D. B. Myopathies. In *Principles and practice of medicine,* eds. A. M. Harvey et al. New York: Appleton-Century-Crofts, p. 1250, 1980.

Fischer, D. S.; Katz, M. E.; and Wiggans, R. G. The therapy of advanced breast cancer. *Conn. Med.* 42:634–639, 1978.

Forsham, P. H., and Thorn, G. W. The adrenals. In *Textbook of endocrinology,* ed. R. H. Williams. Philadelphia: W. B. Saunders, 1955, p. 229.

Fracchia, A. A.; Randall, H. T.; and Farrow, J. H. The results of adrenalectomy for advanced breast cancer in 500 consecutive patients. In *Breast cancer: early and late,* ed. R. L. Clark. Chicago: Year Book, 1970, pp. 369–376.

Glick, J. H. et al. Tamoxifen plus sequential CMF chemotherapy versus tamoxifen alone in postmenopausal patients with advanced breast cancer. *Cancer* 45:735–741, 1980.

Goldenberg, I. S. Testosterone proprionate therapy in breast cancer. *JAMA* 188:1069–1072, 1964.

Griffith, C. T. et al. Preliminary trial of aminoglutethimide in breast cancer. *Cancer* 32:31–37, 1973.

Haagensen, C. D. *Diseases of the breast,* 2nd edition. Philadelphia: W. B. Saunders, 1971.

Haddow, A. et al. Influence of synthetic oestrogens upon advanced malignant disease. *Br. Med. J.* 2:393–398, 1944.

Han, T. et al. Chlorambucil vs. combined chlorambucil corticosteroid therapy in chronic lymphocytic leukemia. *Cancer* 31:502–508, 1973.

Harter, J. G.; Reddy, W. J.; and Thorn, G. W. Studies on an intermittent corticosteroid dosage regimen. *N. Engl. J. Med.* 269:591–596, 1963.

Harvey, H. A. et al. A comparative trial of hypophysectomy and estrogen suppression with aminoglutethimide in advanced breast cancer. *Cancer* 43:2207–2214, 1979.

Heel, R. C. et al. Tamoxifen: a review of its pharmacological properties and therapeutic use in the treatment of breast cancer. *Drugs* 16:1–24, 1978.

Herbst, W. P. Effects of estradiol diproprionate and diethylstilbestrol on malignant prostatic tissue. *Trans. Am. Assoc. Genitourin. Surg.* 34:195–202, 1941.

Heusen, J. Current overview of EORTC clinical trials with tamoxifen. *Cancer Ther. Rep.* 60:1463–1465, 1976.

Hollard, D. et al. High rate of long-term survivals in AML treated by chemotherapy and androgenotherapy. *Cancer* 45:1540–1548, 1980.

Huggins, C., and Bergenstal, D. M. Surgery of the adrenals. *JAMA* 147:101–106, 1951.

Huggins, C., and Scott, W. W. Bilateral adrenalectomy in prostatic cancer; clinical features and urinary excretion of 17-ketosteroids and estrogens. *Ann. Surg.* 122:1031–1041, 1945.

Huggins, C.; Stevens, R. E.; and Hodges, C. V. Studies on prostatic cancer: effects of castration on advanced carcinoma of prostate gland. *Arch. Surg.* 43:209–223, 1941.

Iacobelli, S.; Nehci, I.; and Ranelletti, F. O. Abstracts from the First International Congress on Hormones and Cancer. *Cancer Treat. Rep.* 63:1143–1230, 1979.

Jensen, E. V. Estrogen receptors in hormone-dependent breast cancers. *Cancer Res.* 35:3362–3364, 1975.

Kaiser-Kupser, M. I., and Lippman, M. E. Tamoxifen retinopathy. *Cancer Treat. Rep.* 62:315–320, 1978.

Kelly, R. M., and Baker, W. H. Progestational agents in the treatment of carcinoma of the endometrium. *N. Engl. J. Med.* 264:216–222, 1961.

Kennedy, B. J. Hormonal therapies in breast cancer. *Semin. Oncol.* 1:119–130, 1974.

Kennedy, B. J., and Nathanson, I. T. Effects of intensive sex hormone therapy in advanced breast cancer. *JAMA* 152:1135–1141, 1953.

Kiang, D. T. et al. Comparison of tamoxifen and hypophysectomy in breast cancer treatment. *Cancer* 45:1322–1325, 1980.

Kiang, D. T., and Kennedy, B. J. Tamoxifen (antiestrogen) therapy in advanced breast cancer. *Ann. Intern. Med.* 87:687–690, 1977.

Lawrence, B. V. et al. Influence of estrogen receptor status on response of metastatic breast cancer to aminoglutethimide therapy. *Cancer* 45:786–791, 1980.

Legha, S. S. et al. Tamoxifen: use in treatment of metastatic breast cancer refractory to combination chemotherapy. *JAMA* 242:24–52, 1979.

Legha, S. S., and Carter, S. K. Antiestrogens in the treatment of breast cancer. *Cancer Treat. Rev.* 3:205–216, 1976.

Legha, S. S.; Davis, H. L.; and Muggia, F. M. Hormonal therapy of breast cancer: new approaches and concepts. *Ann. Intern. Med.* 88:69–77, 1978.

Lemon, H. N. Prednisone therapy of advanced mammary cancer. *Cancer* 12:93–107, 1959.

Lerner, H. J. et al. Phase II study of tamoxifen: report of 74 patients with stage IV breast cancer. *Cancer Treat. Rep.* 60:1431–1435, 1976.

Lett, H. Analysis of 99 cases of inoperable carcinoma of breast treated by oophorectomy. *Lancet* 1:227–228, 1905.

Lippman, M. Proceedings of the symposium on antiestrogen therapy for hormone-dependent tumors. *Cancer Treat. Rep.* 64:741–827, 1980.

Manni, A. et al. Antihormone treatment of stage IV breast cancer. *Cancer* 43:444–450, 1979.

Manni, A.; Trujillo, J. E.; and Pearson, O. H. Sequential use of endocrine therapy and chemotherapy for metastatic breast cancer: effects on survival. *Cancer Treat. Rep.* 64:111–116, 1980.

McGuire, W. L. et al. Current status of estrogen and progesterone receptors in breast cancer. *Cancer* 39:2934–2947, 1977.

Miller, T. R. Hypophysectomy. In *Breast cancer: early and late,* ed. R. L. Clark. Chicago: Year Book, 1970, pp. 377–380.

Mouridsen, H. et al. Tamoxifen in advanced breast cancer. *Cancer Treat. Rev.* 5:131–141, 1978.

Nathanson, I. T. Endocrine aspects of human cancer. *Recent Prog. Horm. Res.* 1:261–291, 1947.

Necheles, T. F. *The acute leukemias.* New York: Stratton Intercontinental, 1979.

Newbit, R. M., and Baum, W. C. Endocrine control of prostatic carcinoma. *JAMA* 143:1317–1320, 1950.

Newsome, H. H. et al. Medical and surgical adrenalectomy in patients with advanced breast carcinoma. *Cancer* 39:542–546, 1977.

Nissen-Meyer, R. Prophylactic ovariectomy and ovarian irradiation in breast cancer. *Acta Un. Int. Cancer* 20:527–535, 1964.

Physician's desk reference, 34th edition. Oradell, N.J.: Medical Economics, 1980.

Piver, M. S. et al. Medroxyprogesterone acetate (Depo-Provera) vs. hydroxyprogesterone caproate (Delalutin) in women with metastatic endometrial adenocarcinoma. *Cancer* 45:268–272, 1980.

Plotkin, D. et al. Tamoxifen flare in advanced breast cancer. *JAMA* 240:2644–2648, 1978.

Proceedings of the Annual Spring Meeting of the Primary Breast Cancer therapy group: tamoxifen workshop. *Cancer Treat. Rep.* 60:1409–1466, 1976.

Sanford, E. J. et al. Aminoglutethimide medical adrenalectomy for advanced prostatic carcinoma. *J. Urol.* 115:170–174, 1976.

Santen, R. J. et al. Kinetic, hormonal, and clinical studies with aminoglutethimide in breast cancer. *Cancer* 39:2948–2958, 1977.

Santen, R. J.; Lipton, A.; and Kendall, J. Successful medical adrenalectomy with aminoglutethimide. *JAMA* 230:1661–1665, 1974.

Scott, W. W.; Menon, M.; and Walsh, P. C. Hormonal therapy of prostatic cancer. *Cancer* 45:1929–1936, 1980.

Segaloff, A. Some biochemical and clinical aspects of the action of androgens and estrogens. *Cancer Res.* 23:1459–1464, 1963.

Tagnon, H. J. Antiestrogens in treatment of breast cancer. *Cancer* 39:2959–2964, 1977.

Thorn, G. W. et al. Medical progress: pharmacological aspects of adrenocortical steroids and ACTH in man. *N. Engl. J. Med.* 248:232–245; 284–294; 323–337; 369–378; 414–423; 588–601; 632–646, 1953.

Ulfelder, H. The stilbestrol disorders in historical perspective. *Cancer* 45:3008–3011, 1980.

United States Pharmacopeial Convention. *USP dispensing information.* Easton, Pa.: Mack Publishing Co., 1980.

Wells, S. A. et al. Medical adrenalectomy with aminoglutethimide. *Ann. Surg.* 187:475–484, 1978.

Westerberg, H. Tamoxifen and fluoxymesterone in advanced breast cancer: a controlled clinical trial. *Cancer Treat. Rep.* 64:117–121, 1980.

Wiggans, R. G. et al. Phase II trial of tamoxifen in advanced breast cancer. *Cancer Chemother. Pharmacol.* 3:45–48, 1979.

twenty-nine

Combination Chemotherapy

JOHN C. MARSH
DAVID S. FISCHER

Just as combination antibiotic chemotherapy has been found to be more efficacious in the treatment of tuberculosis and serious Gram-negative sepsis, as compared to single antibiotics, in a similar fashion, combination anticancer chemotherapy has been achieving better results than single agents in many of the tumors tested. Possible exceptions include some of the more sensitive neoplasms such as gestational trophoblastic tumors and African Burkitt's lymphoma where a single agent is often curative. Still, combination regimens seem to have higher response rates and longer durations of disease-free survival in many instances when compared to single agents (DeVita and Schein 1973).

One of the reasons for greater efficacy of combination chemotherapy is that it may prevent or delay drug resistance. Such resistance may develop from increased use of an alternate biochemical pathway (salvage) or rapid repair of a drug-induced lesion. Other possibilities include insufficient uptake of the drug by the neoplastic cells, insufficient drug activation or increased concentration of a target enzyme, or decreased requirement for a specific metabolic product. We are in a very early stage of in vitro testing of tumor cells for drug sensitivity. These techniques may help predict response so that we can rationally select a broad spectrum of effective agents. Until that happy day, we empirically select drugs at random based on their performance in single-dose therapy programs and hope that they work in combination. Nonetheless, there are some guidelines to help in selection.

Some of the rationales for combination chemotherapy are as follows:

1. To block synthetic pathways in sequence or in parallel. The former is when two agents block sequential steps leading to the same product. This usually does not lead to a synergistic response. In concurrent inhibition agents inhibit two or more precursors of the same end product. Complementary inhibition was used to describe a process wherein one agent may inactivate or bind a crucial macromolecule such as DNA, and another agent may prevent its resynthesis or repair (Sartorelli 1969).

2. To interfere with the degradation of antimetabolites, for example, 6-mercaptopurine and allopurinol.

3. To interfere with de novo synthesis of a macromolecule and thus increase the incorporation of analogues entering the macromolecule by preformed pathways; for example, to encourage the synthesis of a fraudulent material whose faulty function may lead to cellular death.

4. To use agents that prevent toxicity selectively in the organ sensitive to the agent. Androgen "protection" of the bone marrow prior to therapy would be such a combination.

Although such theoretical reasons may serve as inspirations for the design of combinations used clinically, it must be admitted that most useful combinations have come about empirically, and they depend on the ability to use them together without too much compromise of optimal dose of any single agent (DeVita and

Schein 1973). Ideally, combinations should consist of drugs without overlapping toxicity. This has led to the great popularity of vincristine and bleomycin, since they do not require a reduction in the dose of myelosuppressive agents as do doxorubicin or cyclophosphamide. Since there is often a steep dose-response curve for the latter agents (versus tumor or bone marrow stem cells), even a modest dose reduction may unfavorably affect the antitumor activity.

Because of its relative lack of marrow toxicity, cisplatin is another favorite agent for combinations. In head and neck cancer, however, attempts to combine high-dose methotrexate and cisplatin can lead to disaster, since both are nephrotoxic and require good renal function to avoid toxicity. The inclusion of bleomycin with radiotherapy in a small cell lung carcinoma regimen (even though the drug has virtually no antitumor activity when used alone) is also unsuccessful because of severe pulmonary fibrosis, probably accentuated by the radiation (Skarin et al. 1975). The dose reduction required in 5-FU and semustine (methyl-CCNU) combinations may cause the lack of advantage in colon cancer over either drug alone.

It is best to select drugs with different mechanisms of cell destruction. One can combine an alkylating agent to kill cells in G_0 or any other phase of the cycle, an antimetabolite to kill rapidly developing tumors, and a corticosteroid or other hormone to control cell growth without definitive cell kill. These agents with differing mechanisms reduce the chances of cell resistance. High-dose intermittent therapy frequently maximizes tumor cell kill while minimizing the side effects on rapidly proliferating tissues such as bone marrow, immune system, hair, and the gastrointestinal mucosa. When selecting drugs with different types of clinical toxicity, one can generally administer full or slightly reduced doses. Such combinations may additively affect the tumor. Even more desirable is a synergistic effect where the response is better than the anticipated sum of the component drug responses. If one combines agents with overlapping toxicities, it is necessary to reduce the dose of drugs with cumulative toxicities by 25% to 50%. In some instances it may be possible to sequence administration so that the marrow and immune system recover before they are again assaulted. Normal tissues usually (but not always) repair themselves and regrow faster than most tumors. When using an active drug in combination with an agent capable of reversing the activity of the former, it is hoped that the normal cells will recover before the tumor cells, such as high-dose methotrexate with folinic acid (leucovorin) rescue.

In the design and evaluation of combination regimens, there are no rigid guidelines. To evaluate drugs adequately is time-consuming. It takes only three or four patients to become convinced of the efficacy of drugs when the response is clear-cut. It may require 30 to 45 patients if the differences between the test group and the controls are not substantial.

To facilitate use of combination chemotherapy, we have compiled some of the more common and useful regimens with their usual dosage, and a reference to the report by the investigators. Sometimes we cite the original report, which may be an abstract, but more often we refer to later but more complete data with possible newer dose modifications. In using one of these combinations, this compilation should serve only as a guide and refresher. *Always* consult the original or cited literature to check dosage, timing, and accuracy before administering one of these potent combinations. Also, remember the synergistic effect of radiation and some chemotherapeutic agents; if combined modality therapy is being used, lower doses may be necessary.

References

DeVita, V. T., Jr., and Schein, P. S. The use of drugs in combination for the treatment of cancer. *N. Engl. J. Med.* 288:998–1006, 1973.

Sartorelli, A. C. Some approaches to the therapeutic exploitation of metabolic sites of vulnerability of neoplastic cells. *Cancer Res.* 29:1019–1032, 1969.

Skarin, A. et al. Combined intensive chemotherapy and radiotherapy in oat-cell carcinoma of the lung. *Proc. Am. Soc. Clin. Oncol.* 16:264, 1975.

Combination Chemotherapy Regimens

Brain Tumors

Procarbazine	100 mg/m^2 p.o. × 14 days
Lomustine (CCNU)	75 mg/m^2 p.o. day 1
Vincristine	1.4 mg/m^2 IV days 1 and 8

Note: Repeat every four weeks. (Higher-dose single-agent lomustine may be just as effective.)

Source: Gutin, P. H. et al. Phase II study of procarbazine, CCNU, and vincristine combination chemotherapy in the treatment of malignant brain tumors. *Cancer* 35:1398–1404, 1975.

Breast Carcinoma

AC

Doxorubicin (Adriamycin)	40 mg/m^2 IV day 1
Cyclophosphamide	200 mg/m^2 p.o. days 3 to 6

Note: Repeat every 21 days.

Sources: Salmon, S., and Jones, S. E. Chemotherapy of advanced breast cancer with a combination of Adriamycin and cyclophosphamide. *Proc. Am. Assoc. Cancer Res.* 15:90, 1974.

Jones, S. E.; Durie, B. G. M.; and Salmon, S. E. Combination chemotherapy with Adriamycin and cyclophosphamide for advanced breast cancer. *Cancer* 36:90–97, 1975.

AC versus ACMF

AC

Doxorubicin (Adriamycin)	40 mg/m² IV day 1
Cyclophosphamide	1 gm/m² IV day 1

Note: Repeat every 21 days.

ACMF

Doxorubicin (Adriamycin)	40 mg/m² IV day 1
Cyclophosphamide	1 gm/m² IV day 1
Methotrexate	30 to 40 mg/m² IV days 21, 28, and 35
5-Fluorouracil	400 to 600 mg/m² IV days 21, 28, and 35

Note: Repeat every 42 days.

Sources: Boston, B. et al. Combination vs. combination sequential non-hormonal chemotherapy in advanced breast cancer. *Proc. Am. Soc. Clin. Oncol.* 17:247, 1976.

Kennealey, G. T., et al. Combination chemotherapy for advanced breast cancer: two regimens containing Adriamycin. *Cancer* 42:27–33, 1978.

AMV

Doxorubicin (Adriamycin)	30 mg/m² IV every 4 weeks
Mitomycin	10 mg/m² IV every 8 weeks
Vinblastine	6 mg/m² IV every 4 weeks

Source: Luikart, S., and Portlock, C. Adriamycin, mitomycin C, and vinblastine in metastatic breast cancer. In *Yale University Research Protocol Y-31181,* New Haven, Conn., 1981.

Ansfield's Modified 5-Drug Regimen

5-Fluorouracil	500 mg/week IV
Methotrexate	25 mg/week IV
Vincristine	1 mg/week IV
Cyclophosphamide	100 mg/day p.o.
Prednisone	45 mg/day p.o. × 2 weeks, then 30 mg/day p.o. × 2 weeks, and 15 mg/day thereafter.

Source: Ansfield, F. J. et al. Five-drug therapy for advanced breast cancer: a phase 1 study. *Cancer Chemother. Rep.* 55:183–188, 1971.

AV

Doxorubicin (Adriamycin)	75 mg/m^2 IV day 1
Vincristine	1.4 mg/m^2 IV days 1 and 8

Note: Repeat every 3 weeks.

Source: Bonadonna, G. et al. Controlled study with multiple drug combination in advanced breast cancer. *Proc. Am. Soc. Clin. Oncol.* 15:176, 1974.

CAF

Cyclophosphamide	500 mg/m^2 IV day 1
Doxorubicin (Adriamycin)	50 mg/m^2 IV day 1
5-Fluorouracil	500 mg/m^2 IV day 1

Note: The regimen differs from FAC only in that 5-fluorouracil is given days 1 and 8 in FAC but is given only once per course in this regimen. Drugs are given every 21 days.

Source: Smalley, R. V. et al. A comparison of cyclophosphamide, Adriamycin, 5-fluorouracil (CAF) and cyclophosphamide, methotrexate, 5-fluorouracil, vincristine, prednisone (CMFVP) in patients with metastatic breast cancer. *Cancer* 40:625–632, 1977.

CMF Adjuvant

Below age 60:

Cyclophosphamide	100 mg/m^2 p.o. days 1 to 14
Methotrexate	40 mg/m^2 IV days 1 and 8
5-Fluorouracil	600 mg/m^2 IV days 1 and 8

Above age 60:

Cyclophosphamide	100 mg/m^2 p.o. days 1 to 14
Methotrexate	30 mg/m^2 IV days 1 and 8
5-Fluorouracil	400 mg/m^2 IV days 1 and 8

Note: Repeat every 28 days.

Source: Bonadonna, G. et al. Combination chemotherapy as an adjuvant treatment in operable breast cancer. *N. Engl. J. Med.* 294:405–410, 1976.

CMFP

Cyclophosphamide	100 mg/m^2 p.o. days 1 to 14
Methotrexate	60 mg/m^2 IV days 1 and 8
5-Fluorouracil	700 mg/m^2 IV days 1 and 8
Prednisone	40 mg/m^2 p.o. days 1 to 14

Note: Repeat course every 28 days.

Source: Canellos, G. P.; Gold, G. L.; and Schein, P. S. Combination chemotherapy for advanced breast cancer: response and effect on survival. *Ann. Intern. Med.* 84:389–392, 1976.

CMFVP

Cyclophosphamide	400 mg/m^2 IV day 1
Methotrexate	30 mg/m^2 IV days 1 and 8
5-Fluorouracil	400 mg/m^2 IV days 1 and 8
Vincristine	1 mg IV days 1 and 8
Prednisone	20 mg p.o., q.i.d. days 1 to 7

Note: Repeat every 28 days.

Source: Smalley, R. V. et al. A comparison of cyclophosphamide, Adriamycin, 5-fluorouracil (CAF) and cyclophosphamide, methotrexate, 5-fluorouracil, vincristine, prednisone (CMFVP) in patients with metastatic breast cancer. *Cancer* 40:625–632, 1977.

Cooper Regimen

5-Fluorouracil	12 mg/kg IV every week × 8 weeks, then every other week for 7 additional months
Methotrexate	0.7 mg/kg/week IV × 8 weeks, then every other week for 7 months
Vincristine	0.035 mg/kg/week IV × 5 weeks, then once a month
Cyclophosphamide	2 mg/kg/day p.o. × 9 months
Prednisone	0.75 mg/kg/day p.o. × 10 days, then ½ above/day × 10 days, then ¼ above/day × 10 days, then 5 mg/day × 20 days and discontinue

Source: Cooper, R. G.; Holland, J. F.; and Glidewell, O. Adjuvant chemotherapy of breast cancer. *Cancer* 44:793–798, 1979.

FAC

5-Fluorouracil	500 mg/m² IV days 1 and 8
Doxorubicin (Adriamycin)	50 mg/m² IV day 1
Cyclophosphamide	500 mg/m² IV day 1

Note: Treatment every 21 days.

Sources: Blumenschein, G. et al. FAC chemotherapy for breast cancer. *Proc. Am. Soc. Clin. Oncol.* 15:193, 1974.

Hortobagyi, G.N. et al. Combination chemoimmunotherapy of metastatic breast cancer with 5-fluorouracil, Adriamycin, cyclophosphamide and BCG. *Cancer* 43:1225–1233, 1979.

FCP

5-Fluorouracil	8 mg/kg/day IV × 5 days
Cyclophosphamide	4 mg/kg/day IV × 5 days
Prednisone	30 mg/day p.o. tapered to 10 mg/day
± Vincristine	1.4 mg/m² IV days 1 and 5

Source: Ahmann, D. L.; Bisel, H. F.; and Hahn, R. G. A phase II evaluation of Adriamycin (NSC 123127) as treatment for disseminated breast cancer. *Proc. Am. Assoc. Cancer Res.* 15:100, 1974.

MV

Mitomycin	20 mg/m² IV day 1
Vinblastine	0.15 mg/kg IV days 1 and 22

Note: Repeat course every 6 to 8 weeks.

Source: Konits, P.H. et al. Mitomycin C and vinblastine chemotherapy for advanced breast cancer. *Proc. Am. Soc. Clin. Oncol.* 21:410, 1980.

Colon Carcinoma

FDVB

5-Fluorouracil	10 mg/kg IV days 1 to 5
Dacarbazine	3 mg/kg IV days 1 and 2
Vincristine	0.025 mg/kg IV day 1
Carmustine (BCNU)	1.5 mg/kg IV day 1

Note: Repeat every 28 days.

Source: Falkson, G.; van Eden, E. B.; and Falkson, H. C. Fluorouracil, imidazole carboxamide dimethyl triazino, vincristine and bis-chloroethyl nitrosourea in colon cancer. *Cancer* 33:1207–1209, 1974.

FMV

5-Fluorouracil	10 mg/kg IV days 1 to 5
Semustine (methyl-CCNU)	175 mg/m^2 p.o. day 1
Vincristine	1 mg/m^2 IV day 1

Note: Repeat every 35 days.

Source: Moertel, C. G. et al. Therapy of advanced colorectal cancer with a combination of 5-fluorouracil, methyl-1, 3-cis(2-chloroethyl)-1-nitrosourea and vincristine. *J. Natl. Cancer Inst.* 54:69–71, 1975.

MOF-Strep

Semustine (Methyl-CCNU)	30 mg/m^2 p.o. days 1 to 5 every 10 weeks
Vincristine (Oncovin)	1 mg IV day 1 every 5 weeks
5-Fluorouracil	300 mg/m^2 IV days 1 to 5 every 5 weeks
Streptozotocin	500 mg/m^2 day 1 and weekly

Source: Kemeny, N. et al. Therapy for metastatic colorectal carcinoma with a combination of methyl-CCNU, 5-fluorouracil, vincristine, and streptozotocin (MOF-Strep.). *Cancer* 45:876–881, 1980.

Ewing's Sarcoma

ACV

Doxorubicin (Adriamycin)	75 mg/m^2 IV days 1 and 43
Cyclophosphamide	40 mg/kg IV day 21
Vincristine	0.04 mg/kg IV day 22

Note: Alternate Adriamycin with cyclophosphamide-vincristine to total Adriamycin dose 300 mg/m^2. Some patients are also given methotrexate 10 to 15 mg intrathecally and whole brain irradiation to 2000 rad in 2 weeks. Radiation is given to primary lesion.

Source: Pomeroy, C., and Johnson, R. E. Combined modality therapy of Ewing's sarcoma. *Cancer* 35:36–47, 1975.

VAC

Vincristine	2 mg/m^2/week IV × 7 weeks
Dactinomycin (actinomycin D)	0.320 mg/m^2/day IV × 7 days every 12 weeks
Cyclophosphamide	300 mg/m^2/day IV × 10 days every 12 weeks, alternating with courses of 7 days when the course coincides with actinomycin D therapy so that cyclophosphamide is given every 6 weeks.

Note: Radiation to primary lesion, 4000 rad, beginning day 1 for 4 weeks, then a cone down-field to a total dose of 5500 to 6000 rad.

Source: Jaffe, N. et al. Improved outlook for Ewing's sarcoma with combination chemotherapy (vincristine, actinomycin D, and cyclophosphamide) and radiation therapy. *Cancer* 38:1925–1930, 1976.

Gastric Carcinoma

FAM

5-Fluorouracil	600 mg/m^2 IV days 1, 8, 28, and 35
Doxorubicin (Adriamycin)	30 mg/m^2 IV days 1 and 28
Mitomycin	10 mg/m^2 IV day 1

Note: Repeat every 56 days.

Sources: Macdonald, J. S. et al. 5-Fluorouracil, mitomycin-C and Adriamycin-FAM: a new combination chemotherapy program for advanced gastric carcinoma. *Proc. Am. Soc. Clin. Oncol.* 17:264, 1976.

Macdonald, J. S. et al. 5-Fluorouracil, doxorubicin, and mitomycin (FAM) combination chemotherapy for advanced gastric cancer. *Ann. Intern. Med.* 93:533–536, 1980.

FAME

5-Fluorouracil	350 mg/m^2/day IV days 1 to 5, 36 to 40
Doxorubicin (Adriamycin)	40 mg/m^2/day IV days 1 and 36
Semustine (methyl-CCNU)	150 mg/m^2/day p.o. day 1

Note: Repeat cycle every 10 weeks.

Source: Gastrointestinal Tumor Study Group. Phase II–III. Chemotherapy studies in advanced cancer. *Cancer Treat. Rep.* 63:1871–1876, 1979.

Head and Neck Carcinoma

BLEO-MTX

Bleomycin	15 units IV 4 to 14 day intervals
Methotrexate	15 mg/m^2 IV 4 to 14 day intervals

Source: Yagoda, A. et al. Combination chemotherapy with bleomycin and methotrexate in patients with advanced epidermoid carcinoma. *Proc. Am. Soc. Clin. Oncol.* 16:247, 1975.

MBD

Methotrexate	40 mg/m^2 IM days 1 and 15
Bleomycin	10 units IM weekly
Cisplatin (cis-dichlorodiammineplatinum)	50 mg/m^2 IV day 4

Note: Repeat every 21 days.

Source: Kaplan, B. H. et al. Chemotherapy of advanced cancer of the head and neck with methotrexate (M), bleomycin (B) and cis-diamminedichloroplatinum (D) in combination-(MBD). *Proc. Amer. Soc. Clin. Oncol.* 20:384, 1979.

M-F

Methotrexate	125 to 250 mg/m^2 IV
5-Fluorouracil	600 mg/m^2 IV 1 hour later
Leucovorin rescue	10 mg/m^2 IV or p.o. at 24 hours, then 10 mg/m^2 p.o. every 6 hours $\times$ 5 doses

Note: Repeat weekly as tolerated. Renal function must be carefully monitored, and leucovorin rescue is imperative.

Source: Pitman, S. W. et al. Sequential methotrexate – 5-fluorouracil: a highly active drug combination in advanced squamous cell carcinoma of the head and neck. *Proc. Am. Soc. Clin. Oncol.* 21:473, 1980.

Leukemia: Acute Lymphocytic (Childhood)

Induction

VP

Vincristine	1.5 mg/m² IV weekly × 4 to 6 weeks
Prednisone	40 mg/m² p.o. daily in divided dose × 4 to 6 weeks

OR

VP plus Daunorubicin

Vincristine and prednisone as above	
Daunorubicin	25 mg/m² IV weekly × 4 to 6 weeks

OR

VP plus L-Asparaginase

Vincristine and prednisone as above	
L-asparaginase	10,000 units/m² IV weekly × 2 weeks

CNS Therapy

Prophylaxis

Begins 1 week after remission is achieved.

Methotrexate	12 mg/m² intrathecally twice weekly × 5 doses

Cranial Irradiation

(age > 2) 2400 rad over 2½ weeks

Maintenance Therapy

Methotrexate	20 mg/m² IV weekly
6-Mercaptopurine	50 mg/m² p.o. daily

Source: Carter, S. K.; Bakowski, M. T.; and Hellman, K. *Chemotherapy of cancer*. New York: John Wiley & Sons, 1977, pp. 234–241.

Leukemia: Acute Myelogenous

AOAP

Doxorubicin (Adriamycin)	40 mg/m^2 IV day 1
Vincristine (Oncovin)	2 mg IV day 1
Cytarabine (ara-C)	100 mg/m^2 IV days 5 to 9 continuous infusion
Prednisone	100 mg/day p.o. days 1 to 5, repeat on day 19

Source: McCredie, K. B. et al. Sequential Adriamycin–Ara-C (A-OAP) for remission induction of adult acute leukemia. *Proc. Am. Soc. Clin. Oncol.* 15:62, 1974.

CD

Cytarabine	100 mg/m^2 IV infusion over 24 hours × 7 days
Daunorubicin	45 mg/m^2 IV days 1, 2, and 3

Note: Repeat courses for further induction or consolidation, with cytarabine for 5 days and daunorubicin for 2 days.

Source: Yates, J. W. et al. Cytosine arabinoside and daunorubicin therapy in acute non-lymphocytic leukemia. *Cancer Chemother. Rep.* 57:485–488, 1973.

COAP

Cyclophosphamide (Cytoxan)	100 mg/m^2/day p.o. × 5 days
Vincristine (Oncovin)	2 mg/week IV day 1
Cytarabine (ara-C)	100 mg/m^2/day IV or SC × 5 days
Prednisone	100 mg/day p.o. × 5 days

Source: Whitecar, J. P. et al. Cyclophosphamide, vincristine, cytosine arabinoside and prednisone (COAP) combination chemotherapy for acute leukemia in adults. *Cancer Chemother. Rep.* 56:543–550, 1972.

CT

Cytarabine	1 to 3 mg/kg IV daily × 8 to 32 days
6-Thioguanine	2.0 to 2.5 mg/kg p.o. daily × 8 to 32 days

Note: Drugs usually given 8 to 10 hours apart with thioguanine in morning and cytarabine in afternoon.

Source: Gee, T. S.; Yu, K-P.; and Clarkson, B. D. Treatment of adult acute leukemia with arabinosylcytosine and thioguanine. *Cancer* 23:1019–1032, 1969.

DAT

Induction

Daunorubicin	60 mg/m^2 IV days 5, 6, and 7
Cytarabine (ara-C)	100 mg/m^2 IV over 30 minutes b.i.d. × 7 days
6-Thioguanine	100 mg/m^2 p.o. every 12 hours × 7 days

Consolidation Therapy

Two cycles of cytarabine (ara-C) and thioguanine every 12 hours for 5 days followed by a single injection of daunorubicin. Consolidation cycles were given at 21-day intervals.

CNS Therapy

Prophylactic 2400-rad cranial irradiation. Cytarabine, 100 mg/m^2 intrathecally divided into 5 doses. The authors did *not* find that this increased survival.

Maintenance Therapy

Monthly 5-day cycles of cytarabine-thioguanine alternating with a single dose of daunorubicin

or

the same chemotherapy plus immunotherapy consisting of twice-monthly intravenous *Corynebacterium parvum*, 2.5 mg/m^2 and 10^9 allogenic irradiated leukemic blast cells on cycle days 14 and 21.

Source: Gale, R. P., and Cline, M. J. High remission-induction rate in acute myeloid leukemia. *Lancet* 1:497–499, 1977.

Low-Dose POMP

Prednisone	150 mg/day p.o. days 1 to 5
Vincristine (Oncovin)	2 mg/day IV day 1
Methotrexate	5 mg/m^2/day IV days 1 to 5
6-Mercaptopurine (Purinethol)	500 mg/m^2/day IV days 1 to 5

Note: Repeat every few weeks as tolerated.

Source: Henderson, E. S., and Serpick, A. The effect of combination drug therapy and prophylactic antibiotic treatment in adult acute leukemia. *Clin. Res.* 15:336, 1967.

TRAMPCOL

6-Thioguanine	100 mg/m^2/day p.o. × 3 days
Daunorubicin (Rubidomycin)	40 mg/m^2/day IV day 1
Cytarabine (ara-C)	100 mg/m^2/day IV days 1 to 3
Methotrexate	7.5 mg/m^2/day IV days 1 to 3
Prednisolone	200 mg p.o. days 1 to 5
Cyclophosphamide	100 mg/m^2/day IV days 1 to 3
Vincristine (Oncovin)	2 mg IV day 1
L-asparaginase	(Optional and for childhood lymphocytic leukemia only) 800 units/m^2/day, days 1 to 28

Note: If blood cell counts are acceptable, some doses are escalated in terms of additional days.

Source: Spiers, A. S. D. et al. Multiple-drug chemotherapy for acute leukemia. *Cancer* 40:20–29, 1977.

TRAP

6-Thioguanine	100 mg/m^2/day p.o. days 1 to 5
Daunorubicin (Rubidomycin)	40 mg/m^2/day IV day 1
Cytarabine (ara-C)	100 mg/m^2/day IV or IM days 1 to 5
Prednisone	30 mg/m^2/day p.o. days 1 to 5

Source: Spiers, A. S. D. A multiple-drug regimen for refractory acute leukemias. *Br. J. Haematol.* 23:262–263, 1973.

Leukemia: Blastic Chronic Granulocytic

VP

Vincristine	2 mg/m² IV weekly
Prednisone	60 mg/m²/day p.o. × 14 days, then tapered

Source: Canellos, G. P. et al. Hematologic and cytogenetic remission of blastic transformation in chronic granulocytic leukemia. *Blood* 38:671–679, 1971.

Ara-C plus 6-TG

Cytarabine (ara-C)	200 mg/m² IV × 5 days
6-Thioguanine	200 mg/m² p.o. × 5 days

Source: Canellos, G. P. et al. Chemotherapy of the blastic phase of chronic granulocytic leukemia. *Proc. Am. Soc. Clin. Oncol.* 16:252, 1975.

Lung Cancer: Non-Small Cell Carcinoma

BACON

Bleomycin	30 units IV day 2, 6 hours after vincristine, weekly × 6 weeks
Doxorubicin (Adriamycin)	40 mg/m² IV day 1 and every 4 weeks
Lomustine (CCNU)	65 mg/m² p.o. day 1 and every 8 weeks
Vincristine (Oncovin)	0.75–1 mg IV day 2 weekly × 6 weeks
Nitrogen mustard (Mechlorethamine)	8 mg/m² day 1 and every 4 weeks

Source: Livingston, R. B. et al. BACON in squamous lung cancer. *Cancer* 37:1237–1242, 1976.

CAMP

Cyclophosphamide	300 mg/m² IV days 1 and 8
Doxorubicin (Adriamycin)	20 mg/m² IV days 1 and 8
Methotrexate	15 mg/m² IV days 1 and 8
Procarbazine	100 mg/day p.o. × 10 days

Note: Repeat every 28 days.

Source: Bitran, J. D. et al. Cyclophosphamide, Adriamycin, methotrexate, and procarbazine (CAMP) effective four-drug combination chemotherapy for metastatic non-oat cell bronchogenic carcinoma. *Cancer Treat. Rep.* 60:1225–1230, 1976.

CAP

Cyclophosphamide	400 mg/m² IV day 1
Doxorubicin (Adriamycin)	40 mg/m² IV day 1
Platinum (cisplatin)	60 mg/m² IV day 1
Mannitol	25 gm IV with cisplatin

Note: Repeat every 4 weeks.

Source: Eagan, R. T. et al. Phase II trial of cyclophosphamide, Adriamycin, and cis-dichlorodiammineplatinum II by infusion in patients with adenocarcinoma and large cell carcinoma of the lung. *Cancer Treat. Rep.* 64:1589–1591, 1979.

CAV

Cyclophosphamide	500 mg/m^2 IV day 1
Doxorubicin (Adriamycin)	50 mg/m^2 IV day 1
Vincristine	1.4 mg/m^2 IV day 1 (not to exceed 2 mg)

Note: Repeat every 28 days.

Source: Mundia, A. et al. Combination of Adriamycin, cyclophosphamide, and vincristine in inoperable lung cancer. *Proc. Am. Soc. Clin. Oncol.* 16:241, 1975.

COMB (No. 3)

Cyclophosphamide	800 mg/m^2 IV day 1 and every 4 weeks
Vincristine (Oncovin)	0.5 to 0.75 mg IV day 2, repeat twice weekly × 48 doses
Semustine (methyl-CCNU)	100 mg/m^2 p.o. day 1 and every 4 weeks
Bleomycin	7.5 units IV day 2, 6 hours after vincristine; repeat twice weekly × 48 doses

Source: Livingston, R., and Einhorn, L. COMB: a four-drug combination in solid tumors. *Cancer* 36:327–332, 1975.

Doxorubicin and Cisplatin

Doxorubicin	60 mg/m^2 IV
Cisplatin	60 mg/m^2 IV

Note: Repeat every 3 weeks.

Source: Morris, R. W. et al. Adriamycin and Cis-dichlorodiammineplatinum in nonresectable and metastatic carcinoma of the lung. *Cancer Clin. Trials* 2:37–41, 1979.

MACC

Methotrexate	30 mg/m^2 IV
Doxorubicin (Adriamycin)	35 mg/m^2 IV
Cyclophosphamide	400 mg/m^2 IV
Lomustine (CCNU)	30 mg/m^2 p.o.

Note: Repeat at 21 days.

Sources: Chahinian, P. A. et al. Chemotherapy with or without immunotherapy in bronchogenic carcinoma. *Proc. Am. Soc. Clin. Oncol.* 18:333, 1977.

Chahinian, P.A. et al. MACC in advanced lung cancer. *Cancer* 43:1590–1597, 1979.

MCC

Methotrexate	10 mg/m^2 p.o. twice weekly
Cyclophosphamide	500 mg/m^2 IV every 3 weeks
Lomustine (CCNU)	50 mg/m^2 p.o. every 6 weeks

Source: Selawry, O. S. The role of chemotherapy in the treatment of lung cancer. *Semin. Oncol.* 1:259–272, 1974.

Vinblastine plus Cisplatin

Vinblastine	0.2 mg/kg IV day 1
Cisplatin	120 mg/m^2 IV day 1
Mannitol	with cisplatin

Source: Bitran, J. D.; Desser, R. K.; and Shapiro, C. M. Velban and cis-platin in the treatment of refractory stage III_m, non-small cell bronchogenic carcinoma (NSBC). *Proc. Am. Soc. Clin. Oncol.* 22:501,1981.

Vindesine plus Cisplatin

Vindesine	3 mg/m^2 IV weekly × 7 then every 2 weeks
Cisplatin	120 mg/m^2 IV day 1, 29 and then every 6 weeks
Mannitol	25 gm IV with cisplatin

Source: Casper, E. S.; Gralla, R J.; and Golbey, R. B. Vindesine (DVA) and cis-dichlorodiammine platinum II (DDP) combination chemotherapy in non-small cell lung cancer. *Proc. Am. Soc. Clin. Oncol.* 20:337, 1979.

Lung Cancer: Small Cell Carcinoma

CAV

Cyclophosphamide	750 mg/m^2 IV days 1 and 22
Doxorubicin (Adriamycin)	50 mg/m^2 IV days 1 and 22
Vincristine	1 mg IV total day 1, then weekly × 12 weeks

Radiation therapy to bulky disease.

After completion of radiation therapy, resume cyclophosphamide, 750 mg/m^2 IV at 12 weeks, and doxorubicin, 50 mg/m^2 IV at 12 weeks, and repeat every 3 weeks to total doxorubicin dose of 450 mg/m^2.

After cessation of doxorubicin, IV cyclophosphamide is given 1000 mg/m^2 every 4 weeks and methotrexate 30 mg/m^2 IV 3 weeks after each cyclophosphamide dose.

Source: Livingston, R. B. et al. Small cell carcinoma of the lung: combined chemotherapy and radiation. *Ann. Intern. Med.* 88:194–199, 1978.

CLMDVP Intensive Therapy

Cyclophosphamide	1500 mg/m^2 IV day 1 and 1000 mg/m^2 IV day 21
Lomustine (CCNU)	100 mg/m^2 p.o. day 1
Methotrexate	15 mg/m^2 IV twice weekly × 5 weeks
Doxorubicin	60 mg/m^2 IV days 42 and 63
Vincristine	2 mg IV days 42 and 63
Procarbazine	100 mg/m^2 p.o. days 42 to 51 and 63 to 72

Sources: Cohen, M. H. et al. Intensive chemotherapy of small cell bronchogenic carcinoma. *Cancer Treat. Rep.* 61:349–354, 1977.

Cohen, M. H. et al. Cyclic alternating combination chemotherapy of small cell bronchogenic carcinoma. *Proc. Am. Soc. Clin. Oncol.* 19:359, 1978.

POCC

Procarbazine	100 mg/m^2 p.o. days 1 to 14
Vincristine (Oncovin)	2 mg IV days 1 and 8
Cyclophosphamide	600 mg/m^2 IV days 1 and 8
Lomustine (CCNU)	60 mg/m^2 p.o. day 1

Note: Repeat cycle every 28 days.

Source: Alexander, M. et al. Combined modality treatment for oat cell carcinoma of the lung: a randomized trial. *Cancer Treat. Rep.* 61:1–6, 1977.

Lymphoma: Hodgkin's Disease

ABVD

Doxorubicin (Adriamycin)	25 mg/m² IV days 1 and 15
Bleomycin	10 units/m² IV days 1 and 15
Vinblastine	6 mg/m² IV days 1 and 15
Dacarbazine (DTIC)	150 mg/m² IV days 1 to 5

Note: Dacarbazine was changed to 350 mg/m² days 1 and 15.

Source: Bonadonna, G. et al. Combination chemotherapy of Hodgkin's disease with Adriamycin, bleomycin, vinblastine, and imidazole carboxamide (ABVD) vs. MOPP. *Cancer* 36:252–259, 1975.

B-CAVe

Bleomycin	5 units/m² IV days 1, 28, and 35
Lomustine (CCNU)	100 mg/m² p.o. day 1
Doxorubicin (Adriamycin)	60 mg/m² IV day 1
Vinblastine	5 mg/m² IV day 1

Note: Cycles repeated every 6 weeks (if blood counts permit) to total of 9 cycles.

Source: Porzig, K. J. et al. Treatment of advanced Hodgkin's disease with B-CAVe following MOPP failure. *Cancer* 41:1670–1675, 1978.

B-DOPA

Bleomycin	4 units/m² IV days 2 and 5
Dacarbazine	150 mg/m² IV days 1 to 5
Vincristine (Oncovin)	1.5 mg/m² IV days 1 and 5
Prednisone	40 mg/m² p.o. days 1 to 6
Doxorubicin (Adriamycin)	60 mg/m² IV day 1

Note: Repeat every 21 days.

Source: Lokich, J. J. et al. New multiple-agent chemotherapy (B-DOPA) for advanced Hodgkin's disease. *Cancer* 38:667–671, 1978.

B-MOPP

Bleomycin	2 units/m^2 IV days 1 and 8
Nitrogen mustard	6 mg/m^2 IV days 1 and 8
Vincristine (Oncovin)	1.4 mg/m^2 IV days 1 and 8
Procarbazine	100 mg/m^2 p.o. days 1 to 14
Prednisone	50 mg/m^2 p.o. days 1 to 14

Note: Repeat every 28 days. Use prednisone in cycles 1 and 4 only.

Source: Coltman, C. A., Jr., and Jones, S. E. MOPP plus low-dose bleomycin (MOPP + LDB) for advanced Hodgkin's disease—a five-year follow-up. *Proc. Am. Soc. Clin. Oncol.* 19:329, 1978.

MOPP

Nitrogen mustard	6 mg/m^2 IV days 1 and 8
Vincristine (Oncovin)	1.4 mg/m^2 IV days 1 and 8
Procarbazine	100 mg/m^2 p.o. days 1 to 14
Prednisone	40 mg/m^2 p.o. days 1 to 14

Note: Prednisone is used in the first and fourth course. Usually 6 courses are given or 2 courses beyond complete remission. C-MOPP simply replaces the nitrogen mustard with cyclophosphamide, 650 mg/m^2 days 1 and 8. Repeat every 28 days.

Source: DeVita, V. T., Jr.; Serpick, A. A.; and Carbone, P. O. Combination chemotherapy in the treatment of advanced Hodgkin's disease. *Ann. Intern. Med.* 73:881–895, 1970.

MVPP

Nitrogen mustard	6 mg/m^2 IV days 1 and 8
Vinblastine	6 mg/m^2 IV days 1 and 8
Procarbazine	100 mg/m^2 p.o. days 1 to 14
Prednisone	40 mg/m^2 p.o. days 1 to 14

Note: Six 14-day courses are given with 28-day rest periods. Usually 6 or more cycles are with prednisone, 40 mg/day in each cycle.

Source: Nicholson, W. M. et al. Combination chemotherapy in generalized Hodgkin's disease. *Br. Med. J.* 3:7–10, 1970.

MVVPP

Nitrogen mustard	0.4 mg/kg IV day 0
Vincristine	1.4 mg/m² IV days 1, 8, and 15
Vinblastine	6 mg/m² IV days 22, 29, and 36
Procarbazine	100 mg/day for 21 days beginning day 22
Prednisone	40 mg/m² p.o. days 1 to 21, then taper to 0 over 2 weeks; omit from course 2 and 4

Note: Repeat every 60 days for 3 courses. Then give low dose of radiation to areas of previously demonstrated bulky tumor and complete with 2 more courses chemotherapy.

Source: Prosnitz, L. R. et al. Long-term remissions with combined modality therapy for advanced Hodgkin's disease. *Cancer* 37:2826–2833, 1976.

Lymphoma: Non-Hodgkin's Disease

BACO

Bleomycin	10 units/m² IM day 2
Doxorubicin (Adriamycin)	40 mg/m² IV day 1
Lomustine (CCNU)	50 mg/m² p.o. day 1
Vincristine (Oncovin)	2 mg IV day 1

Note: Repeat every 3 weeks.

Source: Davis, L. K. et al. Bleomycin, Adriamycin, CCNU, and Oncovin combination chemotherapy (BACO) in advanced and recurrent lymphomas. *Proc. Am. Soc. Clin. Oncol.* 18:273, 1977.

BACOP

Bleomycin	5 units/m² IV days 15 and 22
Doxorubicin (Adriamycin)	25 mg/m² IV days 1 and 8
Cyclophosphamide	650 mg/m² IV days 1 and 8
Vincristine (Oncovin)	1.4 mg/m² IV (maximum 2 mg) IV days 1 and 8
Prednisone	60 mg/m² p.o. days 15 to 28

Note: Cycles repeated every 28 days.

Source: Schein, P. S. et al. Bleomycin, Adriamycin, cyclophosphamide, vincristine, and prednisone (BACOP) combination chemotherapy. *Ann. Intern. Med.* 85:417–422, 1976.

CHOP

Cyclophosphamide (Cytoxan)	750 mg/m^2 IV day 1
Hydroxydaunorubicin (Adriamycin)	50 mg/m^2 IV day 1
Vincristine (Oncovin)	1.4 mg/m^2 IV day 1
Prednisone	100 mg/m^2 p.o. days 1 to 5

Note: Repeat cycle every 3 weeks.

Source: McKelvey, E. M. et al. Hydroxydaunomycin (Adriamycin) combination chemotherapy in malignant lymphoma. *Cancer* 38:1484–1493, 1976.

CHOP-Bleo

Cyclophosphamide	750 mg/m^2 IV day 1
Hydroxydaunorubicin (Adriamycin)	50 mg/m^2 IV day 1
Vincristine (Oncovin)	2 mg IV days 1 and 5
Prednisone	100 mg p.o. days 1 to 5
Bleomycin	15 units IV days 1 and 5

Note: Repeat every 21 or 28 days.

Source: Rodriguez, V. et al. Combination chemotherapy (CHOP-Bleo) in advanced (non-Hodgkin's) malignant lymphoma. *Blood* 49:325–333, 1977.

C-MOPP

Cyclophosphamide	650 mg/m^2 IV days 1 and 8
Vincristine (Oncovin)	1.4 mg/m^2 IV days 1 and 8
Procarbazine	100 mg/m^2 p.o. days 1 to 14
Prednisone	40 mg/m^2 p.o. days 1 to 14

Note: Cycles of 14 days with 14-day rest period. Prednisone is used in the first and fourth course.

Source: DeVita, V. T., Jr. et al. Advanced diffuse histiocytic lymphoma, a potentially curable disease. *Lancet* 1:248–250, 1975.

COMLA

Cyclophosphamide	1500 mg/m^2 IV day 1
Vincristine (Oncovin)	1.4 mg/m^2 IV days 1, 8, and 15
Methotrexate	120 mg/m^2 IV days 22, 29, 36, 43, 50, 57, 64, and 71
Leucovorin	25 mg/m^2 p.o. every 6 hours × 4 doses; start 24 hours after methotrexate
Cytarabine (ara-C)	300 mg/m^2 IV days 22, 29, 36, 43, 50, 57, 64, and 71

Note: Repeat every 91 days.

Source: Berd, D. et al. Long-term remission in diffuse histiocytic lymphoma treated with combination sequential chemotherapy. *Cancer* 35:1050–1054, 1975.

COP

Cyclophosphamide	800 mg/m^2 IV day 1
Vincristine (Oncovin)	2 mg IV day 1
Prednisone	60 mg/m^2/day p.o. days 1 to 5

Note: Repeat day 14.

Source: Luce, J. K. et al. Combined cyclophosphamide, vincristine, and prednisone therapy of malignant lymphoma. *Cancer* 28:306–317, 1971.

COPP

Cyclophosphamide	600 mg/m^2 IV days 1 and 8
Vincristine (Oncovin)	1.4 mg/m^2 IV days 1 and 8
Procarbazine	100 mg/m^2 IV days 1 to 10
Prednisone	40 mg/m^2 IV days 1 to 14

Note: Cycles of 14 days with 14-day rest period.

Source: Stein, R. S. et al. Combination chemotherapy of lymphomas other than Hodgkin's disease. *Ann. Intern. Med.* 81:601–609, 1974.

CVP

Cyclophosphamide	400 mg/m^2 p.o. days 1 to 5
Vincristine	1.4 mg/m^2 IV day 1
Prednisone	100 mg/m^2 p.o. days 1 to 5

Note: Cycle repeated every 21 days.

Source: Bagley, C. M., Jr. et al. Advanced lymphosarcoma: intensive cyclical combination chemotherapy with cyclophosphamide, vincristine, and prednisone. *Ann. Intern. Med.* 76:227–234, 1972.

HOP

Hydroxydaunorubicin (Adriamycin)	80 mg/m^2 IV day 1
Vincristine (Oncovin)	1.4 mg/m^2 IV day 1
Prednisone	100 mg/m^2 p.o. days 1 to 5

Note: Repeat every 3 weeks.

Source: McKelvey, E. M. et al. Hydroxydaunomycin (Adriamycin) combination chemotherapy in malignant lymphoma. *Cancer* 38:1484–1493, 1976.

Melanoma

VBD

Vinblastine	6 mg/m^2 IV days 1 and 2
Bleomycin	15 units/m^2 IV days 1 to 5 in 24 hours (constant infusion)
Cisplatin (cis-dichlorodiammineplatinum)	50 mg/m^2 IV day 5

Note: Repeat every 28 days.

Source: Nathanson, L.; Kaufman, S. D.; and Carey, R. W. Vinblastine-bleomycin-platinum (VBD): a high response rate regimen in metastatic melanoma. *Proc. Am. Soc. Clin. Oncol.* 21:479, 1980.

Multiple Myeloma

CP

Carmustine (BCNU)	150 mg/m² IV day 4
Prednisone	60 mg/m² p.o. days 1 to 4

Note: Repeat every 6 weeks.

Source: Southwest Oncology Group Study. Remission maintenance therapy for multiple myeloma. *Arch. Intern. Med.* 135:147–152, 1975.

Hi-CP

Cyclophosphamide	1000 mg/m² IV day 1
Prednisone	60 mg/m² p.o. days 1 to 4

Note: Repeat every 6 weeks.

Source: Bergsagel, D. E.; Cowan, D. H.; and Hasselback, R. Plasma cell myeloma: response of melphalan-resistant patients to high-dose intermittent cyclophosphamide. *Can. Med. Assoc. J.* 107:851–855, 1972.

M-2

Vincristine	0.03 mg/kg IV day 1
Carmustine (BCNU)	0.5 mg/kg IV day 1
Cyclophosphamide	10 mg/kg IV day 1
Melphalan	0.25 mg/kg p.o. × 4 days
Prednisone	10 mg/kg/day p.o. × 7 days 5 mg/kg/day p.o. × 7 days

Note: Repeat every 35 days.

Source: Case, B. C., Jr.; Lee, B. J.; and Clarkson, B. D. Improved survival times in multiple myeloma treated with melphalan, prednisone, cyclophosphamide, vincristine, and BCNU: M-2 protocol. *Am. J. Med.* 63:897–903, 1977.

MP

Melphalan	10 mg/m^2 p.o. days 1 to 4
Prednisone	60 mg/m^2 p.o. days 1 to 4

Note: Repeat every 6 weeks.

Source: Southwest Oncology Group Study. Remission maintenance therapy for multiple myeloma. *Arch. Intern. Med.* 135:147–152, 1975.

Resistant Myeloma: BCAP

Carmustine (BCNU)	50 mg/m^2 IV day 1
Cyclophosphamide	200 mg/m^2 IV day 1
Doxorubicin (Adriamycin)	20 mg/m^2 IV day 2
Prednisone	60 mg/m^2 p.o. days 1 to 5

Note: Repeat every 4 weeks.

Source: Presant, C. A., and Klahr, C. Adriamycin, 1, 3-bis (2-chloroethyl)-1-nitrosourea (BCNU, NSC # 409962), cyclophosphamide plus prednisone (ABC-P) in melphalan resistant multiple myeloma. *Cancer* 42:1222–1227, 1978.

Neuroblastoma

CDV

Cyclophosphamide	750 mg/m^2 IV day 1
Dacarbazine (DTIC)	250 mg/m^2 IV days 1 to 5
Vincristine	1.5 mg/m^2 IV day 1

Note: Repeat every 22 days.

Source: Finkelstein, J. Z. et al. Combination chemotherapy for metastatic neuroblastoma. *Proc. Am. Assoc. Cancer Res.* 15:44, 1974.

CV

Cyclophosphamide	10 mg/kg IV every other week
Vincristine	0.05 mg/kg IV on the alternate weeks

Note: Treatment to be continued for 12 weeks or longer if there is a favorable response.

Source: James, D. H. et al. Combination chemotherapy for childhood neuroblastoma. *JAMA* 194:123–126, 1965.

Osteogenic Sarcoma

DMC (Investigational)

Doxorubicin (Adriamycin)	2.5 mg/kg/day IV for 3 days
Methotrexate	200 to 750 mg/kg/24 hour IV infusion on day 14
Citrovorum factor	9 mg p.o. starting 12 hours after methotrexate infusion, and repeat every 6 hours for 12 doses

Note: Repeat cycle every 4 weeks.

Source: Rosen, G. et al. High-dose methotrexate with citrovorum factor rescue and Adriamycin in childhood osteogenic sarcoma. *Cancer* 33:1151–1163, 1974.

VMC (Investigational)

Vincristine	2 mg/m² (maximum 2 mg) IV 30 minutes before methotrexate infusion
Methotrexate	3.0 or 6.0 or 7.5 gm/m² by IV infusion over 6 hours
Citrovorum factor (CF)	15 mg IV beginning 3 hours after methotrexate infusion is completed, then repeat CF every 3 hours for 24 hours, followed in 3 hours by 15 mg CF p.o. every 6 hours for additional 48 hours

Note: Therapy repeated every 3 weeks.

Source: Jaffe, N. et al. High-dose methotrexate in osteogenic sarcoma: a five-year experience. *Cancer Treat. Rep.* 62:259–264, 1978.

Ovarian Carcinoma

AP

Doxorubicin (Adriamycin)	50 mg/m² IV every 3 weeks
Cisplatin	50 mg/m² IV every 3 weeks

Source: Bruckner, H. W. et al. Prospective controlled randomized trial comparing combination chemotherapy of advanced ovarian carcinoma. *Proc. Am. Soc. Clin. Oncol.* 20:414, 1979.

CHAP

Cyclophosphamide	150 mg/m² p.o. days 2 to 8
Hexamethylmelamine	150 mg/m² p.o. days 2 to 8
Doxorubicin (Adriamycin)	30 mg/m² IV day 1
Cisplatin (platinum)	50 mg/m² IV day 1

Note: Repeat every 28 days.

Source: Bruckner, H. W. et al. Prospective controlled randomized trial comparing combination chemotherapy of advanced ovarian carcinoma with Adriamycin and cis-platinum and cyclophosphamide and hexamethylmelamine. *Proc. Am. Soc. Clin. Oncol.* 20:414, 1979.

Hexa-CAF

Hexamethylmelamine	150 mg/day p.o. × 14 days
Cyclophosphamide	150 mg/day p.o. × 14 days
Methotrexate (Amethopterin)	40 mg/m² IV days 1 and 8
5-Fluorouracil	600 mg/m² IV days 1 and 8

Note: Repeat every 28 days.

Source: Young, R. C. et al. Advanced ovarian adenocarcinoma: a prospective clinical trial of melphalan (L-PAM) versus combination chemotherapy. *N. Engl. J. Med.* 299:1261–1266, 1978.

PAC-I

Cisplatin (platinum)	50 mg/m^2 IV day 1
Doxorubicin (Adriamycin)	50 mg/m^2 IV day 1
Cyclophosphamide	750 mg/m^2 IV day 1

Note: Repeat every 3 weeks if possible. Severe neutropenia and moderate thrombocytopenia frequently delay subsequent courses.

Source: Ehrlich, C. E. et al. Chemotherapy for Stage III-IV epithelial ovarian cancer with cis-dichlorodiammineplatinum (II), Adriamycin, and cyclophosphamide. A preliminary report. *Cancer Treat. Rep.* 63:281–288, 1979.

VAC

Vincristine	1.5 mg/m^2 IV every week × 10 to 12 weeks
Dactinomycin (actinomycin D)	0.5 mg/day IV × 5 days every 4 weeks
Cyclophosphamide	5 to 7 mg/kg/day IV × 5 days every 4 weeks

Note: Treatment repeated every 4 weeks as tolerated for 2 years.

Source: Smith, J. P., and Rutledge, F. Advances in chemotherapy for gynecologic cancer. *Cancer* 36:669–674, 1975.

Pancreatic Carcinoma

SMF

Streptozotocin	1 gm/m^2 IV days 1, 8, 29, and 35
Mitomycin	10 mg/m^2 IV day 1
5-Fluorouracil	600 mg/m^2 IV days 1, 8, 29, and 35

Note: Repeat every 56 days.

Source: Wiggans, R. G. et al. Phase II trial of streptozotocin, mitomycin-C, and 5-fluorouracil (SMF) in the treatment of advanced pancreatic cancer. *Cancer* 41:387–391, 1978.

Prostatic Carcinoma

CAM

Cyclophosphamide	600 mg/m^2 IV day 1
Doxorubicin (Adriamycin)	40 mg/m^2 IV day 1
Methotrexate	15 mg/m^2 p.o. days 9, 13, 16, and 20

Note: Repeat every 3 weeks.

Source: Straus, M. J. et al. Cytoxan, Adriamycin, and methotrexate (CAM) therapy of stage D prostate cancer. *Proc. Am. Soc. Clin. Oncol.* 19:314, 1978.

CD

Cisplatin	50 to 60 mg/m^2 IV day 1
Doxorubicin	50 to 60 mg/m^2 IV day 1

Note: Repeat every 3 or 4 weeks.

Source: Perloff, M. et al. Adriamycin (ADM) and diamminedichloroplatinum (DDP) in advanced prostatic carcinoma. *Proc. Am. Soc. Clin. Oncol.* 18:333, 1977.

CFD

Cyclophosphamide	500 mg/m^2 IV day 1
5-Fluorouracil	500 mg/m^2 IV day 1
Doxorubicin	50 mg/m^2 IV day 1

Note: Repeat every 3 weeks.

Source: Soloway, M. S., and Tidwell, M. Cytoxan, Adriamycin, and 5-fluorouracil combination chemotherapy in advanced carcinoma of the prostate. *Proc. Am. Assoc. Cancer Res.* 18:2, 1977.

Sarcomas

AD

Adequate Marrow	
Doxorubicin (Adriamycin)	60 mg/m^2 IV day 1
Dacarbazine (DTIC)	250 mg/m^2 IV days 1 to 5
Inadequate Marrow	
Doxorubicin (Adriamycin)	45 mg/m^2 IV day 1
Dacarbazine (DTIC)	200 mg/m^2 days 1 to 5

Note: Repeat every 22 days.

Source: Gottlieb, J. A. et al. Adriamycin used alone and in combination for soft tissue and bony sarcomas. *Cancer Chemother. Rep.* 6:271–282, 1975.

Cy-VA-DiC

Adequate Marrow	
Cyclophosphamide	500 mg/m^2 IV day 1 only
Vincristine	1 mg/m^2 IV days 1 and 5 (maximum 1.5 mg per dose)
Doxorubicin (Adriamycin)	50 mg/m^2 IV day 1 only
Dacarbazine (DTIC)	250 mg/m^2 IV days 1 to 5
Inadequate Marrow	
Cyclophosphamide	400 mg/m^2 day 1
Vincristine	1 mg/m^2 days 1 and 5
Doxorubicin (Adriamycin)	40 mg/m^2 day 1
Dacarbazine (DTIC)	200 mg/m^2 days 1 to 5

Source: Gottlieb, J. A. et al. Adriamycin used alone and in combination for soft tissue and bony sarcomas. *Cancer Chemother. Rep.* 6:271–282, 1975.

Pulse VAC

Vincristine	2 mg/m^2 IV weekly × 12 weeks (maximum 2 mg per dose)
Dactinomycin (actinomycin D)	0.075 mg/kg/course IV over 5 days (maximum 0.5 mg/day) every 3 months × 5 courses
Cyclophosphamide	10 mg/kg/day for 7 days IV or p.o. every 6 weeks

Source: Wilbur, J. R. et al. Chemotherapy of sarcomas. *Cancer* 36:765–769, 1975.

Standard VAC

Vincristine	2 mg/m^2 IV weekly × 12 weeks (maximum 2 mg per dose)
Dactinomycin (actinomycin D)	0.075 mg/kg/course IV over 5 days (maximum 0.5 mg/day) every 3 months × 5 courses
Cyclophosphamide	2.5 mg/kg/day p.o. × 2 years

Source: Wilbur, J. R. et al. Chemotherapy of sarcomas. *Cancer* 36:765–769, 1975.

Testicular Carcinoma

CVB

Cisplatin	20 mg/m^2 IV for 5 consecutive days every 3 weeks × 3 courses
Vinblastine	0.3 mg/kg IV every 3 weeks
Bleomycin	30 units IV weekly × 12 consecutive weeks

Maintenance Therapy

Vinblastine	0.3 mg/kg IV every 4 weeks for 2 years. More recently, authors have tended to give patients not in complete remission a fourth course, and they raise some doubt that maintenance therapy is useful.

Sources: Einhorn, L. H.; Furnas, B. E.; and Powell, N. Combination chemotherapy of disseminated testicular carcinoma with cis-platinum diammine dichloride (CPDD), vinblastine (VBL), and bleomycin (BLEO). *Proc. Am. Soc. Clin. Oncol.* 17:240, 1976 (as modified in *Semin. Oncol.*).

Einhorn, L. H., and Donohue, J. P. Combination chemotherapy in disseminated testicular cancer: the Indiana University experience. *Semin. Oncol.* 6:87–93, 1979.

Triple Therapy

Initial Course

Methotrexate	5 mg p.o. for 16 to 25 days
Chlorambucil	10 mg p.o. for 16 to 25 days
Dactinomycin	0.5 mg IV days 3 to 7, days 12 to 16, and days 21 to 25

After 2-week rest period

Methotrexate	5 mg p.o. × 7 days
Chlorambucil	10 mg p.o. × 7 days
Dactinomycin	0.5 mg IV days 3 to 7

Note: Courses are then repeated every 3 weeks until cure or failure.

Source: Li, M. C.; Whitmore, W. F., Jr.; and Golbey, R. B. Effects of combined drug therapy in metastatic cancer of testis. *JAMA* 174:1291–1299, 1960.

VAB III

Induction

Bleomycin	20 units/m^2/day by continuous IV infusion × 7 days
Vinblastine	4 mg/m^2 IV day 1
Cyclophosphamide	600 mg/m^2 IV day 1
Dactinomycin	1 mg/m^2 IV day 1
Cisplatin	120 mg/m^2 IV day 8 after prehydration and with mannitol diuresis

Consolidation Therapy (treatment every 3 weeks)

Treatments 1 and 4:

Vinblastine	4 mg/m^2 IV
Doxorubicin	30 mg/m^2 IV
Chlorambucil	4 mg/m^2 p.o. daily × 14 days

Treatments 2 and 5:

Vinblastine	4 mg/m^2 IV
Dactinomycin	1 mg/m^2 IV
Chlorambucil	4 mg/m^2 p.o. daily × 14 days

Treatments 3 and 6:

Vinblastine	4 mg/m^2 IV
Cisplatin	50 mg/m^2 IV
Chlorambucil	4 mg/m^2 p.o. daily × 14 days

Maintenance Therapy (every 3 weeks for 2 years)

Vinblastine	4 mg/m^2 IV
Chlorambucil	4 mg/m^2 p.o. daily × 14 days
Dactinomycin	1 mg/m^2 IV

Sources: Cvitkovic, E.; Hayes, D.; and Golbey, R. B. Primary combination chemotherapy (VAB III) for metastatic or unresectable germ cell tumors. *Proc. Am. Soc. Clin. Oncol.* 17:296, 1976.

Golbey, R. B.; Reynolds, T. F.; and Vugrin, D. Chemotherapy of metastatic germ cell tumors. *Semin. Oncol.* 6:82–86, 1979.

VAB IV

Induction

Day 1:	
Cyclophosphamide	600 mg/m^2 IV
Vinblastine	4 mg/m^2 IV
Dactinomycin	1 mg/m^2 IV
Bleomycin	30 units/m^2 IV
Days 2 to 6:	
Bleomycin	20 units/m^2 by continuous infusion
Day 7:	
Cisplatin	120 mg/m^2 IV with mannitol-induced diuresis

Consolidation 1 (treatment every 3 weeks)

Treatments 1 and 3:	
Vinblastine	4 mg/m^2 IV
Doxorubicin	30 mg/m^2 IV
Chlorambucil	4 mg/m^2 p.o. × 7 days
Treatments 2 and 4:	
Vinblastine	4 mg/m^2 IV
Dactinomycin	1 mg/m^2 IV
Chlorambucil	4 mg/m^2 p.o. × 7 days

Reinduction 1

Day 1:	
Cyclophosphamide	600 mg/m^2 IV
Vinblastine	4 mg/m^2 IV
Dactinomycin	1 mg/m^2 IV
Day 7:	
Cisplatin	120 mg/m^2 IV with mannitol

Consolidation 2:

Same as consolidation every 3 weeks.

Reinduction 2:

Same as induction.

Maintenance Therapy (every 3 weeks for 2 years)

Vinblastine	4 mg/m^2 IV
Dactinomycin	1 mg/m^2 IV
Chlorambucil	4 mg/m^2 p.o. × 4 days

Source: Golbey, R. B.; Reynolds, J. F.; and Vugrin, D. Chemotherapy of metastatic germ cell tumors. *Semin. Oncol.* 6:82–86, 1979.

thirty

Regional and Intracavitary Chemotherapy

DAVID S. FISCHER

At the present time, the only chemotherapeutic agent with an exploitable biochemical difference between its effect on normal and cancer cells is L-asparaginase, and so far its use has been limited to a role in hematologic neoplasms, particularly childhood acute lymphoblastic leukemia. Since all other available agents do not have such a biochemical selectivity, different methods and techniques of enhancing the effects of anticancer drugs have been explored.

Several methods of regional drug administration have been studied, including (1) rapid arterial infusion, (2) regional perfusion through an extracorporeal vascular surface, and (3) protracted arterial infusion. These techniques are particularly suitable in the management of patients with advanced but locally confined disease. Some forms of cancer remain localized throughout most of their clinical evolution, and produce symptoms, disability, and finally death by virtue of the relatively localized but uncontrolled growth. This is particularly true of cancers of the head and neck, cervix, primary brain tumors, and sometimes, bladder carcinoma. On the other hand, some neoplasms metastasize to a vital organ such as the liver, although the primary tumor has been totally removed and its only residual is in the liver. This can be the case in some cancers of the colon, pancreas, gallbladder, bile ducts, stomach, and occasionally, the breast. Thus there is an appreciable group of patients whose disease is beyond control with surgical or radiation therapy and is deemed incurable, but who have locally confined cancer in various anatomic sites. Some of these patients may be responsive to a form of regional chemotherapy.

This concept of treatment was first proposed by Klopp and co-workers (1950) as a result of a fortuitous observation of an accident. A patient being treated with mechlorethamine (nitrogen mustard) was inadvertently given the drug into the brachial artery instead of the vein. This resulted in an intense local reaction with erythema, blistering, and subsequent ulceration of the skin over the forearm and hand, with little systemic toxicity. It led to their using this technique with mechlorethamine in a series of treatments through the main arterial blood supply of a number of different tumors, with variable degrees of regression. The potential advantages of this technique are: (1) localization of the drug to give a much higher tissue level in the vicinity of the tumor and thus increased tumor cell kill, and (2) a decreased concentration of the drug in the remainder of the body, resulting in diminished systemic toxicity. Ideally, a drug would have to be used that is either completely absorbed by the tumor on its first passage, or rapidly metabolized in the systemic circulation. Few such ideal agents exist, so methods to limit leakage of the cytotoxic materials to the systemic circulation have been devised, primarily extracorporeal perfusion and intra-arterial infusion.

Regional Perfusion through an Extracorporeal Circuit

Extracorporeal isolated perfusion (Creech et al. 1958; Creech and Krementz 1964) embodies temporary exclusion of the tumor-bearing area from general circulation for a period of 30 to 60 minutes, during which time high concentrations of the drug are perfused in the isolated part. In general, the best results have been obtained with shorter-acting polyfunctional alkylating agents such as mechlorethamine (Clarkson and Lawrence 1961).

The procedure must be carried out in an operating room under general anesthesia. An attempt is made to isolate completely the tumor-bearing region of the body or organ from systemic circulation and to support this area with a pump oxygenator. Best results have been obtained in treatment of a limb for melanoma or sarcoma. One tries to maintain the core temperature of the perfused limb or organ in the range of 102° F. Since the doses of drugs used are potentially lethal, any leak to the systemic circulation is monitored by injecting a radioactive isotope such as iodinated serum albumin into the pump circuit (Stehlin, Clark, and Dewey 1961) and monitoring with a collimator placed over the ventricular blood mass or other remote, highly vascular area. Significant drug leak may occur during femoral, iliac, and pelvic perfusions.

The experience of the M. D. Anderson Hospital with melanoma was published using their staging system (table 30.1) (McBride 1975). In single-drug treatments they used melphalan, 1.5 mg/kg for iliac or femoral perfusions, and 1 mg/kg for popliteal or brachial perfusions. They compared 150 historical controls, treated before 1958 and followed for 10 years, with 282 patients treated with melphalan perfusions starting in 1962. Of the 282 patients, 100 were evaluable with a 10-year follow-up and the majority of the remainder with a 5-year follow-up (table 30.2). Good improvement in survival was demonstrated for those with stages I and II disease. Concomitant with the increase in local control in these patients, the number of both skin grafts and amputations was reduced (table 30.3).

Because of the dissatisfaction with results obtained in single-drug perfusions for patients with advanced stage melanoma, a triple-drug program was initiated using melphalan, dactinomycin, and mechlorethamine (McBride 1970). Of 193 patients treated, 100 are evaluable at five years (table 30.4). A higher percentage of five-year survivals was obtained but one-third of the patients suffered loss of local areas of skin, fibrosis in muscle bundles, postoperative neuritis, and so on. Because dacarbazine (DTIC) has shown good results in systemic treatment of melanoma, it is now being evaluated for regional perfusions (Einhorn et al. 1973; Jönsson et al. 1980). As newer agents are developed, they will no doubt be tried also.

Table 30.1. *M. D. Anderson Hospital Staging for Melanoma*

Stage	*Description*
0	Superficial melanoma
I	Primary melanoma only
IA	Intact primary melanoma
IB	Primary melanoma, locally excised
IC	Multiple primary melanomas
II	Local recurrence or metastases (all disease within 3 cm of primary site)
III	Regional metastases
IIIA	Tissues excluding nodes
IIIB	Node(s)
IIIAB	Skin, etc., plus node(s)
IV	Distant metastases

SOURCE: Modified from McBride 1975.

Arterial Infusion

In this technique, cytotoxic drugs are injected directly into the main arterial blood supply of a tumor, either by open operation or percutaneously, depending on the site and accessibility of the vessel. Either of two strategies is then selected: (1) rapid infusion over a few hours, or (2) protracted infusion over days, weeks, or months.

Rapid Arterial Infusion

This was the method used by Klopp and associates (1950) and developed further by Sullivan and coworkers (1953) and Krakoff and Sullivan (1958). Mechlorethamine was used and exerted profound local effects on normal structures as well as regressive effects on a variety of tumors that had not responded very well to intravenous administration of the drug. The practical use of this therapy was sharply limited, however, by (1) its lack of specificity, (2) its severe destructive effects on normal structures, and (3) the difficulty of preventing its egress to systemic circulation where it damaged the bone marrow. As a result, rapid arterial infusion fell into disuse. It has recently been reinvestigated using cisplatin as the drug of choice (Calvo et al. 1980). Cisplatin has a short initial plasma half-life, in part owing to its high affinity to tissue proteins that are thought to bind this drug during its first passage through the capillary bed. In addition, it has a relatively

Table 30.2. *Raw Survival Rates for Melanoma of the Extremities*

Stage	Historical Controls (%)		Melphalan Perfusions (%)	
	5 years	10 years	5 years	10 years
I	73	61	86	76
II	22	22	55	55
III	16	9	28	16
IV	7	4	13	0
Overall	42	33	66	52

SOURCE: Modified from McBride 1975.

Table 30.3. *Ancillary Treatment*

Treatment	150 Historical Controls (No./%)	282 Melphalan Perfusions (No./%)
Skin grafts	48/32	28/10
Major amputations	12/9	8/3

SOURCE: Modified from McBride 1975.

Table 30.4. *Raw Survival Rates in Advanced Melanoma*

Stage	Historical Controls (%)		Melphalan Perfusions (%)		Triple-Drug Perfusions (%)	
	2 years	5 years	2 years	5 years	2 years	5 years
IIIA	63	13	71	29	80	43
IIIB	30	17	65	30	83	57
IIIAB	25	17	54	23	22	0

SOURCE: Modified from McBride 1975.

low toxic effect on bone marrow. It was infused through a percutaneously placed catheter for three or four hours. Of 19 patients with melanoma treated locally and systemically, 2 had complete remission (CR), 8 had partial remission (PR), 2 remained stable, and 7 progressed. Of 10 cases of regionally confined sarcoma, 1 had CR, 3 had PR, 2 were stable, and 4 progressed. The report is certainly worthy of further study, and may reawaken interest in the technique.

Protracted Intraarterial Chemotherapy

Occasionally, carcinoma of the pancreas, stomach, gallbladder, breast, or colon metastasizes to the liver without evidence of any lymph nodal or other distant spread. In this situation, local resection removes all of the primary malignancy but fails to cure. This carcinoma has usually been treated by systemic chemotherapy. Over the years, however, numerous attempts have been made to treat the liver metastases more directly by intraarterial infusion of chemotherapeutic agents, with quite variable results.

One of the early problems was to determine the blood supply of the metastatic tumor. Most of the time it is by the hepatic artery almost exclusively. Unfortunately, the hepatic artery is frequently anomalous, perhaps as often as 40% of the time. The two most common anomalies are the origin of the right hepatic artery from the superior mesenteric artery, and the origin of the left hepatic artery from the left gastric artery. With the development of the Seldinger technique for percutaneous arterial cannulation, it became possible to do selective celiac and hepatic artery angiography to visualize the anatomy and verify the tumor's blood supply. Then hepatic artery catheters could be placed and chemotherapeutic agents infused.

One of the earliest techniques was developed at the Lahey Clinic (Watkins 1963; Sullivan and Zurek 1964). The catheter was placed at laparotomy, and in the normal anatomic situation it was usually threaded

Table 30.5. *Overall Results of Protracted Hepatic Arterial Infusion Therapy*

Site of Primary Tumor	*Total No. of Patients Infused*	*No. of Patients with Adequate Trial*	*Objective No. of Patients*	*Response of Adequate Trial (%)*
Colorectal with extrahepatic metastases	40	35	17	48
Colorectal without extra-hepatic metastases	66	62	40	64
Gallbladder and bile ducts	18	16	9	56
Hepatoma	8	8	3	37
Stomach	9	7	2	28
Pancreas	19	17	6	35
Miscellaneous	22	19	11	57
Totals	182	164	88	54

SOURCE: Modified from Sullivan 1968.

through the gastroduodenal artery upstream into the hepatic artery. The gastroduodenal artery was then ligated to prevent perfusion of the stomach and duodenum with resulting mucositis; this ligature was also used to secure the catheter in place. Suitable modifications of technique were adapted to anomalous anatomic situations. The catheter was then brought out of the abdomen through a stab wound (to minimize the chance of infection), and was attached by means of a monoflow valve to a chronometric infusion pump. This small pump, worn around the neck, was wound up like a clock, powered by a spring, and contained chemotherapy drug in a sterile bag that was changed periodically (usually daily) by the patient.

In most of these early studies, 5-fluorouracil was used, or occasionally floxuridine (5-fluorouracil-2-deoxyriboside, FUDR) or methotrexate. Patients at the Lahey Clinic with hepatic neoplasms were classified in three stages.

1. Stage I — no symptoms or hepatomegaly, and results of liver function tests (LFTs) were normal. Diagnosis was made at surgery. Some survived two to four years but most developed hepatic insufficiency and died in one year.
2. Stage II — early symptoms of hepatic failure, hepatomegaly, and minor abnormalities of LFTs.
3. Stage III — advanced symptoms of liver failure, massive hepatomegaly, and very abnormal LFTs. This group had a life expectancy of 2.1 months (Sullivan, Norcross, and Watkins 1964).

Most of the patients treated in the early studies had stage III disease.

Of 182 patients accepted for treatment, 164 had an adequate trial of three months or more, and 88 had an objective response. This was defined as a decrease in liver size of 50% or more and the return to normal or near normal of LFTs with associated clinical benefit for a period of at least three months. A breakdown of these results by site of primary tumor is shown in table 30.5.

More recently, there has been a tendency to place the hepatic artery catheter by a percutaneous technique to avoid laparotomy (Tandon et al. 1973; Ansfield et al. 1971). This has the advantage of sparing the patient with advanced disease another surgical procedure. It has the disadvantage that these patients are largely confined to the hospital for the period of their infusion, which is seldom more than two weeks.

With this technique, several new agents have been tried in addition to the standard 5-fluorouracil. Methotrexate has been given intraarterially with leucovorin systemically as rescue shortly afterward, peripherally for melanoma (Oberfield and Sullivan 1969), intracarotid for head and neck tumors, and intrahepatic artery for liver neoplasms (Sullivan, Miller, and Sikes 1959). Percutaneous hepatic artery infusion of mitomycin and floxuridine (FUDR) has been reported to give 83% response rate with a median duration of six to seven months and a median survival of 16 months (Patt et al. 1980). Other drugs (doxorubicin and bleomycin) have also been used intraarterially, but Chen and Gross (1980) question whether there is a significant increase in response compared to systemic use for agents other than 5-FU.

A unique approach used a combination of dichloromethotrexate (DCM) and iododeoxyuridine (IUDR) into the hepatic artery for primary or metastatic neoplasms. The former was selected because it is metabolized by the liver so that systemic toxicity is markedly decreased, and it increases the incorporation of IUDR into DNA with subsequent enhanced radiosensitivity of the DNA (Keiser, Bertino, and Yagoda 1977). A 10-day intrahepatic artery infusion was given to 11 patients, and 1 additional patient also received 1600 rad hepatic irradiation. Toxicity was severe, with mild to moderate mucositis or myelosuppression in 6 of 12 patients, and severe leukopenia with infection and death in 2 of 12 patients. Responses included 1 CR, 1 PR, and 10 showing no response. The patient who also received radiation had no response.

Although this particular study must be judged a therapeutic failure, it suggests two important ideas. Drugs such as dichloromethotrexate that have an effect in the liver and are also metabolized there, can potentially approach the ideal of the drug that acts at the tumor site and is innocuous in the periphery. A search for drugs with a similar dissociation of local cytotoxic effect and minimal remote toxicity should be pursued. In this particular report, only one patient received both DCM and IUDR and then had liver irradiation, but the concept of other radiation potentiators (e.g., metronidazole and misonidazole) is being investigated and may prove useful. Actually, the potentiation of radiation by DCM and IUDR has yet to be evaluated fully.

A totally implantable infusion pump has been developed for intraarterial liver infusions (Buchwald et al. 1980).

Protracted intraarterial chemotherapy for head and neck cancer is discussed in chapter 66.

Intracavitary Chemotherapy

On any active oncology service there is usually at least one patient with a malignant pleural effusion (hydrothorax) or malignant ascites (hydroperitoneum). These patients have advanced disease and are usually symptomatic and require palliative therapy (table 30.6). Hence, in addition to a brief review of principles and some published literature, I will outline approaches that I have found effective.

Malignant Pleural Effusion

Although pleural effusion may occur with any malignancy, it is most frequently associated with carcinomas of the breast, lung, and ovary, lymphoma, and mesothelioma. Except for the last, it usually is a sign of widespread dissemination, although it can occur secondary to obstructing pneumonia or adenopathy. It need not signal a terminal phase, however, as therapy is available (Friedman and Slater 1978).

The most common mechanism leading to formation of an effusion is exudation from scattered tumor implants on the pleural surface from lymphatic or hematogenous dissemination. Rarely, a large malignant pleural plaque is responsible. Occasionally, involvement of the lymph nodes interferes with lymphatic or venous drainage of the pleura and results in serous or chylous effusion. In these cases, pleural fluid cytology is negative, and radiation therapy to the involved nodes may be effective palliation after other potential causes of nonmalignant effusion have been ruled out (table 30.7). Demonstration of malignant cells in sanguineous fluid with specific gravity over 1.016 and protein of 3 gm/dl or more is virtually diagnostic. Pleural mesothelial cells shed into serous fluid may occasionally resemble malignant cells.

When there is doubt about the diagnosis after a simple diagnostic thoracentesis with cytology, cell block, cell count, protein, glucose, specific gravity, LDH, and culture, then a pleural biopsy is indicated by someone skilled in that technique. Hook-type biopsy needles that allow both thoracentesis and pleural biopsy with the same instrument have been devised by Abrams (1958) and Cope (1958). In 1400 cases, adequate specimens were obtained 85% of the time, with a 4% complication rate. Only three patients required therapy for the complication.

Normally, pleural drainage by needle thoracentesis will have only a transient effect, with the fluid rapidly reaccumulating, so a more lasting treatment must be selected (Leff, Hopewell, and Costello 1978). The major goal is relief of symptoms caused by the excess fluid; therefore the pleural space between the visceral and parietal pleural membranes must be obliterated. After establishing by lateral decubitus x-ray that the fluid is not loculated, it can be removed by placing a hard rubber side-draining catheter into the pleural space through an intercostal sterile stab wound. A catheter is then connected to a water-seal suction drainage until x-rays show that the lung has reexpanded and the pleural space is obliterated. Then a sclerosing agent is instilled into the pleural space in 30 to 40 ml sterile saline, and the patient's position rotated to have the fluid run over most of the surfaces. The tube is clamped for four hours, after which time suction is resumed until the lung is again fully expanded and the pleural space obliterated for about 12 to 24 hours. The tube can then be removed.

Various sclerosing agents have been used. Radioactive gold and phosphorus were once popular, but gold has been generally abandoned and phosphorus is gradually losing its popularity because it is expensive

Table 30.6. *Intracavitary Agents*

Generic Name	*Trade or Common Name*	*Major Route(s)*	*Frequent Dose*	*Major Indication(s)*	*Major Toxicities*
Mechlorethamine	Mustargen (HN2) (nitrogen mustard)	Intrapleural Intrapericardial	10–20 mg 10 mg	Hydrothorax Hydropericardium	Marrow
Quinacrine	Atabrine (limited availability)	Intrapleural, intrapericardial	180 mg/day × 5 days	Hydrothorax Hydropericardium	Pleurisy, pericarditis
Tetracycline		Intrapleural	500 mg	Hydrothorax	Pleurisy
Triethylenethio-phosphoramide	Thiotepa	Intrapleural Intraperitoneal	30–60 mg	Hydrothorax Hydroperitoneum	Marrow
5-Fluorouracil	Fluorouracil, Adrucil	Intrapleural Intraperitoneal Intrapericardial Intraarterial	500–1000 mg	Hydrothorax Hydroperitoneum Hydropericardium Liver metastases	Marrow
Bleomycin	Blenoxane	Intrapleural	30 units/m²	Hydrothorax	Fever
Methotrexate	Methotrexate Mexate	Intrapericardial Intraarterial Intrathecal	50 mg Variable 8–12 mg/m²	Hydropericardium Liver metastases, head and neck tumors Carcinomatous meningitis CNS leukemia	Marrow, G.I., pulmonary, renal
Cytarabine	Cytosar-U	Intrathecal	10–30 mg/m²	CNS leukemia, carcinomatous meningitis	Marrow
Floxuridine	FUDR	Intraarterial	4–24 mg/m²/day	Liver metastases	Marrow, G.I.
Melphalan	Alkeran	Arterial perfusion	40–60 mg/m²	Melanoma	Marrow
Cisplatin	Platinol	Arterial perfusion	75–100 mg/m²	Melanoma, sarcoma	Renal, auditory

and difficult to use compared to chemical agents. Mechlorethamine is the most popular antineoplastic agent and has enjoyed wide use in our institution. Mark, Goldenberg, and Montague (1964), using 8 to 40 mg mechlorethamine per instillation, obtained marked improvement in 92% of the patients who lived more than one month after treatment. Of course, the drug is absorbed systemically and may result in some bone marrow depression. Anderson, Philpett, and Ferguson (1974) found 60% of the effusions recurred at three months, 70% at six months, and 83% in one year. Among patients treated with intracavitary triethylenethiophosphoramide (thiotepa), 37% to 57% of 86 patients improved, but follow-up was short (Anderson and Brincker 1978). Single doses of 5-fluorouracil resulted in an improvement in 38% of 55 patients (Suhrland and Weisberger 1965).

Systemic chemotherapy is occasionally effective against effusions caused by metastases from solid tumors. Lymphomatous effusions appear to respond to systemic therapy more readily than to direct intracavitary administration (Weick et al. 1973).

Table 30.7. *Etiologic Characteristics of Pleural Effusions*

Observation	*Malignancy*	*Heart Failure*	*Collagen Disease*	*Pulmonary Embolism*	*Chylothorax*	*Pneumonia*	*Tuberculosis*
Clinical	Cancer	Signs of CHF	Joint problems	Lung scan positive	Malignancy, trauma	Respiratory infection	Positive PPD
Gross	Often sanguineous	Serous	Turbid	Often sanguineous	Chylous	Serous	Serous
Microscopic	50% positive cytology	0	0	0	Fat drops	Bacteria ±	AFB positive 30%–70%
Cells	Erythrocytes, leukocytes, tumor cells, mesothelial cells	Erythrocytes, leukocytes	Lymphocytes	0	Erythrocytes	Granulocytes	Lymphocytes
Culture	0	0	0	0	0	40%–60% positive	10%–70% positive
Specific gravity	75% over 1.016	90% under 1.016	Over 1.016	Over 1.016	Over 1.016	Over 1.016	75% over 1.016
Protein	3 gm or more	Less than 3 gm	3 gm or more	3 gm or more	3 gm or more	3 gm or more	3 gm or more
Sugar	Rarely less than Normal 60 mg/dl		Less than 60 mg/dl	Normal	Normal	Occasionally less than 60 mg/dl	60% less than 60 mg/dl

Although pleurectomy is very effective, complications are frequent and mortality is 10% (Martini, Bains, and Beattie 1975). For many years quinacrine (Atabrine) was used for intrapleural injection with moderate success when there was leukopenia or thrombocytopenia, and one wished to avoid an cytotoxic marrow depressant. Recently, the injectable form of quinacrine has been removed from the market by its manufacturer. Tetracycline has been reported to be effective in 83% to 100% of patients with 6- to 12-month follow-up (Rubinson and Botooki 1972; Wallach 1975). Five hundred milligrams of tetracycline was diluted into 50 ml of saline and administered through a thoracostomy tube in each case. Severe pleuritic pain requiring strong narcotic analgesia, and temperatures over 100° F were not uncommon, but the obliteration of the pleural space was prolonged. This agent appears to be as popular as mechlorethamine and has the advantage of causing no bone marrow suppression.

Bleomycin has been reported to be effective as an intrapleural sclerosing agent (Paladine et al. 1976). In a direct randomized study it was concluded that intrapleural bleomycin and tetracycline were equally effective (54% and 58% respectively) in controlling malignant pleural effusions (Gupta et al. 1980).

Intraperitoneal Chemotherapy

Malignant ascites may occur with carcinoma of the ovary, pancreas, stomach, colon, breast, and testis, and with a variety of sarcomas and lymphomas. Attempts to control the fluid are usually made with chlorthiazides, furosemide, and spironolactone but are frequently unsuccessful. Treatment may lead to abdominal discomfort with elevated diaphragms and diminished respiratory capacity when distention becomes massive.

For many years, abdominal paracentesis was performed with a large-bore hollow trocar to remove 6 to 10 liters of fluid in 10 to 15 minutes. This had the advantage of speed, but occasionally resulted in a precipitous fall in blood pressure and a rare shock-like state. Another technique is to use a needle and tubing connected to a vacuum bottle to aspirate the fluid. This has the advantage of slightly more gradual removal, but requires many vacuum bottles and constant attention by a physician.

During the past several years I have developed a simpler technique that has proved to be very effective (Fischer 1979). Following the usual aseptic preparation of the skin and infiltration with lidocaine, a 14-gauge needle with a 16-gauge catheter is inserted into the free peritoneal cavity. The catheter is advanced as the fluid comes out of the catheter and the needle is withdrawn from the skin. The point of the needle is clamped in a plastic holder with a groove to prevent it from cutting the catheter at its point of exit from the needle. The needle and catheter are then taped to the abdominal wall and an antibiotic ointment and sterile dressing are applied over the puncture site. The needle is connected to a Y-type dialysis drainage tubing and then to three sterile 3000-ml capacity dialysis bags (fig. 30.1). As each bag fills, the tube to the next is opened so that the drainage system can be sterile for up to 9 liters.

With this system I have drained as much as 9 liters from a patient in eight hours without any adverse effects. I usually have 5% dextrose in water running

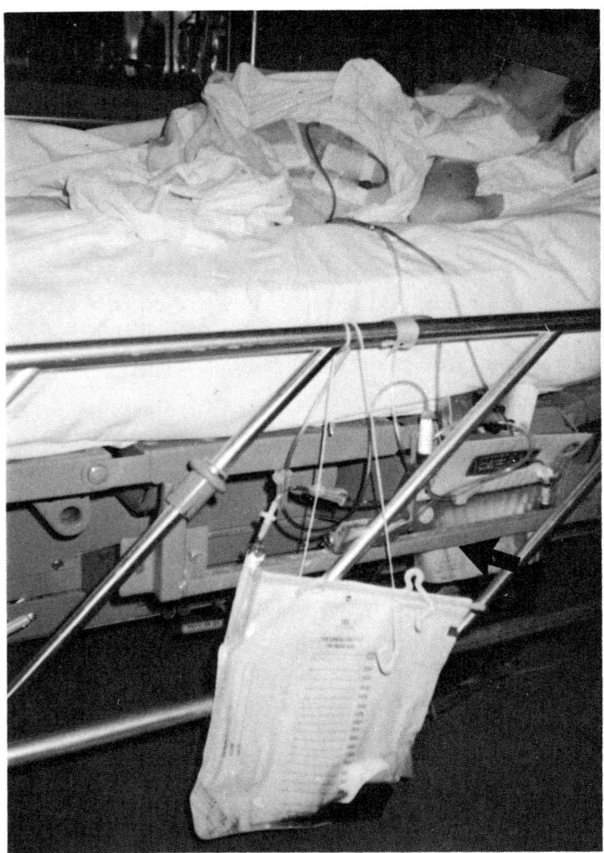

Fig. 30.1. *Paracentesis with Y-type drain showing one of three dialysis bags.*

intravenously to prevent rapid vascular space depletion, but in 300 procedures so far, I have not encountered any serious hypotension. The ascites fluid runs out rapidly when the abdomen is tense, and more slowly later. Less viscous fluids run more rapidly, but those with abundant cellular material occasionally clog the catheter and require that it be flushed with a sterile saline solution. Mucinous or myxomatous fluid will not drain through these small catheters, but they frequently will not drain even with a trocar. This situation is quite different from cirrhotic ascites in which paracentesis may be contraindicated.

Early in my experience I instilled triethylenethiophosphoramide to prevent recurrence, but I have abandoned this. Sclerosing agents such as mechlorethamine hydrochloride (nitrogen mustard) are absolutely contraindicated for instillation into the peritoneal cavity lest they cause adhesions leading to intestinal obstruction. I am unaware of reports of instillation of tetracycline. Cisplatin and 5-fluorouracil have been tried but the reports are not impressive. *Corynebacterium parvum* is being used in a protocol we have just initiated.

In desperate situations a peritoneo-venous shunt (LeVeen et al. 1974) has been placed under local anesthesia to relieve marked ascites (Raaf and Stroehlein 1980). Survivals have been brief, and tumor implantation has been noted on the wall of the superior vena cava in one case.

Intrapericardial Chemotherapy

Although the development of malignant pericardial effusion can lead to life-threatening cardiac tamponade, the gradual onset of symptoms may be so insidious as to escape detection until they are so advanced that the clinician is suddenly faced with an emergency (Theologides 1978). The mechanism of production is almost always tumor implantation on the serosal surface leading to exudation of fluid. Transudation of fluid within the pericardial sac caused by obstruction of the lymphatic flow by mediastinal or hilar neoplastic infiltration requires concomitant obstruction of the coronary sinus and the anterior coronary veins (Lokich 1973), an infrequent association of events.

Diagnosis may be suspected when there is venous distention, distant heart sounds, dyspnea, paradoxical pulse, an enlarged cardiac silhouette on chest x-ray, and poor cardiac pulsation on fluoroscopy. Simultaneous cardiac and lung scans can demonstrate an increased space between the heart blood pool and the lungs or liver. Intravenous carbon dioxide is a rapid and convenient diagnostic test but has its hazards. An EKG showing total electrical alternans is almost diagnostic. The simplest practical method is an echocardiogram, which can be done at the bedside and is usually reliable, noninvasive, and relatively inexpensive. An ultrasound echo from the pericardium distinct from the echo produced by the posterior heart border can be demonstrated in most cases. In difficult cases where the findings are equivocal, cardiac catheterization with angiocardiography is a sophisticated and usually definitive technique.

Pericardiocentesis with an EKG lead attached to the needle can establish the presence of fluid and provide a specimen for cytologic diagnosis with relative safety. While biopsy of the parietal pericardium is possible by those skilled in the technique, histology may not reveal neoplastic tissue in the specimen, as the tumor may be on the visceral pericardium. Instillation of air into the pericardial space during the removal of fluid may outline irregularities of contour, suggest the location of tumor implants, and show fluid reaccumulation if and when it occurs.

The incidence of cardiac and pericardial metastases is relatively high in autopsy series, but antemortem clinical diagnosis is much less frequent. In one series of autopsies of 1082 cancer patients, 7.3% had cardiac involvement, 5.7% had parietal pericardial metastases, and 2% had both (Scott and Garvin 1939). The association is most often seen with acute leukemia, melanoma, and lymphoma, but can occur with almost any primary malignant tumor. In one series, pericardial involvement or its immediate effect was the primary cause of death in 36% of the patients with significant pericardial involvement, and in 49% of the cases it was considered a contributory cause of death. (Thurber, Edwards, and Achor 1962). In this series, only 29% had cardiac symptoms prior to death, and the correct diagnosis was made in only 8.5% of cases antemortem.

Even when a diagnosis was made correctly, some clinicians employed no specific therapy because they regarded the situation as hopeless. Experience dictates a different conclusion. At least 50% or more of these patients can achieve palliation and many may have long survival. In the past, a pleural pericardial window (Hill and Cohen 1970) was the procedure of choice if life-threatening cardiac tamponade was suspected. Otherwise, radiation therapy was used if there had not been previous irradiation to the area, as might occur with Hodgkin's disease or lung or breast cancer. For lymphoma, and especially Hodgkin's disease, rapid responses to chemotherapy frequently occur with total clearing of the pericardial effusion.

At one time, radioactive isotopes were instilled into the pericardial sac, but this technique has fallen into disuse. A variety of chemotherapeutic antineoplastic agents have been employed, including 5-fluorouracil, triethylenethiophosphoramide, mechlorethamine, and methotrexate (Smith, Lane, and Hudgins 1974). The most effective appears to be mechlorethamine, probably because it is also a sclerosing agent. The use of noncytotoxic sclerosing agents has also met with moderate success in palliation. Quinacrine (Atabrine) was used for many years but the sterile powder for solution is no longer commercially available, so tetracycline is now the most widely used agent in this category (Davis et al. 1978). After a review of their own experience and the world literature to 1974, Smith, Lane, and Hudgins concluded: (1) conservative therapy using pericardiocentesis, intrapericardial, and/or systemic chemotherapy or hormonal therapy is associated with a longer symptom-free interval than is creation of a pericardial window accompanied by any combination of other treatment modalities; and (2) duration of survival of patients with malignant pericardial effusion is equivalent when these are secondary to solid tumors or hematologic malignancies, when the effusions are managed with conservative therapy.

What they did not conclude, but seems obvious, is that we need better chemotherapy drugs.

The differential diagnosis of malignant pericardial effusion is sometimes complicated by the presence of radiation pericarditis with effusion. This may occur after exposure to about 4000 rad and can manifest itself during the course of treatment or weeks or months later. Although a few chronic cases have occurred years after the completion of radiation, in the series of Martin and co-workers (1975), 92% occurred in the first 12 months. Of their 81 patients with Hodgkin's disease (stages I to IIIB) who underwent upper mantle radiation therapy, 29.6% met x-ray criteria for the presence of pericardial effusion. In a series of 117 patients with breast cancer who had postoperative radiation therapy, 3.4% developed radiation pericarditis (Stewart et al. 1967).

Although the diagnostic work-up for these patients is the same as for those with malignant pericarditis, the findings may be a little different. The fluid may be bloody and have a high protein content in either situation. The cytology of the pericardial fluid should always be negative in radiation pericarditis, but may be positive or negative with malignant effusions. On chest x-ray, the presence of pneumonitis in areas of the lung demarcated by the radiation field is a strong clue to that diagnosis. In addition, radiation pericarditis is more often self-limiting, but frequently progresses to or presents as constrictive pericarditis.

Treatment for radiation pericarditis has included

the use of systemic steroids most often, and local steroids on occasion. Pericardiocentesis with removal of fluid can be helpful and sometimes instillation of a sclerosing agent is useful, but antineoplastic cytotoxic drugs should be avoided. In cases of constrictive pericarditis with tamponade, pleuropericardial window or pericardiectomy may be necessary.

Intrathecal Chemotherapy

In childhood acute lymphoblastic leukemia, the central nervous system is frequently a sanctuary for leukemic cells during systemic therapy. Hence many groups give prophylactic whole brain radiation and intrathecal methotrexate (Aur et al. 1973; Haghbin et al. 1975). A lyophilized powder should be used and reconstituted with sterile, preservative-free saline for the instillation. It may be that some of the early reports of myelitis were associated with the use of the liquid methotrexate preparation with benzyl alcohol as a preservative, or with excessive doses of methotrexate. Cases of paraplegia continue to occur (Gagliano and Costanzi 1976). A relatively safe dose of methotrexate is 12 mg/m^2 intrathecally twice weekly for five doses.

Extrapolating from the experience in childhood acute leukemia, methotrexate has also been used for treatment of carcinomatous meningitis from melanoma, small cell carcinoma of the lung, and other metastatic tumors. It is also being used in some of the lymphomatous meningitides, and particularly in T-cell convoluted lymphoma.

Cytarabine is an alternate drug that has been used relatively safely and effectively intrathecally in leukemic meningitis, particularly of the granulocytic variety (Wang and Pratt 1970). A case of paraparesis associated with its use has been reported (Breuer et al. 1977).

The use of a subcutaneous cerebrospinal fluid reservoir leading into a lateral ventricle for selected cases of intrathecal chemotherapy provides an alternate to repeated lumbar taps (Ommaya 1963; Ratcheson and Ommaya 1968). Administration of methotrexate by an Ommaya reservoir has been demonstrated to produce adequate cerebrospinal fluid distribution more reliably than lumbar puncture (Shapiro, Young, and Mehta 1975). I used this technique for several years, but abandoned it generally because of the trauma involved in making the neurosurgical placement and because of the frequency of necrotizing encephalopathy (Shapiro, Chernik, and Posner 1973). While still a useful technique in rare cases, the reservoir is no longer popular in many medical centers and is only occasionally implanted in selected special cases.

References

Abrams, L. D. A pleural-biopsy punch. *Lancet* 1:30–31, 1958.

Anderson, A. P., and Brincker, H. Intracavitary thiotepa in malignant pleural and peritoneal effusions. *Acta Radiol.* 7:369–378, 1968.

Anderson, C. B.; Philpett, G. W.; and Ferguson, T. B. The treatment of malignant pleural effusions: a randomized trial. *Cancer* 33:916–922, 1974.

Ansfield, F. J. et al. Intrahepatic arterial infusion with 5-fluorouracil. *Cancer* 28:1147–1151, 1971.

Aur, R. J. et al. Comparison of two methods of preventing central nervous system leukemia. *Blood* 42:349–357, 1973.

Breuer, A. C. et al. Paraparesis following intrathecal cytosine arabinoside. *Cancer* 40:2817–2822, 1977.

Buchwald, H. et al. Intraarterial infusion chemotherapy for hepatic carcinoma using a totally implantable infusion pump. *Cancer* 45:866–869, 1980.

Calvo, D. B., III et al. Phase I-II trial of percutaneous intraarterial Cis-diamminedichloroplatinum (II) for regionally confined malignancy. *Cancer* 45:1278–1283, 1980.

Chen, H-S. C., and Gross, J. F. Intra-arterial infusion of anticancer drugs: theoretic aspects of drug delivery and review of responses. *Cancer Treat. Rep.* 64:31–40, 1980.

Clarkson, B., and Lawrence, W., Jr. Perfusion and infusion techniques in cancer chemotherapy. *Med. Clin. North Am.* 45:689–710, 1961.

Cope, C. New pleural biopsy needle. *JAMA* 167:1107–1108, 1958.

Creech, O., Jr. et al. Chemotherapy of cancer: regional perfusion utilizing an extracorporeal circuit. *Ann. Surg.* 148:616–632, 1958.

Creech, O., Jr., and Krementz, E. T. Regional perfusion in melanoma of limbs. *JAMA* 188:855–858, 1964.

Davis, S. et al. Intrapericardial tetracycline for the management of cardiac tamponade secondary to malignant pericardial effusion. *N. Engl. J. Med.* 299:1113–1114, 1978.

Einhorn, L. H. et al. Intra-arterial infusion therapy with 5-(3, 3-dimethyl-1-triazeno)imidazole-4-carboxamide (NSC 45388) for malignant melanoma. *Cancer* 32:749–755, 1973.

Fischer, D. S. Abdominal paracentesis for malignant ascites. *Arch. Intern. Med.* 139:235, 1979.

Friedman, M. A., and Slater, E. Malignant pleural effusions. *Cancer Treat. Rev.* 5:49–66, 1978.

Gagliano, R. G., and Costanzi, J. J. Paraplegia following intrathecal methotrexate. *Cancer* 37:1663–1668, 1976.

Gupta, N. et al. Intrapleural bleomycin vs. tetracycline for control of malignant pleural effusion. A randomized study. *Proc. Am. Soc. Clin. Oncol.* 21:366, 1980.

Haghbin, M. et al. Treatment of acute lymphoblastic leukemia in children with "prophylactic" intrathecal methotrexate and intensive systemic chemotherapy. *Cancer Res.* 35:807–811, 1975.

Hill, G. J., II, and Cohen, B. I. Pleural pericardial window for palliation of cardiac tamponade due to cancer. *Cancer* 26:81–93, 1970.

Jönsson, P. E. et al. Treatment of malignant melanoma with dacarbazine (DTIC-Dome) with special reference to urinary excretion of 5-s-cysteinyldopa. *Cancer* 45: 245–248, 1980.

Keiser, L. W.; Bertino, J. R.; and Yagoda, A. Phase I trial of intra-hepatic dichloromethotrexate (DCM) and iododeoxyuridine (IUDR) for primary and metastatic hepatic malignancies. *Proc. Am. Soc. Clin. Oncol.* 18:314, 1977.

Klopp, C. T. et al. Fractionated intra-arterial cancer chemotherapy with methyl bisamine hydrochloride; a preliminary report. *Ann. Surg.* 132:811–832, 1950.

Krakoff, I. H., and Sullivan, R. D. Intra-arterial nitrogen mustard in the treatment of pelvic cancer. *Ann. Intern. Med.* 48:839–850, 1958.

Leff, A.; Hopewell, P. C.; and Costello, J. Pleural effusion from malignancy. *Ann. Intern. Med.* 88:532–537, 1978.

LeVeen, H. H. et al. Peritoneovenous shunting for ascites. *Ann. Surg.* 180:580–590, 1974.

Lokich, J. J. The management of malignant pericardial effusions. *JAMA* 224:1401–1404, 1973.

Mark, J. D.; Goldenberg, I. S.; and Montague, A. C. W. Intrapleural mechlorethamine hydrochloride therapy for malignant pleural effusion. *JAMA* 187:858–860, 1964.

Martin, R. G. et al. Radiation-related pericarditis. *Am. J. Cardiol.* 35:216–220, 1975.

Martini, N.; Bains, M. S.; and Beattie, E. J., Jr. Indications for pleurectomy in malignant effusion. *Cancer* 35:734–738, 1975.

McBride, C. M. Advanced melanoma of the extremities: treatment by isolation-perfusion with a triple drug combination. *Arch. Surg.* 101:122–126, 1970.

McBride, C. M. Regional chemotherapy. In *Cancer chemotherapy—fundamental concepts and recent advances.* Chicago: Year Book, 1975, pp. 369–384.

Oberfield, R. A., and Sullivan, R. D. Prolonged and continuous regional arterial infusion chemotherapy in patients with melanoma. *JAMA* 209:75–79, 1969.

Ommaya, A. K. Subcutaneous reservoir and pump for sterile access to ventricular cerebrospinal fluid. *Lancet* 2:983–984, 1963.

Paladine, W. et al. Intracavitary bleomycin in the management of malignant effusions. *Cancer* 38:1903–1908, 1976.

Patt, Y. Z. et al. Percutaneous hepatic arterial infusion (HAI) of mitomycin C and floxuridine (FUDR): an effective treatment for metastatic colorectal carcinoma in the liver. *Cancer* 46:261–265, 1980.

Raaf, J., and Stroehlein, J. R. Palliation of malignant ascites by the LeVeen peritoneo-venous shunt. *Cancer* 45:1019–1024, 1980.

Ratcheson, R. A., and Ommaya, A. K. Experience with the subcutaneous cerebrospinal fluid reservoir. *N. Engl. J. Med.* 279:1025–1031, 1968.

Rubinson, R. M., and Botooki, H. Intrapleural tetracycline for control of malignant pleural effusion. A preliminary report. *South Med. J.* 65:847–849, 1972.

Scott, R. W., and Garvin, C. F. Tumors of the heart and pericardium. *Am. Heart J.* 17:431–436, 1939.

Shapiro, W. R.; Chernik, N. L.; and Posner, J. B. Necrotizing encephalopathy following intraventricular instillation of methotrexate. *Arch. Neurol.* 28:96–102, 1973.

Shapiro, W. R.; Young, D. F.; and Mehta, B. M. Methotrexate: distribution in cerebrospinal fluid after intravenous, ventricular, and lumbar injections. *N. Engl. J. Med.* 293:161–166, 1975.

Smith, F. E.; Lane, M.; and Hudgins, P. T. Conservative management of malignant pericardial effusion. *Cancer* 33:47–57, 1974.

Stehlin, J. S., Jr.; Clark, R. L.; and Dewey, W. C. Continuous monitoring of leakage during regional perfusion. *Arch. Surg.* 83:943–949, 1961.

Stewart, J. R. et al. Radiation-induced heart disease. *Radiology* 89:302–310, 1967.

Suhrland, L. G., and Weisberger, A. S. Intracavitary 5-fluorouracil in malignant effusions. *Arch. Intern. Med.* 116:431–433, 1965.

Sullivan, R. D. Results of protracted ambulatory infusion therapy. In *Protracted cancer chemotherapy by ambulatory arterial infusion,* eds. R. D. Sullivan and E. Watkins, Jr. Boston: Lahey Clinic Foundation, 1968, pp. 317–332.

Sullivan, R. D. et al. The treatment of human cancer with intraarterial nitrogen mustard utilizing a simple catheter technique. *Cancer* 6:121–134, 1953.

Sullivan, R. D.; Miller, E.; and Sikes, M. P. Antimetabolite-metabolite combination cancer chemotherapy: effects of intra-arterial methotrexate-intramuscular citrovorum factor therapy in human cancer. *Cancer* 12:1248–1262, 1959.

Sullivan, R. D.; Norcross, J. W.; and Watkins, E., Jr. Chemotherapy of metastatic liver cancer by prolonged hepatic artery infusion. *N. Engl. J. Med.* 270:321–327, 1964.

Sullivan, R. D., and Zurek, W. Z. Protracted ambulatory infusion cancer chemotherapy by the Watkins chronometric infusor. *Cancer Chemother. Rep.* 37: 47–55, 1964.

Tandon, R. N. et al. The treatment of metastatic carcinoma of the liver by the percutaneous selective hepatic artery infusion of 5-fluorouracil. *Surgery* 73:118–121, 1973.

Theologides, A. Neoplastic cardiac tamponade. *Semin. Oncol.* 5:181–192, 1978.

Thurber, D. L.; Edwards, J. E.; and Achor, R. W. P. Secondary malignant tumors of the pericardium. *Circulation* 26:228–241, 1962.

Wallach, H. W. Intrapleural tetracycline for malignant pleural effusion. *Chest* 68:510–512, 1975.

Wang, J., and Pratt, C. Intrathecal arabinosyl cytosine in meningeal leukemia. *Cancer* 25:531–534, 1970.

Watkins, E., Jr. Chronometric infusor—an apparatus for protracted ambulatory infusion therapy. *N. Engl. J. Med.* 269:850–851, 1963.

Weick, J. K. et al. Pleural effusion in lymphoma. *Cancer* 31:848–853, 1973.

thirty-one

Treatment of Complications

JOHN C. MARSH

Nausea and Vomiting

Nausea and vomiting are probably the most common and troublesome complications of cancer chemotherapy (Knobf et al. 1980). Although not all drugs are associated with these problems, the public perception of chemotherapy is such that these side effects are assumed to be present in any patient who will receive this form of treatment. In some cases nausea and vomiting are so severe that patients refuse what may well be curative treatment with combination chemotherapy programs, for example, in metastatic testicular cancer, advanced lymphoma, or adjuvant therapy in breast cancer.

Nausea and vomiting with chemotherapy depend on many variables (Cadman 1977), including the type of drug(s), the dose, schedule, and the psychological makeup of the patient. Among the agents that most commonly cause vomiting are mechlorethamine, cisplatin, dacarbazine, dactinomycin, cyclophosphamide (especially parenteral), the nitrosoureas, mitomycin, doxorubicin, cytarabine, azacytidine, procarbazine, streptozotocin, mitotane, and high-dose methotrexate. Diethylstilbestrol in the dose used to treat breast cancer (15 mg) often causes unacceptable nausea and vomiting if it is begun at that level.

The mechanism of nausea and vomiting is not known for every agent, but several factors have been implicated. The most important is the chemoreceptor trigger zone (CTZ) located in the area postrema in the floor of the fourth ventricle in the brain (Borison, Brand, and Orkand 1958). It has been postulated that the drug or its metabolites are able to cross the blood-brain barrier and interact with this group of cells (Harris 1978). Mechlorethamine has been shown to do this in experimental animals but also can produce vomiting in animals in which the CTZ has been ablated. It is postulated that peripheral areas can also be activated by the drug and trigger vomiting controlled by the vomiting center located in the reticular formation of the medulla. This is abolished by vagotomy. Some of the peripheral mechanisms of action may actually result from stimulation of non-CTZ areas in the brain. That a strong psychological component exists in many patients is demonstrated by the beginning of vomiting before treatment (usually repeat courses) is even started, and the antiemetic effect that can occur with placebos.

Other causes should not be overlooked, although the time relationship to chemotherapy administration is usually evident. These include intracerebral metastases, adrenal insufficiency, water intoxication, uremia, intestinal obstruction (Harris 1978), or hypercalcemia.

Effective treatment is often possible if small oral intakes on the day of treatment are advised and if antiemetics are begun sufficiently in advance of chemotherapy (table 31.1). The phenothiazines are the drugs most commonly used and include prochlorperazine (Compazine), chlorpromazine (Thorazine), promethazine (Phenergan), fluphenazine (Prolixin), perphenazine (Trilafon), and thiethylperazine (Torecan).

Table 31.1. *Antiemetics*

Drug	*Brand Name*	*Adult Oral Dose (mg)*	*Adult IM Dose (mg)*	*Adult Rectal Dose (mg)*	*Comment*
Prochlorperazine	Compazine	5–10 q 4–6 hr	5–10 q 4–6 hr	25 q 12 hr	The standard phenothiazine
Perphenazine	Trilafon	2–4 q 6–8 hr	5–10 q 6 hr	—	Phenothiazine
Chlorpromazine	Thorazine	10–25 q 4–6 hr	25–50 q 3–4 hr	25–100 q 6–8 hr	Phenothiazine
Thiethylperazine	Torecan	10 q 8 hr	10 q 8 hr	10 q 8 hr	Phenothiazine
Haloperidol	Haldol	1–2 q 12 hr	1–2 q 12 hr	—	Tranquilizer
Droperidol	Inapsine	—	0.5 q 4 hr	—	Anesthetic
Promethazine	Phenergan	25–50 q 12 hr	12.5–25 q 12 hr	25–50 q 12 hr	Antihistaminic phenothiazine
Trimethobenzamide	Tigan	250–400 q 6–8 hr	200 q 6–8 hr	200 q 6–8 hr	Weak
Hydroxyzine	Atarax, Visteril	25–100 q 6–8 hr	25–100 q 4–6 hr	—	Tranquilizer, antihistaminic
Dimenhydrinate	Dramamine	50 q 4 hr	50 q 4 hr	100 q 12 hr	Late nausea and motion sickness
Meclizine	Bonine, Antivert	50 q 12–14 hr	—	—	Late nausea and motion sickness
Delta-9-tetra hydrocannabinol	—	15–20 q 4 hr	—	—	Experimental; marijuana-active constituent

All are available as oral preparations, most of them parenterally, and prochlorperazine, chlorpromazine, and thiethylperazine as rectal suppositories. These agents are thought to block the CTZ, and in high doses, the vomiting center as well. Other effects include sedation, hypotension, extrapyramidal reactions, and, rarely, blood dyscrasias, cholestatic jaundice, skin rash, and lowering of the seizure threshold. Although they are probably the most active agents available and certainly the most widely used, their efficacy is variable and improvements are greatly needed.

Other agents have been evaluated in the nausea and vomiting of cancer chemotherapy. Antihistamines, such as diphenhydramine (Benadryl), are useful in nausea of vestibular origin (for example, motion sickness), but have not found much use in cancer chemotherapy. Butyrophenones such as haloperidol (Haldol) have been reported to be active as antiemetics after chemotherapy (Plotkin, Plotkin, and Okun 1973). Another member of this class, droperidol, has been reported to be useful in ameliorating the nausea and vomiting associated with cisplatin (Grossman, Lessin, and Cohen 1979), which in our experience responds poorly to other agents. Trimethobenzamide (Tigan) does not appear to be as effective as the phenothazines, nor does benzquinamide (Emete-Con), which is available only for parenteral use. Pyridoxine has been reported to reduce nausea and vomiting in patients receiving radiotherapy, but has not achieved any utility in chemotherapy and has not been convincingly shown to be more active than a placebo.

Great interest has developed in recent years in the antiemetic properties of marijuana and its active ingredient, delta-9-tetrahydrocannabinol (THC) (NSC

134454). Following the lead of young marijuana smokers who found that a "high" ameliorated the effects of cancer chemotherapy, several clinical trials have been carried out. Six of seven trials, as summarized by Poster and colleagues (1981), have shown a superior effect of THC compared to placebo or other antiemetics.

In a controlled, double-blind, crossover study of 22 patients (20 of them refractory) undergoing various kinds of chemotherapy, oral THC had an antiemetic effect in 14 of 20 courses, while the placebo was inactive in 22 courses (Sallan, Zinberg, and Frei 1975). This was a young population (median age 29.5 years). The drug was given at a dose of 10 mg/m^2, two hours before, and two and six hours after chemotherapy.

Another positive study is that of Chang and associates (1979) who explored oral and smoked THC in a young (median age 24 years) population receiving high-dose methotrexate. Fourteen of 15 patients had a reduction in nausea and vomiting compared to placebo, and the antiemetic effect correlated with the plasma THC concentration. Some patients treated over a long period of time became less responsive to THC, and five other patients receiving doxorubicin and cyclophosphamide did not respond as well.

In a large study from the Mayo Clinic of 115 patients being treated for gastrointestinal cancer with 5-fluorouracil and semustine (methyl-CCNU), THC was better than placebo but no better than prochlorperazine (Frytak et al. 1979). The THC was given as 15 mg orally three times a day, and phenothiazine, 10 mg orally, three times a day. It may be significant that the median age of this population was 61. Central nervous system toxicity was more severe with THC, and the treatment experience was less pleasant than with prochlorperazine.

In a study from Duke University, 53 patients with "refractory" disease treated with multiple chemotherapy regimens were given THC (Lucas and Laszlo 1980). Seventy-two percent of the patients had either complete or partial (50%) amelioration of their vomiting compared to prior antiemetic therapy. Cisplatin in doses of more than 120 mg caused nausea and vomiting that did not respond to THC, but the symptoms related to lower doses did. The median age was not given.

It was reported that THC was more active than prochlorperazine (in a controlled randomized study in 84 patients, average age 32.5 years) (Sallan et al. 1980). This was a group of patients with refractory disease treated with a variety of chemotherapies but resistant to standard therapy, including phenothiazines. The antiemetic effect of THC was contingent on obtaining a "high."

Adverse effects of THC include drowsiness, disorientation, anxiety, tachycardia, hallucinations, and other psychotic manifestations. The toxicity seems to be worse in older patients. At present, the agent appears to be most active in young patients and should be considered for those who do not respond to other antiemetics. The supply of THC is no problem now that the National Cancer Institute has reclassified it as a group C drug, available to qualified oncologists at many hospitals that will follow the prescribed guidelines.

A new synthetic cannabinoid, nabilone, has been reported to be superior to prochlorperazine in a controlled, double-blind study of 113 patients at two institutions (Herman et al. 1979). Responses were 80% versus 32%, although complete response (absence of symptoms) was rare (8% in the nabilone group). The median age was 33 years, and many of them were receiving cisplatin in combination for testicular cancer. Nabilone is currently unavailable because of some deaths in studies of long-term animal toxicity. Newer agents are being tested. We are participating in a prospective randomized trial of levonantradol. Metoclopramide (Reglan) appears to be effective in mitigating vomiting due to cisplatin (Kahn, Elias, and Mason 1978).

Stomatitis

Mouth ulcerations, often complicated by infection with oral flora, sometimes in association with leukopenia, are often seen after chemotherapy with such drugs as methotrexate, 5-fluorouracil, doxorubicin, dactinomycin, and bleomycin, and somewhat less commonly with 6-mercaptopurine, mitomycin, mithramycin, procarbazine, and daunorubicin. A grading system has been used to describe severity (Capizzi et al. 1970):

Grade 1	Erythema of the oral mucosa
Grade 2	Isolated small ulcerations
Grade 3	Confluent ulcerations
Grade 4	Hemorrhagic ulcerations

When the white patches of *C. albicans* are seen, therapy with oral nystatin is indicated. The oral cavity should be kept clean, and local rinses with 3% hydrogen peroxide (diluted if necessary 1:1 with water or saline) are often effective when used every one to four hours, depending on severity. Cleaning with a soft cotton swab is often helpful, and lidocaine (Xylocaine Viscous) numbs acutely painful mucosal tissues, although the taste is bad. It should be applied just before eating. The diet should be of soft bland foods with avoidance of hot, acidic, or spicy foods.

Diarrhea

Diarrhea occurs commonly with antimetabolites, which have the capability of destroying gastrointestinal mucosa. The most frequent agents producing this symptom are 5-fluorouracil, especially when used in a loading dose as opposed to a weekly one, and methotrexate when used high-dose with leucovorin, in the presence of renal impairment, or on a daily schedule. Mithramycin has also been an occasional cause of diarrhea, as has estramustine, streptozotocin, 5-azacytidine, hydroxyurea, and mitotane. Therapy should focus on discontinuation of the drug, careful attention to repletion of fluid and electrolyte loss, and symptomatic measures. The diarrhea is usually short-lived and responds to opiates such as codeine or paregoric. The most widely used agent is the meperidine congener diphenoxylate with atropine (Lomotil), in a dosage of two tablets (5 mg) four times daily in adults, with dose reduction after control of symptoms. Anticholinergic effects, development of tolerance, and frequent administration are all objections to the use of diphenoxylate, particularly for chronic diarrhea, but it seems suitable for most instances of acute self-limited cases that are encountered with cancer chemotherapy. A newer agent, loperamide (Imodium), has been reported to be more effective than diphenoxylate in both acute (Amery et al. 1975) and chronic (Galambos et al. 1976) diarrhea. It is a piperidine derivative like dephenoxylate, and its major superiority in the acute diarrheas is a more rapid control of symptoms. It acts locally at the bowel wall, is said to be nonaddictive, and does not produce long-term tolerance. Abdominal cramping is sometimes a side effect.

Alopecia

Hair loss is often the most devastating effect of chemotherapy. It is a visible reminder to the patient that he or she has cancer and is undergoing a depersonalizing type of treatment. Although the complication is nearly always reversible, even during the continuation of therapy, it may sometimes be the decisive factor that causes some patients to reject life-saving or life-extending treatment. In recent years, local measures at the time of drug administration have had a significant ameliorating effect.

Cyclophosphamide is one of the agents that most frequently causes alopecia when used in large intravenous doses, and the condition is dose-related. The usual oral doses may result in thinning hair but not the severe alopecia seen with parenteral doses. The hair sometimes returns with a different color or texture. Unfortunately, because of the time required for biotransformation to the active agent, local measures at the time of administration seem to have little protective effect.

Doxorubicin, vincristine, daunorubicin, methotrexate, and mitomycin are probably the most common causes of hair loss; other agents include dactinomycin, 5-fluorouracil, hydroxyurea, vinblastine, etoposide (VP-16-213), and carmustine (BCNU).

Various techniques have been used to prevent this side effect, including scalp tourniquets and scalp cooling. Following an initial report by Simister (1966), a scalp tourniquet was also used by O'Brien and co-workers (1970) to lessen alopecia after vincristine in 30 children. Alopecia developed in three, but was explained by other drugs or causes.

Soukop and colleagues (1978) used a tourniquet that was inflated 10 mm above systolic pressure and left in place for 30 minutes. The chemotherapy was vincristine, cyclophosphamide, and doxorubicin, all given intravenously to 35 women with solid tumors. Delay rather than prevention of alopecia was found, the mean time to hair loss being 10.3 weeks in the treated group and 4.2 weeks in the control group. The results might well have been better if cyclophosphamide had not been used. No scalp metastases were observed during the period of the study.

In one experience (Pesce et al. 1978; Pesce, Cassuto, and Audoly 1978) a scalp tourniquet was used for 20 minutes, with a pressure 50 mm Hg above the patient's systolic pressure, and an average fall of 20 mm Hg during the procedure. Ten percent of patients could not tolerate this. The incidence of alopecia was halved when used with a regimen of doxorubicin, cyclophosphamide, and either vincristine or VM-26 (teniposide).

Various scalp cooling techniques have been used that cause vessel occlusion by pressure and vasoconstriction of scalp by cooling, presumably reduce the metabolic rate of the target tissue, and perhaps reduce cellular uptake of the drug.

Luce and co-workers (1973) demonstrated the protective effect of chilled air directed to the scalp against doxorubicin-induced alopecia. Edelstyn, MacDonald, and MacRae (1977) used cryogel packs held on the scalp and reported good protection in 50% of patients treated with this agent. Dean, Salmon, and Griffith (1979) used plastic bags filled with ice in patients receiving intravenous doxorubicin with oral cyclophosphamide. The ice was applied 5 minutes before and 30 minutes after doxorubicin administration, with 60% of patients having good protection through all cycles of treatment. The effect was dose-related.

We are currently using the Chemo Cap (Therapeutic Products, Inc.), which is a segmented bonnet that contains a cryogel that is frozen in a freezer, but which can then be molded to the shape of a patient's head. It is used 20 minutes before and 30 minutes after drug administration. Our early experience is encouraging. A disposable unit, relying on the cooling produced by the dissolution of an inorganic salt in water in a plastic bag, is also available.

Extravasation of Chemotherapeutic Agents

This problem has been extensively and excellently reviewed by Ignoffo and Friedman (1980). The agents that cause most difficulty when infiltration occurs are the antitumor antibiotics, such as dactinomycin, doxorubicin, daunorubicin, mitomycin, and mithramycin, and the *Vinca* alkaloids, mechlorethamine and streptozotocin. For most of these there is no specific antidote, although empirical therapy with several agents is recommended. Sodium bicarbonate and dexamethasone are suggested for the anthracyclines; sodium bicarbonate for the *Vinca* alkaloids; and sodium thiosulfate for dactinomycin, mithramycin, mitomycin, and mechlorethamine.

One can minimize the chances of extravasation by careful attention to technique. The arm on the side of a mastectomy should be avoided if possible. The best areas for venipunctures (where there is a choice) are in order, the forearm, the dorsum of the hand, the wrist, and the antecubital fossa. This minimizes the chance for damage to nerves and tendons if infiltration occurs. The drug should be well diluted, and in combination chemotherapy the most irritating agent should be given last. Prior radiation therapy to an area of drug administration can exacerbate local reactions after extravasation. Multiple venipunctures should be avoided if possible, and test administration for saline and blood withdrawal should be performed. The time of administration should be at least three minutes or 5 ml per minute, with a 5- to 10-ml saline flush.

If extravasation occurs, the injection should be stopped, several milliliters of blood withdrawn to remove some of the drug, the subcutaneous infiltrate aspirated, the antidote given locally, and warm soaks applied for about an hour. Sometimes plastic surgical repair will be needed (fig. 31.1).

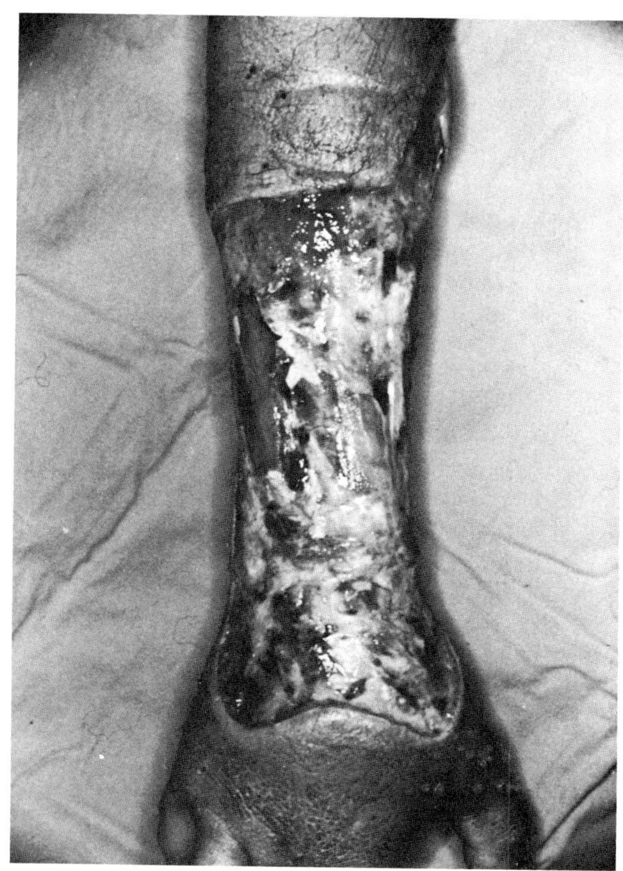

Fig. 31.1. *Arm of patient following extravasation of doxorubicin. Surgical debridement has been performed with exposure of tendons. (Photograph courtesy of Stephen V. Flagg, M.D., Yale University School of Medicine.)*

References

Amery, W. et al. A multicentre double-blind study in acute diarrhoea comparing loperamide (R 18553) with two common antidiarrhoeal agents and a placebo. *Curr. Ther. Res.* 17:263–270, 1975.

Borison, H. L.; Brand, D.; and Orkand, R. K. Emetic action of nitrogen mustard in dogs and cats. *Am. J. Physiol.* 192:410–416, 1958.

Cadman, E. Toxicity of chemotherapeutic agents. In *Cancer, a comprehensive treatise,* vol. 5, ed. F. F. Becker. New York: Plenum, 1977, pp. 59–111.

Capizzi, R. L. et al. Methotrexate therapy of head and neck cancer: improvement in therapeutic index by the use of leucovorin "rescue." *Cancer Res.* 30:1782–1788, 1970.

Chang, A. E. et al. Delta-9-tetrahydrocannabinol as an antiemetic in cancer patients receiving high-dose methotrexate. *Ann. Intern. Med.* 91:819–824, 1979.

Dean, J. D.; Salmon, S. E.; and Griffith, K. S. Prevention of doxorubicin-induced hair loss with scalp hypothermia. *N. Engl. J. Med.* 301:1427–1429, 1979.

Edelstyn, G. A.; MacDonald, M.; and MacRae, K. D. Doxorubicin-induced hair loss and possible modification by scalp cooling. *Lancet* 2:253–254, 1977.

Frytak, S. et al. Delta-9-tetrahydrocannabinol as an antiemetic for patients receiving cancer chemotherapy. A comparison with prochlorperazine and a placebo. *Ann. Intern. Med.* 91:825–830, 1979.

Galambos, J. T. et al. Loperamide: a new antidiarrheal agent in the treatment of chronic diarrhea. *Gastroenterology* 70:1026–1029, 1976.

Grossman, B.; Lessin, L. S.; and Cohen, P. Droperidol prevents nausea and vomiting from cis-platinum. *N. Engl. J. Med.* 301:47, 1979.

Harris, J. G. Nausea, vomiting, and cancer treatment. *CA* 28:194–201, 1978.

Herman, T. S. et al. Superiority of nabilone over prochloperazine as an antiemetic in patients receiving cancer chemotherapy. *N. Engl. J. Med.* 300:1295–1297, 1979.

Ignoffo, R. J., and Friedman, M. A. Therapy of local toxicities caused by extravasation of cancer chemotherapeutic drugs. *Cancer Treat. Rev.* 7:17–27, 1980.

Kahn, T.; Elias, E. G.; and Mason, G. R. A single dose of metoaclopramide in the control of vomiting from cis-dichlorodiammine-platinum (II) in man. *Cancer Treat. Rep.* 62:1106–1107, 1978.

Knobf, M. K. et al. *Cancer chemotherapy: treatment and care.* Boston: G. K. Hall, 1980.

Lucas, V. S., Jr., and Laszlo J. Δ^9-Tetrahydrocannabinol for refractory vomiting induced by cancer chemotherapy. *JAMA* 243:1241–1243, 1980.

Luce, J. K. et al. Prevention of alopecia by scalp cooling of patients receiving Adriamycin. *Cancer Chemother. Rep.* 57:108, 1973.

O'Brien, R. et al. Scalp tourniquet to lessen alopecia after vincristine. *N. Engl. J. Med.* 283:1469, 1970.

Pesce, A. et al. Scalp tourniquet in the prevention of chemotherapy-induced alopecia. *N. Engl. J. Med.* 298:1204–1205, 1978.

Pesce, A.; Cassuto, J. P.; and Audoly, P. Scalp tourniquet in cancer therapy. *N. Engl. J. Med.* 299:606, 1978.

Plotkin, D. A.; Plotkin, D.; and Okun, R. Haloperidol in the treatment of nausea and vomiting due to cytotoxic drug administration. *Curr. Ther. Res.* 15:599–602, 1973.

Poster, D. S. et al. Δ^9-Tetrahydrocannabinol in clinical oncology. *JAMA* 245:2047–2051, 1981.

Sallan, S. E. et al. Antiemetics in patients receiving chemotherapy for cancer: a randomized comparison of delta-9-tetrahydrocannabinol and prochlorperazine. *N. Engl. J. Med.* 302:135–138, 1980.

Sallan, S. E.; Zinberg, N. E.; and Frei, E., III. Antiemetic effect of delta-9-tetrahydrocannabinol in cancer chemotherapy. *N. Engl. J. Med.* 293:795–797, 1975.

Simister, J. M. Alopecia and cytotoxic drugs. *Br. Med. J.* 2:1138, 1966.

Soukop, M. et al. Adriamycin, alopecia, and the scalp tourniquet. *Cancer Treat. Rep.* 62:489–490, 1978.

part five

Specific Malignancies and Their Treatment

thirty-two

Breast Cancer from a Surgeon's Standpoint

FRANK C. SPARKS

What is the place of surgery in treating breast cancer? I frequently am asked, "What operation do you perform?" This chapter presents some of my thoughts on treating patients with breast cancer and what led me to them, and shows why an individualized approach to each patient is appropriate. More detailed analyses to support these conclusions are available (Haskell, Sparks, and Thompson 1980; Sparks 1978).

Our goal as surgeons in treating women with stage I and II breast cancer is to achieve local control and to determine disease stage, that is, remove lymph nodes to determine the risk of recurrence. The best method to achieve local control is determined by a number of ongoing prospective randomized controlled studies that will be discussed subsequently. Clearly, there is a trend away from radical mastectomy and toward smaller operations and radiation therapy. Changing concepts of the biology of the disease have brought about new approaches to its treatment.

Biology

The concept of tumor-doubling time (TDT) is useful in understanding the clinical course of patients with breast cancer. There is a direct correlation between the TDT and the duration of survival after radical mastectomy.

A 1-cm so-called early breast cancer contains 10^9 cells and has already undergone 30 of the 40 doublings that occur prior to the woman's death. The TDT of a primary tumor varies from 23 to 209 days (Haskell, Sparks, and Thompson 1980). Multiplying the TDT times 30 doublings, we see that the 1-cm tumor may have been present from 2 to 17 years prior to diagnosis. Despite the degree of accuracy in applying TDT to such determinations, it seems reasonably certain that months or years pass before a breast cancer can be diagnosed; metastases have adequate time to spread before the primary lesion is detectable; and the concept that early disease is curable may be wishful thinking.

The natural history of untreated breast cancer suggests that it is an acute or chronic disease, depending on the tumor-doubling time. In one study (Haskell, Sparks, and Thompson 1980), average survival from first symptoms was 40 months in 100 untreated patients. Twenty-two percent were alive at the end of 5 years, and 5% after 10 years. This chronic form represents tumors with the longest TDTs. In contrast, about 20% of untreated patients survive less than one year from the onset of first symptoms, and this fraction represents tumors with the more rapid TDTs.

Contrary to previous belief that tumor cells spread in a step-wise fashion from the primary tumor to the lymph nodes and then to distant sites, breast cancer can bypass lymph nodes and spread directly to the blood stream. It can present as a metastasis (Giuliano, Sparks, and Morton 1978). Lymph nodes may act more as a marker of the patient-tumor relationship than as a barrier to tumor dissemination (Pilch et al. 1975).

Microscopic or histologic cancer does not always progress to clinical disease. Although the pathologist can frequently find histologic evidence of multiple lesions, the presence of two or more clinically apparent cancers in one breast is rare. Also, the incidence of cancer developing in the other breast is much lower than that of histologic cancer detected by mirror-image biopsy or autopsy. Finally, the frequency of tumor growing in untreated axillary nodes following total mastectomy is much lower than expected (Fisher et al. 1977).

Breast Cancer as a Systemic Disease

Breast cancer is a systemic disease at the time of first diagnosis in the majority of women (Fisher 1977). Only a small percentage may be fortunate enough to have the biologic variant that does not metastasize and that remains curable by operation or radiation therapy. Surgery does not remove all of the cancer cells in the body, even in women who are thought to be cured of their disease. Mueller and Jefferies (1975) reported that in women undergoing curative operation, 80% to 85% of eventual deaths are from breast cancer, and the death rate is *constant* for as long as 15 years following operation. Because the majority of breast cancer is systemic at the time of diagnosis, it is not surprising that varying the extent of operation or adding one regional modality (postoperative radiation therapy) to another (operation) fails to increase survival.

Local recurrence on the chest wall is a manifestation of systemic disease. Regardless of the treatment of the primary tumor, local recurrence and distant metastases grow simultaneously in almost all patients. This observation serves to emphasize the importance of the patient-tumor relationship (Pilch et al. 1975). Alternative methods of controlling local recurrence, even in an irradiated field, are available and effective (Partridge et al. 1979a, 1979b).

Risk Factors

Davies (1978) has developed a useful method of estimating the quantitative impact of five prognostic factors on the risk of dying from breast cancer during a 10-year period for women of different ages. The method's simplicity and potential clinical value warrant further comment. To use it, one must establish the quantitative value of each of five risk factors (RF) for the patient:

Age, including proximity to menopause
Family history of breast cancer
Patient's pregnancy history
History of benign breast disease
Frequency of breast examinations

Each is a standardized estimate of the relative risk of that factor in the individual compared with that in the general population. The product obtained by multiplying each of these factors is called the composite risk factor, or CRF. Multiplying the CRF by the age-adjusted 10-year risk of death from breast cancer for the normal population results in an estimate of the 10-year incidence of death from breast cancer in women with the characteristics used in the calculation. For example, a 42-year-old menstruating woman (RF 1.11) with a strong family history of breast cancer (RF 3.14), one full-term pregnancy at age 32 (RF 1.49), a history of benign breast disease (RF 3.57), and no breast examination within the last year (RF 1.32) has a CRF of 24.47. The 10-year risk for the patient's age would be 350 per 100,000, but the adjusted risk would be 8564 cases per 100,000 people, or 8.56%. This extremely high risk would suggest a need for especially careful observation of such a patient.

The Trend to Smaller Operations

Radical Mastectomy: Standard, Extended, and Modified

Halsted saw patients with much more advanced breast cancer than we see today. In the case records from the Johns Hopkins Hospital he describes a woman with "a *small* 7 × 8 cm tumor in the upper outer quadrant" (italics mine) (Sparks 1978). To gain local control in such cases, radical mastectomy, frequently with skin grafting, was indeed necessary.

When it became apparent that breast cancer spread to the internal mammary nodes, extended radical mastectomy was devised. In 1963, I believed that breast cancer was a localized or regional disease at diagnosis, and wanted to gain information that would support the use of this operation. I compared the results from radical mastectomy and extended radical mastectomy performed at the Memorial Sloan-Kettering and James Ewing Cancer Hospitals in New York City from 1953 to 1956. I reviewed all cases of primary operable breast cancer and selected only those with infiltrating duct carcinoma located in the inner quadrants or under the nipple. Cases in which there were any unfavorable signs were excluded. All patients had complete five-year follow-up. There was no advantage to resecting the internal mammary lymph nodes in these patients (table 32.1) (Sparks 1978). Analysis according to tumor size or lymph node level in the axilla also failed to show any advantage for the extended radical mastectomy. These data further support the concept that breast cancer is a

Table 32.1. *Results at Five Years*

Status	Radical Mastectomy		Extended Radical Mastectomy	
	No.	%	No.	%
No recurrence	245	59	126	60
Alive with cancer	38	9	22	10
Dead	131	32	62	30

SOURCE: Sparks 1978.

systemic disease and that the regional lymph nodes are merely markers for the patient-tumor relationship (Pilch et al. 1975; Fisher 1977).

The modified radical mastectomy is more correctly termed total mastectomy and axillary dissection. The best study comparing the modified radical and the radical mastectomy is from the Mayo Clinic, where data showed no difference in the local recurrence and survival rates (Robinson et al. 1976). The cosmetic and functional results from modified radical operation are superior to those from radical mastectomy. The former is currently the most frequently performed operation for breast cancer because it achieves local control and removes axillary lymph nodes for accurate pathologic staging.

Total Mastectomy

Total mastectomy, with or without postoperative radiation therapy, has been evaluated in three prospective randomized controlled studies. From the early results, this procedure seems to be adequate primary therapy if followed by radical radiation therapy. In the National Surgical Adjuvant Breast Project (NSABP) study, patients with clinically positive nodes were randomized to either radical mastectomy or total mastectomy plus postoperative radiation therapy. Patients with clinically negative nodes were randomized to radical mastectomy, total mastectomy plus postoperative radiation therapy, or total mastectomy followed by axillary dissection in those patients who subsequently developed positive nodes. With a mean follow-up of three years (range two to six years), Fisher (1977) reports no significant difference in failure or survival rates.

In the King's–Cambridge trial (Cancer Research Campaign 1976), patients with clinical stages I and II breast cancer were randomly assigned to receive total mastectomy with or without postoperative radiation therapy. Axillary node dissection was not performed with simple mastectomy. In the group that was assigned to simple mastectomy alone, a patient's axilla was treated only when evidence of progressive tumor growth occurred. There was no difference in the five-year survival or distant recurrence-free rates. As expected, the local recurrence rate was lower in the group receiving radiation therapy.

In the Cardiff–St. Mary's trial (Forest 1977), patients with both clinical stages I and II breast cancer were randomly assigned to receive either radical mastectomy or total mastectomy and pectoral node biopsy. The biopsy was achieved by sampling nodes that lie within the tail of the breast, and between it and the axillary vein. Postoperative radiation therapy was given to patients in both groups who had histologically positive nodes. There was no difference in the nine-year survival or distant recurrence-free rates. The local recurrence rate was lower in the group undergoing radical mastectomy.

What is the significance of clinically negative, histologically positive axillary lymph nodes? Are they predecessors of distant metastases, or merely manifestations or markers for metastatic disease? Data from both the NSABP and King's–Cambridge trials suggest the latter. In the NSABP trial, only 15% of women with clinical stage I disease who were treated with total mastectomy alone have developed positive axillary nodes requiring delayed axillary dissection. On the basis of findings in patients treated by radical mastectomy, as many as 40% had histologically positive nodes. In the King's–Cambridge trial (Cancer Research Campaign 1976) only 14% of the women followed four or five years have required treatment to the axilla, whereas 32% would have been expected to have histologically positive nodes.

Partial Mastectomy and Radiation Therapy

The Guy's Hospital trial (Hayward 1974) evaluating partial mastectomy and radiation therapy is especially important as it is the only study with a complete 10-year follow-up. Patients over 50 years of age with clinical stages I and II breast cancer were randomly assigned to receive either wide local excision or radical mastectomy. Both groups of patients received radiation therapy, albeit less than would now be considered optimal. The survival rate for patients with stage I disease was the same in both groups, whereas the survival rates for those with stage II disease were higher in women treated by radical mastectomy. The local recurrence rate was higher in patients treated by wide local excision. In many instances local recurrence could be adequately controlled by subsequent therapy.

More recently, Veronesi and others (1981) compared radical mastectomy with partial mastectomy (quadrantectomy), axillary dissection, and radiation therapy in patients with breast cancer measuring less than 2 cm in diameter and with no palpable axillary lymph nodes. From 1973 to 1980, 701 patients were randomized to either of these two primary therapies. From 1973 to 1975, patients with positive lymph nodes were further randomized to receive either postoperative radiation therapy to the supraclavicular and internal mammary nodes or no further therapy. From 1976 to 1980, all patients with positive nodes were treated with adjuvant chemotherapy. Although the median follow-up is relatively short, probably only about three and one-half years, the results are important. There was no difference between the two groups in disease-free or overall survival.

Radiation Therapy

Local excision followed by radiation therapy with doses of 4500 to 5000 rad to the breast and regional nodes gives results that are comparable to those obtained with primary surgery (Levene, Harris, and Hellman 1977). The cosmetic results are superior to those obtained with a modified radical mastectomy. In my experience with a small number of patients treated this way, the breast feels surprisingly normal and the patients have been pleased.

The drawbacks of radiation therapy include the time it takes to complete treatment and the side effects. The entire breast and lymph node areas must be treated five days a week for five to six weeks to deliver the initial 5000 rad. Three to four weeks later, the patient is usually readmitted to the hospital to deliver a booster dose of 2500 to 3000 rad to the site of the excisional biopsy. This is done in the operating room under general anesthesia where radioactive iridium-192 ribbons are carefully placed into the breast tissue.

The side effects of radiation therapy include local effects and long-term carcinogenic effects. Although infrequent, rib or clavicle fracture, radiation pneumonitis, arm edema, pleural effusion, and brachial plexus injury have been reported. Stricture of the esophagus has also been seen.

The long-term carcinogenic effects of radiation therapy are more important. I have personally performed forequarter amputations on two patients who have been "cured" of their primary cancer by radiation therapy, but who developed radiation-induced soft tissue sarcomas. One of these patients (Snyder, Sparks, and Batzdorf 1979) was a 40-year-old woman who had received "routine" postoperative radiation therapy following a radical mastectomy for breast cancer eight years earlier, even though the lymph nodes in her axilla contained no evidence of micrometastases. She developed a radiation-induced malignant schwannoma of the brachial plexus that resulted in a paralyzed, painful, swollen arm. She received significant palliation from the forequarter amputation and was able to return to work following this operation.

Barol, Larsson, and Mallsson (1977) reported that the incidence of breast cancer was increased four times following irradiation of the breast. As is discussed subsequently, there is concern about the carcinogenic effect of irradiation during mammography. If this worry exists, there should certainly be hard questions asked about the use of therapeutic radiation therapy causing breast cancer and osteogenic and soft tissue sarcomas.

Younger women are more likely to choose radiation therapy over mastectomy, especially if they have stage I disease. Mueller, Ames, and Anderson (1978) reported a 60% 20-year survival rate for 1223 women with stage I breast cancer who were under age 50 at the time of diagnosis. The latency period between radiation therapy and the onset of radiation-induced sarcomas varies from 5 to 24 years. Thus the women most likely to choose radiation therapy are also those most likely to suffer from its long-term effects.

The Importance of Staging on Adjuvant Therapy

The stage of the breast cancer determines treatment. The presence of histologically proved metastases in the axillary nodes is the best indicator of whether a patient will ultimately develop recurrence and succumb to her disease (Fisher 1977; Haskell et al. 1977). For pathologic stage I disease (no evidence of metastases in regional nodes), adjuvant chemotherapy is not indicated (Haskell et al. 1977; Bonadonna, Rossi, and Valagussa 1977).

For pathologic stage II disease (metastases in regional nodes), the risk of recurrence is sufficiently high that many oncologists advise adjuvant chemotherapy, especially in premenopausal women. The preliminary results from adjuvant chemotherapy are promising in that the early recurrence rate is decreased (Haskell et al. 1977; Sparks, Wile, and Ramming 1976; Bonadonna, Rossi, and Valagussa 1977). Second-generation adjuvant chemotherapy regimens, perhaps combining chemotherapy and immunotherapy (Sparks, Wile, and Ramming 1976; Sparks, et al. 1977b; Partridge et al. 1979a), may further improve the results. Because adjuvant chemotherapy decreases the quality of life (Meyerwitz, Sparks, and Spears 1979), however, there will have to be a significant increase in survival to make this therapy worthwhile.

If ongoing studies document an improved survival with adjuvant chemotherapy, then accurate staging by axillary and/or internal mammary node dissection will continue to be an important and essential part of the primary treatment of breast cancer. Figure 32.1 shows a woman with a breast cancer in the upper inner quadrant who presented with clinically negative nodes. Because of the high likelihood of metastases to the internal mammary nodes, her medical oncologist wanted to give her adjuvant chemotherapy even if the axillary lymph nodes contained no micrometastases. Following excisional biopsy, the patient selected primary treatment of the breast by radiation therapy. Prior to radiation therapy she underwent axillary and internal mammary node dissections for accurate "staging" or assessment of risk of recurrence, and the need for adjuvant chemotherapy. Both axillary and internal mammary lymph nodes contained no micrometastases. She therefore needed no adjuvant chemotherapy, and by this extended "staging" procedure avoided the side effects of adjuvant chemotherapy. Five years later, she still has no evidence of recurrence.

Recently the author treated another woman with a clinical stage I inner quadrant breast cancer by a total mastectomy and axillary node dissection. When frozen section examination of the axillary lymph nodes showed no micrometastases, an internal mammary node dissection was done during the same operation. There were micrometastases in these internal mammary nodes. Without the internal mammary node dissection, this patient would not have received adjuvant chemotherapy because the permanent section examination of the axillary nodes showed no micrometastases. However, because the extended staging procedure showed metastases in the internal mammary nodes, and therefore a high risk of recurrence, she is receiving adjuvant chemotherapy. This is another example of how accurate staging can determine the necessity of adjuvant chemotherapy.

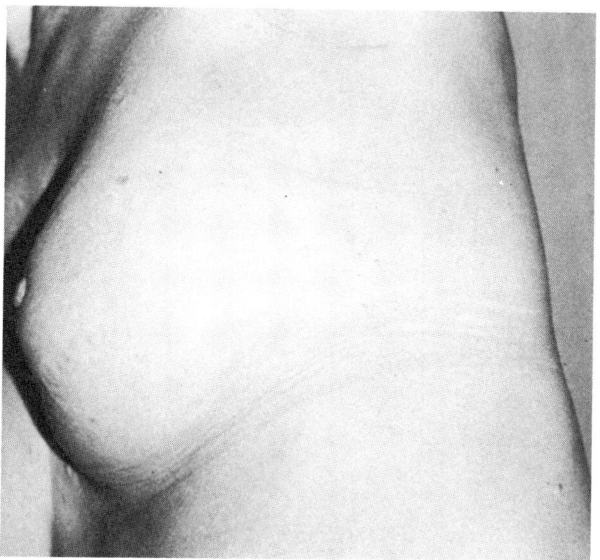

Fig. 32.1. *This patient had a breast cancer excised from the upper inner quadrant of her breast in 1976. Because accurate staging by axillary and internal mammary node dissections showed no evidence of metastases, adjuvant chemotherapy was avoided (see text). The patient received radiation therapy after staging for any residual tumor in the breast.*

An Approach to the Individual Patient

Biopsy

Any woman with a dominant mass in her breast should have either biopsy or aspiration of the mass. Many women do not have a dominant mass and instead have lumpy breasts, either due to physiologic nodularity or varying degrees of mammary dysplasia (fibrocystic disease). To avoid unnecessary biopsies in these women, a combination of skill, judgment, and experience is required on the part of the physician. A skillful examination can on occasion detect a small cancer that can neither be palpated nor seen on mammography. Therefore the breast should first be observed for any signs of skin dimpling while the patient raises her arms and while she tenses her pectoral muscles with her arms at her sides. The breast should then be palpated with the patient in both the sitting and supine positions.

The accuracy of diagnosing a breast cancer on physical examination increases as the patient's age increases; in premenopausal women it may be as low as 30%. In addition to physical findings and age, other factors that enter into the decision of whose breast to biopsy are history (e.g., nipple bleeding), and the composite risk factor previously discussed.

Technique of Biopsy

Aspiration should be considered, as it may remove the need for biopsy should the mass prove to be a cyst. The biopsy itself can almost always be performed through a circumareolar incision that leaves an almost undetectable scar. With adequate sedation and analgesics, most of these procedures can be done on an outpatient basis. Because hormonal assay of the primary tumor can be useful in making subsequent therapeutic decisions if the patient develops metastases, biopsy specimens should be cut up and part sent for permanent section and part frozen for estradiol and progesterone receptor assay if the diagnosis is cancer. If frozen section diagnosis is available by a pathologist, hormonal assay can be performed on only those specimens that are malignant. If a woman has a clinically obvious cancer, a needle biopsy can be obtained in the office, thereby avoiding the more formal excisional biopsy under local analgesia.

Mammography

A mammogram or xerogram should be obtained prior to biopsy of a mass in women over 35 years of age to detect any other areas in either breast that should be biopsied at the same time, and to serve as a baseline for subsequent mammograms. How frequently should such follow-up mammograms be obtained? There is no answer to this question. More important, there is no absolute evidence that mammograms have improved true survival in breast cancer.

Mammograms can diagnose breast cancer earlier and lead to a greater five-year survival *from the time of diagnosis*. There is no clear-cut evidence, however, that survival *from the inception of the cancer* is improved. As an example (fig. 32.2), suppose two identical twins develop breast cancers at the same time (year 0). Both cancers grow identically and metastasize prior to diagnosis by xerography three years later. At that time the tumors are not palpable but measure 0.1 cm^3 and contain a million cells. Twin A is then treated by a modified radical mastectomy. Survival curves begin from treat-

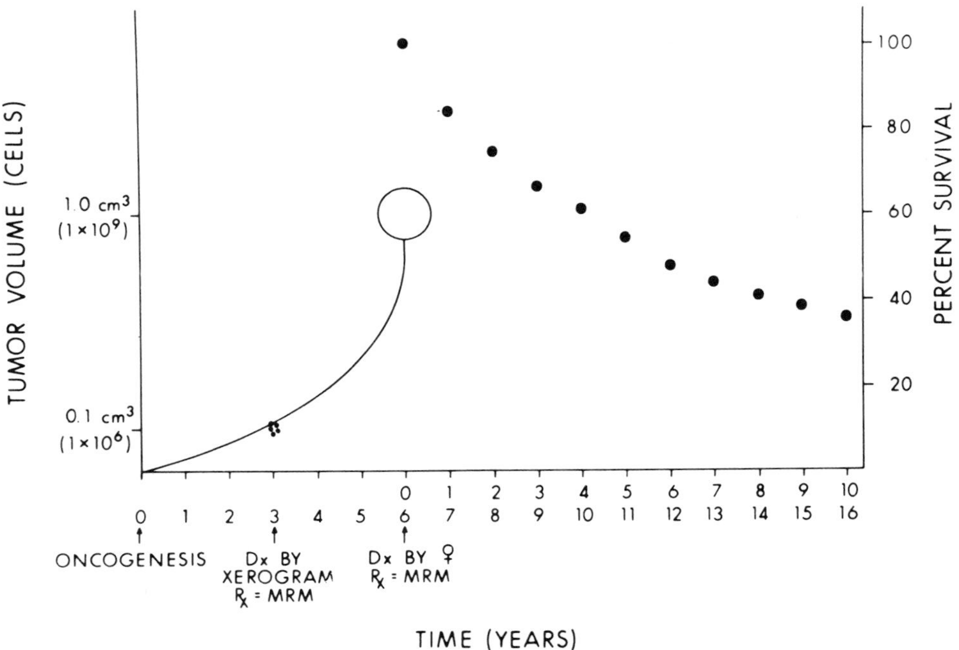

Fig. 32.2. *The benefit of early diagnosis and treatment may be illusory and exist only because the "survival clock" starts at different times (see text).*

ment, and at year 8 the five-year survival would be about 75%. For a variety of reasons twin B is not treated until three years later when she feels a 1 cm^3 lump in her breast. The tumor now contains a billion cells. Treatment again is by a modified radical mastectomy. The five-year survival, now at year 11, would be about 55%. Twin A would seem to benefit from early diagnosis and treatment even though this is only an illusory improvement in the five-year survival that exists because the "survival clock" begins at different times.

In other words, because of a mammogram a physician may tell a woman she has breast cancer and needs an operation several years earlier than if she had found the lump in her breast by herself. If she died from metastases from disease that had occurred prior to its early diagnosis by the mammogram and the subsequent treatment by operation, there would be no benefit from earlier diagnosis. Thus screening procedures may lead to an apparent, but not a real, increase in survival. It may take several decades before the true effect of mammograms becomes apparent.

Bailar (1977) examined the carcinogenic effects of mammography and concluded that there was "a possibility that the routine use of mammography in screening asymptomatic women may eventually take almost as many lives as it saves." Because of the controversy that surrounds the potential value of screening mammograms, the National Cancer Institute carefully considered the wisdom of this diagnostic method, and following an expert panel review, has recommended that in asymptomatic women the procedure be restricted to those over 50 years of age after an initial baseline study at age 35 (Thier et al. 1978). Indications for a mammogram in younger patients include a strong family history of breast cancer, a previous diagnosis of breast cancer, or suspicion of breast disease on the part of the patient or physician. Where available, yearly mammograms after the age of 50 have been recommended. Although this is not always feasible or even advisable, it should be possible to obtain at least a single mammogram on nearly every woman over this age in an attempt to assess whether or not breast disease exists. Wolfe (1976) has suggested that certain patterns of mammographic change may be associated with a high incidence of cancer. If these are found, one would clearly need to follow the patient closely for the development of an occult or early carcinoma. A negative mammogram does not necessarily rule out a breast cancer (Patel et al. 1981).

A sensible approach to assessing the need for a yearly mammogram would be to calculate the adjusted risk of breast cancer in each patient, as described by Davies (1978). If the risk is substantially greater than average, one is probably justified in using every available technique for early diagnosis. If the risk is lower than average, even if the patient is more than 50 years old, yearly mammograms would not be needed.

Choice of Treatment

Most women want to participate in decision making regarding their treatment. A discussion with the woman and her husband, a relative, or close friend is essential to help her reach an intelligent decision that she can live with. In most instances, this should be done when the permanent section results confirm the presence of cancer. There is no need to rush the decision on what treatment she will choose.

Many of my patients who have had primary treatment either by surgery or radiation therapy have volunteered to talk to new patients when they are deciding what treatment to choose. I offer to give the woman who has just had her biopsy diagnosis the names of these volunteers to call should she wish to speak to someone who has already undergone treatment. To make an informed choice, a woman also needs to know about some of the concepts, if not actual clinical trials, previously described in this chapter.

She should be told that the modified radical mastectomy is the standard operation throughout much of the United States, because it achieves good local control and gives accurate pathologic staging that can be used to assess the advisability of adjuvant chemotherapy. She can be reassured that she will have complete use of her arm after this operation, that there is little chance of edema, and that reconstruction of a breast is possible. She should be offered the help of the American Cancer Society's Reach to Recovery program.

She should also be told that there are alternatives to mastectomy, and that there is increasing evidence that the results from radiation therapy are comparable to those obtained with modified radical mastectomy. If a woman with clinical stage I breast cancer wants to avoid mastectomy, the survival data from the Guy's Hospital trial are especially relevant, as this is the only study with a complete 10-year follow-up (Hayward 1974). She should also know the promising results of adjuvant chemotherapy, and thus the importance of sampling the axillary nodes and, in selected cases, the internal mammary lymph nodes to obtain accurate pathologic staging. This is especially important in premenopausal women who choose excisional biopsy and radiation therapy as primary treatment.

Finally, we should help the woman through both the medical and emotional aspects of the disease. Patients can be told of their diagnosis in a truthful manner that they can understand and accept, yet in a way that gives them hope for living as normal a life as possible. We should remember that the breast is not a useless, dispensable organ, but has important psychological and social value. In helping a woman reach an informed decision, we must remember that it is she who must live with or without her breast, with or without the carcinogenic effects of radiation therapy, and with or without the benefits and/or problems of adjuvant chemotherapy.

References

Bailar, J. C., III. Screening for early breast cancer: pros and cons. *Cancer* 39:2783–2795, 1977.

Barol, E.; Larsson, L.; and Mallsson, B. Breast cancer following irradiation of the breast. *Cancer* 40:2905–2910, 1977.

Bonadonna, G.; Rossi, A.; and Valagussa, B. S. The CMF program for operable breast cancer with positive nodes. *Cancer* 39:2904–2915, 1977.

Cancer Research Campaign. Report on an international multicentre trial (1976). Management of early cancer of the breast. *Br. Med. J.* 1:1035–1037, 1976.

Davies, D. F. Estimates of composite risk factors for death from breast cancer. *J. Natl. Cancer Inst.* 60:1519–1524, 1978.

Fisher, B. Biological and clinical considerations regarding the use of surgery and chemotherapy in the treatment of primary breast cancer. *Cancer* 40:574–587, 1977.

Fisher, B. et al. Comparison of radical mastectomy with alternative treatments for primary breast cancer. *Cancer* 39:2827–2839, 1977.

Forest, A. P. M. Conservative local treatment of breast cancer. *Cancer* 39:2813–2821, 1977.

Giuliano, A. E.; Sparks, F. C.; and Morton, D. L. Breast cancer presenting as renal colic. *Am. J. Surg.* 135:842–845, 1978.

Haskell, C. M. et al. Systemic therapy for metastatic breast cancer. *Ann. Intern. Med.* 86:68–80, 1977.

Haskell, C. M.; Sparks, F. C.; and Thompson, R. W. Carcinoma of the breast. In *Cancer treatment: a multidisciplinary approach,* ed. C. M. Haskell. Philadelphia: W. B. Saunders, 1980.

Hayward, J. Conservative surgery in the treatment of early breast cancer. *Br. J. Surg.* 61:770–771, 1974.

Levene, M. B.; Harris, J. R.; and Hellman, S. Treatment of carcinoma of the breast by radiation therapy. *Cancer* 39:2840–2845, 1977.

Meyerwitz, B. E.; Sparks, F. C.; and Spears, I. K. Adjuvant chemotherapy for breast carcinoma: psychosocial implications. *Cancer* 43:1613–1618, 1979.

Mueller, C. B., and Jefferies, W. Cancer of the breast: its outcome as measured by the rate of dying and causes of death. *Ann. Surg.* 182:334–341, 1975.

Mueller, C. B.; Ames, F.; and Anderson, G. D. Breast cancer in 3558 women: age as a significant determinate in the rate of dying and causes of death. *Surgery* 83:123–132, 1978.

Partridge, D. H. et al. Chemoimmunotherapy of stage III breast carcinoma with BCG and a live allogeneic tumor cell vaccine. *Cancer Immunol. Immunother.* 5:217–220, 1979a.

Partridge, D. H. et al. Intratumor bacillus Calmette-Guerin therapy for chest wall recurrence of carcinoma of the breast. *Surg. Gynecol. Obstet.* 148:867–870, 1979b.

Patel, J. et al. Axillary lymph node metastasis from an occult breast cancer. *Cancer* 47:2923–2927, 1981.

Pilch, Y. H. et al. Prospects for the immunotherapy of cancer. *Curr. Probl. Surg.* Part I (January, pp. 3–46); Part II (February, pp. 3–61), 1975.

Robinson, G. N. et al. The primary surgical treatment of carcinoma of the breast: a changing trend toward MRM. *Mayo Clin. Proc.* 51:433–452, 1976.

Snyder, M.; Sparks, F. C.; and Batzdorf, U. Unusual malignant tumors involving the brachial plexus: a report of two cases. *Am. Surg.* 45:42–48, 1979.

Sparks, F. C. Current trends in surgery for breast cancer. *Conn. Med.* 42:629–633, 1978.

Sparks, F. C.; Wile, A. G.; and Ramming, K. P. Immunology and adjuvant chemotherapy of breast cancer. *Arch. Surg.* 111:1057–1062, 1976.

Thier, S. O. et al. NIH/NCI consensus development meeting on breast cancer screening: issues and recommendations. *J. Natl. Cancer Inst.* 60:1519–1521, 1978.

Veronesi, U. et al. Comparing radical mastectomy with quadrantectomy, axillary dissection, and radiotherapy in patients with small cancers of the breast. *N. Engl. J. Med.* 305:6–11, 1981.

Wolfe, J. N. Breast patterns as an index of risk for developing breast cancer. *Am. J. Roentgenol.* 126:1130–1139, 1976.

thirty-three

Radiation Therapy of Breast Cancer

ARTHUR H. KNOWLTON

Recent reports concerning the beneficial effects of adjuvant chemotherapy in breast cancer have caused physicians to view this disease as a systemic problem and led to a general reconsideration of its treatment. There have been controversies regarding this for years, and current ones revolve around the merits of adjuvant chemotherapy and the role of radiation therapy as definitive treatment. Radiation has long been used for its palliative effects and is probably of greatest value here. It has also been traditionally used following mastectomy to decrease local recurrences. More recently, radiation oncologists have become involved in the definitive management of patients with breast cancer.

Preoperative Radiation

Many patients with locally advanced tumors will have a long period of survival, and radiation is beneficial in the treatment of primary disease in these individuals. Often, radiation to the extent of 4000 to 6000 rad over a four- to six-week period, followed by mastectomy, will control locally advanced disease (Stoker and Ellis 1972). Local control was achieved in 20 of 24 patients treated in this fashion. Caldwell (1971) reviewed the literature regarding the value of preoperative radiation as an adjunct to mastectomy. In his opinion, a controlled clinical trial was badly needed. The rationale of preoperative radiotherapy is eradication of tumor cells at the periphery of the lesion, making a complete resection more likely and reducing the possibility of dissemination at the time of surgery. A randomized trial was carried out and included a total of 960 patients (Wallgren et al. 1980). It compared preoperative radiotherapy followed by mastectomy to mastectomy followed by either no further treatment or postoperative radiotherapy. In their series, both preoperative and postoperative radiation increased disease-free survival compared to patients treated by surgery alone. On theoretical grounds, preoperative radiation should have better results than postoperative treatment, since the latter is delivered to cells that are often hypoxic following surgery. Nevertheless, in this series there was no difference in local recurrence rates between the two groups.

Postoperative Radiation

Until recent years, nearly every patient who underwent surgery for breast cancer received postoperative radiation, resulting in marked decrease of local recurrence. The question of whether it increased survival was not generally addressed, but it was assumed by most that it did not. Several excellent reviews are in the literature at this time. Edland and co-workers (1969) reported a local recurrence rate of 9% in patients with stage I disease having only surgery, and 25% of those with stage II disease. In patients treated with surgery and postoperative radiation, the local recurrence in stage I cancer was reduced to 0%, and to 9% in stage II. There was also a modest increase in absolute survival in patients with stage II tumors receiving postoperative radiation, and a striking statistically significant increase in disease-free survival at five years. Distant metastases occurred in those treated with surgery only in 19% of stage I disease and 65% of stage II. Only 5% of stage I and 45% of stage II cancer treated with postoperative radiotherapy progressed in that manner. An increase in survival of patients with stage II cancer treated with megavoltage was also shown in the report from the Department of Surgery of the Norwegian Radium Hospital (Host and Brennhovd 1977). In a randomized trial testing the value of postoperative radiation therapy as an adjuvant to radical mastectomy, those with stage II disease treated with supervoltage radiation showed a significantly reduced relapse rate. The value of radiation in the management of patients having undergone surgery is not yet totally clear.

One looks to this modality to reduce the local recurrence rate and also increase overall survival. It is generally accepted that local recurrence is decreased by postoperative radiation therapy. More difficult, however, is the demonstration of increased overall survival. Not until recently have controlled series been planned and carried out with this as their primary objective, and results are still preliminary. Nevertheless, when stage II disease is adequately treated, increased overall survival seems to be forthcoming. Freedom from local disease is of significant benefit to a patient and greatly improves the quality of life following surgery. Thus withholding postoperative radiotherapy in patients at a high risk for local recurrence appears unacceptable today. When local recurrence does take place the majority of these patients will develop disseminated disease. In patients with a significant risk of local recurrence, elective irradiation diminishes the incidence to 10% (Fletcher 1972), whereas only 50% control is obtained when patients are treatec for already existing chest wall disease. Indications for postoperative radiation therapy are patients with more than three positive axillary lymph nodes or a breast mass measuring greater than 3 cm, or any fixation, skin involvement, edema, erythema, multiple foci of tumor, or invasion of vascular structures, nerves, or lymphatics. Medical oncologists view some of these situations as indications for adjuvant chemotherapy rather than radiation therapy.

Definitive Radiation

Radiation has been traditionally used for inoperable but locally advanced carcinoma of the breast, in a postoperative setting, and in patients in need of palliation. In these situations it has been most effective, and thus it is only natural that eventually the modality would be attempted in local and operable breast cancer as a challenge to other methods of treating early stages of disease. Mastectomy deals with breast cancer on a local basis although the disease may be systemic. Radiation therapy can in selected cases accomplish the same local results as surgery. There are numerous operations dealing with the cancer locally; however, they all seem to accomplish the same end. Definitive radiation following surgical removal of the mass only appears to result in the same survival rate as the more radical operation (Fox 1979). The biologic effect of radiation depends on the total dose and the time over which it is given. Following surgery the number of cells still viable should be small, whereas when radiation is the definitive treatment the likelihood is that a great many more cells need to be eradicated. Thus for local control of operable disease the amount of radiation will be higher and the time period over which it is delivered longer than that of postoperative or even palliative treatment. For definitive treatment the areas at risk (fig. 33.1)—namely, the chest wall and breast itself, the internal mammary chain, the supraclavicular and axillary regions—should receive 4400 to 5000 rad over four and one-half to five and one-half weeks. An additional boost to the area of the tumor itself of 1000 to 2000 rad can be accomplished either by implantation (figs. 33.2 and 33.3) or external beam treatment. The electron beam modality is extremely useful for this.

Patients do better when the radiation is preceded by excisional rather than incisional biopsy (Levene, Harris, and Hellman 1977). There were greater numbers of local failures among patients with T_3 and T_4 cancer who underwent incisional biopsy compared to an excisional one, with only 3 of 19 among those whose mass was completely excised having local recurrence, compared to 20 of 60 who underwent an incisional or needle biopsy only. With fewer cancer cells present, radiation therapy following excisional biopsy should be more effective, and this appears to be the case. Axillary node sampling is also helpful in prognosis and in evaluating the patient for adjuvant chemotherapy.

As mentioned previously, the area that needs to be irradiated includes the entire breast, adjacent chest wall, and the regional lymph nodes. This encompasses the same area that is treated with the more conventional approach of local mastectomy and postoperative therapy. Whether or not all of these areas need to be treated is a question to which no one has the answer, but at this time few radiation oncologists would be willing to compromise.

Patients treated definitively should have the contours of the tumor and the isodose distributions of the radiation plotted out for their treatment. Often, wedges are used in the tangential fields to compensate for the

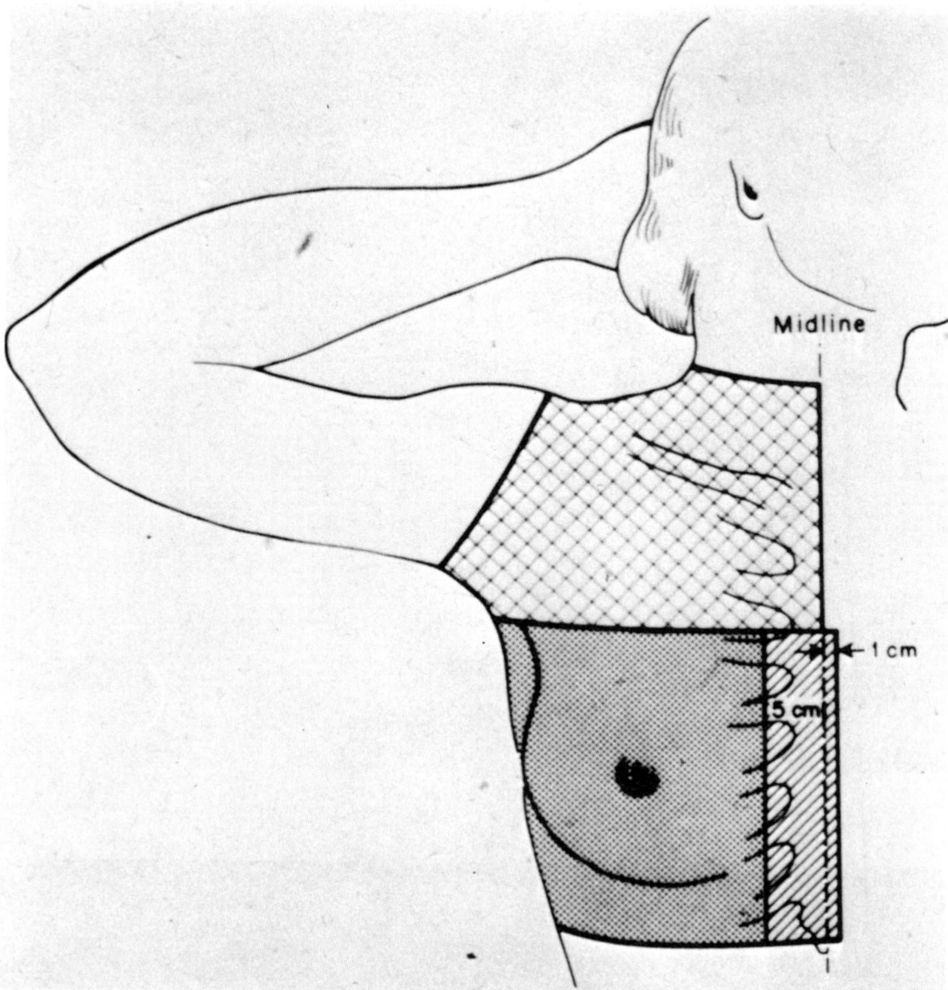

Fig. 33.1. *Areas at risk. (Prosnitz and Goldenberg 1975. Reprinted by permission.)*

sloping surface. A separate internal mammary chain (IMC) port is generally used in patients with a wide separation between tumor and IMC or when the tangential port films include an excessive amount of lung in the field. In patients having an intact breast it is best to avoid a separate internal mammary field if possible. The supraclavicular field is usually angled 15° to avoid the trachea, esophagus, and spinal cord. Blocks are best placed over the head of the humerus and a portion of the shoulder joint. Supervoltage is essential for this type of treatment to achieve a uniform dose to the areas under consideration. The entire procedure is well described in the literature (Prosnitz and Goldenberg 1975).

Side effects of radical radiation for breast cancer are both acute and chronic. The acute reactions are restricted to local skin changes that are transient and vary from a dry desquamation and hyperpigmentation to areas of moist desquamation that heal rapidly. Late reactions that occur many months after therapy have included rib fractures in a few cases. These usually heal without difficulty. Rare cases of radiation-related pulmonary reaction consisting of mild shortness of breath and cough have also been reported. Other complications include pericarditis, chest wall necrosis, brachial plexus problems, arm edema, and fibrosis of the shoulder joint; these are extremely rare and most have been consequences of bad technique. Apical lung fibrosis is commonly seen but has always been asymptomatic.

Local control has been excellent with definitive radiation, reported by Harris, Levene, and Hellman (1978), to be over 95%. At five years the relapse-free survival is 91% for stage I and 56% for stage II disease.

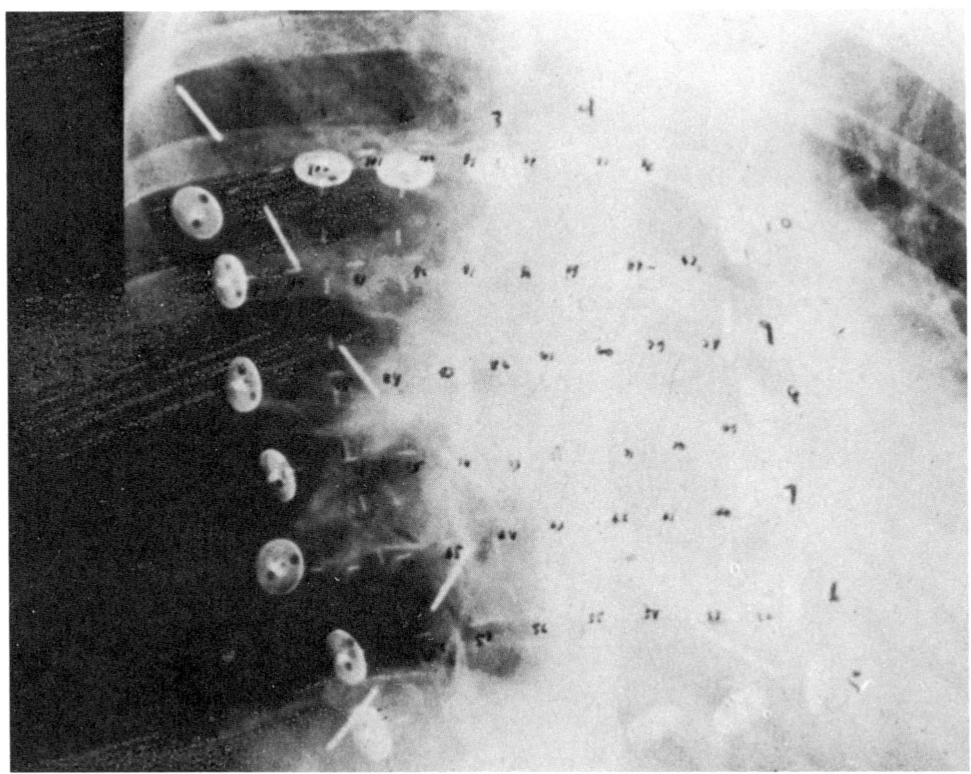

Fig. 33.2. *Radioactive iridium implant of the breast.*

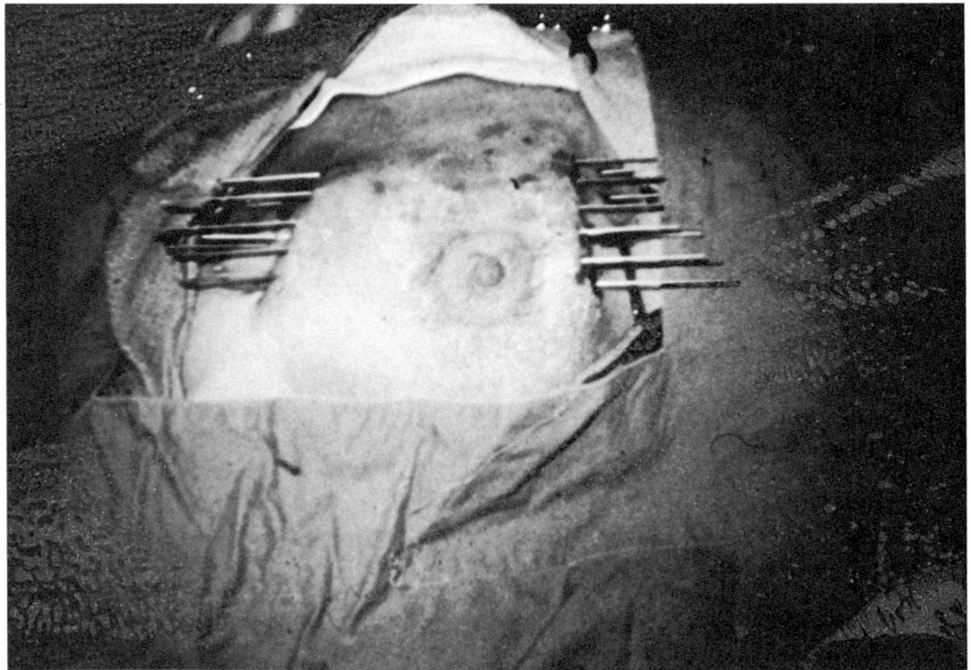

Fig. 33.3. *Hollow implant needles for radioactive iridium.*

Prosnitz (1978), a staunch advocate for definitive radiation therapy, reported on over 250 patients with stage I disease from a multiinstitutional study who had overall survival of 97% and disease-free survival of 92%. Those with clinical stage II disease had overall survival at five years of 80% and disease-free survival of 60%. In this series the patients were staged clinically, they had no axillary dissection, and did not receive adjuvant chemotherapy. When local radical radiation fails the patient still may be salvaged by surgery. Prosnitz and associates (1977) reported on 10 patients who had local recurrence, 5 of whom were disease-free following mastectomy.

As survival appears almost identical regardless of local approach, the psychological, cosmetic, and functional result is what will prove the difference. The overall result with radiation has been most satisfactory. Harris and co-workers (1978) evaluated 29 patients to determine cosmetic results. A 4-point scale was used with excellent being 1. The cosmetic results at 18 months were scored on an average of 1.43 and at 42 months of 1.50, indicative of excellent cosmesis. Careful treatment planning, supervoltage equipment, wedge filters, and judicial use of large fractions have contributed to this. Women with large pendulous breasts are more difficult to treat and have less satisfactory results.

Palliative Radiation

The object of palliative radiation is to provide comfort, not longevity. Most often it takes the form of relief of pain and the maintenance of structural integrity resulting in patient mobility. It must be remembered that retreatment of an area can lead to problems, as one may exceed the normal tissue tolerance.

There are several time-dose combinations that will give excellent palliation for the patient with carcinoma of the breast. Such possibilities are 3000 rad in two weeks, 4000 rad in three weeks, or even 2000 rad in one week. In the very debilitated patient with a limited future the number of fractions should be correspondingly short, as the physical coming and going for treatment can be very difficult. Occasionally, single doses of 1000 rad are extremely effective, although symptomatic relief is not as prolonged as that accomplished when the fractionation is given over a longer period of time. In someone whose life span is extremely short, symptomatic relief can often be accomplished with a single treatment.

Bone pain is one of the most frequent problems requiring palliative therapy in patients with carcinoma of the breast. Other problems seen less often are brain metastases as evidenced by headaches, nausea, vomiting, and weakness, with an accompanying positive brain scan or CT scan. Pulmonary metastasis may cause hemoptysis, cough, and shortness of breath. Occasional esophageal obstruction by hilar adenopathy or other paraesophageal metastasis can be a problem. Recurrent chest nodules following mastectomy are often present, and even when a complete evaluation might indicate that there are no other metastatic deposits, experience will bear out that over 75% of these patients eventually develop systemic disease. Thus they need local treatment to eradicate the chest nodules, as well as systemic therapy. Symptoms such as esophageal obstruction and bleeding are nearly always cleared by palliative radiation, whereas shortness of breath, cough, and hoarseness are virtually impossible to eradicate.

Radiotherapy is the most useful single agent for palliation of local symptoms secondary to breast metastasis. Large fungating tumors of the breast that bleed easily and are extremely malodorous often can be greatly reduced in size and cleaned up considerably; however, they may require a near radical approach to do this. As many of these patients will live for long periods of time, radiotherapy of this nature is justified. Radiation plays little or no role in diffuse lymphangitic spread throughout the lung and in pleural and peritoneal effusions. Although more commonly seen in other cancers, superior vena cava syndrome consisting of obstruction by local adenopathy and resulting in swelling of the head and face is a radiotherapy emergency. These symptoms can usually be resolved quickly within a few days of starting treatment.

Pathologic fractures are relatively common in carcinoma of the breast. One frequently sees impending fractures, and an attempt to sterilize the area locally should be undertaken so the site may heal, although such healing of a postradiation area is slow. An actual pathologic fracture of the femur is best managed by internal fixation followed by radiation therapy. Internal fixation leads to faster mobilization, and that is the aim of palliation. Often, uncertainty exists as to when an orthopedic consultation is necessary in a lytic lesion of the femur. A useful rule is to obtain one in any painful lesion over 2.5 cm in diameter or in any patient whose lesion is over 2.5 cm in diameter and involves the cortex.

Metastatic disease to the brain is also very common, and many of these patients will have short survival. They should be given steroids, and radiation therapy should be initiated immediately. Most often the steroids will relieve the symptoms quickly and radiation can be completed without a great deal of difficulty. In such patients a useful regimen is 100 rad the first day,

200 rad the second day, and then 10 treatments of 300 rad through two lateral fields for a total of 3300 rad. In the patient who appears to have limited disease and is expected to have a longer life, if she has been well evaluated by means of a CAT scan it is often advisable to give an additional three or four treatments to a single area of metastatic cerebral disease.

Physicians must also be alert to early detection of spinal cord metastasis. A myelogram is essential to demonstrate the site of block. Since paraplegia can rapidly develop, early treatment is indicated; again, such patients should be classified as emergencies. In patients who are not already paraplegic our policy is to begin a course of steroids and radiation therapy. The total amount of radiation given will be 3000 rad in two weeks or 4000 rad in four weeks. When paraplegia has already set in or when weakness is apparent, a decompression laminectomy may be indicated.

Occasionally a patient is seen for ablation of the ovaries. Ovarian function can be eradicated with three or four treatments to the pelvis using parallel opposed ports for a total dose of 1200 to 1600 rad. In younger patients, the addition of an extra treatment appears justified.

Thanks to great advances in the field of medical oncology patients are living longer today, and the aim of palliative radiation is not just the relief of symptoms but relief for a prolonged period of time. Although longevity may be increased, the aim is to maximize the quality of patients' remaining days. Prolongation of life without this is not palliation. Most treatments should be carried out on a supervoltage unit with as much thought and care as are given to a patient who can be cured.

There still remain many unanswered questions regarding management of patients with carcinoma of the breast. One issue that needs to be settled is the value of postoperative radiation therapy following mastectomy. Does this increase survival? Is it necessary in view of advances in medical oncology? What patients are suitable for definitive radiation? It is accepted by most that postoperative chemotherapy in premenopausal women increases disease-free survival (Bonadonna et al. 1976). Newer data would indicate that when full-dosage chemotherapy is given even postmenopausal women will have disease-free survival increased (Bonadonna and Valagussa 1980). The size of the primary lesion and status of axillary lymph nodes are the bases on which the decision is made to give adjuvant postoperative chemotherapy. Controversy exists as to whether a patient who will undergo a so-called lumpectomy and be scheduled for definitive radiation should at the time of operation have an axillary lymph node sampling carried out, so that if nodes are positive chemotherapy may be administered. Most medical oncologists feel strongly that they should, since adjuvant chemotherapy has shown an increase in the disease-free survival in patients with multiple positive nodes. Many radiotherapy physicians feel that patients are carefully selected for definitive radiation, resulting in a disease-free survival so high in stage I disease that it would be difficult to improve on it by chemotherapy. This does not appear to be the case, however, in stage II cancer, and hence little doubt remains that axillary sampling should be carried out in these patients. One must always keep in mind that, in general, this disease is systemic. The data on radical radiation for the most part do not go beyond 5 to 10 years.

Another problem not yet settled is the value of postoperative radiation in view of the advances of medical oncology (Holland, Glidewell, and Cooper 1980). I advocate such therapy when the primary tumor is large, namely, stage II or III, and then follow this with chemotherapy. We know for certain that postoperative radiation does decrease the local recurrence rate and that definitive radiotherapy is highly effective in early disease. Data are beginning to accumulate that such treatment of more advanced malignancy will also increase disease-free survival. Better clinical trials addressed to today's problems are presently under way, and in the near future there should be less controversy and more concrete data allowing us to proceed with treatment we know is best, and not treatment we think is best.

References

Bonadonna, G. et al. Combination chemotherapy as an adjuvant treatment in operable breast cancer. *N. Engl. J. Med.* 294:405–410, 1976.

Bonadonna, G., and Valagussa, P. Dose-response effect of CMF in breast cancer. *Proc. Am. Soc. Clin. Oncol.* 21:413, 1980.

Caldwell, W. Preoperative irradiation for locally advanced breast cancer. *Cancer* 28:1647–1650, 1971.

Edland, R. et al. Postoperative irradiation in breast cancer. *Radiology* 93:905–913, 1969.

Fletcher, G. Local results of irradiation in the primary management of localized breast cancer. *Cancer* 29:545–551, 1972.

Fox, M. S. On the diagnosis and treatment of breast cancer. *JAMA* 241:489–494, 1979.

Harris, J.; Levene, M.; and Hellman, S. Results of treating stage I and II carcinoma of the breast with primary radiation therapy. *Cancer Treat. Rep.* 62:985–991, 1978.

Holland, J. F.; Glidewell, O.; and Cooper, R. G. Adverse effect of radiotherapy on adjuvant chemotherapy for carcinoma of the breast. *Surg. Gynecol. Obstet.* 150:817–821, 1980.

Host, H., and Brennhovd, I. The effect of post-operative radiotherapy in breast cancer. *Int. J. Radiat. Oncol. Biol. Phys.* 2:1061–1067, 1977.

Levene, M.; Harris, J.; and Hellman, S. Treatment of carcinoma of the breast by radiation therapy. *Cancer* 39:2840–2845, 1977.

Prosnitz, L. Radiation therapy as initial treatment for breast cancer: is mastectomy necessary? *Conn. Med.* 42:639–641, 1978.

Prosnitz, L. et al. Radiation therapy as initial treatment for early stage cancer of the breast without mastectomy. *Cancer* 39:917–923, 1977.

Prosnitz, L., and Goldenberg, I. Radiation therapy as primary treatment for early stage carcinoma of the breast. *Cancer* 35:1587–1596, 1975.

Stoker, T., and Ellis, H. Post-irradiation toilet mastectomy in the management of locally advanced carcinoma of the breast. *Br. J. Radiol.* 45:851–854, 1972.

Wallgren, A. et al. The value of preoperative radiotherapy in operable mammary carcinoma. *Int. J. Radiat. Oncol. Biol. Phys.* 6:287–290, 1980.

thirty-four

Systemic Therapy of Breast Cancer

JOHN C. MARSH

Breast cancer is an extremely important disease. It is estimated that about 1 out of 15 women in the United States will develop this disease at some time in her life. Each year the diagnosis is made in more than 100,000 women and 35,000 die of it. It is the most common cause of cancer death in women, and it is the single most frequently seen disease in the majority of oncologic practices. The need for systemic therapy is evidenced by the fact that only about 25% to 30% of patients are cured of their disease, which may be present over a long period of time, and in which it is possible to induce either partial or complete regression with many types of agents, both cytotoxic and hormonal. There is beginning to be slight evidence that immunotherapy may also have a role. The definition of the role of estrogen receptors as a guide to treatment, introduction of antiestrogens as a class of useful, relatively nontoxic agents in the therapy of patients with hormonally sensitive tumors, and successful application of adjuvant chemotherapy in high-risk patients, are the major advances that have occurred in the last decade.

Systemic therapy is indicated in basically two situations (Haskell et al. 1977). In the first, the patient is identifiable as having a high risk of recurrence following her initial local treatment, in which case therapy is adjuvant. In the second, the patient has obvious metastatic disease. The two major modalities at the present time are hormonal and cytotoxic. It is now possible to predict the likelihood of patients responding to hormonal therapy by determining the estrogen and progesterone receptor proteins in either the primary tumor or in metastases.

At the time of initial diagnosis 10% of patients have obvious disseminated disease, 45% have localized disease, and 45% regional disease. More than half of all patients with breast cancer will die prematurely within 10 years of their diagnosis, and mortality from the disease may occur more than 20 years after primary treatment.

The historical obsession with patterns of local recurrence has neglected the reality that, for the most part, this is a disseminated disease. Only 20% of patients have their first recurrence in the operative site, while in 45% it is in the skeleton, and in another 12% in the lungs or hilum. In most patients breast cancer is probably disseminated at the time of diagnosis. It may be estimated that to become a palpable mass a tumor cell must have undergone at least 30 doublings, and it is known that even from masses of small size, breast cancer cells may be shed in the circulation. Many, though not all, probably survive as micrometastases. These are initially not detectable, but with the passage of time lead to overt metastatic disease.

Prognostic Factors in Advanced Breast Cancer

Survival in the presence of advanced disease is influenced by the site of metastatic involvement, the total extent of metastases, disease-free interval, performance status, menopausal status, and the presence or absence of

Table 34.1. *Effect of Axillary Lymph Node Involvement on Recurrence and Survival Rates*

Involvement	*Recurrence (%)*			*Survival (%)*	
	18 months	*5 years*	*10 years*	*5 years*	*10 years*
Negative nodes	5	18	24	78	65
Positive nodes	33	65	76	46	25
Positive nodes (1–3)	13	50	64	62	38
Positive nodes (> 3)	52	79	86	32	13
All patients	17	40	50	64	46

SOURCE: Modified from Fisher et al. 1975.

hormonal receptors in tumor tissue. Patients with involvement of the liver or the central nervous system have a very short median survival time—less than six months. For other sites, mortality is related to the number of sites involved rather than to specific areas. Involvement of the bone marrow, which was once thought to be of ominous significance, is not necessarily uncontrollable when patients are treated with modern combination chemotherapy. The time between initial diagnosis and development of recurrent metastatic disease is important in subsequent survival. Patients with a disease-free interval of less than one year have a median survival of less than six months from the time of recurrence, while patients with a disease-free interval greater than five years live a median of 25 months after recurrence. This is an important stratification factor that is sometimes overlooked in comparative clinical trials. As with many other metastatic cancers, the patient who is ambulatory at the time of diagnosis of recurrent disease survives nearly twice as long as one who is bedridden. As a group, postmenopausal women live longer than premenopausal women following relapse of their disease.

Adjuvant Therapy

As shown in table 34.1, the presence or absence of axillary lymph node involvement and the number of such nodes can allow an estimate of the likelihood of disease recurrence and survival. At the extremes, the chance of recurrence is 24% at 10 years in women with negative nodes, while in women with more than three positive nodes, it is 86%. It should be kept in mind that the 5- and 10-year intervals are only convenient measurement points, and that survival continues to decrease over time. Tumor size can also be used as a rough index of prognosis. Because of the dismal results of local therapy in the group with histologically involved nodes, this finding can be used to identify patients as candidates for adjuvant therapy; several studies have already been done. One of the first of these used the alkylating agent thiotepa, given very briefly at the time of operation and shortly thereafter (Fisher et al. 1975). While this had no significant effect for the entire group, it did appear promising in premenopausal women with a large number of involved nodes. Prophylactic castration was also not successful for the overall group with respect to survival, although it did appear to prolong the disease-free interval. These studies were done without knowledge of the estrogen receptors of the patients involved, and it is possible that the outcome would have been different had the study been confined to patients with estrogen receptors in their tumors.

One of the most successful studies was that of the National Surgical Adjuvant Breast Project in which patients with positive axillary nodes were treated with the oral alkylating agent phenylalanine mustard (melphalan) (Fisher et al. 1977). The drug was given over a two-year period intermittently every six weeks. In premenopausal women the disease-free proportion was 79% as compared with 59% in the control group, a statistically significant difference. A significant survival difference was also achieved. No significant survival advantage was achieved in postmenopausal women.

The best known surgical adjuvant study involves the use of the three-drug regimen, cyclophosphamide, methotrexate, and 5-fluorouracil (CMF), and was carried out by the National Cancer Institute in Milan, Italy (Bonadonna et al. 1977). Here too, the results were highly significant with respect both to relapse-free interval and survival in premenopausal but not postmenopausal women. The drugs were given over a one-year period. It is of interest that of the postmenopausal women there was an initial difference in the recurrence rate between the treated and the control groups, but this rapidly disappeared after chemotherapy was discontinued. In a recent analysis of these data it was found that postmenopausal women who were able to receive at least 85% of the planned CMF dose did have a statistically superior five-year relapse-free survival (75%) compared to that of nondrug-treated patients (49%), or those receiving less than 85% of the optimal dose (49% to 56%) (Bonadonna and Valagussa 1981). The efficacy in premenopausal women does not correlate with the development of amenorrhea in these patients. Preliminary results comparing CMF given for 6 months to 12 months show no significant difference.

At present, while the adjuvant chemotherapy of premenopausal women with positive axillary lymph nodes seems to be well established as standard practice, this is not yet true for postmenopausal women. Other studies in progress are suggestive of benefit, but by no means definitive. A study by Cooper, Holland, and Glidewell (1979) without concurrent controls has claimed a dramatic increase in survival over historical high-risk controls in patients given nine months of adjuvant chemotherapy with a five-drug regimen (vincristine, prednisone, cyclophosphamide, methotrexate, and 5-fluorouracil). There was no difference between the disease-free survival of premenopausal and postmenopausal women. Patients given chest wall radiotherapy with a consequent delay before beginning chemotherapy fared much more poorly (Holland, Glidewell, and Cooper 1980). The routine use of postoperative radiotherapy to the chest wall has recently been criticized, since it does *not* improve survival (Lipsett 1981). Additional adjuvant studies to evaluate the role of different chemotherapy, the place of antiestrogens, and the relationship of estrogen-binding proteins are in progress. Yale is participating in the programs of the Eastern Cooperative Oncology Group in hopes of clarifying some of these issues.

Hormonal Therapy of Advanced Breast Cancer

Several endocrine factors are known to be of importance in breast cancer. Estrogens are cocarcinogens in rodents. The incidence of breast cancer is 100-fold greater in women than in men, and occurs after puberty. It is not seen in ovarian dysgenesis. Incidence is diminished after castration, and early pregnancy appears to have a somewhat protective role against the disease (MacMahon, Cole, and Brown 1973). Women with long menstrual lives have more breast cancer than those whose menstrual lives are relatively short (Olch 1937; Wynder, Bross, and Hirayama 1960). Estrogen may induce exacerbations, while both endocrine ablation or the addition of various hormonal agents may induce remissions.

The response rate to various kinds of hormonal treatment in advanced disease, whether ablative (castration, adrenalectomy, hypophysectomy) or additive (estrogen, antiestrogen, progestational agents), is about 30% for all patients and somewhat lower when androgens are used. An objective response is usually defined as at least 50% decrease in the product of the perpendicular diameters of a measurable lesion by either physical examination or chest x-ray. Specific criteria are also available for measuring the response of liver lesions in terms of decreasing hepatomegaly. While some of these endocrine manipulations can and should be used sequentially, there is no specific use for castration in postmenopausal women; estrogens are usually avoided in premenopausal women for fear of exacerbation of disease, although they are usually the first treatment given to women more than five years postmenopausal.

Significant survival advantages are achieved by these treatments, and the duration of remission may sometimes be measured in years. For example, in one experience, responders to oophorectomy had a mean survival of 33 months compared to 9 months for nonresponders (Legha, Davis, and Muggia 1978). Endocrine manipulation is a satisfactory treatment because it is usually more benign than cytotoxic chemotherapy, and the durations of remission when they occur are usually longer. It is not uncommon for a patient to respond to several such hormonal treatments when they are applied sequentially. This is our method as long as it is successful. The response rate to hypophysectomy and adrenalectomy is about the same, and there appears to be no virtue in doing both. The choice between these two procedures is usually dictated by local surgical expertise and experience. With any hormonal treatment, one must be aware of the development of hypercalcemia in patients with bone metastases. It is of interest that many patients will have so-called rebound response when a particular hormonal treatment is discontinued at the time of disease progression (Kaufman and Escher 1961).

Recent studies have shown that patients with tumors containing estrogen receptor proteins are likely to respond to various hormonal treatments with a probability of approximately 50% to 60%, or about twice that observed for patients chosen without regard for this factor. In contrast, in patients whose tumors have low levels of estrogen receptor, response rates are low (generally less than 10%) so as to render hormonal treatments virtually worthless (Legha, Davis, and Muggia 1978). Between 50% and 75% of patients have tumors with significant amounts of estrogen receptor proteins. Normal breast tissue, with the exception of the lactating breast, has a very low content of such protein. The presence of estrogen receptors is not related to histology, tumor size, or site of metastases. They may vary between the primary and metastatic sites in the same patient, although the frequency with which this occurs has been variable (Brennan, Donegan, and Appleby 1979). Experience thus far with regard to predictive value of estrogen receptor proteins is based largely on the content of the primary tumor, and it is not yet clear that measurement of binding protein in the metastatic deposits is any more accurate. The utility of the determination of estrogen receptor protein holds true for all types of hormonal treatment, and is useful for both premenopausal and postmenopausal women. Currently, its chief value is to allow the identification of women who are unlikely to respond to hormonal treatment.

It has recently been reported that the determination of receptors for progestational agents will add to the predictive value of estrogen receptor protein. Patients whose tumor contains both types of receptors are said to have more than an 80% likelihood of responding to hormonal therapy (McGuire et al. 1977).

In my opinion it is mandatory for every patient who has a removal of a breast cancer by biopsy or mastectomy to have a determination of estrogen receptor protein, and if possible, progestational receptor protein, since for about three-quarters of such patients this information will be crucial in making a therapeutic decision. This test now approaches the importance of the pathologic examination. If it is not done on the primary tumor, it should certainly be done on metastatic disease where possible. Indeed, this should probably be done in patients at the time of first relapse if the tissue is easily biopsied, because the presence or absence of estrogen receptors in metastases does not always mirror that in the primary tumor, and may be more pertinent in predicting therapeutic response.

Within the past few years, tamoxifen (Nolvadex), an antiestrogen, has been introduced commercially after several years of clinical trials (Tagnon 1977). It is safe, effective, and nontoxic. It is thought to interfere with binding of endogenous estrogen to estrogen-binding protein in the tumor cell, and thus to inhibit the estrogen-induced transformation of nuclear material, which is finally expressed in RNA and protein synthesis. There is also evidence that tamoxifen interferes with the reversible dissociation of the estrogen-binding protein-steroid complex. The drug inhibits estrogen-induced stimulation of DNA synthesis by breast cancer tissue culture lines in vitro. Its response rate for breast cancer in general, without regard for estrogen-binding protein, is about 35% (Ward 1973). It is about 50% for patients who are known to have estrogen receptor in their tumor.

The likelihood of response is increased in those patients who have a long disease-free interval, prior response to endocrine therapy, and soft tissue disease. Bone and visceral disease respond less frequently than soft tissue disease, but still have an appreciable response rate (Legha, Davis, and Muggia 1978). There is no good evidence for a dose-response curve, and a relatively low dosage of 10 mg twice a day seems adequate. The median duration of response ranges from 7 to 12 months. Although most experience has been with postmenopausal patients, premenopausal women may also respond. Indeed, response to tamoxifen in the premenopausal group has been reported to predict subsequent response to ovarian ablation (Thomson et al. 1980).

Toxicity is uncommon, consisting of nausea, vomiting, or hot flashes, which tend to disappear even though the drug is continued. About 10% of patients have transient bone marrow suppression that usually is of no clinical importance. In some patients a flare of tumor in the skin and increased bone pain may be noted during early days of treatment, but this is not an indication to discontinue therapy (Legha, Davis, and Muggia 1978; Ingle et al. 1981). In fact, it may indicate that response is occurring.

Before the introduction of tamoxifen, diethylstilbestrol (DES) was the treatment of choice in postmenopausal women with metastatic breast cancer. A recent randomized trial showed that the response rates are essentially the same, as are the durations of response, but that toxicity, largely gastrointestinal and fluid retention, is higher with DES (Ingle et al. 1981). In this group, tamoxifen should be the first systemic therapy used, followed by DES in responders when they relapse.

Androgens, progestational agents, and pituitary ablation may also play a role in subsequent treatment of both premenopausal and postmenopausal women. Adrenalectomy has been replaced in many places by a so-called medical adrenalectomy with the drug aminoglutethimide that inhibits the production of adrenal steroids (Santen and Wells 1980). As with other hormonal treatments, response rates are about 30% in unselected patients and about 50% in patients with tumors that have estrogen receptors. Remissions are durable (15 months in the Santen series). The optimal order of hormonal manipulation remains to be determined.

Cytotoxic Chemotherapy

Although there are many drugs that are active when used singly in breast cancer, combination chemotherapy is approximately twice as likely to induce a response and is the preferred treatment. Active agents in approximate order of activity include doxorubicin (Adriamycin), cyclophosphamide, methotrexate, hexamethylmelamine, dibromodulcitol, 5-fluorouracil, melphalan, vincristine, vinblastine, and mitomycin. Response rates to these agents used singly range from 20% to 35%. The disease free interval, site of dominant lesion, and menopausal status can all influence the response to particular agents. Thus in women with a long disease-free interval, doxorubicin seems to be substantially more active than either cyclophosphamide or 5-fluorouracil (Tormey 1977a). Perimenopausal patients are more likely to respond to cyclophosphamide or 5-fluorouracil than than to doxorubicin; whereas the reverse is true in women who are 10 or more years postmenopausal.

Successful combination chemotherapy regimens for advanced metastatic breast cancer have been developed using the principles that the drugs employed should have activity as single agents, that their mechanisms of action should be independent of one another, and that they should have side effects that do not overlap, thus permitting administration of effective doses of the individual agents.

One of the first combination regimens used was that of Greenspan and colleagues (1963), who combined the alkylating agent triethylenethiophosphoramide with the antimetabolite methotrexate, and achieved a response rate of 60%. This was twice that seen with either agent alone, and set the stage for the various combinations that have evolved. In 1969, Cooper reported a response rate of 90% for the five-drug regimen of cyclophosphamide, 5-fluorouracil, methotrexate, vincristine, and prednisone. Many subsequent studies have confirmed the activity of this combination, at an average response rate of about 50% to 60%. Simultaneous use of these drugs has generally given better results than sequential use: one study indicated a six-month increase in remission duration favoring simultaneous administration, due in part to an improved complete remission rate. Dissection of the original five-drug regimen indicated that the three most important drugs are cyclophosphamide, 5-fluorouracil, and methotrexate, with vincristine and prednisone adding relatively little (Davis and Carbone 1978). Thus the response rate is not increased in proportion to the number of agents used. One recent study by the Eastern Cooperative Oncology Group has shown a higher response rate for the four-drug combination cyclophosphamide (Cytoxan), methotrexate, 5-fluorouracil, and prednisone, that for the combination of the first three (63% versus 48%); and a longer duration of response (48 weeks versus 30 weeks) (Band, Tormey, and Bauer 1977). This result is the basis for using the four-drug program in adjuvant chemotherapy trials by this group.

Doxorubicin is probably the most active single agent but is not as effective when used alone as in combination. Combinations that contain doxorubicin are as active as any currently available, and some of the best results obtained occur when it is administered with cyclophosphamide. At Yale we found that such a combination was as effective as the four drugs doxorubicin, cyclophosphamide, methotrexate, and 5-fluorouracil, with a 50% response rate and 10-month median duration of remission with both regimens (Kennealey et al. 1978). Doxorubicin, then, is a very useful drug, and can be given either alone or in combination with vincristine in treating patients who relapse on such combinations as cyclophosphamide, methotrexate, and 5-fluorouracil. This has led to the hope that patients might be treated alternately with noncross-resistant regimens; as yet, this has not yet been shown to be effective in increasing the length of survival (Brambilla et al. 1976; Davis and Carbone 1978).

The serum carcinoembryonic antigen (CEA) is increased in about 50% of patients with metastatic breast cancer. In one study the response rate was much higher in patients who did not have elevated serum CEA than those who did (Tormey 1977b). This may be a function of the amount of disease present, with the response rate expected to be higher in patients with a smaller number of tumor cells and low CEA. This can be as useful a serial test of disease progression or regression in breast cancer as it is in colon cancer.

Because determination of the estrogen receptor protein was useful in predicting a response to hormonal therapy, it was logical to see whether it was also predictive for nonhormonal therapy. Data on this are conflicting. In one study from the National Cancer Institute (Lippman et al. 1978) the response rate to combination chemotherapy was much lower in patients whose tumors contained estrogen receptor protein (12%) as compared with those that did not (76%). At least three other institutions, however, have reported opposite results (Webster, Brown, and Minton 1978; Samal et al. 1978; Kiang et al. 1978). At this time, it would seem premature to choose nonhormonal chemotherapy on the basis of the presence or absence of estrogen receptors. Our current policy for patients who are candidates for hormonal therapy is to treat them so sequentially until failure, and then switch to nonhormonal therapy. In patients with negative estrogen receptors in their tumor, nonhormonal chemotherapy is the initial treatment.

There is beginning to be some evidence that combining hormonal and nonhormonal chemotherapy may be of some benefit. The duration of remission and survival after oophorectomy have been reported by van Dyk and Falkson (1971) to be increased when cyclophosphamide was added. The median survival for the combined group was 37 months after oophorectomy, as compared to 29 months for patients given oophorectomy alone with chemotherapy added at the first sign of relapse. Similar results have been reported from the Mayo Clinic using the three-drug combination of cyclophosphamide, 5-fluorouracil, and prednisone added to oophorectomy, with a median survival of 131 weeks, compared to 88 weeks for oophorectomy alone (Ahmann et al. 1977). The oral androgen fluoxymesterone prolongs the duration of remissions induced by combination chemotherapy, in the experience of one cooperative group (Tormey et al. 1979). Several current studies are evaluating the role of tamoxifen in this regard.

Immunotherapy

As with many other malignancies, it has been reported that patients who still have the ability to respond by skin test to delayed hypersensitivity antigens, such as tuberculin, have a better prognosis than those who do not. The disease-free interval and survival of patients with inoperable breast cancer treated with radiation therapy have been reported to be increased by the addition of the immunostimulant levamisole (Olivari et al. 1980). This and other immunotherapy studies are still investigational and require confirmation.

Summary

Current therapeutic recommendations are as follows. Following primary treatment with either mastectomy or high-dose supervoltage radiation therapy, premenopausal patients with positive axillary lymph nodes are candidates for adjuvant chemotherapy. The place for adjuvant chemotherapy has not yet been fully defined in postmenopausal women who should therefore not be so treated routinely until appropriate therapies have been established by on-going studies. Patients with metastatic disease should be treated with primary hormonal therapy if their tumor contains estrogen receptors or if estrogen receptor status is unknown, and with combination chemotherapy if their tumor does not contain estrogen receptors. Various types of hormonal therapy should be used sequentially until failure, at which time combination chemotherapy should be used. In the future, the role of immunotherapy may be expected to be better defined. The combination of hormonal and nonhormonal treatments will become increasingly important. The efficacy of such new methods of treatments as hyperthermia and interferon may be expected to be clarified.

References

Ahmann, D. L. et al. An evaluation of early or delayed adjuvant chemotherapy in premenopausal patients with advanced breast cancer undergoing oophorectomy. *N. Engl. J. Med.* 297:356–360, 1977.

Band, P. R.; Tormey, D. C.; and Bauer, M. Induction chemotherapy and maintenance chemohormonotherapy in metastatic breast cancer. *Proc. Am. Assoc. Cancer Res.* 18:228, 1977.

Bonadonna, G. et al. The CMF program for operable breast cancer with positive axillary nodes: update analysis on the disease-free interval, site of relapse and drug tolerance. *Cancer* 39:2904–2915, 1977.

Bonadonna, G., and Valagussa, P. Dose-response effect of adjuvant chemotherapy in breast cancer. *N. Engl. J. Med.* 304:16–20, 1981.

Brambilla, C. et al. Response and survival in advanced breast cancer after two non–cross-resistant combinations. *Br. Med. J.* 1:801–804, 1976.

Brennan, J. M.; Donegan, W. L.; and Appleby, D. E. The variability of estrogen receptors in metastatic breast cancer. *Am. J. Surg.* 137:260–262, 1979.

Cooper, R. G. Combination chemotherapy in hormone resistant breast cancer. *Proc. Am. Assoc. Cancer Res.* 10:15, 1969.

Cooper, R. G.; Holland, J. F.; and Glidewell, O. Adjuvant chemotherapy of breast cancer. *Cancer* 44:793–798, 1979.

Davis, T. E., and Carbone, P. P. Drug treatment of breast cancer. *Drug* 16:441–464, 1978.

Fisher, B. et al. Ten-year follow-up results of patients with carcinoma of the breast in a co-operative clinical trial evaluating surgical adjuvant chemotherapy. *Surg. Gynecol. Obstet.* 140:528–534, 1975.

Fisher, B. et al. L-phenylalanine mustard (L-PAM) in the management of primary breast cancer: an update of earlier findings and a comparison with those utilizing L-PAM plus 5-fluorouracil (5-FU). *Cancer* 39:2883–2903, 1977.

Greenspan, E. M. et al. Response of advanced breast carcinoma to the combination of the antimetabolite, methotrexate, and the alkylating agent, thiotepa. *J. Mt. Sinai Hosp.* 30:246–267, 1963.

Haskell, C. M. et al. Systemic therapy for metastatic breast cancer. *Ann. Intern. Med.* 86:68–80, 1977.

Holland, J. F.; Glidewell, O.; and Cooper, R. G. Adverse effect of radiotherapy on adjuvant chemotherapy for carcinoma of the breast. *Surg. Gynecol. Obstet.* 150:817–821, 1980.

Ingle, J. N. et al. Randomized clinical trial of diethylstilbestrol versus tamoxifen in postmenopausal women with advanced breast cancer. *N. Engl. J. Med.* 304:16–21, 1981.

Kaufman, R. J., and Escher, G. C. Rebound regression in advanced mammary carcinoma. *Surg. Gynecol. Obstet.* 113:635–640, 1961.

Kennealey, G. T. et al. Combination chemotherapy for advanced breast cancer: two regimens containing Adriamycin. *Cancer* 42:27–33, 1978.

Kiang, D. T. et al. Estrogen receptors and responses to chemotherapy and hormonal therapy in advanced breast cancer. *N. Engl. J. Med.* 299:1330–1334, 1978.

Legha, S. S.; Davis, H. L.; and Muggia, F. M. Hormonal therapy of breast cancer: new approaches and concepts. *Ann. Intern. Med.* 88:69–77, 1978.

Lippman, M. E. et al. The relation between estrogen receptors and response rate to cytotoxic chemotherapy in metastatic breast cancer. *N. Engl. J. Med.* 298: 1223–1228, 1978.

Lipsett, M. B. Postoperative radiation for women with cancer of the breast and positive axillary lymph nodes: should it continue? *N. Engl. J. Med.* 304:112–114, 1981.

MacMahon, B.; Cole, P.; and Brown, J. Etiology of human breast cancer: a review. *J. Natl. Cancer Inst.* 50:21–42, 1973.

McGuire, W. et al. Current status of estrogen and progesterone receptors in breast cancer. *Cancer* 39:2934–2947, 1977.

Olch, I. Y. Menopausal age in women with cancer of the breast. *Am. J. Cancer* 30:563–566, 1937.

Olivari, A. J. et al. Six years' follow-up in levamisole-treated stage III breast cancer patients. *Proc. Am. Soc. Clin. Oncol.* 21:362, 1980.

Samal, B. et al. Estrogen receptors and response of breast cancer to chemotherapy (correspondence). *N. Engl. J. Med.* 299:604, 1978.

Santen, R. J., and Wells, S. A., Jr. The use of aminoglutethimide in the treatment of patients with metastatic carcinoma of the breast. *Cancer* 46:1066–1074, 1980.

Tagnon, H. J. Anti-estrogens in the treatment of breast cancer. *Cancer* 39:2959–2964, 1977.

Thomson, D. B. et al. Tamoxifen response: a useful guide to subsequent treatment in premenopausal patients with metastatic breast cancer. *Proc. Am. Soc. Clin. Oncol.* 21:407, 1980.

Tormey, D. C. Single agent chemotherapy and comparisons with combination therapy in advanced breast cancer, pp. 790–791 in Young, R. C. (moderator): perspectives in the treatment of breast cancer: 1976. *Ann. Intern. Med.* 86:784–798, 1977a.

Tormey, D. C. Search for marker substances in breast cancer, pp. 794–796 in Young, R. C. (moderator): perspectives in the treatment of breast cancer: 1976. *Ann. Intern. Med.* 86:784–798, 1977b.

Tormey, D. C. et al. Impact of chemohormonal therapy upon maintenance in advanced breast cancer. *Proc. Am. Soc. Clin. Oncol.* 20:356, 1979.

van Dyk, J. J., and Falkson, G. Extended survival and remission rates in metastatic breast cancer. *Cancer* 27:300–303, 1971.

Ward, H. W. C. Anti-oestrogen therapy for breast cancer: a trial of tamoxifen at two dose levels. *Br. Med. J.* 1:13–14, 1973.

Webster, D. J. T.; Brown, D. G.; and Minton, J. P. Estrogen receptors and response of breast cancer to chemotherapy (correspondence). *N. Engl. J. Med.* 299:604, 1978.

Wynder, E. L.; Bross, I. J.; and Hirayama, T. A study of the epidemiology of cancer of the breast. *Cancer* 13:559–601, 1960.

thirty-five

Reconstruction after Mastectomy

PHILIP F. CORSO

Over 90,000 women in the United States will undergo mastectomy this year for cancer (Leis 1977; Schmitz 1979). Of this number only a small proportion, 5% to 7%, will eventually seek and undergo reconstruction (Robson 1978; Synderman 1974, 1977, 1978). This chapter attempts to determine why such a small fraction ultimately seek correction of the deformity, and discusses the current techniques available and prevailing attitudes regarding management of the uninvolved breast.

Although statistics regarding breast cancer are frequently mentioned, they deserve reemphasis. Approximately one woman dies of breast cancer every 15 minutes in the United States, and 7% of women will develop the disease. Almost 10% of women who live to the age of 85 years will develop breast cancer. Of the over 90,000 women treated with mastectomy annually in this country, most will undergo a so-called modified radical operation, while a minority will undergo a so-called Halsted classical radical procedure (Schmitz 1979). The absolute five-year survival rates for patients with the more common lobular and infiltrating carcinomas are in the range of 70% (Anderson and Pallesen 1979; Donegan and Perez-Mesa 1972; Foote and Stewart 1945).

It would be unfair and unrealistic to suppose that every patient with breast cancer could or should have a modified mastectomy that would preserve the pectoralis major and thereby present the plastic surgeon with an ideal situation for reconstruction. Although there may be some truth in the theory that a bigger operation is not necessarily a better operation, I do believe there is wisdom in the attitude that a living patient cured of her disease with a major defect is preferable to a dead patient with a minor defect (Robson 1978; Synderman 1977, 1979).

In the past, similar to the attitude that surrounded reconstructive surgery of the head and neck, the feeling was that reconstructive surgery could alter the course of breast cancer following mastectomy. I believe there is an adequate volume of statistical information to show that reconstructive surgery in no way alters the ultimate outcome of breast cancer (Bostwick, Vasconez, and Jurkiewicz 1978; Lynch, Madden, and Franklin 1978). It is not and should not be the role of the plastic surgeon to dictate or direct the method of treatment of this disease. There cannot, however, be a cavalier attitude on the part of the general surgeon to discourage, deny, or dissuade the patient postmastectomy from considering reconstructive surgery (Guthrie 1978; Guthrie and Imber 1979; Hartwell et al. 1976).

Premastectomy Consultation with a Plastic Surgeon

This topic has provoked some understandable friction between general surgeons and plastic surgeons. Experience has shown that the majority of patients who are offered the opportunity of preoperative consultation with a plastic surgeon and advised by their general surgeon that opportunities for reconstruction are definitely possible actually do not request the consultation. They appear to be satisfied and adequately reassured to have the general surgeon perform their mastectomy (Bostwick, Vasconez, and Jurkiewicz 1978; Cronin and Upton 1978; Synderman 1979).

Just knowing that the possibility of reconstructive surgery exists enables a patient to face the prospect of losing the breast with greater equanimity. It has been suggested that the more completely she is informed preoperatively regarding reconstruction, the less likely she is actually to consider it postoperatively (Synderman 1977, 1979). I have made it a practice to emphasize that the first goal in the treatment of all patients with breast cancer is cure—the removal of all cancerous and potentially cancerous tissue of the breast and the surrounding structures (Hicken 1940). If the patient chooses to initiate a discussion concerning incisions and preservation of various structures such as the pectoralis muscle or the areola-nipple complex, I usually say that I will discuss these aspects of surgery with her general surgeon. I refrain from making commitments or indulging in long explanations that would commit the general surgeon to principles that may not be consistent with good cancer surgery. In this regard, it is desirable for a general surgeon to be familiar with the philosophy and attitudes of the particular plastic surgeon to whom a premastectomy patient, or indeed a postmastectomy patient, may be referred. It will answer most of the patient's questions and avoid conflicting statements by the two physicians (Hauschild 1970; Lynch, Madden, and Franklin 1978; Robson 1978).

The Postmastectomy Patient and Reconstructive Surgery

There are many factors to consider in evaluating the postmastectomy patient seeking reconstructive surgery. Age should be no reason for denial. Patients as old as 75 or 80 will frequently seek reconstruction and for extremely valid reasons, one of them being severe discrepancy between the size of the mastectomy side and the remaining breast, difficulty in finding clothing that fits, and reluctance to participate in physical activities when the mastectomy appears quite obvious. Presuming there are no medical contraindications and that the patient can tolerate anesthesia satisfactorily, age should not be a barrier.

The stage of the disease can be a major consideration. It is my feeling that in patients with stage III disease, it is desirable to wait a minimum of 6 months and preferably 12 to 18 months, since these are patients with the poorest prognosis (Hauschild 1970; Lynch, Madden, and Franklin 1978). As is well known, the majority of recurrences, about 80%, will appear within the first 18 to 24 months, and it seems reasonable to be assured that the patient is free of disease for at least that period of time (Leis 1977).

Ideally, most plastic surgeons feel that six months should elapse between the mastectomy and subsequent reconstructive surgery. During this time the patient is usually able to regain total motion of her shoulder and arm, and this should be one prerequisite prior to reconstruction. Also, there should be complete healing of the flaps and a reasonable degree of mobility of the flaps overlying either the pectoralis or chest wall. Interestingly, it has been observed that patients who have preservation of the pectoralis muscles (both major and minor) may require a longer period of time for total rehabilitation of shoulder-arm motion because of the associated pain, injury, and scarring caused by the surgery overlying that muscle. Patients who have undergone a classical Halsted mastectomy with removal of the pectoralis major and minor frequently show earlier rehabilitation of the shoulder-arm area (Guthrie 1978; Guthrie and Imber 1979).

Chemotherapy and/or radiation therapy can delay reconstructive surgery. Most plastic surgeons feel that if postoperative irradiation is to be given, a period of three to six months following completion of therapy should be observed.

There exist two philosophies regarding chemotherapy. One subscribes to the theory that reconstructive surgery can be done during chemotherapy, since there is no evidence to indicate that the low dosages normally used interfere with wound healing. Conventionally, the reconstruction will be done during the quiescent interval of the therapy program. The second attitude is that reconstructive surgery should be withheld until chemotherapy is completed; however, this may be as long as two years. The patient need not be turned down out of hand, and generally it is appropriate for the plastic surgeon to discuss the surgery with the chemotherapist and arrive at a decision most appropriate for the patient.

Advances in the past few years have made it possible to reconstruct the breasts of virtually every mastectomy patient regardless of the original procedure that was carried out. Obviously, the extent of the original operation has a direct bearing on the type and magnitude of reconstruction. It is apparent that preservation of the pectoralis major makes it infinitely easier to perform subsequent reconstructive procedures. Sacrifice of the muscle frequently necessitates a major operation for the purpose of bringing up adequate tissue to the pectoral area for coverage of the implant that is to be inserted simultaneously or subsequently (Bostwick, Vasconez, and Jurkiewicz 1978).

Although many general surgeons do preserve the pectoralis major, occasionally the nerve to the muscle is injured, ultimately resulting in neurogenic atrophy of the pectoralis, thereby simulating a condition in which the muscle was actually removed. Therefore it should be emphasized that if the muscle is to be preserved, its nerve supply should also be. The Halsted radical mastectomy is by far the most difficult type to reconstruct because of the hollowness below the clavicular area. In a large series of patients who were surveyed regarding their mastectomy defects, it was found that the infraclavicular defect was the most disturbing (Robson 1978).

Type of Mastectomy

As previously stated, a plastic surgeon can only suggest to the general surgeon those mastectomy incisions that make subsequent reconstruction easier. Perhaps the easiest way for a general surgeon to appreciate the problems facing a plastic surgeon regarding the placement of incisions, would be to look at the patient with her brassiere on and then plan the incision so that it would be concealed by the brassiere (Cronin and Upton 1978). Consequently, the ideal incisions would be oblique or horizontal, would not extend below the inframammary fold or up into the axillary hair-bearing skin, and would not extend across the midline of the chest. The most popular incisions are oblique and horizontal, and most plastic surgeons would prefer the oblique one that goes along the lateral border of the pectoralis muscle, since reconstruction is infinitely simplified if the muscle can be used.

Preoperative Evaluation

Where the interval of time is six months or more, I believe every patient should have at least a mammogram of the remaining breast and a bone scan in addition to the usual blood counts and chemistries. Although local recurrence is an early sign of recurrent carcinoma, lesions seen on bone scans may be the first sign of metastatic disease. Reconstructive surgery in the face of either problem is difficult to justify.

Once the patient has survived a six-month interval following mastectomy and laboratory tests indicate she is free of disease, what is to be discussed and what are the possibilities for reconstructive surgery? There are three major considerations: reconstruction (1) of the breast mound itself, (2) of the areola-nipple complex, and (3) of the subclavicular defect, if necessary, in those patients who have had a Halsted mastectomy.

In addition, several considerations must be discussed with the patient regarding the other breast. First of all would be the possibility of some type of surgery to remove the remaining breast tissue in the opposite breast, for example, subcutaneous mastectomy with immediate reconstruction. Statistics indicate the opposite breast carries a risk of 3% to 30% of developing carcinoma, depending on the age of the patient, the type of carcinoma in the original tumor (intralobular malignancy carrying the highest incidence of bilaterality), whether or not the patient is premenopausal or postmenopausal, and family history (Leis 1977). The role of subcutaneous mastectomy for the opposite breast will be discussed subsequently. Another consideration is that frequently the opposite breast would eventually require some type of procedure, most commonly a reduction mammaplasty to achieve symmetry with the reconstructed breast (Amaacki et al. 1979; Donegan and Parez-Mesa 1972; Pennisi and Capozzi 1975).

It should be emphasized to the patient that there are two goals in reconstructing breasts: *volumetric* equality and *geometric* equality. Volumetric equality—creating a breast mound on the reconstructed side that will equal the opposite un-operated breast—is easier to achieve. Geometric equality, in which the appearance of the breasts is similar, is more difficult (figs. 35.1 and 35.2). It has been the experience of virtually every plastic surgeon that as improvements in technique develop, expectations of the patient develop equally as rapidly (Birnbaum and Olsen 1978). If the patient has had a conventional modified mastectomy in which there has been preservation of the pectoralis major, the conventional technique to reconstruct the mound is to insert a silicone prosthesis below the muscle. Frequently, it is necessary also to elevate portions of the serratus anterior muscle as well as a portion of the rectus to achieve an adequate pocket to insert a prosthesis of sufficient size. It is remarkable how large a prosthesis can be inserted subpectorally, with 230- to 300-cc prostheses not uncommon on the postmastectomy side (Birnbaum and Olsen 1978). In those patients in whom there is an inadequate amount of skin for insertion of a prosthesis and creation of a mound, the possibility of developing a flap on the lateral thoracic aspect and subsequently rotating it into the wound must be considered. This type of flap—the so-called thoracoepigastric flap—is quite useful. It can be elevated and inserted as a one-stage procedure. If it is unusually long, however, a delayed proce-

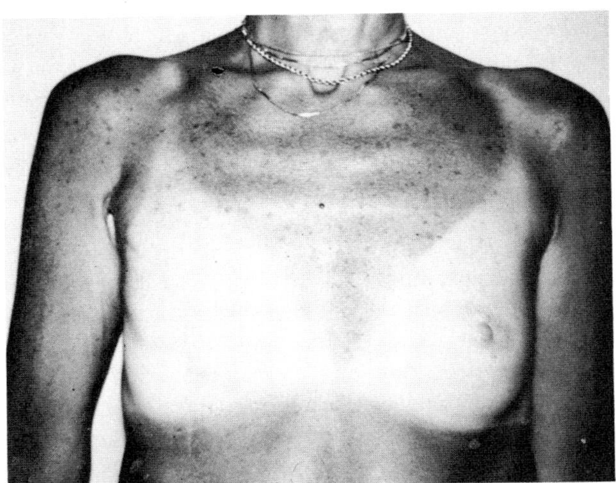

Fig. 35.1. *A 49-year-old woman seven years following modified mastectomy on right.*

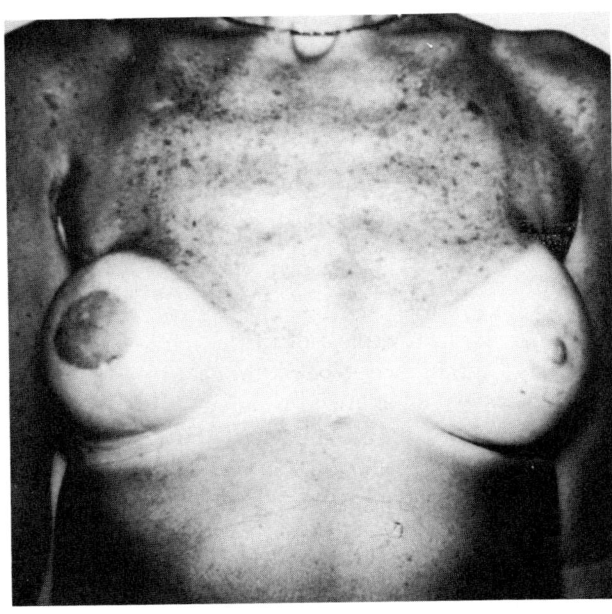

Fig. 35.2. *Same patient as in figure 35.1 one year postoperative after subcutaneous silicone prosthesis insertion and areolar reconstruction with a labial graft on right side. Some degree of capsular contracture can be seen. Left side was augmented also.*

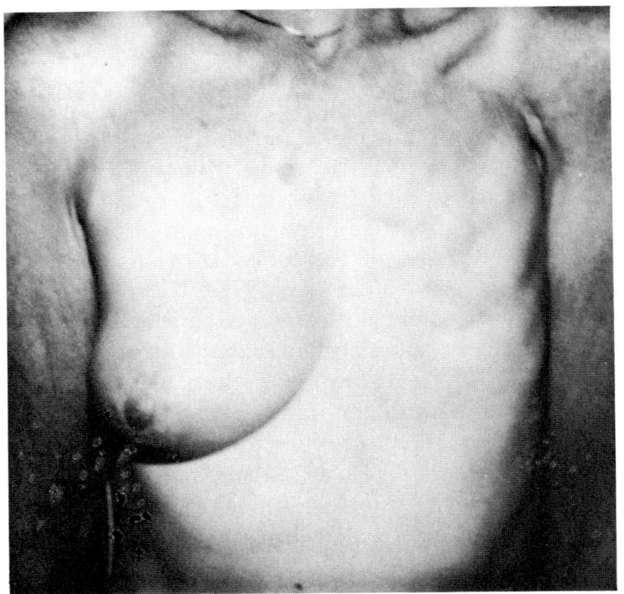

Fig. 35.3. *Frontal view of a 51-year-old woman 11 years after left Halstead mastectomy. Note very thin chest wall skin and subclavicular defect.*

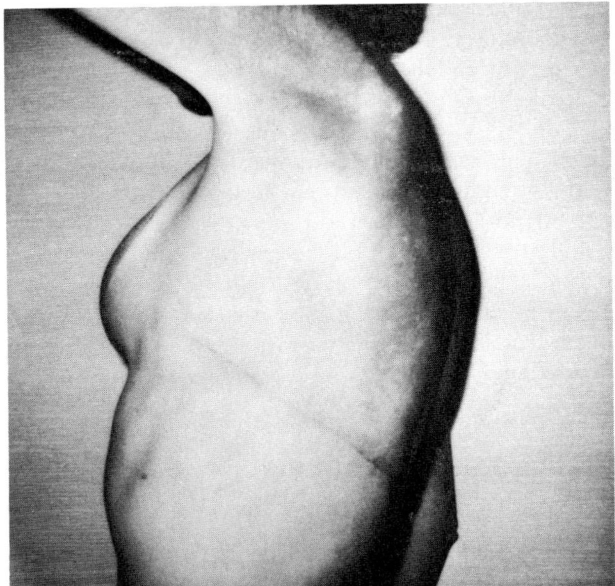

Fig. 35.4. *Lateral view of same patient in figure 35.3.*

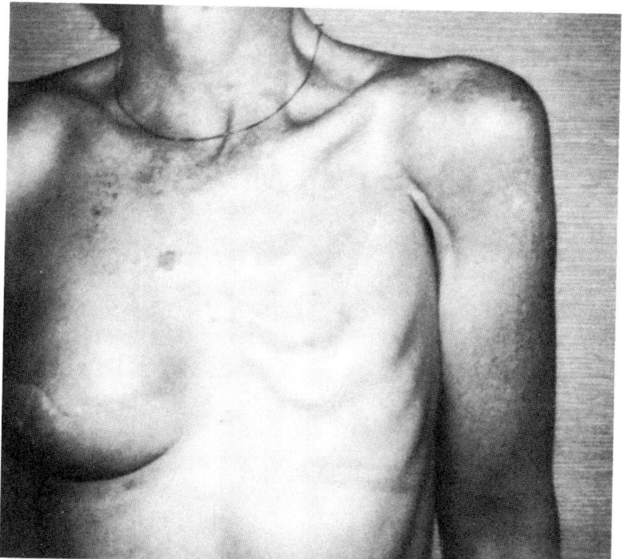

Fig. 35.5. *Same patient as in figures 35.3 and 35.4, nine months after right subcutaneous mastectomy and immediate subpectoral silicone implant reconstruction.*

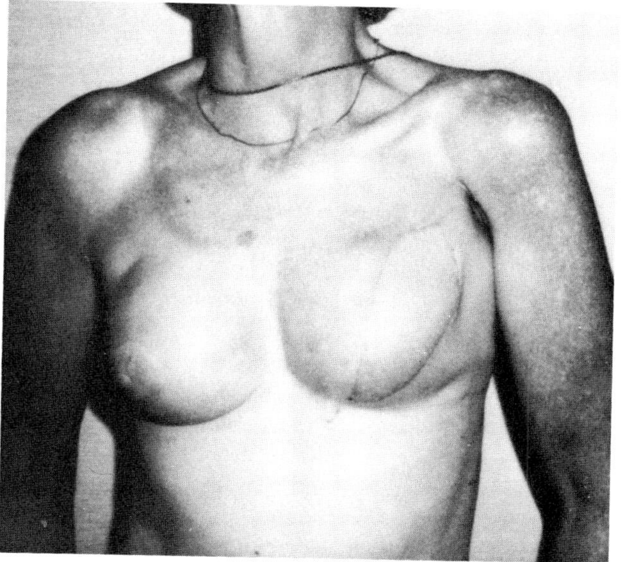

Fig. 35.6. *Same patient as in figure 35.5 four months after left breast reconstruction using a latissimus dorsi myocutaneous flap for coverage and immediate silicone prosthesis placement below the latissimus. Areolar reconstruction followed.*

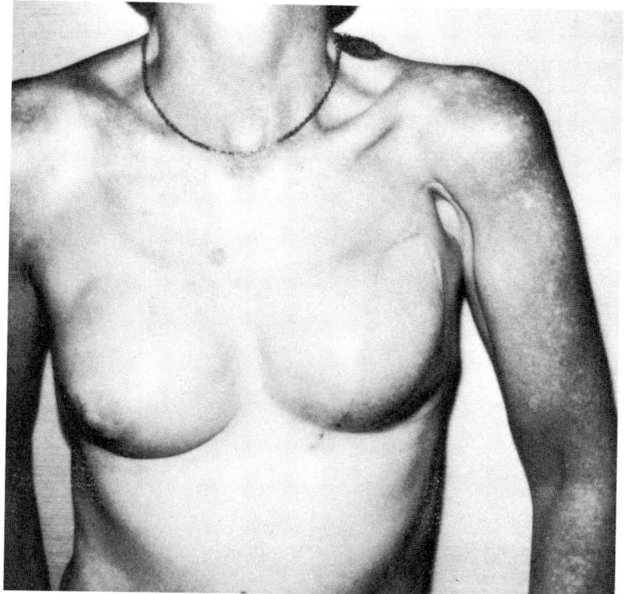

Fig. 35.7. *Anterior view of reconstructed left breast to show donor scar from thoracoepigastric flap.*

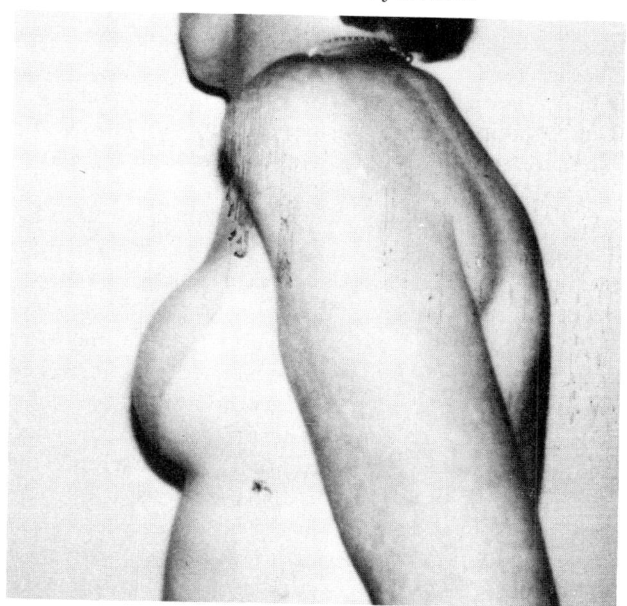

Fig. 35.8. *Lateral view of patient in figure 35.7 to show breast profile.*

dure may be necessary. Insertion of the prosthesis is usually accomplished at the time the flap is placed at its new position over the mastectomy area.

For the patient who has had a Halsted mastectomy it is frequently necessary to consider reconstructive surgery using a so-called myocutaneous, or latissimus dorsi flap (Synderman 1979). This is a one-stage procedure in which the myocutaneous flap, including a portion of the skin from the infrascapular area on the same side, with underlying latissimus dorsi is rotated anteriorly to provide coverage and bulk over the mastectomy area. Usually, the prosthesis can be inserted at the same time. In explaining this operation to the patient it is useful to show diagrams and photographs of previous patients so that the magnitude of the operation and the resulting posterior scar can be appreciated. This operation requires four to six hours and precise planning; however, in those cases where the planning has been careful and the execution uncomplicated, results are extremely dramatic and gratifying to both the patient and the plastic surgeon. It should be emphasized again that the oblique incision, which goes in the direction along the lateral border of the pectoralis, is almost ideal, as it permits easy access to the subpectoral pocket. Also, its direction is suitable for those patients who may require a thoracoepigastric flap for additional coverage or those who may require a latissimus dorsi myocutaneous flap (Bostwick, Vasconez, and Jurkiewicz 1978) (figs. 35.3–35.8).

Subpectoral placement of a silicone prosthesis has become by far the most popular and the most common technique by which breasts are reconstructed. Its advantages are many, including the softness of the mound, diminished incidence of capsular contracture, increased volume of prosthesis that can be inserted into the pocket, and reduction of postoperative complications, since any thinness of the overlying skin is protected by the underlying pectoral muscle. Additionally, recurrences of tumor can be easily felt, as the prosthesis in its retro position would be behind any probable metastases that are most likely to develop in the skin and the incision (Synderman 1979).

The Prosthesis

Over the years, I have preferred the use of a prefabricated, prefilled silicone prosthesis on the basis of increased incidence of leakage being reported in the inflatable type. There are situations, however, in which the inflatable silicone prosthesis has a definite place in constructive surgery, particularly in those patients in whom the size that would be necessary for reconstruction cannot be determined precisely (Birnbaum and Olsen 1978). Accordingly, it is necessary to have a wide selection of both types of implants available in the operating room.

Nipple-Areola Reconstruction

The time for nipple-areola reconstruction can be variable; however, it is my preference to wait a minimum of three months to permit the previously reconstructed mound to achieve its final position so that placement of the areola-nipple complex can be more precisely determined. Nothing could be more embarrassing than to place a nipple-areola complex at the same time as mound reconstruction, and then with the passage of time find that the reconstructed complex had shifted to an inferior position creating "strabismus" with the opposite side (Anderson and Pallesen 1979).

At the present time there are many techniques available for nipple-areola reconstruction, including the following: use of the banked nipple-areola from the mastectomy side, use of half of the opposite complex, split-thickness or full-thickness skin from the groin or the inner aspect of the thigh, a graft from the labia majora or minora, or a split-thickness graft from the inner aspect of the upper arm (Gryber 1977). There is less and less enthusiasm for use of tissue banked from the removed breast in view of several new procedures that

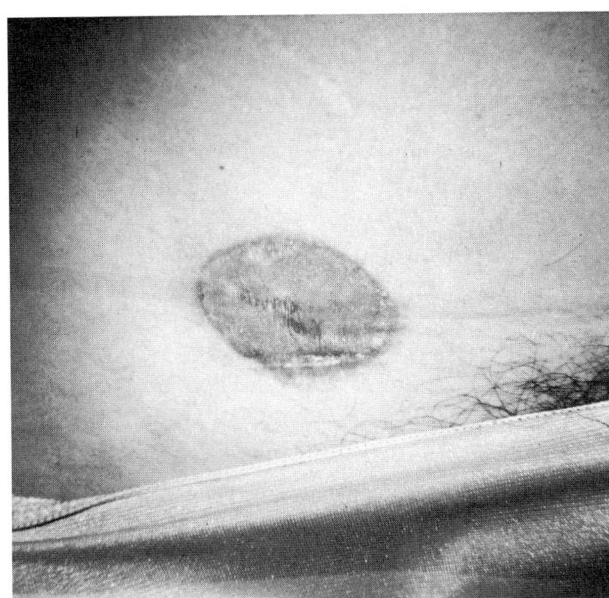

Fig. 35.9. *Nipple-areola complex banked in patient's opposite groin seen six months postoperatively. Usually, true nipple projection is lost in banking and subsequent breast regrafting. The procedure is becoming less popular with development of other suitable procedures.*

have become available and the relative similarity in results that can be achieved (Anderson and Pallesen (1979). Banking (fig. 35.9) and subsequent reimplantation have given results not too different from or any better than the other techniques that have been mentioned (Gryber 1977). Additionally, the risk of carcinoma below the nipple-areola complex itself is something that must be considered, since 52% of breast carcinomas occur in the upper outer quadrant, 17% in the upper inner quadrant, and 2% in the area directly below the areola (Leis 1977). Specifically, any carcinoma within 3 cm of the areolar border is too close to consider the banking technique.

Use of either the labia or split-thickness skin graft from the groin or thigh area both have produced acceptable results (figs. 35.10 and 35.11). The grafts from the labia tend to become more deeply pigmented in contrast to those from the thigh or the groin. In some situations it is possible to deepen the pigmentation of a grafted areola with a sun lamp. Using half of the opposite areola has both advantages and disadvantages. Obviously, it uses tissue identical to the previously removed areola; however, it does necessitate surgery on the opposite breast that some patients may object to. Additionally, there are many patients who will have an areola smaller than 4.5 cm from which it would be difficult to harvest an adequate amount of tissue to reconstruct a new one. In those patients who are to have a subcutaneous mastectomy on the opposite side done at the same time as the reconstruction, the situation can often be ideal for harvesting adequate areolar tissue.

By far the most difficult problem has been construction of a true nipple. The projection of a normal nipple on its areolar base is a unique anatomic feature not easily duplicated. Techniques using various types of incisions in the areola or diced cartilaginous implants below the areolar skin or dermis have been tried with varying degrees of success. A feature often not observed in making a new areola is the fact that the one on the opposite breast may not be perfectly round. In fact, in many patients, particularly those with large pendulous breasts, the opposite nipple is often elliptical in a horizontal direction, so that if reconstructive surgery is to be considered this should be noted.

Reconstruction of the nipple-areola complex is often *not* desired by the patient who has already had reconstruction of the mound. When the patient demonstrates this attitude I have taken the position of offering the possibility of areolar reconstruction as an out-patient procedure. Reconstruction of the nipple-areola complex often represents a desire for perfection on the part of the plastic surgeon; however, it should not be forced on the patient, since creation of the mound may fulfill her expectations.

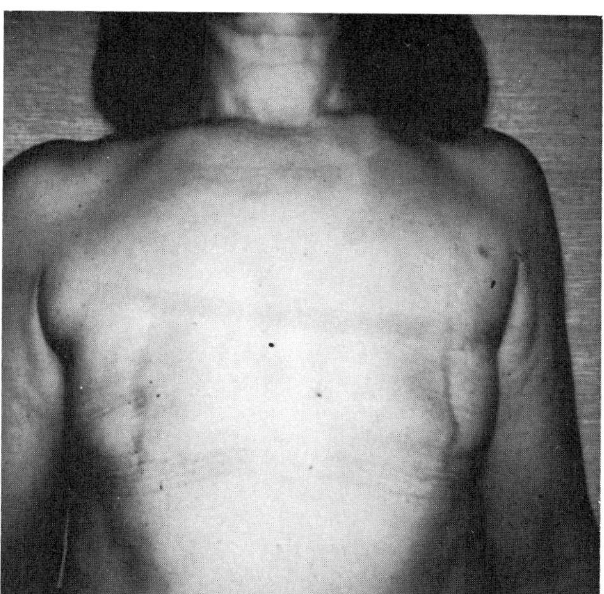

Fig. 35.10. *A 52-year-old woman 13 years after simple mastectomies for bilateral "early" cancer.*

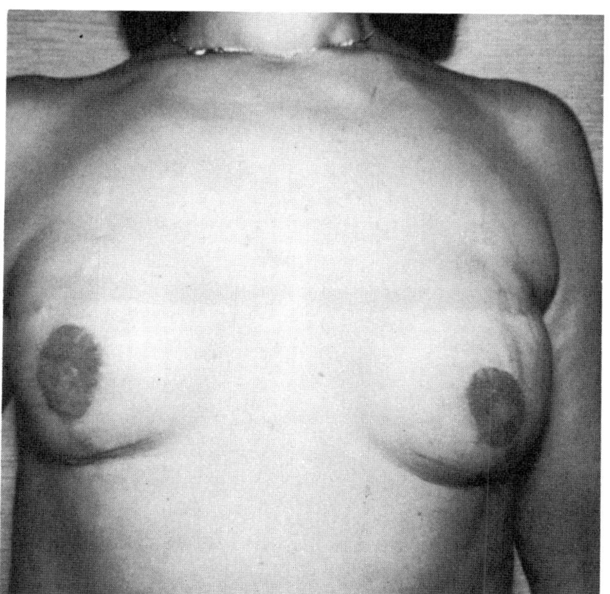

Fig. 35.11. *Same patient as in figure 35.10 one year after bilateral silicone subcutaneous implants and bilateral nipple-areola reconstruction using labia.*

The Contralateral Breast

With the passage of time and accumulation of statistical evidence (Urban 1969), it becomes evident that there is a group of high-risk patients in whom it is desirable to remove all contralateral breast tissue (Donegan and Perez-Mesa 1972). Arguments do not seem to center around the need for the operation, but rather the technique that is to be employed (Hoffman, Simon, and Kahn 1979). It is a procedure that often is difficult to explain to the patient; however, when the facts, figures, and reasons are presented, there are few who object to considering this procedure. Indeed, in my own practice the majority of these were done on the recommendation of the general surgeon who had carried out the original mastectomy (Corso 1974; Redfern and Hoopes 1978; Synderman 1978) (figs. 35.12 and 35.13).

Situations in which contralateral mastectomy is desirable include: (1) a suspicious mammogram on the opposite side, (2) positive family history of breast cancer, (3) patients who are under the age of 50 when they develop their primary lesion, (4) multicentric primary lesion, (5) patients with extensive fibrocystic disease in the opposite breast who have had one or two previous biopsies, and in whom it is difficult to determine the seriousness of their fibrocystic disease or rule out the possibility of carcinoma, and (6) patients with a severe phobia of developing cancer in the opposite breast. This is not purely an emotional problem but must be viewed as a realistic consideration, since cancer developing in the contralateral breast reduces survival time (McAvoy 1979).

Although there has been some criticism regarding the techniques of subcutaneous mastectomy, it is fair to say that there is increasing awareness on the part of the plastic surgeon that mastectomy on the opposite breast must be complete and adequate (Synderman 1978). The only tissue that should be saved is the areola-nipple complex, and under these circumstances there should be a separate biopsy of the subareolar area to be certain of the absence of carcinoma (Corso 1978; Corso and Zubiri 1975). Ideally, all specimens should have radiologic evaluation first and subsequently pathologic analysis. It is my practice to advise the patient that if a suspicious or a frank carcinoma is found on the contralateral side, a simple closure of the wound will be carried out and the entire matter discussed postoperatively. Thus if any additional surgery is necessary or desirable the patient can be appraised of it and participate in decision making. The newer techniques of subcutaneous mastectomy make it possible to do immediate reconstruction subpectorally with very good results (Corso 1978; Corso and Zubiri 1975).

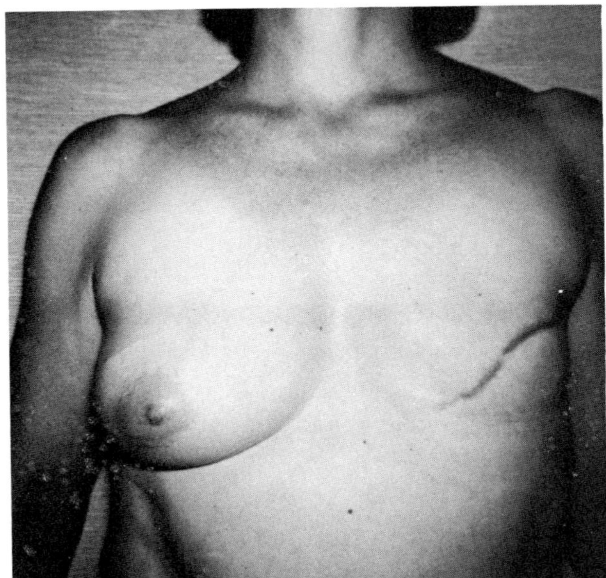

Fig. 35.12. *A 54-year-old woman six months after a left modified mastectomy through an oblique scar. Patient still had extensive fibrocystic disease on the right, with suspicious mammogram.*

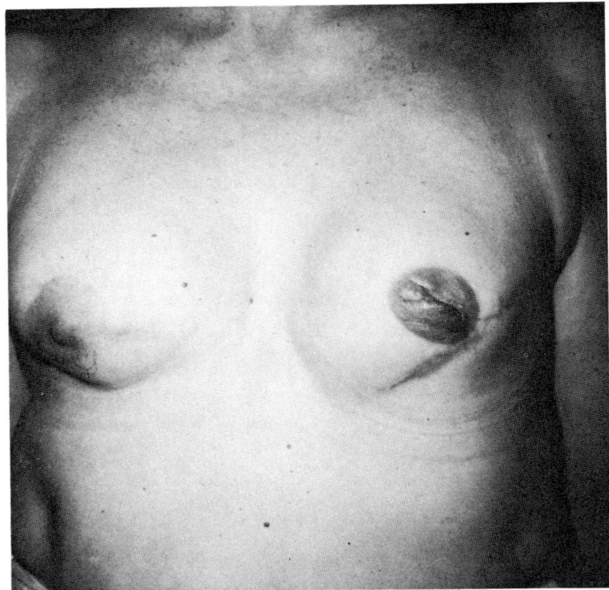

Fig. 35.13. *Same patient as in figure 35.12 one year after left subpectoral silicone implant and labial graft for areola. A subcutaneous mastectomy with immediate subpectoral silicone reconstruction was done on the right at same time.*

Complications

As with all surgery, one is never free of the possibility of complications, and this is true of reconstructive surgery after mastectomy. The most common complications are: (1) related to skin healing such as erosion, necrosis, and atrophy, and (2) those with flaps, such as scarring of the recipient and donor areas, sloughs, and inadequacy and/or nodularity of the flaps (Lewis 1979). Those related to the prosthesis include movement, poor positioning, capsular contracture, and erosion through the skin. Complications in the nipple-areola complex include eccentric positioning, asymmetry, inequality of color, and flatness.

A list of complications would not be complete without mentioning those related to dissatisfaction of the patient in terms of expectations and emotional considerations (Synderman 1974). These perhaps could be the easiest to avoid by engaging in a complete and thorough explanation of the operative procedures that are to be performed and the possible difficulties that can be associated with them. It has been my own experience that the patient no longer is focusing on the mastectomized side but, indeed, is looking at her entire chest in the hope that she can have both volumetric and geometric equality. The emotional factor I believe is frequently associated with that patient who has had reconstructive surgery immediately at the time of the mastectomy. In these situations, it is not unusual for the patient to awaken from surgery with the highest expectation of having a breast totally similar to the one that was removed. Obviously, this is completely unrealistic and justifiably leads to emotional problems. This is another reason that I recommend both to my patients and to my general surgery colleagues that an interval of at least six months should pass before reconstruction is recommended (Synderman 1977). This time interval allows the patient to recognize the seriousness of the surgical defect following mastectomy and the difficulties involved in reconstruction.

Insurance Coverage

At the present time, patients in Connecticut are fortunate that the 1979 legislature passed a law that now makes it mandatory that some payment for reconstructive breast surgery be included in all health insurance policies. Prior to 1979, a substantial number of patients gave no consideration to reconstructive surgery since the prevailing attitude had been that it was "cosmetic" and therefore would not be covered by conventional insurance policies. The terminology and the attitudes regarding these procedures have been clarified, and indeed, court decisions have been rendered in other states that now specifically state that postmastectomy breast surgery is to be regarded as reconstructive or restorative, and not as cosmetic.

References

Amaacki, T. et al. Prophylactic subcutaneous total glandectomy for mammary cystic disease with immediate primary breast reconstruction. *Ann. Plast. Surg.* 3:420–424, 1979.

Anderson, J. A., and Pallesen, R. M. Spread to the nipple and areola in carcinoma of the breast. *Ann. Surg.* 189:367–372, 1979.

Birnbaum, L., and Olsen, J. A. Breast reconstruction following radical mastectomy using custom-designed implants. *Plast. Reconstr. Surg.* 61:355–363, 1978.

Bostwick, J., III; Vasconez. L. O.; and Jurkiewicz, J. M. Breast reconstruction after a radical mastectomy. *Plast. Reconstr. Surg.* 61:682–693, 1978.

Corso, P. F. Subcutaneous mastectomy: indications and technique. *Conn. Med.* 38:159–161, 1974.

Corso, P. F. Subcutaneous mastectomy with a breast-halving incision: technique and modifications. In *Symposium on aesthetic surgery of the breast,* eds. J. Q. Owsley, Jr. and R. Peterson. St. Louis: C. V. Mosby, 1978, pp. 174–179.

Corso, P. F., and Zubiri, J. A breast-halving incision for subcutaneous mastectomy. *Plast. Reconstr. Surg.* 56:1–4, 1975.

Cronin, T. D., and Upton, J. Reconstruction of the breast after mastectomy. In *Symposium on aesthetic surgery of the breast,* eds. J. Q. Owsley, Jr. and R. Peterson. St. Louis: C. V. Mosby, 1978, p. 202.

Donegan, W., and Perez-Mesa, C. Lobular carcinoma: an indication for elective biopsy of the second breast. *Ann. Surg.* 176:178–189, 1972.

Foote, F., and Stewart, F. Comparative studies of cancerous versus noncancerous breast: role of so-called chronic cystic mastitis in mammary carcinogenesis. *Ann. Surg.* 121:197–222, 1945.

Gryber, R. Method to produce better areolae and nipples on reconstructed breasts. *Plast. Reconstr. Surg.* 60: 505–513, 1977.

Guthrie, R. The case for breast reconstruction after mastectomy. *CA* 28:218–224, 1978.

Guthrie, R., and Imber, G. Breast reconstruction after mastectomy. *Ann. Plast. Surg.* 2:273–285, 1979.

Hartwell, S., Jr. et al. Reconstruction of the breast after mastectomy for cancer. *Plast. Reconstr. Surg.* 57:152–157, 1976.

Hauschild, W. Reconstruction of the female breast after bilateral simple mastectomy. *Br. J. Plast. Surg.* 23:54–57, 1970.

Hicken, N. A clinical pathologic study demonstrating why most mastectomies result in incomplete removal of the mammary gland. *Arch. Surg.* 40:6–14, 1940.

Hoffman, S.; Simon, B.; and Kahn, S. Alternatives to subcutaneous mastectomy. *Plast. Reconstr. Surg.* 64:214–220, 1979.

Leis, H. The diagnosis of breast cancer. *CA* 27:209–232, 1977.

Lewis, J. R. Use of a sliding flap from the abdomen to provide cover in breast reconstruction. *Plast. Reconstr. Surg.* 64:491–497, 1979.

Lynch, J.; Madden, J.; and Franklin, J. Breast reconstruction following mastectomy for cancer. *Ann. Surg.* 187:490–501, 1978.

McAvoy, J. Subcutaneous mastectomy in the treatment of high-risk female. Is emotionalism obscuring the facts? *Ann. Plast. Surg.* 3:219–223, 1979.

Pennisi, V., and Capozzi, A. The incidence of obscure carcinoma in subcutaneous mastectomy: results of a national survey. *Plast. Reconstr. Surg.* 56:9–12, 1975.

Redfern, A., and Hoopes, J. Subcutaneous mastectomy: plea for conservatism. *Plast. Reconstr. Surg.* 62:706–707, 1978.

Robson, M. Breast reconstruction following ablation for cancer. *Conn. Med.* 42:642–646, 1978.

Schmitz, R. The breast cancer survey of the commission on cancer. *Bull. Am. Coll. Surg.* 64:15–19, 1979.

Synderman, R. Subcutaneous mastectomy with immediate prosthetic reconstruction: an operation in search of patients. *Plast. Reconstr. Surg.* 56:582–589, 1974.

Synderman, R. Reconstruction of the breast after mastectomy. *CA* 27:360–366, 1977.

Synderman, R. Subcutaneous mastectomy. In *Symposium on aesthetic surgery of the breast,* eds. J. Q. Owsley, Jr. and R. Peterson. St. Louis: C. V. Mosby, 1978, p. 149.

Synderman, R. The present status of breast reconstruction following mastectomy in the female. *Aesth. Plast. Surg.* 64:214–218, 1979.

Urban, J. Bilateral breast cancer. *Cancer* 24:1310–1313, 1969.

thirty-six

Esophageal Cancer: Diagnosis and Treatment

ELLIOT M. LIVSTONE

Squamous cell carcinoma of the esophagus is relatively rare, accounting for only 1.1% of all cancers (Mason, Bailar, and Eisenberg 1964). Its mortality closely parallels incidence, as the yield from available therapies is rather dismal. Esophageal cancer occurs most frequently in persons over 55 years of age, and is seen three times more commonly in men than in women (Cliffton 1970). While mortality has been stable among Caucasians, it has risen steadily for black men since 1940 (Cutler and Young 1975). The risk factors (Auerbach et al. 1965; Tuyns 1970; Wychulis et al. 1971) are as follows, in order:

- Non-white population
- Excessive alcohol use
- Excessive tobacco use
- Plummer-Vinson syndrome
- Hot beverage ingestion
- Lye ingestion
- Geographic factors
- Genetic factors
- Achalasia

Aside from the genetic, geographic, and racial factors, risk for acquiring esophageal cancer results from metabolic destabilization or intense irritation of the esophageal mucosa.

Symptoms

The most common symptom of esophageal cancer is dysphagia—the sensation of food sticking in the throat or retrosternal area. Dysphagia should be considered pathognomonic until proved otherwise, and it should never be ignored in any patient. The sensation is progressive and persistent. It is progressive in the sense that the patient first notices difficulty swallowing solid foods, later semisolids, and ultimately, liquids. The progressive occlusion of the esophageal lumen by tumor may be masked if the patient subconsciously restricts intake to avoid such unpleasant sensations; therefore careful attention should be paid to the consistency of ingested foods when inquiring about esophageal capacity. Dysphagia will usually be persistent in the sense that it is present at all meals rather than intermittently, as it might be in esophageal spasm, achalasia, or other motility disorders.

The pain associated with esophageal cancer is usually steady, dull, and substernal, occasionally radiating to the back. The level at which pain is experienced, however, does not necessarily correlate with the location of the tumor. Sometimes patients report odynophagia (painful swallowing), which may be related to a tumor of the upper one-third of the esophagus. Pain is an unfavorable prognostic symptom because it may represent perineural growth of tumor in the mediastinum.

Hoarseness may indicate vocal cord paralysis from laryngeal nerve involvement with tumor, or chronic laryngitis. A chronic cough is also an unfavorable prognostic symptom as it may indicate an esophagobronchial or tracheoesophageal fistula, a lung abscess, or chronic "overflow" aspiration of saliva or food into the lungs resulting from esophageal lumen obstruction. Pulmonary involvement is not uncommon, as nearly half of patients with esophageal cancer have findings of bronchopneumonia at autopsy.

Anorexia and weight loss are nonspecific symptoms related both to the presence of the disease in general and the problems it creates with eating. Most patients thus are cachectic (defined by convention as a 10% loss in body weight within six months).

Patients with esophageal cancer may develop iron deficiency anemia. Bleeding is usually a slow occult process; fewer than 5% experience frank hemorrhage.

Rare signs of the disease include esophagopleural fistulas, hypercalcemia (unrelated to bone metastases), and ectopic hormone production (gonadotropins, corticotropins) (Stephens, Hansen, and Muggia 1973; McKechnie and Fechner 1971; Lohrenz and Custer 1965).

Physical findings are rarely specific for this malignancy. Occasionally, supraclavicular lymphadenopathy or hepatomegaly secondary to metastases is noted.

Diagnosis

Esophageal cancer is customarily diagnosed by radiographic, endoscopic, or cytologic techniques. Radiography, however, is usually the first method employed (fig. 36.1). These tumors usually encroach on the esophageal lumen, but they may take the form of thickening or rigidity of one wall of the esophagus. Cineradiography or double-contrast studies using barium followed by water, with the patient in the upright position, may better uncover the more subtle lesions (Suzuki et al. 1972). Alternatively, the radiologist may use a marshmallow dipped in barium to serve as a radiopaque bolus to locate the specific site of the problem.

Endoscopy allows an observer to view esophageal lesions directly, photograph them, and obtain biopsy samples and brushings for cytologic examination. Because many epidermoid tumors stimulate an inflammatory response and scar formation at their advancing margins, an endoscopic biopsy may only demonstrate the chronic inflammatory tissue; single biopsies yield positive results in only 70% to 80% of cases. When multiple biopsies and endoscopic brushings are obtained for cytology, the diagnostic accuracy of endoscopy increases in most reported series to 96% to 100% (Winawer et al. 1975; Winawer, Sherlock, and Hajdu 1976).

Lavage exfoliative cytology is an alternative to endoscopic brush cytology. The technique involves inserting a radiopaque nasogastric tube through the esophageal stricture using fluoroscopic guidance and aspirating fasting gastric contents, with prompt fixation and immediate processing. After this, washings of the stomach and esophageal lesion are obtained and processed immediately. The diagnostic yield of this procedure exceeds 95% when it is done by properly trained personnel and when specimens are selected carefully and processed with meticulous attention to detail.

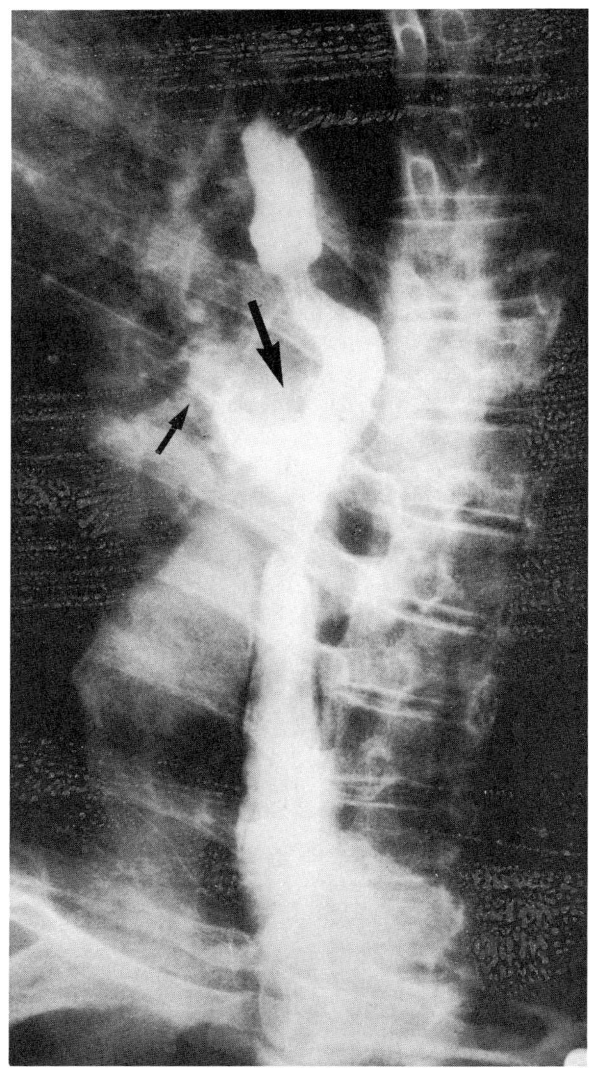

Fig. 36.1. *An oblique radiograph from a barium swallow demonstrates a malignant esophageal stricture at the junction of the lower and middle third of the esophagus* (large arrow). *Barium is seen in an esophagobronchial fistula* (small arrow).

It should be noted that negative results on biopsy or cytologic examination, by whatever technique, do not rule out the diagnosis of esophageal cancer. Conversely, false positive results are extremely rare for this disease: a positive biopsy or cytology usually means cancer.

Differential diagnosis includes benign peptic stricture, cancer of the gastric fundus or esophagogastric junction, and achalasia. Patients with peptic stricture usually have a long history of heartburn or have had an indwelling nasogastric tube for more than five days following surgery or during a severe illness. X-ray films show a long smooth stricture, and endoscopy reveals scar tissue and inflammation. The diagnosis is confirmed by biopsy and cytology.

When adenocarcinoma is found on esophageal biopsy, the tumor usually arises from the gastric fundus. With the exception of columnar epithelial remnants from embryonal development and a few mucus glands scattered through the esophagus, there are no structures in the normal esophagus that can produce a glandular cancer (Lortat-Jacob et al. 1968; Raphael, Ellis, and Dockerty 1966). Chronic reflux of gastric acid into the esophagus, however, leads to columnar metaplasia (Barrett's syndrome) of the esophageal epithelium, a premalignant condition that may lead to adenocarcinoma. It is important to distinguish epidermoid esophageal cancer from the adenocarcinoma in Barrett's epithelium and from the esophageal encroachment of gastric fundal cancer, because adenocarcinomas follow the natural history of gastric cancer, responding better to certain chemotherapy regimens and less well to radiation.

In the patient with achalasia, dysphagia is usually intermittent and nonprogressive. On x-ray the esophagus may be dilated, but the lower end tapers into a "bird beak" configuration. Endoscopy and biopsy should be performed in every new case of achalasia so that the narrowed area in the distal esophagus may be examined and the correct diagnosis made.

Treatment

The treatment of esophageal cancer requires correct staging as well as a tissue diagnosis. The use of surgery, radiation therapy, or chemotherapy depends on the location of the tumor within the esophagus and the presence of localized resectable disease, regional disease, or widespread disease with distant metastases. Because the connective tissue covering the esophagus is loose, malignant cells spread quite readily to the lungs and mediastinum. Chest x-rays and tomography or thoracic computerized axial tomography should therefore be part of the staging evaluation. Because the liver is also a common site for esophageal cancer metastases, a liver scan or ultrasound examination should be obtained.

Approximately 50% of esophageal cancers are operable, based on their location in the lower one-third of the esophagus and in the absence of regional or distant metastases determined by noninvasive methods of diagnosis. Of these, slightly less than half are actually resectable for an overall rate of 22% (Gunnlaugsson et al. 1970). Older studies have suggested a benefit for resection of lower third lesions, but no such benefit over the yield from radiation therapy of middle and upper third lesions (Pearson 1974). The problem with both forms of therapy is that long-term results are poor, with most patients dying within one year and fewer than 5% living five years. Reports primarily in the Japanese literature have recommended two-stage and three-stage surgical procedures in combination with radiation therapy. Such efforts, however, have not generated widespread enthusiasm in this country as they have not demonstrated convincing evidence of prolonged ambulatory life outside the hospital. Colonic interposition techniques have been described for esophageal bypass or for reconstruction following cervical or total esophagectomy. Similarly, "gastric pull-up" techniques have been described for esophagogastric anastomoses at the level of the aortic arch and for reconstruction after resection of middle third lesions. The ability to perform such surgical gymnastics requires a skilled thoracic surgeon who should be consulted when there is no radiographic or scan evidence of metastases.

As a result of the low resectability rate, treatment is directed primarily at palliation. Radiation therapy provides a good deal of relief for esophageal obstruction, although it is temporary and subject to local as well as distant failure (progression of disease). During the first two weeks of radiation therapy there is a period of edema in which the obstruction of the esophageal lumen is accentuated and dysphagia is more pronounced. Some gastroenterologists feel that esophageal bougienage should be performed at this time and thereafter to maintain the caliber of the esophageal lumen and to prevent radiation-induced stricture formation (Heit et al. 1978). Radiation therapists, on the other hand, argue that this practice is unnecessary and possibly dangerous.

When the problem is a tracheoesophageal or esophagobronchial fistula, relief from aspiration sometimes can be provided with an esophageal prosthesis or stent. The prothesis (stent) is a semisolid plastic funnel-shaped tube that can be seated in the tumor, and that serves to occlude the esophageal orifice of the fistula. The prosthesis may be inserted surgically or, in some instances, by a gastroenterologist by means of a peroral technique (Palmer 1973). Without such a stent, radiation or chemotherapy (if effective) may enlarge the fistula and increase the amount of food or saliva that is aspirated.

When metastases are widespread or when there is a failure of primary forms of therapy (surgery or radiation), one is tempted to use chemotherapy. Unfortunately, there is no effective standard chemotherapy for advanced esophageal cancer. This disease really should be considered a clinical situation appropriate for investigational forms of therapy. The American literature contains little in the way of acceptable information about the effectiveness of chemotherapeutic agents. Single-agent activity has been reported for 5-FU, mitomycin, bleomycin, cisplatin, and vindesine with response rates in small series approximating 15% to 19%. A recent report (Kelsen, Chapman, and Bains 1981) of six partial responses in 14 advanced esophageal cancer patients treated with cisplatin, vindesine, and bleomycin is the most encouraging study to date. It would seem, then, that a patient unfortunate enough to be in this situation should participate in a clinical trial.

Summary

Epidermoid carcinoma of the esophagus is an uncommon but lethal disease. The best opportunity for improved survival is the alertness of patient and physician to its characteristic symptoms so that earlier detection and the chance for surgical resection are magnified. Usually, however, the available therapeutic options constitute support and palliation.

References

Auerbach, O. et al. Histologic changes in the esophagus in relation to smoking habits. *Arch. Environ. Health* 11:4–15, 1965.

Cliffton, E. E. Treatment of cancer of the esophagus. *Mod. Treat.* 7:1261–1283, 1970.

Cutler, S. J., and Young, J. L., Jr. *Third national cancer survey: incidence data.* Bethesda, Md.: National Cancer Institute, 1975.

Gunnlaugsson, G. H. et al. Analysis of the records of 1657 patients with carcinoma of the esophagus and cardia of the stomach. *Surg. Gynecol. Obstet.* 130:997–1005, 1970.

Heit, H. A. et al. Palliative dilatation for dysphagia in esophageal carcinoma. *Ann. Intern. Med.* 89:629–631, 1978.

Kelsen, D. P.; Chapman, R.; and Bains, M. Cisplatin, vindesine, and bleomycin combination chemotherapy of esophageal cancer. *Proc. Am. Soc. Clin. Oncol.* 22:454, 1981.

Lohrenz, F. N., and Custer, G. S. ACTH-producing metastases from carcinoma of the esophagus. *Ann. Intern. Med.* 62:1017–1022, 1965.

Lortat-Jacob, J. L. et al. Primary esophageal adenocarcinoma: report of 16 cases. *Surgery* 64:535–543, 1968.

Mason, M. J.; Bailar, J. C., III; and Eisenberg, H. Geographic variations in the incidence of esophageal cancer. *J. Chron. Dis.* 17:667–676, 1964.

McKechnie, J. C., and Fechner, R. E. Choriocarcinoma and adenocarcinoma of the esophagus with gonadotropin secretion. *Cancer* 27:694–702, 1971.

Palmer, E. D. Peroral prosthesis for the management of incurable esophageal carcinoma. *Am. J. Gastroenterol.* 59:487–498, 1973.

Pearson, J. G. Value of radiation therapy. Current concepts in cancer, #42. II. Esophagus: treatment — localized and advanced. *JAMA* 227:181–183, 1974.

Raphael, H. A.; Ellis, F. H.; and Dockerty, M. B. Primary adenocarcinoma of the esophagus: 18-year review and review of the literature. *Ann. Surg.* 164:785–796, 1966.

Stephens, R. L.; Hansen, H. H.; and Muggia, F. M. Hypercalcemia in epidermoid tumors of the head and neck and esophagus. *Cancer* 31:1487–1491, 1973.

Suzuki, H. et al. Diagnosis of early esophageal cancers. *Surgery* 71:99–103, 1972.

Tuyns, A. J. Cancer of the esophagus: further evidence of the relation to drinking habits in France. *Int. J. Cancer* 5:152–156, 1970.

Winawer, S. J. et al. Endoscopic brush cytology in esophageal cancer. *JAMA* 232:1358, 1975.

Winawer, S. J.; Sherlock, P.; and Hajdu, S. I. The role of upper gastrointestinal endoscopy in patients with cancer. *Cancer* 37(suppl.):440–448, 1976.

Wychulis, A. R. et al. Achalasia and carcinoma of the esophagus. *JAMA* 215:1638–1641, 1971.

thirty-seven

Gastric Cancer: Diagnosis and Treatment

ELLIOT M. LIVSTONE

Gastric cancer was once the leading cause of cancer death in the United States. Over the last half century, however, mortality from this disease has declined to the sixth-ranked position, with 14,100 deaths predicted for 1982. This apparent improvement has not resulted from any dramatic advance in detection or therapy, but rather from declining incidence of disease. When mortality is defined in terms of five-year survival, no significant improvement has occurred during the same half-century (Comis and Carter 1974). In 1982, 24,200 new cases of stomach cancer will be diagnosed (Silverberg 1982), four-fifths with disease that is not curable by surgery. Any major impact on survival and cure will therefore depend on earlier detection and advances in other modes of therapy.

Gastric cancer is primarily a disease of men more than women, and nonwhites more than whites. It is seen most commonly in Japan, Finland, Poland, and Chile. It has a predilection for people with blood group A, pernicious anemia, gastric polyps, atrophic gastritis, acanthosis nigricans, dermatomyositis, patients with prior gastric resection, or the members of so-called "cancer families" (Sleisenger and Fordtran 1978). The symptoms are vague and nonspecific, leading many patients to believe that they are suffering from acid peptic disease or other digestive disorders. Relative frequencies of symptoms among patients with advanced gastric cancer (McNeer and Pack 1967) are as follows:

Weight loss	96%
Pain	70%
Vomiting	50%
Bowel changes	35%
Anorexia	25%
Early satiety	10%
Dysphagia	9%
Hematemesis	8%

Occult bleeding, weakness, and fatigue are also common, but their incidence is not precisely defined. Physical findings such as palpable mass, hepatomegaly, cachexia, and abdominal tenderness are common but not pathognomonic for this disease.

Achlorhydria is an important laboratory finding, but the presence of stomach acid does not exclude the possibility of gastric cancer. Anemia associated with stomach cancer may be caused by blood loss, intrinsic factor deficiency, folate deficiency, or any combination of these factors. Occult blood is commonly found in the stool. Liver function tests may or may not be abnormal, depending on the amount of functioning liver tissue available. Carcinoembryonic antigen levels are rarely elevated in early gastric cancer, and are of only limited value for managing recurrent or metastatic tumor.

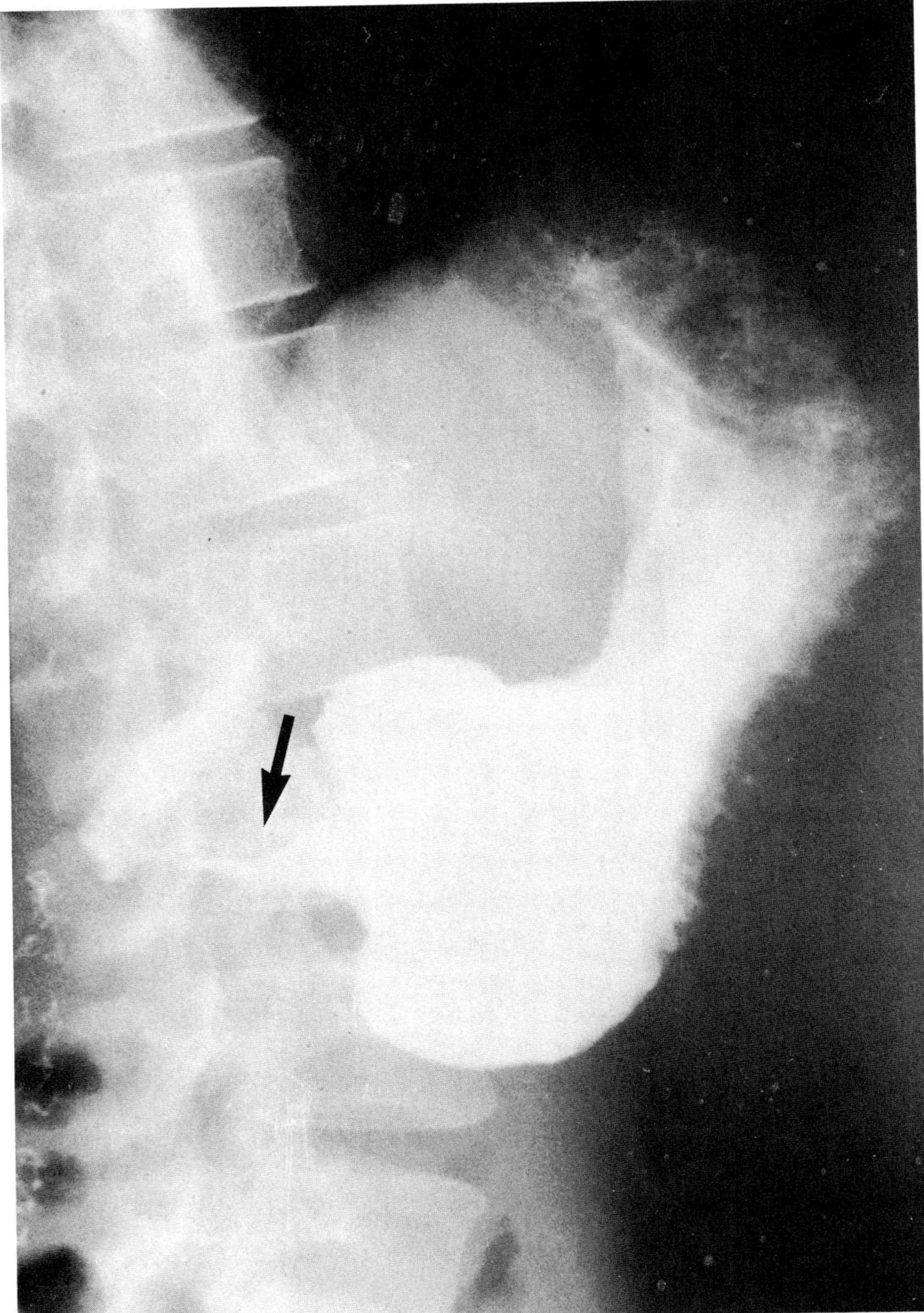

Fig. 37.1. *Adenocarcinoma of the pre-pyloric antrum. This oblique view from an upper gastrointestinal series demonstrates a "napkin ring" concentric stricture of the distal antrum.*

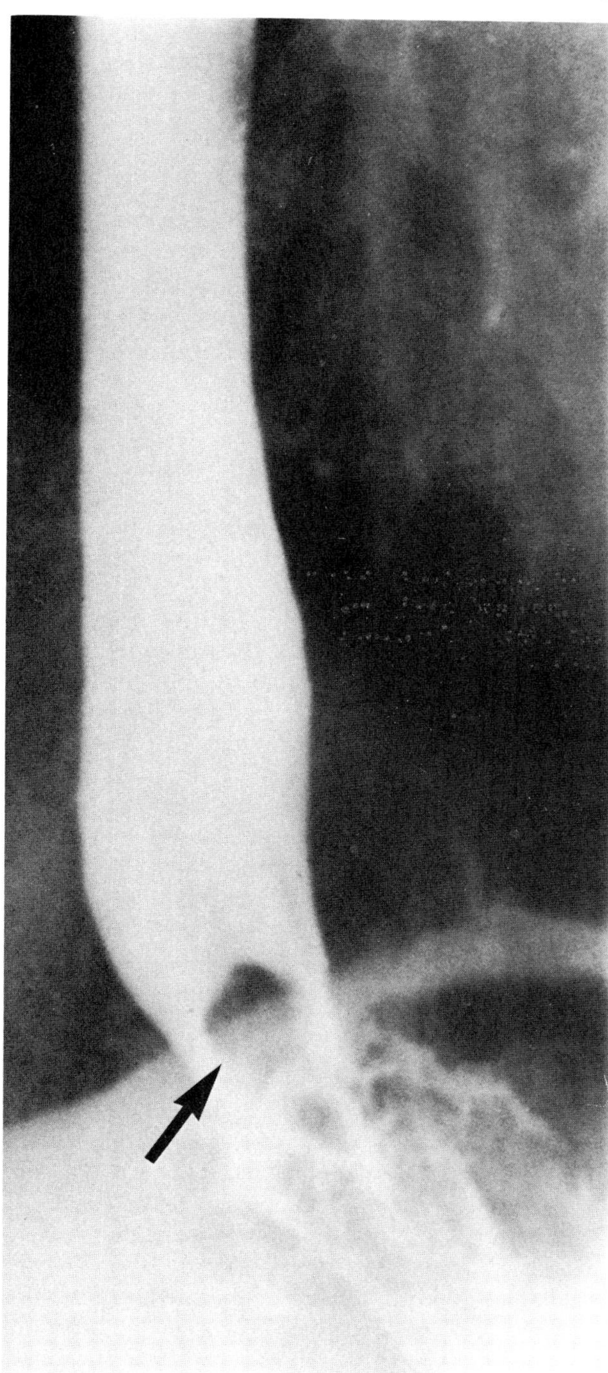

Fig. 37.2. *Adenocarcinoma of the gastric fundus. The gastric tumor is growing cephalad in the submucosa of the esophagus. It is seen as a filling defect in the lower end of the esophagus* (arrow). *This radiolucency is sometimes mistaken for a squamous tumor of the esophagus.*

Diagnosis

The upper gastrointestinal barium x-ray is the keystone of gastric cancer diagnosis (figs. 37.1 and 37.2). Other tests include barium meal or double-contrast x-ray studies, endoscopy with biopsy or brush cytology, and lavage cytology. To demonstrate the small, early, noninvasive, potentially curable lesions, a bas relief of the gastric mucosal folds is essential. Accordingly, the Japanese, for whom stomach cancer is the leading killer, have developed techniques for air contrast barium studies of the upper digestive tract with excellent accuracy (Shirakabe 1971). Although the incidence of early disease is less in the West, the double-contrast examination provides detection and characterization of benign and malignant gastric disease to a degree not possible with conventional barium techniques.

With the development of several generations of thin flexible fiberscopes in the 1970s, gastroscopy has become an important procedure in the diagnosis of stomach cancer (Morrissey 1971). The diagnostic yield of visually directed gastroscopic biopsies increases with the number of biopsies taken and approximates 85%; the combination of endoscopic biopsy and brush cytology raises this to 90%.

If exfoliative lavage cytology is added to these diagnostic maneuvers the yield may exceed 96%; however, there are some limitations and pitfalls to the use of this technique. Lavage cytology is not helpful for diagnosing submucosal tumors that do not penetrate the gastric epithelium. Furthermore, the random, casually obtained gastric aspirate sent to the laboratory labeled "gastric cytology" is totally useless. False positive results are rare, but bizarre ballooned gastric mucosal cells may be exfoliated in atrophic gastritis and in treated or untreated pernicious anemia. Nonetheless, proper technique leads to highly accurate results. The patient should be well hydrated, have fasted for 8 hours, and should not have taken antacids for 24 hours before the test. A trained technician should centrifuge the gastric aspirate promptly, following which the centrifuged pellet should be immediately chilled, fixed in alcohol, and sent to the laboratory for analysis by an experienced cytopathologist. At Yale, the cytopathology laboratory exceeds 99.8% accuracy. Thus the test is widely used at this institution to evaluate the possibility of gastric cancer in high-risk situations such as all gastric ulcers, narrow antrum or thickened gastric folds on x-ray, gastric polyps, pernicious anemia, and achlorhydria, and for cell typing of overt tumors.

Treatment

Treatment planning logically should be related to the extent or stage at which the disease is diagnosed. A patient with localized disease is a potential candidate for a curative surgical resection. A patient with unresected (or unresectable) regional disease is a candidate for palliative bypass surgery and potentially, for chemotherapy, radiation therapy, or a combination. A patient with distant metastatic disease will derive little survival benefit from palliative surgery or radiation therapy, but may experience tumor shrinkage and/or prolongation of life with single-drug or multiple-drug therapy.

To study the various treatment options among these three clinical stages of disease, the National Cancer Institute has established several multiinstitutional cooperative groups. The Gastrointestinal Tumor Study Group (GITSG) is a small, relatively homogeneous confederation of universities that has conducted multidisciplinary studies of new gastric cancer therapies for the last eight years. These studies have derived as logical extensions of the prevailing literature or from the prior investigations of individual group members.

In 1972–1973, during the formative years of the GITSG, 5-fluorouracil (5-FU) was the mainstay of gastric cancer therapy. The English literature subsequent to 1960 suggested a 22% overall response rate (97 of 448) in advanced measurable disease for 5-fluorouracil given as a single agent (Comis and Carter 1974). Similarly, mitomycin (Mutamycin) as a single agent was associated with a 30% response rate (63 of 211). If one eliminated the optimistic early Japanese reports, the response rate fell to 24% (24 of 98), and the average duration of a response was one to three months compared to four to five months attributed to 5-fluorouracil.

During this same period, studies from the Mayo Clinic and elsewhere suggested a role for nitrosoureas in the chemotherapy of this disease. Kovach and colleagues (1974) demonstrated a 41% (14 of 34) response rate for the combination of 5-fluorouracil and carmustine (BiCNU) with survival advantage over patients treated with either drug singly. Oral nitrosoureas were unimpressive used as single agents, but uncontrolled data from the Mayo Clinic suggested that semustine might be the best nitrosourea for gastric cancer therapy when given in combination with 5-fluorouracil (Moertel 1973). Certainly, if therapeutic equivalency were assured, the oral route was preferable because of ease of administration and diminished toxicity, especially elimination of the consequences of nitrosourea extravasation. A subsequent Eastern Cooperative Oncology Group (ECOG) study confirmed this contention with a 40% response rate among all patients with advanced measurable disease (Moertel et al. 1976) and a 48% response rate (14 of 29) among a subpopulation of patients with advanced disease with an ECOG status of zero to one. Most noteworthy in this study was a 50% improvement in median survival (20 weeks versus 13 weeks) among patients responding to 5-fluorouracil and semustine combination compared to those responding to semustine alone. At that point, it was apparent that the combination deserved extensive investigation by controlled randomized prospective trials in all stages of gastric cancer.

At the same time, doxorubicin (Adriamycin) emerged as a promising antineoplastic agent that had been undergoing investigation in the treatment of many solid tumors. At the Mayo Clinic, four of eight ambulatory, previously treated patients with advanced gastric cancer experienced a partial objective response with acceptable toxicity; these responses lasted 2½ to 10½ months and suggested activity for this drug against gastric cancer (Frytak et al. 1975). Although this was a selected population entered into an uncontrolled trial, the result warranted further study of doxorubicin as a single agent and possibly as part of a combination regimen.

With this information as a background, in 1974, the GITSG undertook studies of adjuvant therapy in patients who had undergone an allegedly curative resection, and studies of combined modality therapy in patients with locally unresectable disease (defined as surgically confirmed residual disease confined to the stomach, local lymph nodes, local omentum, and/or local peritoneum within an area 20 × 20 cm). Because of conflicting data from single-institution trials and from the large cooperative groups, the GITSG also developed its own advanced disease chemotherapy protocols to provide its own data base for the choice of therapies in the more localized stages of disease.

In 1974, the GITSG began a phase III clinical trial (protocol 8174) designed to evaluate the effectiveness of adjuvant therapy prospectively by means of a randomized study of patients with alleged surgical cure. The protocol specified that the control group would receive no therapy other than surgery. Originally, 5-fluorouracil plus carmustine was designated as the adjuvant therapy to be tested. After 14 patients had been randomized into the study it was apparent that the combination was not being tolerated well. Based on the Mayo Clinic and ECOG data regarding semustine, the 5-fluorouracil plus carmustine was terminated, and 5-fluorouracil plus semustine was activated in its place. Drug dosages were reduced from the ECOG regimen in an effort to reduce toxicity to a level that was appro-

Table 37.1. *5-FU plus Semustine as an Adjuvant to Allegedly Curative Surgical Resection for Gastric Cancer*

	Control	*Treated*	*Totals*
Evaluable patients	71	71	142
Recurrences	38	29	67
% recurred	54	41	
Mean weeks disease-free*	30	> 54	
Deaths	46	31	77
% dead	65	44	
Mean weeks to death†	33	> 54	

SOURCE: Livstone et al. 1981.
* $P < 0.01$.
† $P < 0.02$.

priate for the adjuvant setting. Semustine, 150 mg/m^2, was given every 70 days, and 5-fluorouracil was given for five days every five weeks, 325 mg/m^2/day in courses with semustine, and 375 mg/m^2/day five weeks later.

To date 165 patients have been randomly entered into the control arm and into treatment with 5-FU and semustine. One hundred forty-two patients are available for analysis, 71 in each group. Selected data from the evaluable patients are presented in table 37.1.

Chemotherapy, as given in this protocol, delayed the recurrence of gastric cancer and prolonged survival by more than 50% in treated patients compared to untreated control patients. When survival probabilities were analyzed, the odds of a treated patient living one, two, three, and four years were 89%, 69%, 62%, and 52% respectively, compared to odds of 87%, 55%, 45%, and 33% for control subjects. This study, then, was the first North American research program to show a survival benefit for gastric cancer adjuvant therapy.

In patients with locally unresectable disease, the GITSG designed a prospective, randomized phase III clinical trial (protocol 8274) to compare the relative effectiveness of chemotherapy alone versus chemotherapy administered in combination with radiotherapy. Data from the Mayo Clinic (Moertel et al. 1969) had previously suggested that a combination of 5-fluorouracil plus 3500 rad was superior to radiation alone. To improve local control of disease extension, the radiation dosage in the present study was increased to 5000 rad given in four weeks. The study was designed as a comparison between 5-fluorouracil plus semustine alone versus 5000 rad followed by 5-fluorouracil plus semustine. Because of concerns about drug toxicity, especially in conjunction with radiation therapy, dosages were decreased from those used in the ECOG study.

Patient accession into this study was stopped in January 1977, and the data codes were broken following detection of a statistically significant difference in survival between the two treatments. Ninety-six patients had been entered into the study, and as of January 1978, 87 of these were evaluable. The projected mean survival time of patients treated with combination chemotherapy alone was 71 weeks compared to 42 weeks for those treated with 5000 rad and the two drugs (P less than 0.005). Sixty-four percent of patients treated with combined modality therapy experienced grade 3 or worse toxicity compared to 42% of patients receiving chemotherapy alone (P less than 0.05). Specifically, vomiting, other gastrointestinal toxicities, and leukopenia (WBC below 2000) were worse among patients treated with the combined modality, especially during the first 10 weeks of therapy (P less than 0.01) when radiation was being given. During these first 10 weeks, patients treated with combined therapy tended to experience greater declines in performance status and more rapid weight loss than their counterparts treated with chemotherapy alone. A case-by-case analysis of early deaths showed disease progression within the local area, sepsis, or nutritional deficiencies as contributory factors.

Although it was tempting to question the role of radiation therapy, the median survival of patients on both treatment arms was greater than the median survival of any other treatment ever reported in locally unresectable disease. Furthermore, an updated analysis of this study in September 1979 (Schein and Novak 1980) demonstrated a 21% three-year survival probability in both treatment arms, an intersection of the survival curves at three years, and the probability that long-term survival advantage will shift to the combined treatment arm. Far from condemning radiation therapy in gastric cancer, continued analysis of this study has suggested a possible role in future studies for a lower radiation dose in combined modality treatment, a change in the sequence of delivering radiation and chemotherapy, and/or hyperalimentation as nutritional support during the radiation part of a combined modality program.

In the area of advanced gastric cancer, the GITSG first studied in phase II and III comparative trials the relative effectiveness of doxorubicin given as a single agent and in combination with 5-fluorouracil and semustine (FAMe), and the MIFUCA regimen—mitomycin plus 5-fluorouracil plus cytarabine (Cytosar)—popularized at Memorial Sloan-Kettering (DeJager et al. 1974). Between June 1975 and July 1976, 174 patients entered this protocol.

Among previously untreated patients with measurable disease, response rates associated with each treatment group were: doxorubicin, 24%; FAMe, 35%; and MIFUCA, 21%. Among previously treated patients the response rate was 19% for doxorubicin and 8% for MIFUCA; previously treated patients were not eligible to receive FAMe. Thus activity was established for doxorubicin in this study. In addition, those treated with FAMe lived significantly longer than patients receiving MIFUCA (*P* less than 0.01), with a median survival of 22 weeks compared to 17 weeks for the latter (O'Connell et al. 1978).

As a result of its high response rate and apparent survival benefit, the FAMe treatment arm was retained in the GITSG second-generation study (protocol 8376) for advanced gastric cancer; however, because FAMe was the most toxic as well as the "best" treatment arm in protocol 8375, the 5-fluorouracil and semustine dosages of this regimen were reduced. For comparison, the 5-fluorouracil and semustine regimen was given in the same dosage schedule as previously reported by the ECOG (Moertel et al. 1976). Similarly, the GITSG elected to study 5-fluorouracil plus doxorubicin plus mitomycin (FAM) combination based on a 55% response rate among 29 patients with advanced gastric cancer studied at Georgetown University (MacDonald et al. 1976). Most encouraging was the reported 9.5-month median duration of response and the 13-month median survival. As a fourth treatment arm, ICRF-159 (Razoxane), a drug with reputed activity in gastrointestinal cancer (Bellet et al. 1975; Marciniak et al. 1975), was added to 5-fluorouracil and semustine to produce the so-called FIMe regimen.

By January 1979, 205 patients had been randomized into this study, of whom 183 were evaluable. Progression-free survival and overall survival were significantly longer (*P* less than 0.05) for patients receiving the FAMe and FAM regimens compared to those associated with the FIMe and 5-fluorouracil plus semustine regimens. Among a subpopulation of patients

Table 37.2. *Combination Chemotherapy Responses in Advanced Gastric Cancer*

Treatment	*Response Fraction*	*Objective Response Rate (%)*
FAMe	3/11	27
FAM	3/12	25
FIMe	4/19	21
5-Fluorouracil plus semustine	1/17	6

SOURCE: O'Connell et al. 1980.

with measurable lesions and without active heart disease, objective tumor response fractions and rates were observed as noted in table 37.2. Although the absolute values of objective tumor response rates were disappointingly lower than in other recent reports, the superiority of the FAMe and FAM regimens was confirmed while benefit from the ECOG dosage of 5-fluorouracil plus semustine was not. Preliminary analysis of this study suggests that the response rate values may be related to patient selection factors not adequately described by ECOG status, or to the relatively small number of patients with measurable lesions and with active heart disease who were available for analysis in each treatment group.

The GITSG continues its search for active regimens in advanced disease in a series of phase II and phase III trials. Currently, the value of 5-fluorouracil and doxorubicin in the two active regimens (FAM and FAMe) is being tested by comparing the two drugs in common to the FAM and FAMe regimens. In a second study (protocol 8477), the value of ICRF-159 and the antifols methotrexate and triazinate is being tested in patients with measurable lesions who have had prior treatment with 5-fluorouracil, doxorubicin, mitomycin, or semustine.

In summary, the best chance to cure gastric cancer results from early diagnosis and surgical removal of the lesion. If the tumor is unresectable, bypass surgery provides good palliation. If the lesion is unresectable, extending a noncurative resection does not necessarily improve survival. If the tumor is resected, the value of adjuvant therapy for gastric cancer seems to be of value. For locally residual gastric cancer, the role of radiation therapy is limited and dose-dependent; it requires further study. Finally, combination chemotherapy provides the best palliation and survival for advanced disease: 5-fluorouracil, doxorubicin, mitomycin, and semustine are active agents. Future studies will hopefully identify other active drugs, optimum doses, and better means of delivering therapy.

References

Bellet, R. E. et al. Phase II study of ICRF-159 (NSC 129943) in human solid tumors. *Proc. Am. Assoc. Cancer Res.* 16:224, 1975.

Comis, R. L., and Carter, S. K. A review of chemotherapy in gastric cancer. *Cancer* 34:1576–1586, 1974.

DeJager, R. et al. Mitomycin C, 5-fluorouracil, and cytosine arabinoside (MFC) in gastrointestinal cancer. *Proc. Am. Assoc. Cancer Res.* 15:178, 1974.

Frytak, S. et al. Adriamycin (NSC 123127) therapy for advanced gastrointestinal cancer. *Cancer Chemother. Rep.* 59:405–409, 1975.

Kovach, J. S. et al. A controlled study of combined 1,3 bis-(2-chlorethyl)-1-nitrosourea and 5-fluorouracil therapy for advanced gastric and pancreatic cancer. *Cancer* 33:563–567, 1974.

Livstone, E. et al. Adjuvant chemotherapy with 5-FU and methyl-CCNU prolongs recurrence free interval and survival following curative resection for gastric adenocarcinoma. *Gastroenterology* 80:1215, 1981.

MacDonald, J. et al. 5-Fluorouracil, mitomycin C, and Adriamycin—FAM: a new combination chemotherapy program for advanced gastric carcinoma. *Proc. Am. Assoc. Cancer Res.* 17:264, 1976.

Marciniak, T. A. et al. Phase II study of ICRF-159 (NSC 129943) in advanced colorectal carcinoma. *Cancer Chemother. Rep.* 59:761–763, 1975.

McNeer, G., and Pack, G. T. *Neoplasms of the stomach.* Philadelphia: J. B. Lippincott, 1967.

Moertel, C. G. Therapy of advanced gastrointestinal cancer with the nitrosoureas. *Cancer Chemother. Rep.* 4:27–34, 1973.

Moertel, C. G. et al. Combined 5-fluorouracil and supervoltage radiation therapy of locally unresectable gastrointestinal cancer. *Lancet* 1:865–867, 1969.

Moertel, C. G. et al. Sequential and combination chemotherapy of advanced gastric cancer. *Cancer* 38:678–682, 1976.

Morrissey, J. F. Gastrointestinal endoscopy. *Gastroenterology* 62:1241–1268, 1971.

O'Connell, M. J. et al. Adriamycin, 5-fluorouracil + mitomycin C + cytosine arabinoside, and 5-fluorouracil + Adriamycin + methyl-CCNU in advanced gastric carcinoma. *Proc. Am. Assoc. Cancer Res.* 19:343, 1978.

O'Connell, M. J. et al. A comparative assessment of combination chemotherapy in advanced gastric cancer. *Proc. Am. Assoc. Cancer Res.* 21:420, 1980.

Schein, P., and Novak, J. Combined modality therapy versus chemotherapy alone for locally unresectable gastric cancer. *Proc. Am. Assoc. Cancer Res.* 21:419, 1980.

Shirakabe, H. *Double contrast studies of the stomach.* Tokyo: Bunkodo, 1971.

Silverberg, E. Cancer statistics, 1982. *CA* 32:15–31, 1982.

Sleisenger, M. H., and Fordtran, J. S. *Gastrointestinal disease,* 2nd edition. Philadelphia: W. B. Saunders, 1978.

thirty-eight

Pancreatic Cancer: Diagnosis and Treatment

R. GLEN WIGGANS

Carcinoma of the pancreas has been increasing in incidence in the United States during the past three decades. It is presently the fourth most common cause of cancer deaths in this country, exceeded only by lung, large bowel, and breast cancer. Approximately 22,000 new cases of pancreatic cancer are diagnosed each year, and essentially all patients can be expected to die of their disease (Silverberg 1981).

Risk Factors and Incidence

The available epidemiologic data suggest several potential risk factors. Cigarette smoking, especially among men, carries an increased risk (although not to the same degree as with lung cancer), whereas alcohol does not (Wynder et al. 1973). The role of diet as an etiologic factor remains unclear, although there is some information suggesting an association with high fat intake (Wynder et al. 1973). A recent report of a possible association of coffee and cancer of the pancreas (MacMahon et al. 1981) has aroused interest and controversy. The importance of chemical carcinogens is suggested by the fact that there is a higher incidence of pancreatic cancer among engineers and nonferrous metal workers, coke and gas plant employees, and workers exposed to beta-naphthylamine and benzidine, and chemists (Wynder et al. 1973). Animal studies have demonstrated that N-methyl-N-nitrosourea and di-N-propylnitrosamine can produce adenocarcinoma of the pancreas in rats (Pour et al. 1975).

In women, an association with early-onset diabetes mellitus and cholecystectomy has been seen. Pancreatic adenocarcinoma is much more common in men, especially those under 50 years of age, probably in large part a reflection of their excess cigarette smoking. Blacks have a somewhat higher rate of pancreatic carcinoma than whites. It has also been noted that pancreatic carcinoma is relatively infrequent among the native Japanese population and increases in incidence among Japanese immigrants to the United States. This has also been observed for breast carcinoma, suggesting an environmental factor.

Survival statistics remain dismal in this disease, reflecting in large part late detection and also the relative ineffectiveness of current therapy. The most common presenting symptoms are weight loss (75% of patients averaging 20 pounds) and abdominal pain (72%) with radiation of pain to the back in 25% to 30%. Anorexia (47%), nausea and vomiting (33%), and jaundice (25%) are other frequent presenting manifestations. Physical findings include hepatomegaly in approximately 50%, icterus in 40%, abdominal mass in only 15% to 20%, and ascites in 10% (Gudjonsson, Livstone, and Spiro 1978). The organ's retroperitoneal location makes early diagnosis by physical examination exceptionally difficult.

Diagnosis

The conventional upper gastrointestinal series (UGI) most often detects only a large carcinoma of the head of the pancreas that has infiltrated surrounding structures. Hypotonic duodenography has been reported to have a diagnostic accuracy of 75% in lesions of the pancreatic head and about 90% in ampullary carcinoma; unfortunately, it is not helpful in evaluating lesions of the body and tail of the pancreas (Macdonald, Widerlite, and Schein 1976).

The Mayo Clinic performed a prospective study of diagnostic tests in 70 patients suspected of having pancreatic carcinoma. After all studies had been performed, diagnosis was made by laparotomy in 68 cases and liver biopsy in 2. Of the 70 cases there were 30 pancreatic carcinomas (17 of the head or head and body, 12 of the body or body and tail, 1 ampullary) with 4 cases of localized disease, 10 with regional metastases, and 16 with intraabdominal metastases. The following conclusions were noted in this prospective study: pancreatic selenomethionine scan is nonspecific, with a false positive rate of over 30%. Ultrasonography, endoscopic retrograde pancreatography (ERCP), and pancreatic function tests were found to detect 90% of all pancreatic disease and 80% of pancreatic cancer. Computerized tomographic scanning was used in 15 cases and was felt to be similar to ultrasonography in its diagnostic accuracy. Results with arteriography were similar to those with ERCP when positive (85% to 90% accurate). Among 44 cases in which arteriography did not show carcinoma, however, 8 were found to have carcinoma whereas with ERCP there was less than a 5% false negative interpretation (DiMagno et al. 1977).

In assessing the diagnostic accuracy of two of the most widely used noninvasive procedures—ultrasound and CT scan—for their evaluation of the pancreas, a few conclusions can be noted. A good prospective comparison is not yet available. From the literature, however, diagnostic accuracy appears equivalent (ranging from 75% to 95% in most series). With lesions of the tail of the pancreas, CT appears preferable. With body lesions both modalities are accurate, and with head lesions ultrasonography is better (Sample and Sarti 1979). Small lesions causing biliary or pancreatic duct obstruction are noted on both studies, whereas nonobstructing solid abnormalities are best seen on ultrasound.

The role of circulating markers in the early detection of malignant disease has been under careful investigation. Carcinoembryonic antigen (CEA) has been noted to be elevated (greater than 2.5 ng/ml) in 85% of patients with pancreatic carcinoma; in 71% of those with metastatic disease CEA was greater than 10 ng/ml (Ona et al. 1973). Unfortunately, CEA lacks specificity. In one study of pancreatitis, CEA was elevated in 43% of patients (18 of 42) (Delwiche, Zamcheck, and Marion 1973). In nonjaundiced patients with known pancreatic disease a CEA above 9.0 ng/ml is highly suggestive of malignancy rather than inflammatory disease (Kalser et al. 1978). Elevation of both pancreatic juice and plasma CEA is felt by some to be more supportive of a diagnosis of pancreatic carcinoma than elevation of pancreatic juice or plasma CEA alone (Sharma et al. 1976). Alpha-fetoglobulin is a fetal protein that may be elevated in patients with hepatomas or embryonal cell carcinoma of the testes. It is very nonspecific, and in one study was elevated in 25% of patients with pancreatic carcinoma (McIntire et al. 1975).

Treatment

The treatment results in pancreatic carcinoma remain dismal. Surgery is still the only present modality with a potential for cure. Lesions at the head of the pancreas producing early obstructive jaundice may be amenable to radical resection for cure (10% to 25% of explored patients); however, operative mortality in these procedures is high—10% to 40%—and five-year survival remains low—less than 5% (Gudjonsson, Livstone, and Spiro 1978). Biliary diversion and gastroenterostomy can alleviate the symptoms of jaundice and bowel obstruction and may increase survival slightly when compared with no palliative operation. With general supportive care and surgical palliation the median survival is 3.5 months, with 8% alive at one year and 2% at two years (Carter and Comis 1975). The need to identify an effective therapy is obvious.

In patients with locally unresectable carcinoma of the pancreas (defined as tumor extension to regional nodes or encasing a vital blood vessel) the combination of radiation and 5-fluorouracil (Fluorouracil, Adrucil) (15 mg/kg intravenously on first three days of irradiation) has improved survival from a mean of 6.3 months with radiation alone to 10.4 months with combination therapy (Moertel et al. 1969). The Gastrointestinal Tumor Study Group (GITSG) undertook a controlled prospective evaluation of three treatment regimens for locally advanced disease: 6000 rad alone, 4000 rad and 5-fluorouracil, and 6000 rad and 5-fluorouracil. Survival in patients treated with radiation alone was inferior to that observed in the other two arms: median 18 weeks compared to 35 weeks in patients treated with combined modalities (Moertel et al. 1976a). Presently, there appears to be a slight advantage for patients treated with 6000 rad and 5-fluorouracil (median survival 39 weeks) compared to 4000 rad and 5-fluorouracil (31 weeks). Despite this slight improvement in median survival, less than 10% are projected to be alive at two years (Lokich et al. 1979). In addition to conventional irradiation with photons, investigators at the Vincent T. Lombardi Cancer Research Center have used fast neutron therapy in combination with 5-fluorouracil for locally unresectable disease. In 13 patients with followable disease treated with 1716 rad of 15 MeV fast neutrons, there were partial responses in six patients with median duration of survival of 13 months (6 to over 22) in responders versus 4 months in nonresponders. Toxicity in terms of myelosuppression and gastrointestinal side effects was severe (Macdonald et al. 1978).

The role of chemotherapy alone in metastatic pancreatic carcinoma at the present time remains undefined. Of the currently available drugs, few have undergone extensive evaluations in this disease (table 38.1). The most intensively investigated drug has been 5-fluorouracil, and the range of response rates varies from 0% to 67% (Hurley and Ellison 1960); however, most studies show responses of around 20%. Intravenous administration has a 21% response rate compared to 0% for orally treated patients at the same dosage in one study (Solinsky, Pugh, and Bateman 1973). Mitomycin has produced a similar response rate to 5-fluorouracil, although it has been tested in a much smaller group of patients (Carter and Comis 1975). Of the chloroethyl nitrosoureas (carmustine, lomustine, and semustine), lomustine (CeeNU) and semustine have shown a response rate of around 10% and carmustine (BiCNU) was found to be inactive when tested at the Mayo Clinic (Moertel et al. 1976b). Streptozotocin, a naturally occurring methylnitrosourea noted to be effective in islet cell carcinomas, has also demonstrable activity in pancreatic adenocarcinomas (DuPriest et al. 1975). One other drug, doxorubicin, has undergone single-agent testing with responses noted in 2 of 15 previously untreated patients (Schein et al. 1978).

Combination chemotherapy in adenocarcinoma of the pancreas is in its infancy. In a number of studies good response rates have been obtained (table 38.2), but further investigation with controlled studies needs to be done to confirm the superiority of combination therapy over single-agent therapy and to assess the actual impact on patient survival.

The combination of 5-fluorouracil and carmustine as reported by Kovach and co-workers (1974) had a 33% response rate (10 of 30) compared to 16% with 5-fluorouracil alone and 0% for carmustine alone. The combination did not produce any survival advantage compared to treatment with single agents alone *or* to untreated historical controls. The median duration of survival of all patients was six months. Another study with 5-fluorouracil and carmustine had a 20% response rate with an overall median survival of five months (Lokich et al. 1974).

Combination therapy with 5-fluorouracil and testolactone with or without spironolactone was reported to produce a median survival in excess of 21 months in 13 patients with advanced pancreatic carcinoma (Waddell 1973). The Eastern Cooperative Oncology Group (ECOG) evaluated the effectiveness of the 5-fluorouracil and spironolactone combination with or without streptozotocin in a large controlled prospective randomized trial (Moertel and Lavin 1977). This group's conclusions were that neither spironolactone nor streptozotocin improved survival; median duration was 15 weeks.

In a phase II trial at the Vincent T. Lombardi Cancer Research Center, we evaluated the three-drug combination of streptozotocin, mitomycin, and 5-fluorouracil (SMF) in patients with advanced measurable pancreatic cancer (Wiggans et al. 1978). Ten of 23 cases (43%) responded—9 PR and 1 CR, with 1 patient alive and free of disease three and one-half years after biopsy-proved liver metastases. The median survival of all cases was 6 months; responders had a median survival of 10 months as compared to 3 months for nonresponders. Toxicity consisted of nausea and vomiting, experienced by all patients and felt to be related to streptozotocin; mild myelosuppression; median leukocyte nadir of 2900 and platelet nadir of 73,000; and nephrotoxicity consisting of mild proteinuria and renal insufficiency in 2 of 23 patients, with creatinine elevations to 2.7 mg/dl and 4.8 mg/dl. The same three drugs in another study produced a response rate of 31% (5 of 16 cases) compared to 21% for 5-fluorouracil and streptozotocin.

Another three-drug combination regimen (FAM)—5-fluorouracil, doxorubicin (Adriamycin), and mitomycin—with previously documented effectiveness in gastric carcinoma has been tested in a phase II trial of patients with pancreatic carcinoma (Smith et al. 1979). Ten of 25 patients with advanced measurable disease have attained a partial response with median survival for responders in excess of nine months. Both the SMF and FAM regimens are now undergoing randomized prospective trials in the GITSG.

Conclusions

The overall role of chemotherapy in patients with pancreatic carcinoma is under evaluation, but hopefully some of the optimism generated by these early reports

Table 38.1. *Single-Agent Chemotherapy in Pancreatic Cancer*

Drug	*Response Rate (%)*	*Reference*
5-Fluorouracil (5-FU)	21	Solinsky, Pugh, and Bateman 1973
Mitomycin	27	Carter and Comis 1975
Carmustine (BCNU)	0	Moertel et al. 1976
Lomustine (CCNU)	10	Moertel et al. 1976
Semustine (Methyl-CCNU)	10	Moertel et al. 1976
Streptozocin	36	DuPriest et al. 1975
Doxorubicin (Adriamycin)	13	Schein et al. 1978

Table 38.2. *Combination Chemotherapy in Pancreatic Cancer*

Combination	*Response Rate (%)*	*Reference*
5-FU + carmustine	33	Kovach et al. 1974
5-FU + carmustine	20	Lokich et al. 1974
5-FU + testolactone	77	Waddell 1973
5-FU + spironolactone ± streptozocin	(12 weeks median survival)	Moertel and Lavin 1977
Streptozocin + mitomycin + 5-FU	43	Wiggans et al. 1978
5-FU + doxorubicin + mitomycin	40	Smith et al. 1979

will be translated into significant increases in survival.

One final point in the management of these patients that deserves mention is nutritional status. They tend to lose significant amounts of body weight, and one investigator found that in 12 cases of pancreatic carcinoma (8 of head and 4 of body lesions) there was a significant decrease in fat absorption in 9 patients (DiMagno 1979). He noted that malabsorption rather than decreased food intake was the most important factor in the weight loss, and that fat absorption was improved with the ingestion of eight tablets of pancreatin at each meal. In addition to enzyme replacements, the use of high-protein, high-caloric liquid supplements and adequate analgesia is routinely encouraged.

It is hoped that with further refinement of presently available diagnostic tools such as CT scan and ultrasonography, earlier diagnosis and therapy of this disease might be accomplished. Radiation therapy along with 5-fluorouracil has a proved role in locally advanced disease. In advanced metastatic disease effective drug combinations have been identified; further testing of existing combinations as well as identification of new drugs is eagerly awaited.

References

Carter, S. K., and Comis, R. L. Adenocarcinoma of the pancreas: current therapeutic approaches, prognostic variables, and criteria of response. In *Cancer therapy: prognostic factors and criteria of response,* ed. M. J. Staquet. New York: Raven Press, 1975.

Delwiche, R.; Zamcheck, N.; and Marion, M. Carcinoembryonic antigen in pancreatitis. *Cancer* 31:328–330, 1973.

DiMagno, E. P. Report on nutrition in pancreatic cancer. Presented at the Gastrointestinal Tumor Study Group, San Diego, February 1979.

DiMagno, E. P. et al. A prospective comparison of current diagnostic tests for pancreatic carcinoma. *N. Engl. J. Med.* 297:737–742, 1977.

DuPriest, R. W. et al. Streptozotocin therapy in 22 cancer patients. *Cancer* 35:358–367, 1975.

Gudjonsson, B.; Livstone, E. M.; and Spiro, H. M. Cancer of the pancreas—diagnostic accuracy and survival statistics. *Cancer* 42:2494–2506, 1978.

Hurley, J. D., and Ellison, E. H. Chemotherapy of solid cancer arising from the gastrointestinal tract. *Ann. Surg.* 152:56–82, 1960.

Kalser, M. H. et al. Circulating carcinoembryonic antigen in pancreatic carcinoma. *Cancer* 42:1468–1471, 1978.

Kovach, J. S. et al. A controlled study of combined 1,3-bis-(2-chloroethyl)-1-nitrosourea and 5-fluorouracil therapy for advanced gastric and pancreatic cancer. *Cancer* 33:563–567, 1974.

Lokich, J. J. et al. Chemotherapy in pancreatic carcinoma: 5-fluorouracil (5-FU) and 1,3-bis-(2-chloroethyl)-1-nitrosourea (BCNU). *Ann. Surg.* 179:450–453, 1974.

Lokich, J. J. for GITSG. A multi-institutional comparative trial of radiation therapy alone and in combination with 5-fluorouracil for locally unresectable pancreatic carcinoma. *Ann. Surg.* 189:205–208, 1979.

Macdonald, J. S. et al. Phase I–II trial of fast neutron radiation with and without 5-fluorouracil for locally advanced pancreatic and gastric adenocarcinoma. *Proc. Am. Soc. Clin. Oncol.* 19:377, 1978.

Macdonald, J. S.; Widerlite, L.; and Schein, P. S. Current diagnosis and management of pancreatic carcinoma. *J. Natl. Cancer Inst.* 56:1093–1099, 1976.

MacMahon, B. et al. Coffee and cancer of the pancreas. *N. Engl. J. Med.* 304:630–633, 1981.

McIntire, K. R. et al. Serum α-fetoprotein in patients with neoplasms of the gastrointestinal tract. *Cancer Res.* 35:991–996, 1975.

Moertel, C. G. et al. Combined 5-fluorouracil and supervoltage radiation therapy of locally unresectable gastrointestinal cancer. *Lancet* 2:865–867, 1969.

Moertel, C. G. et al. An evaluation of high-dose radiation and combined radiation and 5-fluorouracil therapy for locally unresectable pancreatic carcinoma. *Proc. Am. Soc. Clin. Oncol.* 17:244, 1976a.

Moertel, C. G. et al. Therapy for gastrointestinal cancer with nitrosoureas alone and in drug combination. *Cancer Treat. Rep.* 60:729–732, 1976b.

Moertel, C. G., and Lavin, P. T. An evaluation of 5-FU, nitrosourea and lactone combinations in therapy of upper gastrointestinal cancer. *Proc. Am. Soc. Clin. Oncol.* 18:344, 1977.

Ona, F. et al. Carcinoembryonic antigen (CEA) in the diagnosis of pancreatic cancer. *Cancer* 31:324–327, 1973.

Pour, P. et al. A new approach for induction of pancreatic neoplasms. *Cancer Res.* 35:2259–2268, 1975.

Sample, W. F., and Sarti, D. A. Diagnosis of pancreatic disease by ultrasound and computed tomography. In *Diagnostic ultrasound in gastrointestinal disease*, ed. K. J. W. Taylor. New York: Churchill Livingstone, 1979.

Schein, P. S. et al. Randomized phase II clinical trial of Adriamycin in advanced measurable pancreatic carcinoma—a gastrointestinal tumor study group report. *Cancer* 42:19–22, 1978.

Sharma, M. P. et al. Carcinoembryonic antigen (CEA) activity in pancreatic juice of patients with pancreatic carcinoma and pancreatitis. *Cancer* 38:2457–2461, 1976.

Silverberg, E. Cancer statistics, 1981. *CA* 31:13–28, 1981.

Smith, F. P. et al. Phase II evaluation of FAM in advanced pancreatic cancer. *Proc. Am. Soc. Clin. Oncol.* 20:415, 1979.

Solinsky, D. C.; Pugh, R. P.; and Bateman, J. R. 5-fluorouracil (NSC 19893) therapy for pancreatic carcinoma: comparison of oral and intravenous routes. *Cancer Treat. Rep.* 4:27–34, 1973.

Waddell, W. R. Chemotherapy for carcinoma of the pancreas. *Surgery* 74:420–429, 1973.

Wiggans, R. G. et al. Phase II trial of streptozotocin, mitomycin C and 5-fluorouracil (SMF) in the treatment of advanced pancreatic cancer. *Cancer* 41:387–391, 1978.

Wynder, E. L. et al. A case control study of cancer of the pancreas. *Cancer* 31:641–648, 1973.

thirty-nine

Primary Cancer of the Liver

MARTIN E. KATZ

Epidemiology

Primary carcinoma of the liver (hepatoma) has widely varying incidence in different regions of the world. In the United States it accounts for only 1.7% of all malignancies of the digestive tract, as compared to much higher incidence in eastern and southern Africa where it may represent up to 20% to 50% of all cancer deaths (Seidman, Silverberg, and Holleb 1976; Dunham and Bailar 1968). Cancer of the liver is two to four times more frequent in men than in women, with peak incidence in the fifth and sixth decades. In autopsy series 0.1% to 1% of livers have been found to contain hepatomas (Lopez-Corella, Ridaura-Sanz, and Albores-Saavedra 1968). The term hepatoma encompasses the common variant hepatocellular carcinoma as well as the less frequent hepatoblastomas and mixed carcinomas (with hepatocellular and cholangiocarcinoma elements). In this chapter, unless stated otherwise, hepatoma and hepatocellular carcinoma will be used interchangeably.

The wide variation in incidence has led to a search for environmental carcinogens (table 39.1). Cirrhosis and/or fibrosis is present in the majority of livers containing hepatocellular carcinoma. Cirrhosis is usually of the macronodular (postnecrotic) type (Curutchat et al. 1971), but hepatocellular carcinomas have been reported to develop in livers involved by micronodular cirrhosis, biliary cirrhosis, and hemochromatosis. In the United States a history of alcoholism and alcoholic liver disease is often obtained from the patient with hepatocellular carcinoma (Ihde et al. 1974), but prior exposure to hepatitis B virus seems to be of greater importance in non-American series (Altman 1980). The percentage of patients with detectable hepatitis B surface antigen and concomitant hepatoma varies widely, with reported figures of 3% to 41% in Africa, 15% to 40% in Japan, and 80% in Taiwan, although these figures do not take into account variations in the detection methods for the antigen. It has been suggested that there is a latent period between the acquisition of hepatitis B virus and development of hepatoma, and that the chronic carrier state may place an individual at 22.6

Table 39.1. *Conditions Predisposing to Hepatoma*

1. Cirrhosis due (related) to:
   a. Macronodular (postnecrotic)
   b. Micronodular (Laennec's)
   c. Primary biliary
   d. Hemochromatosis
2. Chemical agents
   a. Aflatoxin
   b. Thorotrast
   c. Semisynthetic androgens and estrogens
   d. ? Oral contraceptives
   e. Alcohol
3. Hepatitis B virus

times increased risk for developing primary liver carcinoma (Szmuness 1978). Whether hepatitis B virus leads directly to the development of cancer in an otherwise normal liver or whether there must be a transition from chronic hepatitis to cirrhosis to hepatocellular carcinoma is unknown. Clearly, some livers do not show changes of cirrhosis or fibrosis.

Hemochromatosis may be associated with a 7% to 14% incidence of hepatoma (Locker et al. 1979). Subsequent tumor development is apparently not affected by attempts at vigorous phlebotomy to reduce iron overload. Thorotrast, a contrast agent used between 1917 and 1930 in the United States and until the 1950s in Europe, has been associated with the development of several types of cancer including hepatomas and hepatic angiosarcomas, as are arsenic and vinyl chloride (Berk 1976). There is an estimated 400-fold risk in people chronically exposed to vinyl chloride. (Clinical features, diagnosis, and treatment of hepatic angiosarcoma are reviewed by Locker and associates, 1979.) Both semisynthetic androgens and estrogens have also been connected with primary liver cancer (Hernandez-Nieto et al. 1977; Boyd and Mark 1977).

Over the past six years extensive literature has accumulated detailing benign hepatic lesions in premenopausal women taking oral contraceptives with the very serious complication of hemoperitoneum from tumor rupture (Klatskin 1977). Also of major concern is reported primary hepatocellular carcinoma arising with the use of these drugs (Boyd and Mark 1977; Stauffer and Hill 1976). It has been suggested that some of these tumors may develop into hepatic adenomas, but a clear-cut cause and effect relationship between them has not been established (Klatskin 1977; Christopherson and Mays 1977).

Aflatoxin, a potent carcinogen produced by the fungus *Aspergillus flavus,* has been linked to hepatocellular carcinoma by the observation that the incidence of primary liver cancer parallels the intake of aflatoxin (Altman 1980). The fungus grows in moist areas where grain is stored, for example, in Africa where dietary intake of aflatoxin is substantial. Africa, however, is also an area of high hepatitis B virus infection, making it difficult to discern the relative role of each factor. Specific mechanisms of hepatocarcinogenesis are unknown despite extensive epidemiologic data.

Signs and Symptoms

The clinical findings in patients with hepatocellular carcinoma (table 39.2) fall into three major categories: (1) those attributable to the primary tumor, (2) related to metastases, and (3) related to paraneoplastic syndromes. Initial complaints often include right upper quadrant and/or epigastric fullness with or without associated pain, abdominal swelling, general malaise, and anorexia (Ihde et al. 1974; Okuda 1976). Pruritus, fever, weight loss, and change of skin color (jaundice) are usual complaints at initial diagnosis. Physical findings usually reflect primary liver involvement by tumor and may include hepatomegaly, a palpable right upper quadrant mass, and ascites, and less frequently, hepatic bruits, spider angiomata, splenomegaly, jaundice, and gynecomastia. Frequent sites of metastases include regional nodes, the inferior vena cava and portal venous system, and the lungs, although involvement of virtually all organs, both intraabdominal and extraabdominal has been reported. Physical findings may thus also reflect distant spread of the cancer.

Table 39.2. *Presenting Symptoms of Patients with Hepatoma*

Common	*Unusual*
Abdominal pain	Fever
Abdominal fullness	Weight loss
Abdominal swelling	Jaundice
General malaise	Pruritus
Anorexia	

Several interesting paraneoplastic syndromes have been reported in patients with hepatoma, including erythrocytosis (secondary polycythemia), hypercalcemia, hypoglycemia, and gynecomastia and feminization (Margolis and Homey 1972). Erythrocytosis may be secondary to increased erythropoietin production by the kidney, perhaps modulated by a factor derived from the primary liver cancer. Hypercalcemia may reflect extraparathyroidal hormone production, skeletal metastases, or a coincidental functioning parathyroid adenoma. Hypoglycemia may be a result of nearly total replacement of glycogen stores by the tumor in terminal disease, and less frequently, a liver in which there are poorly understood abnormalities in glycogen metabolism not explained by increases in insulin or inhibitory effects of counter-regulatory hormones. Acquired glucose-6-phosphatase deficiency leading to decreased glycogenolysis has been suggested as a possible mechanism. Gynecomastia usually reflects markedly elevated levels of beta subunit of human chorionic gonadotropin produced by the tumor, while feminization may be a manifestation of increased conversion of dehydroepiandrosterone to estrone and estradiol by the cancer tissue (Kew et al. 1977; Braunstein et al. 1973).

Diagnostic Methods

Abnormalities of liver-related chemistries are frequent in patients with primary carcinoma of the liver, but they are nonspecific and do not show a typical or diagnostic pattern (Van der Walt, Gomperts, and Kew 1977). The alkaline phosphatase, 5′-nucleotidase and albumin are usually abnormal at the time of initial diagnosis, while hyperbilirubinemia, transaminasemia, and abnormalities of clotting proteins are less often noted. Hemostasis in hepatocellular carcinoma has been studied in detail and is characterized by a pattern of prolonged prothrombin time, partial thromboplastin time, and reptilase time, increased levels of fibrinogen, fibrin-fibrinogen degradation products, factor VIII-related antigen and procoagulant factor VIII activity, moderately decreased levels of factors V, IX, and X, antithrombin III and plasminogen, and markedly decreased levels of factors II and VII. Factors XI, XII, and XIII and quantitative platelet counts are usually normal (Van der Walt, Gomperts, and Kew 1977).

Serum alpha-fetoprotein (AFP), a serum alpha-1 globulin synthesized during fetal development and present in only minute quantities in the healthy adult (30 to 40 ng/ml) is elevated in 70% to 80% of patients with hepatocellular carcinoma when radioimmunoassay techniques are used (Waldman and McIntire 1974; McIntire et al. 1975). Elevation of AFP is not diagnostic for hepatocellular carcinoma and may occur in patients with viral hepatitis, testicular and ovarian germ cell tumors containing endodermal sinus (yolk sac) elements, malignancies of the bile ducts, gallbladder, pancreas, and stomach, and a variety of non-neoplastic gastrointestinal diseases. Levels above 200 to 300 ng/ml are highly suggestive of malignancy. The fall (and disappearance) of elevated AFP levels may be useful as a guide to effective antineoplastic therapy.

Although both abdominal ultrasonography (Kamin, Bernardino, and Green 1979) and computerized axial tomography (Itai, Nishikawa, and Tasaka 1979) have been used tentatively to diagnose hepatoma, these techniques have occasionally failed because the tumor has been of similar radiographic density as surrounding normal liver tissues. Hepatic arteriography still remains a more definitive technique for diagnosis but cannot be used for screening (Okuda et al. 1977a). Typical findings include hypervascularity and abnormal tumor vasculature, often with evidence for inferior vena cava or portal venous obstruction. Histologic diagnosis must rest on biopsy material, however.

Pathology

From a histopathologic viewpoint, primary cancer of the liver is not a uniform disease. Numerous growth patterns have been described and include microtrabecular, pseudoglandular, adenoid, macrotrabecular, pelioid, and eosinophilic hepatocarcinoma with lamellar fibrosis. Some liver cell carcinomas will demonstrate evidence for cholangiolar differentiation, the so-called mixed carcinomas (Peters 1976; Edmundson 1958). Similarly, there are several cytologically recognizable variants: clear cell, giant cell, eosinophilic cell, and four well-defined grades of differentiation. Encapsulated hepatocellular carcinoma may be associated with a distinct clinicopathologic pattern, including intrinsic slow growth and associated long-term survival (Okuda et al. 1977b). Hence any clinical trial needs to stratify for cytologic, histologic, and grade variants of primary liver cell carcinoma because there may be significantly different responses to new treatment modalities.

Treatment

The median duration of survival following diagnosis of hepatoma is one to seven months (Curutchat et al. 1971; Bengmark, Borjesson, and Hafstrom 1971; Raffucci and Ramirez-Schon 1970). Age, sex, cirrhosis, and the extent of liver involvement do not appear to correlate with survival, although hyperbilirubinemia and marked weight loss at the time of initial diagnosis portend a poor prognosis (Primack et al. 1975).

Surgical Resection

Surgical resection remains the only available therapeutic modality with the potential for cure. Unfortunately, in most series less than 10% to 20% of patients are candidates for aggressive surgery because the tumor may be multicentric in origin, may involve both the right and left lobes of the liver by direct extension, or may be diagnosed in a setting of severe hepatic dysfunction secondary to underlying cirrhosis (Lee 1977). Following an attempt at curative resection a small fraction of patients will achieve long-term survival (and presumably cure), although many will subsequently have relapse in the remaining liver or develop distant metastases. Operative mortality remains high.

Radiation Therapy

Despite the use of external supervoltage radiotherapeutic techniques, survival of treated patients with nonresectable hepatomas has been dismal. It is difficult to deliver a tumoricidal dose of radiation to the tumor bed without inducing severe radiation hepatitis and nephritis (Lee 1977).

Systemic Chemotherapy

With the exception of systemically administered doxorubicin (Adriamycin), there are no well-established drugs available for the treatment of patients with hepatocellular carcinoma. Table 39.3 summarizes recently reported clinical trials involving both single-agent and combination chemotherapy using standard definitions of clinical complete and partial response. In a limited phase II trial, zinostatin (neocarzinostatin) demonstrated a 20% objective response rate (Falkson, Von Hoff, and Carbone 1979) and is currently being compared to amsacrine (AMSA) and doxorubicin in an Eastern Cooperative Oncology Group Study.

Hepatic Artery Infusional Chemotherapy

Infusional chemotherapy has the potential advantages of achieving higher local concentrations of the antineoplastic agent, prolonging the contact time of the drug with the cancer cells, and of reducing systemic toxicity. As there are no large randomized prospective studies using strict response criteria comparing it with systemic treatment, it is difficult to know whether infusional therapy offers any clear-cut advantages. Mulitple anecdotal reports of prolonged response are available in the literature suggesting that intraarterial 5-fluorouracil, mitomycin, and doxorubicin may each have a role in treating patients with primary carcinoma of the liver (Misra et al. 1977; Ramming et al. 1977).

Table 39.3. *Recent Trials of Systemic Chemotherapy in Advanced Hepatoma*

Investigators	*Drug Regimen*	*CR/PR (%)**
LAC-USC (Link et al. 1977)	5-FU (oral)	0/12
	5-FU (IV)	0/9
Baylor (Kennedy et al. 1977)	5-FU (oral)	6/12 (50)
London (Cochrane et al. 1977)	5-FU (IV) + CTX + MTX + VCR	0/10
	Radiation, followed by 5-FU + CTX + MTX + VCR	0/8
Miami/Bangkok (Umsawasdi, Chainuvati, and Viranuvatti 1978)	5-FU (IV) + mitomycin	5/13 (38)
Mayo Clinic (Moertel 1975)	5-FU (IV) + BCNU	7/19 (37)
ECOG (Falkson et al. 1978)	5-FU (oral)	0/48
	5-FU (oral) + streptozotocin	4/33 (12)
	5-FU (oral) + methyl-CCNU	2/47 (4)
	Doxorubicin	9/57 (16)
NCI-VAH (Ihde et al. 1977)	Doxorubicin	2/13 (15)
SEG (Vogel et al. 1977)	Doxorubicin	7/41 (17)
Uganda (Olweny et al. 1975)	Doxorubicin	11/11 (100)
SWOG (Baker et al. 1977)	5-FU (IV) + doxorubicin	5/38 (13)
NCI-VAH (Ihde, Bunn, and Cohen 1979)	Doxorubicin + streptozotocin	2/13 (15)
SEG (Ravry and Hester 1980)	Doxorubicin + bleomycin	5/26 (19)
MSKCC (Lightdale et al. 1980)	Amsacrine	0/9
ECOG (Falkson et al. 1979)	Zinostatin	6/30 (20)

NOTES: 5-FU = 5-fluorouracil; CTX = cyclophosphamide; MTX = methotrexate; VCR = vincristine; carmustine (BCNU) = 1,3-bis(2-chloroethyl)-1-nitrosourea; semustine (methyl-CCNU) = 1-(2-chloroethyl)-3-(4-methylcyclohexyl)-1-nitrosourea; amsacrine (AMSA) = 4′-9(acridinylamino)-methanesulfan-m-anisidide; LAC-USC = Los Angeles County–University of Southern California; ECOG = Eastern Cooperative Oncology Group; NCI-VAH = National Cancer Institute–Veterans Administration Hospital; SEG = Southeast Oncology Group; SWOG = Southwest Oncology Group; MSKCC = Memorial Sloan-Kettering Cancer Center.

*CR + PR = complete plus partial response rate (number of patients responding divided by the number of patients adequately treated) using standard response criteria.

The Northern California Oncology Group recently reported treating 13 patients with intraarterial infusions of doxorubicin and 5-fluorouracil plus whole-liver radiation (Friedman et al. 1979). Six of 13 patients (46%) had objective tumor regression, with 9 patients obtaining subjective benefit. Median survival, however, was still measured in months for the group as a whole. Toxicity was tolerable and there were no catheter-associated complications.

Catheters can be placed into the hepatic artery either percutaneously or directly at the time of celiotomy. There are significant risks associated with placement, including a 5% to 15% operative mortality with directly placed catheters, bacteremia and sepsis from the catheter acting as a foreign body, extravasation of the chemotherapy drug, hepatic artery thrombosis, and catheter migration (Lee 1977).

Hepatic Artery Ligation with Infusional Chemotherapy

Ligation of the hepatic artery has its scientific basis in the fact that most primary and metastatic tumors involving the liver obtain their blood supply almost exclusively through the hepatic arterial system, whereas the normal liver has a dual blood supply through the hepatic artery (25%) and the portal venous system (75%). Complete dearterialization of the liver may, however, result in significant hepatic necrosis without improving the response rate. Similarly, it has been suggested that cirrhosis should be a contraindication for hepatic artery ligation, as the liver will become rearterialized.

Nevertheless, this procedure can result in selective tumor necrosis. Since viable tumor cells will always be left behind in the outer margins of the necrotic area, and since collateral blood flow will develop to the damaged area, some investigators have suggested subsequent infusional chemotherapy (Lee and Irwin 1978). Review of the literature indicates that reduction in tumor size may occur, but long-term survival is unusual (Lee 1977). There are no large prospective randomized studies comparing hepatic artery ligation with infusional chemotherapy to infusional therapy or systemic chemotherapy.

Summary

Approximately 2500 persons in the United States die each year from hepatoma. In some parts of the world (Africa, Asia) this is the most common cause of cancer death. Surgical resection remains the treatment of choice whenever possible, although most patients are candidates only for palliative therapy. Systemic chemotherapy is currently under intense investigation with the regrettably few active single agents. These can also be important in combined modality approaches with radiation therapy, which used alone has little role in the treatment of hepatoma. Regional chemotherapy with or without hepatic artery ligation will result in occasional objective and subjective responses, and should be compared prospectively to systemic chemotherapy in carefully controlled trials.

References

Altman, D. Hepatoma. *West. J. Med.* 132:514–520, 1980.

Baker, L. W. et al. Adriamycin and 5-fluorouracil in the treatment of advanced hepatoma: a Southwest Oncology Group study. *Cancer Treat. Rep.* 61:1595–1597, 1977.

Bengmark, S.; Borjesson, B.; and Hafstrom, L. The natural history of primary carcinoma of the liver. *Scand. J. Gastroenterol.* 6:351–355, 1971.

Berk, P. D. Vinyl chloride-associated liver disease. *Ann. Intern. Med.* 84:717–731, 1976.

Boyd, P. R., and Mark, G. J. Multiple hepatic adenomas and a hepatocellular carcinoma in a man on oral methyltestosterone for eleven years. *Cancer* 40:1756–1770, 1977.

Braunstein, G. D. et al. Ectopic production of human chorionic gonadotropin by neoplasms. *Ann. Intern. Med.* 78:39–45, 1973.

Christopherson, W. M., and Mays, E. T. Liver tumors and oral contraceptive steroids: experience with the first one hundred registry patients. *J. Natl. Cancer Inst.* 58:167–170, 1977.

Cochrane, A. M. G. et al. Quadruple chemotherapy versus radiotherapy in the treatment of primary hepatocellular carcinoma. *Cancer* 40:609–614, 1977.

Curutchat, H. P. et al. Primary liver cancer. *Surgery* 70:467–479, 1971.

Dunham, L. J., and Bailar, J. C., III. World maps of cancer mortality rates and frequency ratios. *J. Natl. Cancer Inst.* 41:155–203, 1968.

Edmunson, H. A. Tumors of the liver and intrahepatic bile ducts. In *Atlas of tumor pathology,* section VII, Fascicle 25. Washington, D.C.: Armed Forces Institute of Pathology, 1958.

Falkson, G. et al. Chemotherapy studies in primary liver cancer. *Cancer* 42:2149–2156, 1978.

Falkson, G.; Von Hoff, D.; and Carbone, P. P. A phase II study of neocarzinostatin (NSC 157365) in patients with hepatocellular carcinoma. *Proc. Am. Soc. Clin. Oncol.* 20:296, 1979.

Friedman, M. A. et al. Therapy for hepatocellular cancer with intrahepatic arterial Adriamycin and 5-fluorouracil combined with whole-liver irradiation: a Northern California Oncology Group study. *Cancer Treat. Rep.* 63:1885–1888, 1979.

Hernandez-Nieto, L. et al. Benign liver cell adenoma associated with long-term administration of an androgenic anabolic steroid (methandienone). *Cancer* 40:1761–1764, 1977.

Ihde, D. C. et al. Clinical manifestations of hepatoma. *Am. J. Med.* 56:83–90, 1974.

Ihde, D. C. et al. Adriamycin therapy in American patients with hepatocellular carcinoma. *Cancer Treat. Rep.* 61:1385–1387, 1977.

Ihde, D. C.; Bunn, P. A.; and Cohen, M. H. Combination chemotherapy of hepatocellular carcinoma with Adriamycin and streptozotocin. *Proc. Am. Soc. Clin. Oncol.* 20:410, 1979.

Itai, Y.; Nishikawa, J.; and Tasaka, A. Computed tomography in the evaluation of hepatocellular carcinoma. *Radiology* 131:165–170, 1979.

Kamin, P. D.; Bernardino, M. E.; and Green, B. Ultrasound manifestations of hepatocellular carcinoma. *Radiology* 131:459–461, 1979.

Kennedy, P. S. et al. Oral 5-fluorouracil therapy of hepatoma. *Cancer* 39:1930–1935, 1977.

Kew, M. C. et al. Mechanism of feminization in primary liver cancer. *N. Engl. J. Med.* 296:1084–1088, 1977.

Klatskin, G. Hepatic tumors: possible relationship to use of oral contraceptives. *Gastroenterology* 73:386–394, 1977.

Lee, Y. N. Systemic and regional treatment of primary carcinoma of the liver. *Cancer Treat. Rev.* 4:195–212, 1977.

Lee, Y. N., and Irwin, L. Hepatic artery ligation and Adriamycin infusion chemotherapy for hepatoma. *Cancer* 41:1249–1255, 1978.

Lightdale, C. et al. Phase II trial of AMSA in primary liver cancer. *Proc. Am. Soc. Clin. Oncol.* 21:417, 1980.

Link, J. S. et al. 5-fluorouracil in hepatocellular carcinoma. *Cancer* 39:1936–1939, 1977.

Locker, G. Y. et al. The clinical features of hepatic angiosarcoma: a report of four cases and a review of the English literature. *Medicine* 58:48–64, 1979.

Lopez-Corella, E.; Ridaura-Sanz, C.; and Albores-Saavedra, J. Primary carcinoma of the liver in Mexican adults. *Cancer* 22:678–685, 1968.

Margolis, S., and Homey, C. Systemic manifestations of hepatoma. *Medicine* 51:381–391, 1972.

McIntire, K. R. et al. Serum alpha-fetoprotein in patients with neoplasms of the gastrointestinal tract. *Cancer Res.* 35:991–996, 1975.

Misra, W. C. et al. Intrahepatic arterial infusion of combination of mitomycin C and 5-fluorouracil in treatment of primary and metastatic liver carcinoma. *Cancer* 39:1425–1429, 1977.

Moertel, C. G. Clinical management of advanced gastrointestinal cancer. *Cancer* 36:675–682, 1975.

Okuda, K. Clinical aspects of hepatocellular carcinoma — analysis of 134 cases. In *Hepatocellular carcinoma,* eds. K. Okuda and R. L. Peters. New York: John Wiley & Sons, 1976, pp. 387–436.

Okuda, K. et al. Angiographic assessment of gross anatomy of hepatocellular carcinoma: comparison of celiac angiograms and pathology in 100 cases. *Radiology* 123:21–29, 1977a.

Okuda, K. et al. Clinicopathologic features of encapsulated hepatocellular carcinoma. *Cancer* 40:1240–1245, 1977b.

Olweny, C. L. M. et al. Preliminary communication: treatment of hepatocellular carcinoma with Adriamycin. *Cancer* 36:1250–1257, 1975.

Peters, R. L. Pathology of hepatocellular carcinoma. In *Hepatocellular carcinoma,* eds. K. Okuda and R. L. Peters. New York: John Wiley & Sons, 1976, pp. 107–168.

Primack, A. et al. A staging system for hepatocellular carcinoma: prognostic factors in Ugandan patients. *Cancer* 35:1357–1364, 1975.

Raffucci, F. L., and Ramirez-Schon, G. Management of tumors of the liver. *Surg. Gynecol. Obstet.* 130:371–385, 1970.

Ramming, K. P. et al. Management of hepatic metastases. *Semin. Oncol.* 4:71–80, 1977.

Ravry, M. J. R., and Hester, M. Combination chemotherapy of hepatocellular and biliary tract carcinoma with Adriamycin and bleomycin. *Proc. Am. Soc. Clin. Oncol.* 21:366, 1980.

Seidman, H.; Silverberg, E.; and Holleb, A. I. Cancer statistics, 1976—a comparison of white and black population. *Cancer* 26:2–30, 1976.

Stauffer, J. Q., and Hill, R. B. Systemic contraceptives and liver tumors. *Ann. Intern. Med.* 85:122–124, 1976.

Szmuness, W. Hepatocellular carcinoma and hepatitis B virus—evidence for a causal association. *Progr. Med. Virol.* 24:40–69, 1978.

Umsawasdi, T.; Chainuvati, T.; and Viranuvatti, V. Combination chemotherapy of hepatocellular carcinoma with 5-fluorouracil and mitomycin C. *Proc. Am. Assoc. Cancer Res.* 19:193, 1978.

Van der Walt, J. A.; Gomperts, E. D.; and Kew, M. C. Hemastatic factors in primary hepatocellular cancer. *Cancer* 40:1593–1603, 1977.

Vogel, C. L. et al. A phase II study of Adriamycin (NSC 123127) in patients with hepatocellular carcinoma from Zambia and the United States. *Cancer* 39:1923–1929, 1977.

Waldmann, T. A., and McIntire, K. R. The use of a radioimmunoassay for alpha-fetoprotein in the diagnosis of malignancy. *Cancer* 34:1510–1515, 1974.

forty

Cancer of the Gallbladder and Bile Ducts

HUGH F. LENA
RICHARD P. BENTON
DAVID S. FISCHER

Carcinoma of the gallbladder and bile ducts is the sixth most common neoplasm of the gastrointestinal tract (table 40.1) in the United States. Among the southwestern American Indians it is the third most common malignant tumor of women (Black et al. 1977). Incidence seems to be related to the frequency of cholecystitis and cholelithiasis in the population studied.

Although 75% of gallbladder cancer is reported in women, 60% of bile duct cancer is seen in men. Because of the differing populations afflicted and the somewhat different surgical approach, these two related disorders are discussed separately.

Carcinoma of the Gallbladder

Carcinoma of the gallbladder is unusual but not rare, being the most common malignancy of the biliary tract (54%). Approximately 3200 cases are reported in the United States each year. Incidence, 1.5 cases per 100,000 of population, generally parallels that of cholelithiasis so it is not surprising that this cancer predominates in women with a sex ratio of over 3:1. Incidence in Southwest American Indians where gallstones are common is six times that of the non-Indian population In this group, gallstones were present in 93% of cases. The older age groups predominate, with a mean age of 65 years and 60% of patients over 50 years.

Although nearly all gallbladder cancers are associated with preexisting gallstones, the etiologic relationship is unclear. Possible factors include chronic mechanical irritation from stones, chronic inflammation (especially with calcification of the gallbladder wall), carcinogens derived from altered bile acids (which are structurally similar to the known carcinogen, methylcholanthrene), and preexisting benign neoplasms (Piehler and Crichlow 1978).

Adenocarcinoma of the columnar cell variety is by far the most common type of cancer. It is usually infiltrative rather than papillary. In the Mayo Clinic series, only 3% were squamous cell carcinomas, 12% were adenoacanthomas (mixed adenocarcinoma and squamous), and 85% adenocarcinoma (Adson 1973). A disproportionately high incidence of squamous cell type was found in southwestern Indians. The tumor usually arises in the fundus or neck of the viscus, and occasionally in the cystic duct. It infiltrates the wall at the site of involvement and frequently involves the entire organ. Spread is usually to the regional lymph nodes and by direct extensions to the liver, common bile duct, stomach, duodenum, and colon. Distant metastases are most commonly to peritoneum, ovaries, and pleura. The mode of lymphatic spread is of special interest to surgeons. Mural lymphatics of the gallbladder drain to the cystic duct nodes and to nodes along the common duct. Lymphatic channels then drain to superior pancreaticoduodenal nodes and from there to posterior pancreaticoduodenal and to celiac nodes.

Table 40.1. *Annual Incidence of Gastrointestinal Neoplasms in the United States*

Site	*Incidence/100,000 Population*	
Colon excluding rectum	32.3	
Sigmoid		11.4
Cecum		6.6
Transverse colon		4.1
Ascending colon		3.9
Descending colon		2.7
Large intestine, NOS*		1.8
Splenic flexure		0.8
Hepatic flexure		0.7
Appendix		0.3
Rectum and rectosigmoid	14.7	
Rectosigmoid junction		4.6
Rectum		10.1
Stomach	9.8	
Pancreas	9.7	
Esophagus	3.6	
Gallbladder and bile ducts	2.8	
Gallbladder		1.5
Other biliary		1.3
Liver	2.1	
Small intestine	0.8	
Anus, anal canal	0.6	
Retroperitoneum	0.5	
Other digestive	0.4	
Peritoneum, omentum	0.2	

SOURCE: Compiled from Young et al. 1978.
*NOS = not otherwise specified.

Symptoms are usually nonspecific and mimic benign gallbladder disease. The diagnosis should be considered in an elderly woman with a history of biliary complaints who has a change in frequency or severity of pain, a right upper quadrant mass, hepatomegaly, or constitutional symptoms of malignant disease. In a study of 75 patients (Perpetuo et al. 1978), 97% had a preexisting clinical history of recurrent right upper quadrant pain suggestive of cholecystitis for a median duration of three years, and 98% had gallstones. Loss of 10% or more of body weight occurred in 77%, hepatomegaly in 65%, nausea and vomiting in 64%, jaundice in 44%, and a palpable abdominal mass in 35%. Diagnostic procedures such as upper gastrointestional x-rays were abnormal in 39% of cases, liver scan in 55%, oral cholecystogram in 81%, intravenous cholecystogram in

67%, liver function tests in 67%, and carcinoembryonic antigen in 100%. Nonetheless, these abnormal tests did not establish the diagnosis. Newer procedures such as abdominal ultrasound, computerized axial tomography, and selective angiography rarely are successful in confirming the diagnosis at an early stage. Laparotomy is ultimately the diagnostic procedure that most closely approximates 100% accuracy when performed by experienced surgeons.

The results of surgical treatment are discouraging. The majority of reported series show a cure rate of 3% or less. The disease often causes no symptoms in its early stages. Since most cases are associated with gallstones, some are discovered incidentally at the time of cholecystectomy for cholelithiasis. In a series of 26 such occult carcinomas of the gallbladder, 25 were discovered by chance and most were cured by cholecystectomy (Nevin et al. 1978). Unfortunately, the majority of cases are discovered late, and the tumor has already invaded the liver and lymph nodes or encased the gallbladder, pancreas, or major vessels. Surgical options then are very limited (Strauch 1960; Beltz and Condon 1974).

Surgical Procedures

Biopsy only

Because of the extent of the disease most cases are suitable for laparotomy and biopsy only. At times it is even difficult to determine whether the primary tumor is in the gallbladder, bile ducts, or elsewhere.

Simple cholecystectomy

This is occasionally necessary not only in those cases where the tumor seems to be confined to the gallbladder itself, but also in more advanced cases with associated acute cholecystitis.

Cholecystectomy

The procedure includes local resection of the adjacent liver substance and regional lymphadenectomy. Experience with this operation has been somewhat limited. In addition to removal of the gallbladder, it consists of a deep wedge resection of the gallbladder bed and skeletonization of the portal triad. There seems to be little enthusiasm for hepatic lobectomy in carcinoma of the gallbladder.

Transcutaneous biliary drainage under radiologic guidance

For debilitated patients, this may be the best way to alleviate itching and jaundice with minimal morbidity (Pereiras 1978; Pollock et al. 1979) in patients whose life expectancy is only two to five months (Piehler and Crichlow 1978; Perpetuo et al. 1978).

When surgery has failed to produce cure or prolonged survival, radiation therapy and chemotherapy have been attempted. The results are palliative at best, and the incidence and duration of response are of a low order. Specific details are given in the discussion of carcinoma of the bile ducts, since the cases are usually grouped together for consideration of these therapies.

Carcinoma of the Extrahepatic Bile Ducts

Carcinoma of the extrahepatic bile ducts is nearly as common as carcinoma of the gallbladder in the United States—1.3 per 100,000 of population (Young et al. 1978). Incidence in men is slightly greater than that in women (table 40.2). The highest frequency is in the sixth and seventh decades of life, except in cases associated with ulcerative colitis where the median age is 40 years (Morowitz et al. 1971; Ritchie et al. 1974). Incidence in the Orient is significantly higher, probably due to liver fluke infections with *Clonorchis sinensis*, *Opisthorchis felineus*, and *O. viverrini*. The simplest explanation for the action of these flukes is that they incite an inflammatory reaction in the bile ducts, potentiating the action of carcinogenic agents excreted in the bile, most likely nitrosoamines (Bismuth and Malt 1979).

Unlike gallbladder carcinoma, gallstones are present in only 30% of cases. Ulcerative colitis would appear to be a predisposing condition (Akwari et al. 1975). In a series of 103 cases of bile duct carcinoma reported at the Lahey Clinic, 8 patients had associated ulcerative colitis; their average age was between 20 and 30 years (Moorhead and Warren 1976). Other predisposing conditions include regional enteritis, sclerosing cholangitis, the typhoid carrier state, and choledochal cysts. The significance of all these associations remains unclear. Carcinogens such as methylcholanthrene bear a close structural resemblance to chemicals derived from bile acids. Ingested materials such as dimethylnitrosoamines in the diet may also play a role (Bhamarapravati 1978).

Most cancers of the bile ducts are adenocarcinomas, with squamous cell carcinomas, adenoacanthomas, embryonal rhabdomyosarcomas, melanomas, and leiomyosarcomas much less frequent (Braasch 1973; Davis, Kissane, and Ishak 1969). The adenocarcinomas have a decided tendency to be sclerosing and infiltrate for long distances beneath the mucosa. This not only makes surgical cure less likely but may even make the diagnosis difficult as there may be no discernible

Table 40.2. *Differential Character of Peribiliary Lesions*

Patient Information	*Cancer of the Gallbladder*	*Cancer of the Bile Ducts*	*Cancer of the Head of Pancreas*	*Cholelithiasis*	*Choledocholithiasis*
Age	50 to 70 yrs	50 yrs (peak)	60 yrs (peak)	30 to 50 yrs	40 to 60 yrs
Sex	Women 3:1	Men 1.5:1	Men 3:1	Women 4:1	Women 2:1
Type jaundice	Late	Early, incomplete	Complete	Incomplete	Incomplete
Percentage with jaundice	About 50%	About 95%	About 75%	About 20%	About 70%
Pain	About 70%	About 65%	About 85%	High	About 75%
Palpable	About 50%	Variable	About 65%	Rare	Rare
Blood in stool	Rare	About 80%	Rare	Almost never	Rare
X-ray	Nonvisualization	Ulceration	Nonspecific	Nonvisualization	Nonvisualization
Ultrasound	Variable	Ducts dilated	Sometimes see tumor	Stones detected	Ducts dilated

SOURCE: Modified from Ackerman and del Regato 1970.

tumor. There is often an intense fibroblastic reaction and tumor cells may be few and far between, causing the surgeon to consider this to be sclerosing cholangitis instead of a malignancy (Altemeir and Culbertson 1973).

The extrahepatic bile ducts consist of the right and left hepatic ducts, the common hepatic duct, and the common duct. Although the cure rate in general is extremely poor, the chance of a good result is somewhat better in the distal duct. Unfortunately, in most series incidence of these carcinomas is higher in the proximal ducts. Moorhead and Warren (1976) reported that 70% of these cases were at or above the bifurcation of the common hepatic duct, 22% in the central bile ducts, 8% in the distal common duct, and 8% were spread throughout the extrahepatic ductal system.

Symptoms are primarily caused by bile duct obstruction, with jaundice, weight loss, chills, fever, pruritus, upper abdominal pain, nausea, and vomiting. A palpable gallbladder (Courvoisier's sign) is noted in one-third of patients. In establishing the diagnosis, oral cholecystogram and intravenous cholangiograms are of little help especially if the serum bilirubin level is over 3.5 mg/dl. The serum alkaline phosphatase and 5'-nucleotidase are elevated in 95% of cases. Upper gastrointestinal series, hypotonic duodenogram, duodenal cytology, and radioactive liver scans with technetium Tc 99m sulfur colloid or rose bengal sodium I 131 also contribute very little. Ultrasound and computer tomography may identify the site of obstruction in some instances. Celiac arteriography is also occasionally used. Percutaneous transhepatic cholangiography employing the Chiba "skinny" needle can often indicate the site and character of the bile duct obstruction (Tabrisky et al. 1976; Redeker et al. 1975). Serious complications of bile leak with peritonitis and hemorrhage have occurred. The surgeon must be prepared to proceed with prompt laparotomy should either of these complications arise. Some surgeons have recommended a minilaparotomy under local anesthesia to perform the test under direct vision. A bile leak or hemorrhage from the site of the liver puncture can thus be visualized and corrected. Endoscopic retrograde cholangiography in the hands of an experienced endoscopist is usually successful and is probably the most helpful diagnostic tool (Elias et al. 1974). Even though bile leaks and hemorrhage did not occur, some patients have developed cholangitis following the procedure. This again might require immediate surgery with decompression of the biliary tree. Cholangiography is also usually done during surgery to delineate the site and extent of tumor. Occasionally, intraoperative choledochoscopy may be required to identify multifocal or radiologically inapparent neoplasms (Tompkins et al. 1976).

The prognosis for bile duct carcinoma is as dismal as for gallbladder carcinoma, with five-year survival of less than 3%. Surgery offers the only hope of cure as well as providing the best form of palliation. With rare exceptions, only those lesions occurring in the distal common duct have been amenable to radical resection (Iwasaki et al. 1977; Ross, Braasch, and Warren 1973).

Surgical Procedures

Laparotomy, biopsy, and frozen section

Occasionally, multiple biopsies are necessary, and curettage may also be required to obtain an adequate specimen.

Palliative dilatation of malignant stricture

This may be splinted with a buried Y-tube or a T-tube to maintain patency and hopefully to relieve the jaundice and pruritus.

Cholecystojejunostomy

This is a poor palliative procedure for low common duct lesions. There may be a temporary decrease in jaundice but the carcinoma tends to spread upward and obstruct the cystic duct.

Hepaticojejunostomy or hepaticoduodenostomy

Carcinomas of the mid-duct may be amenable to these types of palliative procedures.

Pancreaticoduodenectomy

This is useful in some lesions of the low common duct. The majority of long-term survivors has occurred in this group. The pancreatic duct is usually not dilated or thick-walled, which makes anastomosis to the duodenum difficult and hazardous.

Intrahepatic cholangiojejunostomy of Longmire

This procedure has not been advocated by many surgeons in the treatment of high-lying lesions (Longmire et al. 1973).

The aim in treatment of carcinoma of the bile ducts is to do a curative resection, but this is rarely possible. A palliative bypass procedure should relieve jaundice and pruritus and may even prolong life, since the patient is less likely to die of hepatic failure and biliary cirrhosis if the bypass remains open.

For patients who are too old or too debilitated for surgery, transcutaneous tubes can be the definitive therapy. A tube may be passed through the neoplasm and manipulated so that its proximal end lies in an intrahepatic duct while its distal end rests in the duodenum or drains externally through the skin. While it is esthetically more pleasing to have the tube drain into the duodenum, this situation frequently leads to obstruction of the tube and of the duodenum, and produces reflux cholangitis. Exterior tubes can be cleaned or replaced. This procedure may be safer and more economical than surgical drainage for the majority of elderly patients with limited prognosis.

Radiation and Chemotherapy

For the patient who has residual tumor after surgery, further palliation may sometimes be obtained with radiation therapy, especially in bile duct carcinoma (Green, Mikkelsen, and Kernen 1973). In the small series reported by Smoron (1977), 20% (one of five) of patients with gallbladder carcinoma had evidence of palliation, while 50% (four of eight) of those with bile duct carcinoma had a palliative response. This type of therapy warrants further experience in a more structured prospective cooperative group setting.

Results with chemotherapy are sporadic and hard to evaluate. As with most adenocarcinomas of the gastrointestinal tract, response rates to single-agent chemotherapy are low, and the tumors are generally non-measurable and hence difficult to follow. Few institutions have large numbers of patients available for clinical trials, therefore most available information is based on patients handled therapeutically on an individual basis.

Of 36 patients treated with 5-FU, there were no significant responses (Perpetuo et al. 1978), but 3 of 5 patients treated with combined 5-FU, doxorubicin, and a nitrosourea had responses graded as less than partial remission but more than just stabilization. Of 62 patients treated with 5-FU, only 3 (5%) achieved partial remission while 7 of 15 (47%) did with mitomycin (Ramming, Haskell, and Tesler 1980).

Combination chemotherapy with FAM (5-fluorouracil, Adriamycin [doxorubicin], and mitomycin) was used to treat 17 patients with cholangiocarcinoma. Only 13 patients had measurable disease, and of these 4 (31%) had an objective partial remission. The median duration of response was 8.5 months (range 5 to 16 months). An additional 6 of the 13 had stabilization of tumor growth for a median duration of six months (range three to nine months). Median survival of responders was 10 months and of those with stabilization, 8.5 months, while nonresponders died in 3 months. Of the three patients without measurable disease, the median survival is 10 months. One patient with tumor obstructing the left hepatic duct at exploration remains free of detectable disease at over three years (Cambareri et al. 1980).

A group of eight patients with biliary tract carcinoma was treated with doxorubicin and bleomycin over a six-week period. Of the three evaluable patients, one had a partial remission and two were worse (Ravry et al. 1980). The authors felt that the response was solely to doxorubicin.

Intraarterial perfusion for hepatic metastases has been tried with 5-FU, 5-FUdR, mitomycin, doxorubicin, and most recently with cisplatin. In a study reported by Wu and co-workers (1979), one patient with bile duct carcinoma had a fall in bilirubin from 25 to 1.5 mg/dl with improved angiogram after therapy with cisplatin, while a patient with gallbladder carcinoma had a bilirubin decrease from 45 to 7.5 mg/dl.

A rare biliary tract tumor, embryonal rhabdomyosarcoma, was treated in six children with a combination of radiation therapy and chemotherapy including vincristine, dactinomycin, cyclophosphamide, and sometimes doxorubicin. Responses included four complete remissions, one partial remission, and one early death (Ruymann et al. 1980). Doxorubicin was not felt to be active in three. Median survival for responders was 28 months. Two survivors continue in remission at longer than 39 and 45 months.

In an effort to obtain prospective data on randomized patients, cooperative group studies are in progress. One by the Eastern Cooperative Oncology Group (ECOG) is comparing the response of advanced gallbladder and bile duct cancer to oral 5-FU, oral 5-FU plus intravenous streptozocin, and oral 5-FU plus semustine (methyl-CCNU). Patients who received 5-FU therapy prior to going on this study will be randomized to streptozocin or semustine.

Clearly, the results in gallbladder and biliary duct carcinoma are unsatisfactory with any and all modalities of treatment, and there must be improvement in the future.

References

Ackerman, L. V., and del Regato, J. A. *Cancer, diagnosis, treatment and prognosis,* 4th edition. St. Louis: C. V. Mosby, 1970, p. 603.

Adson, M. A. Carcinoma of the gallbladder. *Surg. Clin. North Am.* 53:1203–1216, 1973.

Akwari, O. E. et al. Cancer of the bile ducts associated with ulcerative colitis. *Ann. Surg.* 181:303–309, 1975.

Altemeir, W. A., and Culbertson, W. R. Scirrhous carcinoma of the hepatic bile ducts. *Surg. Clin. North Am.* 53:1229–1243, 1973.

Beltz, W. R., and Condon, R. E. Primary carcinoma of the gallbladder. *Ann. Surg.* 180:180–184, 1974.

Bhamarapravati, N. Animal studies on liver fluke infestation, dimethylnitrosoamine, and bile duct carcinoma. *Lancet* 1:206–207, 1978.

Bismuth, H., and Malt, R. A. Carcinoma of the biliary tract. *N. Engl. J. Med.* 301:704–706, 1979.

Black, W. C. et al. Carcinoma of the gallbladder in a population of Southwestern American Indians. *Cancer* 39:1267–1279, 1977.

Braasch, J. W. Carcinoma of the bile duct. *Surg. Clin. North Am.* 53:1217–1227, 1973.

Cambareri, R. J. et al. FAM, 5-fluorouracil (F), Adriamycin (A) and mitomycin-C (M) in cholangiocarcinoma. *Proc. Am. Soc. Clin. Oncol.* 21:419, 1980.

Davis, G. L.; Kissane, G. M.; and Ishak, K. G. Embryonal rhabdomyosarcoma (sarcoma botyroides) of the biliary tree: report of 5 cases and a review of the literature. *Cancer* 24:333–342, 1969.

Elias, E. et al. Endoscopic retrograde cholangiopancreatography in the diagnosis of jaundice associated with ulcerative colitis. *Gastroenterology* 67:907–911, 1974.

Green, N.; Mikkelsen, W. P.; and Kernen, J. A. Cancer of the common bile ducts—palliative radiotherapy. *Radiology* 109:687–689, 1973.

Iwasaki, Y. et al. Treatment of carcinoma of the biliary system. *Surg. Gynecol. Obstet.* 144:219–224, 1977.

Longmire, W. P., Jr. et al. Carcinoma of the extrahepatic biliary tract. *Ann. Surg.* 178:333–345, 1973.

Moorhead, D., and Warren, K. Changing patterns of surgery of the gallbladder, bile ducts, and liver. *Surg. Clin. North Am.* 56:649–666, 1976.

Morowitz, D. A. et al. Carcinoma of the biliary tract complicating chronic ulcerative colitis. *Cancer* 27:356–361, 1971.

Nevin, J. E. et al. Carcinoma of the gallbladder: staging, treatment, and prognosis. *Cancer* 37:141–148, 1978.

Pereiras, R. V., Jr. Relief of malignant obstructive jaundice by percutaneous insertion of a permanent prosthesis in the biliary tree. *Ann. Intern. Med.* 89:589–593, 1978.

Perpetuo, M. D. C. et al. Natural history study of gallbladder cancer. *Cancer* 42:330–335, 1978.

Piehler, J. M., and Crichlow, R. W. Primary carcinoma of the gallbladder. *Surg. Gynecol. Obstet.* 147:929–942, 1978.

Pollock, T. W. et al. Percutaneous decompression of benign and malignant biliary obstruction. *Arch. Surg.* 114:148–151, 1979.

Ramming, K. P.; Haskell, C. M.; and Tesler, A. S. Extrahepatic bile ducts. In *Cancer treatment,* ed. C. M. Haskell. Philadelphia: W. B. Saunders, 1980, pp. 336–342.

Ravry, M. J. R. et al. Combination chemotherapy of hepatocellular (HC) and biliary tract carcinoma (BC) with Adriamycin (Adr) plus bleomycin (Bleo). *Proc. Am. Soc. Clin. Oncol.* 21:366, 1980.

Redeker, A. et al. Percutaneous transhepatic cholangiography. *JAMA* 231:386–387, 1975.

Ritchie, J. K. et al. Biliary tract carcinoma associated with ulcerative colitis. *Q. J. Med.* 43:263–279, 1974.

Ross, A. P.; Braasch, J. W.; and Warren, K. W. Carcinoma of the proximal bile ducts. *Surg. Gynecol. Obstet.* 136:923–928, 1973.

Ruymann, F. B. et al. Extrahepatic biliary rhabdomyosarcoma. *Proc. Am. Soc. Clin. Oncol.* 21:388, 1980.

Smoron, G. L. Radiation therapy of carcinoma of gallbladder and biliary tract. *Cancer* 40:1422–1424, 1977.

Strauch, G. O. Primary carcinoma of the gallbladder. *Surgery* 47:368–383, 1960.

Tabrisky, J. et al. Chiba percutaneous cholangiography. *Am. J. Roentgenol.* 126:755–760, 1976.

Tompkins, R. K. et al. Operative endoscopy in the management of biliary tract neoplasms. *Am. J. Surg.* 132:174–182, 1976.

Wu, S. J. et al. Short-term intra-arterial infusion of Cisplatinum diamminedichloride (CPDD) for regional control of cancer. *Proc. Am. Soc. Clin. Oncol.* 20:443, 1979.

Young, J. L., Jr. et al. *SEER program: cancer incidence and mortality in the United States, 1973–1976*. Bethesda, Md.: National Cancer Institute, 1978.

forty-one

Cancer of the Colon and Rectum

DAVID S. FISCHER
J. SCOTT NYSTROM

Cancer of the colon and rectum is the most common internal malignancy today. It afflicts more than 120,000 Americans each year and kills about 55,000 annually (Silverberg 1981). The five-year survival rate from the time of diagnosis for all stages of disease is 45%, but survival in localized disease is 71%.

Colorectal cancer is unusual below age 40 years, except for patients with inflammatory bowel disease and inherited polyposis syndromes. The peak incidence is at age 75 and the median at age 60. Men and women are affected equally. Patients with a prior colorectal neoplasm, breast cancer, or female genital tract cancer have a higher risk of developing colorectal cancer. In addition, there is a higher incidence of this neoplasm in some families. Although its cause is unknown, some clues are available from the study of polyps, polyposis syndromes, inflammatory bowel disease, and dietary factors.

Polyps

A polyp is a growth or tumor raised up above its surrounding mucous membrane. A nomenclature for polyps that correlates with their neoplastic potential is shown in table 41.1, from Katz, Wiggans, and Fischer (1979) based on studies of Morson (1976). About 75% of all polyps are adenomatous and 10% are villous.

Table 41.1. *Histopathologic Type of Epithelial Colorectal Polyp and Probability of Associated Carcinoma*

Histology	*Synonyms*	*Percentage with Associated Carcinoma*
Hyperplastic polyp	Metaplastic	0
Adenomatous polyp	Tubular; glandular adenomas	4.8
Villoglandular polyp	Tubulovillous; papillary; mixed adenomas	22.5
Villous adenoma	Villous papilloma	40.7
Polypoid cancer		100

SOURCE: Katz, Wiggins, and Fischer 1979.

NOTE: Adenomatous and villoglandular polyps and villous adenoma have neoplastic potential.

Although polyps less than 1 cm in diameter have a small chance of containing a carcinoma, villous adenomas are 10 times more likely to be malignant compared to adenomatous polyps. Indeed, some authors are not convinced that adenomatous polyps less than 2 cm are premalignant (Rawson 1976). We believe that villous adenomas of any size and all polyps greater than 2 cm should be removed for histologic examination, and not simply fulgerated. There is some evidence to suggest that for those polyps that eventually give rise to car-

Table 41.2. *Inherited Gastrointestinal Polyposis Syndromes*

Polyposis Syndrome	*Inheritance*	*Location of Polyps*	*Pathology of Polyps*	*Population at Risk of Cancer*	*Extraintestinal Manifestations*
Familial polyposis	Autosomal dominant	Colon, rectum	Adenomatous	> 80 % of untreated patients	None
Gardner's syndrome	Autosomal dominant	Colon, rectum; rarely in small intestine, stomach	Adenomatous	High as in familial polyposis; increased risk of pancreatic, ampullary, duodenal carcinoma as well	Osteomas, fibromas, lipomas, desmoids
Juvenile polyposis	Autosomal dominant	Colon, rectum; occasionally in small intestine, stomach	Hamartomatous	Probable increased risk of stomach, duodenal, pancreatic, colonic carcinoma	None
Peutz-Jehgers	Autosomal dominant	Small intestine; commonly in stomach, colon, rectum	Hamartomatous	Probable increased risk of cancer often involving stomach and duodenum	Melanin spots on eyelids, lips, buccal mucosa, digits, anus

SOURCE: Katz, Wiggans, and Fischer 1979.

cinoma, an average of at least 4 to 5 years is involved in the adenoma—carcinoma sequence, and possibly as long as 10 to 15 years. This makes timely diagnosis possible, as perhaps two-thirds of invasive cancer arises from neoplastic polyps. Presumably the remainder originate de novo from colonic epithelium.

Premalignant Polyposis Syndromes

There are several inherited gastrointestinal polyposis syndromes (table 41.2). Familial polyposis (familial adenomatous colonic polyposis) is an autosomal dominant syndrome with incomplete penetrance, characterized by hundreds to thousands of small adenomatous polyps in the colon and rectum and without extracolonic manifestations. On the average a diagnosis of polyposis is made at age 27 and carcinoma and polyps at an average age of 39 years. At the time of diagnosis of invasive cancer half of the patients have multicentric lesions.

Therapy is controversial, but most surgeons recommend either total proctocolectomy or total colectomy with an ileorectal anastomosis. In the latter instance, routine proctoscopy at six-month intervals is indicated, with removal or destruction of developing polyps.

Gardner's syndrome is an autosomal dominant colonic polyposis with incomplete penetrance but with extracolonic benign soft tissue and osseous tumors and a high incidence of malignant neoplasms arising in the pancreaticoduodenal region. Treatment is similar to that of the familial polyposis syndrome but with closer follow-up of the upper tract.

Juvenile polyposis is an autosomal dominant syndrome with a high degree of penetrance characterized by hamartomatous polyps in the colon and rectum, and less commonly in the stomach and small intestine. Stemper and co-workers (1975) suggest an associated high risk of development of carcinoma in the stomach, duodenum, pancreas, and proximal colon. Management is difficult but usually involves resection of polyps as indicated by the individual's clinical condition.

Turcot syndrome is a rare familial autosomal recessive disease characterized by colonic adenomatous polyps and gliomas of the brain.

Peutz-Jeghers syndrome is a rare autosomal dominant disease characterized by hamartomatous polyposis always involving the small intestine and frequently involving the stomach, colon, and rectum. The lesions usually have an epithelial lining of goblet cells that secrete mucus into the polyp, and they are generally considered nonmalignant; however, a few patients have coexistent adenomatous polyps. The usual extraintestinal manifestation is melanin spots on the eyelids, lips, buccal mucosa, digits, and anus. Tumors of the ovary have also been reported in this syndrome. The risk of associated gastrointestinal cancer is 2% to 3%, with malignancy frequently arising in the stomach or duodenum. Treatment includes resection of all gastric and duodenal polyps, and those that are symptomatic and of large size.

Table 41.3. *Signs and Symptoms of Colorectal Cancer*

Signs	*Right Colon*	*Left Colon*	*Rectum*
Pain	Vague, dull, uncharacteristic	Gas pain; cramps	A late feature
Bleeding, gross	None seen, or dark red blood mixed in stool	Bright red blood coating surface of stool	Bright red blood coating surface of stool
Lumen	Large, not likely to obstruct	Small, frequent obstruction	Large, obstruction rare
Peristalsis	Good	Slow	Good
Complaints	Nonspecific	Alternating constipation and diarrhea	Tenesmus
	Abdominal pain	Decrease in caliber of stools	Incomplete evacuation
	Anemia		Mucous diarrhea
	Abdominal mass		

Inflammatory Bowel Disease

Ulcerative colitis ultimately progresses to carcinoma in 3% to 5% of cases. Incidence increases significantly 10 years after initial diagnosis in patients with extensive colitis and chronic continuous disease. The role of total proctocolectomy in the management of these patients remains controversial (Devroede et al. 1971).

Regional enteritis or Crohn's disease of both the small and large intestine is associated with an increased risk of adenocarcinoma, especially in patients with long-standing disease. The degree of increased risk is unknown but it may be as high as 20 times that of a control population (Weedon et al. 1973).

Diet

Some clues to the possible etiology of colorectal carcinoma are provided by epidemiologic studies (Reddy 1976):

1. The highest incidence is in western Europe and the United States, while the lowest incidence is in Africa, Asia, and South America (except Uruguay and Argentina). In general, the more economically developed a society is, the greater is its incidence of colon cancer.
2. A negative correlation exists between gastric and colon cancers and there is a positive association between colon cancer and malignancies of the breast and prostate.
3. Significant differences in incidence have been found between Japan and the United States and between Puerto Rico and the United States.
4. Seventh Day Adventists who consume less meat and fat than most Americans have a significantly lower incidence of disease.
5. There is a higher incidence among American blacks than African blacks and among Japanese in Hawaii and California as compared to Japanese in Japan.

From these facts it has been surmised that a diet emphasizing beef and in particular a high-fat intake correlates with a higher incidence of colon cancer. Correlation with dietary deficiency of fiber, excess of refined carbohydrates, transit time of stool, and consistency of stool has been controversial, but these are probably not important factors.

The results of experiments in several laboratories indicate that dietary intake high in fat affects the metabolic activity of the intestinal microflora as well as levels of certain fecal steroids that can act as tumor promoters for the colon. Populations on a high-fat, mixed western diet and with a high rate of large bowel cancer excreted cholesterol and bile acid metabolites to a greater degree than did those people with a relatively low rate and different dietary habits.

Diagnosis

The clinical picture of colorectal cancer is changing (table 41.3). Forty years ago the typical patient was a man in his sixties with rectal bleeding. The diagnosis could be made with digital examination. In the 1940s, 82% of colorectal cancer was in the sigmoid colon or lower and could be diagnosed by sigmoidoscopy or digital examination. By 1975, 40% of tumors were higher than the sigmoid colon (Rhodes et al. 1977); in Vermont, 35% now occur in the right colon (Abrams and Reines 1979). With this changing pattern digital examination and proctosigmoidoscopy are inadequate alone for diagnosis of the symptomatic and screening of the asymptomatic patient.

Early diagnosis is clearly the key to improving survival and cure rates (Sherlock and Winawer 1977). Nearly all asymptomatic patients in whom colorectal cancer is detected have localized disease (less than 4% have distant metastases) and therefore are potentially curable with surgery. In fact the five-year survival rate in this group approaches 90% (Miller 1976). This compares favorably with the overall five-year survival rate of only 44%, and even the 71% rate for all patients with localized disease. Thus the key to better results lies in making the diagnosis while the patient is asymptomatic, and this means some form of screening.

Screening

The fact that colorectal cancer is a slowly progressive disease with a long asymptomatic period means that early diagnosis is possible with periodic examinations (Dean 1977). This may take the form of organized mass screening (Hastings 1974), a cancer detection clinic (Hertz et al. 1960), or the periodic complete health examination by one's primary physician.

A variety of techniques have been evaluated for screening (fig. 41.1). The most economically sound is the test for occult blood in the stool. In selecting from among the available tests one wants a test (Stroehlein et al. 1978) that is both highly specific and reproducible, and limited in sensitivity so that false positives are minimized. Compared to ^{51}Cr-labeled red cells, guaiac reagent and orthotolidine (Hematest) tablets were extremely sensitive but yielded false positive reaction rates of 72% and 76% respectively on the 240 specimens compared (Morris et al. 1976). A modified guaiac test (Hemoccult) exhibited a false positive rate of 12%. Hemoccult is approximately one-fourth as sensitive as guaiac and Hematest, but can miss lesions with low rates of bleeding unless multiple stools are tested. A positive Hemoccult test usually indicates significant gastrointestinal bleeding, and at present seems to be the test of choice provided that at least three stools are tested to minimize false negative results. Some authors find that detection is improved by the ingestion of dietary roughage during the four-day period of stool collection (Greegor 1974). False positives may be reduced by the use of a meat-free diet whenever a positive result is detected (Miller and Knight 1977). The manufacturer is now offering, in addition, Hemoccult as a card with three double slides and sticks and a mailing envelope. The patient is instructed to prepare two stool specimens from different parts of the stool from three consecutive bowel movements. Thus the physician will receive and develop six slides. Since the test really detects the peroxidase enzyme associated with hemoglobin, the patient is advised to eat no "red" meat, turnips, or horseradish during the test period.

It should be unnecessary to remind physicians that a physical examination is not complete if digital exploration of the rectum has been omitted, which is too often the case. This examination can detect a tumor in the prostate, rectal mucosa, or in other pelvic organs, and it usually yields a specimen of stool for another test for occult blood. Abdominal palpation reveals a tumor only when it is very large and widespread.

Proctosigmoidoscopy

There is a large and controversial literature regarding the utility and cost-effectiveness of routine proctosigmoidoscopy. For the asymptomatic patient with no increased risk factors, the recommendation for this examination every year after age 40 is being discontinued because the cost is between \$10,000 and \$70,000 spent per case of cancer found. A more realistic recommendation is proctosigmoidoscopy every two years after age 50 (Corman et al. 1975). In the high-risk patient, that is, one with a positive family history for colorectal carcinoma, known polyps, a family polyposis syndrome, or inflammatory bowel disease, proctosigmoidoscopy is indicated at a much younger age and on a yearly basis. The value of a routine procedure must be evaluated on a risk-benefit basis for each patient. A study at the University of Minnesota (Gilbertsen 1971) picked up 11 asymptomatic carcinomas of the colon in 103,645 routine examinations. Unfortunately, there were five perforations above the peritoneal reflection that required abdominal exploration and repair. The procedure was beneficial to the 11 patients with unsuspected colon cancer, but it was a disaster for the 5 asymptomatic patients who suffered the perforation. With the new flexible fiberoptic colonoscope it is hoped that a greater part of the colon can be visualized at less risk to the patient.

Barium Enema

Although some executive screening programs still employ a barium enema as a routine study, it is extremely costly and time-consuming. It is often of suboptimal value because of poor patient preparation or omission of air contrast techniques. Its value is realized in the high-risk or symptomatic patient, or in one scheduled for colonoscopy. Blind areas occur on every colonoscopy, especially in the rectosigmoid and the splenic and hepatic flexures. The barium enema is an uncomfortable and unesthetic procedure, but one of low risk and moderately high specificity and accuracy (fig. 41.2).

Colonoscopy

The advent of the flexible fiberoptic colonoscope has revolutionized diagnostic and therapeutic capabilities in the evaluation of high-risk and symptomatic patients. It extends the area of direct observation from 25 cm to the entire colon, which can be visualized in 80% of patients (Winawer et al. 1976). Through the colonoscope diagnostic or excisional biopsy can be performed, as can target brushing and cytology.

Colonic lavage cytology gained popularity in only a few institutions that set up specific programs directed to that diagnostic modality. It has proved to be tedious, expensive, and not esthetically pleasing. Now, however, interest in and popularity of jet stream lavage cytology through the colonoscope for an already prepared bowel is being revived, as it is simple and effective (Katz et al.

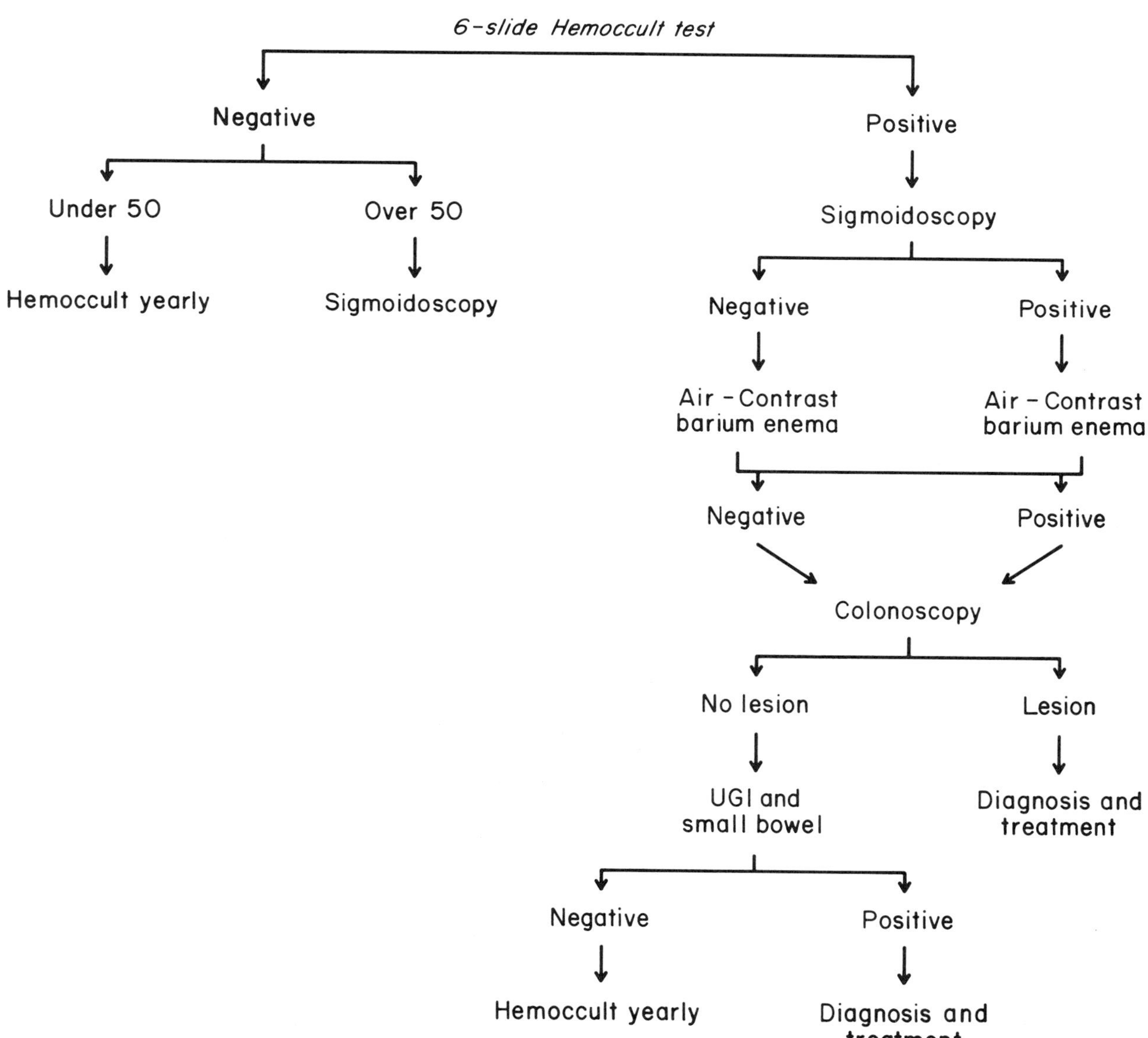

Fig. 41.1. *Screening for colorectal cancer. (Katz, Wiggans, and Fischer 1979. Reprinted by permission.)*

1972). It is particularly useful in patients with premalignant lesions like ulcerative colitis or familial polyposis where single or multiple biopsies are negative. Rare false positives occur in less than 1% of patients.

CEA and Tumor Markers

The introduction of the test for carcinoembryonic antigen (CEA) in 1965 heralded an extensive study of tumor-associated antigens as clinically useful diagnostic markers in human cancer (Gold and Freedman 1965). Unfortunately, that promise has not yet been realized. It is now known that the antigen is found in normal serum, normal adult colon tissue, other primary gastrointestinal malignancies, cirrhosis, pancreatitis, inflammatory bowel disease, and in heavy smokers. It is not a sensitive test for the early detection of colonic cancer (Holyoke and Cooper 1976). It may be related more to vascular invasion or tumor necrosis than to the amount of tumor present. The test correlates roughly with the response to surgery, radiation, and/or chemotherapy and is useful as a diagnostic adjuvant (Mayer et al. 1978). It is twice as sensitive as alkaline phosphatase for liver metastases from colonic carcinoma; however, it is not clear how reliable the test is in following patients for recurrence. Some groups find it inadequate for early detection of recurrent tumor (Moertel et al. 1978), and others use it for long-term follow-up to predict tumor recurrence with a lead time of several months (Mach et al. 1978).

Preoperative CEA levels have been found to be useful as prognostic indicators in colorectal carcinoma. The recurrence rate was higher in patients with localized and regional disease who had preoperative CEA levels greater than 5 ng/ml. There was a linear inverse correlation between preoperative levels and estimated mean time to recurrence, ranging from 30 months for a level of 2 ng/ml to only 9.8 months for a level of 70 ng/ml (Wanebo et al. 1978). Some authors even use the CEA as a guide to the need for a second-look operation or as an indication to begin chemotherapy (Herrera et al. 1976). Thus the CEA is useful for following colorectal cancer, but not for its diagnosis in the asymptomatic person.

Clinical Manifestations

Patients being evaluated for colorectal cancer may be grouped into four categories:

- Symptomatic
- Asymptomatic but with a premalignant condition
- Asymptomatic but at high risk
- Asymptomatic with a normal risk

The symptomatic patient may have rectal bleeding, diarrhea, rectal discharge of mucus, tenesmus, abdominal pain, nausea, obstruction, anemia, distention, and/or constipation. The evaluation of such a

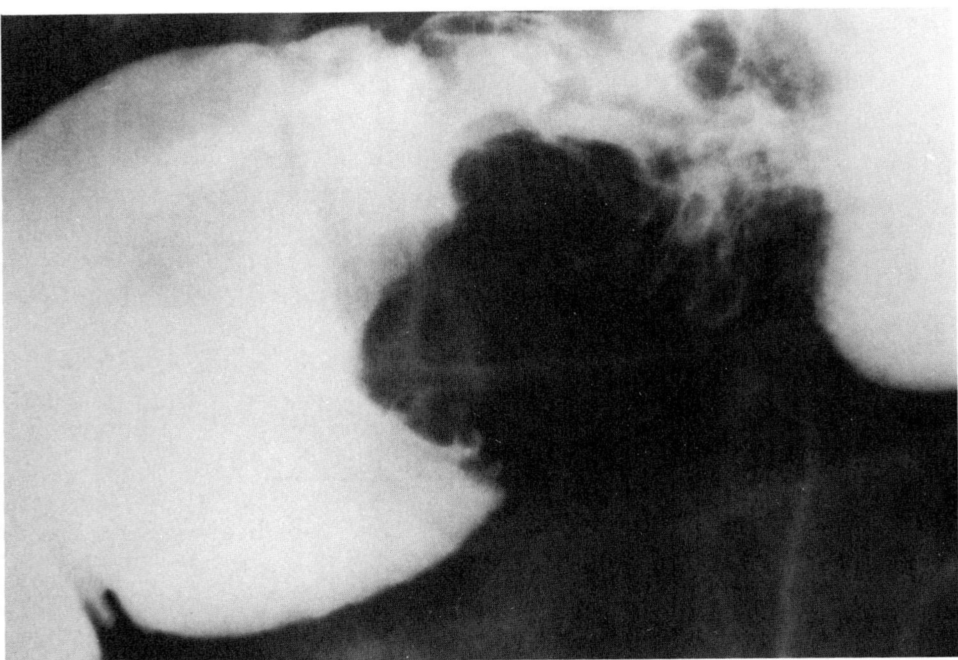

Fig. 41.2. *Typical carcinoma of the colon as revealed by barium enema.*

patient should be expeditious and should include a test for occult blood, digital rectal examination, sigmoidoscopy, air contrast barium enema, and if any doubt remains about the diagnosis or location of lesions, a colonoscopy with biopsy or brushings. If carcinoma is found, attempts to document metastases are indicated and might include a liver scan, ultrasound of the liver, chest x-ray, CEA, and liver-associated chemistries. Surgery may be indicated for cure or palliation depending on staging.

The asymptomatic patient with a premalignant condition could have the test for occult blood omitted, as it is usually positive. Such a patient should have sigmoidoscopy, barium enema, and colonoscopy, possibly with lavage cytology at appropriate intervals, depending on the length of time the underlying premalignant condition has been present.

The asymptomatic patient at high risk is one who has a family history of single or multiple primary carcinomas of the colon, has had multiple cancers in different anatomic sites (ovary, breast, colon, uterus), is a relative of patients with polyposis syndromes, or who has had previous colon polyps or cancers. These individuals should be followed at intervals with Hemoccult slide testing, a digital rectal examination, and sigmoidoscopy. Those with polyps or cancers should have a barium enema yearly after age 35 years if they have no plans for child-bearing. A colonoscopy should be done only if one of the earlier tests is positive or unsatisfactory.

The asymptomatic adult patient with no risk factors should have a yearly Hemoccult test with six slides on three separate specimens. A digital examination is also indicated. Over the age of 50, a sigmoidoscopy is probably indicated every second or third year. Further testing would depend on the findings and any index of suspicion.

Surgery

Surgery is the only means by which colorectal carcinoma is now cured. The depth of cancerous invasion into the bowel wall and the presence of nodal metastases directly affect the surgeon's ability to prevent recurrent disease. The Dukes' pathologic staging system (table 41.4) as modified by Kirklin and co-workers (1949) and later Astler and Coller (1954) has provided a useful classification for predicting recurrence and survival.

Dukes' stage A disease has a five-year survival ranging from 74% to 100% (Copeland et al. 1968). Stage B1 has a five-year survival of 60% to 65%, while for stage B2 it is 40% to 60% (Hoth and Petrucci 1976). Regional lymph node involvement (stage C) is seen in over 50% of cases at surgery (Gilbertsen 1967) and further reduces five-year survival to approximately 30%. The number and location of lymph nodes (Dukes and Bussey 1958) has also been shown adversely to affect prognosis. Location of the primary tumor influences prognosis, with survival being 10% to 15% less in extraperitoneal rectal lesions as compared to similarly staged lesions above the peritoneal reflection (Silverberg and Holleb 1974).

Table 41.4. *Modified Dukes' Staging System for Colorectal Carcinoma*

A	Limited to mucosa or submucosa
B1	Extension into but not through the muscularis; negative nodes
B2	Extension to or through the serosa; negative nodes
C1	Extension into but not through the muscularis; positive nodes
C2	Extension into or through the serosa; positive nodes
D	Distant metastases or liver involvement by tumor

SOURCE: Astler and Coller 1954.

Unlike other solid tumors such as breast carcinoma and melanoma that may have late relapses, recurrences in colorectal carcinomas usually occur within five years from definitive treatment. Death is related to local recurrences in one-half the patients and to distant metastases in the other half (Carter 1976). Liver metastases are present at initial surgery in 15% to 25% (Ranson et al. 1973) and at autopsy in 64% of patients. The other frequent sites of distant spread include lung (20% to 30%), bone, ovaries, and brain (10% or less).

Survival from proof of recurrence or unresected primary is usually short. Moertel (1969) reported a median time of 7 months, with 10% of patients alive at 18 months. In patients with liver metastases the median survival is approximately five months (Jaffe et al. 1968). As can be seen from these survival figures, once there has been a recurrence the chances of cure are small.

Radiation Therapy

Radiation therapy has been proved effective for symptomatic palliation in inoperable or recurrent rectal carcinoma (Wang and Schultz 1962). The role of radiation in resectable tumors also appears promising. A study conducted by Kligerman and associates (1972) at Yale randomized patients with potentially curable adenocarcinoma of the rectum or rectosigmoid to 4400 to 4600 rad over four and one-half weeks followed by resection four weeks later, or to resection alone. Patients given preoperative irradiation had nodal involvement in only

3 of 13 cases versus 11 of 16 treated by surgery alone. Survival in this small series was improved in the irradiated group. The Veterans Administration Surgical Adjuvant Group's randomized study of preoperative irradiation (2000 to 2500 rad in two weeks) (Higgins et al. 1975) showed a survival advantage at five years for the irradiated group (40.8% versus 28.4%), only in those patients undergoing an abdominoperineal resection. There are numbers of ongoing cooperative group studies evaluating the role of preoperative and postoperative radiation alone and in combination with chemotherapy in the treatment of resectable rectal carcinoma (Davis and Kisner 1978). It is certainly hoped that current studies will substantiate the effectiveness of radiation as an adjunct to surgical resection.

Adjuvant Therapy

The only acceptable curative therapy for invasive adenocarcinoma of the large bowel continues to be radical surgical excision. Unfortunately, newer surgical techniques and manipulations have not improved five-year survival rates for more than two decades. It is now believed that adjuvant therapies may be effective in subgroups of disease defined by the presence or absence of risk factors. If so, the role of immunomanipulation also holds promise of significance.

One of the pitfalls that plagued early surgical adjuvant chemotherapy trials was a lack of awareness of those patient characteristics associated with a high probability of disease recurrence, regardless of the adequacy of the surgical resection. These include microscopic blood vessel invasion, perineural involvement, lymph node or serosal involvement, and microscopic tumor in the resected margin.

In one review (Polk and Spratt 1971), first disease recurrence within 18 months of surgical operation was observed in more than 75% of patients in whom one of the poor prognostic factors was seen.

Adjuvant Chemotherapy

Historically, adjuvant chemotherapy was used in an attempt to destroy cells left in the operative field and to prevent spread through the blood stream or lymphatics during operation. Therefore early studies employed short-duration adjuvant therapy to eradicate the small pool of locally residual cancer cells. At first, local irrigation of the bowel ends with half-strength Dakin's solution or 1:500 perchloride of mercury was advocated (Cole 1965).

Systemic chemotherapy began with early randomized controlled studies testing effects of nitrogen mustard, triethylenethiophosphoramide (thiotepa) and fluorodeoxyuridine (FUDR). Various routes of administration were used (intraperitoneal, mesenteric vein, and intravenous) but were unsuccessful (Holden et al. 1967) in prolonging survival or preventing recurrence.

Increased survival in patients with lymph node involvement was shown compared with a retrospective untreated control group when intraluminal 5-FU and systemic administration of 5-FU two days postoperatively were used (Rousselot et al. 1968).

These observations motivated the initiation of randomized cooperative studies comparing 5-FU (given by various routes, schedules, and doses) to patients treated by surgery alone. The considerable benefits claimed for adjuvant 5-FU in nonrandomized trials may be erroneous in view of the variations reported in strictly surgical series (Rousselot et al. 1972; Li and Ross 1976). Thus only studies that are randomized prospective trials and involve concurrent surgical controls will be discussed.

In 1971 the Veterans Administration Surgical Adjuvant Group (VASAG) reported on a randomized study of patients with colon cancer given no treatment compared with those treated with 5-FU (Higgins et al. 1971). The drug was given in the immediate postoperative period (14 days postresection) for 5 successive days intravenously at 12 mg per kg of body weight. Treatment assignment was not stratified by Dukes' classification or other prognostic variables influencing recurrence, but by the surgeon's opinion regarding potential for cure. All patients were followed for the extent of their survival. Those who underwent surgical procedures termed clinically palliative and clinically curative received a second course of 5-FU seven weeks later (standard therapy would be three weeks later). There was no statistically significant difference in the five-year survival rate or the disease-free interval between treated and untreated populations in any of the patient groups. Furthermore, retrospective analysis by Dukes' classification again failed to show that therapy with 5-FU achieved survival rates superior to those of control populations. The five-year survival rate for patients undergoing curative resection was 58.2% for treated patients versus 48.0% for controls. The trend of this study appears to favor chemotherapy, but statistical significance is lacking. Thus findings in early trials with Thiotepa, FUDR, and 5-FU have failed to show significant prolongation in survival. Doses, schedules, route of administration, the short duration of adjuvant treatment, and disregard for prognostic factors in treatment assignment may be important factors in the failure.

The advocacy of *prolonged* intermittent systemic adjuvant chemotherapy came about with the realization that (1) occult metastatic cancer sites can exist at the time of operation and do not result exclusively from surgical manipulation, and (2) repeated courses of treatment are necessary to eradicate this small residual tumor cell burden.

The VASAG has also investigated prolonged intermittent chemotherapy (5-FU) in colon cancer. Chemotherapy was given in the manner as in their previous study but was repeated every 6 weeks for 18 months (again, most give it every 4 weeks). Case accrual terminated in August 1973. To date no significant difference has been shown in patient survival associated with prolonged 5-FU treatment (Higgins et al. 1978).

Prolonged intermittent 5-FU adjuvant therapy has been tested in a randomized prospective study by the Central Oncology Group (Grage et al. 1977, 1979). Before random assignment to groups receiving 5-FU or no treatment, patients with poor prognosis were classified as having had curative or palliative resection. Poor prognosis in those undergoing curative operation included the following factors: (1) positive lymph nodes, (2) serosal penetration or invasion of perirectal fat, (3) blood vessel invasion, (4) lymphatic invasion, and (5) cancer in other organs removed as part of the resection.

In this study, 5-FU was given intravenously at 12 mg per kg of body weight per day for four days, and then 6 mg per kg of body weight every other day for five doses or to toxicity. Following this induction course, 5-FU was given weekly at 12 mg per kg of body for one year. Endpoints were first disease recurrence and death.

The follow-up period is still relatively short, but at last report (Grage et al. 1979) 54 of 97 patients (56%) classified as having had curative resection for colon or rectal cancer were disease-free after treatment with 5-FU, as compared with 57 of 113 patients (50%) similarly classified and assigned to no treatment. This difference is not significant. When the 61 rectal cancer patients were considered separately, a benefit was seen for disease-free interval ($P = 0.06$) and survival ($P = 0.011$) in the chemotherapy treated group. For patients with both curative and palliative resection, 5-FU has not shown statistically significant superiority over no treatment with respect to disease-free interval or five-year survival, but the trend is in favor of the group receiving drug therapy.

The recent reports of regression rates higher than anticipated in metastatic disease with combination chemotherapy using drugs with low individual activity have prompted the use of these combinations as adjuncts to surgery (Falkson et al. 1974). This adds further risk of systemic toxicity, difficult patient management, interference with quality of life, and potentially greater immune "paralysis" with (tolerance to) residual tumor burden. In spite of these difficulties several cooperative groups have initiated studies using combination chemotherapy (namely Me-CCNU plus 5-FU) as an adjuvant to operation (Moertel et al. 1975).

A recent colon cancer study by the GITSG of more than 600 patients compared (1) chemotherapy with 5-FU and semustine, (2) immunotherapy with the methanol-extractable residue of BCG (MER), (3) both modalities, and (4) no therapy. No significant difference has yet been found (Killen et al. 1981).

The same group, however, has found a positive effect of treatment in surgically "curable" rectal cancer (Mittelman et al. 1981). Over 200 patients were entered into a study comparing (1) 5-FU and semustine, (2) radiotherapy (4000 to 4800 rad), (3) both modalities, and (4) no additional therapy after surgery. A greater recurrence rate (P greater than 0.001) was found in the control arm compared to the combined modality treatment arm; survival of the control arm was significantly inferior to all the treatment arms combined. The combination modality arm was the best, but the differences between the three treatment arms are not yet significant.

Immunotherapy as Adjuvant Treatment

Many investigators have theorized that the clinical use of immunomanipulation may be effective only at the time of minimal tumor burden because host-immune paralysis increases with increasing tumor burden (Smith 1972). Reactive regional lymph node hyperplasia with germinal center proliferation draining a primary malignancy has been observed in both breast and colon cancer. This suggests a host immune response to the tumor.

Recent preliminary results have shown increased disease-free interval for patients with colon cancer treated with BCG (Dukes' C stage) compared with historical controls (Mavligit et al. 1975). Even though historical controls have been used for treatment comparison, such data help substantiate early implementation of immunotherapy in this disease. Clinical trials of specific immunotherapy (for example, with transfer factor, immune ribonucleic acid [RNA], modified tumor antigens, cell wall extracts) are chiefly limited to studies in single institutions with small numbers of patients because of procurement and logistic problems.

Studies using immunotherapy alone in a surgical adjuvant study for colon cancer are in progress based on several reasons: (1) there are no conclusive data that

Table 41.5. *Combination Chemotherapy of Advanced Colon Cancer*

Drugs	*Partial Response (%)*	*Median Survival (Weeks)*	*Severe Toxicity (%)*
ECOG #4275—no prior therapy			
F, M	10	26	34
F, M, V	12	33	34
F, M, D	14	41	16
F, M, D, V	15	40	13
F, H	21	33	23
ECOG #4275—prior F therapy			
M, V	2	17	39
M, D	15	32	23
M, D, V	7	24	46
M, dT	2	20	31
ECOG #4273			
F alone	16	31	11

SOURCE: Engstrom et al. 1978

NOTE: Drugs and abbreviations as follows: F = 5-fluorouracil; M = methyl-CCNU; V = vincristine; D = dacarbazine; H = hydroxyurea; dT = deoxythioguanosine.

single or combination adjuvant chemotherapy prolongs disease-free interval or survival for large bowel cancer; (2) chemotherapy may entail additional systemic toxicity and potential for impairment of quality of life; (3) while chemotherapy may enhance host immunoreactivity to large volume malignancies, it may also paralyze established nodal defense systems against minimal tumor cell numbers; (4) combination chemotherapy when used in an adjuvant setting leaves few alternative chemotherapeutic drugs available at first disease recurrence; (5) chemotherapy could potentially be antagonistic to immunomanipulation; (6) information about dose, routes, and single-agent effectiveness for immunostimulants should be established prior to combination with chemotherapeutic regimens.

Treatment of Advanced Disease

Since the late 1950s, the major drug used for treatment of colorectal carcinoma has been 5-FU, introduced by the Wisconsin group (Ansfield et al. 1962). Most reports since then have used their criteria for response:

1. Measurable reduction of at least 25% in the size of a measurable lesion
2. Subjective improvement
3. Leveling off or reversal of a downward weight curve
4. Improvement in performance status
5. Presence of all these criteria for not less than two months

A summation of reports of over 2000 patients treated with 5-FU alone indicates an overall response rate of 21% (Wasserman et al. 1975). Of the many drugs thought to be effective in colorectal cancer, including mitomycin C, ftorafur, 5-fluoro-2-deoxyuridine, BCNU, CCNU, methyl-CCNU, triazinate, and ICRF-159, none has exceeded 5-FU in response rate (Moertel 1978). Hence combination chemotherapy was investigated.

Falkson and co-workers (1974) reported a 42% response rate with a four-drug combination of vincristine, 5-FU, dacarbazine, and BCNU. Moertel and associates (1975) reported a 43% response rate with a combination of 5-FU, methyl-CCNU, and vincristine. Macdonald and colleagues (1976) reported a 40% response rate with the same drugs on a slightly different schedule. Spurred by these early reports suggesting a 100% improvement in response, several cooperative groups launched prospective randomized trials of combination chemotherapy. We participated in Eastern Cooperative Oncology Group (ECOG) study #4275 that randomized patients with measurable disease to five combination drug treatment groups if they were previously untreated, or to four such groups if they had received prior 5-FU. In table 41.5 results are compared to ECOG protocol #4273 where 5-FU alone was used weekly (Engstrom et al. 1978). It can be seen that only 5-FU plus hydroxyurea gave a higher response rate than 5-FU alone, and that all treatment arms had more toxicity. Slightly greater median survival even in those arms is probably not significant.

Thus at the present time, both adjuvant and palliative therapy of colorectal cancer should be in well-designed and well-managed prospective randomized clinical trials in order to ascertain the best treatment modalities. When this is not feasible, therapy should be structured to give the least toxicity with the best chance of response, which is 5-FU alone.

Rectal Carcinoma

In general, the chemotherapy and immunotherapy of adenocarcinoma of the rectum is the same as for adenocarcinoma of the colon. In the former there appears to be a role for adjuvant radiation and chemotherapy, which has already been detailed.

Anal Cancer

In contrast to adenocarcinoma of the colon and rectum, cancer of the anus is relatively rare. Histologically, it is usually a poorly differentiated epidermoid, basosquamous, or basaloid carcinoma. It is more common in women than men. Drainage of the upper anal canal is toward the rectum and the perirectal and pelvic lymph nodes, while the lower anus drains to the inguinal nodes. Inguinal dissection is indicated only if there is palpable tumor there. Therapy is usually surgical with an abdominoperineal resection indicated if there are no demonstrable metastases. If spread is confined to the nodes mentioned or if the tumor is bulky, radiation therapy may be worthwhile for palliation. If there are liver or lung metastases chemotherapy may be indicated. There is little chemotherapy experience, randomized or otherwise, with this tumor. We have tended to use a chemotherapy combination of methotrexate plus cyclophosphamide, but will be exploring the efficacy of newer agents and combinations in the future.

References

Abrams, J. S., and Reines, H. D. Increasing incidence of right-sided lesions in colorectal cancer. *Am. J. Surg.* 137:522–526, 1979.

Ansfield, F. J. et al. Five years' clinical experience with 5-fluorouracil. *JAMA* 181:295, 1962.

Astler, U. B., and Coller, E. A. The prognostic significance of direct extension of carcinoma of the colon and rectum. *Ann. Surg.* 139:846–851, 1954.

Carter, S. K. Large bowel cancer—the current status of treatment. *J. Natl. Cancer Inst.* 56:3–10, 1976.

Cole, W. H. et al. Carcinoma of the colon. *Arch. Surg.* 91:547–557, 1965.

Copeland, E. M. et al. Prognostic factors in carcinoma of the colon and rectum. *Am. J. Surg.* 116:875–881, 1968.

Corman, M. L. et al. Proctosigmoidoscopy—age criteria for examination in the asymptomatic patient. *CA* 25:286–290, 1975.

Davis, H. L., and Kisner, D. L. Analysis of adjuvant therapy in large bowel cancer. *Cancer Clin. Trials* 1:273–287, 1978.

Dean, T. M. Carcinoma of the colon and rectum: a perspective for practicing physicians with recommendations for screening. *West. J. Med.* 126:431–440, 1977.

Devroede, G. J. et al. Cancer risk and life expectancy of children with ulcerative colitis. *N. Engl. J. Med.* 285:17–21, 1971.

Dukes, C. E., and Bussey, H. J. R. The spread of rectal cancer and its effect on prognosis. *Br. J. Cancer* 12:309–320, 1958.

Engstrom, P. et al. Combination chemotherapy of advanced bowel cancer. *Proc. Am. Soc. Clin. Oncol.* 19:384, 1978.

Falkson, G. et al. Fluorouracil, imidazole carboxamide dimethyltriazeno, vincristine and bischloroethyl nitrosourea in colon cancer. *Cancer* 33:1207–1209, 1974.

Gilbertsen, V. A. Improving the prognosis for patients with intestinal cancer. *Surg. Gynecol. Obstet.* 124:1253–1259, 1967.

Gilbertsen, V. A. The earlier diagnosis of adenocarcinoma of the large intestine. *Cancer* 27:143–149, 1971.

Gold, P., and Freedman, S. O. Demonstration of tumor-specific antigens in human colonic carcinoma by immunologic tolerance and absorption techniques. *J. Exp. Med.* 121:439–462, 1965.

Grage, T. B. et al. Adjuvant chemotherapy with 5-fluorouracil after surgical resection of colorectal carcinoma (COG protocol 7041). A preliminary report. *Am. J. Surg.* 133:59–66, 1977.

Grage, T. B. et al. Adjuvant chemotherapy in large bowel cancer. Updated analysis of single agent chemotherapy. In *Adjuvant therapy of cancer II,* eds. S. E. Jones and S. E. Salmon. New York: Grune & Stratton, 1979, pp. 587–594.

Greegor, D. H. Occult blood testing for detection of asymptomatic colon cancer. *Cancer* 28:131–134, 1974.

Hastings, J. B. Mass screening for colorectal cancer. *Am. J. Surg.* 127:228–233, 1974.

Herrera, M. A. et al. Carcinoembryonic antigen (CEA) as a prognostic and monitoring test in clinically complete resection of colorectal carcinoma. *Ann. Surg.* 183: 5–9, 1976.

Hertz, R. E. et al. Value of periodic examination in detecting cancer of the rectum and colon. *Postgrad. Med.* 27:290–294, 1960.

Higgins, G. A. et al. 5-fluorouracil as an adjuvant to surgery in carcinoma of the colon. *Arch. Surg.* 102:339–343, 1971.

Higgins, G. A. et al. Preoperative radiotherapy for colorectal cancer. *Ann. Surg.* 181:624–631, 1975.

Higgins, G. A. et al. The case for adjuvant 5-fluorouracil in colorectal cancer. *Cancer Clin. Trials* 1:35–41, 1978.

Holden, W. D. et al. The use of triethylenethiophosphoramide as an adjuvant to the surgical treatment of colorectal carcinoma. *Ann. Surg.* 165:481–503, 1967.

Holyoke, E. D., and Cooper, E. H. CEA and tumor markers. *Semin. Oncol.* 3:377–385, 1976.

Hoth, D. F., and Petrucci, P. E. Natural history and staging of colon cancer. *Senin. Oncol.* 3:331–336, 1976.

Jaffe, B. M. et al. Factors influencing survival in patients with untreated hepatic metastases. *Surg. Gynecol. Obstet.* 127:1–11, 1968.

Katz, S. et al. Rectocolonic exfoliative cytology; a new approach. *Am. J. Digest. Dis.* 17:1109–1116, 1972.

Katz, M. E.; Wiggans, R. G.; and Fischer, D. S. Colorectal cancer: current diagnostic approaches and strategies for management. *Conn. Med.* 43:613–620, 1979.

Killen, J. Y. et al. Adjuvant therapy of adenocarcinoma of the colon following clinically curative resection: an interim report from the GITSG. In *Adjuvant therapy of cancer III*, eds. S. E. Jones and S. E. Salmon. New York: Grune & Stratton, 1981, pp. 527–538.

Kirklin, J. W. et al. The role of the peritoneal reflection in the prognosis of carcinoma of the rectum and sigmoid colon. *Surg. Gynecol. Obstet.* 88:326–331, 1949.

Kligerman, M. M. et al. Preoperative irradiation of rectosigmoid carcinoma including its regional lymph nodes. *Am. J. Roentgenol.* 114:498–503, 1972.

Li, M. C., and Ross, S. T. Chemoprophylaxis for patients with colorectal cancer—prospective study with five-year follow-up. *JAMA* 235:2825–2828, 1976.

Macdonald, J. et al. 5-Fluorouracil (5-FU), methyl-CCNU and vincristine in the treatment of advanced colorectal cancer: phase II study utilizing weekly 5-FU. *Cancer Treat. Rep.* 60:1597–1600, 1976.

Mach, J. P. et al. Long-term follow-up of colorectal carcinoma patients by repeated CEA radioimmunoassay. *Cancer* 42:1439–1447, 1978.

Mavligit, G. M. et al. Adjuvant immunotherapy and chemo-immunotherapy in colorectal cancer of the Dukes' C classification. *Cancer* 36:2421–2427, 1975.

Mayer, R. J. et al. Carcinoembryonic antigen (CEA) as a monitor of chemotherapy in disseminated colorectal cancer. *Cancer* 42:1428–1433, 1978.

Miller, D. G. The early diagnosis of cancer. In *Physiopathology of cancer,* vol. 2, ed. F. Homburger. Basel: S. Karger, 1976, pp. 5–64.

Miller, S. F., and Knight, A. R. The early detection of colorectal cancer. *Cancer* 40:945–949, 1977.

Mittelman, A. et al. Adjuvant chemotherapy and radiotherapy following rectal surgery: an interim report from the GITSG. In *Adjuvant therapy of cancer III*, eds. S. E. Jones and S. E. Salmon. New York: Grune & Stratton, 1981, pp. 547–558.

Moertel, C. G. Natural history of gastrointestinal cancer. In *Advanced gastrointestinal cancer clinical management and chemotherapy,* eds. C. G. Moertel and R. J. Reitemeier. New York: Harper and Row, 1969, pp. 3–14.

Moertel, C. G. Current concepts in cancer — chemotherapy of gastrointestinal cancer. *N. Engl. J. Med.* 299:1049–1052, 1978.

Moertel, C. G. et al. Brief communication: therapy of advanced colorectal cancer with a combination of 5-fluorouracil, methyl-1, 3-cis (2 chlorethyl)-1-nitrosourea and vincristine. *J. Natl. Cancer Inst.* 54:69–71, 1975.

Moertel, C. G. et al. Carcinoembryonic antigen test for recurrent colorectal carcinoma: inadequacy for early detection. *JAMA* 239:1065–1066, 1978.

Morris, D. W. et al. Reliability of chemical tests for fecal occult blood in hospitalized patients. *Am. J. Digest. Dis.* 21:845–852, 1976.

Morson, B. C. Genesis of colorectal cancer. *Clin. Gastroenterol.* 5:505–525, 1976.

Polk, H. C., and Spratt, J. S. Recurrent colorectal carcinoma: detection, treatment and other considerations. *Surgery* 69:9–23, 1971.

Ranson, J. H. et al. Preoperative assessment for hepatic metastases in carcinoma of the colon and rectum. *Surg. Gynecol. Obstet.* 137:435–438, 1973.

Rawson, R. W. Colonic polyps: antecedent or associated lesions of large bowel cancer. *Semin. Oncol.* 3:361–367, 1976.

Reddy, B. A. Dietary factors and cancer of the large bowel. *Semin. Oncol.* 3:351–359, 1976.

Rhodes, J. B. et al. Changing distribution of primary cancers in the large bowel. *JAMA* 238:1641–1643, 1977.

Rousselot, L. M. et al. A five-year progress report on the effectiveness of intraluminal chemotherapy (5-fluorouracil) adjuvant to surgery for colorectal cancer. *Am. J. Surg.* 115:140–147, 1968.

Rousselot, L. M. et al. Adjuvant chemotherapy with 5-fluorouracil in surgery for colorectal cancer: a clinical cooperative multihospital trial. *Dis. Colon Rectum* 10:169–174, 1972.

Sherlock, P., and Winawer, S. J. The role of the early diagnosis in controlling large bowel cancer. *Cancer* 40:2609–2615, 1977.

Silverberg, E. Cancer statistics–1981. *CA* 31:13–28, 1981.

Silverberg, E., and Holleb, A. I. Cancer statistics–1974. Worldwide epidemiology. *CA* 24:2–21, 1974.

Smith, R. T. Possibilities and problems of immunologic intervention in cancer. *N. Engl. J. Med.* 287:439–450, 1972.

Stemper, T. J. et al. Juvenile polyposis and gastrointestinal carcinoma. *Ann. Intern. Med.* 83:639–646, 1975.

Stroehlein, J. R. et al. Hemoccult detection of fecal occult blood quantitated by radioimmunoassay. *Am. J. Digest. Dis.* 21:845–852, 1978.

Wanebo, H. J. et al. Preoperative carcinoembryonic antigen level as a prognostic indicator in colorectal cancer. *N. Engl. J. Med.* 299:448–451, 1978.

Wang, C. C., and Schultz, M. D. The role of radiation therapy in management of carcinoma of the sigmoid, rectosigmoid and rectum. *Radiology* 79:1–5, 1962.

Wasserman, T. H. et al. Tabular analysis of the clinical chemotherapy of solid tumors. *Cancer Chemother. Rep.* 6:399–419, 1975.

Weedon, D. D. et al. Crohn's disease and cancer. *N. Engl. J. Med.* 289:1099–1103, 1973.

Winawer, S. J. et al. Screening for colon cancer. *Gastroenterology* 70:783–789, 1976.

forty-two

Surgical Treatment of Genitourinary Cancers

ROBERT M. WEISS

Treatment of genitourinary cancers has evolved into employment of the combined modalities of surgery, chemotherapy, and radiotherapy. No attempt is made in this chapter to provide an encyclopedic review of renal, bladder, prostatic, and testicular cancers; rather, attention is concentrated on the surgical aspects of a few of the more frequently observed malignancies.

Renal Carcinoma

Diagnosis of Renal Masses

The diagnosis of renal carcinomas involves differentiation of neoplastic disease from other masses:

- Cysts
  - single
  - multiple
  - bilateral
- Hydronephrosis
- Tumors
  - renal cell carcinoma
  - adenoma
  - transitional cell carcinoma
  - Wilms' tumor
  - metastatic tumor
- Renal pseudotumors
  - column of Bertin
- Inflammatory
  - renal carbuncle
  - tuberculosis
- Traumatic
  - hematoma
  - aneurysm
- Hamartoma
  - angiomyolipoma
- Pseudotumor
  - retroperitoneal
  - suprarenal
  - pancreatic

The most frequent lesion that must be differentiated from renal cell carcinoma is a renal cyst. These may be single, multiple, or may occur in both kidneys. When they are multiple or bilateral they usually are cysts; however, a cyst and a tumor may occur within the same kidney, and in rare instances a tumor may form within the wall of a cyst. Renal cysts in themselves are not premalignant.

With the advent of modern excretory urographic techniques, it became evident that in the elderly individual the ratio of cyst to tumor was approximately 20:1. Since patients of this age group can least afford the risks of exploration for benign disease, the importance of preoperative differentiation of benign from malignant disease is evident. Using a combination of excretory urography, renal ultrasonography, renal cyst puncture, and renal arteriography, it usually is possible to differentiate cystic lesions from neoplasms.

Hydronephrosis may present as a renal mass lesion and can usually be diagnosed with appropriate modalities. The most common tumor to involve the kidney is the renal cell carcinoma or renal clear cell adenocarcinoma. Renal pelvic transitional cell carcinomas frequently present as filling defects within the renal pelvis; however, at times they may be renal masses. The treatment of renal cell carcinomas is nephrectomy, whereas therapy for transitional cell carcinomas of the renal pelvis is nephroureterectomy with removal of a cuff of bladder surrounding the involved ureteral orifice. These carcinomas of the renal pelvis represent one manifestation of a diffuse urothelial abnormality that may also involve the ureters and bladder.

Wilms' tumor occurs most frequently in children, but may occur in adults. Metastatic lesions to the kidney, especially from the lung, have been described. In addition, lesions histologically similar to renal carcinomas of less than 2 cm in diameter have been classified as benign renal adenomas. It is possible, although never proved, that a renal adenoma represents the earliest developmental stage of renal clear cell carcinoma.

Normal benign variants are the renal pseudotumors (column of Bertin). At times these may be difficult to differentiate from renal carcinomas. They usually are intrarenal, and situated between the midcalices and the calices to the upper or lower pole. Although they lack neoplastic-appearing tortuous vessels on arteriography, there is an increased flush on the nephrographic phase of the arteriogram. The most useful modality in differentiating this from the typical renal carcinoma is the renal scan. A carcinoma or cyst should cause a negative filling defect on a renal scan, whereas the column of Bertin, since it represents functioning renal tissue, will not cause such a defect.

Renal carbuncles represent another form of mass that at times needs to be differentiated from a renal carcinoma. The renal carbuncle may be preceded by a cutaneous inflammatory process, and *Staphylococcus aureus* is the most common organism involved. In a series of renal carbuncles recently treated at Yale, urine and blood cultures were negative in the majority of instances. Abnormal vessels seen on arteriography tend to be stretched and attenuated, rather than cork-screwing as seen with the more classic renal carcinomas. Although standard treatment was exploration with drainage, recent evidence suggests that intravenous oxacillin followed by oral dicloxacillin will be sufficient in the treatment of many of these lesions.

Other renal masses include hematomas and renal artery aneurysms. Angiomyolipomas when bilateral are frequently associated with tuberosclerosis, although in middle-aged women there may be a unilateral distribution. These lesions contain fat and small aneurysmal dilatations and thus can be differentiated from renal adenocarcinomas with nephrotomography, arteriography, and computerized axial tomography. Fatal hemorrhage has been reported; however, a conservative approach is required when the tumors are bilateral. Retroperitoneal adrenal and pancreatic lesions may also require differentiation from renal carcinomas.

Evaluation

Intravenous pyelography, nephrotomography, ultrasonography, renal arteriography, radioisotope scanning, and at times, percutaneous needle aspirations have all been used to distinguish between benign lesions of the kidney and carcinomas. Intravenous pyelography (excretory urography) itself will define whether a mass exists, but will not in itself differentiate benign from malignant disease. Nephrotomography should be routinely incorporated with intravenous pyelogram when a mass is evident. After defining the presence of a mass with excretory urography, a renal ultrasound is indicated (fig. 42.1). If the lesion is sonolucent (fig. 42.2), one usually proceeds to a percutaneous puncture with the aid of either fluoroscopic monitoring or ultrasonography. Injection of contrast material into the cyst may define aspects suggestive of neoplasia. A renal cyst

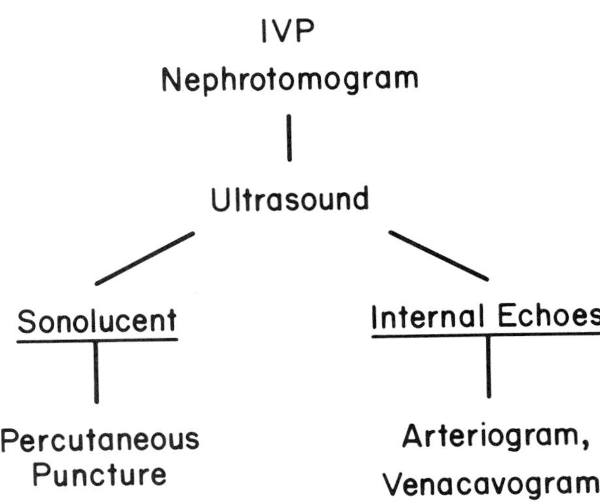

Fig. 42.1. *Indications for diagnostic procedures to identify renal masses.*

should have smooth margins; its fluid is clear, lacks neoplastic cells, and has no increase in fat or lactic dehydrogenase (LDH).

If the ultrasound shows echos within the lesion, an arteriogram is indicated. Renal carcinomas frequently have abnormal vessels (fig. 42.3), although some are avascular. A histologic variant referred to as a papillary-tubular adenocarcinoma is frequently avascular, but can be differentiated from cystic disease with arteriography and ultrasonography (Weiss et al. 1969). Exploration is indicated for any lesion that appears to be neoplastic or in which proof of benignity is not obtained from the diagnostic studies. Preoperative diagnosis of renal cyst usually precludes the necessity of exploration. A venogram aids in determining whether the renal vein or vena cava is involved with tumor and thus affects the extent of surgery.

Systemic Effects

Renal carcinoma has been referred to as the internist's tumor because of its many systemic effects. Elevation of the sedimentation rate, anemia, and polycythemia have been described. Anemia occurs more frequently than polycythemia. Other signs and symptoms may include hypertension, weight loss, fever, hypercalcemia with production of parathormone, and neuromyopathy. The classic triad of hematuria, pain, and renal mass is observed only in a minority of cases. Significant numbers of patients with renal carcinomas have abnormal liver function tests. These in themselves do not necessarily indicate the presence of metastatic disease. The acute onset of a right-sided varicocele should suggest the possibility of a lesion with impingement on the vena cava.

Surgical Treatment

The surgical treatment for a primary renal carcinoma is radical nephrectomy (Robson, Churchill, and Anderson 1969) aimed at early ligation of the vascular pedicle, complete excision of the kidney and its surrounding Gerota's fascia, and removal (fig. 42.4) of the regional lymph nodes. The approach may be either transperitoneal or thoracoabdominal, and a flank approach may be used at times. Although radical nephrectomy is the usual treatment, a partial nephrectomy may be indicated in the presence of a solitary kidney with or without the

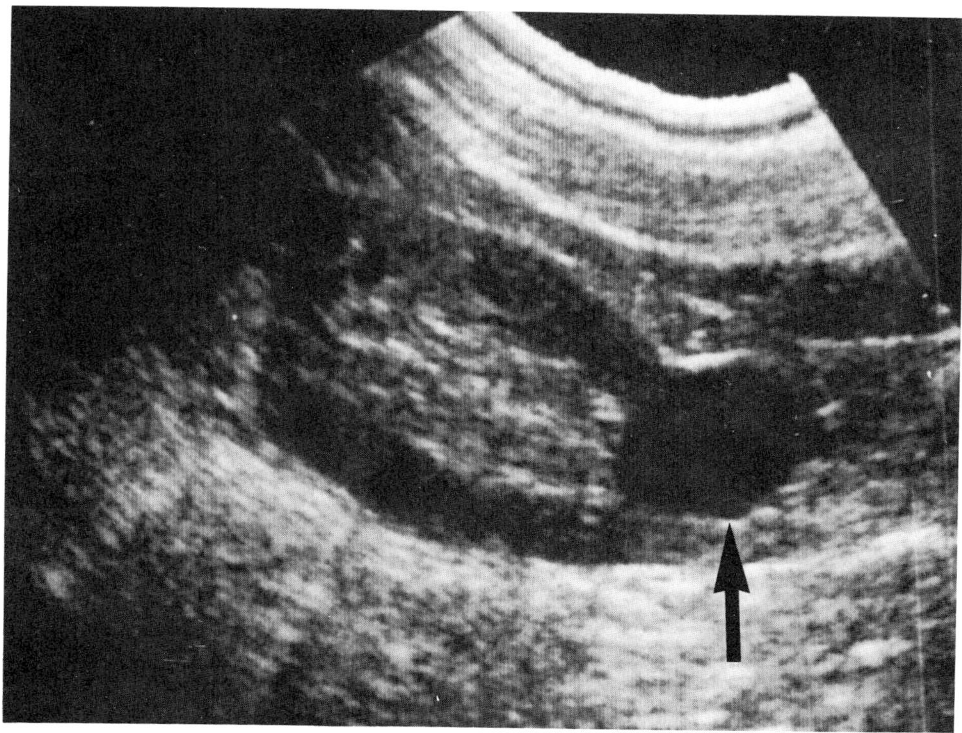

Fig. 42.2. *Longitudinal ultrasound visualization of renal cyst* (arrow). *Normal kidney is to the left. (Photograph courtesy of Kenneth Taylor, M.D., Department of Diagnostic Radiology, Yale–New Haven Hospital, New Haven, Conn.)*

employment of so-called bench surgery, in which the kidney is removed and perfused through its renal artery while leaving its ureter intact (Novick et al. 1977). Microdissection is used to free the kidney of tumor, and the kidney is subsequently autotransplanted into the iliac region, leaving the ureterovesical junction intact. The survival of selected patients treated with partial nephrectomy approximates that of radical nephrectomy.

The extent of spread and histologic degree of pleomorphism influences survival. Data suggest that nephrectomy is indicated in the presence of a single, potentially treatable metastatic site (Middleton 1970). Surgical removal is deferred in those with multiple metastases, unless local complications related to the tumor, such as uncontrollable pain or hemorrhage, are present.

Wilms' Tumor

Wilms' tumor (nephroblastoma) is the most common renal malignant neoplasm of childhood (fig. 42.5). It occurs once in every 10,000 to 50,000 live births, and the average age at diagnosis is approximately three years. Initially, therapy was nephrectomy. With the advent of radiotherapy and the addition of dactinomycin to treatment protocols, survival of patients with Wilms' tumor has markedly improved.

It became evident several years ago that those children whose diagnosis was made before the age of two did significantly better than those with diagnosis at an older age. It also was realized that the complications of both radiotherapy and chemotherapy were significant, and the question arose as to whether both modalities

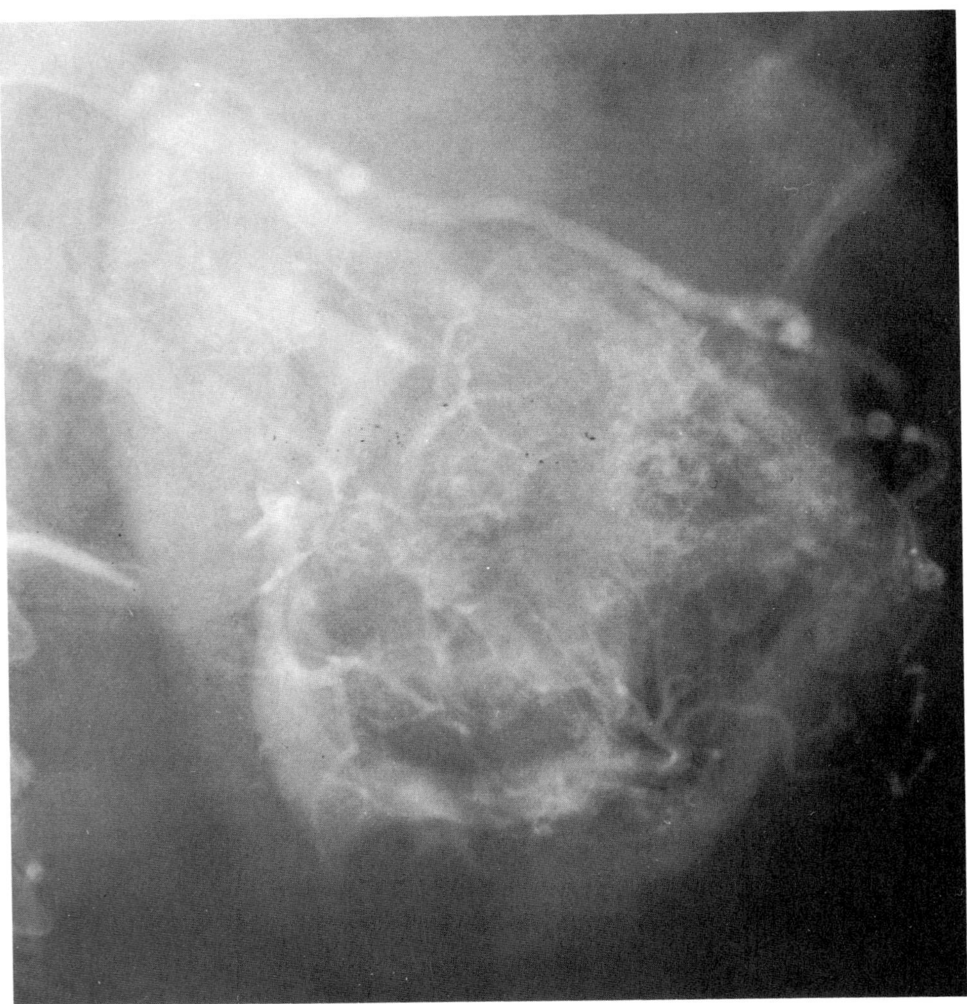

Fig. 42.3. *Arteriogram showing neovascularity of renal cell carcinoma.*

were needed as adjuvant treatment of all patients with Wilms' tumor. Dactinomycin has significant hematologic and gastrointestinal toxicity, and radiotherapy causes growth disturbances.

A combined modality national Wilms' tumor program was thus instituted to establish optimum treatment (D'Angio et al. 1976). The following defines staging of the disease, which is an important determinant of prognosis and therefore of therapy:

Stage I — limited to kidney and completely resected
Stage II — extension beyond kidney but completely resected
Stage III — residual nonhematogenous tumor in the abdomen
Stage IV — hematogenous metastases
Stage V — bilateral renal involvement

The first national protocol set up specific treatment groups for patients with stage I disease. All patients underwent nephrectomy and received dactinomycin. Some received radiotherapy while others did not. The data showed that radiotherapy did not influence the survival of children under two years of age. For those over the age of two, radiotherapy caused a slight improvement in percentage of survival. Thus for children under age two with stage I disease radiotherapy is no longer employed.

Patients with stage II and stage III disease were divided into several treatment groups. All underwent surgery and all received radiotherapy. Some received dactinomycin alone, some vincristine alone, and others a combination of those agents. It should be noted that the primary complications of dactinomycin are hematologic, whereas those of vincristine are neurologic; thus the toxicities are not additive. The data from the first protocol showed that patients with stages II and III

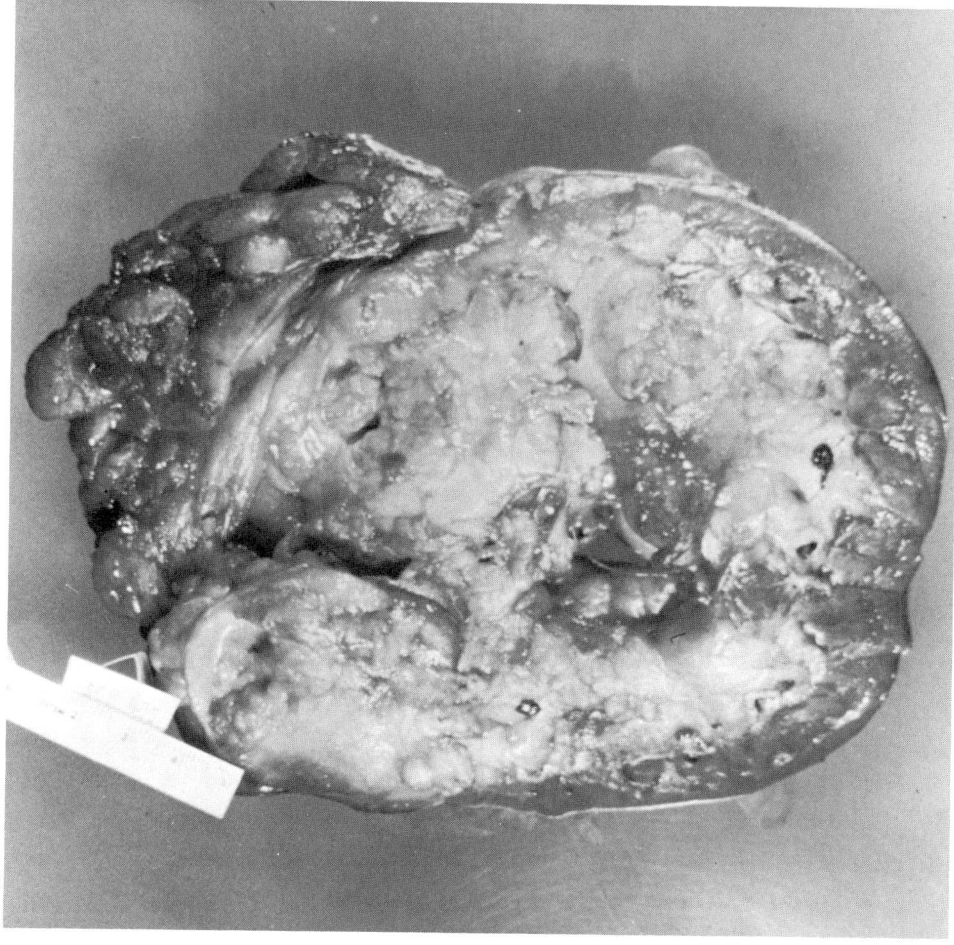

Fig. 42.4. *Cut section of renal cell carcinoma.*

disease who received both drugs did significantly better than those receiving either one alone. Preliminary data from a more recent study suggest that the addition of doxorubicin (Adriamycin), an agent whose primary toxicity is cardiac, to dactinomycin and vincristine may further increase survival rate.

An aggressive approach is indicated in patients with metastatic Wilms' tumor. Significant lengthening of survival has occurred in patients treated by nephrectomy, and then either radiotherapy or surgical excision of metastatic disease. With bilateral disease, nephrectomy on the most involved side and partial nephrectomy on the least involved side seems to be the treatment of choice.

Congenital mesoblastic nephroma, a solid tumor observed in the neonate, has a significantly better prognosis than Wilms' tumor. Although histologically similar to Wilms' tumor, these are a benign form of hamartoma. It is important to note that a solid mass in the neonate may not be true Wilms' tumor, so that nephrectomy need not be performed on an emergency basis. Time may be allowed until the infant is old enough or strong enough to tolerate surgical exploration. In addition, adjuvant radiotherapy or dactinomycin is not required in these patients. It should be emphasized, however, that nephrectomy is necessary, as these lesions may become malignant with time.

Carcinoma of the Bladder

Transitional cell carcinomas are the most common histologic neoplasm affecting the bladder (Miller 1977). Adenocarcinomas are rare, and when present are usually located at the dome of the bladder in relation to a persistent urachal remnant, or near the trigone where they probably arise from the periurethral Albarran's glands. Neoplasms associated with extrophy of the blad-

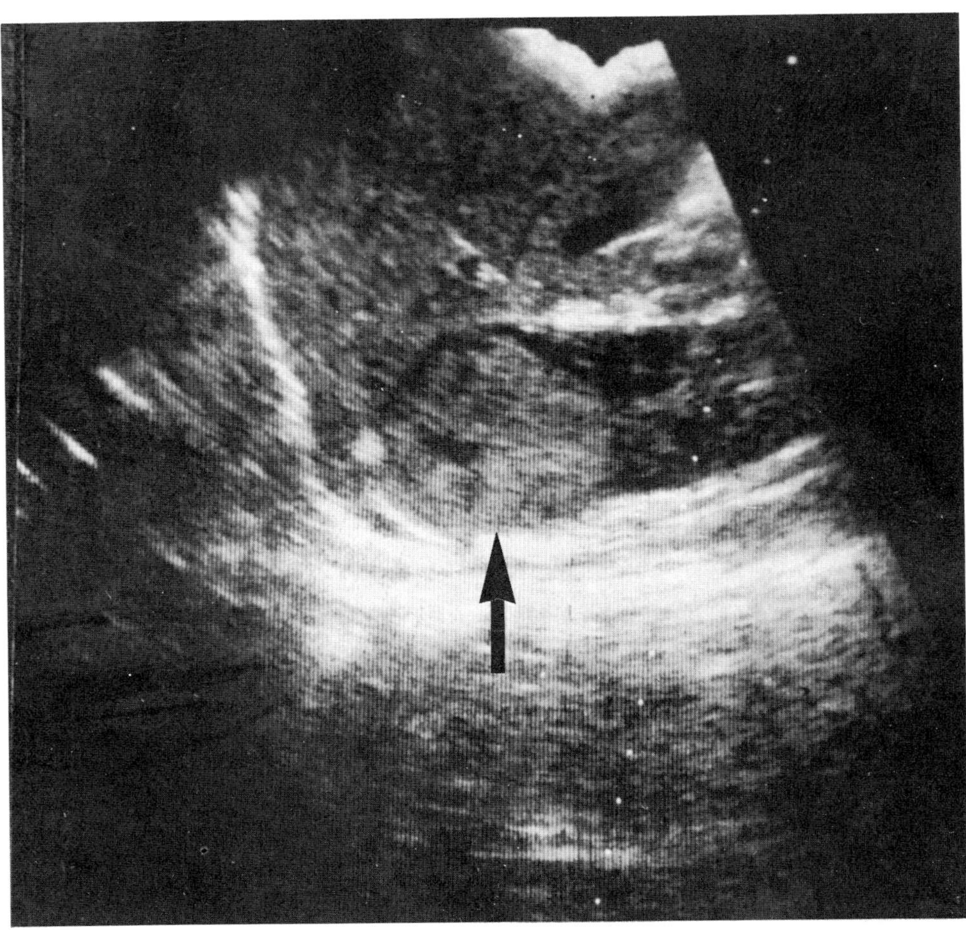

Fig. 42.5. *Ultrasound of Wilms' tumor* (arrow). *Normal kidney is also shown. (Photograph courtesy of Kenneth Taylor, M.D., Department of Radiology, Yale–New Haven Hospital, New Haven, Conn.)*

der tend also to be adenocarcinomas. Squamous cell carcinomas, which are frequently associated with inflammatory disease, represent a highly anaplastic form of transitional cell carcinoma.

Management of these tumors is predicated on their high recurrence rates and on the finding that they represent only one aspect of a diffuse abnormality of the urothelium. Once a transitional cell carcinoma has been diagnosed and treated, follow-up cystoscopies and periodic evaluation of the upper urinary tract for associated ureteral and renal pelvic transitional cell carcinomas are required for the remainder of the patient's life.

Staging

Management of these carcinomas depends on staging the lesion. Stage 0 (in situ) and A (invasion of submucosa) lesions are confined to the urothelium. Stage B1 tumors invade the superficial musculature; stage B2 disease extends more than halfway through the musculature; stage C lesions extend through the muscle and into the surrounding serosa. Stage D refers to metastatic disease: D1 within the pelvis; D2 beyond the pelvis. Histologic grading is also a prognostic factor. Grades I and II are the less pleomorphic; grades III and IV are more pleomorphic. Higher stages tend to be lesions of higher grade, although the relationship is not absolute.

Etiology

Several etiologic factors have been identified, the most important of which is cigarette smoking. In addition, certain industrial carcinogens, tryptophan metabolites, schistosomias, and chronic inflammatory conditions have been related to the development of bladder carcinomas.

Diagnosis

Cystoscopy, endoscopic biopsy, and bimanual examination are the main modalities for the diagnosis, staging, and grading of bladder tumors. Urine cytology is of value in surveillance, especially of patients with high-grade lesions. Ultrasonography, computerized axial tomography, arteriography, and lymphangiography are of less value and should be reserved for specific indications.

Treatment

Treatment for bladder tumors may consist of a combination of surgery, radiotherapy, and chemotherapy. This discussion is confined to their surgical treatment (Prout 1976).

Endoscopic excision and fulguration is the modality of choice for low-grade and low-stage lesions. Suprapubic excision and fulguration is rarely indicated, and should be limited to the unusual case of a superficial tumor in which endoscopic therapy is not feasible.

Recently, the Helmstein distention therapy that provides for pressure necrosis of superficial and low-grade tumors has been added to the surgical modalities (England et al. 1973). It provides a means of endoscopically treating some low-grade and low-stage lesions that previously required open excision and fulguration. A balloon is inserted into the bladder and the pressure within the balloon is raised to halfway between the diastolic and systolic pressure. Continuous epidural anesthesia is employed and the distention is continued for four to six hours. The results with superficial lesions have been promising, and complications have not been frequent.

In general, high-stage and high-grade lesions have required total cystectomy, either simple or radical, with excision of regional lymph nodes. Survivals with simple and radical cystectomy have not been shown to be significantly different, although some patients with regional nodal involvement might be cured with the more radical procedure. Lesions on the dome in which wide surgical margins can be obtained probably can be treated as effectively with partial as with total cystectomy (Novick and Stewart 1976).

Indications for cystectomy are high-grade and high-stage lesions that do not lend themselves to partial cystectomy because of their location or their multicentricity. In addition, the procedure is indicated for low-grade lesions that have become so profuse and so multicentric that endoscopic therapy is no longer feasible.

At our institution, the treatment for high-grade, high-stage bladder carcinomas has consisted of preoperative radiotherapy plus cystectomy (Barzell and Whitmore 1978). Survivals appear to be greater than with radiation alone, and at least theoretically the combined modality treatment appears to be preferable to the use of surgery alone.

Carcinoma of the Prostate

Carcinoma of the prostate is the most frequent genitourinary tumor of men. Peak incidence is in the sixth and seventh decade, and if one meticulously takes stepwise sections of prostatic specimens from elderly individuals, incidence may exceed 80%. In recent years, as the therapy for carcinoma of the prostate has evolved, the use of surgery as primary approach has declined in many institutions (VA Cooperative Group 1967).

Diagnosis

As the majority of carcinomas of the prostate arise in the posterior capsule, rectal examination provides the most important modality for diagnosis. In many instances percutaneous transperineal needle biopsy will provide histologic confirmation of the clinical impression. The standard enzymatic methods of assaying for serum acid phosphatase have aided in determining the extent of spread. A normal serum acid phosphatase does not rule out spread of disease; however, an elevated value using enzymatic methodologies provides evidence that the tumor has at least extended out of the capsule. More recently, immunoassays have been developed for evaluation of serum acid phosphatase levels and it is hoped that these highly specific assays, which can detect minute quantities of acid phosphatase, may provide a means of detecting earlier disease (Foti et al. 1977).

Bone marrow acid phosphatase is another means of detecting spread of this carcinoma. Data in the literature are conflicting, which may be due to inaccuracies in the assay methods available. Bone marrow acid phosphatase determinations may prove to be of more value as immunoassays are perfected.

In addition, these patients require intravenous pyelogram, chest x-ray, bone scan, and cystoscopy. The intravenous pyelogram will detect evidence of obstruction of the upper urinary tract secondary to local extension of disease. The bone scan has proved to be a more accurate method of detecting bone metastases than the standard skeletal survey.

Staging

The staging nomenclature for prostatic cancer is as follows:

Stage A refers to carcinoma detected incidentally at the time of a procedure performed for the management of clinically suspected benign prostatic hypertrophy or disease noted at autopsy.

Stage B disease refers to a carcinoma confined to the prostate without extension beyond the capsule. Some investigators subdivide stage B lesions into B1 and B2 depending on the extent of involvement within the gland.

Stage C carcinoma is local disease that has extended beyond the capsule and perhaps into the fascial planes around the seminal vesicles.

Stage D disease refers to metastatic involvement; D1 within the pelvis and D2 beyond the pelvis.

Surgical Therapy

Evaluation of any treatment of carcinoma of the prostate is difficult because of the slow progression of the disease (Whitmore 1973). Whereas one can discuss therapeutic modalities for most cancers in terms of 5-year survival rates, 10-year and 15-year survival rates are required before one can make significant interpretations of therapy in prostate cancer.

There is no universally accepted treatment protocol for any stage of this disease. Stage A disease that is detected at the time of surgery for benign prostatic hypertrophy should be reclassified into two groups. When only a single focus of well-differentiated carcinoma is detected, probably no further therapy is required. Chances of the disease spreading appear to be small, and the potential complications of surgery and radiotherapy are outweighed by the relatively benign course of the disease (Khalifa and Jarman 1976). When stage A disease consists of either a poorly differentiated carcinoma or more extensive involvement of the prostate, some form of curative therapy is indicated. Some centers recommend radical prostatectomy; however, it must be remembered that the incidence of incontinence following this operation is higher in patients who previously have had surgery for benign disease. Technical difficulties may also be encountered when implantation of ^{125}I seeds is attempted in patients who have undergone either open prostatectomy or extensive transurethral resection. For these reasons, I have usually employed external beam radiation.

Stage B carcinoma of the prostate is the only stage in which there has been widespread employment of radical surgery (Jewett 1970). Survival percentages are dependent on whether these clinically localized tumors are indeed histologically localized to the prostate or whether positive nodes and extension outside the capsule is present. If they are microscopically localized to the gland, survival following radical prostatectomy approaches expected survival of the normal population. If there is evidence of microscopic extension, survival drops off precipitously. Recent data obtained during staging pelvic lymphadenectomy at the time of either surgical or radiation therapy have revealed that approximately 20% to 25% of patients with clinically localized lesions have positive nodes (Dahl et al. 1974).

Because the survivals with radiation therapy approximate those with radical prostatectomy, and because the morbidity encountered after pelvic lymphadenectomy and implantation of ^{125}I seeds has been less than that following radical prostatectomy, we have employed the isotope implantation for the treatment of localized disease. Radical prostatectomy results in approximately 10% associated incontinence and nearly 100% impotence. These side effects appear to be negligible with ^{125}I implantations (Whitmore, Hilaris, and Grabstald 1972). It should be emphasized, however, that whether operation or radiotherapy is planned, a staging lymphadenectomy aids in determining the extent of management and the ultimate prognosis. Lymphadenectomy, however, also presents the risk of impotence.

The management of stage C and stage D disease has in general been hormonal manipulation, which includes bilateral orchiectomy (Blackard, Byar, and Jordan 1973). In many patients with stage C disease, a staging lymphadenectomy and implantation of ^{125}I seeds has proved effective. Depending on the extent of nodal involvement, adjuvant radiotherapy has been employed. Another form of surgical therapy has been transurethral resection of the prostate. This should be reserved for patients with significant voiding complaints who do not respond to hormonal manipulation. This operation, of course, is not curative.

Testicular Carcinomas

The most common histologic type of testicular carcinoma is seminoma. It has been subclassified into (1) typical, (2) anaplastic, and (3) spermatocytic categories. This is the most frequent testicular tumor in individuals with undescended testes, and has the best prognosis. The nonseminomatous germinal cell carcinomas involving the testes are (1) embryonal, (2) teratocarcinomas, and (3) choriocarcinomas. The last have the worst prognosis. Appreciable numbers of testicular tumors are of mixed histology (Culp, Boatman, and Wilson 1973).

Approximately 65% are painless swellings within the scrotum, although swelling may be painful and tender and at times is first detected following trauma. A small percentage of patients develop hormonal effects such as gynecomastia. The first evidence of a testicular tumor may be related to its metastatic spread.

These are a rather uncommon form of genitourinary tumors; however, incidence in patients who have had an undescended testis is approximately 20 times that of the general population. There is no definite evidence to suggest that orchiopexy decreases incidence of this malignancy, although most urologists recommend that the procedure be done before the age of five, since testicular tumors are not frequently seen in patients so treated. A longer period of observation is required before the issue is clearly answered.

Diagnosis

In addition to a chest x-ray, serum for alpha-fetoprotein and beta subunit of human chorionic gonadotropin (HCG) should be obtained prior to surgical exploration. Elevation of one or both of these tumor markers is highly suggestive of a nonseminomatous tumor, and comparison with postorchiectomy values may aid in management (Lange et al. 1976). It is possible although not proved that a small percentage (less than 5%) of patients with pure seminoma also may have elevation of the beta subunit of HCG (Javadpour et al. 1978).

Staging

Stage I tumors are those confined to the testes, stage II have metastasized to the retroperitoneal lymph nodes, and stage III are tumors that have metastasized beyond the retroperitoneal nodes. In addition to histologic type, the stage of the lesion influences ultimate prognosis and determines the extent of therapy.

Surgical Treatment

Once the suspicion of a testicular tumor is present, the patient should undergo inguinal exploration and probable orchiectomy (Staubitz et al. 1968; Skinner 1976). It is not necessary to await the report of the tumor markers prior to exploration. After establishing histologic proof, further metastatic work-up is indicated with an intravenous pyelogram, lymphangiogram, and bone scan.

Exploration should be through the inguinal region for all forms of testicular tumors. A clamp is placed on the spermatic cord at the internal inguinal ring prior to mobilization of the testis. If there is gross evidence of a tumor it is usually best to remove the testis without performing a biopsy.

Subsequent management depends on the histologic findings. It should be noted that with germinal cell tumors in which there is more than one cell type, management is usually dependent on the most malignant histologic configuration. That is, if one finds a seminoma with embryonal elements, the patient is treated for embryonal carcinoma.

In addition to inguinal orchiectomy, patients with seminoma should receive retroperitoneal radiation. The extent of radiation is determined by the findings at lymphangiography. Continued elevation of tumor markers following orchiectomy provides presumptive evidence of residual nonseminomatous germ cell disease in the retroperitoneal nodes. These patients should be treated in a manner similar to those with nonseminomatous germ cell tumors.

Retroperitoneal lymphadenectomy in addition to inguinal orchiectomy is indicated for patients with nonseminomatous germ cell lesions (Ray, Hajdu, and Whitmore 1974). Dissection should begin at least at the level of the renal pedicle and extend to the internal inguinal ring on the ipsilateral side and to the bifurcation of the aorta on the contralateral side. Although there is variation in different centers concerning the need for further adjuvant therapy, it has been our policy to employ chemotherapy only in those patients whose retroperitoneal lymph nodes are positive or in whom there is a persistent elevation in tumor markers. The five-year survival for patients with stage I nonseminomatous germ cell tumors is approximately 85% to 90%, and for stage II approximately 60% to 70%.

Tumor Markers

In recent years the detection of tumor markers has aided in the management of patients with testicular tumors. In one study, elevations after inguinal orchiectomy provided clear evidence of the presence of residual tumor in the retroperitoneal lymph nodes. In addition, patients who have positive tumor markers following orchiectomy appear to have a poorer prognosis than those with negative markers. These also have provided a means of following patients for recurrent disease and for assessing response to therapy.

References

Barzell, W., and Whitmore, W. F., Jr. Radical cystectomy with or without planned preoperative irradiation in the treatment of bladder cancer. *Urol. Res.* 6:249–251, 1978.

Blackard, C. E.; Byar, D. P.; and Jordan, W. P. Orchiectomy for advanced prostatic carcinoma: a reevaluation. *Urology* 1:553–560, 1973.

Culp, D. A.; Boatman, D. L.; and Wilson, V. B. Testicular tumors: 40 years' experience. *J. Urol.* 110:548–553, 1973.

Dahl, D. S. et al. Pelvic lymphadenectomy for staging localized prostatic cancer. *J. Urol.* 112:245–246, 1974.

D'Angio, G. J. et al. The treatment of Wilms' tumor—results of the national Wilms' tumor study. *Cancer* 38:633–646, 1976.

England, H. R. et al. Evaluation of Helmstein's distension method for carcinoma of bladder. *Br. J. Urol.* 45:593–599, 1973.

Foti, A. G. et al. Detection of prostatic cancer by solid-phase radioimmunoassay of serum prostatic acid phosphatase. *N. Engl. J. Med.* 297:1357–1361, 1977.

Javadpour, N. et al. The role of the radioimmunoassay of serum alpha-fetoprotein and human chorionic gonadotropin in the intensive chemotherapy and surgery of metastatic testicular tumors. *J. Urol.* 119: 759–762, 1978.

Jewett, H. J. The case for radical perineal prostatectomy. *J. Urol.* 103:195–199, 1970.

Khalifa, N. M., and Jarman, W. D. A study of 48 cases of incidental carcinoma of the prostate followed 10 years or longer. *J. Urol.* 116:329–331, 1976.

Lange, P. H. et al. Serum alpha-fetoprotein and human chorionic gonadotropin in the diagnosis and management of nonseminomatous germ cell cancer. *N. Engl. J. Med.* 295:1237–1240, 1976.

Middleton, R. G. Surgery for metastatic renal cell carcinoma. *J. Urol.* 97:973–977, 1970.

Miller, L. S. Bladder cancer. *Cancer* 39:973–980, 1977.

Novick, A. C. et al. Partial nephrectomy in treatment of renal adenocarcinoma. *J. Urol.* 118:932–936, 1977.

Novick, A. C., and Stewart, B. H. Partial cystectomy in the treatment of primary and secondary carcinoma of the bladder. *J. Urol.* 116:570–574, 1976.

Prout, G. R. The surgical management of bladder carcinoma. *Surg. Clin. North Am.* 3:149–175, 1976.

Ray, B.; Hajdu, S. I.; and Whitmore, W. F., Jr. Distribution of retroperitoneal lymph node metastases in testicular germinal tumors. *Cancer* 33:340–348, 1974.

Robson, C. J.; Churchill, B. M.; and Anderson, W. The results of radical nephrectomy for renal cell carcinoma. *J. Urol.* 101:297–301, 1969.

Skinner, D. G. Non-seminomatous testis tumors: a plan of management based on 96 patients to improve survival in all stages by combined therapeutic modalities. *J. Urol.* 115:65–69, 1976.

Staubitz, W. J. et al. Surgical management of testes tumors. *Trans. Am. Assoc. Genitourinary Surg.* 60:65–70, 1968.

Veterans Administration Cooperative Urological Research Group. Treatment and survival of patients with cancer of the prostate. *Surgery* 124:1101–1017, 1967.

Weiss, R. M. et al. Angiographic appearance of renal papillary-tubular adenocarcinomas. *J. Urol.* 102: 661–664, 1969.

Whitmore, W. F., Jr. The natural history of prostatic cancer. *Cancer* 32:1104–1112, 1973.

Whitmore, W. F., Jr.; Hilaris, B.; and Grabstald, H. Retropubic implantation of iodine 125 in the treatment of prostatic cancer. *J. Urol.* 108:918–920, 1972.

forty-three

Radiation Therapy of Urologic Malignancies

BERNARD PERCARPIO

Kidney

At present the role of radiotherapy in the management of renal carcinoma is chiefly palliation of symptomatic metastases. Prospective randomized trials have studied the use of prenephrectomy irradiation with 3000 rad (van der Werf-Messing 1973) and postnephrectomy with 5500 rad (Finney 1973). Neither study was able to demonstrate survival advantage with combined therapy. Patients with known residual tumor following nephrectomy, extensive regional lymph node involvement, or perinephric involvement are at risk for local tumor recurrence and its resultant morbidity (Riches 1968), and should be considered for postnephrectomy irradiation of the renal fossa with doses of at least 4000 rad over four weeks.

Bladder

The precise role of radiotherapy in the management of bladder carcinoma has been debated because of the natural history of the disease and inaccuracy of staging (Caldwell 1974). Many patients are considered for more definitive treatment such as cystectomy or radical irradiation only after multiple fulgurations have failed to control the disease. Obviously, this group of patients is a selected one and would be expected to do less well than those chosen for definitive treatment at the time of initial diagnosis. Current staging classifications attempt to predict prognosis on the basis of the depth of invasion of the tumor into or through the bladder wall (Caldwell 1974). Frequently, however, biopsies are superficial and do not permit adequate assessment of the depth of invasion. Understaging is common.

Results of primary irradiation for bladder carcinoma reflect the selection of previously treated patients, inaccuracy of staging based on biopsy, and inclusion of patients ineligible for surgery on a medical basis. Following delivery of 6000 to 7000 rad to the bladder in seven weeks, five-year survival (Caldwell et al. 1967; Frank 1970; Miller 1977) of 50% to 60% is seen in patients with stage A disease and 40% to 50% in those with stage B1 disease. With more advanced lesions the five-year survival rates are poor, with 20% to 30% in stage B2 and 15% to 20% in stage C, and less than 10% in stage D1. In general, these results are poorer than with radical cystectomy, and thus primary irradiation should be recommended only for patients who are medically unfit for operation. Pretreatment lymphangiography and/or computed tomography of the pelvis are recommended to delineate better the extent of pelvic involvement.

The high incidence of pelvic lymph node involvement and local failure for patients with stage B2 or C bladder carcinoma treated by radical surgery have prompted the investigation of additional treatments. Preoperative pelvic irradiation has been recommended by some to sterilize microscopic tumor not removed at cystectomy (Whitmore et al. 1977). Pelvic doses of 4000 to 5000 rad given over four to five weeks have been studied. This combined therapy for patients with stages B2 and C tumors has improved five-year survival statistics to approximately 50% (van der Werf-Messing 1975). A randomized prospective study at M. D. Anderson Hospital compared radical irradiation to preoperative irradiation with radical cystectomy (Miller 1977). Five-year survival (46%) was significantly better for the group receiving combined therapy. For those patients who actually underwent the proposed cystectomy, five-year survival was 53%.

In an attempt to expedite treatment, a shorter course of preoperative irradiation using 2000 rad in five days has been proposed (van der Werf-Messing 1975). Similar survival with conventional irradiation has been claimed, but the comparison suffers from using a retrospective control group with a higher percentage of advanced lesions. A national prospective randomized trial is currently investigating the effect of 2000 rad in five days versus 5000 rad in five weeks preoperatively for advanced disease. Until the results of that study are available, pelvic doses of 4500 to 5000 rad in five weeks are recommended as preoperative irradiation for stages B2 and C.

Prostate

Until the mid-1960s, adenocarcinoma of the prostate was considered to be a radioresistant tumor. This impression was based on the poor results following attempted treatment of early lesions by the injection of radioactive colloidal gold into the prostatic bed or external irradiation of the prostate by poorly penetrating orthovoltage x-rays. Both methods were unable to deliver the uniform doses in excess of 6000 rad necessary to sterilize localized prostatic carcinoma. In the past 15 years several groups have reported their experience with radical external beam irradiation using cobalt 60 units or high-energy linear accelerators (Bagshaw et al. 1975; Harisiadis et al. 1978; Perez et al. 1977; Ray, Cassady, and Bagshaw 1973).

Prior to therapy patients are evaluated for metastases by chest x-ray, bone scan, IVP, acid phosphatase determination, and bone marrow aspirate and biopsy. More recently, lymphangiography has assisted in staging these patients prior to treatment. The Stanford University series of patients staged by laparotomy indicated an overall accuracy of 76% for lymphangiography (Ray et al. 1976). The incidence of lymph node metastases is approximately 20% for stage B and 50% for stage C lesions (Ray et al. 1976). In general, patients with prostatic tumors limited to the pelvis are given doses of 6500 to 7000 rad to the known tumor volume over seven weeks' time. Five-year disease-free survival rates are about 85% for stage A (Harisiadis et al. 1978) and 70% for stage B disease (Harisiadis et al. 1978; Perez et al. 1977; Ray, Cassady, and Bagshaw 1973), comparable to most surgical series. Stage C tumors are generally considered inoperable, but radical irradiation results in five-year disease-free survival rates of about 40% (Harisiadis et al. 1978; Perez et al. 1977; Ray, Cassady, and Bagshaw 1973). Although some patients eventually develop distant metastases, the local control rate of tumor within the pelvis for all stages is about 80% (Perez et al. 1977).

Clinically, these tumors respond slowly to irradiation and it may take 6 to 12 months in some instances before the gland returns to normal size. Biopsies following irradiation tend to parallel the gross response to treatment. In one series, patients with stage C prostatic carcinoma had serial biopsies up to three years following radical irradiation (Cox and Stoffel 1977). The percentage of positive results correlated only with the interval following treatment and did not predict ultimate prognosis. Therefore prostatic biopsies should only be done to document obvious tumor recurrence following irradiation. Interestingly, serum or bone marrow acid phosphatase levels have not correlated with the prognosis of patients receiving radiotherapy (Harisiadis et al. 1978; Ray, Cassady, and Bagshaw 1973).

The complications of external irradiation are acceptable. Less than 10% of treated patients have persistent significant gastrointestinal problems such as prolonged diarrhea or intermittent rectal bleeding. Most of these complications resolve within one year of therapy. Urethral stricture is seen more frequently following multiple transurethral resections but occurs in less than 5% of patients. Potency is maintained in approximately 70% of patients who were potent prior to irradiation (Ray, Cassady, and Bagshaw 1973).

The addition of orchiectomy or estrogen therapy to irradiation has not been shown to be of benefit in any study (Perez et al. 1977) and should be reserved for patients with demonstrated metastases or recurrence. Patients with poorly differentiated tumors or ureteral obstruction have significantly poorer survival following irradiation (Harisiadis 1978). They might represent a subgroup of patients who should be included in future clinical trials of adjuvant chemotherapy.

The development of encapsulated sources of iodine 125 in 1965 prompted its use in the treatment of various solid tumors. The main advantage of this isotope over others is the low energy of its emitted gamma ray, thus allowing a great reduction in the dose of radiation to surrounding normal tissue. Since 1970, over 200 patients with adenocarcinoma of the prostate have been treated with iodine 125 at Memorial Sloan-Kettering Cancer Center in New York (Whitmore 1976). Patients eligible for this treatment have had stage B or limited stage C disease with moderately or well-differentiated histology. Following metastatic evaluation, bilateral extraperitoneal pelvic lymph node dissection is performed. If no obvious lymph node involvement is noted, hollow 17-gauge stainless steel needles are inserted retropubically into the prostate. These are then used to guide the insertion of iodine seeds in a geometrical pattern designed to encompass all of the known tumor. The insertion of approximately 20 mC results in a dose to the tumor of at least 8000 rad in two months and 16,000 rad in one year. Because of the low energy of this isotope, the dose to the remaining pelvic contents is very low (usually less than 2000 rad in one year). Complications have been minimal, and early survival calculations indicate an excellent rate of local control. This technique should still be considered experimental and limited to investigational use until further follow-up determines the long-term rates of morbidity and survival.

Other important uses of irradiation for prostatic carcinoma are the palliation of symptomatic osseous metastases and the prevention of painful gynecomastia in patients treated with estrogens. Doses of 3000 rad in two weeks to bone metastases offer a high rate of pain relief. Prior to the institution of estrogen therapy, 1500 rad to both breasts in two or three sessions will prevent symptomatic gynecomastia in the majority of patients. Similar treatment is ineffective once gynecomastia has developed.

Testis

Testicular tumors include some of the most satisfying and frustrating clinical situations seen in radiation oncology. The spectrum of histologic neoplasms extends from classical seminoma easily controlled by relatively low doses of radiation, to choriocarcinoma that frequently presents with disseminated disease. Probably the most important initial step in management of these tumors is adequate review of the histology by an experienced pathologist. From 15% to 20% of testicular tumors may be mixed cell types. Thus the entire testis and spermatic cord must be serially sectioned to determine the most malignant component. A mixed tumor containing seminoma and embryonal elements would be incorrectly treated, and with catastrophic results, if a diagnosis of pure seminoma were made on the basis of a few histologic sections.

Following diagnosis, the minimum clinical evaluation for a patient with a testicular tumor includes lymphangiography, intravenous pyelogram, chest x-ray with pulmonary tomography, and alpha-fetoprotein and beta subunit human chorionic gonadotropin (HCG) determinations. The lymphatic drainage of the testis is directly to the ipsilateral paraaortic lymph nodes in the middle and upper lumbar regions. A lymphangiogram is essential to: (1) determine the location of radiotherapy portals if the patient requires irradiation, (2) assess the adequacy of retroperitoneal lymphadenectomy if the patient requires surgery, and (3) measure the response to chemotherapy if the patient has disseminated disease. Conventional pulmonary tomography or computed tomography of the lungs is important to exclude small metastases that might be missed by a routine chest x-ray. Alpha-fetoprotein and HCG elevations are seen in the majority of patients with advanced nonseminomatous testicular tumors and may indicate an unsuspected mixed cell type or the presence of occult metastatic disease.

The clinical staging system commonly used in this country was developed at Walter Reed Army Medical Center (Maier and Mittemeyer 1977). Disease limited to the testis is classified as stage I, paraaortic or pelvic lymph node metastasis is stage II, and supradiaphragmatic or visceral metastasis is stage III. This simple system accurately predicts survival and allows the intelligent application of different therapeutic modalities.

Patients with stage I or stage II pure seminoma are treated with irradiation following inguinal orchiectomy. Patients with stage I disease should receive 2000 to 2500 rad to the paraaortic and ipsilateral pelvic lymph nodes. Such treatment without lymphadenectomy or chemotherapy results in five-year survival rates of 95% to 100%. Those with stage II tumors should receive doses of at least 3000 rad to the same regions with subsequent irradiation of the next most likely areas of lymphatic involvement—the mediastinal and supraclavicular lymph nodes. Five-year survival rates of 80% to 90% are reported for patients treated in this manner (Earle, Bagshaw, and Kaplan 1973; Maler and Sulak 1973). Anaplastic seminoma has been suggested by some authors to behave in a more aggressive manner, but a recent review of patients with this histology has demonstrated that its reponse to irradiation and prognosis are similar to the more commonly encountered classical seminoma (Percarpio et al. 1979). Patients with stage III seminoma should receive irradiation if their metastases can safely be encompassed by radiotherapy portals. Otherwise, combination chemotherapy is indicated. The treatment results of stage III seminoma vary greatly with selection of patients.

Few other topics in urologic oncology remain as controversial as the optimal treatment for patients with stages I and II nonseminomatous carcinoma of the testis.

Table 43.1. *Radiation Therapy (RT) of Urologic Malignancies*

Disease Site and Stage		*5-Year Disease-Free Survival (%)*	*Reference*
TESTIS:			
Seminoma	Stage I	95–100	Earle, Bagshaw, and Kaplan 1973; Maier and Sulak 1973
	Stage II	80–90	Earle, Bagshaw, and Kaplan 1973; Maier and Sulak 1973
Nonseminomatous carcinoma	Stage I (primary radiation)	70–90	Maier and Mittemeyer 1977; Peckham and McElwain 1974; van der Werf-Messing 1976
	Stage II (combined radiation and lymphadenectomy)	80	Maier and Mittemeyer 1977
PROSTATE:			
Stage A		85	Harisiadis 1978
Stage B		70	Harisiadis 1978; Perez et al. 1977; Ray, Cassady, and Bagshaw 1973
Stage C		40	Harisiadis 1978; Perez et al. 1977; Ray, Cassady, and Bagshaw 1973
BLADDER:			
Stage A		50–60	Caldwell et al. 1967; Frank 1970
Stage B1		40–50	Caldwell et al. 1967; Frank 1970
Stage B2 and C (primary RT)		15–30	Caldwell et al. 1967; Frank 1970; Miller 1977
Stage B2 and C (preop RT and cystectomy)		45–55	Miller 1977; van der Werf-Messing 1975

Surgery, radiotherapy, and chemotherapy in various combinations have been proposed by several authors. Because of the relative rarity of these tumors, very few controlled studies have been reported and most therapeutic proposals have been based on retrospective selected series.

To sterilize paraaortic micrometastases of nonseminomatous testicular tumors, doses of at least 4000 to 4500 rad are required (Maier and Lee 1977). Such treatment for stage I tumors has been reported by several European and American medical centers (Maier and Mittemeyer 1977; Peckham and McElwain 1974; van der Werf-Messing 1976). The five-year survival rates of 70% to 90% following orchiectomy and irradiation alone are comparable to those in most surgical series. Because of the ejaculatory, fertility, and gastrointestinal complications of lymphadenectomy, radical irradiation alone represents a sound therapeutic alternative with a low complication rate for the patient with stage I nonseminomatous testicular tumor and negative tumor markers (Percarpio et al. 1979).

The patient with a clinical stage II tumor represents a greater therapeutic dilemma. Lymphadenectomy alone has been recommended by some (Staubitz et al. 1973) but has numerous deficiencies. Although the procedure can frequently handle the large paraaortic masses of metastatic testicular cancer, it is inadequate to deal with residual microscopic disease left in the paraaortic region. As revealed by postsurgical x-rays, lymphadenectomy rarely results in the removal of all lymph nodes from the region. Following surgery alone, five-year survival averages only about 50%. Radiotherapy alone for stage II disease is also deficient. While effective for microscopic disease, irradiation is frequently unable to control large (greater than 2 cm) metastatic deposits in paraaortic lymph nodes. The doses necessary to increase the control rate of such metastases may surpass the tolerance levels of overlying small and large intestine. Average survival figures following radiation therapy alone have been poor.

The combination of lymphadenectomy to control large paraaortic metastases and irradiation to sterilize microscopic tumor cells not removed by surgery is attractive in theory. A randomized prospective trial at Walter Reed Army Medical Center from 1968 to 1973 compared radical irradiation to the combination of lymphadenectomy and irradiation for 91 patients with stages I and II nonseminomatous testicular cancer (Maier and Mittemeyer 1977). For those who received combined therapy, lymphadenectomy was preceeded by 3000 rad of irradiation to the paraaortic and pelvic lymph nodes. Following surgery, an additional 1500 rad were delivered to the same regions. The results revealed no significant survival difference between the treatment modalities for patients with stage I carcinoma. For stage II disease the results also seemed comparable; that is, 81% three-year disease-free survival for combined treatment and 82% for radiation. On analyzing the results, it was found that the randomization had not been strictly followed and several patients with more advanced disease, as evidenced by large metastatic deposits noted on lymphangiogram, had been entered on the combined treatment arm. Nonetheless, even with the selection seemingly biased against combined treatment, survival rates were similar. In any case, an 81% cure rate in stage II tumors represents a significant improvement over surgical and radiotherapeutic approaches used previously. Furthermore, when the treatment failures were studied, 5 of 11 patients had elements of choriocarcinoma in the original tumor or had persistent HCG elevation following orchiectomy. These two prognostic factors probably indicate the need for adjuvant combination chemotherapy in these patients.

National cooperative trials of the addition of chemotherapy to lymphadenectomy are currently at an early stage. Until these studies are completed, control rates in excess of 80% can be expected for stage II disease by the combination of irradiation and lymphadenectomy, with adjuvant chemotherapy added for those patients with elements of choriocarcinoma in the tumor or persistent HCG elevation following orchiectomy. At present, radiotherapy is only of benefit for patients with stage III cancer as palliation of symptomatic metastases.

Summary

Current results of radiation therapy of urologic cancer are summarized in table 43.1.

References

Bagshaw, M. A. et al. External beam radiation therapy of primary carcinoma of the prostate. *Cancer* 36:723–728, 1975.

Caldwell, W. L. Carcinoma of the urinary bladder. *JAMA* 229:1643–1645, 1974.

Caldwell, W. L. et al. Efficacy of linear accelerator x-ray therapy in cancer of the bladder. *J. Urol.* 97:294–303, 1967.

Cox, J. D., and Stoffel, T. J. The significance of needle biopsy after irradiation for stage C adenocarcinoma of the prostate. *Cancer* 40:156–160, 1977.

Earle, J. D.; Bagshaw, M. A.; and Kaplan, H. S. Supervoltage radiation therapy of the testicular tumors. *Am. J. Roentgenol.* 117:653–661, 1973.

Finney, R. An evaluation of postoperative radiotherapy in hypernephroma treatment—a clinical trial. *Cancer* 32:1332–1340, 1973.

Frank, H. G. Policy and results of treatment by radiotherapy of carcinoma of the bladder in Leeds. *Clin. Radiol.* 21:425–430, 1970.

Harisiadis, L. et al. Carcinoma of the prostate: treatment with external radiotherapy. *Cancer* 41:2131–2142, 1978.

Maier, J. G., and Lee, S. N. Radiation therapy for nonseminomatous germ cell testicular cancer in adults. *Urol. Clin. North Am.* 4:477–493, 1977.

Maier, J. G., and Mittemeyer, B. Carcinoma of the testis. *Cancer* 39:981–986, 1977.

Maier, J. G., and Sulak, M. H. Radiation therapy in malignant testis tumors. I. Seminoma. *Cancer* 32:1212–1216, 1973.

Miller, L. S. Bladder cancer. *Cancer* 39:973–980, 1977.

Peckham, M. J., and McElwain, T. J. Radiotherapy of testicular tumors. *Proc. R. Soc. Med.* 65:14–17, 1974.

Percarpio, B. et al. Anaplastic seminoma: an analysis of 77 patients. *Cancer* 43:2510–2513, 1979.

Perez, C. A. et al. Radiation therapy in the definitive treatment of localized carcinoma of the prostate. *Cancer* 40:1425–1433, 1977.

Ray, G. R. et al. Operative staging of apparently localized adenocarcinoma of the prostate: results in fifty unselected patients. *Cancer* 38:73–83, 1976.

Ray, G. R.; Cassady, J. R.; and Bagshaw, M. A. Definitive radiation therapy of carcinoma of the prostate. *Radiology* 106:407–418, 1973.

Riches, E. The place of irradiation. *JAMA* 204:230–231, 1968.

Staubitz, W. J. et al. Surgical treatment of nonseminomatous germinal testes tumors. *Cancer* 32:1206–1211, 1973.

van der Werf-Messing, B. H. P. Carcinoma of the kidney. *Cancer* 32:1056–1061, 1973.

van der Werf-Messing, B. H. P. Carcinoma of the bladder treated by preoperative irradiation followed by cystectomy. *Cancer* 36:718–722, 1975.

van der Werf-Messing, B. H. P. Radiotherapeutic treatment of testicular tumors. *Int. J. Radiat. Oncol. Biol. Phys.* 1:235–248, 1976.

Whitmore, W. F., Jr. et al. A comparative study of two preoperative radiation regimens with cystectomy for bladder cancer. *Cancer* 40:1077–1086, 1977.

Whitmore, W. F., Jr.; Hilaris, B.; and Grabstald, H. Retropubic implantation of I^{125} in the treatment of prostatic cancer. *J. Urol.* 109:918–920, 1972.

forty-four

Chemotherapy of Renal, Bladder, and Prostate Cancer

GERARD T. KENNEALEY

Renal Carcinoma

Renal cell carcinoma is an important cause of morbidity and mortality in this country, with 15,000 new cases each year, and 7000 deaths. It is more common in men than in women, with a ratio of approximately 1.5:1. The 10-year survival varies widely from series to series, but the range is between 20% and 30%. There has been a slight increase in five-year survival in the past few years, although the reason for this is not known. The sites most frequently involved by metastatic disease are lungs, bone, brain, and liver. Cure is a function of adequate surgical removal, tumor size, and invasion of perinephric tissues and the renal vein. No role for adjuvant systemic therapy has been established.

Treatment

Treatment of advanced renal cell carcinoma with chemotherapy has been very disappointing, with no consistent improvement in response rate or survival in the last three decades. Given the fact that this is a fairly common illness, the results of chemotherapy are perhaps the most dismal of those for any solid tumor. The mainstay of treatment has been hormonal manipulation. This has been used for over 15 years since it was first shown that estrogen-induced renal tumors of hamsters regressed when the animals were treated with testosterone or progesterone (Bloom 1973). Since that time, several workers have used derivatives of these hormones in human subjects with renal cell carcinoma and the response rates have been as high as 20%. These have all been small series. The overall response to hormonal manipulation is thought to be more in the range of 5% to 10%. Unfortunately, at this point very little else is effective in this disease. Thus most patients with advanced tumors are treated initially with progestational agents such as medroxyprogesterone (Provera) and megestrol (Megace), which fortunately have only minimal side effects. These include fluid retention, increased appetite, mild hypertension, and in men, impotence.

The usual chemotherapeutic agents have been disappointing in renal cell carcinoma. As with other tumors, combination chemotherapy has also been tried. Several small studies in the literature claim that combinations of a nitrosourea, such as lomustine (CCNU), with vinblastine (VBL) have some effect. One such chemotherapy program for advanced disease is as follows (Davis and Manale 1978):

> CCNU, 120 mg/m^2 p.o. day 1; and VBL, 0.1 mg/kg days 1 and 15 every 6 to 8 weeks.
> In 29 patients there were 2 CR, 5 PR, 7 no change (NC), and 15 disease progressions.

Progestational agents have not been shown to add to the efficacy of nonhormonal treatments such as vinblastine or semustine (methyl-CCNU) (Hahn et al. 1978) in which the response rate was 10% or less. The antiestrogen tamoxifen has similarly shown either no activity (Glick et al. 1980) or minimal activity (5%) (Al-Sarraf 1979). Methyl-glyoxal bis-guanylhydrazone (methyl-GAG) produced objective responses in 3 of 14 patients in one study (Knight et al. 1980) and 4 of 25 in another (Todd, Garnick, and Canellos 1980). Moderately high-dose methotrexate with citrovorum factor rescue, either alone or with other agents, resulted in responses in 4 of 15 patients (27%) (Baumgartner et al. 1980).

In summary, the treatment of metastatic renal cell carcinoma at this point is not very promising. Single-agent chemotherapy is essentially useless. Progesterone and probably testosterone are most likely harmless, but they are probably not particularly useful. The approach in the future should be controlled clinical trials of new agents and combinations.

Metastases

Not all patients with advanced renal cell carcinoma have a rapidly progressive downhill course. This disease can be extremely variable, and length of survival from the original nephrectomy or from the onset of metastatic disease can be quite lengthy. Many will have pulmonary metastases as their first sign of metastatic disease. If there is no evidence of disease outside the chest and the lung lesion can be encompassed surgically, then pulmonary resection is justified. The approach to these patients has been improved with the widespread availability of the computerized tomographic scan that allows one to look very carefully at the thorax. In addition to the commonly seen isolated pulmonary metastases, there is a rare patient with renal cell carcinoma who will have an isolated brain metastasis. If the metastatic focus is in the nondominant hemisphere or in the cerebellum and the patient is otherwise in good health, certainly a resection of the metastatic nodule should be considered. In summary, this illness is quite variable and it is often worthwhile to treat recurrences with an aggressive surgical approach.

Carcinoma of the Bladder

Carcinoma of the bladder is more common than renal carcinoma and fortunately is a tumor for which the therapeutic options are not as limited. There are 36,000 new cases annually in the United States, with 10,000 deaths. Basically, early tumors are treated with surgery and radiation, and at each stage of the disease it is controversial as to whether one or both modalities should be used.

Chemotherapy has a role at both ends of the disease spectrum. In early disease—stage 0 or stage A—intravesical chemotherapy has been used for a quarter of a century. The trifunctional alkylating agent triethylenethiophosphoramide (Thiotepa) is the standard agent. It is instilled directly into the bladder, usually in a dose of 60 to 90 mg, and left for several hours. Most urologists use it once or twice a week initially and then less and less often until it is used monthly. It is quite effective in patients with either low-grade tumors or early disease. Systemic side effects from intravesical administration are rare, and the regimen is well tolerated. More recently, other drugs have been used intravesically for the treatment of early stage bladder cancer. Mishina and colleagues (1975) instilled mitomycin into the bladders of 50 patients in the following schedule: 20 mg three times a week, for 20 courses. Seventy-six percent responded, with 22 (44%) patients having CR, 16 (32%) with PR, and 12 (24%) showing no response. Doxorubicin (Adriamycin), another antitumor antibiotic, has also been used intravesically with a similar response rate. More recently, Nakazono and Iwata (1978) injected doxorubicin directly into the bladder tumor through a 21-gauge needle passed through the cystoscope. They claimed that this treatment was effective when intravesical thiophosphoramide or doxorubicin had failed. While thiophosphoramide still remains the mainstay of intravesical chemotherapy, there is evidence that other drugs are effective in the treatment of this disease. Unfortunately, to date there has been no study comparing the efficacy of thiophosphoramide to mitomycin or doxorubicin. Hopefully, this will be done in the near future. Again, even with the antitumor antibiotics, systemic toxicity is rarely seen with intravesical administration.

Advanced stage D carcinoma of the bladder has historically been considered resistant to treatment with chemotherapy. Until recently it was viewed with the same pessimism with which we still approach treatment of advanced renal cell carcinoma. The advent of newer agents and more aggressive treatments in the 1970s is beginning to change this (de Kernion 1977). Table 44.1 represents a combination of several series of patients treated with standard chemotherapeutic agents for carcinoma of the bladder. The first three agents, methotrexate, 5-fluorouracil, and cyclophosphamide, have been used for over 20 years and these early studies show responses; however, duration of response in most of these studies has been extremely brief. The largest published experience with this disease is with doxorubicin (Yagoda 1980). The response rate is respectable and represents an advance in treatment. Mitomycin has been used with a response rate of 16% to 33% (de Kernion, Stewart, and Yagoda 1978). Early studies with cisplatin (Platinol) have shown that this too may be a useful drug (Merrin 1978; Yagoda 1980). Its advantage in patients with carcinoma of the bladder is that it does not cause bone marrow suppression. Since most patients have had

Table 44.1. *Response of Advanced Bladder Cancer to Systemic Chemotherapy*

Agent	*Number of Patients*	*Objective Response (%)*	
		Average	*Range*
Methotrexate	88	24	17–36
5-FU	56	39	0–75
Cyclophosphamide	41	41	0–53
Doxorubicin	235	23	0–37
Mitomycin	50	20	16–33
Cisplatin	42	40	

substantial pelvic radiation prior to chemotherapy, the availability of a nonmyelotoxic drug becomes very important. The myelotoxic drugs such as doxorubicin and cyclophosphamide must be given with substantial dosage reduction in patients who have received radiation therapy to the bone marrow in the pelvis; however, they can tolerate standard doses of cisplatin. For this reason it has been viewed with great enthusiasm in the treatment of a variety of advanced genitourinary tract malignancies.

As with most other tumors, combination chemotherapy has also been tried in patients with advanced carcinoma of the bladder. Williams and associates (1978) achieved 10 partial responses out of 17 patients treated with the following regimen: cisplatin, 50 to 75 mg/m^2; doxorubicin, 50 mg/m^2; and 5-fluorouracil, 500 mg/m^2, given in combination intravenously every three to four weeks. They combined three of the most effective agents in carcinoma of the bladder at fairly high doses. Toxicity was acceptable and the response rate was substantial. For advanced bladder cancer, Steinberg and co-workers (1977) of the M. D. Anderson Hospital used the following schedule: cyclophosphamide, 650 mg/m^2 on day 1; doxorubicin, 50 mg/m^2 on day 1; and cisplatin, 100 mg/m^2 on day 2, and a repeat course every 21 days. Ten patients responded out of 12 treated. At Memorial Sloan-Kettering Cancer Center, Yagoda (1977) combined cisplatin and cyclophosphamide for a 60% (12 of 20 patients) response rate (CR and PR). The dose of cisplatin in this study was high (1.6 mg/kg IV; and cyclophosphamide, 250 to 1000 mg/m^2 every three to four weeks) and the toxicity, as expected, was substantial, in many cases leading to discontinuation of treatment by patients even in the presence of a response. In a controlled clinical trial, the response rate for the combination of doxorubicin and cisplatin was higher (36%) than for doxorubicin alone (20%) (Gagliano 1980).

It now appears that we have several drugs that are effective either alone or in combination, in the treatment of advanced carcinoma of the bladder. Within the next few years we hope to see reports of combination chemotherapy that provide acceptable toxicity, increased response rates, and more importantly, increased quality and quantity of life as a result of treatment.

With the availability of moderately active drugs for advanced disease and the ability to identify patients at high risk for recurrence, it is natural to consider adjuvant chemotherapy. A typical group at risk would be patients with invasive tumors treated with preoperative irradiation, urinary diversion, and total cystectomy, but with residual involvement of paraaortic nodes. Controlled clinical trials are in progress but no definitive information is yet available.

Carcinoma of the Prostate

The most common genitourinary malignancy is carcinoma of the prostate (Catalona and Scott 1978). The annual incidence in the United States is approximately 65,000 with 21,000 deaths. The treatment of early stage disease is covered in chapters 42 and 43, and this discussion is confined to the treatment of stage D or metastatic carcinoma, which unfortunately is present in about 50% of patients at the time of diagnosis.

The initial treatment of stage D disease has not changed appreciably in almost 40 years. In 1941, Huggins and Hodges demonstrated that these patients often responded to orchiectomy. They noted that treatment with estrogens would also produce a response. Their basic discovery was that many prostatic cancers are hormonally dependent, that is, they will respond either to ablative or additive hormonal manipulation. The timing of initial hormonal manipulation, whether orchiectomy or estrogen treatment, continues to be controversial. On one side are those who feel that the presence of metastatic disease is an indication for treatment. On the other are those who believe that endocrine manipulation should be reserved until there is evidence of advancing or symptomatic disease such as anemia or bone pain.

The overall response rate to initial endocrine therapy is in the range of 80%. Most patients will experience subjective evidence of response with relief of bone pain, improvement in sense of well-being, weight gain, and relief of anorexia. Objective evidence is less common. A decrease in the serum acid phosphatase may occur, but this is not always an active reflection of tumor burden. Metastatic disease in lymph nodes and in the lungs will often shrink following endocrine manipulation. Bone metastases, the most common manifestation of advanced prostatic cancer, often do not change radiologically even when there is substantial subjective evidence of improvement. Ninety-five percent of the bone metastases from this disease are blastic and in most patients do not change either by bone scan or by x-ray. Improvement of anemia often does occur. The response is often rapid and there are many anecdotes that refer to patients with painful bone metastases who awaken pain-free following orchiectomy.

While there is no doubt that most patients with advanced carcinoma of the prostate will respond to initial hormonal manipulation, there is some question as to whether survival is improved. The largest study to address this question is the Veterans Administration Hospital study in the late 1960s that showed no increase in survival in patients treated with diethylstilbestrol compared to those who received no treatment (Bailar and Byar 1970). Most urologists and oncologists, however, feel that endocrine manipulation will prolong useful life in the majority of patients. According to the literature there is little if any difference in the response rate between estrogen therapy or orchiectomy; most urologists will recommend castration if the patient will permit it and estrogen treatment if he will not. There is no evidence that castration followed by immediate institution of oral estrogen is more efficacious than treatment with either modality alone; in addition, patients who respond to one form of treatment and then relapse have only a small chance (10% or less) of responding to the other.

The most frequently used oral estrogen is diethylstilbestrol (DES). Fortunately, there does not appear to be a dose-response curve to this drug. The Veterans Administration study showed that there was no difference in response rate when patients were treated with 5 mg or 1 mg of DES. Those who received 5 mg daily had a very substantial increase in cardiovascular morbidity and mortality. Heart attacks, congestive failure, pulmonary edema, and claudication were seen more often in patients who received the higher dose. As a result of this study, most physicians use a dose of DES in the range of 1 to 3 mg daily, or an equivalent dose of another form of estrogen.

Our experience over the years with prostatic cancer and with another hormonally dependent tumor, carcinoma of the breast, is that when patients do respond to initial hormonal manipulation and then relapse, there is some likelihood that they will respond to further hormonal manipulation. The most common secondary therapy is diethylstilbestrol diphosphate (Stilphostrol), given intravenously daily for five days and then weekly or biweekly thereafter (Band et al. 1973). It has been our experience that substantial numbers of patients who have initially responded to other endocrine manipulations and then relapsed will respond to this drug. Patients who did not respond to initial endocrine manipulation are unlikely to respond to this agent.

Other forms of secondary hormonal manipulation that have been tried include adrenalectomy and hypophysectomy. The latter was tried extensively many years ago and then fell into disuse because of the substantial morbidity and mortality associated with the procedure. With recent perfection of surgical techniques there has been a revival of interest in this form of endocrine manipulation. Silverberg (1977) published the results of 17 patients who underwent hypophysectomy for advanced symptomatic metastatic disease. Seven had a subjective response, and an additional five had an objective response as well. The mean response duration in the former group was 3.8 months (range 1 to 6), while in the latter it was 11 months (range 5 to 20). As expected, patients with hepatic metastases and those who had not responded to previous endocrine manipulation did not respond to hypophysectomy. Unfortunately, at this point we cannot predict who will respond to hormonal manipulation and who will not. A search for androgen receptors in prostatic carcinoma has been beset by many technical difficulties, but it is hoped that in the 1980s we will be able to examine prostatic malignancy with an eye toward predicting the likelihood of response to hormonal manipulation, as we can do now with carcinoma of the breast.

Nonhormonal chemotherapy has always had a secondary role in carcinoma of the prostate, and appropriately so in a tumor that has such a high response rate to hormonal manipulation. Unfortunately, by the time many of these patients have failed conventional endocrine manipulation and are considered for chemotherapy, their functional status has deteriorated to the point where response to any form of treatment is unlikely. In many cases these patients are bedridden, racked with pain, uremic, and in need of catheter drainage. As must be expected, they do not respond well to chemotherapy.

Recently, however, patients with higher performance status have been treated with chemotherapy. The National Prostatic Cancer Project (NPCP) (Schmidt et al. 1980) has been instrumental in encouraging early chemotherapy trials. Attempts have been made by this group to standardize criteria for evaluation of therapy, including the category of disease stabilization. The first study, begun in July 1973, randomized patients to treatment with 5-fluorouracil, cyclophosphamide, or so-called standard therapy—that is, no chemotherapy. For the first time, chemotherapy was shown to have some advantage over observation alone (Johnson et al. 1977). The Eastern Cooperative Oncology Group published data comparing two agents that were thought to be effective in this disease—doxorubicin and 5-fluorouracil (DeWys and Begg 1978). Nine of 37 patients (24%) treated with doxorubicin, 60 mg/m^2 intravenously every 21 days, demonstrated objective response; 3 of 40 patients (8%) showed objective response when given 5-FU, 600 mg/m^2 intravenously every week. The response rate to doxorubicin was significant; with 5-fluorouracil it was low. It is important to note that these are objective response rates and do not include the substantial number of patients with subjective responses. Other agents that have been shown to be effective in careful studies, where only objective response rates were measured, include doxorubicin, hydroxyurea, cisplatin, lomustine (CCNU), dacarbazine (DTIC), and estramustine (Torti and Carter 1980).

With the excellent response rate to hormonal manipulation and the improved response rate to chemotherapy, the next logical step would be that patients with advanced disease should be treated with a combination of hormonal manipulation and chemotherapy. A pilot study of this combined modality treatment was carried out in Connecticut (Kennealey et al. 1978). Estramustine, a synthetic combination of nitrogen mustard and estradiol, was used as the hormonal manipulation. The original theory behind the synthesis of this drug was that the estrogen moiety would lead to increased uptake by the prostate, where the alkylating agent would be in close proximity to the malignant cells, a theory that has been recently questioned. This drug was combined with the antimetabolite 5-fluorouracil. Twenty-five patients were treated with estramustine, 14 mg/kg/day orally; plus 5-FU, 600 mg/m^2/week IV. Objective regression was demonstrated in 3 of the 25 patients (12%), and subjective regression in 8 (32%). The results are very similar to those reported with the use of estramustine alone, and it is unlikely that 5-fluorouracil contributed anything to this regimen. The approach of combining hormonal agent with chemotherapy is promising, however, and needs to be tested with agents that are more effective than 5-fluorouracil. The side effects from this experimental estrogen were well tolerated and were basically toxicities expected from standard estrogens, although less severe.

Summary

Secondary and primary endocrine manipulations are quite effective in the treatment of advanced carcinoma of the prostate. The newer chemotherapeutic agents such as doxorubicin and cisplatin appear to be useful alone. The combination of hormonal treatment and chemotherapeutic agents should be further evaluated, as should combinations of other chemotherapeutic agents.

References

Al-Sarraf, M. The clinical trial of tamoxifen in patients with advanced renal cell cancer. A Southwest Oncology Group study. *Proc. Am. Soc. Clin. Oncol.* 20:378, 1979.

Bailar, J. C., III, and Byar, D. P. Estrogen treatment for cancer of the prostate—early results with three doses of diethylstilbestrol and placebo. *Cancer* 26:257–261, 1970.

Band, P. R. et al. High-dose diethylstilbestrol diphosphate therapy of prostatic cancer after failure of standard doses of estrogens. *Can. Med. Assoc. J.* 109:697–699, 1973.

Baumgartner, G. et al. Methotrexate–citrovorum factor used alone and in combination chemotherapy for advanced hypernephromas. *Cancer Treat. Rep.* 64: 41–46, 1980.

Bloom, H. J. G. Hormone-induced and spontaneous regression of metastatic renal cancer. *Cancer* 32:1066–1071, 1973.

Catalona, W. J., and Scott, W. W. Carcinoma of the prostate: a review. *J. Urol.* 119:1–8, 1978.

Davis, T. E., and Manale, F. B. Combination chemotherapy of advanced renal cell cancer with CCNU and vinblastine. *Proc. Am. Soc. Clin. Oncol.* 19:316, 1978.

de Kernion, J. B. The chemotherapy of advanced bladder carcinoma. *Cancer Res.* 37:1771–1774, 1977.

de Kernion, J. B.; Stewart, B. H.; and Yagoda, A. Treatment of advanced bladder cancer. In *Genitourinary cancer,* eds. D. G. Skinner and J. B. de Kernion. Philadelphia: W. B. Saunders, 1978, pp. 284–294.

DeWys, W. D., and Begg, C. B. Comparison of Adriamycin and 5-fluorouracil in advanced prostatic cancer. *Proc. Am. Soc. Clin. Oncol.* 19:394, 1978.

Gagliano, R. Adriamycin versus Adriamycin plus cis-platinum in transitional cell bladder carcinoma. *Proc. Am. Soc. Clin. Oncol.* 21:347, 1980.

Glick, J. H. et al. Phase II study of tamoxifen in patients with advanced renal cell carcinoma. *Cancer Treat. Rep.* 64:343–344, 1980.

Hahn, R. G. et al. Phase II study of vinblastine, methyl-CCNU, and medroxyprogesterone in advanced renal cell cancer. *Cancer Treat. Rep.* 62:1093–1095, 1978.

Huggins, C., and Hodges, C. F. Studies on prostatic cancer. I. The effect of castration, of estrogen and androgen injection on serum phosphatase in metastatic carcinoma of the prostate. *Cancer Res.* 1:293–297, 1941.

Johnson, D. E. et al. National randomized study of chemotherapeutic agents in advanced prostatic carcinoma: a progress report. *Cancer Treat. Rep.* 61:317–323, 1977.

Kennealey, G. T. et al. Treatment of advanced carcinoma of the prostate with estramustine and 5-fluorouracil. *Proc. Am. Soc. Clin. Oncol.* 19:394, 1978.

Knight, W. A., III et al. Methyl-glyoxal bis-guanylhydrazone (methyl-GAG, MGBG) in advanced renal carcinoma. *Proc. Am. Soc. Clin. Oncol.* 21:367, 1980.

Merrin, C. Treatment of advanced bladder cancer with cis-diaminedichloroplatinum II (NSC 119875): a pilot study. *J. Urol.* 119:493–495, 1978.

Mishina, T. et al. Mitomycin C bladder instillation therapy for bladder tumors. *J. Urol.* 114:217–219, 1975.

Nakazono, M., and Iwata, S. A preliminary study of chemotherapeutic treatment for bladder tumors. *J. Urol.* 119:598–600, 1978.

Prout, G. R., Jr. Bladder carcinoma. *N. Engl. J. Med.* 287:86–90, 1972.

Schmidt, J. D. et al. Chemotherapy programs of the National Prostatic Cancer Project (NPCP). *Cancer* 45:1937–1946, 1980.

Silverberg, G. D. Hypophysectomy in the treatment of disseminated prostatic cancer. *Cancer* 39:1727–1731, 1977.

Steinberg, J. J. et al. Combination chemotherapy (CISCA) for advanced urinary tract carcinoma. *JAMA* 238:2282–2287, 1977.

Todd, R. F., III; Garnick, M. B.; and Canellos, G. P. Chemotherapy of advanced renal adenocarcinoma with methyl-glyoxal-bis-guanylhydrazone (methyl-GAG). *Proc. Am. Soc. Clin. Oncol.* 21:340, 1980.

Torti, F. M., and Carter, S. K. The chemotherapy of prostatic adenocarcinoma. *Ann. Intern. Med.* 92:681–689, 1980.

Williams, S. D. et al. Chemotherapy of bladder cancer with cis-diaminedichloroplatinum (DDP), Adriamycin (ADR) and 5-fluorouracil (5-FU). *Proc. Am. Soc. Clin. Oncol.* 19:316, 1978.

Yagoda, A. Future implications of phase II chemotherapy trials in ninety-five patients with measurable advanced bladder cancer. *Cancer Res.* 37:2775–2780, 1977.

Yagoda, A. Chemotherapy of metastatic bladder cancer. *Cancer* 45:1879–1888, 1980.

forty-five

Testicular Tumors

WILLIAM D. MEDINA
ED CADMAN

There has been dramatic progress in the management of testicular tumors in the last 10 years. Greatest strides have occurred in the detection of tumor markers and in the evolution of more effective combination chemotherapy. Sensitive assays for human chorionic gonadotropin and alpha-fetoprotein are now widely available. These tests have improved the accuracy of clinical staging and allow earlier detection of recurrent disease. Many investigators have shown that the majority of patients with advanced disease can now be cured with chemotherapy. The challenge facing physicians in the 1980s is to find optimal management of the patient with a testicular tumor. This will require the close cooperation of surgeons, radiation oncologists, and medical oncologists.

Epidemiology

The annual incidence of testicular tumors in the United States is 3.1 per 100,000 males. They account for 1% of all malignancies seen in males. (For comparison, Hodgkin's disease represents 1.3% of tumors in males.) These tumors have attained a notoriety disproportionate to their numbers because they occur most often in the prime of life—they are the most common malignancy in men between the ages of 20 and 34. Testicular neoplasms occur more than four times as frequently in whites as in blacks (Cutler and Young 1975).

The age distribution of testicular tumors shows three peaks—infancy, 20 to 40 years, and 70 to 80 years. The proportions of the various types of germ cell tumors vary with age. In infancy, the endodermal sinus tumor (yolk sac tumor, embryonal carcinoma, infantile type) is most common. In young adulthood, all types of tumors are seen. In old age, seminomas are most common (Mostofi 1973).

The number of testicular tumors has been slowly increasing over the past 20 years. This is due not only to demographic changes consisting of an increase in the number of men aged 20 to 35 but also to a significant and unexplained rise in the age-adjusted incidence rate. Data from the Connecticut Tumor Registry (Sullivan 1981) show a steady increase in the age-adjusted incidence rate per 100,000 males, from 2.78 in 1960–1964 to 3.71 in 1975–1979.

There are three principal risk factors for testicular tumors. First, cryptorchidism increases the risk tenfold to 14-fold. It is reported that an abdominal testis is more likely to become malignant than an inguinal testis. Orchiopexy does not protect against the development of a neoplasm. In a review of the literature, however, Martin (1979) found that of 97 well-documented cases of a tumor developing in a testis following orchiopexy, only 6 occurred if the procedure was performed before the age of 10 years, and none following orchiopexy before age 5. Second, patients who have had a tumor in one testis are more likely to develop a tumor in the remaining testis. Third, a person whose brother or father had a testicular tumor is more likely to have a tumor.

Pathology

In a review of over 7000 testicular tumors, Mostofi (1973) found that 94% were the germ cell variety, the remainder were chiefly Sertoli cell or Leydig cell tumors and lymphomas. For men over 50, however, lymphomas may comprise as many as 25% (Duncan et al. 1980). Only germ cell tumors are discussed in this chapter.

Unfortunately, there has not been general agreement on the classification of germ cell tumors (GCT). One system, proposed by Willis (1960) and later modified by Collins and Pugh (1964), is based on the theory that seminomas arise from germ cells but that all other testicular tumors arise from totipotential embryonic cells. They recognized three types of GCT: seminoma, spermatocytic seminoma, and teratoma. This classification has been popular in Britain but has never gained acceptance in the United States, and is not discussed further.

The other system of classification is based on the theory, now in the ascendancy, that all germ cell tumors arise from germ cells. These classifications place greater emphasis on different histologic patterns. This theory was the basis for the first comprehensive classification of GCT proposed in 1946 by Friedman and Moore. They recognized four so-called pure tumor patterns—seminoma, embryonal cell carcinoma, choriocarcinoma, and teratoma—and a number of mixed patterns all of which were lumped under the term teratocarcinoma. (A word of caution: teratocarcinoma as used by most authors today refers to the specific combination of teratoma and embryonal carcinoma.) Dixon and Moore (1952) accepted these histologic patterns, but divided the tumors into five groups based on survival data.

In the past 10 years several modifications of the Friedman and Moore classification have been proposed (Mostofi 1973, 1980; Mostofi and Sobin 1976; Hajdu and Hajdu 1976) that seek a more precise delineation of histologic differences among GCT. It should be emphasized that the different schemes are in accord for the vast majority of GCT. They all accept the same four single histologic patterns described by Friedman and Moore and agree that many GCT (40%) have mixed patterns. Disagreement concerns whether several uncommon variants of the pure types should themselves be considered pure types. These variants include a subtype of seminoma—spermatocytic seminoma, and two subtypes of embryonal carcinoma—yolk sac tumor and polyembryoma. All of the classifications also require a description of the patterns seen in a mixed tumor. (The pathologic characteristics of GCT are discussed briefly; for a more detailed discussion the reader is referred to the above references.)

Seminomas are the single most common type of GCT, comprising 40% to 48% of the group. The majority are diagnosed between the ages of 30 and 50 years; they are seen very rarely before puberty, and 2% are bilateral (Smith 1978). The testis is enlarged in 85% of cases, usually diffusely. Three histologic patterns have been described: typical, anaplastic, and spermatocytic (Mostofi 1973). Typical seminoma is the pattern seen in over 85% of cases. Anaplastic seminoma contains more than three mitoses per high-power field and comprises 10% of seminomas. Despite its more malignant appearance, anaplastic seminoma is felt to have the same natural history and response to treatment as typical seminoma (Percarpio et al. 1979). Spermatocytic seminoma, on the other hand, has a different natural history (Smith 1978; Talerman 1980). Seventy percent of the cases occur beyond age 50 years and there have been no documented instances of metastasis.

Embryonal carcinomas comprise 15% to 20% of all GCT. The majority are diagnosed between the ages of 20 and 40 years. They tend to be somewhat smaller than seminomas, with an average diameter of 5 to 6 cm. Three histologic patterns have been described for this tumor also: adult, infantile, and polyembryoma. The adult pattern makes up nearly all the embryonal carcinomas seen beyond infancy. The infantile type (yolk sac and endodermal sinus tumors) is the most common testicular tumor of infancy, remains localized to the testis for long periods of time, and if it metastasizes, tends to do so through the blood stream, resulting in pulmonary metastases without regional nodal involvement (Exelby 1980). Pure yolk sac tumor is seen very rarely in adults; when it occurs it is usually in association with teratocarcinoma (Mostofi 1973). Polyembryoma is a rare variant of yolk sac tumor about which little has been written.

Teratomas constitute 7% to 10% of the GCT and are seen most frequently in the first three decades of life. They are comprised of mesodermal, endodermal, and ectodermal elements. The testis is usually enlarged. All teratomas should be considered malignant even if their histology appears benign.

Choriocarcinomas comprise only 1% of GCT. Most pure choriocarcinomas are seen between the ages of 15 and 30 years. The testis is usually small or of normal size; as a result, the presenting manifestation is often related to a metastasis. Both the primary lesion and metastases have a remarkable propensity for hemorrhage.

The remainder of GCT are composed of mixtures of the various pure types. The single most common combination is teratoma and embryonal carcinoma (24% of all GCT). Most are mixtures of two types, a few contain elements of three.

The GCT are peculiar in that metastases may have a histologic pattern different from that of the primary. In a few cases a pure pattern will transform to another pure pattern. Much more commonly, a mixed GCT will give rise to metastases with different proportions of tumor elements.

Lymphatic dissemination is the most common route of spread. The retroperitoneal lymph nodes are both the initial and most common sites of metastasis. In addition, since over half the patients with involvement of these nodes are cured by lymphadenectomy (Whitmore 1979), it can be concluded that the retroperitoneal nodes are often the only sites of metastasis. According to Ray, Hajdu, and Whitmore (1974) 29% of those found to have involvement of this area at surgery have only a single positive node. Left testicular tumors most frequently involve the paraaortic and preaortic nodes near the junction of the left testicular vein and the left renal vein. This is at the level of L1 to L2. Right testicular tumors most frequently involve the paracaval and interaortocaval nodes near the junction of the right testicular vein and the inferior vena cava. This is at the level of L1 to L3 (Watson 1979).

After the retroperitoneal nodes, the next most common site of involvement is the lung. This is especially true for the nonseminomatous GCT. Of 963 patients with germ cell tumors of the testis seen at Memorial Sloan-Kettering Cancer Center from 1949 to 1974, 163 had distant metastasis at initial diagnosis. In 85% of these patients the lungs were the only sites of metastasis (Batata et al. 1980). In the same series, one-third of the patients with distant metastases had no clinical or radiographic evidence of nodal involvement. Choriocarcinomas are the exception to the rule of primary lymphatic spread; hematologic dissemination occurs early and may in fact be the principal route of spread (Mostofi 1973; Fraley, Lange, and Kennedy 1979).

In an autopsy study of 78 patients who died with GCT, Johnson and colleagues (1976) found that approximately 90% had lung metastases, 80% had positive retroperitoneal lymph nodes, 70% had hepatic metastases, and 65% had tumor in the mediastinal nodes. In addition, 25% to 30% had involvement of the brain, kidney, and gastrointestinal tract. In 80% of the patients, death could be attributed to organ failure. The organs involved were lung, brain, liver, and gastrointestinal tract (in that order). Thirteen percent died of hemorrhage, and 7% died of sepsis.

The GCTs are often divided into seminomatous and nonseminomatous tumors (NSGCT). Although distinctions have been blurred somewhat by the development of more effective radiotherapy and chemotherapy, the dichotomy still has useful prognostic and therapeutic implications. The overall five-year survival for seminomas is 83% and for the NSGCT 44%. Survival falls to less than 25% if choriocarcinomatous elements are present (Smith 1978; Maier and Sulak 1973; Batata and Unal 1979). Nearly all of the patients in these series were treated before 1970. With the therapeutic advances of the past decade, current survival rates should be approximately 90% for seminomas and 80% for NSGCT. Radiation therapy is the principal treatment modality for seminomas; surgery and chemotherapy play much more important roles in the management of NSGCT.

Clinical Manifestations

The most common symptom is enlargement of the testicle. Although this may take the form of a discrete nodule, diffuse enlargement of the entire testicle is seen in 50% to 75% of patients. This enlargement is usually painless; however, since pain is described by 18% to 47% of patients its presence by no means should exclude the diagnosis of a testicular tumor. Some patients may complain of a heavy sensation in the scrotum without actual enlargement of the testis (MacKay and Sellers 1966; Borski 1973; Sandeman 1979).

With more advanced disease involving the retroperitoneal nodes, ureters, or inferior vena cava, patients may complain of flank or low back pain, radiculopathy, edema of the lower extremities, or symptoms of obstructive uropathy. Pulmonary metastases may cause cough, dyspnea, or chest pain. Brain metastases cause neurologic symptoms.

A careful examination of the scrotum will reveal either diffuse or nodular enlargement in 75% to 90% of patients with GCT. Occasionally, a difference in weight of the two testes can be detected by the examiner even if the testes are of equal size. In addition to testicular tumors, the differential diagnosis of scrotal masses includes orchitis, hydrocele, spermatocele, varicocele, hematocele, and torsion. Orchitis is nearly always painful, the testis is quite tender, and the patient often will have pyuria. If it is elected to give a course of antibiotics and prompt resolution does not occur, a urologic consultation should be obtained. The presence of a hydrocele can be confirmed by transillumination, but it should be recalled that testicular tumors can also occur in patients with hydroceles. Therefore even if transillumination is observed, if the mass is of recent origin the patient should be referred to a urologist for further examination.

During physical examination, particular attention should be paid to the lungs, supraclavicular regions (5% to 10% of patients will have a positive left supraclavicular node), breasts (5% of patients will have gynecomastia), abdomen (enlarged retroperitoneal nodes may be palpable and the liver should be measured). One-quarter of patients with seminoma and nearly two-thirds of those with NSGCT have either nodal involvement or more distant metastases at the time of diagnosis (Maier and Sulak 1973; Batata and Unal 1979; Smith 1978). Half of the nonseminomatous metastases consist only of microscopic retroperitoneal nodal involvement (Maier and Sulak 1973).

Regrettably, there is often a delay of six or more months from initial symptoms to diagnosis. Fortunately, two studies (MacKay and Sellers 1966; Sandeman 1979) have shown that the delay does not correlate with stage of the disease.

Tumor Markers

The two most important markers for GCT are human chorionic gonadotropin (HCG) and alpha-fetoprotein (AFP).

The name HCG was coined in 1928 by Ascheim and Zondek, who devised a bioassay to detect its presence in the urine. In 1930, Zondek reported the presence of HCG in the urine of a man with a testicular tumor. It is a glycoprotein with a molecular weight of about 45,000 (Waldmann 1979). It is normally secreted by the placenta during pregnancy. It is composed of two subunits designated α and β. The smaller subunit is identical to the α subunit of the glycoprotein hormones of the pituitary—luteinizing (LH), follicle-stimulating (FSH), and thyroid-stimulating (TSH). Antibodies directed against HCG or α-HCG cross-react with these hormones. It was not until 1972, when Vaitukaitis, Braunstein, and Ross reported the development of a sensitive radioimmunoassay for detection of the β subunit, that low concentrations of HCG could be measured and distinguished from LH, FSH, and TSH. Levels are normally less than 1 ng/ml.

The presence of AFP was first described in humans in 1956 by Bergstrand and Czar. Abelev (1970) was the first to report its presence in a man with a testicular tumor. It is also a glycoprotein with a molecular weight of about 70,000. It is normally present in high concentrations in the fetus but by the time of birth has fallen to levels of around 50,000 ng/ml (Catalona 1979). Waldmann and McIntire (1974) developed a sensitive radioimmunoassay and showed that normal levels are less than 40 ng/ml.

Catalona (1979) reviewed the results of 11 series and found that of patients with NSGCT, 65% had an elevated AFP, 63% an elevated HCG, and 84% had an elevation of either AFP or HCG or both. These data are nearly identical to those in the single largest series reported by Javadpour (1980a). He found that 100% of choriocarcinomas produced HCG, that 88% of embryonal carinomas produced HCG or AFP or both, but that only 44% of teratomas produced one of these markers. In addition, three of four yolk sac tumors were associated with elevated levels of AFP (one also produced HCG).

Unfortunately, these markers are not as helpful for seminomas. The estimated incidence of elevated HCG ranges from 7% to 17% (Catalona 1979; Javadpour 1980a; Lange et al. 1980). An elevated HCG in a patient believed to have a pure seminoma should prompt a search for nonseminomatous elements that may be present in either the primary tumor or metastases. It is now accepted that a small number of pure seminomas contain syncytiotrophoblastic cells that produce HCG. An elevated level of AFP essentially rules out a diagnosis of pure seminoma. There has been only a single case reported in the literature (Javadpour 1980b) of a patient with a pure seminoma and an elevated AFP. Here the AFP was thought to be related to regeneration of the liver surrounding a hepatic metastasis. (Even in this case, the hepatic metastasis was examined by only a needle biopsy, so nonseminomatous elements could not be completely excluded.)

The biologic half-lives of these markers must be taken into consideration following resection of tumor. They are: AFP, 5 days; HCG, 12 to 24 hours; α-HCG, 20 minutes; β-HCG, 60 minutes. The short half-life of α-HCG makes it of potential value in localizing a tumor by selective venous catheterization (Javadpour 1980a).

HCG and AFP are not specific for germ cell tumors. Vaitukaitis (1975) states that over 20% of patients with pancreatic and gastric carcinoma, and lesser numbers of patients with other tumors may have elevated HCG. The AFP (Catalona 1979) may be elevated in association with hepatomas and other gastrointestinal neoplasms as well as hepatitis and regenerating hepatic necrosis; however, these conditions are rarely part of differential diagnosis.

In a number of patients with widespread disease, lactic dehydrogenase (LDH) is elevated. This can be helpful in following the response to treatment particularly in patients with seminoma who usually have normal levels of HCG and AFP.

The principal uses of these markers are detection of residual disease after orchiectomy following a response to chemotherapy or radiation therapy, and early detection of recurrent disease. Since the markers are made by different types of cells, and since the proportion of tumor patterns within a mixed germ cell tumor can change, levels of HCG and AFP will not necessarily parallel one another. Therefore both markers should be measured. It should be emphasized that they are only additional tools to be used in close follow-up of these patients, and that there is a significant false negative rate. To turn around what was stated previously, 15% of patients with NSGCT do not have an elevated HCG or AFP. This should be considered a minimum estimate. The error is probably greater in patients with microscopic nodal involvement. In a group of 10 patients with clinical stage I disease and normal marker levels, 7 had pathologic stage II disease (Fraley et al. 1980). Scardino and co-workers (1977), in a small group of patients with recurrent disease, found that 33% had normal marker levels.

Evaluation and Staging

The cornerstone of evaluation (and management) of all testicular tumors is inguinal orchiectomy. A testicular mass in a young man is a tumor until proved otherwise. A biopsy of the mass should never be done. The tumor may be missed and violation of the tunica albuginea increases the likelihood and changes the pattern of tumor dissemination.

Once the diagnosis has been established blood tests should include the routine studies (including LDH) plus HCG and AFP. (Although they play no role in the decision to perform an orchiectomy, it would be helpful to know the level of these markers prior to operation.) A chest roentgenogram should be obtained. Several authors recommend chest tomography because it will reveal metastases not seen on the plain chest film in 10% to 15% of patients with pulmonary involvement (Fraley et al. 1980). Computerized axial tomography will reveal even smaller lesions, but it may be difficult to distinguish metastases from benign lesions.

The retroperitoneal lymph nodes have traditionally been evaluated using bipedal lymphangiograms. These tests have a false negative rate of around 25% in most series, however, and a false positive rate of 12% to 22% (Fraley et al. 1980; Smith 1978). In addition, they sometimes cause inflammation that makes subsequent lymphadenectomy more difficult. The majority of patients with NSGCT will undergo node dissection regardless of the results of the lymphangiogram; thus this test is no longer part of the evaluation in many centers. It is still widely accepted in the staging of seminomas, most of which are treated not by lymphadenectomy but with radiation. Computed tomography and ultrasonography are being used more widely to evaluate retroperitoneal lymph nodes. Studies by Hutschenreiter, Aiken, and Schneider (1979) and Williams and co-workers (1980a) on a total of 50 patients found that ultrasonography was 82% accurate. For 32 patients who underwent computed tomography, the accuracy was 87%.

Intravenous pyelography is usually performed prior to surgery, although it is not as sensitive as the other radiographic studies.

Paterson, Peckham, and McReady (1976) observed positive gallium scans in 13 of 15 patients with widespread seminoma. They are of little value in NSGCT. Brain, bone, or liver and spleen scans should not be obtained unless metastases to those areas are suspected.

Routine left supraclavicular node biopsy has been advocated by some authors, but the yield is so low and treatment so infrequently changed that it is no longer recommended (Donohue et al. 1977; Fowler, McLead, and Stutzman 1979; Lynch and Richie 1980).

The traditional staging system for testicular tumors has been:

Stage I — tumor confined to the scrotum
Stage II — tumor involving the retroperitoneal lymph nodes
Stage III — tumor beyond the retroperitoneal lymph nodes

This system had definite therapeutic and prognostic value. Most patients with stage I or II disease underwent surgery and/or radiation therapy, and those with stage III disease received chemotherapy. Table 45.1 shows the percentage of patients with seminomas and NSGCT in each stage at the time of diagnosis, and five-year survival by stage. The majority of patients with seminoma were staged clinically; the majority with NSGCT were staged surgically. As stated before, current survival rates are much higher.

A good staging system should reflect the natural history of the disease and distinguish categories of disease that require different forms of treatment. As our understanding of a tumor improves, staging should evolve to take new knowledge into consideration. In addition, new forms of treatment may cut across traditional stages and require their revision. This is nowhere more true than in testicular germ cell tumors.

Although this evolution of the staging system is healthy and even a cause for enthusiasm since it reflects dramatic improvements in the management of these tumors, it is nonetheless a source of confusion for both the specialist and the nonspecialist. This is especially true because there is no consensus over how the stages should be modified. A partial review of the literature of the last few years reveals at least seven proposed systems.

There is agreement that stage II needs to be subdivided to distinguish microscopic or minimal disease

Table 45.1. *Distribution and Five-Year Survival of Patients with Testicular Tumors by Stage*

Stage	% Patients at Presentation*		% 5-Year Survival†	
	Seminoma	NSGCT	Seminoma	NSGCT
I	75	36	93	77
II	20	38	69	37
III	5	26	22	9

SOURCE: Maier and Sulak 1973; Batata and Unal 1979; Smith 1978.

* Data from 2346 patients with seminoma reported in 26 series (Smith 1978) and 1162 patients with NSGCT seen at Walter Reed General Hospital and Memorial Sloan-Kettering Cancer Center (Maier and Sulak 1973; Batata and Unal 1979).

† All patients in these series were diagnosed and treated prior to 1974.

from bulky disease, since patients with bulky disease clearly have the worst prognosis (Tyrrell and Peckham 1976; Maier and Sulak 1973; Doornbos, Hussey, and Johnson 1975; Quivey et al. 1977; Einhorn 1979; Smith 1978; DeWys 1979; Vugrin et al. 1979; Lange et al. 1980). There is disagreement over what the subdivisions should be. Some authors have suggested that the number of nodes and whether involvement is microscopic or gross be used to separate divisions. A difficulty in using the number of nodes to divide substages is that the number obtained during a retroperitoneal node dissection varies widely among surgeons. Others have advocated using lymph node size as the criterion. All agree that bulky disease (usually not defined) should be placed in a separate category. Several believe that serum markers should be part of the staging system (Javadpour 1980a; Fraley, Lange, and Kennedy 1979).

None of the proposals is clearly better than the others. In the experience of each investigator the system used has been of prognostic value. As more knowledge is gained, evolution will continue. The burden will be on the reader to know which system an author is using.

The staging system about which the greatest amount of information is known is the tumor-node-metastasis (TNM) classification proposed by the American Joint Committee for Cancer Staging and End-Results Reporting in 1977 (table 45.2). Batata and co-workers (1980) reviewed the records of 963 patients with germ cell tumors treated at Memorial Sloan-Kettering Cancer Center from 1949–1974 and retrospectively staged them using this method. They correlated the stages with five-year survival (table 45.3).

They found that the T stage did not correlate with either recurrence or survival. The data indicated that the few patients (22) with involvement of a single retroperitoneal lymph node did just as well as those without nodal involvement. Patients with microscopic nodal disease had a survival rate between that of patients with no disease and patients with gross nodal involvement. (Similar results were seen by Maier and Sulak in 1973.) Survival of patients with juxtaregional node involvement was comparable to that of patients with positive regional nodes. Patients with positive mediastinal or supraclavicular nodes and those with abdominal disease palpable on physical examination had the same five-year survival as patients with distant metastases—10%.

Two points should be made. Ideally, it should be stated whether stage assignment was clinical or surgical. Second, survival figures given in this report do not reflect the improvements in combination chemotherapy made since 1974.

Management

Everyone agrees that the initial management of testicular tumors consists of an inguinal orchiectomy. That having been done, consensus is more difficult to find. The area of greatest controversy is the proper management of patients with regional (stage II) disease. Specifically, with combination chemotherapy capable of curing over 60% of the patients with advanced disease, what is the role of chemotherapy for patients with nodal disease whose survival rates have ranged from 10% to 80%? This question has not yet been answered, but guidelines are beginning to emerge. We will consider first the treatment of seminomas, then that of NSGCT.

Seminomas

Because of their sensitivity to radiation, radiotherapy is the mainstay of treatment for seminomas. Patients with local disease (stage I) should receive 2500 rad in three weeks to the ipsilateral inguinal-iliac and bilateral paraaortic-caval nodes as high as the crura of the diaphragm. This should be curative in over 95% of pa-

Table 45.2. *TNM Classification of Testicular Cancer*

T—Primary Tumor	*N—Regional or Juxtaregional Lymph Nodes*	*M—Distant Metastases*
T0 – no evidence of primary tumor	N0 – no evidence of nodal involvement	M0 – no distant metastases
T1 – tumor limited to testis	N1 – microscopic or gross involvement of a single node	M1 – distant metastases
T2 – tumor extending beyond tunica albuginea	N2 – involvement of multiple retroperitoneal nodes, microscopic or gross	
T3 – tumor involving rete testis or epididymis	N3 – palpable abdominal mass	
T4 – tumor involving spermatic cord or scrotum	N4 – juxtaregional (pelvic, inguinal, mediastinal, supraclavicular) nodes involved	

SOURCE: American Joint Committee for Cancer Staging and End-Results Reporting 1977.

Table 45.3. *Five-Year Survival According to NM Classification in Testicular Germ Cell Tumors*

Extent	*Seminoma (%)*	*Nonseminomatous Germ Cell Tumors (%)*	
Local			
N0M0	88	76	
Regional*	64	36	
N1			82
N2			
microscopic			57
gross			28
N3			11
Juxtaregional			
N4	53	30†	
Distant			
M1	27	11	
Total	(243/304)80	(295/659)45	

SOURCE: Batata et al. 1980.

* Too few patients with seminoma underwent retroperitoneal lymph node dissection to allow comparison of N substages.

† Survival was 42% for pelvic or inguinal node involvement (14 of 33) and 10% for mediastinal or supraclavicular node involvement (2 of 20).

tients. (As many as 75% of the patients would be cured with orchiectomy alone, but these results are so excellent and the morbidity so low that any recommendation to discontinue radiation is unlikely.)

Patients with minimal (certainly microscopic, probably nodes smaller than 2 cm) regional (stage II) disease are also satisfactorily treated with radiation. It should be administered to the same areas as in patients with local disease, with an additional 1000 rad to areas of known nodal disease. In addition, the mediastinal and supraclavicular nodes should receive 2500 rad over three weeks. Although data for minimal disease are hard to come by (most series do not distinguish minimal and extensive stage II disease), this treatment should be curative in 80% to 90% of patients (Tyrrell and Peckham 1976; Doornbos et al. 1975).

The management of bulky (again, usually not defined) retroperitoneal disease is in a state of flux. Doornbos and associates (1975) believe that bulky disease can be adequately treated by whole abdominal radiation followed by the same treatment used for minimal regional disease. This has not been the experience of others (Smith, de Kernion, and Skinner 1979; Lange et al. 1980), who found the five-year survival of these patients to be below 50%. They believe chemotherapy should be a part of management. The approach used by Smith and colleagues (1979) was to give dactinomycin, vincristine, and cyclophosphamide two to four weeks before conventional radiation therapy. Eight weeks after the completion of radiotherapy patients are started on chlorambucil and dactinomycin, which is continued intermittently for two years. Since beginning this regimen, five of five patients have been free of disease with a minimum follow-up of 18 months. Lange and co-workers (1980) recommend lymphadenectomy followed by chemotherapy for patients with bulky disease or with an elevated HCG after orchiectomy. They have no results at this time. Another approach would be to treat these patients as though they had NSGCT. Optimal management is not yet known. Physicians who have patients with bulky abdominal disease are encouraged to enter these patients into trials designed to answer this question.

Patients with distant metastases should be managed in a fashion similar to those with metastatic NSGCT. If a patient with seminoma who receives irradiation has persistent disease or develops recurrent disease, a search for nonseminomatous elements should be made, including a review of the histology of the primary tumor as well as repeat determinations of β-HCG and AFP. If nonseminomatous elements are discovered, and perhaps even if they are not, the patient should receive combination chemotherapy.

Nonseminomatous Germ Cell Tumors

Orchiectomy alone would be sufficient treatment for one-third of patients with stage I NSGCT, but our inability to identify this subgroup requires adjuvant therapy for all patients who clinically have local disease. In the United States this treatment has traditionally been bilateral retroperitoneal lymph node dissection, and in England it is radiation therapy. Both methods are successful about 87% of the time. The chief morbidity of the lymphadenectomy is aspermia secondary to loss of sympathetic innervation to the seminal vesicles and ejaculatory ducts. Fewer than 10% of the patients irradiated (4000 to 4500 rad in four to five weeks) will have complications including enteritis and intestinal stricture formation. A poorly defined number will have diminished bone marrow reserve. For a discussion of the type of operation and relative benefits, the reader is referred to several excellent articles (Whitmore 1979; Glatstein 1979; Fraley, Lange, and Kennedy 1979). A factor in the decision between surgery and radiation is whether the results of the lymphadenectomy would change subsequent treatment. In other words, one reason for a dissection would be the use of adjuvant chemotherapy if nodes were positive.

Regional (stage II) disease has traditionally been treated by either retroperitoneal node dissection or irradiation. Cure rates for both ranged from 45% to 80%, with an average of 60%. Patients with bulky disease were sometimes treated with both modalities, and their poorer response did not appear in the statistics of either treatment alone. Combined therapy was found to offer no advantage. Failure was usually due to distant metastases. Evidence accumulated that bulky abdominal disease did much more poorly. Therefore, treatment for minimal and extensive disease should be considered separately.

Tyrrell and Peckham (1976) found that 85% of patients with nodes smaller than 2 cm could be cured by radiation, whereas only 33% of patients with greater disease survived. Batata and co-workers (1980) observed that 67% of patients with N_1 or N_2 microscopic disease were free of disease at five years, but only 25% of patients with N_2 or N_3 disease were alive at five years. Assuming that 70% of patients with minimal regional disease can be cured with lymphadenectomy or radiation, and that 60% of those who relapse can be salvaged by chemotherapy, it should be possible to cure nearly 90% of this group and expose only 30% to the morbidity of chemotherapy. Data from Williams, Einhorn, and Donohue (1980) suggest that the salvage rate may be in excess of 85% when recurrences are detected early.

Survival of patients with extensive disease is so poor that chemotherapy should be used as part of their initial management. This modality could replace, or be used prior to or after surgery. The only published report of preoperative chemotherapy is that of Donohue, Einhorn, and Williams (1980). Twenty-six patients with bulky stage II or III disease were given four cycles of vinblastine, bleomycin, and cisplatin (VBP) and then underwent retroperitoneal lymph node dissection. Twenty-one of these patients had no evidence of disease with a minimum follow-up of one year. These authors believe that chemotherapy should be the initial treatment of patients with bulky disease. If there is no evidence of residual disease after four cycles of VBP they recommend that lymphadenectomy not be done, and carry out monthly check-ups including markers. If residual disease is present it should be resected. In the experience of these investigators, one-third of the patients have only fibrosis, one-third have benign teratoma, and one-third have persistent tumor. Patients with persistent tumor have all relapsed, and this subset should probably receive additional postoperative chemotherapy.

Skinner and Scardino (1980) reported the results of a study of 35 patients with stage II disease who received both preoperative and postoperative chemotherapy. Patients with minimal disease received dactinomycin before and for two years after surgery. Patients with bulky disease received a seven-drug combination including vinblastine and bleomycin before surgery and vinblastine, bleomycin, and dactinomycin afterward. At a minimum follow-up of one year, 88% had no evidence of disease. Despite this result, these authors are now using three cycles of vinblastine, bleomycin, and cisplatin as preoperative treatment of bulky disease.

The most extensive adjuvant data were reported by Vugrin and colleagues (1979). In a nonrandomized study, patients with stage II disease (stage determined at surgery) received chemotherapy after complete resection of tumor. Thirty-three patients with minimal disease (five or fewer positive nodes, all smaller than 2 cm, and negative markers) were treated with "mini-VAB" (vinblastine, dactinomycin, bleomycin, and chlorambucil). All 33 had no evidence of disease at a median follow-up of longer than 19 months. Of 29 patients with more extensive disease treated with the same regimen, only 19 were free of disease at over 25 months. A similar group of 22 patients with extensive disease was treated with full doses of VAB III (vinblastine, dactinomycin, bleomycin, cyclophosphamide, cisplatin, and chlorambucil). At a median follow-up of more than 10 months there were no relapses. Their conclusion was that for patients with extensive regional disease, intensive adjuvant chemotherapy was necessary to prevent recurrence.

Thus chemotherapy clearly has a role in the management of regional disease. More patients will need to take part in studies before that role can be sharply defined. A randomized intergroup trial is now in progress studying the use of modified versions of VBP and VAB IV as adjuvant therapy (Carter 1979; DeWys et al. 1979). A reasonable approach for patients with microscopic disease in only a few nodes who do not participate in trials would be watchful waiting (monthly physical examinations, chest roentgenograms, and marker levels). For patients with more extensive disease, either preoperative chemotherapy with VBP followed by resection of residual disease (if any), or postoperative adjuvant chemotherapy with VAB III or IV or VBP would be acceptable.

Finally, patients with seminomas or nonseminomatous germ cell tumors and distant metastases require chemotherapy. The two most widely used induction regimens are VBP and VAB III or IV. The former (Einhorn and Donohue 1977, 1979; Einhorn 1979) consists of vinblastine, bleomycin, and cisplatin given for 12 weeks, followed by maintenance vinblastine every four weeks for 2 years. (Recently this has been modified by omitting the maintenance vinblastine.) Including a small number of patients who had residual disease resected after induction chemotherapy, the complete response rate is about 70%. Most of these patients have been free of disease for over three years and are presumably cured. The principal morbidity of the regimen is myelosuppression. Nausea and vomiting may also be severe. (We have had some success in lessening this by slowing the cisplatin infusion and by using droperidol as an antiemetic.) Hydration is very important to prevent nephrotoxicity. This has the virtue of being a simpler regimen than VAB III or VAB IV. The VAB (Golbey, Reynolds, and Vugrin 1979) regimens were developed at Memorial Sloan-Kettering Cancer Center (see chapter 29). Both are seven-drug regimens that include cyclophosphamide, vinblastine, dactinomycin, bleomycin, cisplatin, doxorubicin, and chlorambucil. The VAB IV has a more intensive reinduction phase. Like VBP, they both have a two-year maintenance phase. The prolonged CR rate for VAB III is 45%, for VAB IV 60%.

It is not clear that maintenance chemotherapy is necessary. Bosl and co-workers (1980) reported on 28 patients treated with VBP for four to six cycles followed by one year of maintenance vinblastine. Their results were just as good as with the usual VBP regimen. Sturgeon and colleagues (1980) reported on 37 patients treated with cyclophosphamide, vinblastine, dactinomycin, bleomycin, and cisplatin. Thirty-one entered complete remission and were given no maintenance therapy at all. At a median follow-up of 14 months, only one had relapsed. Finally, Vugrin and colleagues (1981) have reported very good results with the newest VAB regimen, VAB VI, a five-drug program (doxorubicin and chlorambucil deleted from earlier regimens) in which chemotherapy is given for only one year. Twenty-one of 25 patients remain in complete remission with a median follow-up of 16 months. An additional feature of VAB VI is the resection of residual disease after the first three cycles of chemotherapy.

Patients refractory to VBP have not fared well. Fortunately, the epipodophylotoxin etoposide (VP-16-213) has activity against germ cell tumors. Williams and associates (1980b) recently reported that of 30 refractory patients treated with etoposide, cisplatin, and doxorubicin or bleomycin or both, 12 are free of disease at 16 to 32 months.

References

Abelev, G. I. Alpha-fetoprotein in ontogenesis and its association with malignant tumors. *Adv. Cancer Res.* 14:295–358, 1970.

American Joint Committee for Cancer Staging and End-Results Reporting. *Manual for staging of cancer.* Chicago: American Joint Committee, 1977.

Ascheim, S., and Zondek, B. Die Schwangerschaftsdiagnose aus dem Harn durch nachweis des hypophysenvorderlappen Hormons. *Klin. Wochenschr.* 7:1404–1441, 1928.

Batata, M. A. et al. TNM staging of testis cancer. *Int. J. Radiat. Oncol. Biol. Phys.* 6:291–295, 1980.

Batata, M. A., and Unal, A. The role of radiation therapy in relation to stage and histology of testicular cancer. *Semin. Oncol.* 6:69–73, 1979.

Bergstrand, C. G., and Czar, B. Demonstration of a new protein fraction in serum from the human fetus. *Scand. J. Clin. Lab. Invest.* 8:174, 1956.

Borski, A. A. Diagnosis, staging, and natural history of testicular tumors. *Cancer* 32:1202–1205, 1973.

Bosl, G. J. et al. Vinblastine, bleomycin, and cis-diamminedichloroplatinum in the treatment of advanced testicular carcinoma. *Am. J. Med.* 68:492–496, 1980.

Carter, S. K. A perspective on adjuvant chemotherapy of testicular cancer. *J. Cancer Res. Clin. Oncol.* 95:1–9, 1979.

Catalona, W. J. Tumor markers in testicular cancer. *Urol. Clin. North Am.* 6:613–638, 1979.

Collins, D. J., and Pugh, R. C. B. *Pathology of testicular tumors.* Edinburgh and London: E. S. Livingstone, 1964.

Cutler, S. J., and Young, J. L., Jr., eds. *Third national cancer survey: incidence data.* Bethesda, Md.: National Cancer Institute, 1975.

DeWys, W. D. Basis for adjuvant chemotherapy for stage II testicular cancer. *Cancer Treat. Rep.* 63:1693–1695, 1979.

DeWys, W. D. et al. Chemotherapy for advanced germinal cell neoplasms: preliminary report of an ECOG study. *Cancer Treat. Rep.* 63:1675–1680, 1979.

Dixon, F. J., and Moore, R. A. Tumors of the male sex organs. In *Atlas of tumor pathology.* Washington, D.C.: Armed Forces Institute of Pathology, 1952, pp. 48–103.

Donohue, J. P.; Einhorn, L. H.; and Williams, S. D. Cytoreductive surgery for metastatic testis cancer: considerations of timing and extent. *J. Urol.* 123:876–880, 1980.

Donohue, R. E. et al. Supraclavicular node biopsy in testicular tumors. *Urology* 9:546–549, 1977.

Doornbos, J. F.; Hussey, D. H.; and Johnson, D. E. Radiotherapy for pure seminoma of the testis. *Radiology* 116:401–404, 1975.

Duncan, P. R. et al. Extranodal non-Hodgkin's lymphoma presenting in the testicle. *Cancer* 45:1578–1584, 1980.

Einhorn, L. H. Combination chemotherapy with cis-dichlorodiammineplatinum (II) in disseminated testicular cancer. *Cancer Treat. Rep.* 63:1659–1662, 1979.

Einhorn, L. H., and Donohue, J. P. Cis-diamminedichloroplatinum, vinblastine, and bleomycin, combination chemotherapy in disseminated testicular cancer. *Ann. Intern. Med.* 87:293–298, 1977.

Einhorn, L. H., and Donohue, J. P. Combination chemotherapy in disseminated testicular cancer: the Indiana University experience. *Semin. Oncol.* 6:87–93, 1979.

Exelby, P. R. Testicular cancer in children. *Cancer* 45:1803–1809, 1980.

Fowler, J. E., Jr.; McLead, D. G.; and Stutzman, R. E. Critical appraisal of routine supraclavicular lymph node biopsy in staging of testicular tumors. *Urology* 14:230–232, 1979.

Fraley, E. E. et al. Staging of early nonseminomatous germ cell testicular cancer. *Cancer* 45:1762–1767, 1980.

Fraley, E. E.; Lange, P. H.; and Kennedy, B. J. Germ cell testicular cancer in adults. *N. Engl. J. Med.* 301:1370–1377; 1420–1426, 1979.

Friedman, N. B., and Moore, R. A. Tumors of the testis: a report on 922 cases. *Mil. Surgeon* 99:573–593, 1946.

Glatstein, E. Radiotherapy in the management of nonseminomatous testicular carcinomas. *Cancer Treat. Rep.* 63:1649–1651, 1979.

Golbey, R. B.; Reynolds, T. F.; and Vugrin, D. Chemotherapy of metastatic germ cell tumors. *Semin. Oncol.* 6:82–86, 1979.

Hajdu, S. I., and Hajdu, E. O. *Cytopathology of sarcomas and other nonepithelial malignant tumors.* Philadelphia: W. B. Saunders, 1976.

Hutschenreiter, G.; Aiken, P.; and Schneider, H. M. The value of sonography and lymphography in the detection of retroperitoneal metastases in testicular tumors. *J. Urol.* 122:766–769, 1979.

Javadpour, N. The role of biologic tumor markers in testicular cancer. *Cancer* 45:1755–1761, 1980a.

Javadpour, N. Significance of elevated serum alpha-fetoprotein (AFP) in seminoma. *Cancer* 45:2166–2168, 1980b.

Johnson, D. E. et al. Metastases from testicular carcinoma. *Urology* 8:234–239, 1976.

Lange, P. H. et al. Serum alpha-fetoprotein and human chorionic gonadotropin in patients with seminoma. *J. Urol.* 124:472–478, 1980.

Lynch, D. F., Jr., and Richie, J. P. Supraclavicular node biopsy in staging testis tumors. *J. Urol.* 123:39–40, 1980.

MacKay, E. N., and Sellers, A. H. A statistical review of malignant testicular tumors based on the experience of the Ontario Cancer Foundation Clinics, 1938–1961. *Can. Med. Assoc. J.* 94:889–899, 1966.

Maier, J. G., and Sulak, M. H. Radiation therapy in malignant testis tumors. *Cancer* 32:1212–1226, 1973.

Martin, D. C. Germinal cell tumors of the testis after orchiopexy. *J. Urol.* 121:422–424, 1979.

Mostofi, F. K. Testicular tumors: epidemiologic, etiologic, and pathologic features. *Cancer* 32:1186–1201, 1973.

Mostofi, F. K. Pathology of germ cell tumors of testis. A progress report. *Cancer* 45:1735–1754, 1980.

Mostofi, F. K., and Sobin, L. H. *Histological typing of testicular tumors.* Geneva: World Health Organization, 1976.

Paterson, A. H. G.; Peckham, M. J.; and McReady, V. R. Value of gallium scanning in seminoma of the testis. *Br. Med. J.* 1:1118–1121, 1976.

Percarpio, B. et al. Anaplastic seminoma. *Cancer* 43:2510–2513, 1979.

Quivey, J. M. et al. Malignant tumors of the testis: analysis of treatment results and sites and causes of failure. *Cancer* 39:1247–1253, 1977.

Ray, B.; Hajdu, S. I.; and Whitmore, W. F. Distribution of retroperitoneal lymph node metastasis in testicular germinal tumors. *Cancer* 33:340–348, 1974.

Sandeman, T. F. Symptoms and early management of germinal tumours of the testis. *Med. J. Aust.* 2:281–284, 1979.

Scardino, P. T. et al. The value of serum tumor markers in the staging and prognosis of germ cell tumors of the testis. *J. Urol.* 118:994–999, 1977.

Skinner, D. G., and Scardino, P. T. Relevance of biochemical tumor markers and lymphadenectomy in management of non-seminomatous testis tumors: current perspective. *J. Urol.* 123:378–382, 1980.

Smith, R. B. Management of testicular seminoma. In *Genitourinary cancer,* eds. D. G. Skinner and J. B. De Kernion. Philadelphia: W. B. Saunders, 1978, pp. 460–469.

Smith, R. B.; De Kernion, J. B.; and Skinner, D. G. Management of advanced testicular seminoma. *J. Urol.* 121:429–431, 1979.

Sturgeon, J. F. G. et al. Advanced non-seminomatous testicular tumors: maintenance chemotherapy is unnecessary. *Proc. Am. Assoc. Cancer Res.* 21:153, 1980.

Sullivan, P. Connecticut Tumor Registry, personal communication, 1981.

Talerman, A. Spermatocytic seminoma. *Cancer* 45:2169–2176, 1980.

Tyrrell, C. J., and Peckham, M. J. The response of lymph node metastases of testicular teratoma. *Br. J. Urol.* 48:363–370, 1976.

Vaitukaitis, J. L. Chorionic gonadotropin and its subunits. Placental proteins and their subunits as tumor markers. *Ann. Intern. Med.* 82:71–83, 1975.

Vaitukaitis, J. L.; Braunstein, G. D.; and Ross, G. T. A radioimmunoassay which specifically measures human chorionic gonadotropin in the presence of human luteinizing hormone. *Am. J. Obstet. Gynecol.* 113:751–758, 1972.

Vugrin, D. et al. Adjuvant chemotherapy in resected non-seminomatous germ cell tumors of testis: stages I and II. *Semin. Oncol.* 6:94–98, 1979.

Vugrin, D. et al. Combination chemotherapy in disseminated cancer of the testis. *Ann. Intern. Med.* 95:59–61, 1981.

Waldmann, T. A. Tumor markers in the diagnosis and management of patients with testicular germ cell neoplasms. Testicular germ cell neoplasms: recent advances in diagnosis and therapy. *Ann. Intern. Med.* 90:373–385, 1979.

Waldmann, T. A., and McIntire, K. R. The use of a radioimmunoassay for alpha-fetoprotein in the diagnosis of malignancy. *Cancer* 34:1510–1515, 1974.

Watson, R. C. Lymphography of testicular carcinoma. *Semin. Oncol.* 6:31–36, 1979.

Whitmore, W. F., Jr. Surgical treatment of adult germinal testis tumors. *Semin. Oncol.* 6:55–68, 1979.

Williams, S. D. et al. Abdominal staging of testicular tumors using ultrasonography and computed tomography. *J. Urol.* 123:872–875, 1980a.

Williams, S. D. et al. VP-16-213 salvage therapy for refractory germinal neoplasms. *Cancer* 46:2154–2158, 1980b.

Williams, S. D.; Einhorn, L. H.; and Donohue, J. P. High cure rate of stage I or II testicular cancer with or without adjuvant therapy. *Proc. Am. Assoc. Cancer Res.* 21:421, 1980.

Willis, R. A. *Pathology of tumors,* 3rd edition. London: Butterworth, 1960.

Zondek, B. Versuch einer biologischen (hormonalen) Diagnostik beim malignen Holdentumor. *Chirurg.* 2:1072–1073, 1930.

forty-six

Endometrial Cancer

ERNEST I. KOHORN

Epidemiology

There is a reported epidemic of endometrial cancer associated with the administration of estrogen to perimenopausal women. Great controversy rages whether this estrogen causes the carcinoma.

That endometrial hyperplasia, anaplasia, and eventual carcinoma are associated with prolonged exposure to estrogen has been known for many years. Association with anovulation, Stein-Leventhal syndrome, and granulosa cell tumor of the ovary bears witness to this phenomenon. In the 1960s and early 1970s it was fashionable to maintain women on fairly high doses of estrogen for prolonged periods of time in spite of the warnings that the medication for menopausal symptoms should be cut to the minimum. A minimal dose suffices to control not only vasomotor symptoms but vulvar and vaginal atrophy. Studies from King's College, London (Whitehead and Campbell 1978) have demonstrated that Premarin, 1.25 mg, may induce hyperplasia in women with a previously normal endometrial biopsy. There is no statistically increased incidence of hyperplasia in women given 0.625 mg. The incidence of hyperplasia was diminished if progestogens were given concomitantly with the increased amount of Premarin. The dose of progesterone given with estrogen needs to be adequate. Sequential oral contraceptive ("Pill") medication has also been associated with the development of endometrial carcinoma in some patients with anovulation.

Numerous statistical analyses have placed the risk factor for endometrial carcinoma following administration of estrogen at three to seven times that of controls (Hoogerland et al. 1978; Horowitz and Feinstein 1978). Only one study (Gambrell 1978) quarrels with the statistics but unfortunately this argument has gained no support. Although we must accept that there is a risk factor from estrogen therapy, only rarely does endometrial cancer associated with estrogen therapy cause metastases and death. It is likely that fractures of the hip and complications from osteoporosis carry a higher mortality than endometrial carcinoma. A good many physicians deny women low-dose estrogen for fear that endometrial cancer may develop. Yet they have no good alternative for symptoms that are miserable and physically debilitating. Probably the woman herself should be allowed to make the decision whether or not to take estrogen and thus take the risk of developing endometrial hyperplasia and carcinoma. It is the responsibility of the physician and gynecologist to make sure that she receives the lowest dose of medication for the shortest possible time to control her symptoms and to prevent irremediable vaginal stenosis or osteoporosis. On occasion it may even be justified to perform hysterectomy to permit estrogen administration. There is at present no evidence that estrogen increases the risk of breast carcinoma (Gambrell 1978).

There are two cohorts of patients with endometrial carcinoma. The first is the younger obese woman who gives a history of anovulation or Stein-Leventhal syndrome for many years, and who usually develops a well-differentiated tumor localized to the uterus and easily treated by hysterectomy. The second cohort is the older patient, frequently childless, but quite often with a normal menstrual history, who after the menopause develops endometrial carcinoma. It is remarkable that these older patients tend to have a histologically more poorly differentiated, and therefore frequently a higher stage of tumor. The administration of estrogen for menopausal symptoms increases the risk of endometrial cancer in the perimenopausal woman otherwise not at risk, over that of the anovular obese woman of the first cohort.

Diagnosis

The cardinal symptom of endometrial carcinoma is perimenopausal or postmenopausal bleeding. Any abnormal bleeding in this age group must be investigated. Intermenstrual bleeding in a younger woman who has been anovular should be investigated by endometrial biopsy, as even in that age group endometrial carcinoma is not as rare as was once thought. In most patients a diagnosis can be established satisfactorily by outpatient endometrial sampling using a small curette. This is better that 90% accurate, far more than endometrial washing, brushing, or vaginal cytology, procedures that are significantly less sensitive. In only a few women will inpatient diagnostic curettage under anesthesia be necessary.

It is well known that obesity, diabetes, and hypertension or other vascular problems are common in patients with endometrial cancer. In spite of this, surgery remains the mainstay of therapy, as untreated patients usually die not from their medical problems but from their carcinoma. If hysterectomy is not possible at the time of diagnosis because of coexisting medical problems, the uterus should be removed as soon as the patient is well enough, to avoid later recurrence of unmanageable tumor.

Management

Surgery and Radiotherapy

Endometrial carcinoma has always been regarded as a "better" type of cancer to have. The clinical impression that most patients were cured is due to the fact that 70% of patients have stage I disease and 70% of these are grade 1. This impression is reflected in the report of therapy for endometrial carcinoma from Stockholm (Kottmeier 1979) that shows that the overall cure rate is 65%. These are the positive results; what about the 35% who do poorly? Neophytes of oncology, the gynecologic oncologists, deserve credit for defining the high-risk groups who do poorly (Creasman et al. 1976).

The most important risk factor in this disease is tumor grade. Well-differentiated tumors tend to invade the uterine musculature slowly, tend not to involve lymph nodes, and not to spread to the cervix frequently (Creasman et al. 1976). The incidence of lymph node involvement with stage I grade 1 disease that has not invaded the myometrium is 0.5%. As the tumor becomes more anaplastic it invades the uterine musculature more frequently and metastasizes to pelvic and paraaortic lymphatics. With a grade 3 carcinoma that invades the myometrium deeply, incidence of positive pelvic lymph nodes is 40% and of paraaortic involvement is 20%, which explains why patients with grade 3 tumors do poorly. This does not mean that all patients with endometrial carcinoma require lymph node dissection or radical hysterectomy. It does mean that the patient with a high-grade tumor and deep myometrial invasion requires more therapy than the patient with a stage I grade 1 tumor with no such invasion.

It has been known for many years that surgical removal of involved lymph nodes is rarely curative. Among one group, 9 of 15 patients with positive pelvic nodes survived, and all these had radiation therapy (Lewis, Stallworthy, and Cowdell 1970). Survival with positive nodes without radiation is rare and anecdotal. Patients with either myometrial invasion or those with grade 3, and possibly even grade 2, tumor require radiation to the node-bearing areas. If grade 3 histology coexists with myometrial invasion, radiation of the paraaortic nodes should be considered. Management planning is thus becoming much more complicated. It is the responsibility of the gynecologist making the primary diagnosis to stage and grade the tumor precisely so that treatment based on that information can be implemented.

The other risk factor, besides tumor grade and myometrial invasion, is cervical involvement. In most cases, spread to the cervix occurs through tissue spaces and lymphatics and is actually a sign of myometrial invasion rather than a risk factor in itself. It can be easily established by outpatient endocervical biopsy, and the procedure should be routine.

While endocervical biopsy is mandatory for staging, another useful investigation is hysterography. The radiologic pattern within the uterus may significantly correlate with the degree of myometrial invasion.

While these recent findings have led to more treatment for patients at risk, we can also say that patients with an early well-differentiated tumor may not require the radical radiation that was frequently previously offered. What is important is to obtain a precise assessment of the disease. Should all patients have some form of radiation therapy? We think the answer is yes, because treatment with vaginal radium has significantly reduced the incidence of vault recurrence from some 10% to 2%.

From all this information a treatment plan may be drawn up. Patients with well-differentiated early carcinoma of the endometrium in a small uterus may be treated with hysterectomy and postoperative vaginal radium. In other cases of stage I disease intrauterine radium is followed by immediate surgical removal of the uterus and exploration of the node-bearing areas. Precise pathologic information is thus obtained. External radiation therapy is added to the plan if myometrial invasion is found or if the tumor is poorly differentiated, or more particularly, if positive nodes are found.

It still needs to be shown that these new treatment philosophies will improve survival among the patients with more advanced disease and poorly differentiated tumors.

Systemic Therapy

Progestational agents have been known to be effective in metastatic endometrial carcinoma for more than two decades (Kohorn 1976). Why then, should they not be used as an alternative to surgery and irradiation with primary disease? High-dose progestational agents are effective only in the well-differentiated tumor and then only control disease in some 50% of these. With poorly differentiated tumors the response is 15%. These drugs should therefore be reserved for use in recurrent disease or metastases, both of which are better first treated with radiation or surgery.

There may be a place for primary progestational therapy in patients whose medical problems preclude surgical intervention. Uterine instillation produces tumor necrosis and conversion of neoplastic to normal endometrium. This technique may find a place as an alternative to intracavitary uterine radium therapy.

Progestational agents used with recurrent or metastatic endometrial carcinoma offer excellent therapy There is no toxicity even with high doses. A high loading dose is required and at least 3 gm of medroxyprogesterone (Depo-Provera or oral Provera) need to be given in the first two weeks of therapy. If megestrol is used, 160 mg should be given daily. Once a loading dose has been accomplished a full dose of gestagen should be continued for at least two years. The dose of oral Provera is 200 mg daily. Depo-Provera is given by two injections of 400 mg per week and the dose of megestrol is 160 mg daily. Lesser doses do not produce effective blood levels. Some progesterone therapy should be continued as long as response is maintained.

No data are presently available about the use of estrogens adjuvant to progesterone. The antiestrogen, tamoxifen, has been used and is reported to produce some response; perhaps it should be given with progesterone.

Measurement of estrogen and progesterone receptors in endometrial carcinoma has led to the hope of better means of predicting which patients would be sensitive to progestational therapy. Estrogen receptors are present in most endometrial carcinoma tissue while the presence of the progesterone receptor is related to histologic differentiation of the tumor (Pollow, Robel, and Vilko 1978). The well-differentiated tumor tends to have significantly higher levels of progesterone receptor than the poorly differentiated tumor (Pollow, Robel, and Vilko 1978; Kohorn 1980). Little is known at present about the induction of progesterone receptors with estrogen or with tamoxifen, but it does appear that progestogens diminish both estrogen and progesterone receptors. At the present time, unfortunately, knowledge of the amount of receptor gives no more useful information than tumor grade. Some well-differentiated tumors do not respond to progestational agents while some poorly differentiated tumors not exhibiting progesterone receptors do respond clinically to high-dose progestogens.

We need to continue our studies of receptors to learn more about the mechanism of action of steroid hormones in this disease. We need to study particularly the mechanism of translating the steroid hormone from the cytoplasm to the nucleus and in what manner estrogen and progesterone are dependent on each other in making the cells more sensitive to gestagens. The question also arises whether progesterone in fact de-differentiates the endometrial carcinoma cells to normal cells.

From a clinical point of view, however, the question is not whether progestational agents should be given; they should always be given because there is no toxicity and a response may be obtained. The question is whether cytotoxic chemotherapy should be given to patients with poorly differentiated tumors, taking into consideration that in these patients the response to progesterone is no better than 15%.

Unfortunately, there are no very effective drugs for use in metastatic endometrial carcinoma at the present time (Kohorn 1980). The most effective single one is doxorubicin (Adriamycin), which has an objective response rate of 34%. Because of cardiovascular toxicity this drug cannot be used in many patients. Cyclophosphamide, 5-fluorouracil, and methotrexate have a response rate of some 20%, equal to that of gestagens in poorly differentiated tumors. Good results have been reported with combinations of an alkylating agent with 5-fluorouracil and methotrexate, but in most of these trials a progestational agent was given as well. Trials by the Gynecologic Oncology Group and by various individual centers in the United States are now in progress. We need to wait for the results of these to determine the most efficacious combination.

Endometrial carcinoma is an endocrine-dependent disease with some potential for endocrine palliative therapy. The best hope for cure remains early diagnosis and individualized surgery with irradiation.

References

Creasman, W. T. et al. Adenocarcinoma of the endometrium: its metastatic lymph node potential. A preliminary report. *Gynecol. Oncol.* 4:239–243, 1976.

Gambrell, R. D., Jr. The role of hormones in endometrial cancer. *South. Med. J.* 71:1279–1286, 1978.

Hoogerland, D. L. et al. Estrogen use, risk of endometrial carcinoma. *Gynecol. Oncol.* 6:451–458, 1978.

Horowitz, R. I., and Feinstein, A. R. Alternative analytic methods for case control studies of estrogens and endometrial cancer. *N. Engl. J. Med.* 299:1089–1094, 1978.

Kohorn, E. I. Gestagens and endometrial cancer. *Gynecol. Oncol.* 4:398–411, 1976.

Kohorn, E. I. Hormonal and non-hormonal chemotherapy of endometrial carcinoma. In *Gynecology and obstetrics,* vol. 4, *Oncology,* ed. H. Buchsbaum. New York: Harper & Row, 1980.

Kottmeier, H. L. Annual report on the results of treatment in gynecologic cancer 1969–1972. *Radiumhemmet* S-104 01, p. 45, Stockholm, 1979.

Lewis, B. U.; Stallworthy, J. A.; and Cowdell, R. Adenocarcinoma of the body of the uterus. *J. Obstet. Gynecol. Br. Cwlth.* 77:343–348, 1970.

Morrow, C. P.; DiSaia, P. J.; and Townsend, D. E. Current management of endometrial carcinoma. *Obstet. Gynecol.* 42:399–406, 1973.

Pollow, K.; Robel, P.; and Vilko, R. Steroid receptors and the human endometrium. In *Hormonal biology of endometrial cancer,* eds. G. S. Richardson and D. I. Machaughlin. Geneva: UICC Technical Report, 1978.

Whitehead, H. L., and Campbell, S. Endometrial histology, uterine bleeding, and estrogen levels in menopausal women receiving estrogen therapy and estrogen-progesterone therapy. In *Endometrial cancer,* eds. M. G. Brush, R. J. B. King, and R. W. Taylor. London: Bailliere Tindall, 1978, p. 65.

forty-seven

Ovarian Cancer

PETER E. SCHWARTZ

Ovarian cancer is the second most common cancer of the female reproductive organs in the United States today, but has the highest mortality associated with the common reproductive organ malignancies. The American Cancer Society estimates that 18,000 new ovarian cancers will be diagnosed in the United States this year and over 11,000 patients will die of the disease (Silverberg 1981). It is estimated that 1 of every 70 women born in the United States today will develop ovarian cancer (Barber 1978). This chapter reviews current developments in its management.

Symptoms

Ovarian cancer generally causes vague, nonspecific symptoms including lower abdominal discomfort, progressive abdominal distention, and weight loss. It is unusual to find this disease associated with severe pain except for the relatively infrequently occurring nonepithelial cancers (Katz et al. 1981). In general, the risk of epithelial ovarian cancer increases as women reach age 35, and the peak incidence is reached at about age 70 years. The nonepithelial cancers of the ovary are infrequent, and most often occur in the second and third decades of life.

Unlike the other common cancers involving the female reproductive organs, ovarian cancer does not give early warning signals such as postmenopausal bleeding and is not readily diagnosed by a routine screening test such as the Pap smear. Multiple attempts to develop routine serum screening procedures have yet to establish a technique for early diagnosis. As a result, the differential diagnosis of pelvic masses includes functional ovarian cysts, congenital anomalies such as pelvic kidney and urachal cysts, inflammatory changes such as tubo-ovarian abscesses and diverticular disease, and changes associated with pregnancy including intrauterine gestations and ectopic pregnancies. It must also include neoplasms such as leiomyomas and carcinomas involving the sigmoid colon, cecum, fallopian tubes, and rare retroperitoneal tumors.

A patient with a pelvic mass should undergo diagnostic evaluation consistent with her history and physical findings. Ovarian cancer is extremely unusual in women under age 25 years, and elaborate diagnostic procedures for a pelvic mass that persists through menstrual periods and is greater than 10 cm in diameter are usually not necessary. In older women, however, the presence of a pelvic mass requires more extensive evaluation, including a chest x-ray to rule out widespread metastases, and intravenous pyelogram to eliminate the possibility of congenital anomalies of the kidneys, ureter, bladder, as well as obstruction or deviation of the ureters or infiltration of the bladder by a malignancy. A barium enema is appropriate to eliminate the possibility of carcinoma arising from within the large bowel itself, and to rule out the presence of diverticular disease that may present as a pelvic mass. If the patient has a history of prior carcinoma, before definitive therapy one must also include an upper gastrointestinal series, liver and spleen scan, and a bone scan.

Table 47.1. *FIGO Staging For Primary Carcinoma of the Ovary*

Stage	*Extent of Disease*
I	Growth limited to the ovaries
IA	Growth limited to one ovary; no ascites i No tumor on the external surface; capsule intact ii Tumor present on the external surface and/or capsule ruptured
IB	Growth limited to both ovaries; no ascites i No tumor on the external surface; capsule intact ii Tumor present on the external surface and/or capsule(s) ruptured
IC	Tumor either stage IA or stage IB, but with ascites* present or positive peritoneal washings
II	Growth involving one or both ovaries with pelvic extension
IIA	Extension and/or metastases to the uterus and/or tubes
IIB	Extension to other pelvic tissues
IIC	Tumor either stage IIA or stage IIB, but with ascites present or positive peritoneal washings
III	Growth involving one or both ovaries with intraperitoneal metastases outside the pelvis and/or positive retroperitoneal nodes. Tumor limited to the true pelvis with histologically proved malignant extension to small bowel or omentum
IV	Growth involving one or both ovaries with distant metastases. If pleural effusion is present there must be positive cytology to allot a case to stage IV. Parenchymal liver metastases equals stage IV
Special category	Unexplored cases that are thought to be ovarian carcinoma

SOURCE: American Joint Committee for Cancer Staging and End-Results Reporting 1978.

*Ascites is peritoneal effusion that in the opinion of the surgeon is pathologic and/or clearly exceeds normal amounts.

Recent developments in diagnostic radiology including gray-scale ultrasonography and computed tomography have resulted in direct assessment of the composition of pelvic masses (Schwartz and Weiner 1979). Unfortunately, when a mass is obviously present, the value of these examinations is frequently limited. However, in situations where the pelvic examination is equivocal (for example, in children who are unable to tolerate routine pelvic examinations, women who have had prior irradiation and have intense fibrosis of the abdominal wall, obese patients, and those with vaginal or anal stenosis precluding adequate bimanual examination) ultrasound and computed tomography may be extremely useful.

Once the decision has been made in favor of surgical exploration, staging is extremely important in determining subsequent therapy. The current International Federation of Gynecology and Obstetrics (FIGO) staging system for ovarian cancer is shown in table 47.1. It should be noted that stage I cancer is confined to the ovary with substaging for involvement of one or both ovaries, the presence of excrescences on the surface of the tumor, rupture of the tumor, and the presence of ascites. Stage II disease involves other pelvic organs with substaging for involvement of the reproductive organs as opposed to other pelvic organs and the presence of ascites. Stage III cancer has spread to the upper abdomen and stage IV represents distant spread, that is, beyond the abdominal cavity or involvement of parenchymal liver disease. Malignant pleural effusions are considered to be stage IV; however, the presence of pleural effusion without documented malignant cells is insufficient evidence for stage IV disease.

Ovarian cancer appears to spread by direct extension and by shedding cells into the peritoneal cavity. It would appear that implantation occurs on all the peritoneal surfaces, as the disease frequently involves the omentum, and preferentially involves the right diaphragm. Ovarian cancer does not routinely spread hematogenously, as the presence of parenchymal liver disease is quite unusual at the time of initial examination. Parenchymal liver disease in a patient with a pelvic mass should lead one to suspect that a nonovarian malignancy is present.

Epithelial Cancers of the Ovary

The common epithelial neoplasms represent approximately 50% of the benign tumors and 80% of malignancies of the ovary. These tumors appear to arise from the surface epithelium of the ovary, and result in serous, mucinous, endometrioid, clear cell, Brenner, and adenofibromatous tumors. Such neoplasms may be benign, in which case they are called cystomas or cystadenomas; they may be obviously malignant in which case they are referred to as carcinomas, but at times they may be of borderline malignant potential. It is important to be aware of the last category, as these tumors represent changes that are capable of spreading beyond the ovary and seeding onto peritoneal surfaces, but do not infiltrate the stroma of the ovary. The prognosis even for advanced stages of borderline malignant potential tumors is far better than that of the common epithelial cancers (Aure, Hoeg, and Kolsted 1971).

Principles of surgical management are (1) careful intraabdominal staging, which requires inspection and palpation of all peritoneal surfaces including the diaphragms and the retroperitoneal areas such as the paraaortic area; (2) aspiration for cytologic assessment of any fluid that may be present at the time of the initial surgery; and (3) removal whenever possible of all gross tumor. Failure to inspect the diaphragm properly, and to evaluate the entire large and small bowel and mesentery, paracolic spaces, pelvic peritoneum, retroperitoneum, and paraaortic areas can lead to misstaging and possibly to inadequate treatment.

Patients with stage I disease, that is, confined to the ovaries, should undergo a total abdominal hysterectomy and bilateral salpingo-oophorectomy. The only exception is when the stage I lesion is confined to one ovary and is of borderline malignant potential, and fertility is desired. Common epithelial cancers of the ovary are frequently bilateral, and when a frankly invasive cancer is present it is in the patient's best interest to have both ovaries removed at the initial operation. In addition to hysterectomy, patients with stage I cancer should undergo removal of the grossly normal omentum from the level of its attachment to the transverse colon. The reason for this is twofold: microscopic disease may be present in the omentum, and this may change staging and postoperative management. The omentum is the second most common site of residual cancer at second-look surgery following completion of adjuvant chemotherapy. Therefore removing it is of some therapeutic benefit. If the patient does not have ascites, irrigating the pelvic and paracolic spaces with normal saline and sending the irrigant for cytology and cell block will help in staging and demonstrate occult spread of microscopic disease. Recent reports have suggested that ovarian cancer may spread to the diaphragm and not be clinically obvious. A biopsy of the diaphragmatic peritoneum should be obtained after inspecting it for any irregularities.

When the cancer has spread beyond the ovary, as much bulk tumor as possible should be resected. The minimum goal in the presence of advanced disease is to remove both ovaries and the omentum. This is often inadequate to remove all cancer, however, and an aggressive attempt should be made to excise any seedings greater than 1 cm in diameter. Aggressive surgery requires meticulous postoperative treatment or its benefits will be lost.

Postoperative adjuvant therapy has generally been either radiation therapy or more recently, chemotherapy. If the former is chosen it must be administered to the whole abdomen. Various techniques are available. The open-field procedure results in the entire abdomen being irradiated at one time; this is generally taken to a maximum dosage of 2000 to 2500 rad followed by an additional 2000 rad to the pelvis. Dosages to the upper abdomen are determined by the radiation tolerance of the liver and the kidneys rather than by radiosensitivity of the tumor. It is quite clear that the field must include the entire diaphragm to treat the malignancy adequately.

In the past, management of ovarian cancer with postoperative radiation has resulted in five-year survivals of patients with stage I disease of approximately 70%. Those with stage II disease with all residual tumor removed have approximately a 55% five-year survival, but if any residual tumor is present it is approximately 20%. Patients with stage III disease without residual have about a 30% five-year survival, whereas with residual present five-year survival is generally between 5% and 8%. Stage IV cancers have been reported to have less than a 5% five-year survival (Aure, Hoeg, and Kolsted 1971). Recent data suggest that if one employs the moving-strip technique, irradiates the entire abdomen, does not use a liver shield, and makes every effort to be sure that the radiation field extends above the diaphragm, patients who have no residual tumor and have had the ovaries and uterus completely removed have a significantly increased five-year survival (Dembo et al. 1979).

Chemotherapy has been employed as adjuvant therapy in both early and advanced cancer. Data from a

Table 47.2. *Prospective Randomized Studies Comparing Radiation Therapy to Chemotherapy After Surgical Staging in Patients with Ovarian Cancer*

Institution	*Patient Selection*	*Treatment*	*Results*
M.D. Anderson Hospital	Stages I, II, limited stage III (residual tumor masses 2 cm)	Melphalan (12 cycles) versus whole abdominopelvic radiation 2600 to 2800 rad plus pelvic boost 2000 rad	No differences in disease-free overall survival at 6 years between two treatment groups
Gynecologic Oncology Group	Stage IA, IB	Observation versus melphalan (18 cycles) versus pelvic radiation 5000 rad	No differences in overall survival among three treatment groups
Princess Margaret Hospital	Stage IA	Observation versus pelvic radiation 4500 rad	No differences in disease-free or overall survival at 5 years between two treatment groups
	Stages IB, II, asymptomatic III	Pelvic radiation 4500 rad versus pelvic radiation 4500 rad plus chlorambucil (daily for 2 years) versus whole abdominal radiation 2250 rad plus pelvic boost 2250 rad	Significant survival advantage at 5 years for group receiving abdominopelvic radiation provided that initial total abdominal hysterectomy—bilateral salpingo-oophorectomy was surgically complete
Gynecologic Oncology Group	Stage III stratified by extent of residual disease	Melphalan (18 cycles) versus whole abdominal radiation plus pelvic boost versus radiation followed by melphalan versus melphalan followed by radiation	No differences in survival among four treatment groups

SOURCE: Modified from Katz et al. 1981.

prospective randomized study employing single-agent therapy suggests that the results with melphalan for stage I and stages II and III cancer without any residual tumor is not statistically different than the results with moving-strip irradiation to the whole abdomen with additional radiation to the pelvis (Smith, Rutledge, and Delclos 1975). Several randomized prospective studies comparing radiation therapy to chemotherapy are shown in table 47.2.

Recent advances in chemotherapy have demonstrated agents that are active when used alone in the management of advanced ovarian cancer. Some response rates are tabulated in table 47.3. It appears that they have an increased activity when used in combination, as illustrated in table 47.4. A prospective randomized study comparing melphalan, hexamethylmelamine, and 5-fluorouracil as single-agent therapy for advanced disease revealed that melphalan and hexamethylmelamine each have approximately a 30% objective response rate, that is, complete disappearance of tumor and control of effusions (complete response), or a reduction in volume of persisting tumor to less than half the initial diameters (partial response) for at least three months (Fisher and Young 1978). It was found that 5-fluorouracil was relatively inactive, with the objective response rate only 12%. A subsequent prospective study comparing melphalan, hexamethylmelamine, and doxorubicin as single agents to combination therapy with hexamethylmelamine plus cyclophosphamide established that doxorubicin is active as a single agent with the same response rate as the other two single agents, approximately 30% (Fisher and Young 1978). The most important finding, however, was that the response rate with hexamethylmelamine and cyclophosphamide in combination was approximately 50%, with two-thirds of the responses being complete.

Recent data have demonstrated that cisplatin is extremely active in advanced ovarian cancer as a single agent, and when combined with doxorubicin has enhanced activity over cisplatin alone (Bruckner et al. 1978). Studies at Yale—New Haven Hospital comparing doxorubicin in combination with cyclophosphamide to hexamethylmelamine in combination with cyclophosphamide have established an increased response rate for these combinations compared to single-agent therapy (table 47.5); that is, approximately 50% of objective response rates with combinations compared to 30% response rates with single agents (Schwartz, Lawrence,

Table 47.3. *Chemotherapy in Stages III and IV Ovarian Cancer in Both Untreated and Treated Patients*

Agent	Patients Treated (number)	Clinical Responses (number)	Response (%)
Melphalan	541	252	47
Cyclophosphamide (conventional dose)	335	144	43
Cyclophosphamide (high dose)	36	22	61
Chlorambucil	388	196	51
Triethylene thiophosphoramide	337	162	48
Mechlorethamine (nitrogen mustard)	99	31	31
Carmustine (BCNU)	34	2	6
Lomustine (CCNU)	74	14	19
Semustine (methyl-CCNU)	26	0	0
Cisplatin	237	73	31
Hexamethylmelamine	142	36	25
Doxorubicin (Adriamycin)	224	34	14
5-Fluorouracil	92	18	20
Methotrexate (conventional dose)	25	5	20
Methotrexate plus leucovorin rescue	27	5	18
6-Mercaptopurine	19	1	5
Vinblastine	10	2	20
Vincristine	22	0	0
Etoposide (VP-16-213)	38	2	5
Teniposide (VM-26)	16	0	0
Amsacrine (m-AMSA)	24	2	8
Dianhydrogalactitol	39	6	15

SOURCE: Modified from Katz et al. 1981.

and Katz 1981). It was also demonstrated that doxorubicin may be particularly active against poorly differentiated cancers. It appears that the most active combination available today is doxorubicin and cisplatin, and the addition of agents such as cyclophosphamide and hexamethylmelamine may enhance response rates in advanced disease. Some prospective randomized trials compared single agent to combinations (table 47.6). No results are currently available using doxorubicin and cisplatin in early-stage ovarian cancer, but if the results in advanced stages are confirmed in other trials, this combination may also be more active than single-agent therapy in controlling early disease.

Second-Look Surgery

When radiation therapy to the whole abdomen and pelvis is employed for managing ovarian cancer, the patient is treated over a short period of time with the maximum dose possible. Studies combining chemotherapy with radiation therapy have failed to demonstrate any benefit (Dembo et al. 1979). Once the patient has received whole abdominal irradiation with additional radiation to the pelvis, to reoperate on completion of this therapy is probably more hazardous than simply to follow her for clinical evidence of recurrent disease. When using chemotherapy, however, it is possible to

Table 47.4. *Prospective Randomized Trials of Combination Chemotherapy in Previously Untreated Patients with Stages III and IV Ovarian Cancer*

Institution	*Drug Regimen**	*Responders†* (%)	*Responders†* (number)	*Complete Responders* (%)	*Median Survival of All Patients* (mos)	*Comments*
Indiana	CPDD + DOX + CTX (PAC V)	88	(22/25)	44	23	No difference in response rates or survival but more negative
Roswell Park	CPDD + DOX + CTX (PAC I)	75	(24/31)	40	23	Second-look operations in PAC I group
Mt. Sinai	CPDD + DOX	70	(13/18)	30	19+	
	CPDD + DOX + CTX + HMM	80	(29/36)	40	19+	
Milan	CPDD + DOX + CTX	71	—	43	—	
	HMM + DOX + CTX	62	—	31	—	
Royal Marsden	CLB	25	(4/16)	0	—	Chlorambucil arm statistically inferior to other two treatments
	CLB + CPDD	59	(18/34)	32	—	
	CLB + CPDD + DOX	67	(16/24)	41	—	
Yale	CTX + HMM	44	(10/23)	26	14	No difference to response rates or survival
	CTX + DOX	50	(10/20)	20	16	
Gynelogic Oncology Group	Melphalan + HMM	52	(50/97)	27	—	No difference in response rates or survival
	CTX + DOX	49	(35/72)	23	—	
Southwest Oncology Group	CTX + DOX	36	(22/61)	—	13	Statistically better survival in chemo-immunotherapy group
	CTX + DOX + BCG	53	(30/57)	—	24	

SOURCE: Modified from Katz et al. 1981.

*CPDD = cis-diamminedichloroplatinum; DOX = doxorubicin; CTX = cyclophosphamide; HMM = hexamethylmelamine; CLB = chlorambucil; BCG = bacillus Calmette-Guérin.

†Percentage of responders and, in parentheses, complete plus partial responders/number of patients treated.

treat the patient for a longer period of time than necessary and thereby expose her to the toxic side effects of these agents when cancer is no longer present.

It has been suggested that when a patient on chemotherapy has achieved a complete response, that is, when no cancer is clinically detectable, chemotherapy may be discontinued and second-look operations are unnecessary. Unfortunately, when ovarian cancer recurs and is clinically obvious it often fails to respond to retreatment with agents to which it was initially sensitive. An alternative is simply to treat the patient indefinitely because of the very low incidence of cures with chemotherapy. It is now recognized, however, that using alkylating agents and exposing patients to prolonged treatment may result in their being cured of ovarian cancer, but a small percent will develop acute non-lymphocytic leukemia (Reimer et al. 1977). Another suggestion has been to examine the patient by laparoscopy at the time of com-

Table 47.5. *Response to Treatment by Grade*

	No. of Patients		
	A–C	*H–C*	*Total*
Well-differentiated and moderately differentiated combined			
Response	0	6	6
No response	6	6	12
Total	6	12	18
Response rate	0.0	0.50	$P = 0.05$*
Poorly differentiated			
Response	9	4	13
No response	1	4	5
Total	10	8	18
Response rate	0.90	0.50	$P = 0.09$*

SOURCE: Schwartz, Lawrence, and Katz 1981.

NOTES: Complete or partial response. Three patients in each treatment group were not evaluable for response; one patient in the A–C group did not have primary cancer biopsied. A = doxorubicin (Adriamycin), C = cyclophosphamide, H = hexamethylmelanine.

*Fisher's exact test.

Table 47.6. *Prospective Randomized Trials of Single Agent versus Combination Chemotherapy in Previously Untreated Patients with Stages III and IV Ovarian Cancer (**continued on page 530**)*

Institution	*Drug Regimen**	*Responders†* (%)	*Responders†* (number)	*Complete Responders‡* (%)	*Median Survival of All Patients* (mos)	*Comments*
Gynecologic Oncology Group	Melphalan	29	(28/96)	17	9	No differences in response rates or survival among four treatment groups
	Melphalan + 5-FU	27	(21/77)	16	13	
	Melphalan + 5-FU + Dact	32	(24/85)	17	13	
	CTX + 5-FU + Dact	26	(13/45)	9	8	
Gynecologic Oncology Group	Melphalan	38	(24/64)	13	—	No differences in response duration or survival among three treatment groups
	Melphalan + HMM	52	(50/97)	27	—	
	CTX + DOX	49	(35/72)	23	—	
Northern California Oncology Group	Melphalan	30	(7/23)	3	14	No difference in survival
	CTX + DOX	71	(17/24)	8	14	
Milan	DOX	25	(3/12)	—	—	No difference in response rates
	DOX + Melphalan	22	(3/14)	—	—	
Mayo Clinic	CTX	31	(11/35)	—	12	No difference in response rates or survival
	CTX + DOX	36	(13/36)	—	12	

Table 47.6. *(Continued)*

Institution	Drug Regimen*	Responders† (%)	Responders† (number)	Complete Responders‡ (%)	Median Survival of All Patients (mos)	Comments
M.D. Anderson Hospital	Melphalan	25	(9/31)	11	—	
	DOX	27	(9/34)	12	—	
	HMM	29	(9/31)	13	—	
	HMM + CTX	40	(13/32)	34	—	
Eastern Cooperative Oncology Group	Melphalan	26	(30/114)	17	28	No difference in survival
	CTX + MTX + 5-FU	41	(45/110)	19	17	
National Cancer Institute	Melphalan	54	(20/37)	16	17	Combination regimen resulted in statistically significant better response rate and survival
	CTX + MTX + 5-FU + HMM	75	(30/40)	33	29	
Princess Margaret Hospital	Melphalan	43	(9/21)	10	—	No differences in survival among three treatment groups, but study still ongoing
	CTX + MTX + 5-FU + HMM	37	(9/24)	8	—	
	CTX + DOX + CPDD	59	(13/22)	22	—	
Mt. Sinai	CPDD	20	(4/18)	—	20	Higher response rate with CPDD + DOX combination but no survival advantage
	CPDD + DOX	76	(14/18)	—	20	
	Thiotepa ± MTX	20	(3/17)	—	10	

SOURCE: Katz et al. 1981.

*5-FU = 5-fluorouracil, Dact = dactinomycin, CTX = cyclophosphamide, DOX = doxorubicin, CPDD = cisplatin, HMM = hexamethylmelamine, MTX = methotrexate.

†Percentage of responders and, in parentheses, complete plus partial responders/number of patients treated.

‡Includes both clinically and surgically restaged complete responders.

plete response or on completion of a planned program of chemotherapy, and if no cancer is present, to discontinue therapy. Laparoscopic assessment of the abdomen and pelvis, however, is inadequate for evaluating metastases to retroperitoneal lymph nodes and the posterior peritoneal surfaces. Thus one may have a negative laparoscopy but still have residual ovarian cancer present. It appears that the only objective way to assess the absence of ovarian cancer following completion of a program of chemotherapy is to perform second-look surgery.

This is a carefully planned laparotomy at which time any cancer that may be present is removed. If no gross disease is present, cytologic washings are obtained from the pelvis and each lateral paracolic space. Biopsies are obtained from the diaphragm, paracolic spaces, bowel serosa, mesentery, pelvic peritoneum including the particular areas where the ovary may have been adherent such as the pelvic sidewall, the infundibulopelvic ligaments, the round ligaments, bladder peritoneum, and cul-de-sac peritoneum. Any retroperitoneal nodules in the pelvis and paraaortic region are routinely biopsied, as these may be the only sites of persistent cancer. In general, 20 to 30 biopsies should be obtained from areas where ovarian cancer frequently metastasizes, and any adhesions or nodularities should be carefully assessed. If the omentum has not been previously resected it should be removed. In general, at second-look surgery the entire omentum should be removed; if a partial omentectomy was performed at the original operation, remnants between the transverse colon and stomach should be excised. If all biopsies are negative, chemotherapy may be discontinued.

The risk of recurrence following a negative second-look operation is greatest in those patients who had the most advanced stages and the largest amount of residual cancer left at the initial operation. In general, patients with stages I and II disease with no residual left at the original surgery, followed by a planned program of chemotherapy and a negative second-look operation, have extremely low incidences of recurrence, whereas those with advanced disease may have approximately a 30% chance of recurrence following a negative second-look operation (Schwartz and Smith 1977). Patients with gross cancer left at second-look surgery have a much worse prognosis than those who had all gross cancer removed during the procedure. Following a positive second-look operation, if the cancer has clearly decreased in volume but is persisting, it is best to continue with the preoperative form of therapy. Chemotherapy should be changed if the patient has an increased amount of cancer compared to that left at the initial surgery. Third-look surgery has been performed in those patients who have had a complete response to second-line chemotherapy; however, the likelihood of recurrent disease following a negative third-look operation is probably higher than after a second-look procedure.

Germ Cell Tumors of the Ovary

Germ cell tumors of the ovary represent the second most common type of ovarian neoplasm. The mature teratoma is the most common tumor arising from the germ cell, and is composed of histologically adult tissue that is almost always benign. This tumor is usually a benign cystic teratoma, a neoplasm with elements derived from each of three germ cell layers. At times it may be pure thyroid-like tissue, in which case it is called struma ovarii. Malignant degeneration occurs in less than 2% of benign cystic teratomas and usually is found in those removed from perimenopausal and postmenopausal women (Genadry, Parmley, and Woodruff 1979). The most common malignant degeneration is squamous cell cancer.

The immature teratoma represents a rare cancer that contains fetal tissue. The presence of fetal neuroectoderm is particularly ominous, and a grading system has been devised based on the volume of this tissue. The presence of fetal neuroepithelium involving four or more low-power fields on any slide from an immature teratoma is associated with two-year survival of approximately 30% prior to the introduction of effective combination chemotherapy. The majority of immature teratomas are stage I. The addition of radiation to the management of immature teratomas does not appear to enhance response. Recent developments, however, have resulted in a change from this being a tumor with a terrible prognosis to one that has an excellent prognosis when treated with combination chemotherapy such as vincristine, dactinomycin, and cyclophosphamide (VAC). Experience at our institution suggests that complete remissions are maintained for prolonged periods of time using this combination in stage I disease (Schwartz, Merino, and LiVolsi 1979).

Prognosis of immature teratoma can also be based on grading metastases. Rarely one finds benign fetal elements metastatic throughout the abdominal cavity. This condition is called gliomatosis peritonei. Metastatic implants may also contain fetal neuroepithelium. Indeed, in a series from the Armed Forces Institute of Pathology (Norris, Zirkin, and Benson 1976), no patients were alive following the diagnosis of grade 3 immature teratoma with grade 3 immature teratoma metastases. Our recent experience has demonstrated that when these patients are treated with VAC chemotherapy, metastases may undergo a maturation and at the time of second-look surgery may be found to be benign cystic teratomas (Schwartz, Merino, and LiVolsi 1979). These patients no longer need chemotherapy. It is believed that this redifferentiation to benign tissue is nonreversible.

The dysgerminoma is another tumor that may develop from germ cells. It has a tendency to spread by way of the lymphatics and represents the only ovarian neoplasm that is exquisitely radiation-sensitive. It is extremely important to evaluate the pelvic and paraaortic lymph nodes in patients with dysgerminoma, and to include the paraaortic area in radiation portals if this therapy is required. In general, dysgerminomas are stage I cancers and in young women in whom fertility is a factor, unilateral salpingo-oophorectomy is satisfactory management provided the abdominal cavity has been adequately evaluated intraoperatively, biopsies have been obtained from the omentum and the opposite ovary, and the paraaortic and pelvic lymph nodes have been adequately assessed. In the event that the diagnosis is made postoperatively, a lymphangiogram may be very useful in deciding whether radiation fields to include the paraaortic area are necessary. It has been advocated that when the patient is no longer fertile, reexploration be performed and the residual ovary removed.

Germ cell tumors may also give rise to the very rare endodermal sinus tumor, a lesion that has been reported to have a 12% to 19% two- to three-year survival despite adjuvant radiation therapy (Kurman and Norris 1976). This tumor generally occurs in the second and third decades of life and is associated with alpha-fetoprotein (AFP) production. Recent advances in managing these tumors with combination chemotherapy have demonstrated that the VAC regimen is very active in controlling early stage tumors, while our experience employing cisplatin, vinblastine, and bleomycin has suggested that this combination is extremely active in managing advanced disease. Using a radioimmunoassay for AFP, this marker is a sensitive way of determining the response of the tumor to chemotherapy. A unilateral salpingo-oophorectomy is adequate surgical management for stage I disease, as these tumors are not reported to occur bilaterally and removing the contralateral ovary does not enhance response. Postoperatively, VAC should be administered for 12 months with serial AFP determinations. This chemotherapy in young women does not necessarily interfere with ovulation and they must be cautioned that they may become pregnant while on therapy. It appears that women over age 30 are more sensitive to the effects of this combination chemotherapy and fertility may cease when they are exposed to it for longer than one year.

Ovarian choriocarcinoma is a rare cancer that is best treated with combination chemotherapy consisting of methotrexate, dactinomycin, and cyclophosphamide. Serial radioimmunoassay determinations for the beta chain of human chorionic gonadotropin (HCG) may be used to monitor response.

Embryonal carcinoma has been described in the ovary (Schwartz and Smith 1976). It is associated with the production of both AFP and HCG. It appears to have a better prognosis than the endodermal sinus tumor or choriocarcinoma, at least in stage I disease. It may be successfully managed with surgery and combination chemotherapy.

It is not uncommon to have mixed tumors of the ovary composed of dysgerminoma, endodermal sinus tumor, immature teratoma, and choriocarcinoma in various combinations. Important prognostic factors include the size of the tumor, and the percentage of grade 3 immature teratoma, choriocarcinoma, and endodermal sinus tumor. The presence of these neoplasms in greater than one-third of the tumor means a very poor prognosis. Our experience again suggests that these tumors are exquisitely sensitive to combination chemotherapy. One of our patients with a mixed dysgerminoma and endodermal sinus tumor who was treated with VAC has had one successful pregnancy following a negative second-look operation and is currently pregnant with her second child.

The last germ cell tumors to be considered are the gonadoblastomas. These are benign, and occur in patients who are phenotypically females but karyotypically have a Y chromosome. The tumors may undergo malignant degeneration and form the rare germ cell tumors. Fifty percent will form pure dysgerminomas, while the remainder will form mixed tumors composed of immature teratomas, dysgerminoma, endodermal sinus tumor, and choriocarcinoma. The presence of a Y chromosome in a phenotypic female with hypoplastic external genitalia and primary amenorrhea should lead the physician to recommend removal of the internal genitalia.

Functioning Stromal Tumors (Sex Cord Mesenchyme Tumors)

Functioning ovarian tumors may be either feminizing or masculinizing. The feminizing group includes granulosa cell and theca cell tumors. The masculinizing series includes Sertoli-Leyig cell tumor (arrhenoblastoma) and the lipid or lipoid tumors. In general, granulosa cell tumors are stage I lesions. They can be extremely friable and may rupture prior to or during surgical extirpation. In young women they may be present with findings compatible with ruptured ectopic pregnancies or bleeding ovarian cysts. Young women with tumor confined to one ovary are generally treated by removing the ovary and careful follow-up. With advanced stage cancer, bulk tumor reduction surgery is appropriate, followed by adjuvant therapy. It appears that when maintenance of fertility is a factor, patients with stage I disease may be followed clinically without adjuvant therapy.

Granulosa cell tumors are the classic late recurring cancer of the ovary. Many patients have developed recurrences more than five years from the original diagnosis. Therefore any patient with this diagnosis requires long-term follow-up. Advanced disease that has been completely removed may be controlled by adjuvant radiation therapy; however, if gross tumor is left behind, combination chemotherapy employing VAC appears to be active (Waxman et al. 1979). Localized recurrences should be managed with aggressive surgery, and if completely removed, selective radiation to the tumor bed may be appropriate; if incompletely removed, VAC chemotherapy appears to control this disease for long periods. Thecomas are rarely malignant, and some authors have questioned the existence of a malignant thecoma (Smith and Rutledge 1975). In general, they are treated surgically simply by removing the ovary.

Sertoli-Leydig cell tumors usually occur in the second and third decades of life, but have been diagnosed in perimenopausal and postmenopausal women. These tumors are usually stage I cancer and can be successfully treated simply by removing the ovary. Advanced disease should be treated with aggressive debulking surgery and combination chemotherapy with VAC (Waxman et al. 1979).

The combination of Sertoli-Leydig cell and granulosa-theca cell tumor is called a gynandroblastoma. It is extremely rare. A unilateral salpingo-oophorectomy appears to be satisfactory therapy for stage I cancer, but advanced disease should be treated aggressively with debulking surgery and combination chemotherapy.

Second-look surgery should be employed following completion of a program of VAC therapy for all germ cell tumors of the ovaries.

Nonfunctioning Ovarian Stromal Tumors

Nonfunctioning ovarian stromal tumors derive from the nonspecific mesenchyme, the most common tumor of which is the fibroma. It has been associated with Meig's syndrome, which is unilateral pleural effusion, ascites, and a pelvic mass. Fibromas are benign tumors that are treated by simple excision. Rarely, one can find leiomyomas, lipomas, and other benign connective tissue tumors of the ovary. The most disconcerting ones, however, are those that appear to undergo malignant degeneration and form sarcomas. They are extremely rare, quite aggressive, and generally spread in the same fashion as epithelial cancers.

A sarcoma variant is the mixed mesodermal tumor that tends to occur in women over age 60 and is composed of both malignant epithelial and stromal elements. Mixed mesodermal tumors have been divided into a histologically homologous type in which the sarcomatous element contains traces of mesenchyme normally found in the ovary, and a heterologous type that contains elements not routinely found in ovarian stroma such as cartilage, bone, and striated muscle. Management of these tumors is aggressive chemotherapy with VAC. It has been suggested that the combination of VAC plus irradiation may enhance the response rate (Smith and Rutledge 1975). Our experience suggests that this combination probably increases toxicity without providing significant improvement of response rate, and is therefore avoided.

Metastatic Cancer

The ovary is a common site of metastatic cancer. A peculiar variant is called a Krukenberg tumor. It is characterized by bilateral ovarian involvement, and retention of the general shape of the ovaries so that the tumor appears to be multilobulated, and is freely mobile. Histologically, signet ring cells are present as well as hyperplasia of the ovarian stroma. Other tumors metastasize to the ovary. The management of a metastatic lesion is first to remove the ovaries to prevent bowel or ureteral obstruction and then to treat the primary cancer.

Summary

Ovarian cancer represents the second most common cancer of the female reproductive organs. It is usually not associated with significant warning signals that would lead to early diagnosis. Management is based on adequate surgical staging, removal of as much of the bulk tumor as possible, careful histologic assessment of the primary cancer and its metastases, and appropriate postoperative adjuvant therapy. Stage I cancer confined to one ovary and with a very favorable histology such as borderline malignant epithelial cancers, dysgerminoma, granulosa cell tumor, and Sertoli-Leydig cell tumor may be treated with surgery alone. Stage I epithelial cancers are best treated with total abdominal hysterectomy, bilateral salpingo-oophorectomy, and adjuvant chemotherapy or radiation therapy. Stage I nonepithelial tumors are best treated with a unilateral salpingo-oophorectomy followed by aggressive combination chemotherapy. Advanced ovarian cancers, regardless of histologic origin, should be treated with aggressive surgery including complete removal of the tumor whenever possible, followed by adjuvant therapy selected on the basis of histology. Complete remission should be confirmed by second-look operation prior to discontinuing adjuvant therapy.

References

American Joint Committee for Staging and End-Results Reporting. *Manual for staging of cancer.* Chicago: Whiting Press, 1978.

Aure, J. C.; Hoeg, J.; and Kolsted, P. Clinical and histological studies of ovarian carcinoma. Long-term follow-up of 990 cases. *Obstet. Gynecol.* 37:1–9, 1971.

Barber, H. R. K. *Ovarian carcinoma—etiology, diagnosis, and treatment.* New York: Masson, 1978, p. 1.

Bruckner, H. W. et al. Cis-platinum (DDP) for combination chemotherapy of ovarian carcinoma: improved response rates and survival. *Proc. Am. Assoc. Cancer Res.* 19:373, 1978.

Dembo, A. J. et al. The Princess Margaret Hospital study of ovarian cancer: stage I, II, and asymptomatic II presentations. *Cancer Treat. Rep.* 63:249–254, 1979.

Fisher, R. I., and Young, R. C. Chemotherapy of ovarian cancer. *Surg. Clin. North Am.* 58:143–150, 1978.

Genadry, R.; Parmley, T.; and Woodruff, J. D. Secondary malignancies in benign cystic teratomas. *Gynecol. Oncol.* 8:246–251, 1979.

Katz, M. E. et al. Epithelial carcinoma of the ovary: current strategies. *Ann. Intern. Med.* 95:98–111, 1981.

Kurman, R. J., and Norris, H. J. Embryonal carcinoma of the ovary—a clinicopathologic entity distinct from endodermal sinus tumor resembling embryonal carcinoma of the adult testis. *Cancer* 38:2420–2433, 1976.

Norris, H. J.; Zirkin, H. J.; and Benson, W. L. Immature (malignant) teratoma of the ovary—a clinical and pathologic study of 58 cases. *Cancer* 37:2359–2372, 1976.

Reimer, R. R. et al. Acute leukemia after alkylating agent therapy of ovarian cancer. *N. Engl. J. Med.* 297:177–181, 1977.

Schwartz, P. E.; Lawrence, R.; and Katz, M. Combination chemotherapy for advanced ovarian cancer: a prospective randomized trial comparing hexamethylmelamine–cyclophosphamide to Adriamycin–cyclophosphamide. *Cancer Treat. Rep.* 65:137–141, 1981.

Schwartz, P. E.; Merino, M. J.; and LiVolsi, V. A. Immature ovarian teratomas: maturation following chemotherapy. *Am. J. Diag. Obstet. Gynecol.* 1:361–366, 1979.

Schwartz, P. E., and Smith, J. P. Treatment of ovarian stromal tumors. *Am. J. Obstet. Gynecol.* 125:402–408, 1976.

Schwartz, P. E., and Smith, J. P. The role of second-look surgery in ovarian cancer management. Presented at the Eighth Annual Meeting of the Felix Rutledge Society, Los Angeles, July 24–27, 1977.

Schwartz, P. E., and Weiner, M. Ultrasound in gynecology: a clinician's viewpoint. *Clin. Diag. Ultrasound* 2:183–190, 1979.

Silverberg, E. Cancer statistics, 1981. *CA* 31:13–28, 1981.

Smith, J. P., and Rutledge, F. N. Advances in chemotherapy for gynecologic cancer. *Cancer* 36:669–674, 1975.

Smith, J. P.; Rutledge, F. N.; and Delclos, L. E. Results of chemotherapy as an adjunct to surgery in patients with localized ovarian cancer. *Semin. Oncol.* 2:277–281, 1975.

Waxman, M. et al. Ovarian low-grade stromal sarcoma with thecomatous features—a clinical reappraisal of the so-called "malignant thecoma." *Cancer* 44:2206–2217, 1979.

forty-eight

Cancer of the Uterine Cervix

MURRAY JOSEPH CASEY

It is estimated that 61,000 women in the United States will develop cervical carcinoma in 1982; 16,000 will have invasive cancer, 7200 will die of the malignancy, and 45,000 will be discovered in the situ stage (Silverberg 1982). At the present rate, 3% of American women will develop some form of this disease (Silverberg 1975). Since 1935, there has been a steady decrease in the incidence of invasive cervical carcinoma, accompanied by an increasing proportion of carcinomas diagnosed in situ (Silverberg 1975). This has been associated with declining death rates from uterine cancer from 28 per 100,000 in 1930 to 8 per 100,000 in 1975. A better understanding of cervical neoplastic disease and the development of improved modalities for therapy account for some of this, but more important is the accessibility of the cervix for observation, study, and detection of disease in its earliest stages (Silverberg 1975; Dickinson 1975).

Preinvasive Cervical Epidermoid Carcinoma

The concept of epidermoid carcinoma in situ as a preinvasive form of cervical cancer was slow in developing, but now most gynecologic oncologists and pathologists agree that the earliest forms of cervical neoplasms can be discovered in intraepithelial states even more limited than in situ carcinoma (Reagan and Hamonic 1956). Nearly 100 years of investigative pathology have culminated in the current theory that dysplastic cells arising in areas of repair and metaplasia at or near the squamocolumnar junction progress from proliferation of atypical basal cells to full-thickness involvement of the cervical epithelium. Thus mildly dysplastic lesions result in preinvasive tumors of progressively greater thickness and advancing area until a full-thickness lesion or in situ carcinoma results (Richart 1968). To emphasize the spectrum of this process, the designation cervical intraepithelial neoplasia—mild, moderate, severe (CIN I, II, or III)—has been proposed and is the accepted terminology of most gynecologic oncologists and pathologists today (Richart 1968). Until recently, all epidermoid neoplastic transformations from benign metaplasia to intraepithelial neoplasms were believed to occur only at the squamocolumnar junction; now the entire area is considered susceptible to transformation, and is termed the transformation zone (TZ) (Richart 1968) (figs. 48.1–48.4).

Early reports of several investigators indicated that a large proportion of dysplastic lesions regressed completely while under study, but these overlooked the potentially therapeutic effects of diagnostic biopsies that may remove smaller lesions and induce inflammatory responses that might lead to rejection of some others (Koss et al. 1963). Several authors have observed progression of intraepithelial neoplasms to more advanced lesions, and at times, to invasive carcinomas (Fox 1967; Christopherson 1977). Progression is unpredictable;

The author thanks Katharine Granquist for her diligent research and technical assistance.

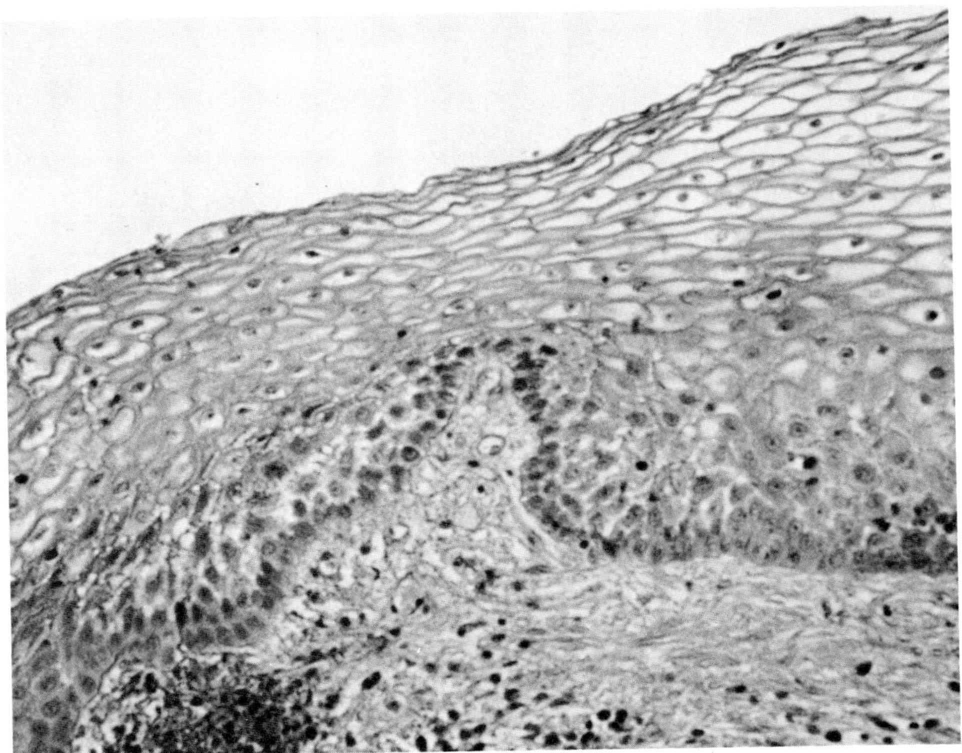

Fig. 48.1. *Normal stratified squamous epithelium of ectocervix showing maturation of parabasal, intermediate, and superficial cells with underlying connective tissue stroma.*

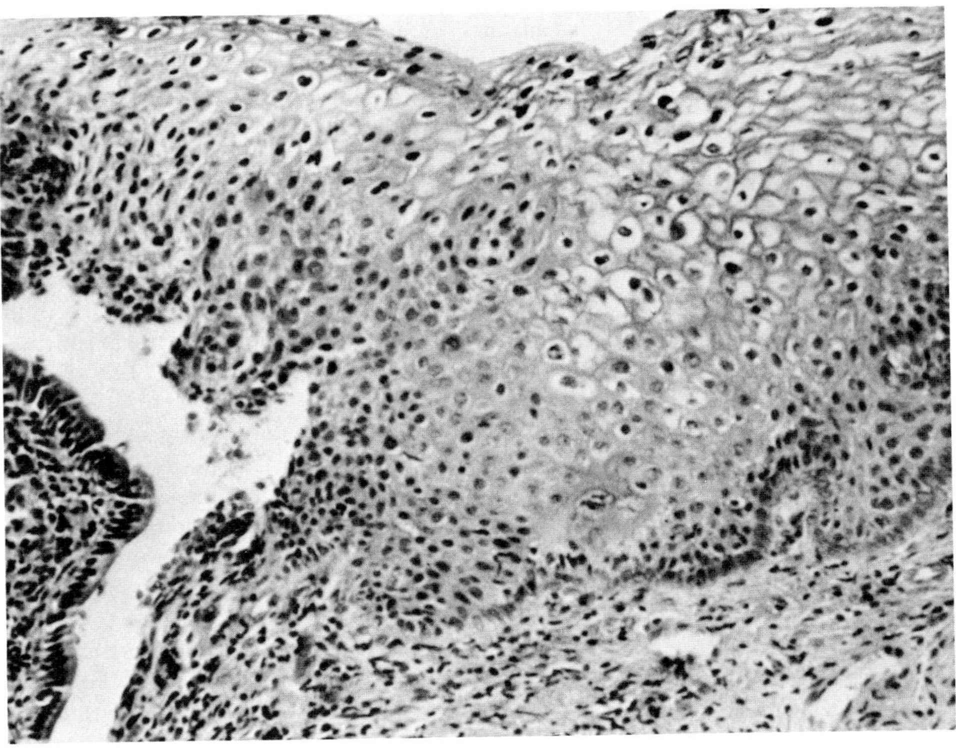

Fig. 48.2. *Dysplastic squamous epithelium of CIN I–II showing loss of polarity and abnormalities of parabasal and intermediate cell differentiation.*

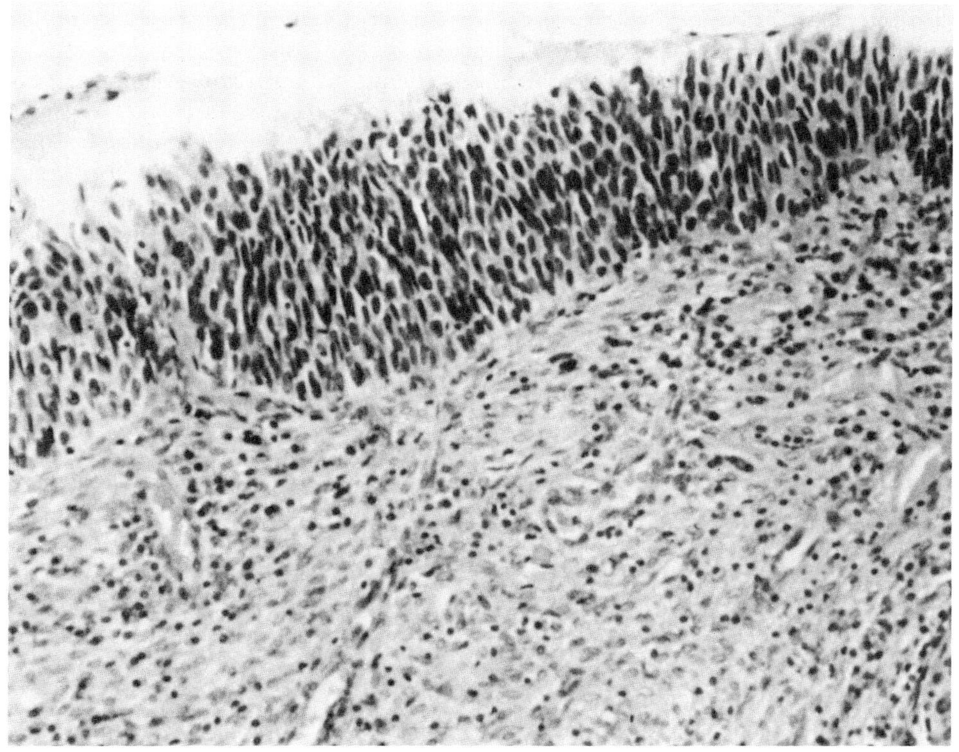

Fig. 48.3. *In situ carcinoma with immaturity throughout entire thickness of the epithelium, with apparent basement membrane intact. Note capillary-like spaces in nearby stroma.*

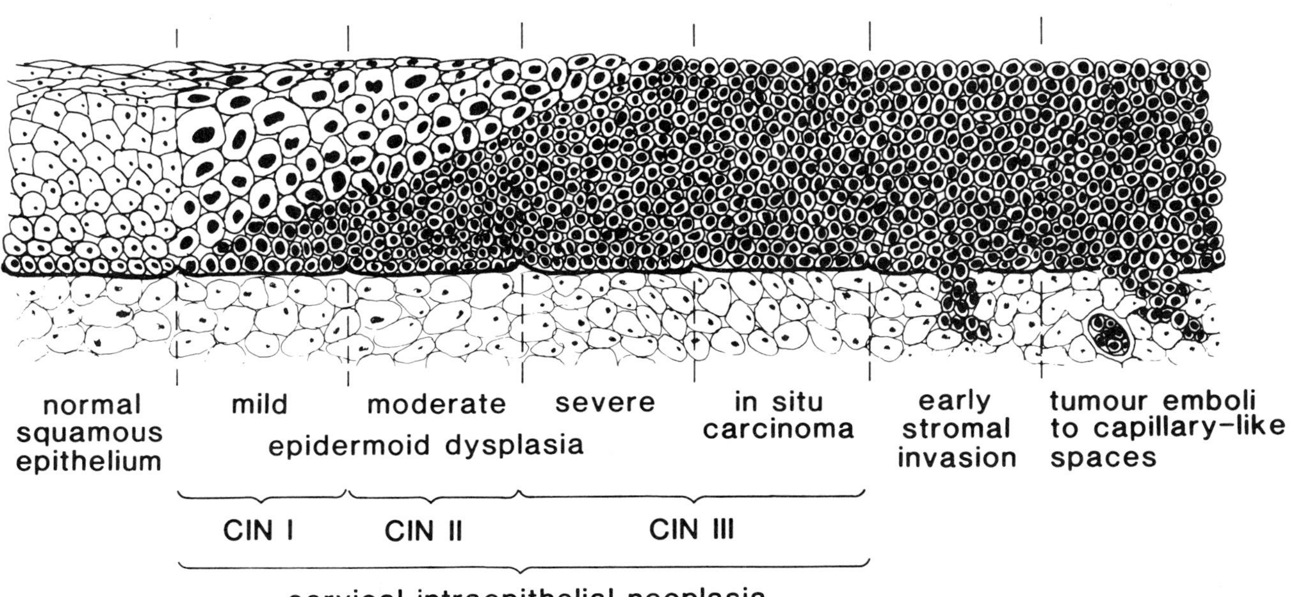

Fig. 48.4. *The spectrum and nomenclature of cervical squamous cell neoplasms from mild dysplasia through carcinoma in situ and microinvasion.*

while intraepithelial lesions may regress or remain unchanged for long periods, progression to invasive carcinomas may occur in less than two to three years (Dunn 1953; Barron, Cahill, and Richart 1978). From these experiences studies evolved that followed these lesions with colposcopy, colpomicroscopy, and several cytologic techniques without biopsy. In one historic study, mild to moderate neoplasms regressed to normal in 30% of 278 patients who were followed, while 60% progressed to severe disease, and 3 patients to invasive carcinomas (Fox 1967). Intraepithelial lesions that were severe at the commencement of this study progressed rapidly to geographically larger lesions and rarely regressed. Although stepwise progression from mild to moderate and then severe dysplasia usually occurred, there was no way of predicting how long a lesion might remain unchanged. This was in spite of the fact that during observation of over 500 women 3 intraepithelial lesions progressed to invasive carcinomas (Barron and Richart 1968; Richart and Barron 1969).

Further evidence of the malignant potential of these tumors is provided by studies that have demonstrated persistent aneuploidy in cells cultured from dysplasias, carcinomas in situ, and invasive carcinomas of the cervix (Kirkland 1969). These observations were confirmed by studies using microspectrophotometric techniques indicating that cells from mildly dysplastic lesions more frequently demonstrated diploid DNA distribution than cells from cervical carcinomas in situ, and aneuploid DNA distribution was more frequently found in cells from the more severe lesions (Wilbanks et al. 1967).

Epidemiology

Etiology

In the past, carcinoma of the cervix has been associated with patients of low economic status, poor hygiene, and high parity. Voluminous data have linked the disease with early and frequent sexual intercourse with more than one partner (Gusberg 1978), and it was extremely rare or nonexistent among Catholic nuns (Gagon 1952). Recent British studies surveying the partners of patients with cervical cancer have shown association of disease with male occupations at the lower economic level and those requiring extensive travel (Wakefield et al. 1973). Furthermore, many investigations have demonstrated an association of cervical cancer with genital infections of venereal origin, such as syphilis, gonorrhea, wart virus, and other microbial agents, leading to the conclusion that it follows the pattern of sexually transmitted diseases (Schachter et al. 1975). In spite of the positive association, however, no consistent pattern has yet emerged.

Recognition by kinetic neutralization tests of two major *Herpesvirus hominus* subtypes allowed epidemiologic studies of this virus in the 1960s, which have since related serotype I (HV I) to oral-pharyngeal infections and transmission; serotype II (HV II) was related to sexual infections and transmission (Dowdle et al. 1967). Changing patterns of sexual behavior may begin to blur these distinctions (Willcox 1972).

Sero-epidemiologic studies have consistently shown a higher incidence of HV II antibodies in patients with invasive epidermoid carcinoma of the cervix in the United States than in their matched controls (Naib et al. 1969; Simon 1976); however, it is important to interpret these data. While most patients with invasive carcinomas showed serologic evidence of previous HV II infections, those with earlier disease were less likely to demonstrate serum antibody titers against this virus. Given a hypothesis of the continuous spectrum of this carcinoma from early dysplasia through invasive cancer, a prevalent etiologic factor should be expected. Furthermore, the incidence of HV II antibodies increased with age in both controls and patients, and a difference of incidence between the groups was less apparent in some non-American population studies. Nonetheless, evidence continues to accumulate linking cervical carcinoma to a possible latent neoplastic infection by this DNA virus, which shows so many similarities to proved oncogenic viruses in experimental and natural animal models (Kessler 1974). Recently, apparently specific antigens have been demonstrated with immunofluorescence in exfoliated cells from cervical cancer using antisera raised by animal inoculation with herpesvirus-induced antigens (Aurelian 1974). Whether HV II proves to be a causative factor or whether the association is fortuitous, this is a fertile field for research, and no doubt a far better understanding of the process of latent virus infection and its pertinence to human, animal, and plant diseases will result.

Studies from the United Kingdom have shown variations in cervical cells caused by sperm histone, and an increased histone:protamine ratio has been demonstrated in the sperm of men from the same occupational areas that have been associated with cervical cancer in their partners (Singer and Reid 1979). A New York study (Melamed et al. 1969) showed an increased prevalence of severe intraepithelial neoplasms in women who were taking oral contraceptives compared with those using a barrier method. A cause and effect relationship could not be established from this or from another study (Stern et al. 1971). There was no significant difference in the characteristics of those who preferred oral contraceptives to intrauterine devices (IUDs) (Sandmire et al. 1976). The matter is not settled as to whether mechanical barriers might offer some protection from cervical malignancy.

Although it is doubtful that oral steroidal contraceptives are the initiating factor of cervical transformation (Ory et al. 1976), some epidemiologic studies indicate that their use was associated with more rapid progression of established lesions (Stern et al. 1977). This brings up other possibilities of operating cofactors in cervical carcinogenesis. As bits and pieces of information are fit together, a clearer picture of the etiology and relationship of genetics and immunity will unfold. Sexual activity would seem important to the induction of this disease; however, in the future this may prove not to be the case with regard to all cervical carcinomas.

Age

Several investigators have concluded that there has been an increasing incidence of abnormal cytologic findings consistent with preinvasive cervical malignancy among American teenagers in recent years (Kaufman et al. 1970); others disagree (Nealon and Christopherson 1979). The major increase in incidence has been attributed to sexual activity. In this population, one study reported that the cytologic diagnosis of cervical cancer precursors was made in 188 of 2655 sexually active 13-year-old to 19-year-old young women; 71 showed CIN II to III, a rate of 26 of 1000, nearly half of which were confirmed with biopsies (Feldman et al. 1976). Others reported lower but significant rates of 5.9 to 23 per 1000 teenagers with Papanicolaou (Pap) smears consistent with intraepithelial neoplasms (Kaufman et al. 1970; Wallace and Slankard 1973) including a large number of parous younger women in their teens who had abnormal smears (Kling and Buchsbaum 1973). A number of epidemiologic investigations, including carefully cross-matched control studies, implicated a young age of first coitus as the single most important risk factor for cervical cancer (Barron and Richart 1971; Rotkin 1973). The significance of this is not yet determined, but the frequent colposcopic finding of abnormal transformation zones in adolescent women engaging in frequent sexual activity may be relevant (Coppleson 1969).

The experience of many gynecologists and data generated by some studies (Kling and Buchsbaum 1973; Snyder et al. 1976) led to the guarded conclusion that both preinvasive and invasive cervical carcinomas are present in younger patients. Between initiation of the neoplastic process and the development of severe intraepithelial and invasive disease, a latent period is likely; if disease prevalence in two separate groups is the same, previously unscreened populations should have the highest rate of detection (Dunn 1953; Barron, Cahill, and Richart 1978). Yet the total detection for both in situ and invasive carcinoma of the cervix in women younger than 20 years remains lower than in women in their fourth and fifth decades who were not screened previously. Prevalence of dysplasia seems to be increasing in younger women, however (Kaufman et al. 1970). A study of young women living in a low-income housing project noted that first contact with HV II peaked at ages 15 to 19 years in parous women; whereas antibodies were absent in 38 nulliparous women of this age group from the same population, and a strong association between dysplasia and prevalence of HV II antibodies was demonstrated (Ory et al. 1975). Perhaps the young metaplastic cervix is unusually susceptible to transformation by herpesvirus infection or by some other sexually transmitted agent.

Screening and Evaluation

The success of the past 20 years in detection of early cervical neoplasms and thus the lowering of death rates from invasive carcinomas had led the American Cancer Society to recommend that all sexually active women undergo cervical screening with Papanicolaou (Pap) cytology (American Cancer Society 1979). False negative rates may exceed 30% when sampling is from the ectocervix alone by means of an Ayers spatula; adequate samples of the endocervix may well reduce this rate to as little as 1% (Richart and Vaillant 1965). The false negative rate may be higher in patients who have been recently screened. Although only 82% of patients referred for evaluation for abnormal Pap smears were found to have subsequent abnormal cytology in one series, colposcopy with biopsies and endocervical curettage demonstrated neoplastic tissues in 95% of these patients (Shingleton et al. 1975). Thus a subsequent negative smear in a patient who has had a recent abnormal test should not be considered firm evidence of no disease.

Severe intraepithelial and even invasive carcinomas may produce only mildly abnormal smears (Figge et al. 1970; Jafari 1978). Furthermore, as the interval of progression of individual lesions is not predictable (Barron and Richart 1968; Koss 1969), all abnormal smears must be evaluated. Visible lesions should be biopsied and vaginal infections specifically treated. Colposcopic examination should be performed for evaluation as well as directed biopsies of abnormal epithelium. Virtually every gynecologic oncologist has seen patients referred for the treatment of invasive cervical cancer whose worst Pap smear has been reported as class II, and in some cases the cytology has been negative (Figge et al. 1970).

There is a question as to how frequently cervical Pap smears should be performed. This can be approached from at least two different perspectives: that of expected yield from screening programs, and that of the individual physician caring for patients. The first approach is more concerned with cost-effectiveness (Spriggs and Husain 1977); the second with ascertaining good health and freedom from disease (Dickinson 1975). Regrettably, cervical carcinoma is capable of progressing from an undetectable lesion to a significantly invasive cancer within alarmingly short periods of time. In one series, five patients (aged 27, 30, 45, 52, and 58 years) with invasive carcinomas had normal Pap smears 8 to 36 months earlier; three were obtained less than 24 months before diagnosis, and two of these women subsequently died with cancer (Figge et al. 1970). Even disease progression from its earliest intraepithelial stages to in situ carcinoma may require more extensive therapy than mild to moderate dysplasia. The physician will do well to consider all that is known of epidemiology and etiology in recommending a regimen for reexamination and Pap smears. From the individual standpoint, the yield and detection of cancer is improved and false negative rates are diminished by reexamination (Gad and Koch 1978); the effectiveness of repeated screening to further reduce mortality rates may be impossible to demonstrate.

Certain high-risk factors, such as are associated with the sexually active teenager, can be readily identified; others may be operative that have not yet been delineated or those such as multiple sexual partners may not be divulged if patient-doctor communication is poor. Conservative treatment suggests a recommendation for more frequent evaluations and early therapy.

One difficulty expressed by directors of large screening programs, and confirmed by the experiences of many engaged in evaluating and treating patients with abnormal Pap smears, has been a tendency of some of these patients to be unreliable in keeping appointments and continuing follow-up (Kaufman et al. 1970). Programs must be established to induce patients to undergo screening and ensure follow-up. Serious resources must be devoted to patient education and the social services to accomplish this.

Treatment of Cervical Intraepithelial Epidermoid Carcinoma

CIN I-II

A histologically verified intraepithelial neoplasm in its earliest, mildest form dictates evaluation of the cervix and upper vagina by careful endocervical aspiration and smears, contracervical-vaginal smears for further cytologic examination, colposcopy with directed biopsies of the most significant lesions, and in most cases, endocervical curettage. When colposcopy and biopsies agree on a diagnosis of CIN I-II cancer, and the lesion is confined to the transformation zone, fully visible by colposcopy without extension to the endocervix, the lesion can be treated in any manner that ensures total local eradication. It is imperative that endocervical curettings show no neoplastic tissue before locally directed therapy is undertaken. Invasive carcinoma involving the endocervix is often underrated as intraepithelial disease (Townsend et al. 1970), whereas negative curettage together with mild to moderate intraepithelial neoplasm by cytology and biopsies virtually assures the absence of invasive carcinoma.

Excisional biopsies and electrocoagulation or cryosurgical cautery have all been effective and each has its proponents (Chanen and Hollyock 1971; Creasman et al. 1973). A versatile approach to clearly defined early lesions is the key to treatment. Presently, cryosurgery is the most popular. Undoubtedly this is because it is so easy to perform and is virtually free from serious side effects so long as reasonable precautions are observed. Good results can be achieved and defined lesions completely treated within the ice ball created by a temperature lowered to at least $-50°$ C for two three-minute freeze-thaw cycles (Townsend and Ostergard 1971).

The CO_2 laser has also been adapted to the treatment of colposcopically defined lesions (Stafl et al. 1977). Its chief disadvantage is capital expense, and consequently the necessarily high fee for individual treatments. These techniques are just emerging, and considerably more investigative work and follow-up need to be done before they can be generally recommended (Upton 1975). If the endocervical curettage is positive for neoplastic tissues or the lesion cannot be fully visualized by colposcopy, as may occur in older women when the squamocolumnar junction regresses to within the endocervix (Shingleton et al. 1977), it is necessary to resort to cervical conization to further confirm the diagnosis (Townsend et al. 1970).

CIN III

Cytohistologic diagnosis of advanced intraepithelial disease, severe dysplasia, or carcinoma in situ leads us to recommend colposcopically defined cervical conization for both diagnostic and therapeutic purposes. Cryosurgical procedures have been attended by a failure rate of up to 30% when cervical neoplasms have reached this stage (Tredway et al. 1972). Although its results are improved by negative endocervical curettage and diligent colposcopy confirming that the lesion is confined to the ectocervix (Underwood et al. 1976), even the most experienced colposcopists report satisfactory examinations when their diagnosis is within one degree of the histologically confirmed lesion (Stafl and Mattingly 1973). The next step following severe full-thickness intraepithelial malignancy is early invasive carcinoma.

Reports of advanced invasive cervical carcinomas occurring after failure to observe approved diagnostic techniques or failed cryosurgery are beginning to appear in the literature (Sevin et al. 1979). Clearly, local incision and cautery have no place in the treatment of invasive carcinoma. On the other hand, all lesions up to invasive carcinoma can be effectively treated and controlled by carefully designed wide and deep excisions, such as are carried out with colposcopically directed conization (Kolstad and Klem 1976). When used alone, Schiller's test is not reliable for defining the extent of dysplastic tissues (Rubio and Thomassen 1976), and poor results leaving residual CIN may occur when colposcopy is not used rigorously to define the lesion to ensure wide excision (Garcia et al. 1975).

We feel that outpatient colposcopy should be carried out on all patients with abnormal smears predictive of severe intraepithelial or early invasive disease to define and biopsy the worst focus and delineate any visible lesion, thus circumventing cervical conization (Kolstad and Klem 1976). In the majority of well screened patients biopsy will show no invasion, and conization under colposcopic direction should then be performed. During the procedure care should be taken to include all abnormal tissue within the circumferential incision, extending it, if necessary, to encompass the defined lesion. Following this, biopsy of the residual endocervix above the apex of the cone and curettage of the internal os and lower uterine segment should always be carried out. It is appropriate to schedule a hysterectomy 48 hours following conization. Should early invasive cancer be detected, one may then proceed to extrafascial or extended hysterectomy before development of severe inflammatory parametritis, which is likely to follow cervical cone biopsies by several days. If meticulous sectioning and pathologic review of the tissues delivered by cone excision show clear surgical margins and no evidence of invasive disease, and if the biopsies and curettings taken from above the apex of the cone are negative, therapy is complete and there is no need for more extensive surgery (Ahlgren et al. 1975).

Microinvasion, Stage IA

Surgery

In redefining early invasive cervical cancer, the International Federation of Gynecology and Obstetrics classified tumors showing early stromal invasion as microinvasive carcinomas, stage IA, but chose not to involve itself in the definition of microinvasive. Complete staging as established by the American College of Obstetricians and Gynecologists (1977) is shown in table 48.1.

Review of the accumulated clinical and histologic data from many series of early cervical carcinomas confirmed the good results that were obtained in patients who were treated with simple hysterectomies alone for microinvasive disease (Fennell 1978). In a large series of 162 patients treated with simple hysterectomies and bilateral pelvic lymphadenectomies, there were no recurrences and there were no metastases to lymph nodes when the primary invasive lesions extended less than 1 mm beneath the epithelial surface and there was no evidence of tumorous involvement of microscopic lymphatic channels in the adjacent stroma (Averette et al. 1976). When the depth of tumor invasion is 2 to 5 mm, pelvic lymph nodes may be involved with metastases in 2% to 5% of patients (Savage 1972; Fennell 1978). Although early observations demonstrated pelvic node metastases in 63% of patients with stages I and II disease who were found to have invasion of the local lymphatic vessels (Cherry and Glücksmann 1955), the significance in microinvasion of tumor emboli within apparent lymphatic capillaries lying as close as 1.5 mm to the surface has not as yet been determined (Roche and Norris 1975; Sedlis et al. 1979).

Considering available data we favor treatment by transabdominal extrafascial hysterectomy. Cure rate is excellent and there are minimal untoward effects when

Table 48.1. *Staging of Carcinoma of the Uterine Cervix*

Stage	*Extent of Disease*
0	Carcinoma in situ
I	Carcinoma confined to cervix (extension to the corpus is disregarded)
IA	Microinvasive carcinoma (early stromal invasion)
IB	All other cases of stage I; occult cancer should be marked "occ"
II	Carcinoma involves vagina, but not lower one-third or infiltrates parametrium, but has not reached pelvic wall
IIA	No obvious parametrial involvement
IIB	Obvious parametrial involvement
III	Carcinoma involves lower one-third of vagina or extends to pelvic wall
IIIA	No extension to pelvic wall
IIIB	Extension to pelvic wall and/or hydronephrosis or nonfunctioning kidney
IV	Carcinoma involves mucosa of bladder or rectum or extends beyond true pelvis
IVA	Involves mucosa of bladder or rectum, but not beyond true pelvis
IVB	Extension beyond true pelvis

SOURCE: American College of Obstetricians and Gynecologists 1977.

NOTE: Recommended by the General Assembly of the International Federation of Obstetricians and Gynecologists, 1976.

microinvasive carcinoma up to 1 mm is diagnosed following study of multiple sections from intact cervical conization with colposcopy and Schiller's stain. Conization alone is often inadequate to eradicate even the earliest invasive carcinomas, and should not be relied on (Sedlis et al. 1979). When metastases to pelvic nodes have advanced beyond 1 mm we carry out bilateral pelvic lymphadenectomies. When tumor extends to 1 to 3 mm or when tumorous involvement of capillary-like spaces is found, we favor extended hysterectomies with removal of the entire cervix and adjacent proximal parametria with small vaginal cuff. Tumors that involve the surgical margins of the conization and those that have advanced beyond 3 mm deserve to be treated as more advanced tumors by radical hysterectomies and bilateral pelvic lymphadenectomies to ascertain removal of all potentially involved paracervical tissues and pelvic nodes.

Radiotherapy

Microinvasive cervical carcinomas may be effectively treated with radiation therapy when there are serious contraindications to surgery (Marcial 1977), but radiotherapy does not improve prognosis beyond the good results achieved with surgery and may be associated with significant side effects as well as the loss of ovarian function, which may be preserved by surgical management. Conservation of gonadal hormone production is advocated in the treatment of young women in whom ovarian metastases do not seem to be a danger (Webb 1975). With these approaches to the treatment of microinvasive cervical carcinoma up to 5 mm in depth, one should expect cure rates approaching 100% (Savage 1972; Sedlis et al. 1979).

Early Invasive Carcinoma, Stages IB and IIA

When smaller cervical carcinomas are confined to the cervix (stage IB) or extend minimally to the upper vagina (stage IIA), comparable cure rates of 85% to 90% are obtained with radical surgery (Masubuchi et al. 1969; Morley and Seski 1976; Webb and Symmonds 1979) or radical radiotherapy (Kottmeier 1964; Marcial 1977). When larger tumors are encountered in these stages cure rates diminish with both modalities (Pilleron et al. 1974; Burghardt and Pickel 1978). It is these larger tumors that are more frequently associated with occult involvement of the parametria and pelvic lymph nodes. Adjuvant radical irradiation with radical surgery in the past led to no improvement in cure rates obtained with either treatment alone, but was associated with significant increases in morbidity (Burch and Chalfant 1970; Adcock 1979). Combined therapy is being reassessed (Easley and Fletcher 1971; Surwit et al. 1978).

Historically, five-year survival rates of 20% to 50% have been achieved in patients with positive pelvic nodes treated with radical hysterectomies and bilateral pelvic lymphadenectomies for stages IB to IIA disease. Recent surveys have shown less residual disease and a significantly lower percentage of positive lymph nodes in patients who underwent similar operations following irradiation (Rutledge et al. 1964; Surwit et al. 1976). In view of these findings it has been disquieting that no improvement in survival rates was achieved in one randomized prospective series by postoperative radiotherapy for those patients who were found to have positive pelvic nodes at the time of surgery (Lagasse et al. 1974). Furthermore, although radiotherapy is capable of reducing the mass and sterilizing the central tumor (Fletcher 1971), and thus perhaps achieving greater frequency of central control, no significant increase in survival rates has been realized (Burch and Chalfant 1970; Surwit et al. 1978).

Considering the accumulated data and growing experience with cervical carcinoma, treatment of patients with tumors confined to the cervix and upper vagina should be individualized. Young women who might have life-long untoward effects of radiation therapy, but who are better able to withstand radical hysterectomy and pelvic node dissection, may be managed with primary surgery, while older patients are assigned to radiation therapy. Because tumor emboli in vascular capillaries on biopsies (Cherry and Glücksmann 1955; Barber et al. 1978) and larger cervical tumors (Pilleron et al. 1974; Burghardt and Pickel 1978) are associated with pelvic node metastases, these patients are also assigned to radiation therapy. While the data are as yet inconclusive, radical radiotherapy may better eliminate metastatic disease from pelvic lymph channels than surgery (Kolbenstvedt and Kolstad 1976). Because of the increase in complications with combined radical radiation and radical surgery (Burch and Chalfant 1970; Adcock 1979) adjunctive use of these modalities with some modification (Rampone et al. 1973; Surwit et al. 1978) in early cervical cancer should be reserved for bulky central tumors with free parametria and those with extension to the uterine corpus (Perez et al. 1975). Better local control and thus improved prognosis for cure of these very unfavorable tumors can be expected (Perez et al. 1975).

Advanced Cervical Tumors: Stages IIB, III, and IV

Massive extension of cervical carcinoma into the parametria (stage IIB) or lower vagina (stage IIIA), tumorous fixation of the pelvic sidewalls (stage IIIB), and metastatic disease to the pelvic nodes (stage IIIB) or beyond the pelvis (stage IV) preclude surgical therapy. Many relatively large epidermoid carcinomas of the cervix, clinically confined to the pelvis, may be treated with radical radiation therapy with good control of the central tumor (Paunier et al. 1967; Fletcher 1971). A skillful combination of megavoltage external radiation therapy and brachytherapy with placement of sources guided by intraoperative roentgenography is necessary to achieve such good results while minimizing injuries (Stockbine et al. 1970).

Endophytic Tumors

Endophytic tumors that extend to involve the endometrium (Perez et al. 1975) and those that expand the cervix and lower uterine segment bilaterally to take a barrel shape (Lu et al. 1976) fare poorly with radiation therapy (Marcial 1977). Expansion of these tumors into the proximal parametria and the associated poor prognosis has led to the inclusion of barrel-shaped tumors greater than 6 cm in substage IIB (Nelson et al. 1975). Possible improvement of results in treating these tumors using combined external radiation and brachytherapy followed by conservative extrafascial hysterectomy is being investigated. Preliminary reports are encouraging both with regard to survival and control of local disease (Nelson et al. 1975). Unfortunately, the poor prognosis of these endophytic tumors appears in large measure to be due to their association with rather early and widespread metastatic disease (Perez et al. 1975).

Pelvic Nodes

While it is clear that radiotherapy is capable of sterilizing metastases in pelvic lymph nodes (Rutledge et al. 1964; Lagasse et al. 1974) when effective doses are administered (Kottmeier 1964; Marcial 1977), massive cancerous involvement of nodes in the lateral pelvis may escape control because of the rapid exponential fall-off of dosage from centrally placed radiation sources (Paunier et al. 1967). In the hands of skilled radiation oncologists, deaths from pelvic recurrences most often result from inability to control massive tumor at the pelvic side-walls. Although more intensive radiation therapy has resulted in better tumor control and fewer deaths from cancer, this was accomplished at the cost of increasing numbers and severity of postirradiation complications. Since a large proportion of advanced cervical cancers are accompanied by metastases to pelvic lymph nodes, adjunctive pelvic lymphadenectomies following radiotherapy were performed, but this practice failed to improve survival rates and complications were increased (Rutledge et al. 1964). The occurrence of metastatic disease beyond the field of effective surgery or radiation therapy thus may account for many losses to cancer in spite of local and regional control.

Extrapelvic Nodes

Metastatic involvement of the higher common iliac and paraaortic nodes beyond the nodes of the parametria and the hypogastric and obturator groups heralds a poor prognosis (Nelson et al. 1977). The relatively high incidence of unsuspected metastases to extrapelvic nodes that has been demonstrated by preirradiation celiotomy requires a rethinking of management of this disease, since 20% to 40% of patients surgically evaluated now have been shown to have cancers beyond the scope of any therapy that is limited to the pelvis (Buchsbaum 1972; Nelson et al. 1977). In spite of observations that radical radiotherapy was capable of controlling metastatic disease to pelvic lymph nodes (Fletcher and Rutledge 1972), extension of the external radiotherapy ports to encompass the common iliac and paraaortic node groups, as originally advocated, has added little to the cure rate and was accompanied by extreme incidences of seriously disabling and fatal complications (Piver et al. 1975; Nelson et al. 1977). Tumorous involvement of small extrapelvic lymphatics can be sterilized by extended-field supervoltage external radiotherapy in those who survive the complications of treatment. This has been verified by reports of long-term survival without evidence of metastatic disease, and by reports of negative node dissections following paraaortic irradiation for biopsy-proved metastases (Fletcher and Rutledge 1972; Wharton et al. 1977). Analysis of time and site of cancer recurrences following extended-field external radiation revealed high incidences of uncontrolled pelvic tumors and metastases, even when disease was apparently controlled within the paraaortic ports (Fletcher and Rutledge 1972). Unless control of the primary cancer is achieved, and presence of metastases to the paraaortic nodes along with absence of distant dissemination have been assured, it would not be reasonable to undertake extended-field radiotherapy with its attendant high morbidity.

Lymphangiography

Lymphangiography to evaluate the status of extrapelvic nodes has been attempted with mixed success (Benninghoff, Herman, and Nelson 1966; Brown et al. 1979). For this reason and because of the high rate of complications, gynecologic oncologists have been reluctant to undertake external irradiation to paraaortic fields without histologic confirmation of treatable metastatic tumor within the extended ports. Complications of both surgery and radiation have been reduced by confining exploration of the pelvis and paraaortic areas to retroperitoneal approaches (Schellhas 1975) or by means of lymphangiographic screening and percutaneous needle biopsies of suspicious nodes (Zornoza et al. 1977). Lymphangiography, of course, may be less valid because of significantly common false negative nodes (Benninghoff, Herman, and Nelson 1966; Brown et al. 1979). Large primary tumors, those most often associated with metastases to pelvic nodes (Berman et al. 1977), are also associated with paraaortic and distant metastases (Casey and Watson 1974; Nelson et al. 1977).

Radiotherapy Techniques

In view of the current understanding of this disease and available therapeutic modalities, we prefer irradiation using supervoltage external therapy and brachytherapy with meticulously placed and balanced sources (Fletcher 1971; Marcial 1977) to cover the lymphatics of the parametria, obturator, hypogastric, external iliac, and lower common iliac node groups, and fully encompass the pelvic tumor as determined by examination under anesthesia. Following external radiotherapy of 4000 to 5000 rad over four to six weeks, radium or cesium after-loading applicators are operatively places using roentgenographic control with the patient under anesthesia, with optimal application ascertained by physical examination and x-ray. Usually, two brachytherapy applications are used at two- to three-week intervals, but individualization is the rule.

Follow-up and Surgical Salvage

When posttreatment examinations reveal complete response of the primary tumor, total reevaluation is carried out at about three months. In the absence of metastatic disease determined by physical examination, biochemistry, scanning, and roentgenographs (Casey and Watson 1974), examination under anesthesia with endoscopy and biopsies may be used to corroborate the clinical impression. Although central residual cervical carcinomas can be extirpated, the postirradiation prognosis is not good (Barber 1967; Pilleron et al. 1974). Nonetheless, the 20% to 40% survival results with radical surgery in these patients still exceeds expectations from primary therapy of many other tumors. Therefore surgical exploration to determine resectability should be done in the rare event of persistent central tumor without evidence of extrapelvic dissemination. Furthermore, there may be a place for early surgical exploration by the retroperitoneal approach (Schellhas 1975) several months after primary therapy in those patients in whom work-up reveals excellent response of the central tumor. Removal of paraaortic nodes with microscopic metastases and subsequent paraaortic external irradiation (Lepanto et al. 1975; Piver and Barlow 1977) or application of newer techniques of intraoperative irradiation, currently being investigated (Goldson et al. 1978), may salvage some of these patients, and the risks would seem to be worth taking.

Glandular Carcinomas

Fewer than 10% of cervical cancers are adenocarcinomas (Tasker and Collins 1974); the majority of these are of the endocervical cell type. Mixed adenosquamous carcinomas, clear cell, and mesonephric tumors and even more unusual varieties of glandular tumors combine to make up only 10% of all primary adenocarcinomas. Some investigators have called attention to a decreasing ratio of epidermoid carcinomas to adenocarcinomas as the proportion of the latter appears to be rising.

Clear Cell Carcinomas

Epidemiology

Astute observations, clinicopathologic correlation, and a carefully designed epidemiologic study led to the discovery of an association between maternal ingestion of nonsteroidal estrogens during the first trimester of pregnancy and the subsequent development of clear cell vaginal and cervical adenocarcinomas in their young offspring (Herbst et al. 1971, 1979a). The drugs had been prescribed in the belief that they could be beneficial in saving pregnancies threatened by spontaneous abortion in patients with medical histories of low fertility. This information (Herbst et al. 1971) placed the medical community and the population on the alert to avoid the use of estrogenic hormones during pregnancy, although subsequent findings have resulted in the diagnoses of a very small proportion of this disease among the offspring of the many women who used these medications (Herbst et al. 1974).

Prognosis

Fifty-seven percent of clear cell adenocarcinomas were diagnosed while they were still confined to the cervix or vagina (Herbst et al. 1979a); retrospective analysis of all cervical carcinomas in a large series disclosed that only 38% were confined to the cervix when first discovered (Tasker and Collins 1974). Prognosis for survival of patients with this tumor and the likelihood of lymph node metastases are related to tumor diameter and depth of invasion. Although lymphatic metastases may occur with small tumors and with superficial invasion less than 3 mm, pelvic node metastases were usually associated only with the larger, more deeply infiltrating tumors. Tumors confined to the cervix and vagina were associated with at least 17% pelvic nodes positive for tumor emboli, and when tumors invaded underlying tissues, more than one-third were found to have metastases to the pelvic lymph nodes (Herbst et al. 1974). When lymph nodes are involved the prognosis is grave.

Nonestrogen-Associated Tumors

Interviews and reviews of past medical records disclosed that clear cell adenocarcinomas may develop also in the absence of evidence for in utero gestational exposure to nonsteroidal estrogens (Herbst et al. 1974; Noller et al. 1976). While increased numbers of clear cell carcinomas have been noted at the Mayo Clinic since 1960, most were not related to known exposure to exogenous estrogens (Noller et al. 1974). These tumors usually cause abnormal vaginal bleeding, but they may be asymptomatic and associated with normal Pap smears (Herbst et al. 1974). They are rare before age 14 years, have a peak incidence at 17 to 21 years of age, and are not influenced by the use of hormonal birth control medications (Herbst et al. 1979b).

Detection and Management

Case findings and management of clear cell vaginal and cervical carcinomas should begin with the thorough gynecologic evaluation of all premenarchal children with symptoms of vaginal bleeding. A maternal history of steroidal medications during pregnancy should lead to examination of female offspring at menarche or around 13 years of age. Careful visualization and palpatory examination may be more revealing than cytology or colposcopy. Biopsy should be taken of any questionable lesion, and abnormal Pap smears should lead to further evaluation. Surgery is favored if resection by radical hysterectomy with or without partial or complete vaginectomy could be expected to extirpate the primary tumor with good margins. While small tumors may be controlled with radiation (Wharton et al. 1975), poor results have generally been achieved with radiotherapy alone (Nordquist et al. 1976; Herbst et al. 1979a). On the other hand, excellent results and ovarian conservation have been achieved with surgery (Herbst et al. 1974, 1979a; Nordquist et al. 1976). Because of the propensity of this tumor to metastasize to regional lymphatics, pelvic lymphadenectomies should be included until their worth can be determined. The small amount of analyzable material available at this time indicates little if any hope for survival when lymphatic spaces or nodes are involved (Noller et al. 1976). Advanced tumors beyond the scope of surgical resectability may be treated with radiation, but the prognosis for control is poor (Noller et al. 1976; Herbst et al. 1979b). Fortunately, the discovery of many of these tumors at an early stage allows potentially curative surgery.

Risk of Clear Cell and Epidermoid Cancer after Estrogen Exposure

The likelihood of developing a glandular cervicovaginal carcinoma is very low for young women exposed in utero to nonsteroidal estrogens (Lanier et al. 1973; Herbst et al. 1974). As a better understanding of the embryologic development of the Müllerian system emerges through clinical and experimental animal studies, the natural history of vaginal adenosis unfolds (Ng et al. 1977). The extensive areas of squamous metaplasia noted in the cervixes of these young women have been proposed by some as fertile fields for the development of epidermoid carcinomas, and an increased risk for intraepithelial neoplasms has been suspected (Mattingly and Stafl 1976). Others, however, have found no increased incidence of squamous cell neoplasms among these young women (Robboy et al. 1977; Burke, Antonioli, and Rosen 1978). Whether or not young women exposed in utero to nonsteroidal estrogens are at greater risk for squamous dysplasia because of the apparent necessity of transforming factor(s) for the genesis of these neoplasms, it is expected that the probability of developing this disease will closely parallel the patient's sexual practices (Kessler 1976).

Endocervical Adenocarcinoma

Adenocarcinomas of the cervix of endocervical type are present in about the same distribution by stage as epidermoid carcinomas (Tasker and Collins 1974). Increasing tumor size has been associated with poor prognosis (Wheeless et al. 1970; Rutledge et al. 1975). Excellent results have been achieved in early tumors using radical surgery, with little further gained by adjuvant radiotherapy. Endocervical adenocarcinomas, as distinguished from clear cell carcinomas, occurred in older age groups who also had the highest incidence of cervical squamous cell carcinomas. Prognosis for survival in this disease was related to histologic differentiation of the tumor; anaplastic cancers had the poorest outlook. It remains to be seen whether a combination of modified radiotherapy and extrafascial hysterectomy will improve prognosis and diminish central recurrences beyond the rather poor results that were obtained by radiation therapy alone for large barrel-shaped endophytic adenocarcinomas (Kagan et al. 1973). As with squamous carcinomas, advanced endocervical adenocarcinomas must be treated with radiation therapy, but the results have not been favorable (Rutledge et al. 1975; Hurt et al. 1977).

Adenoepidermoid Carcinoma

Rarer types of glandular malignancy such as adenoepidermoid carcinoma and its poorly differentiated variety, the so-called glassy-cell carcinoma, and adenoid cystic carcinoma are associated with poor prognoses whether treated with surgery or radiation therapy (Wheeless et al. 1970; Seltzer et al. 1979; Hoskins et al. 1979). A radical approach with extensive resection and lymphadenectomies followed by postoperative radiation therapy might improve the outlook.

Cervical Cancer in Pregnancy

The experience of one of the major cancer centers of the United States showed that the prognosis for patients whose diagnosis of cervical cancer was made while pregnant was no worse than for those who were not pregnant (Creasman et al. 1970). More advanced tumors were diagnosed in the later phases of pregnancy and in the immediate postpartum period than earlier in pregnancy. This led to the conclusion that diagnosis during pregnancy resulted from failure to screen and detect early and preinvasive neoplasms in sexually active women. The more advanced tumors found in later pregnancy and postpartum were, of course, associated with poorer prognoses than were those diagnosed at an earlier stage. Treatment using radiotherapy led to a disease-free survival for 43 of 47 patients (91%) with stage I carcinomas and 27 of 37 patients (73%) with stage II disease. These results were similar to those achieved in the treatment of cervical cancer in nonpregnant patients.

Surgical management of early cancers of the cervix in pregnancy has also led to excellent results. Three separate series reported survival without evidence of cancer in nearly 100% of pregnant patients who were treated with radical surgery for carcinomas confined to the cervix (Kelso and Funnell 1973; Sall et al. 1974; Thompson et al. 1975). It appeared that only patients with neglected tumors had a poor prognosis. One group of oncologists followed a policy of treating cervical cancers in pregnancy with external radiotherapy followed by radical surgery, and reported a five-year survival of nine of nine patients with stage I and five of five patients with stage II disease (Kelso and Funnell 1973). Although radical radiotherapy alone proved as effective as surgery when employed for cancers confined to the cervix (Creasman et al. 1970; Thompson et al. 1975), each group used radiotherapy for more advanced cancers and reported rather poor results with the small number of patients treated. Patients with intraepithelial carcinoma detected during pregnancy fared well when treated conventionally during the postpartum period, with no apparent compromise by vaginal delivery (Boutselis 1972).

Based on these observations, management of pregnancy should include careful visualization and cytologic screening of the cervix early in pregnancy if not already done. High-risk patients should be considered for reevaluation of the cervix later in their pregnancy. All abnormal lesions should be biopsied and if cytology deviates from normal the patient should be evaluated by colposcopy and directed biopsies. By these procedures virtually all invasive tumors will be detected (Abitabol, Benjamin, and Gastillo 1973a). The everted cervix of pregnancy lends itself to colposcopic examination; thus preinvasive lesions may be safely followed throughout pregnancy. Unless colposcopy and selected punch biopsies reveal very extensive severe intraepithelial neoplasms with suspicion of microinvasive disease, cervical conization with its risks for serious complications should be avoided during pregnancy. In the unlikely event that conization is required care must be taken to prevent disruption of the endocervical canal by designing a shallow cone to encompass the lesion. Once the pregnancy is completed the carcinoma can be safely treated in the puerperium by conventional means. If a cesarean section is indicated, hysterectomy can be carried out at the same time with little or no increase in postoperative morbidity (Abitabol, Benjamin, and Gastillo 1973b). Before undertaking this operation, the lesion must be well defined so that it will be encompassed by the surgery. Otherwise, cesarean section may be done for obstetrical indications and conization or hysterectomy, as indicated, may be delayed until the postpartum period.

When the diagnosis of microinvasive or early invasive cancer is made during pregnancy, consideration of fetal viability is important in determining therapy. Radical surgery or radiotherapy may be chosen (Creasman et al. 1970; Thompson et al. 1975). In most cases, surgery with ovarian conservation would be favored (Webb 1975). Advanced tumors of any stage should be managed with radiation therapy. Vaginal delivery may be followed by postpartum radical surgery in women with very early invasion; because of the danger of serious hemorrhage, patients with larger tumors should be delivered by cesarean section. The mode of delivery has no deleterious effects on either maternal or fetal survival (Creasman et al. 1970; Thompson et al. 1975). Postpartum treatment should proceed along the lines of management already discussed for nonpregnant patients.

Management of Recurrent Carcinoma

The pioneering work at the Memorial Sloan-Kettering Cancer Center has given a second opportunity to many women who failed to have their primary cervical cancers controlled by surgery or radiation (Barber 1967). Radical surgery for patients who had failed primary treatment with surgery resulted in 20% five-year survival rates among 222 patients at that institution (Barber and O'Neil 1971). Surgery following failure of radiation resulted in five-year survival rates of less than 20% when exenteration was needed to encompass the recurrent tumor to over 40% when resection could be accomplished by a lesser procedure (Barber 1967; Symmonds et al. 1975). The results of exenterative surgery for recurrent cancer can be improved by strict adherence to criteria for indications and contraindications and through improvements in techniques.

A higher incidence of malignant nodal disease was found in patients treated for recurrent cervical cancer (26.5%) compared with those who were being primarily treated (40%) (Barber and O'Neil 1971). In turn, survival was extremely rare in patients found to have metastatic tumor to lymph nodes when they were treated with surgery for postirradiation recurrences. Patients treated with exenteration for postsurgical recurrences fared no better when measured by five-year survival rates than those who were treated after radiation failure (Symmonds et al. 1975); however, morbidity secondary to loss of bowel integrity and fistulization was considerably more frequent in patients having operation after heavy irradiation to the pelvis.

As with most solid tumors, the first treatment of cervical cancer is the best. In one recent large series, an 87% five-year survival rate was accomplished with radical surgery for primary stage I carcinomas only, and 22.5% of the patients survived five years after being treated with surgery for postirradiation recurrences (Collins and Allen 1970). Although in the United States surgery has been the preferred treatment for recurrent disease after irradiation, elsewhere re-irradiation has been advocated. When performed by one group with an aim to cure, results rivaled those achieved with pelvic exenterations (Kitchen 1975). Some hope for survival may be achieved even when radiation is delivered with a palliative intent. Most postsurgical recurrences are not amenable to surgical resection; however, modern high-energy radiation with brachytherapy by applications or implants may be effective in the control of some of these tumors (Kitchen 1975; Marcial 1977).

As yet, no prospective comparison has been made between surgery and radiotherapy in the management of postsurgical central recurrences. Because of the implications of re-irradiation for the development of serious necrotic complications, a surgical approach to post-irradiation failures is currently indicated. At times it is impossible to ascertain the presence of cancer in the midst of massive radiation necrosis (Barber and Brunschwig 1970; Symmonds et al. 1975). Occasionally, these patients may be palliated by definitive resection. Survival of patients following exenteration is poor even in the absence of recurrent cancer. Furthermore, although careful histologic examinations of the removed tissues may show only radionecrosis with no malignancy, some patients may eventually succumb to metastatic disease. Therefore diligent preoperative search must be made to lessen the chances of this (Casey and Watson 1974). The psychological, financial, and social costs, debility, and functional disability following exenterative surgery can be staggering. This operation should be done only when the central mass can be widely resected; it has no place in palliative management.

Persistent or recurrent intraepithelial carcinoma following surgical treatment usually represents incomplete removal of the lesion, and can be effectively treated by means of simple resective surgery (Jimerson and Merrill 1976). Dysplasia arising in the cervix following radiation treatment of invasive disease may have different implications (Wentz and Reagan 1970). The prognosis for these lesions is as yet uncertain; but in one clinical series, this diagnosis within the first three months after treatment was associated with a 70% rate of tumor recurrence and an extremely poor five-year survival rate of 33.8%, with only 7% of patients surviving at eight years (Wentz and Reagan 1970). Postirradiation dysplasia that developed after three years was followed by a 44% recurrence rate and an eight-year survival rate of 84.6%. These figures are of great interest, as the occasional isolated experiences of many gynecologists have led to the expectation of a relatively benign course for these lesions. While biopsy is mandatory to rule out the presence of recurrent invasive cancer, surgical treatment has been frustrating because these tumors tend to be multicentric and may recur after simple surgical excisions. Furthermore, the danger of fistulization and necrosis is always possible with surgical approach to these intraepithelial tumors in the irradiated mucosa. The established effectiveness of topical 5-fluorouracil cream (Ballon, Roberts, and Lagasse 1979) led to a trial of this medication, which has proved effective in treatment of postirradiation dysplasia as well (Daly and Ellis 1980).

Antineoplastic Chemotherapy

An intensive review of the literature and studies reported to the National Cancer Institute, Division of Cancer Treatment concluded that the alkylating agents, bleomycin, mitomycin, and vincristine all showed cytotoxic activity against cervical carcinoma (Wasserman and Carter 1977). Subsequently, others have reported activity as measured by objective responses for 5-fluorouracil in the treatment of these tumors (Malkasian et al. 1977). A comparison of doxorubicin (Adriamycin) with moderate-dose methotrexate or high-dose methotrexate and citrovorum factor rescue showed objective responses with each regimen ranging from 29% to 42% measured by partial regressions in tumor sizes (Cavins and Geisler 1978). Responses were short-lived, lasting only two to six months, and complete responses were rare. Doxorubicin and methotrexate were used in combination in two studies that reported dissimilar results. One group (Haid et al. 1977) reported partial responses in only 2 of 16 patients (12.5%) treated, while the other (Guthrie and Way 1978) claimed a response rate of 66% (partial responses 26 of 59, complete responses 13 of 59) with higher but tolerable dosages. Doxorubicin alone in one large series gave a response rate of only 6%; when used in combination with 5-fluorouracil and cyclophosphamide, objective responses were achieved in four of seven patients treated (Piver et al. 1978). Clinical trials with newer drugs such as cisplatin (DDP) (Cohen et al. 1978) and newer combinations such as doxorubicin and methyl-CCNU (Day et al. 1978) have led to encouraging reports of objective responses. Polychemotherapy has been associated with response rates no better than those achieved with simpler, less toxic combination therapies (Forney et al. 1975). Perhaps the most encouraging results have been achieved with regimens containing sequential combinations of bleomycin and mitomycin, with objective response rates of over 50% and improvement in survival curves (Miyamoto et al. 1978; Baker et al. 1978). Progestational agents have been ineffective (Malkasian et al. 1977).

Although treatments with cytotoxic agents have been followed by tumor regressions with relief of obstruction and pain, no cures have been credited to these drugs. Attempts to deliver high tumor doses and reduce systemic toxicities led to a number of experiments in the 1960s with intraarterial infusions with mixed results. Recently, pelvic arterial infusion of methotrexate with folinic acid (citrovorum factor) and vincristine was reported to be of limited if any value, giving partial responses in only 3 of 14 patients and no demonstrable increase in survival (Lifshitz et al. 1978). Development of drugs that may localize in squamous cell tumors, better understanding of the cell cycle, and safer management of toxicities may lead to more effective chemotherapy for recurrent cancer by systemic administration or arterial infusion, and perhaps as an adjunct to surgery and/or radiation therapy.

Conclusions

The solution to cervical carcinoma lies in prevention. Avoidance of drugs in pregnancy that may result in congenital deformities of the reproductive tract has been made possible by the astute observations of investigators over the past decade. Screening methods by cytology and colposcopy allow diagnosis of cervical neoplasms in their earliest preinvasive forms, when they may be eliminated by simple cauterization or excision. An understanding of the epidemiology and natural history of the disease may one day lead to the elimination of a transmissable etiologic agent. The development of higher-energy radiation sources, sophisticated computerized dosimetry, and greater clinical skills in radiotherapy and patient support are leading to improvement in survival rates, not only for early but for more advanced tumors.

References

Abitabol, M. M.; Benjamin, F.; and Gastillo, N. Management of the abnormal cervical smear and carcinoma in situ of the cervix during pregnancy. *Am. J. Obstet. Gynecol.* 117:904–908, 1973a.

Abitabol, M. M.; Benjamin, F.; and Gastillo, N. Cesarian hysterectomy in the treatment of carcinoma in situ of the cervix diagnosed during pregnancy. *Am. J. Obstet. Gynecol.* 117:909–912, 1973b.

Adcock, L. A. Radical hysterectomy preceded by pelvic irradiation. *Gynecol. Oncol.* 8:152–163, 1979.

Ahlgren, M. et al. Conization as treatment of carcinoma in situ of the uterine cervix. *Obstet. Gynecol.* 46:135–139, 1975.

American Cancer Society. *Cancer-related checkup: guidelines for site tests and examinations.* New York: American Cancer Society, 1979.

American College of Obstetricians and Gynecologists. *Technical bulletin no. 47.* Chicago: American College of Obstetricians and Gynecologists, 1977.

Aurelian, L. Persistence and expression of herpes simplex virus type 2 genome in cervical tumor cells. *Cancer Res.* 34:1126–1135, 1974.

Averette, H. E. et al. Diagnosis and management of microinvasive (stage IA) carcinoma of the uterine cervix. *Cancer* 38:414–425, 1976.

Baker, L. H. et al. Mitomycin C, vincristine, and bleomycin therapy for advanced cervical cancer. *Obstet. Gynecol.* 52:146–150, 1978.

Ballon, S. C.; Roberts, J. A.; and Lagasse, L. D. Topical 5-fluorouracil in the treatment of intraepithelial neoplasia of the vagina. *Obstet. Gynecol.* 54:163–166, 1979.

Barber, H. R. K. Results of surgical treatment of cancer of the cervix at the Memorial–James Ewing Hospitals, New York. In *Advances in obstetrics and gynecology,* eds. S. L. Marcus and C. C. Marcus. Baltimore: Williams & Wilkins, 1967, pp. 622–632.

Barber, H. R. K. et al. Vascular invasion as a prognostic factor in stage IB cancer of the cervix. *Obstet. Gynecol.* 52:343–348, 1978.

Barber, H. R. K., and Brunschwig, A. Definitive treatment of radiation necrosis. Five-year results in 77 patients. *Obstet. Gynecol.* 35:344–350, 1970.

Barber, H. R. K., and O'Neil, W. H. Recurrent cervical cancer after treatment by a primary surgical program. *Obstet. Gynecol.* 37:165–172, 1971.

Barron, B. A.; Cahill, M. C.; and Richart, R. M. Statistical model of natural history of cervical neoplastic disease. Duration of carcinoma in situ. *Gynecol. Oncol.* 6:196–205, 1978.

Barron, B. A., and Richart, R. M. Statistical model of the natural history of cervical carcinoma based on a prospective study of 557 cases. *J. Natl. Cancer Inst.* 41:1343–1353, 1968.

Barron, B. A., and Richart, R. M. Epidemiologic study of cervical neoplastic disease. Based upon a self-selected sample of 7000 women in Barbados, West Indies. *Cancer* 27:978–986, 1971.

Benninghoff, D. L.; Herman, P. G.; and Nelson, J. H., Jr. Clinicopathologic correlation of lymphangiography and lymph node metastases in gynecologic neoplasms. *Cancer* 19:885–888, 1966.

Berman, J. L. et al. Operative evaluation of patients with cervical carcinoma by an extraperitoneal approach. *Obstet. Gynecol.* 50:658–664, 1977.

Boutselis, J. G. Intraepithelial carcinoma of the cervix associated with pregnancy. *Obstet. Gynecol.* 40:657–666, 1972.

Brown, R. C. et al. Accuracy of lymphangiography in the diagnosis of paraaortic lymph node metastases from carcinoma of the cervix. *Obstet. Gynecol.* 54:571–575, 1979.

Buchsbaum, H. J. Paraaortic lymph node involvement in cervical carcinoma. *Am. J. Obstet. Gynecol.* 113:942–947, 1972.

Burch, J. C., and Chalfant, R. L. Preoperative radium irradiation and radical hysterectomy in the treatment of cancer of the cervix. *Am. J. Obstet. Gynecol.* 106:1054–1064, 1970.

Burghardt, E., and Pickel, H. Local spread and lymph node involvement in cervical cancer. *Obstet. Gynecol.* 52:138–145, 1978.

Burke, L.; Antonioli, D.; and Rosen, S. Vaginal and cervical squamous cell dysplasia in women exposed to diethylstilbestrol in utero. *Am. J. Obstet. Gynecol.* 132:537–544, 1978.

Casey, M. J., and Watson, R. C. Roentgenographic techniques in the evaluation of epidermoid carcinoma of the cervix uteri. *Surg. Obstet. Gynecol.* 139:367–369, 1974.

Cavins, J. A., and Geisler, H. E. Treatment of advanced unresectable cervical carcinoma already subjected to complete irradiation therapy. *Gynecol. Oncol.* 6: 256–260, 1978.

Chanen, W., and Hollyock, V. E. Colposcopy and electrocoagulation-diathermy for cervical dysplasia and carcinoma in situ. *Obstet. Gynecol.* 37:623–628, 1971.

Cherry, C. P., and Glücksmann, A. Lymphatic emboli and lymph node metastasis in cancers of the vulva and uterine cervix. *Cancer* 8:564–575, 1955.

Christopherson, W. M. Dysplasia, carcinoma in situ and microinvasive carcinoma of the uterine cervix. *Hum. Pathol.* 8:489–501, 1977.

Cohen, C. J. et al. Treatment of advanced squamous cell carcinoma of the cervix with Cis-platinum (II) diamminedichloride (NSC 119875). *Am. J. Obstet. Gynecol.* 130:853–854, 1978.

Collins, J. A., and Allen, H. H. Surgical management of carcinoma of the cervix. *Am. J. Obstet. Gynecol.* 108:441–444, 1970.

Coppleson, M. Carcinoma of the cervix, epidemiology and aetiology. *Br. J. Hosp. Med.* 2:960–980, 1969.

Creasman, W. T. et al. Carcinoma of the cervix associated with pregnancy. *Obstet. Gynecol.* 36:495–501, 1970.

Creasman, W. T. et al. Efficacy of cryosurgical treatment of severe cervical intraepithelial neoplasia. *Obstet. Gynecol.* 41:501–506, 1973.

Daly, J. W., and Ellis, G. F. Treatment of vaginal dysplasia and carcinoma in situ with topical 5-fluorouracil. *Obstet. Gynecol.* 55:350–352, 1980.

Day, T. G., Jr. et al. Chemotherapy for squamous carcinoma of the cervix: doxorubicin-methyl-CCNU. *Am. J. Obstet. Gynecol.* 132:545–548, 1978.

Dickinson, L. E. Control of cancer of the uterine cervix by cytologic screening. *Gynecol. Oncol.* 3:1–9, 1975.

Dowdle, W. R. et al. Association of *Herpesvirus hominus* to site of recovery. *J. Immunol.* 99:974–980, 1967.

Dunn, J. E. Relationship between carcinoma in situ and invasive cervical carcinoma. *Cancer* 6:873–886, 1953.

Easley, J. D., and Fletcher, G. H. Analysis of the treatment of stage I and stage II carcinomas of the uterine cervix. *Am. J. Roentgenol.* 111:243–248, 1971.

Feldman, M. J. et al. Abnormal cervical cytology in the teen-ager: a continuing problem. *Am. J. Obstet. Gynecol.* 126: 418–421, 1976.

Fennell, R. H., Jr. Microinvasive carcinoma of the uterine cervix. *Obstet. Gynecol. Surv.* 33:406–411, 1978.

Figge, D. C. et al. Cervical cancer after initial negative and atypical vaginal cytology. *Am. J. Obstet. Gynecol.* 108:422–428, 1970.

Fletcher, G. H. Cancer of the uterine cervix: Janeway lecture, 1970. *Am. J. Roentgenol.* 111:225–242, 1971.

Fletcher, G. H., and Rutledge, F. N. Extended-field technique in the management of the cancers of the uterine cervix. *Am. J. Roentgenol.* 114:116–122, 1972.

Forney, J. P. et al. Seven-drug polychemotherapy in the treatment of advanced and recurrent squamous carcinoma of the female genital tract. *Am. J. Obstet. Gynecol.* 123:748–752, 1975.

Fox, C. H. Biological behavior of dysplasia and carcinoma in situ. *Am. J. Obstet. Gynecol.* 99:960–984, 1967.

Gad, C., and Koch, F. Limitation of screening effect. A review of cervical disorders in previously screened women. *Acta Cytol.* 21:719–722, 1978.

Gagon, F. Lack of occurrence of cervical carcinoma in nuns. *Proceedings of the Second National Cancer Conference.* 1:625–638, 1952.

Garcia, R. L. et al. Evaluation of cone biopsy in the management of carcinoma in situ of the cervix. *Gynecol. Oncol.* 3:32–39, 1975.

Goldson, A. L. et al. Intraoperative radiation of the paraaortic nodes in cancer of the uterine cervix. *Obstet. Gynecol.* 52:713–717, 1978.

Gusberg, S. B. Cancer of the cervix. Diagnosis and principles of treatment. In *Corscaden's gynecologic oncology,* 5th edition, eds. S. B. Gusberg and H. C. Frick II. Baltimore: Williams & Wilkins, 1978, pp. 152–153.

Guthrie, D., and Way, S. Use of Adriamycin and methotrexate in carcinoma of the cervix. The development of a safe effective regimen. *Obstet. Gynecol.* 52:349–354, 1978.

Haid, M. et al. Adriamycin-methotrexate combination chemotherapy of advanced carcinoma of the cervix. *Obstet. Gynecol.* 50:103–105, 1977.

Herbst, A. L. et al. Adenocarcinoma of the vagina. Association of maternal stilbestrol therapy with tumor appearance in young women. *N. Engl. J. Med.* 284:878–881, 1971.

Herbst, A. L. et al. Clear cell adenocarcinoma of the vagina and cervix in girls: analysis of 170 registry cases. *Am. J. Obstet. Gynecol.* 119:713–726, 1974.

Herbst, A. L. et al. Analysis of 346 cases of clear cell adenocarcinoma of the vagina and cervix with emphasis on recurrence and survival. *Gynecol. Oncol.* 7:111–122, 1979a.

Herbst, A. L. et al. Epidemiologic aspects and factors related to survival in 384 registry cases of clear cell adenocarcinoma of the vagina and cervix. *Am. J. Obstet. Gynecol.* 135:876–886, 1979b.

Hoskins, W. J. et al. Adenoid cystic carcinoma of the cervix uteri: report of six cases and review of the literature. *Gynecol. Oncol.* 7:371–384, 1979.

Hurt, W. G. et al. Adenocarcinoma of the cervix: histopathologic and clinical features. *Am. J. Obstet. Gynecol.* 129:304–315, 1977.

Jafari, K. False-negative Pap smear in uterine malignancy. *Gynecol. Oncol.* 6:76–82, 1978.

Jimerson, G. K., and Merrill, J. A. Cancer and dysplasia of the posthysterectomy vaginal cuff. *Gynecol. Oncol.* 4:328–334, 1976.

Kagan, A. R. et al. Adenocarcinoma of the uterine cervix. *Am. J. Obstet. Gynecol.* 117:464–468, 1973.

Kaufman, R. H. et al. Cervical cytology in the teenage patient. *Am. J. Obstet. Gynecol.* 108:515–519, 1970.

Kelso, J. W., and Funnell, J. D. Combined surgical and radiation treatment of invasive carcinoma of the cervix. *Am. J. Obstet. Gynecol.* 116:205–213, 1973.

Kessler, I. I. Perspectives on the epidemiology of cervical cancer with special reference to the herpes virus hypothesis. *Cancer Res.* 34:1091–1110, 1974.

Kessler, I. I. Human cervical cancer as a venereal disease. *Cancer Res.* 36:783–791, 1976.

Kirkland, J. A. Study of chromosomes in cervical neoplasia. *Obstet. Gynecol. Surv.* 24:784–794, 1969.

Kitchen, D. H. Treatment of recurrent cervical cancer. *Aust. N.Z.J. Obstet. Gynecol.* 14:125–133, 1975.

Kling, T. G., and Buchsbaum, H. J. Cervical carcinoma in women under twenty-one years of age. *Obstet. Gynecol.* 42:205–207, 1973.

Kolbenstvedt, A., and Kolstad, P. Difficulties of complete pelvic lymph node dissection in radical hysterectomy for carcinoma of the cervix. *Gynecol. Oncol.* 4:244–254, 1976.

Kolstad, P., and Klem, V. Long-term follow-up of 1121 cases of carcinoma in situ. *Obstet. Gynecol.* 48:125–129, 1976.

Koss, L. G. Concept of genesis and development of carcinoma of the cervix. *Obstet. Gynecol. Surv.* 24:850–860, 1969.

Koss, L. G. et al. Some histological aspects of behavior of epidermoid carcinoma in situ and related lesions of the uterine cervix. *Cancer* 16:1160–1211, 1963.

Kottmeier, H. L. Surgical and radiation therapy of invasive carcinoma of the uterine cervix. *Acta Obstet. Gynecol. Scand.* 43(suppl. 2):1–48, 1964.

Lagasse, L. D. et al. Effect of radiation therapy on pelvic lymph node involvement in stage I carcinoma of the cervix. *Am. J. Obstet. Gynecol.* 119:328–334, 1974.

Lanier, A. P. et al. Cancer and stilbestrol. A follow-up of 1719 persons exposed to estrogens in utero and born 1943–1959. *Mayo Clin. Proc.* 48:793–799, 1973.

Lepanto, P. et al. Treatment of para-aortic nodes in carcinoma of the cervix. *Cancer* 35:1510–1513, 1975.

Lifshitz, S. et al. Intraarterial pelvic infusion chemotherapy in advanced gynecologic cancer. *Obstet. Gynecol.* 52:476–480, 1978.

Lu, T. et al. Barrel-shaped cervical carcinoma. *Am. J. Obstet. Gynecol.* 124:596–600, 1976.

Malkasian, G. D., Jr. et al. Chemotherapy of carcinoma of the cervix. *Gynecol. Oncol.* 5:109–120, 1977.

Marcial, V. A. Carcinoma of the cervix. Present status and future. *Cancer* 39:945–958, 1977.

Masubuchi, K. et al. Five-year cure rate for carcinoma of the cervix uteri. With special reference to the comparison of surgical and radiation therapy. *Am. J. Obstet. Gynecol.* 103:566–573, 1969.

Mattingly, R. F., and Stafl, A. Cancer risk in diethylstilbestrol-exposed offspring. *Am. J. Obstet. Gynecol.* 126:543–548, 1976.

Melamed, M. R. et al. Prevalence rates of uterine cervical carcinoma in situ for women using the diaphragm or contraceptive oral steriods. *Br. Med. J.* 3:195–200, 1969.

Miyamoto, T. et al. Effectiveness of a sequential combination of bleomycin and mitomycin C on an advanced cervical cancer. *Cancer* 41:403–414, 1978.

Morley, G. W., and Seski, J. C. Radical pelvic surgery versus radiation therapy for stage I carcinoma of the cervix (exclusive of microinvasion). *Am. J. Obstet. Gynecol.* 126:785–789, 1976.

Naib, Z. M. et al. Genital herpetic infection. Association with cervical cysplasia and carcinoma. *Cancer* 23: 940–945, 1969.

Nealon, N. A., and Christopherson, W. M. Cervical cancer precursors in young offspring of low-income families. *Obstet. Gynecol.* 54:135–139, 1979.

Nelson, A. J., III. et al. Indications for adjunctive conservative extrafascial hysterectomy in selected cases of carcinoma of the uterine cervix. *Am. J. Roentgenol.* 123:91–99, 1975.

Nelson, J. H., Jr. et al. Incidence, significance and follow-up of para-aortic lymph node metastases in late invasive carcinoma of the cervix. *Am. J. Obstet. Gynecol.* 128:336–340, 1977.

Ng, A. B. P. et al. Natural history of vaginal adenosis in women exposed to diethylstilbestrol in utero. *J. Reprod. Med.* 18:1–13, 1977.

Noller, K. L. et al. Mesonephric (clear cell) carcinoma of the vagina and cervix. *Obstet. Gynecol.* 43:640–644, 1974.

Noller, K. L. et al. Clear-cell adenocarcinoma of the vagina and cervix: survival data. *Am. J. Obstet. Gynecol.* 124:285–288, 1976.

Nordquist, S. R. B. et al. Clear cell adenocarcinoma of the cervix and vagina. A clinicopathologic study of 21 cases with and without a history of maternal ingestion of estrogens. *Cancer* 37:858–871, 1976.

Ory, H. W. et al. Epidemiology and interrelationship of cervical dysplasia and type 2 herpesvirus in a low income housing project. *Am. J. Obstet. Gynecol.* 123:269–274, 1975.

Ory, H. W. et al. Contraceptive choice and prevalence of cervical dysplasia and carcinoma in situ. *Am. J. Obstet. Gynecol.* 124:573–577, 1976.

Paunier, J. P. et al. Causes, time of death and sites of failure in squamous cell carcinoma of the uterine cervix on intact uterus. *Radiology* 88:555–562, 1967.

Perez, C. A. et al. Prognostic significance of endometrial extension from primary carcinoma of the uterine cervix. *Cancer* 35:1493–1504, 1975.

Pilleron, J. P. et al. Prognostic value of node metastases in cancer of the uterine cervix. *Am. J. Obstet. Gynecol.* 119:458–462, 1974.

Piver, M. S. et al. Paraaortic lymph node irradiation for carcinoma of the uterine cervix using split-course technique. *Gynecol. Oncol.* 3:168–175, 1975.

Piver, M. S. et al. Adriamycin alone or in combination in 100 patients with carcinoma of the cervix or vagina. *Am. J. Obstet. Gynecol.* 131:311–313, 1978.

Piver, M. S., and Barlow, J. J. High-dose irradiation to biopsy-confirmed aortic node metastases from carcinoma of the uterine cervix. *Cancer* 39:1243–1246, 1977.

Rampone, J. F. et al. Combined treatment of stage IB carcinoma of the cervix. *Obstet. Gynecol.* 41:163–167, 1973.

Reagan, J. W., and Hamonic, M. J. Dysplasia of the uterine cervix. *Ann. NY Acad. Sci.* 63:1–36, 1956.

Richart, R. M. Natural history of cervical intraepithelial neoplasia. *Clin. Obstet. Gynecol.* 10:748–784, 1968.

Richart, R. M., and Barron, B. A. Follow-up study of patients with cervical dysplasia. *Am. J. Obstet. Gynecol.* 105:389–393, 1969.

Richart, R. M., and Vaillant, H. W. Influence of cell collection techniques upon cytological diagnosis. *Cancer* 18:1474–1478, 1965.

Robboy, S. J. et al. Squamous cell neoplasia controversy in the female exposed to diethylstilbestrol. *Hum. Pathol.* 8:483–485, 1977.

Roche, W. D., and Norris, H. J. Microinvasive carcinoma of the cervix. *Cancer* 36:180–196, 1975.

Rotkin, I. D. Comparison review of key epidemiological studies in cervical cancer related to current searches for transmissable agents. *Cancer Res.* 33:1353–1367, 1973.

Rubio, C. A., and Thomassen, P. Critical evaluation of the Schiller test in patients before conization. *Am. J. Obstet. Gynecol.* 125:96–99, 1976.

Rutledge, F. N. et al. Pelvic lymphadenectomy as an adjunct to radiation therapy in treatment for carcinoma of the cervix. *Am. J. Roentgenol.* 93:607–614, 1964.

Rutledge, F. N. et al. Adenocarcinoma of the uterine cervix. *Am. J. Obstet. Gynecol.* 122:236–245, 1975.

Sall, S. et al. Surgical management of invasive carcinoma of the cervix in pregnancy. *Am. J. Obstet. Gynecol.* 118:1–5, 1974.

Sandmire, H. F. et al. Carcinoma of the cervix in oral contraceptive steroid and IUD users and nonusers. *Am. J. Obstet. Gynecol.* 125:339–345, 1976.

Savage, E. W. Microinvasive carcinoma of the cervix. In *Obstetrics and gynecology annual,* vol. 1, ed. R. M. Wynn. New York: Appleton-Century-Crofts, 1972, pp. 453–476.

Schachter, J. et al. Chlamydial infection in women with cervical dysplasia. *Am. J. Obstet. Gynecol.* 123: 753–757, 1975.

Schellhas, H. F. Extraperitoneal para-aortic node dissection through an upper abdominal incision. *Obstet. Gynecol.* 46:444–447, 1975.

Sedlis, A. et al. Microinvasive carcinoma of the uterine cervix: a clinical pathologic study. *Am. J. Obstet. Gynecol.* 133:64–74, 1979.

Seltzer, V. et al. Glassy cell cervical carcinoma. *Gynecol. Oncol.* 8:141–151, 1979.

Sevin, B.-U. et al. Invasive cancer of the cervix after cryosurgery. Pitfalls of conservative management. *Obstet. Gynecol.* 53:465–471, 1979.

Shingleton, H. M. et al. Contribution of endocervical smears to cervical cancer detection. *Acta Cytol.* 19:261–264, 1975.

Shingleton, H. M. et al. Significance of age in the colposcopic evaluation of women with atypical Papanicolaou smears. *Obstet. Gynecol.* 49:61–62, 1977.

Silverberg, E. *Gynecologic cancer: statistical and epidemiological information.* New York: American Cancer Society, 1975.

Silverberg, E. Cancer statistics, 1982. *CA* 32:15–31, 1982.

Simon, J. W. Association of Herpes simplex virus and cervical cancer: a review. *Gynecol. Oncol.* 4:108–116, 1976.

Singer, A., and Reid, B. L. Does the male transmit cervical cancer? *Contemp. Ob/Gyn.* 13:173–180, 1979.

Snyder, R. N. et al. Dysplasia and carcinoma in situ of the uterine cervix: prevalence in very young women (under age 22). *Am. J. Obstet. Gynecol.* 124:751–756, 1976.

Spriggs, A. I., and Husain, O. A. N. Cervical smears. *Br. Med. J.* 1:1516–1518, 1977.

Stafl, A. et al. Laser treatment of cervical and vaginal neoplasia. *Am. J. Obstet. Gynecol.* 128:128–136, 1977.

Stafl, A., and Mattingly, R. F. Colposcopic diagnosis of cervical neoplasia. *Obstet. Gynecol.* 41:168–176, 1973.

Stern, E. et al. Contraceptive methods: selective factors in a study of dysplasia of the cervix. *Am. J. Pub. Health* 61:553–558, 1971.

Stern, E. et al. Steroid contraceptive use and cervical dysplasia: increased risk of progression. *Science* 196:1460–1462, 1977.

Stockbine, M. F. et al. Complications in 831 patients with squamous cell carcinoma of the intact uterine cervix treated with 3000 rad or more whole-pelvis irradiation. *Am. J. Roentgenol.* 108:293–304, 1970.

Surwit, E. A. et al. Radical hysterectomy with or without preoperative radium for stage IB squamous cell carcinoma of the cervix. *Obstet. Gynecol.* 48:130–133, 1976.

Surwit, E. A. et al. Radical hysterectomy with preoperative intracavity therapy for stage IB squamous cell carcinoma of the cervix. *Int. J. Roentgenol.* 4:865–871, 1978.

Symmonds, R. E. et al. Exenterative operations: experience with 198 patients. *Am. J. Obstet. Gynecol.* 121: 907–918, 1975.

Tasker, J. T., and Collins, J. A. Adenocarcinoma of the uterine cervix. *Am. J. Obstet. Gynecol.* 118:344–348, 1974.

Thompson, J. D. et al. Surgical management of invasive cancer of the cervix in pregnancy. *Am. J. Obstet. Gynecol.* 121:853–863, 1975.

Townsend, D. E. et al. Abnormal Papanicolaou smears, evaluation by colposcopy, biopsies, and endocervical curettage. *Am. J. Obstet. Gynecol.* 108:429–434, 1970.

Townsend, D. E., and Ostergard, D. R. Cryocauterization for preinvasive cervical neoplasia. *J. Reproduct. Med.* 6:171–176, 1971.

Tredway, D. R. et al. Colposcopy and cryosurgery in cervical intraepithelial neoplasia. *Am. J. Obstet. Gynecol.* 114:1020–1024, 1972.

Underwood, P. B., Jr. et al. Cryosurgery. Its use for the abnormal Pap smear. *Cancer* 38(suppl.):546–552, 1976.

Upton, R. Carbon dioxide laser surgery in the management of cervical intraepithelial neoplasia. Presented at the Sixth Annual Meeting of the Felix Rutledge Society, Charleston, S.C., April 6–9, 1975.

Wakefield, J. et al. Relation of abnormal cytologic smears and carcinoma of the cervix uteri to husband's occupation. *Br. Med. J.* 2:142–143, 1973.

Wallace, D. L., and Slankard, J. E. Teenage cervical carcinoma in situ. *Obstet. Gynecol.* 41:697–700, 1973.

Wasserman, T. H., and Carter, S. K. Integration of chemotherapy into combined modality treatment of solid tumors. VIII. Cervical cancer. *Cancer Treat. Rev.* 4:25–46, 1977.

Webb, G. A. Role of ovarian conservation in the treatment of carcinoma of the cervix with radical surgery. *Am. J. Obstet. Gynecol.* 122:476–484, 1975.

Webb, M. J., and Symmonds, R. E. Wertheim hysterectomy: a reappraisal. *Obstet. Gynecol.* 54:140–145, 1979.

Wentz, W. B., and Reagan, J. W. Clinical significance of postirradiation dysplasia of the uterine cervix. *Am. J. Obstet. Gynecol.* 106:812–817, 1970.

Wharton, J. T. et al. Treatment of clear cell adenocarcinoma in young females. *Obstet. Gynecol.* 45:365–368, 1975.

Wharton, J. T. et al. Preirradiation celiotomy and extended field irradiation for invasive carcinoma of the cervix. *Obstet. Gynecol.* 49:333–338, 1977.

Wheeless, C. R. et al. Prognosis and treatment of adenoepidermoid carcinoma of the cervix. *Obstet. Gynecol.* 35:928–932, 1970.

Wilbanks, G. D. et al. DNA content of cervical intraepithelial neoplasia studied by two-wavelength Feulgen cytophotometry. *Am. J. Obstet. Gynecol.* 98:792–799, 1967.

Willcox, R. R. World look at venereal diseases. *Med. Clin. North Am.* 56:1057–1071, 1972.

Zornoza, J. et al. Percutaneous retroperitoneal lymph node biopsy in carcinoma of the cervix. *Gynecol. Oncol.* 5:43–51, 1977.

forty-nine

Radiation Therapy of Gynecologic Malignancies

FRANCIS S. CARDINALE

Radiation therapy has played an important role in the treatment of gynecologic malignancies since shortly after the isolation of radium by Marie Curie. Cancers of the cervix and endometrium served as models for determining radiation effects and for refining techniques that later became applicable to other human cancers. This chapter presents an understanding of the basic principles of radiation as applied to gynecologic cancer, what acute and chronic reactions it produces, and what future developments hold promise for extending its capabilities.

Intracavitary Therapy

Shortly after the isolation of radium, capsulated sources were applied in various fashions for the treatment of gynecologic cancers. This was the beginning of the development of brachytherapy or intracavitary techniques. Common to nearly all of these applicators was a central intrauterine source most commonly referred to as a tandem, which was used in conjunction with a wide variety of sources placed in the vagina. There are thus two components to nearly all intracavitary systems.

From this empiric beginning the science of brachytherapy evolved in two major centers, the names of which became associated with the two major philosophies of treatment—the Paris and Stockholm techniques. The former involved application of small amounts of radium for long periods of time, for example, four days. By contrast, the Stockholm technique advocated application of larger amounts of radium for shorter periods of time, on the order of 36 hours. In both systems, radiation exposure and the tolerance of pelvic organs were described in milligram-hours. This was simply the amount of radium used for a given length of time. For example, 10 mg radium used for 100 hours is equal to 1000 mg-hours (10 mg × 100 hours).

As more experience was gained it became apparent that while this uniform expression of exposure was related to the radiation dose delivered, it was not adequate for understanding the dose to pelvic structures in patients with distorted anatomy or with other factors that affected placement of the applicators. In Manchester, England these problems were recognized and refinements were developed that provided a more solid understanding of doses and other factors related to radiation complications. At the Holt Radium Institute in Manchester, Tod and Meredith (1953) defined the concepts of points A and B. Point A is defined as a point in the paracervical triangle 2 cm cephalad to the external os or the lateral vaginal fornix, and 2 cm lateral to the central uterine source. Point B was defined as a point 3 cm lateral to point A, thus placing it near the pelvic side wall (fig. 49.1). These points do not correspond to any anatomic structure, but were arbitrarily chosen by the physicist Meredith. This was the first accepted attempt to relate radiation dosage to standard points within the pelvis and to understand more clearly the radiation tolerance of pelvic organs. From observations of the doses at points A and B the principal advantage of intracavitary or brachytherapy can be seen, namely the inverse square effect. By this we mean that the radiation intensity from small or point sources decreases inversely with the square of the distance. Thus moving 2 cm will decrease the radiation exposure by a factor of 4. This means a large radiation dose can be delivered to cancer-containing tissues in the vicinity of the applicators with a great reduction in the dose to normal organs located a short distance away. Computer-assisted dosimetry has greatly assisted the ability to calculate the precise doses in rad (radiation-absorbed dose) to both normal pelvic organs and tumor tissues (fig. 49.2).

There are many applicators available today for gynecologic brachytherapy. Indications depend largely on the clinical situation and the preference of the radiation oncologist or gynecologist. Most modern applicators use after-loading principles, that is, applicators that are placed within the patient and do not contain radioactive sources. Following placement, the patient may pass through the recovery room and appropriate dosimetry films can be obtained without any exposure to hospital personnel. Radioactive sources are then loaded when the patient is returned to her room (Fletcher 1980; Moss, Brand, and Battifora 1979).

Isotopic Radiation Sources

A further recent improvement in safe handling and decreased personnel exposure has been the substitution of radioactive cesium 137 for radium 226. Radium sources consist of hollow tubes containing radium salts and gases that are produced in the radioactive decay of radium. Trauma from normal usage makes these tubes subject to leakage, which can create contamination problems. The gamma rays produced by radium are also highly penetrating, with an energy of approximately 1 million eV. Cesium 137 is less energetic, with an energy of approximately 600 keV; it is a solid radioactive source, making it much less susceptible to trauma and thus much easier to handle and to shield, further reducing the personnel exposures (table 49.1).

External Beam Therapy

When radiotherapy is the primary treatment modality, brachytherapy is rarely used alone. External or teletherapy is used to boost the radiation dose to areas that lie

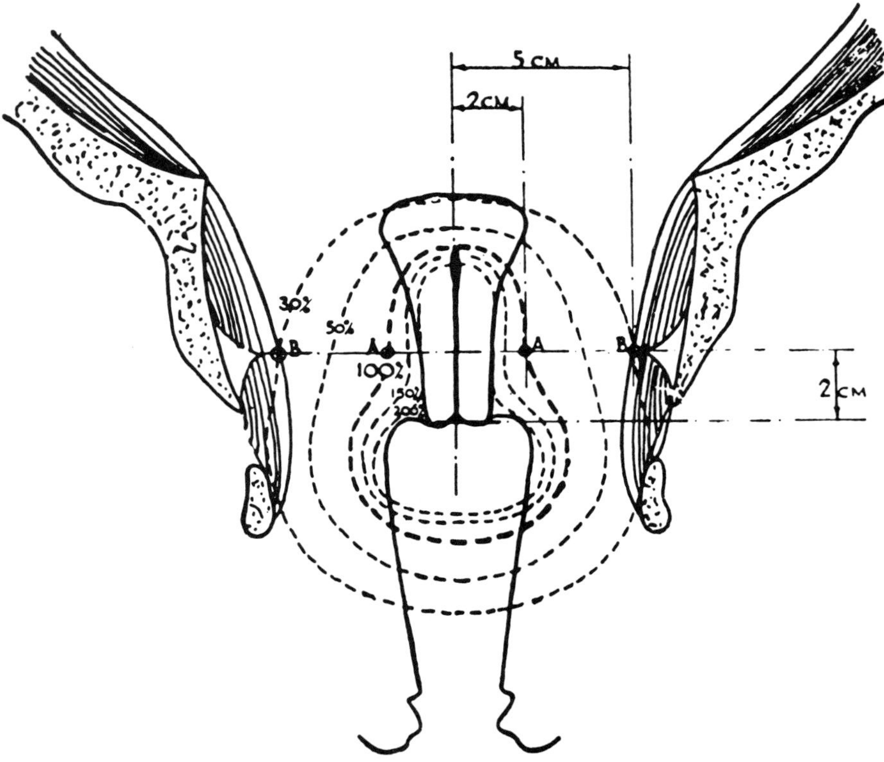

Fig. 49.1. *Relation of radiation dosage to standard points within the pelvis.*

Table 49.1. *Comparison of Physical Characteristics of Most Commonly Used Isotopes in Gynecologic Brachytherapy*

Cesium 137	*Radium 226*
600 kV gamma ray	1000 kV gamma ray
27-year half-life	1500-year half-life
Solid source	Salt and gases in hollow tube
Available from fission reactors	Rare natural mineral

at some distance from the primary tumor site such as the lymph nodes along the pelvic side walls. These areas would be undertreated if intracavitary methods were used alone. The standard for external beam therapy today is megavoltage or supervoltage units such as linear accelerators or cobalt 60 machines. Megavoltage refers to radiation energies greater than 600 kV. Radiations above this energy level have the advantage of providing penetration of the x-ray beam below the skin, producing a skin-sparing effect and greatly reducing skin reactions. These high-energy beams also penetrate the body more deeply, giving a greater depth of dose and greater homogeneity of the radiation throughout the treatment volume. With sharply defined beams the area treated can be limited to an exact volume. Precise control of the radiation dose within this volume has a direct relation to the prevention of side effects and complications.

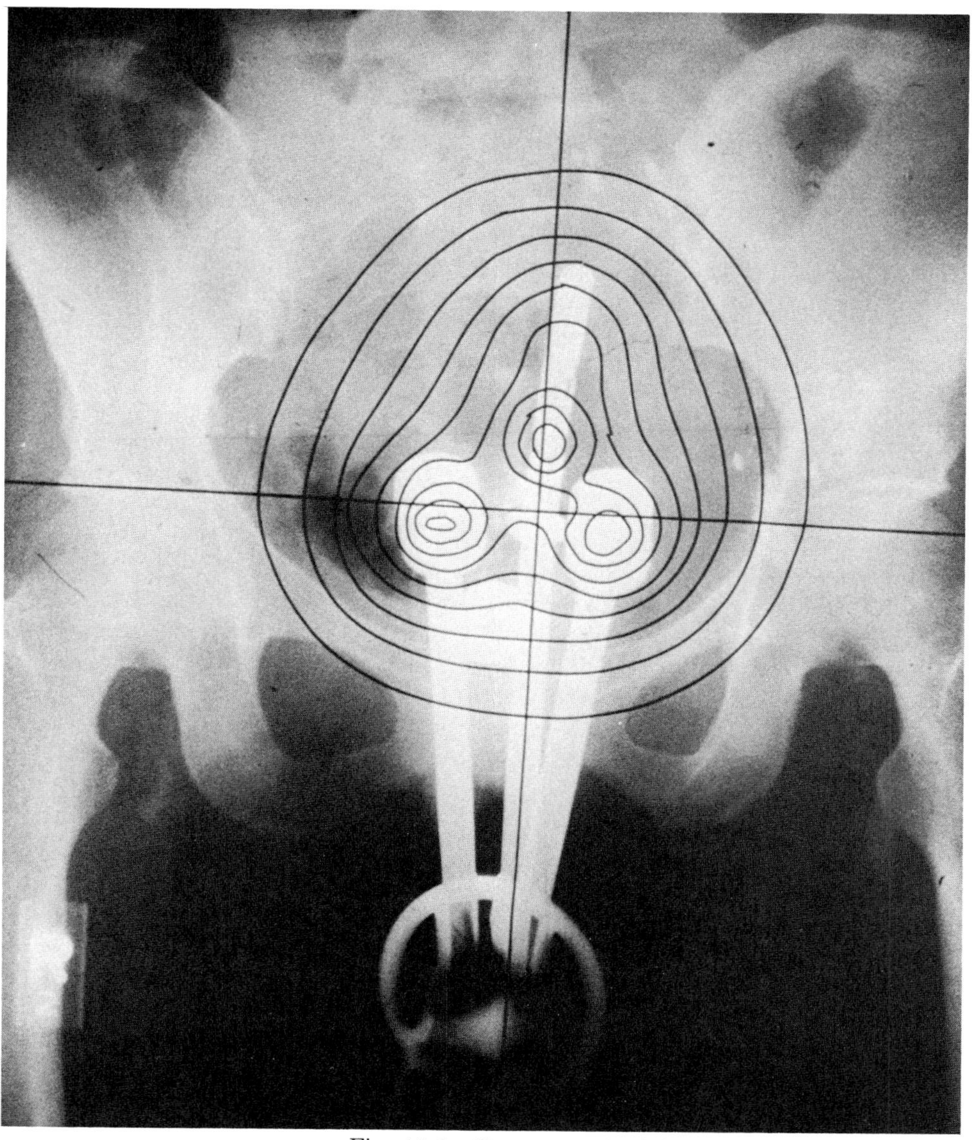

Fig. 49.2. *Computer-assisted dosimetry to normal pelvic organs and tumor tissues.*

Side Effects

Side effects of irradiation of the pelvic region can be divided into generalized and local reactions. They are directly related to several factors including the total dose of radiation delivered, volume of tissue treated, the dose rate from intracavitary applicators, dose distribution within the treated volume, the stage of disease, and the history of treatments including prior radiation or surgery. The most common acute reactions include fatigue, anorexia, nausea, dysuria, diarrhea, skin erythema, and leukopenia and/or thrombocytopenia. Not all these reactions are exhibited by all patients, and their intensity varies greatly. Fatigue and anorexia can be treated simply by careful counseling and reassurance. Nausea and diarrhea can be alleviated to a great extent by the use of medications and by diet counseling. Nausea, for example, responds to a variety of phenothiazine antiemetics such as prochlorperazine (Compazine), promethazone (Phenergan), or trimethobenzamide (Tigan). Diarrhea from acute proctitis can be successfully controlled by a combination of low-fiber or low-residue diet and antidiarrheal drugs such as Paregoric, diphenoxylate (Lomotil), or loperamide (Imodium). Skin reactions are usually self-limited and do not require active treatment unless moist desquamation is seen. When this develops, usually in the gluteal crease, gentle debridement, moist to dry soaks, and antiinflammatory creams are useful.

Careful monitoring of the blood is necessary during radiation treatments to the pelvis. Blood counts should be monitored weekly. Severe drops in the white blood cell and platelet counts are not usually seen, however, unless there is some predisposing factor such as prior chemotherapy or radiation therapy that influences the radiation tolerance of the marrow.

Progressive or chronic side effects are principally due to the sensitivity of midline structures, namely the rectum, bladder, and small bowel. The uterus and cervix themselves can tolerate extremely high radiation doses, such as those delivered by intracavitary applicators. Doses in the range of 20,000 to 30,000 rad are delivered in the vicinity of the intracavitary applicators and are well tolerated by the uterus and the cervix (Kottmeier 1953). Necrosis of the vaginal vault is seen infrequently and is often difficult to differentiate from tumor recurrence. These are most often seen with extensive cancers involving the vaginal fornices (Barber 1979). The majority heal without sequelae. In a very small percentage they may be precursors of fistulas.

Although acute reactions in the rectum and sigmoid resulting in diarrhea are almost universal, late progressive bowel complications are rare and generally seen in patients with advanced central disease (Fletcher 1980). Late reactions can occur several months up to two years after therapy. They become manifest as a gradual thickening of the bowel wall due to edema and fibrosis. Patients may experience diarrhea, bleeding, and severe tenesmus. If symptoms become severe enough, obstruction can occur and surgical intervention with resection of bowel or colostomy may be required to obtain relief. The small bowel has radiation tolerance similar to the rectosigmoid. Because of the motility of the small bowel, however, there is less danger of injury unless larger extended radiation ports are used or unless there is history of previous pelvic surgery. In the latter case, adhesions may cause a loop of bowel to maintain close proximity to a brachytherapy applicator, with resultant injury.

Other complications such as ureteral stricture are exceedingly rare (Slater and Fletcher 1971) and are most often secondary to recurrence in the parametria.

Enhancing Effects

With advances in technology and the ability to deliver irradiation to deep-seated tumors, radiotherapists have begun to look at factors that may account for the failure of a planned course of treatment. Gray and associates (1953) and Tomlinson and Gray (1955) described the oxygen effect and its possible implications for radiotherapy. Their observations showed that hypoxic cells were less susceptible to the lethal effects of radiation than well-oxygenated cells. Hierlihy, Jenkin, and Stryker (1969) and Bush and co-workers (1978) described a poorer prognosis for patients with carcinoma of the cervix with anemia secondary to hemorrhage. This worsening of the prognosis was attributed to hypoxic cells within the cancer. Radiobiologists and radiotherapists have focused on ways to decrease the proportion of hypoxic cells in the tumors and thus increase the oxygen enhancement ratio. Attempts at using hyperbaric oxygen chambers with treatment at high oxygen pressures have shown no significant improvements in the results (Glassburn, Bradley, and Plenk 1977). Other more promising methods have included the use of radiation sensitizers that mimic the action of oxygen within tissues and increase radiation sensitivity. These substances include metronidazole (Flagyl) and several of its analogues. These substances have shown the ability to specifically sensitize hypoxic cells to the effects of irradiation, and they are now entering active clinical trials. Other substances such as hydroxyurea have been reported to improve the results of treatment of advanced cervical carcinoma although its mechanism of action is unclear (Hreshchyshyn et al. 1979). Radiation by means of heavy particles including neutrons and negative pi-mesons also show damaging effects on hypoxic cells and less dependence on the oxygen tension within tissues. These modalities are also currently in active clinical trial (Caderao et al. 1976).

With advances in the technology to deliver radiation in precisely determined volumes and with further understanding of the nature of the cancer cell, new strategies will continue to be developed for radiation treatment of gynecologic malignancies.

References

Barber, H. R. K. Management of failures and complications of cancer of the cervix. *Int. J. Radiat. Oncol. Biol. Phys.* 5:2143–2145, 1979.

Bush, R. S. et al. Definitive evidence for hypoxic cells influencing cure in cancer therapy. *Br. J. Cancer* 37:302–306, 1978.

Caderao, J. F. et al. Fast neutron radiotherapy for locally advanced pelvic cancer. *Cancer* 35:2620–2629, 1976.

Fletcher, G. H. *Textbook of radiotherapy,* 3rd edition. Philadelphia: Lea & Febiger, 1980, pp. 720–834.

Glassburn, J. R.; Bradley, L. W.; and Plenk, H. P. Hyperbaric oxygen in radiation therapy. *Cancer* 39:751–765, 1977.

Gray, L. H. et al. The concentration of oxygen dissolved in tissues at the time of radiation as a factor in radiotherapy. *Br. J. Radiol.* 26:638–648, 1953.

Hierlihy, P.; Jenkin, R. D. T.; and Stryker, J. A. Anemia as a prognostic factor in carcinoma of the cervix. *Can. Med. Assoc. J.* 100:1100–1102, 1969.

Hreshchyshyn, M. M. et al. Hydroxyurea or placebo combined with radiation to treat stage IIIB and IV cervical cancer confined to the pelvis. *Int. J. Radiat. Oncol. Biol. Phys.* 5:317–322, 1979.

Kottmeier, H. L. *Carcinoma of the female genitalia.* Baltimore: Williams & Wilkins, 1953.

Moss, W. T.; Brand, W. N.; and Battifora, H. *Radiation oncology—rationale, techniques, results,* 5th edition. St. Louis: C. V. Mosby, 1979, pp. 440–505.

Slater, J. M., and Fletcher, G. H. Ureteral strictures after radiotherapy for carcinoma of the uterine cervix. *Am. J. Roentgenol.* 3:269–272, 1971.

Tomlinson, R. H., and Gray, L. H. The histological structure of some human lung cancers and the possible implications for radiotherapy. *Br. J. Cancer* 9:539–549, 1955.

Tod, M., and Meredith, W. J. Treatment of cancer of the cervix uteri—a revised "Manchester Method." *Br. J. Radiol.* 26:252–257, 1953.

fifty

Gestational Trophoblastic Disease

ERNEST I. KOHORN

Postmolar gestational trophoblastic disease remains the human malignancy that if treated early is nearly 100% responsive to cycle-specific agents (Hatch 1979; Kohorn 1979). Even advanced metastatic disease is extremely responsive to chemotherapy. Trophoblastic disease is a malignancy in which the number of malignant cells is directly proportional to the tumor marker, human chorionic gonadotropin (HCG). It is known from tissue culture experiments and from projections from clinical situations that 5 mIU of the beta subunit of HCG per ml of serum represent a tumor load of some 10^7 cells. A minimum of 10^9 cells must be present to detect clinically demonstrable disease. Trophoblastic disease may therefore be recognized at a subclinical level. Such information becomes important during therapy when it may be necessary to give an additional course of drugs to obliterate those cells that are not detectable even by this very sensitive assay.

Gestational trophoblastic disease is a malignancy the recognition and management of which are fairly well worked out, but the etiology of which is still uncertain. It is known that molar pregnancy occurs more frequently in Oriental races, and that among Orientals who migrate to Western societies this high incidence decreases. Associations with particular blood grouping and with HLA spectra have not been substantiated. It has lately been suggested that the frequent XX configuration of the mole may be wholly derived from paternal genetic material.

Diagnosis and Local Therapy

The incidence of hydatidiform mole in the eastern United States is about 1 in 1500 pregnancies. The diagnosis is made positively by ultrasound examination of women with symptoms of first trimester threatened abortions who may have an enlarged uterus for dates, hyperemesis gravidarum, or possibly early preeclamptic toxemia. Ultrasound distinguishes the condition from threatened miscarriage of a normal pregnancy, blighted ovum, or multiple gestation. When a positive diagnosis has been made, the uterus should be evacuated by suction curettage. Early detection and therapy obviate the major previous complications of the condition—hemorrhage and infection. Embolization of molar tissue to the lungs following evacuation is a serious complication that occurs particularly if the uterine size is excessive considering dates (Kohorn 1978). Following evacuation of the mole, the patient requires effective contraception, as a further pregnancy cannot be differentiated from persistence or recurrence of trophoblastic disease. It has recently been suggested that the use of oral contraceptives following evacuation is associated with more frequent persistence of human chorionic gonadotropin, leading to more frequent therapy for trophoblastic disease (Stone et al. 1976). This issue needs to be settled, and the Gynecologic Oncology Group will soon perform a prospective randomized study. As an alternative to hormonal contraception, effective mechanical contraception with the intrauterine device, diaphragm, or condom should be prescribed.

Follow-up

The patient must be followed by serial human chorionic gonadotropin titers. These should be performed by a trophoblast center laboratory, as there is variation among laboratories and some of the speedy radioimmunoassays for HCG give values at very high or very low levels. Chorionic gonadotropin receptor assays also give values that do not fully correlate with precise values of HCG. Trophoblast centers have now moved wholly away from measurement of urinary chorionic gonadotropin (UCG) to measurement of the beta subunit of HCG (β-HCG). It should be noted that 1000 international units (IU) of UCG per 24 hours is approximately equivalent to 500 milli-international units (mIU) of β-HCG per ml of serum. The assay performed should be cross-reactive at less than 5 mIU of β-HCG. A value should be obtained immediately post-evacuation and then at weekly intervals until three nondetectable levels have been obtained. Subsequent to this, the test should be performed monthly for six months, and every two months for a further six months. After this, the patient may be allowed to become pregnant. In the patient in whom the HCG value falls to a nondetectable level in four to six weeks and in whom the initial value was below 10,000 mIU/ml of β-HCG, and who has no other contraindicating factors, pregnancy may be allowed following six months of contraception. The mean time to nondetectable levels of human chorionic gonadotropin is 8 to 12 weeks. On occasion this time period is longer, but provided successive values are falling there is no reason to intervene with chemotherapy. So far trophoblastic disease without detectable HCG β-subunit has been described only as a rarity. Even in those cases, the beta subunit was eventually detected, with initial disease reappearing in the presence of only the alpha subunit (Quigley, Tyrey, and Hammond 1980).

Systemic Management

Prophylactic chemotherapy is now used only very rarely. Even in United States centers where 20% to 30% of patients are given chemotherapy for persistently elevated titers following hydatidiform mole evacuation, prophylactic chemotherapy would necessitate giving drugs unnecessarily to seven out of eight patients. Morbidity and mortality have attended the use of such prophylactic chemotherapy. The fact that patients treated within the first 16 weeks following mole evacuation have a nearly universal successful response to single-agent chemotherapy obviates the use of prophylactic chemotherapy. It has been suggested that a uterus enlarged four weeks in excess of dates associated with theca-lutein cysts represents a high risk for trophoblastic disease. Only 40% to 60% of such patients may require chemotherapy. Because β-HCG is such an excellent discriminator for therapy, and since the cure rate with early chemotherapy is so high, it would seem that β-HCG should be the only discriminator.

For patients who have completed childbearing, hysterectomy provides an alternative to suction evacuation. Most patients have difficulty in deciding whether or not to sacrifice their fertility at that time, and there is really no need to make the decision then. If sterilization is required within the first year following evacuation, hysterectomy rather than tubal ligation should be performed.

In most American centers, the indication for chemotherapy following hydatidiform mole is a plateau of β-HCG of three values over two weeks, or a progressive rise over a similar period of time. British clinics are more conservative and tend to watch HCG values longer. Prior to effective chemotherapy very few patients with molar disease, in fact, developed clinical choriocarcinoma, certainly less than 5%. Thus there is a gap between the number of patients who receive therapy in American clinics and the number who would in fact develop clinical choriocarcinoma. The basis for diagnosis in prechemotherapy days was development of metastases or the diagnosis of choriocarcinoma in the uterus in those few patients who had a timely hysterectomy. Today there is more interest in preserving the reproductive function of these women and returning them to good health if HCG titers persist, rather than in making a precise pathologic diagnosis. Since early treatment is so effective, however, one can wait for four to five weeks, particularly at lower values of HCG (that is, those below 1000 mIU/ml) before treatment. At the Yale Trophoblastic Disease Center, it is now our practice to treat patients only if a plateau of HCG persists over four to five weeks or if there is a rising titer. Treatment may be instituted earlier if values plateau at levels above 100,000 mIU/ml or if there is clinical evidence of persistent or particularly metastatic trophoblastic disease. Experience throughout the United States has demonstrated that patients with gestational trophoblastic disease should be treated at a trophoblast center and that mortality and morbidity associated with treatment by an occasional therapist are significantly greater.

Trophoblastic disease is defined clinically as persistently elevated HCG titers. It is called metastatic if there is evidence of metastases by clinical examination, radiologic investigations, CT scan, liver scan, and similar studies. Cerebral angiography is contraindicated for fear of precipitating cerebral hemorrhage. In the absence of metastases, a diagnosis of nonmetastatic disease is made. Trophoblastic disease is also divided into low-risk and high-risk categories (Hammond et al. 1973):

- Low risk
  - Disease less than four months
  - Titer less than 100,000 IU/24 hours urinary chorionic gonadotropin or 50,000 mIU/ml β-HCG
  - Lung metastases only
- High risk
  - Disease longer than four months
  - Titer greater than 100,000 IU/24 hours urinary chorionic gonadotropin or 50,000 mIU/ml β-HCG
  - Brain metastases
  - Liver metastases
  - Bowel metastases
  - Previous full-term pregnancy
  - Previous inadequate therapy

Chemotherapy

Postmolar trophoblastic disease and low-risk metastatic disease are treated with single-agent chemotherapy. This may be either methotrexate or dactinomycin, the choice depending on the individual institution. An adequate dose must be given. The first attempt at chemotherapy provides the best chance for control of the disease. Morbidity must therefore be avoided. High-risk trophoblastic disease has been found to be so frequently unresponsive to single agents that therapy with three drugs is used from the onset. Previously these were dactinomycin, methotrexate, and chlorambucil, but most trophoblast centers have replaced chlorambucil with cyclophosphamide. Patients who fail this regimen have responded successfully to the seven-drug regimen initially designed by Bagshawe (Surwit et al. 1979). This, in fact, appears to present a lower toxicity than the triple-drug regimen and it has been suggested that it should be tried as primary treatment. A randomized trial is likely to be performed by the Gynecologic Oncology Group in the near future.

With metastatic trophoblastic disease certain sites will require special attention in addition to chemotherapy. Patients with cerebral metastases will require head irradiation to a total dose of 2000 to 3000 rad. Liver metastases are usually treated with 2000 rad to the liver. In both instances, radiation is given more to control the potential bleeding than to control the cancer. With persistent liver and pelvic metastases, there is a place for arterial infusion chemotherapy. Surgery plays a part only in excision of pelvic or lung metastases resistant to treatment.

It has been our practice to administer single-agent chemotherapy to outpatients providing that they live nearby. Patients living any distance from the center should be admitted to the hospital to guard against morbidity from chemotherapy. Patients receiving triple therapy should be hospitalized, and it is essential that they be carefully supervised during the subsequent nadir of granulocytopenia and platelet depression.

This account has so far related essentially to postmolar gestational trophoblastic disease. It should be emphasized, however, that the most dangerous form follows previous full-term pregnancy or previous miscarriage or termination of pregnancy. Under such conditions the disease may present as an obscure pneumonia, as an ill-defined malaise, or even as a cerebral tumor. The investigation of any illness in a woman of childbearing age that is at all suggestive of a malignancy should include an HCG estimation. This test is now so universally available that an immediate diagnosis can be made and long investigations including inappropriate surgery or biopsy may be avoided. The internist and general surgeon should be alert to this diagnosis, as it is one they will rarely encounter. When early diagnosis is made a potentially disastrous situation will be converted into a therapeutic success.

References

Hammond, C. G. et al. Treatment of metastatic trophoblastic disease; good and poor prognosis. *Am. J. Obstet. Gynecol.* 115:451–457, 1973.

Hatch, K. D. Gestational trophoblastic disease. *J. C. E. Obstet. Gynecol.* 21:17–27, 1979.

Kohorn, E. I. Gestational trophoblastic disease: diagnosis and management. *Contrib. Gynecol. Obstet.* 13: 165–176, 1979.

Kohorn, E. I. et al. Pulmonary embolization of trophoblastic tissue in molar pregnancy. *Obstet. Gynecol.* 51:165–205, 1978.

Quigley, M. M.; Tyrey, L.; and Hammond, C. B. Subunit in sera of choriocarcinoma patients in remission. *J. Clin. Endocrinol. Metab.* 50:98–102, 1980.

Stone, M. et al. Relationship of oral contraception to development of trophoblastic tumor after evacuation of a hydatidiform mole. *Br. J. Obstet. Gynecol.* 83:913–916, 1976.

Surwit, E. A. et al. A new combination chemotherapy for resistant trophoblastic disease. *Gynecol. Oncol.* 8: 110–118, 1979.

fifty-one

Acute Lymphocytic and Childhood Leukemias

DAVID S. FISCHER
DIANE M. KOMP

Within little more than a decade, the treatment of acute leukemia has progressed to such an extent that many children with this disease now lead a comfortable life for months, and, in some instances, even years. Although leukemia continues to be invariably fatal, the importance of the advances made in its treatment can hardly be overestimated. (Avery 1959)

These editorial comments alerted the practicing pediatrician to the advances in treatment that signaled new hope for the child with leukemia. Contrast them with the following:

Since approximately 50% of all patients treated by modern standards are able to have their therapy stopped, and approximately 70 to 80% of this group will remain in complete remission for at least four years thereafter, the best estimate of the overall proportion of all newly diagnosed patients treated by modern therapy who will ultimately be cured is just under 40%. (George et al. 1979)

The startling contrast between the two statements occurs in the phrases *invariably fatal* and *ultimately cured*.

While researchers debate the merits and relative success rates of various regimens, a single unifying theme is heard: children with acute lymphocytic leukemia enjoy a far better prognosis than was dreamed possible two decades ago, and length of survival has been measurably improved. These advances have been made by intensification of treatment (Pinkel 1979) over the palliative approaches of previous years. They can be better appreciated in the overall context of leukemia in children and young adults.

Demography

Acute lymphocytic leukemia (ALL) is a disease of children and young adults. In the United States in the age group 1 to 14 years, cancer causes 11.3% of all deaths and is the second commonest cause of death, exceeded only by accidents. Of the 2364 children in this age group who died of cancer in 1977 (Silverberg 1980), 45% died of leukemia. In people aged 15 to 34 years leukemia remains the leading cause of cancer death in men, although it slipped from first to second in women between 1976 (Silverberg 1979) and 1977, when it was exceeded by breast cancer (Silverberg 1980).

Definition and Classification

Acute leukemia in its natural history is a malignant neoplasm of the blood-forming organs characterized by a majority of primitive, or blast, cells in the bone marrow. It is usually fatal within two and one-half months when untreated; the three-year survival rate is

Table 51.1. *French-American-British Morphologic Classification of Acute Lymphocytic Leukemia*

Cytologic Features	*L-1*	*L-2*	*L-3*
Cell size	Small	Large, heterogeneous	Large, homogeneous
Nuclear chromatin	Homogeneous	Variable, heterogeneous	Homogeneous, finely stippled
Nuclear shape	Regular	Clefting and indentation	Regular, oval to round
Nucleoli	Inconspicuous	Prominent	Prominent
Cytoplasm	Scanty	Moderately abundant	Moderately abundant
Cytoplasmic basophilia	Slight	Variable	Very deep
Vacuolization	Variable	Variable	Often prominent

SOURCE: Modified from Bennett et al. 1976.

less than 1%. Subacute leukemia runs a somewhat longer course and exhibits more cellular differentiation and clinically is managed as the acute forms (Linman 1975). Lymphocytic leukemia is a leukemic proliferation of lymphocytes and lymphoblasts (hence often called acute lymphoblastic leukemia), and frequently includes the undifferentiated-cell leukemias. In an attempt to create some order from the antecedent chaos in morphologic diagnosis, Bennett and associates (1976) proposed a standardized classification for the acute leukemias agreed on by the French-American-British cooperative group (FAB) (table 51.1).

Acute myelocytic leukemia (AML) is a malignant proliferation of granulocytes and their precursors. The terminology here has become confused and has tended to include erythroleukemia, monocytic, myelomonocytic, eosinophilic, basophilic, promyelocytic, megakaryocytic, and subacute myelocytic leukemias as well as myelodysplastic syndromes. We now use the inclusive label acute non-lymphocytic leukemia (ANLL) for this group and therefore the FAB classification for myeloid leukemias is discussed in chapter 52, on ANLL.

The relative incidence of acute lymphocytic versus acute myelocytic leukemia in childhood is difficult to define because of the lack of clarity of (1) morphologic definition in the literature and (2) the precise ages of childhood. Thus Wintrobe (1974) indicates that more than 80% of cases of leukemia in children were lymphoblastic in his clinic, and Linman (1975) gives a figure of 90% under the age of 14 years. At the Children's Cancer Foundation in Boston, 32% of patients were considered to have AML (Fraumeni, Manning, and Mitus 1971) and in the National Cancer Institute (NCI) End-Results Group (ERG) survey, 54% of leukemias in children under 15 years of age were of the acute lymphocytic type. Other forms of acute leukemia accounted for 41%, and 5% were considered to be a form of chronic leukemia (Myers et al. 1976). For people in their teens and early twenties ALL and AML are about equal in frequency, and as age increases AML tends to predominate. After the age of 45 years ALL is rare. The sex frequency is approximately three males to two females for both conditions.

Etiology

Thus far no etiologies have been linked directly to specific cases of leukemia; however, several exceptionally high-risk groups have been defined. Persons exposed to therapeutic doses of ionizing radiation for ankylosing spondylitis and Hodgkin's disease are at increased risk for AML. There is no evidence that diagnostic radiation exposure carries similar risk. Persons within 1000 meters of the hypocenter of the Hiroshima nuclear explosion have a 1 in 60 risk of leukemia in 12 years. Most of the leukemias associated with nuclear weapons exposure have been acute or chronic myelocytic types, with only occasional cases of acute lymphocytic and few or no cases of chronic lymphocytic leukemia.

Chromosomal abnormalities are seen frequently in acute leukemia, but in general are thought to be secondary to the disease rather than causative. The changes include hypodiploidy, hyperdiploidy, translocations (Oshimura and Sandberg 1977), and the presence of the Philadelphia chromosome (Ph^1), which is generally a poor prognostic sign (Priest et al. 1980). Other genetic factors include the increased risk of leukemia in children with Down's and Bloom's syndromes and Fanconi's anemia (Mauer 1969).

Chemical leukemogenesis has been established for benzene and is suspected for a few other substances. The most frequent sequence of events is an exposure to benzene followed by a period of aplastic anemia with survival, and later development of acute nonlymphocytic leukemia.

Viral leukemogenesis is being actively investigated. The clear demonstration that RNA viruses cause and transmit leukemia in fish, birds, mice, cats, chickens, cattle, and nonhuman primates must have some relation to human leukemia. So far, there has been no demonstration of such a relationship but viral markers have been found in human cells (Gallo and Meyskens 1978). The bulk of the evidence has been obtained in myelogenous leukemia and suggests a role as a cocarcinogen along with chemicals, radiation, and hereditary factors.

Diagnostic Clinical Manifestations

The onset of ALL is usually abrupt, with fatigue, bone pain, and fever with or without infection. Frequently, hemorrhage or purpura without trauma is the first sign of abnormality, since pallor with anemia is sometimes not appreciated early. Unexplained weight loss or failure to thrive may precipitate the visit to a physician where examination may reveal lymphadenopathy, hepatosplenomegaly, bone tenderness, and petechiae or purpura.

Laboratory screening with a complete blood count (CBC) and platelet count may reveal leukocytosis, anemia, thrombocytopenia, and abnormal cells in the differential count. About 25% of patients have white cell counts below 4000 and 15% have normal counts; the latter have a more favorable prognosis. About 15% have white cell count (WBC) in excess of 100,000 and their prognosis is poor (Simone, Verzosa, and Rudy 1975).

Frequently, the peripheral blood has increased primitive cells (blasts), often to the exclusion of significant numbers of normal cells. At one time these blasts were characterized only morphologically (Bennett et al. 1976) (fig. 51.1), then by both morphology and cytochemistry (Hayhoe and Cawley 1972) (fig. 51.2), surface markers (Brouet and Seligmann 1978; Sallan et al. 1980), by biochemical determinants (McCaffrey et al. 1975; Shaw et al. 1978), and finally by some combination of two or more such factors (Coleman et al. 1978). The following summarizes methods for characterizing blast cells as modified from Catovsky (1977):

- Morphology
  - French-American-British group classification
  - Hayhoe classification
- Cytochemistry
  - Peroxidase
  - Sudan black B
  - Periodic acid-Schiff
  - Lysozyme *(continued on p. 568)*

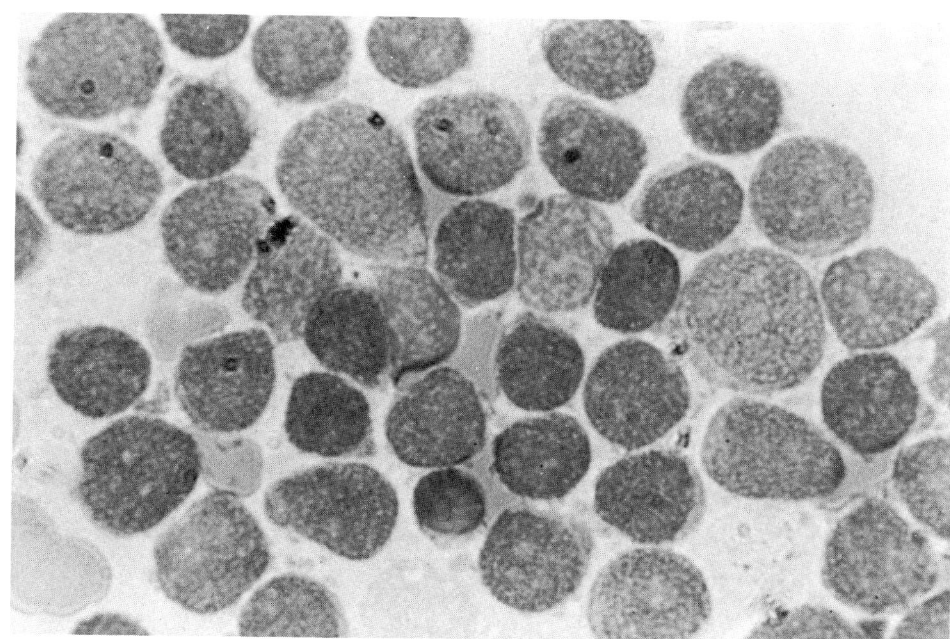

Fig. 51.1. *Sheets of blast cells with acute lymphocytic leukemia in a 15-year-old patient. Type L-2 in the FAB classification, as shown in table 51.1.*

Electron microscopy
- Morphology and cytochemistry

Surface markers
- E rosettes (T cell)
- Membrane immunoglobulin (B cell)
- Cytoplasmic immunoglobulin (pre-B cell)
- Antilymphocytic leukemia serum (Greaves)
- Fc receptors (B cell) (some T cells)
- C3 receptors (EAC) (B cell) (some T cells)
- Epstein-Barr virus receptor (B cell)
- Measles virus receptors (LM rosettes) (T cells)

Biochemistry
- Terminal deoxynucleotidyl transferase
- Adenosine deaminase
- Serum lysozyme

Cytogenetics
- Ph^1 chromosome
- Hyper- and hypodiploidy
- Translocations

While diagnosis is often clear-cut from the peripheral WBC and differential, bone marrow aspiration and often, needle biopsy, are indicated to verify the diagnosis, estimate cellularity, and obtain additional material for cytogenetic, biochemical, immunologic, and cell antigen typing studies. It is desirable to determine the patient's HLA type in anticipation of the potential need for leukocyte and platelet transfusions.

Treatment Principles

Almost everything we know about acute leukemia is relatively new. Less than half a century ago, when the therapy and results in carcinoma of the stomach and lung (non-small cell) were not much different than they are today, leukemia was not considered a neoplasm and was not included in the first national cancer survey in 1937 (Myers et al. 1976). It was included in the second survey in 1947, but there was no effective therapy. It was not until later that year that Farber first treated a child with aminopterin (Farber 1947) and was later able to report some palliation of symptoms and prolongation of survival (Farber et al. 1948; Farber 1949). These observations stimulated intense laboratory and clinical studies of acute leukemia.

It has been clearly demonstrated in L 1210 mouse leukemia that the response to chemotherapy generally follows first-order kinetics (Skipper, Schabel, and Wilcox 1964). Human ALL is probably the closest human analogue to the experimental situation.

The objective of therapy is cure. The best current strategies to achieve that objective have been worked out in several cooperative group studies and in some individual studies in large cancer centers. The most widely accepted strategy is to induce complete remission (CR) in bone marrow and peripheral blood. At the time of diagnosis the average patient has 10^{12} leukemic cells, about a trillion, equal to 1 kg of tumor. Induction of remission can be achieved in about 20% to 50% of

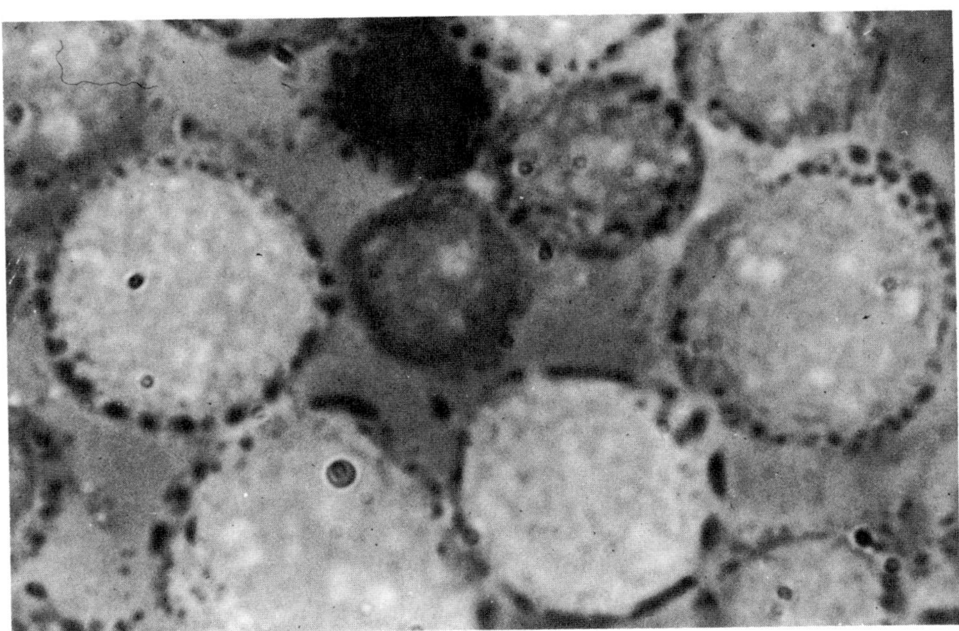

Fig. 51.2. *Lymphoblasts showing positive periodic acid-Schiff (PAS) stain in periphery of cells.*

patients with a single drug, but it does not last long. Combination chemotherapy is used to induce CR by reducing the cell burden by at least 99% to 10^{10} cells. At this level blasts are minimal in the bone marrow and absent in the blood; however, if no further treatment is given relapse soon occurs. If only a single drug is used thereafter, a drug-resistant clone emerges after a variable period and relapse follows. Only with continued multiple-drug maintenance to reduce the tumor burden to a level where body defenses are effective, perhaps 10^4 cells, can long-term relapse-free survival be achieved (fig. 51.3). Then, and only then, can therapy be stopped with a reasonable expectation that the continued disease-free state might eventually be vouchsafed a cure.

Induction Therapy

Although various combinations of two or more drugs have been used for remission induction, the most effective has been vincristine and prednisone (VP). In addition to a good level of activity, these drugs are not myelosuppressive and their toxicity is not additive (Frei and Sallan 1978). Remission is induced by this combination in about 80% to 90% of cases (Mauer and Simone 1976), compared to prednisone-6-mercaptopurine (6-MP), 86%; prednisone-cyclophosphamide, 81%; prednisone-daunomycin, 81%; and prednisone-methotrexate (oral), 80%.

Three-drug and four-drug combinations produce slightly higher response rates of questionable significance: prednisone-vincristine-L-asparaginase, 97%; prednisone-vincristine-daunomycin, 94% to 98%; and prednisone-vincristine-6-MP-methotrexate, 88% to 94%. A prednisone-vincristine-asparaginase-cyclophosphamide regimen produced 81% CR but with greater toxicity (Komp et al. 1976). Indeed, the toxicity of L-asparaginase, although not myelosuppressive, is multiple and severe (Land et al. 1972). Nonetheless, it is widely used because it seems to achieve CR sooner and the remissions achieved seem more durable.

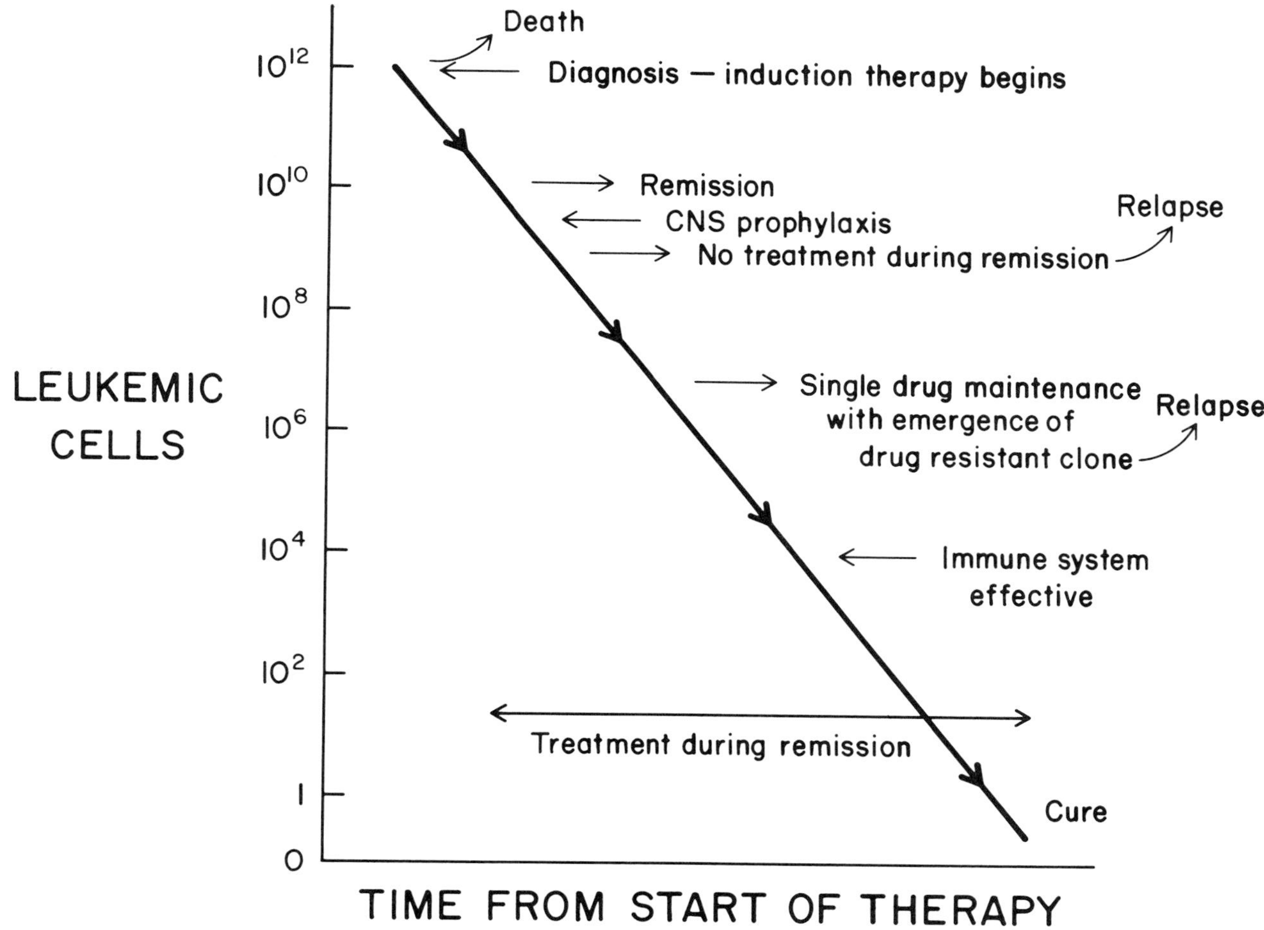

Fig. 51.3. *Course of acute lymphocytic leukemia. (Modified from Frei and Sallan 1978.)*

For patients who relapse on chemotherapy, reinduction is possible with combinations of two, three, or four drugs. Their prognosis is uniformly poor, however, and few achieve prolonged CR. For patients who relapse after chemotherapy has been discontinued, reinduction is successful three-quarters of the time, and many have gone on to prolonged CR and eventually had therapy discontinued a second time and remained relapse-free (Chessells and Cornbleet 1979; Herson et al. 1979). Patients failing initial remission induction with vincristine, prednisone, an anthracycline, or L-asparaginase in combination, may achieve remission with a combination of teniposide (VM-26) and cytarabine (cytosine arabinoside) in about one-third of cases (Rivera et al. 1980).

Central Nervous System Prophylaxis

As induction regimens succeeded in putting most patients into CR, recurrence in the central nervous system (CNS) emerged as the major limiting factor in disease control (Mauer 1980). Fully one-half of all relapses began in the CNS, which served as a sanctuary for leukemic cells that infiltrated the arachnoidea and were protected from effective drug concentrations by the blood-brain barrier (Price and Johnson 1973).

In the late 1960s, the St. Jude Hospital group began studies of CNS prophylaxis with craniospinal irradiation. This proved too toxic, but eventually, a program of cranial irradiation with 2400 rad and five intrathecal injections of methotrexate during the period of irradiation evolved as safe and effective (Hustu et al. 1973). In many institutions this is now a standard part of therapy (fig. 51.4) and is begun as soon as the patient is in complete remission. It should not be done if there is residual disease lest that residua serve to repopulate the body and the CNS with leukemic cells, and the cerebral irradiation, which is not innocuous, will have been wasted.

Undesirable side effects of cranial irradiation in a small subset of patients include leukoencephalopathy and diminution of intellectual function and short-term memory (Simone 1978). The leukoencephalopathy seemed to occur mostly in patients who had 2000 rad or more of cranial irradiation followed by intravenous methotrexate (Price and Jamieson 1975). Brain irradiation and intrathacal methotrexate showed little or no association. It is presumed that irradiation increased the permeability of the membranes to high doses of methotrexate given intravenously so that very high local concentrations were achieved. Intrathecal methotrexate never achieved high concentrations in the brain because it was diffusing against the flow of the cerebrospinal fluid (CSF). Similarly, oral methotrexate had no association with leukoencephalopathy because large doses could not be ingested, and hence high CSF concentrations were never achieved. On the other hand, high-dose methotrexate with leucovorin rescue would be extremely hazardous after cranial irradiation.

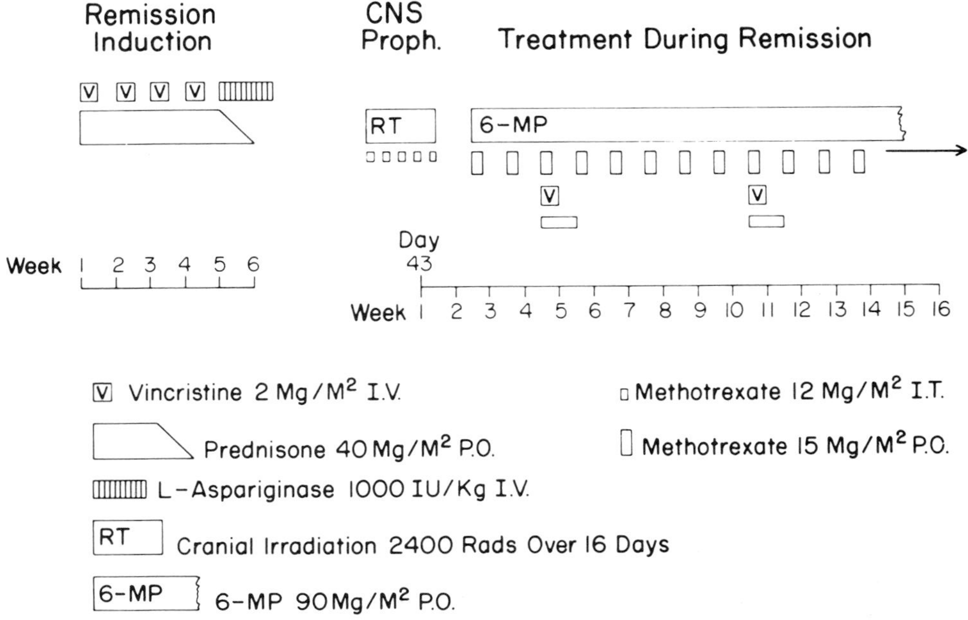

Fig. 51.4. *ALL: "standard" treatment protocol. (Frei and Sallan 1978. Reprinted by permission.)*

In a prospective evaluation of the chronic neurologic disturbances of children following therapy, McIntosh and co-workers (1976) found neurologic symptoms in 12 of 23 patients. All had received 2400 rad of cranial irradiation, intrathecal methotrexate, and intermittent maintenance therapy with intravenous methotrexate, cyclophosphamide, and cytarabine. All 12 of those affected had intermittent limping and incoordination, and five sustained seizures; four of these had subsequent abnormalities in motor, perceptual, behavioral, or language development. Three school-age children had learning disability and perceptual-motor defects.

Other late side effects include ataxia, drowsiness, and Lhermitte's sign (sudden electric shock-like tingling down the spine and paresthesias of the fingers and toes on sharp flexion of the neck) that has been associated with demyelinization (Kirs and Herman 1980). Another consequence is a mineralizing vasculopathy (Price and Birdwell 1978), but the functional effect of this is unknown. Radiation effects on the large and small vessels of the brain have been reported but their significance is unknown, as is mild dilatation of the ventricles and decreased attenuation of the brain substance reported on computed tomography (CT) studies.

The need for cranial irradiation for CNS prophylaxis has been questioned (Komp et al. 1975; Gee et al. 1976; Haghbin 1976). These investigators achieved the same low CNS relapse rate using intrathecal methotrexate with intensive systemic chemotherapy and no cranial irradiation, which certainly challenges the current orthodoxy. The schema of the L-2 protocol of Memorial Sloan-Kettering Cancer Center in figure 51.5 shows the intensity of therapy using 11

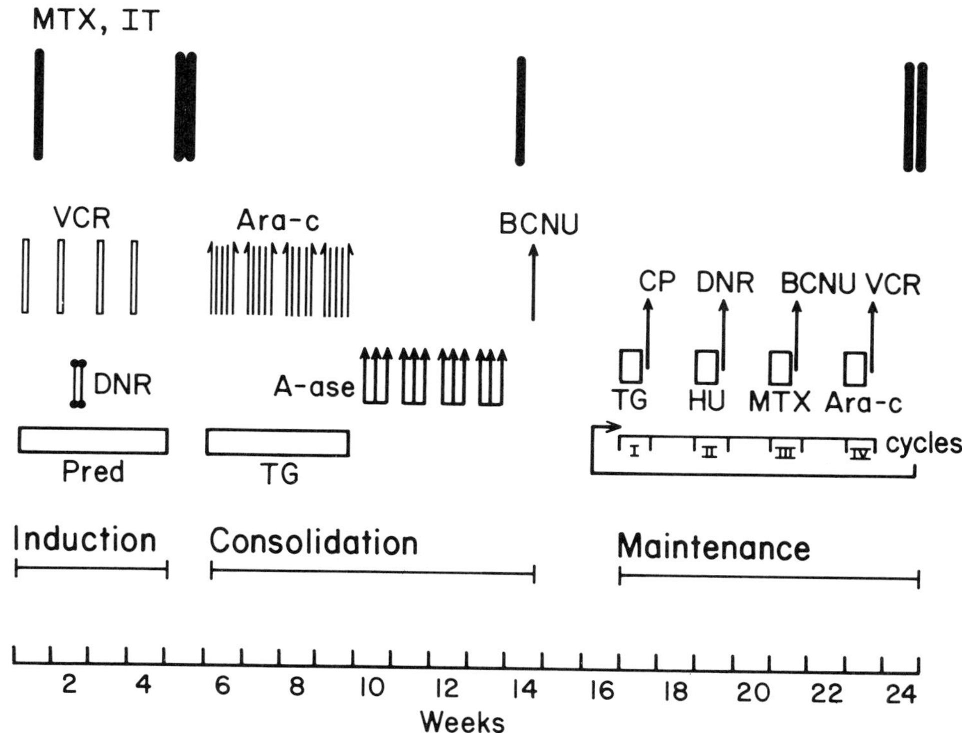

Fig. 51.5. *Outline of the L-2 protocol. (Haghbin et al. 1980. Reprinted by permission.)*

Induction: *VCR (vincristine) 1.5 to 2 mg/m² IV*
Pred (prednisone) 60 mg/m² p.o.
DNR (daunorubicin) 60 mg/m² IV

Consolidation: *Ara-C (cytarabine) 150 mg/m² IV*
TG (thioguanine) 75 mg/m² p.o.
A-ase (L-asparaginase) 60,000 IU/m² IV
BCNU (carmustine) 60 mg/m² IV

Maintenance: *TG (thioguanine) 300 mg/m² p.o.*
CP (cyclophosphamide) 600 mg/m² IV
HU (hydroxyurea) 2400 mg/m² p.o.
DNR (daunorubicin) 45 mg/m² IV
MTX (methotrexate) 10 mg/m² p.o.
BCNU (carmustine) 60 mg/m² IV
Ara-C (cytarabine) 150mg/m² IV
VCR (vincristine) 2 mg/m² IV
MTX (methotrexate) 6.25 mg/m² IT

drugs (Haghbin et al. 1980). In spite of this treatment and an even more intense 11-drug protocol (L-10), CNS relapses occurred in about 10% of cases. In an intermittent combination regimen with doxorubicin, vincristine, prednisone, L-asparaginase, intrathecal methotrexate, and 2400 rad cranial irradiation, there were no primary CNS prophylaxis failures in 137 children (Sallan et al. 1978) at the time of that report, but there have been some since then.

Consolidation and Intensification

After achieving bone marrow remission patients still have a large tumor burden that will surely proliferate if given an opportunity. Therefore the strategy in a number of protocols (as in fig. 51.5) is to have a consolidation or intensification phase. This usually consists of a combination of noncross-resistant drugs, not previously used, to avoid the development of drug resistance. Both cell cycle phase-specific and nonspecific agents are used to destroy cells that are proliferating but that may be resting. The advantage of this therapeutic maneuver is that it further reduces the leukemic cell population and moves it toward the level at which immune body defenses might be adequate to contain it (fig. 51.3). The danger is that if it is too aggressive it may wipe out the normal stem cell line so that recovery is delayed or impossible. In addition, a prolonged period of granulocytopenia predisposes to infection with opportunistic organisms in addition to the ubiquitous bacterial flora. Hemorrhage secondary to prolonged and severe thrombocytopenia is another risk during this period.

Maintenance Therapy

In the L-2 protocol shown in figure 51.5 the demarcation of maintenance from consolidation therapy is clear. In many other protocols it is a gray area with one shading into the next. In the protocol in figure 51.4 maintenance is simply called therapy during remission, and no consolidation phase is listed separately, unless the CNS prophylaxis is so interpreted.

Just as there are many approaches to induction, there are many programs of maintenance. Probably the most popular is that illustrated in figure 51.4 with daily oral 6-mercaptopurine (6-MP) and oral methotrexate once or twice weekly. In a controlled study to test the efficacy and toxicity of one-, two-, three-, and four-drug regimens for maintenance, patients in CR were randomized to intravenous methotrexate, oral 6-MP plus oral methotrexate, cyclophosphamide plus 6-MP plus methotrexate, or cyclophosphamide and L-asparaginase plus 6-MP and methotrexate (Aur et al. 1978). In the group receiving intravenous methotrexate alone, 14 of 20 patients relapsed and 9 developed leukoencephalopathy without antecedent CNS leukemia, apparently due to the high dose of methotrexate. In the other three groups the results were equivalent, but there was no leukoencephalopathy. The addition of cyclophosphamide or L-asparaginase increased toxicity and complications without demonstrably increasing the leukemocidal effect.

Cessation of Therapy

Since the development of induction, consolidation, and maintenance therapy, the majority of patients with ALL now survive more than five years. Even maintenance therapy has some morbidity and potential mortality, so it is desirable to stop treatment at some point at which cure seems likely. The St. Jude Hospital group policy is to stop all antileukemic therapy for patients who have remained in initial complete remission for two and one-half years; have remained in initial hematologic remission for at least two and one-half years and at least one year after successful treatment of relapse in an extramedullary site (CNS or testis); or have attained a second complete remission after one or more hematologic relapses and then met the first two requirements. Of 278 children in whom therapy was stopped after meeting these criteria, 55 (20%) have relapsed, mainly in the bone marrow (Simone et al. 1978; George et al. 1979). The relapse rate, as in most series, was higher for the first year than for the next three years. Boys had twice as high a relapse rate as girls. None of the 79 patients who remained in complete remission for at least four years off therapy has relapsed yet.

In a study of testicular relapse by the Childrens Cancer Study Group (CCSG), 20 (5%) of 395 male patients developed testicular infiltration prior to or concomitant with their first bone marrow relapse (Nesbit et al. 1980). Fourteen occurred as an isolated relapse and six were concurrent with bone marrow and/or CNS relapse. Nine of the patients had discontinued therapy after three years of continuous complete remission. There were no relapses in a group of 76 who received presymptomatic gonadal irradiation immediately after achieving an initial marrow remission.

Prognosis

In spite of the gratifying results achieved in the last few years, failures of therapy continue to plague us. Our early assumption that ALL was a relatively homoge-

Table 51.2. *Classification of ALL by Membrane Phenotype*

Surface Markers	*Type ALL*	*Classification*	*Morphology*	*Antinull ALL Serum*
T markers	T	Childhood—20%	Variable, L-1 or L-2	Negative
B markers	B	Burkitt's, lymphosarcoma	L-3 L-2, rarely L-1	Negative
Absent or minimal (cytoplasmic IgM)	Pre-B	Childhood	L-2	Positive
Absent	Null	Childhood, adult	L-1 (75%) L-2 (68%)	Positive (72%) Positive (50%)

SOURCE: Modified from Catovsky 1977.

neous disease appears to have been naive. As we search for the causes of some of our failures we see that there are qualitatively different subgroups with different responses.

If we look at ALL cell surface markers (table 51.2), we see at least four separate groups. Patients with T cell markers constitute about 20% of cases and tend to be a little older, have higher initial WBCs, and generally have poorer responses with shorter remissions and a higher relapse rate. A T cell variant called suppressor cell leukemia is rare (Broder et al. 1978). Patients with B cell ALL are much less common, but have a high cellular proliferative rate, a high initial WBC, and the shortest remissions. The pre-B cell leukemia is a new phenotype of ALL with cytoplasmic IgM and little or no surface marker, but with a relatively good response to therapy (Vogler et al. 1978). An immunologic classification based in part on these and other markers is correlated with age, sex, WBC, and so on (table 51.3).

Other prognostic factors include morphologic cell type, initial hemoglobin and platelet count, and status of lymph nodes, liver, and spleen. In general, a poor prognosis seems to correlate with a child being black, older than 15 years, male, having enlarged lymph nodes, hepatosplenomegaly, and especially, a mediastinal mass and CNS involvement at time of diagnosis (table 51.4) (Shaw et al. 1976).

In addition to the better prognosis in ALL, females have fewer problems with puberty and reproductive function after chemotherapy for leukemia. In a study of 35 girls and women (Siris, Leventhal, and Vaitukaitis 1976), 28 (80%) had normal pubertal progression during a median of 74 months after diagnosis of leukemia and 49 months of chemotherapy. Seven patients were abnormal; four exhibited hypothalamic-pituitary dysfunction, and three others had evidence of primary ovarian dysfunction that was reversible in two. Normal development is further enhanced in patients who are prepubertal at onset of leukemia.

Marrow Transplantation

For those who are doomed to fail all chemotherapy regimens for leukemia, so-called supralethal chemo-radiation therapy designed to eradicate the leukemic cell population, followed by marrow transplantation to obviate the marrow toxicity, is an attractive concept. Thomas and co-workers (1979) treated 26 patients with ALL who were in relapse with cyclophosphamide, 60 mg/kg on each of two days, total-body irradiation of 920 rad, and a marrow transplant from an HLA-identical sibling. Four of the patients are alive 15 to 35 months after transplantation. By way of contrast, 11 of 22 patients with ALL who underwent transplantation in second or subsequent remissions were alive 15 to 35 months later. Thus marrow transplantation works best for those who need it least, and is worst for those who need it most. The limitations of the technique even for those fortunate enough to have an HLA-matched sibling are long hospitalization, significant expense, and only a 50% survival rate for those who have already achieved remission. For the identifiable high-risk group, however, marrow transplantation offers the best chance for long-term survival.

Adult ALL

Essentially all adolescents over age 15 and adults with ALL have a poor prognosis. About 5% to 10% have a Burkitt-type ALL, which has the worst prognosis and shortest remissions. At least an additional 10%, and probably many more, have T cell ALL that carries a

Table 51.3. *Immunologic Classification of ALL*

Factor	*Common*	*Null Cell*	*T Cell*	*B Cell*		*B–T Cell*
				Burkitt's/Non-Burkitt's		
Frequency (%)	58	20	20		2	< 1
Sex ratio	M = F	?	M > F	M = F	?	?
Age	2–6	?	> 8	?	?	?
Origin	Marrow	?	Thymus	Nasopharynx	?	?
Mitoses	Low	?	High	High	?	?
Initial WBC	Low	High	High	High	High or low	High
Remission	Long	Long	Short	Shortest	?	?
Surface Ig	0	0	0	+	+	+
E rosettes	0	0	+	0	0	+
Thymic antigens	0	0	+	0	0	+(?)
Common ALL antigen	+	0	0	?	+	?
Ia antigen	+	±	0	+	+	+(?)

SOURCES: Modified from Pinkel 1979 and Necheles 1979.

Table 51.4. *Prognostic Factors in Childhood ALL*

Factor	*Good Prognosis*	*Intermediate Prognosis*	*Poor Prognosis*
Race	Caucasian		Black
Age	3–7 years	< 3, > 7 years	> 15 years
Sex	Female		Male
Morphologic	L-1		L-2, L-3
Immunologic	Common antigen, pre-B cell		T cell, B cell
Cytogenic	Hyperdiploidy		Ph^1+
WBC	< 10,000/mm^3	10–50,000/mm^3	> 50,000/mm^3
Hemoglobin	> 12 gm/dl		< 7 gm/dl
Platelets	> 100,000/mm^3		< 25,000/mm^3
Immunoglobulins	Normal, increased		Decreased
Lymph nodes	Normal		Enlarged
Liver	Normal		Enlarged
Spleen	Normal		Enlarged
Response time	Within 2 weeks	Within 4 weeks	No remission
CNS involvement	Absent		Present
Mediastinal mass	Absent		Present

SOURCE: Modified from Smithson, Gilchrist, and Burgert 1980.

poor prognosis. An as yet unknown proportion of adults have Ph^1 plus ALL with a high incidence of meningeal leukemia and a poor prognosis (Woodruff 1978).

Therapy employs the same drugs used in childhood ALL, with combinations of two, three, and four drugs. The response rates range from 43% with 14.5 months median CR with COAP (cyclophosphamide, vincristine, cytarabine, and prednisone) (Bodey and Rodriguez 1978), to 78% with 25 months median CR using vincristine, prednisone, and daunorubicin and intrathecal methotrexate (Gee et al. 1976). Vigorous consolidation and maintenance therapy are necessary. In some institutions, adults who are poor-risk ALL patients receive one-third higher doses in an attempt to increase the remission rate and duration. These patients in particular must be screened for cardiac toxicity and need supportive care with fluids, diuretics, allopurinol, and if they receive methotrexate, with urinary alkalinization. Central nervous system prophylaxis, management of infection and hemorrhage, and blood component therapy all play essential roles if the outcome is to be satisfactory.

Childhood Acute Myeloblastic Leukemia (AML)

The diagnosis of AML in childhood is not always immediately clear-cut. The diagnostic Auer rod is often difficult to see. Morphology sometimes presents problems although the experienced hematologist should be able to separate ALL and AML about three-quarters of the time on morphologic grounds alone; cytochemical studies should raise the level of accuracy to 90%. With the other modalities shown on pages 567–568 accuracy should eventually approach 100%.

Therapy for AML or ANLL is not as successful as in ALL. A combination of cytarabine and 6-thioguanine resulted in a 66% CR lasting 4 to 68 months (Moreno, Castleberry, and McCann 1977). Although CNS prophylaxis was not employed, there was only one CNS relapse in the group of 20 children. A series of 163 children from the CCSG reported a 59% remission rate (less than 15% blasts) with a survival rate of 55.4% at 12 months for the entire group (Chard 1978).

In another study, 21 children were treated with cytarabine, 6-thioguanine, and doxorubicin (Haghbin, Murphy, and Tan 1977). The CR rate was 74%. For consolidation additional courses of cytarabine and 6-thioguanine were given, followed by L-asparaginase. The maintenance program was the same as for the L-2 protocol (fig. 51.5), including intrathecal methotrexate for CNS prophylaxis. Of 16 evaluable patients, 8 went into CR for 9 to 72 months. In five of eight, chemotherapy was terminated after 3 years and all continue in remission for 11 to 32 months posttreatment. While these results are not as gratifying as those in ALL, they demonstrate that prolonged relapse-free survival is possible in AML of childhood.

Conclusions

In addition to the duration of survival in acute leukemia, or any neoplastic disease, the quality of that survival is important. If a child lives a long time, but half of life is in the hospital, that is an unsatisfactory result. Currently, less than 10% of total days from diagnosis are spent in the hospital and even that proportion should be reduced.

Successful integration of a child with leukemia into the community and the school requires meeting the rehabilitation needs of the child and the family. There must be cooperation among the educators, nurses, social workers, psychologists (or psychiatrists), and the primary physician and oncologist. Working together, the results can only improve to the ultimate benefit of the patient, the family, and society.

References

Aur, R. J. A. et al. Childhood acute lymphocytic leukemia, study VIII. *Cancer* 42:2123–2134, 1978.

Avery, J. B. Advances in the control of cancer in infants and children. *J. Pediatr.* 54:406–408, 1959.

Bennett, J. M. et al. Proposals for the classification of the acute leukemias. French-American-British (FAB) cooperative group. *Br. J. Haematol.* 33:451–458, 1976.

Bodey, G. P., and Rodriguez, V. Approaches to the treatment of acute leukemia and lymphoma in adults. *Semin. Hematol.* 15:221–261, 1978.

Broder, S. et al. Characterization of a suppressor-cell leukemia. *N. Engl. J. Med.* 298:66–72, 1978.

Brouet, J. C., and Seligmann, M. The immunological classification of acute lymphoblastic leukemia. *Cancer* 42:817–827, 1978.

Catovsky, D. Immunologic cell markers in acute leukemia, pp. 743–746 in Gralnick, H. R., moderator. Classification of acute leukemia. *Ann. Intern. Med.* 87:740–753, 1977.

Chard, R. Increased survival in childhood ANLL after treatment with prednisone, cytosine arabinoside, 6-thioguanine, cyclophosphamide, and Oncovin (PATCO) combination chemotherapy. *Med. Pediatr. Oncol.* 4:263–273, 1978.

Chessells, J. M., and Cornbleet, M. Combination chemotherapy for bone marrow relapse in childhood lymphoblastic leukemia (ALL). *Med. Pediatr. Oncol.* 6:359–365, 1979.

Coleman, M. S. et al. Adenosine deaminase, terminal deoxynucleotidyl transferase (TdT), and cell surface markers in childhood acute leukemia. *Blood* 52:1125–1131, 1978.

Farber, S. Action of pteroylglutamine conjugates on man. *Science* 106:619–621, 1947.

Farber, S. Some observations on the effect of folic acid antagonists on acute leukemia and other forms of incurable cancer. *Blood* 4:160–167, 1949.

Farber, S. et al. Temporary remissions in acute leukemia in children produced by folic acid antagonist, 4-aminopteroyl glutamic acid (aminopterin). *N. Engl. J. Med.* 238:787–793, 1948.

Fraumeni, J. F., Jr.; Manning, M. D.; and Mitus, W. J. Acute childhood leukemia: epidemiologic study by cell type of 1263 cases at the Children's Cancer Research Foundation in Boston, 1947–1965. *J. Natl. Cancer Inst.* 46:461–470, 1971.

Frei, E., III, and Sallan, S. E. Acute lymphoblastic leukemia: treatment. *Cancer* 42:828–838, 1978.

Gallo, R. C., and Meyskens, F. L. Advances in the viral etiology of leukemia and lymphoma. *Semin. Hematol.* 15:379–398, 1978.

Gee, T. S. et al. Acute lymphoblastic leukemia in adults and children: differences in response with similar therapeutic regimens. *Cancer* 37:1256–1264, 1976.

George, S. L. et al. A reappraisal of the results of stopping therapy in childhood leukemia. *N. Engl. J. Med.* 300:269–273, 1979.

Haghbin, M. Chemotherapy of acute lymphoblastic leukemia in children. *Am. J. Hematol.* 1:201–209, 1976.

Haghbin, M. et al. A long-term clinical follow-up of children treated with intensive chemotherapy regimens. *Cancer* 46:241–252, 1980.

Haghbin, M.; Murphy, M. L.; and Tan, C. T. C. Treatment of acute non-lymphoblastic leukemia in children with a multiple-drug protocol. *Cancer* 40:1417–1421, 1977.

Hayhoe, F. G. J., and Cawley, J. C. Acute leukaemia: cellular morphology, cytochemistry and fine structure. *Clin. Haematol.* 1:49–94, 1972.

Herson, J. et al. Vincristine and prednisone vs vincristine, L-asparaginase, and prednisone for second remission induction of acute lymphocytic leukemia in children. *Med. Pediatr. Oncol.* 6:317–323, 1979.

Hustu, H. O. et al. Prevention of central nervous system leukemia by irradiation. *Cancer* 32:585–597, 1973.

Kirs, P. J., and Herman, R. M. Neuromotor and neuropsychological manifestations of "total therapy" in children with acute lymphoblastic leukemia. *Cancer Treat. Rev.* 7:85–94, 1980.

Komp, D. M. et al. Is cranial radiation necessary for CNS prophylaxis in ALL childhood? *Proc. Am. Soc. Clin. Oncol.* 16:232, 1975.

Komp, D. M. et al. Cyclophosphamide-asparaginase-vincristine-prednisone induction therapy in childhood acute lymphocytic and non-lymphocytic leukemia. *Cancer* 37:1243–1247, 1976.

Land, V. J. et al. Toxicity of L-asparaginase in children with advanced leukemia. *Cancer* 30:339–347, 1972.

Linman, J. W. *Hematology: physiologic, pathophysiologic, and clinical principles.* New York: Macmillan, 1975.

Mauer, A. M. *Pediatric hematology.* New York: McGraw-Hill, 1969.

Mauer, A. M. Therapy of acute lymphoblastic leukemia in childhood. *Blood* 56:1–10, 1980.

Mauer, A. M., and Simone, J. V. The current status of the treatment of childhood acute lymphoblastic leukemia. *Cancer Treat. Rev.* 3:17–41, 1976.

McCaffrey, R. et al. Terminal deoxynucleotidyl transferase activity in human leukemic cells and in normal human thymocytes. *N. Engl. J. Med.* 292:775–780, 1975.

McIntosh, S. et al. Chronic neurologic disturbance in childhood leukemia. *Cancer* 37:853–857, 1976.

Moreno, H.; Castleberry, R. P.; and McCann, W. P. Cytosine arabinoside and 6-thioguanine in the treatment of childhood acute myeloblastic leukemia. *Cancer* 40:998–1004, 1977.

Myers, M. H. et al. *Cancer incidence survival and mortality for children under 15 years of age.* New York: American Cancer Society, 1976.

Necheles, T. F. *The acute leukemias.* New York: Stratton Intercontinental, 1979.

Nesbit, M. E., Jr. et al. Testicular relapse in childhood acute lymphoblastic leukemia: association with pretreatment patient characteristics and treatment. *Cancer* 45:2009–2016, 1980.

Oshimura, M., and Sandberg, A. A. Chromosomes and causation of human cancer and leukemia. Significance of the Ph^1 (including unusual translocations) in various acute leukemias. *Cancer* 40:1149–1160, 1977.

Pinkel, D. The ninth annual David Karnofsky lecture. Treatment of acute lymphocytic leukemia. *Cancer* 43:1128–1137, 1979.

Price, R. A., and Birdwell, D. A. The central nervous system in childhood leukemia. III. Mineralizing microangiopathy and dystrophic calcification. *Cancer* 42:717–728, 1978.

Price, R. A., and Jamieson, P. A. The central nervous system in childhood leukemia. II. Subacute leukoencephalopathy. *Cancer* 35:306–318, 1975.

Price, R. A., and Johnson, W. W. The central nervous system in childhood leukemia. I. The arachnoid. *Cancer* 31:520–533, 1973.

Priest, J. R. et al. Philadelphia chromosome-positive childhood acute lymphoblastic leukemia. *Blood* 56:15–22, 1980.

Rivera, G. et al. Combined VM-26 and cytosine arabinoside in treatment of refractory childhood lymphocytic leukemia. *Cancer* 45:1284–1288, 1980.

Sallan, S. E. et al. Intermittent combination chemotherapy with Adriamycin for childhood acute lymphoblastic leukemia: clinical results. *Blood* 51:425–433, 1978.

Sallan, S. R. et al. Cell surface antigens: prognostic implications in childhood acute lymphoblastic leukemia. *Blood* 55:395–402, 1980.

Shaw, M. et al. Prognostic factors in acute leukemia. *Semin. Oncol.* 3:199–325, 1976.

Shaw, M. T. et al. Terminal deoxyribonucleotidyl transferase activity in B-cell acute lymphocytic leukemia. *Blood* 51:181–187, 1978.

Silverberg, E. Cancer statistics. 1979. *CA* 29:6–21, 1979.

Silverberg, E. Cancer statistics. 1980. *CA* 30:23–38, 1980.

Simone, J. V. Childhood leukemia as a model for cancer research: the Richard and Hinda Rosenthal Foundation award lecture. *Cancer Res.* 39:4301–4307, 1978.

Simone, J. V. et al. Three to ten years after cessation of therapy in children with leukemia. *Cancer* 42:839–844, 1978.

Simone, J. V.; Verzosa, M. S.; and Rudy, J. A. Initial features and prognosis in 363 children with acute lymphocytic leukemia. *Cancer* 36:2099–2108, 1975.

Siris, E. S.; Leventhal, B. G.; and Vaitukaitis, J. L. Effects of childhood leukemia and chemotherapy on puberty and reproductive function in girls. *N. Engl. J. Med.* 294:1143–1146, 1976.

Skipper, H. E.; Schabel, F. M.; and Wilcox, W. S. Experimental evaluation of potential anticancer agents. XII. On the criteria and kinetics associated with "curability" of experimental leukemias. *Cancer Chemother. Rep.* 35:1–111, 1964.

Smithson, W. A.; Gilchrist, G. S.; and Burgert, E. O. Childhood acute lymphocytic leukemia. *CA* 30:158–181, 1980.

Thomas, E. D. et al. Marrow transplantation for patients with acute lymphoblastic leukemia in remission. *Blood* 54:468–476, 1979.

Vogler, L. B. et al. Pre-B-cell leukemia. A new phenotype of childhood lymphoblastic leukemia. *N. Engl. J. Med.* 298:872–878, 1978.

Wintrobe, M. M. *Clinical hematology,* 7th edition. Philadelphia: Lea & Febiger, 1974.

Woodruff, R. The management of adult lymphoblastic leukemia. *Cancer Treat. Rev.* 5:95–113, 1978.

fifty-two

Adult Acute Non-Lymphocytic Leukemias

MARTIN E. KATZ

The adult acute non-lymphocytic leukemias (ANLL) are a group of diseases characterized by the malignant proliferation and accumulation of immature hematopoietic cells with subsequent bone marrow replacement and visceral organ infiltration leading to infection, bleeding, organ failure, and eventually death. This chapter summarizes kinetic abnormalities of the acute leukemias, reviews a new international classification system, highlights the relationships of ANLL to other hematologic disorders, and discusses the current chemotherapeutic and immunotherapeutic strategies of treatment.

Cell Kinetics

At the time of diagnosis of human acute leukemia, the total body burden of leukemic cells has been estimated to be between 10^{11} and 10^{13} (average 10^{12}) cells. A three-log reduction from 10^{12} (one trillion equals 1 kilogram) to 10^{9} (one billion equals 1 gram) cells results in clinical remission. If one assumes that human leukemia is uniclonal in origin and that a single leukemic cell can reproduce to a lethal number, to achieve cure it is necessary to eradicate all leukemic cells that have the potential to reproduce. If the cell doubling time is four to five days, 10 doublings would bring the number of cells from 10^{9} (remission) back to 10^{12} (relapse) in 40 to 50 days. Since the doubling time increases and the growth fraction (that fraction of the cell population actively proliferating and thus progressing through the cell cycle) decreases as the leukemic cell population expands, the reappearance of 10^{12} cells might take two to four months. This seems to be the case in the unmaintained patient who achieves clinical remission (Thompson, Hall, and Moloney 1965).

Although a prolonged course of antileukemic therapy may be "curative" in terms of eradicating all leukemic cells, it is necessary that a sufficient number of hematopoietic pluripotent stem cells survive. Current chemotherapy schedules all reflect the use of short intensive courses of drug treatment with rest periods to allow normal cells to recover. One hopes that normal cells will recover more rapidly than the leukemic cells so that with each course of treatment a further relatively selective log kill of leukemic cells will result in the elimination of the last viable cell. The three main obstacles to achieving eradication of all leukemic cells are drug resistance, sanctuary sites of disease (leptomeninges and testes), and the small fraction of leukemic cells that stay in an extended dormant or resting phase (G_0) and hence are unaffected by drugs.

The differences in clinical manifestations of ANLL (fulminant disease versus smoldering leukemia versus myelodysplastic states) represent a complex interaction of several factors: the fraction of the leukemic population actively proliferating (growth fraction), the time required for each cell to pass from one mitosis to the next (generation time), the fraction of cells that have the capacity for unlimited reproduction (clonogenic fraction), and the fraction of cells that leaves the proliferating pool to mature or die (rate of spontaneous loss).

Comparing the duration of the phases of the cell cycle (G_1, S, G_2, M) of human acute leukemic myeloblasts to normal myeloblasts, the generation time of normal myeloblasts averages 40 hours as opposed to an average of 45 hours (range 25 to 360 hours) for leukemic myeloblasts. In other words, it takes longer for the leukemic blast to traverse the cell cycle than for the normal blast (Clarkson and Fried 1971; Arlin et al. 1978). The variability of the G_1 portion of the cell cycle (16 hours in normal myeloblasts versus 10 to more than 200 hours in leukemic myeloblasts) accounts for this surprising observation. Kinetic measurements suggest that the growth fraction of the leukemic cell population is smallest at the time of clinical diagnosis. As leukemic cells are destroyed by chemotherapy, cells in the resting phase (G_0) of the cell cycle are capable of returning to active proliferation. Thus in "early" leukemia (10^9 to 10^{10} cells) as compared to "late" leukemia (10^{12} cells), the population doubling times have been estimated at 106 hours versus 264 hours, labeling indices at 38% versus 19%, and mitotic indices 2% versus 0.9% (Clarkson and Fried 1971; Arlin et al. 1978).

Antileukemic therapy should include agents that exert their effects in different phases of the cell cycle, as drugs that are maximally cytotoxic in the same phase may not provide additive effects. In addition, the effectiveness of sequencing combinations may be influenced by using an agent that arrests (blocks) cells at one stage of the cycle followed by one that kills them maximally at the point of the block itself or in the phase immediately succeeding the block.

Treatment programs in clinical practice often make use of an induction phase to reduce the number of leukemic cells from 10^{12} to 10^9 (clinical remission), a consolidation phase to provide further cytoreduction, a maintenance or late intensification phase to kill any remaining resting or slowly proliferating cells, and often, central nervous system prophylaxis to kill any cells sequestered in the leptomeninges.

Great difficulty still remains in defining the optimal sequence of antileukemic drugs as can be seen with cytarabine (cytosine arabinoside), and the anthracycline antibiotics, daunorubicin (Cerubidine) and doxorubicin (Adriamycin). There are no differences in complete remission rates when the two most active antileukemic drugs, cytarabine and an anthracycline, are given sequentially or simultaneously (Arlin et al. 1978). Anthracyclines given first do not cause a consistent increase in the growth fraction of leukemic cells to make them ready for the killing effect of cytarabine in the S phase. In fact, the number of cells in the S phase is often decreased. Similarly, cytarabine given first may cause an accumulation of cells in the S phase, but increased killing in the S phase by the anthracycline is not seen.

Classification of ANLL

The acute leukemias represent a heterogeneous group of diseases with different clinical signs and symptoms, responses to therapy, and prognoses. Methods for characterizing blast cells have included morphology, cytochemistry, electron microscopy, immunology, biochemistry, and cytogenetics. A French-American-British (FAB) classification system was proposed in 1976 (Bennett et al. 1976; Gralnick et al. 1977). This was designed to allow workers more accurately to identify subgroups of leukemia and thus relate treatment modalities to clinical features of disease and prognosis more effectively. The FAB classification (table 52.1) defines six myelocytic variants, designated M1 through M6. The M1 through M3 variants show predominantly granulocytic differentiation.

M1 (myeloblastic without differentiation)—minimal evidence of granulocyte differentiation but no maturation along the granulocytic pathway.

M2 (myeloblastic with differentiation)—clear evidence of maturation to the promyelocyte stage and beyond; the promyelocytes appear morphologically normal. It is often seen with Auer rods (figs. 52.1 and 52.2).

M3 (promyelocytic)—form in which the abnormal cells are packed with Auer rods or abnormal azurophilic granules; also called hypergranular promyelocytic leukemia; this form is regularly associated with disseminated intravascular coagulation.

The FAB classification defines two variants that include a monocytic component.

M4 (myelomonocytic, Naegeli type)—granulocytic and monocytic components exist in varying proportions with different degrees of maturation along each cell line.

M5 ("pure" monocytic, Schilling type)—almost all cells in the bone marrow are monoblasts with the peripheral blood containing either monoblasts (monoblastic without differentiation) or a preponderance of promonocytes and monocytes (monoblastic with differentiation).

One variant is defined with an erythrocytic component.

M6 (erythroleukemia, Di Guglielmo's syndrome)—diagnosed when a high proportion of cells in the marrow are erythroblasts; severe dyserythropoiesis is present; erythroblasts are present in the peripheral blood.

Table 52.1. *FAB Classification of Acute Myelocytic Leukemia*

Variant	*Classic Terminology*	*Predominant Cell Type*
M1	Undifferentiated	Granulocytes
M2	Myeloblastic	Granulocytes
M3	Promyelocytic	Progranulocytes
M4	Myelomonocytic	Granulocytes and monocytes
M5	Monocytic	Monocytes
M6	Erythroleukemia	Erythrocytes and granulocytes

SOURCES: Bennett et al. 1976 and Gralnick et al. 1977.

Histochemical identification of leukemic cells is illustrated in table 52.2. Of note are the peroxidase and Sudan black B stains used in the identification of myeloblastic and myelomonocytic leukemias; the specific esterase stain, naphthol-ASD-chloroacetate esterase, used to identify myeloblastic leukemia; the nonspecific esterase stain, naphthol-ASD-acetate esterase, used to separate myeloblastic from pure monoblastic leukemias; and the PAS stain used to identify lymphoblastic leukemia (Gralnick et al. 1977).

With a uniform program of intensive antileukemic therapy no correlation between the FAB subclass of ANLL and response to therapy, remission duration, or survival has been noted (Foon, Naeim, and Gale 1978).

Relationship of ANLL to Other Diseases

Current theories of the etiology of the acute leukemias have been reviewed in detail by Necheles (1979) and are not discussed here. The incidence of acute myelogenous leukemia in the United States is 2.2 cases per 100,000 people per year (Sieber 1975). Acute leukemia has been reported as a terminal event in a wide variety of hematologic disorders and in association with solid tumors, renal transplantation, and connective tissue diseases (Casciato and Scott 1979). The disease as a consequence of nonleukemic hematologic disorders has recently been summarized, and is outlined as follows (Bloomfield and Brunning 1976):

1. Hereditary disorders
   a. Fanconi's anemia (constitutional aplastic anemia with characteristic physical anomalies)
   b. Ataxia telangiectasia
   c. Bloom's syndrome
2. Acquired nonmalignant hematopoietic disorders
   a. Idiopathic aplastic anemia
   b. Chemical or drug-associated—benzene, chloramphenicol, alkylating agents
   c. Ionizing radiation *(continued on p. 582)*

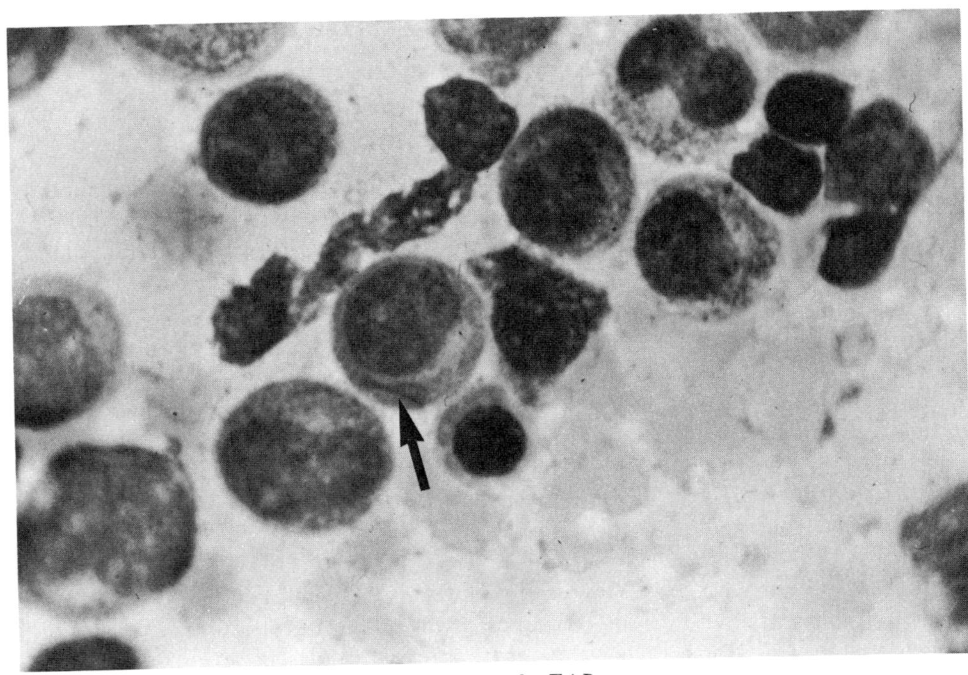

Fig. 52.1. *Acute myeloblastic leukemia (M2 in the FAB classification) with characteristic Auer rod* (arrow).

Table 52.2. *Histochemical Features of the Acute Leukemias*

Histochemical Stain	*AML* *M1*	*M2, M3*	*AMML* *M4*	*AMoL* *M5*	*Erythroleukemia* *M6*	*ALL*
Peroxidase	1+	3+	2+	1+ or 0	1+	0
Sudan black B	1+	3+	2+	1+ or 0	1+	0
Naphthol-ASD-chloroacetate esterase	1+	2+	1+	0	0	0
Naphthol-ASD-acetate esterase						
(without NaF)	1+	2+	3+	3+	1+ or 0	1+ or 0
(with NaF)	1+	2+	3+	0	1+ or 0	1+ or 0
Alpha naphthyl acetate or butyrate esterase	0	0	1+	3+	3+	0
Periodic acid-Schiff (PAS)	1+ or 0	1+	2+	2+	2+	3+
Lysozyme	0	1+	2+	3+	—	0

SOURCE: Gralnick et al. 1977.

NOTES: 0 = no reaction, 1+ = weakly positive, 2+ = positive, 3+ = strongly positive.

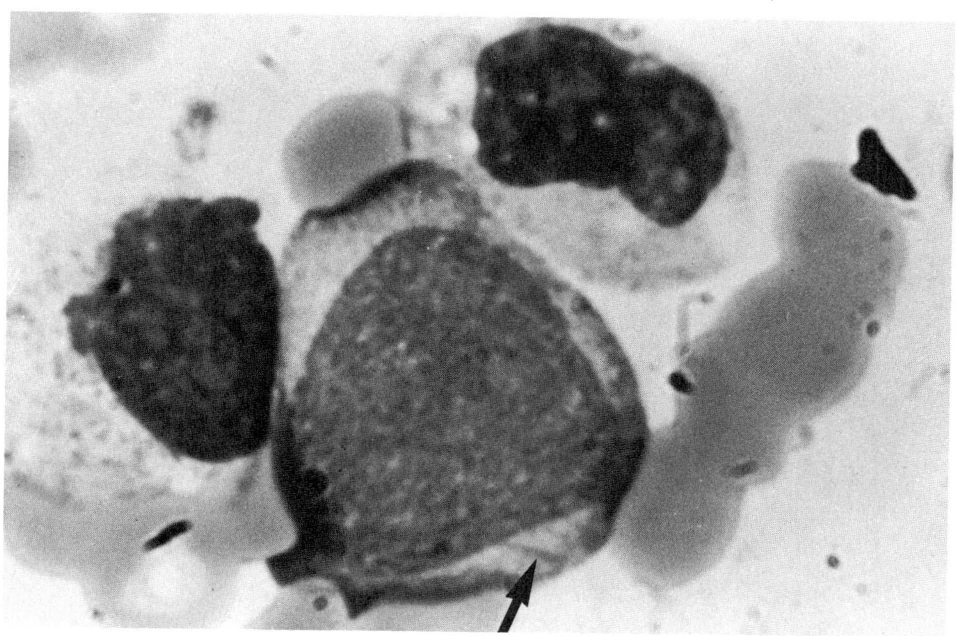

Fig. 52.2. *Typical myeloblast with diagnostic Auer rod* (arrow).

   d. Paroxysmal nocturnal hemoglobinuria
   e. Idiopathic sideroblastic anemia
   f. Polycythemia rubra vera
3. Acquired malignant hematopoietic disorders
   a. Multiple myeloma
   b. Hodgkin's disease (fig. 52.3)
   c. Malignant non-Hodgkin's lymphomas

In view of the potential for long-term disease-free survival and possible cure following treatment for Hodgkin's disease (DeVita, Lewis, and Rosencweig 1978), malignant lymphoma (Lewis and DeVita 1978), and ovarian carcinoma (Young et al. 1978), the increased risk of late development of acute leukemia is disturbing. A number of reviews from cooperative oncology groups and from large cancer centers indicate that there is an excessive risk for the development of acute myelogenous leukemia after treatment for Hodgkin's disease (Toland, Coltman, and Moon 1978; Cadman, Capizzi, and Bertino 1977; Coleman et al. 1977), malignant lymphomas (Collins et al. 1977; Zarrabi, Rosner, and Bennett 1978); and ovarian cancer (Reimer et al. 1977; Einhorn 1978). The common features noted are a long latent period (usually greater than three years) following diagnosis and initial treatment of the primary malignancy, a prolonged exposure to alkylating agents, or procarbazine, and the use of radiation therapy (especially total nodal fields) (Casciato and Scott 1979). The literature suggests that combined modality therapy may be associated with the highest risk, especially in the older age group. It is difficult to define the denominator at the present time. It has been argued that acute leukemia may be a "natural" outcome for some long-term survivors of otherwise fatal neoplasms, especially those of a hematologic nature. The associations of ionizing radiation and leukemia in the Japanese during World War II (Liu et al. 1973) and immunosuppressive agents and leukemia in nonneoplastic disorders (Bukowski et al. 1977; Silvergleid and Schrier 1974; Alexson and Brandt 1977) make this hypothesis unlikely as the sole explanation for the increased risk of leukemia following treatment for lymphoma and ovarian cancer.

Myelodysplastic Syndromes

Idiopathic myelodysplastic syndromes are a group of disorders that have in common defective red cell production unresponsive to specific treatment, often in association with disordered granulopoiesis and thrombopoiesis. These conditions may presage the development of acute myelocytic leukemia.

Refractory anemia with an excess of blasts (RAEB) is the most frequent of these syndromes and has often been called preleukemia or smoldering leukemia (fig. 52.4). These terms imply that all patients will

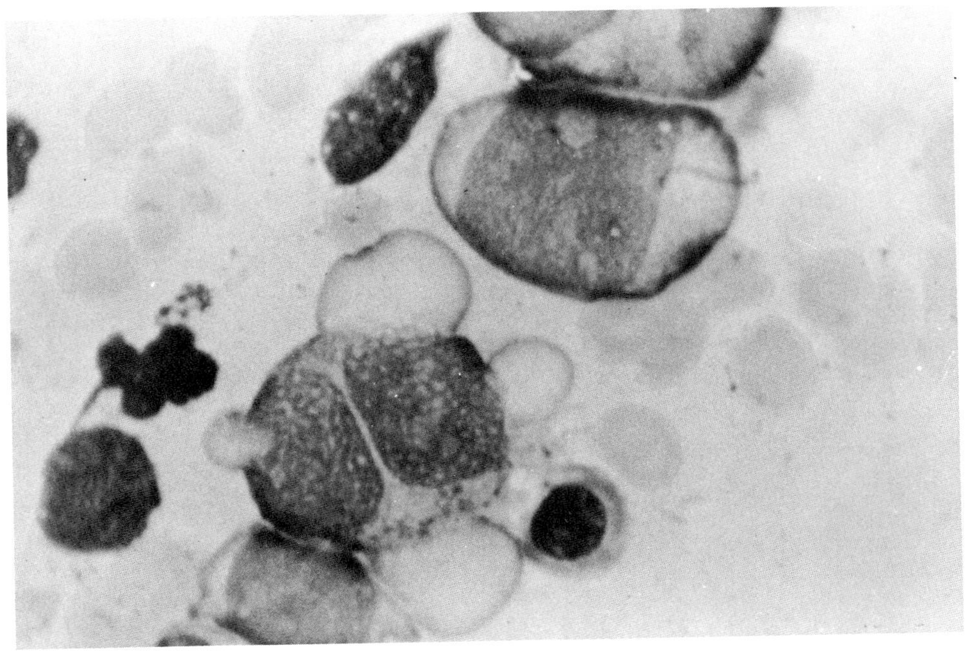

Fig. 52.3. *Typical acute blastic leukemia (M2 in the FAB classification) developing in patient with Hodgkin's disease after combination of radiation therapy and sequential chemotherapy.*

eventually develop leukemia, yet only about 30% do even with long-term follow-up. Hence "preleukemia" should be used only in retrospective fashion. Differentiation between RAEB and acute myelocytic leukemia may require repeated bone marrow examinations to assess the stability of the blast and promyelocytic cell populations. Myeloblastic proliferation is often but not invariably present quite early in the disease.

These syndromes appear to represent a spectrum of disorders that often cause unexplained cytopenic states and progress through RAEB, smoldering leukemia, and acute leukemia. Early diagnostic clues in the peripheral blood may include variable degrees of anemia, neutropenia, thrombocytopenia, monocytosis, oval macrocytosis, nucleated red cells, hyposegmented granulocytes (Pelger-Huet), and bizarre platelets. Bone marrow examination is always hypercellular and may reveal sideroblasts, megaloblastoid erythropoiesis, abnormal or increased megakaryocytes, a left shift in the myeloid series, and the absence of overt leukemia (including the absence of Auer rods) (Saarni and Linman 1973; Linman and Bagby 1978).

Antileukemia therapy is contraindicated in "preleukemic" states, RAEB, smoldering leukemia, and chronic (subacute) myelomonocytic leukemia because patients often remain stable without treatment for many months or years (Linman and Bagby 1978). There is no information to demonstrate that early treatment modifies the natural outcome of this spectrum of disorders (Foucar et al. 1979; Cohen et al. 1979; Najean and Pecking 1979). In a prospective trial conducted by the Cooperative Group for the Study of Aplastic and Refractory Anemias, there was no difference in overall survival or incidence of frank leukemia among groups of patients receiving supportive care only, metenolone (an oral androgen), or low-dose cytarabine (Najean and Pecking 1979).

Treatment

Single-agent chemotherapy has not resulted in durable remissions, but has defined a group of active drugs (table 52.3) from which combinations could be more rationally constructed. Current regimens to induce remission of adult ANLL employ both cytarabine and an anthracycline antibiotic (daunorubicin or doxorubicin) and are capable of achieving complete remission rates of 50% to 82% (Wiernik 1978; Bodey and Rodriguez 1978). Results appear additive when compared to studies using each agent alone. Two studies suggest that the use of 6-thioguanine may add slightly to complete

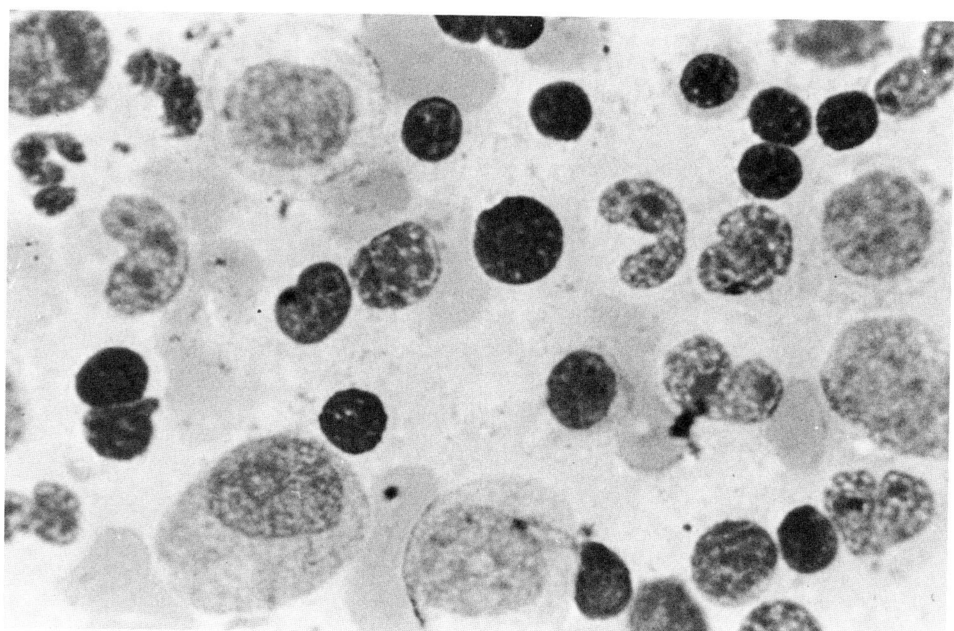

Fig. 52.4. *Patient, originally diagnosed as acute myelomonocytic leukemia with excellent response to one year of therapy, has now survived eight years (seven years off therapy). He is best classified now as either refractory anemia with excess blasts or chronic myelomonocytic leukemia.*

Table 52.3. *Single-Agent Therapy for Acute Myelocytic Leukemia*

Drug	*Approximate Complete Remission Rates (%)*
Daunorubicin	25–50
Doxorubicin (Adriamycin)	10–25
Cytarabine (Ara-C)—standard dose	15–45
Cytarabine (Ara-C)—high dose	25–45
5-Azacytidine	8–30
Amsacrine (m-AMSA)	20–30
6-Thioguanine	< 5
6-Mercaptopurine	< 5
Cyclophosphamide	< 5
L-asparaginase	< 5
Methotrexate	< 5
Vincristine	< 5
Prednisone	< 5

SOURCES: Compiled from Gale 1979; Legha et al. 1980; Von Hoff, Slavik, and Muggia 1976.

remission (Gale and Cline 1977; Peterson et al. 1978). Whether daunorubicin is superior to doxorubicin for induction is unclear at the present time. Doxorubicin regimens are capable of achieving complete remissions of 70% to 82%, thus rivaling those containing daunorubicin (Bodey and Rodriguez 1978; Peterson et al. 1978; Preisler et al. 1978). Cancer and Acute Leukemia Group B is currently in the process of a prospective three-arm study comparing seven- and three-day courses of cytarabine and an anthracycline antibiotic respectively. Cytarabine is administered in a dosage of 100 mg/m^2 continuous intravenous infusion days one to seven in all arms. The anthracycline antibiotics being compared are doxorubicin, 30 mg/m^2 intravenous push days one to three; daunorubicin, 30 mg/m^2 intravenous push days one to three; and daunorubicin, 45 mg/m^2 intravenous push days one to three. Preliminary results show no obvious differences in complete remission rates, but toxicity data illustrate the need to reduce the dosage of anthracycline in patients with impaired hepatic function (Benjamin, Wiernik, and Bachur 1974; Katz and Cassileth 1977).

The relative roles of consolidation and maintenance therapy in prolonging the length of initial remission and overall survival remain unclear. Median initial remissions in various programs using consolidation and/or maintenance therapy appear to last on the order of 5 to 13 months (Wiernik et al. 1976; Glucksberg et al. 1975; Manaster et al. 1975; Cassileth and Katz 1977). In a study from Stanford University using cytarabine, daunorubicin, and 6-thioguanine induction therapy, the investigators randomly compared cytarabine plus 6-thioguanine maintenance to no maintenance at all in the patients showing complete response (Embury et al. 1977). Although median remission duration was prolonged in the maintained group, overall survival results were not statistically significant between the two. In a study from Johns Hopkins University, patients achieving a complete remission after treatment with cytarabine and daunorubicin were followed without further therapy until relapse (Vaughan, Karp, and Burke 1980). Median duration of unmaintained remission was 10 months for the group of complete responders following induction. The Eastern Cooperative Oncology Group is presently conducting a prospective study of the relative roles of intensive consolidation plus maintenance chemotherapy versus maintenance chemotherapy alone in patients achieving complete remission following induction therapy with cytarabine, daunorubicin, and 6-thioguanine.

A novel approach has been taken at the M. D. Anderson Hospital in an attempt to prolong initial remission status. Following initial induction of complete remission and one year of maintenance therapy, patients in continuous complete remission were treated with a combination chemotherapy regimen different from the one that had been used in initial induction, and then with bacillus Calmette-Guerin (BCG) for an additional year (Bodey et al. 1976; Freireich et al. 1978). Of 62 patients entered into the program of late intensification, 29 (47%) are still in complete remission, 12 of whom have been off chemotherapy for more than four years. Of major importance is the observation that 94% of relapses occurred within the first two years of completion of late intensification.

Of several newer chemotherapeutic agents, only 5-azacytidine and amsacrine (m-AMSA; 4′-[9-acridinylamino] methanesulfon-m-anisidide monochloride) have been shown to have significant antileukemic activity. Complete remission rates of 20% to 30% have been produced by 5-azacytidine in patients refractory to "standard" treatment (Von Hoff, Slavik, and Muggia 1976; Vogler, Miller, and Keller 1976; Saiki et al. 1978; Van Echo, Wiernik, and Aisner 1978). Since remission durations have been short, the role of 5-azacytidine as part of initial induction therapy needs to be explored. In a pilot study for initial remission induction therapy testing the efficacy of 5-azacytidine in consolidation therapy, a disappointing 53% complete remission rate was obtained when cytarabine and daunorubicin were combined in a five-day plus three-day combination (Cassileth et al. 1979).

Amsacrine is an exciting new drug with significant single-agent activity in adult acute myeloid leukemia. It is a rationally synthesized aminoacridine with DNA-intercalating properties that has been under clinical study since 1976. Phase I and II studies in patients with acute leukemia refractory to cytarabine and anthracyclines suggest a complete remission rate of 20% to 30% when dose schedules of 75 to 90 mg/m^2/day for seven days, or 120 mg/m^2/day for five days are used (Issell 1980; Weiss, Charles, and MacDonald 1980; Legha et al. 1980). Drug-related side effects include marrow aplasia often prolonged for four to six weeks at the higher dose schedule, mild to moderate hyperbilirubinemia without transaminasemia, and occasionally, a local phlebitis minimized by dilution of amsacrine in large volumes of 5% dextrose (Issell 1980; Winton, Vogler, and Rose 1980; Lawrence et al. 1980). Other reported side effects include fatal cardiac arrhythmias often seen in the setting of hypokalemia, transient stocking and glove paresthesias, and rarely, grand mal seizures. Phase III studies will address the role of amsacrine as a first-line agent in conjunction with anthracycline and/or cytarabine, its role in maintenance therapy, and in combination with 5-azacytidine.

The immunotherapy of acute myelogenous leukemia is reviewed in detail by Murphy and Hersh (1978) and by Alexander and Powles (1978), and is discussed in chapter 15. The results of trials incorporating BCG alone, allogeneic cells plus BCG, methanol-extractable residue (MER) of BCG, and allogeneic cells plus MER-BCG have yielded inconsistent results in terms of increasing overall survival, remission duration, and survival after initial relapse, when compared to chemotherapy alone. Differences in study design, lack of prospective randomized controls, and small numbers of patients are major factors accounting for some of these differences. Despite initial complete remission rates of greater than 60%, a major impediment to the improvement of survival of adults with ANLL is a lack of effective treatment after initial relapse.

Acute promyelocytic leukemia (M3) is almost always associated with disseminated intravascular coagulation. Clinically, patients have symptoms of hemorrhage and historically have a rapidly fatal course with terminal gastrointestinal or central nervous system hemorrhage. A tissue factor that initiates intravascular coagulation appears to be present in the malignant promyelocyte (Gralnick and Sultan 1975). Treatment involves both a chemotherapeutic attack on the leukemia and control of hemorrhagic manifestations. Continuous infusion of heparin at a dose of 100 to 200 units per kilogram per 24 hours begun shortly before or at the time of initial induction chemotherapy has been advocated, and continuing until the tumor load of promyelocytic cells is drastically reduced in the bone marrow or there has been marked improvement in the hypofibrinogenemia, decreased factor V level, prolonged prothrombin time, and prolonged partial thromboplastin time, as well as decrease in the titer of fibrin split products (Gralnick and Sultan 1975; Collins et al. 1978; Valdivieso et al. 1975; Jones and Saleem 1978). Patients should receive platelet transfusions to maintain the platelet count greater than 5000 cells/mm^3. The role of fresh-frozen plasma and cryoprecipitate is undefined (Collins et al. 1978). Long-term survival is certainly possible with early recognition and appropriate management.

Supportive Care

Red Cell Transfusions

Red cell replacement therapy is necessary for almost all patients with acute leukemia to prevent the adverse consequences of anemia and hypoxemic organ damage. With the exception of massive gastrointestinal hemorrhage requiring whole blood, red cell replacement should be in the form of packed red cells made buffy coat-poor, or frozen cells that are washed during deglycerolization and thus separated from most of the leukocytes and almost all of the plasma components. Packed red cells minimize the hazard of volume overload in patients with borderline cardiac reserve, while removal of leukocytes minimizes febrile reactions to pyrogens and leukocyte antigens. The cost of frozen red cells is high but offers the advantage of infrequently being associated with urticarial, anaphylactic, and leukoagglutinin reactions. Red cell transfusions have been associated with transmission of infection (viral hepatitis, cytomegalovirus, infectious mononucleosis, toxoplasmosis, and malaria), sudden intravascular hemolysis secondary to ABO incompatibility, delayed intravascular hemolysis due to Rh incompatibility, and delayed intravascular hemolysis secondary to minor blood group incompatibility. Rarely, posttransfusion purpura in PlA^1-negative recipients may occur (Howard, Glassberg, and Perkins 1979). Red cell transfusions should be given as needed to maintain the hemoglobin greater than 8 gm/dl or whenever the patient is symptomatic at any hemoglobin level above 8 gm/dl.

Platelet Transfusions

The availability of platelet transfusions has reduced the incidence of hemorrhagic death in leukemia from 70% to 80% to 20% to 30%. The risk of hemorrhage climbs markedly when platelet counts are below 20,000 cells/mm^3 (Gaydos, Freireich, and Mantel 1962), although hemorrhagic phenomena may be evident at higher counts in the presence of bacterial sepsis, gastrointestinal bleeding, or disseminated intravascular coagulation. In general, platelets are transfused prophylactically when the platelet count is less than 15,000 plus or minus 5000 cells/mm^3, or at any level if microscopic hematuria, positive stools for occult blood, or fresh fundal hemorrhages are noted (Lister and Yankee 1978).

Platelets lack Rh antigens but have A antigens. Platelet sources may include random donors, HLA-matched donors (related or unrelated to the patient), and frozen autologous platelets obtained from the patient when in remission (Levine and Deisseroth 1978). In general, one unit (approximately 5 to 10×10^{10} platelets) of random-donor platelets yields a 5000-cell to 10,000-cell/mm^3 increment with a half-life of three to four days when transfused into the nonsensitized recipient. About 30% of each unit is immediately sequestered in the spleen. Sensitization due to isoantibodies and alloantibodies, bacterial sepsis, bleeding, and disseminated intravascular coagulation all tend to decrease the expected increment. Usually, 6 to 10 platelet units are transfused from a random donor source. Donors who are HLA-compatible are used when alloimmunization to platelet antigens results in refractoriness to the transfusions (Levine and Deisseroth 1978). Interestingly, prior random-donor platelet transfusion does not prejudice the subsequent utility of HLA-matched platelets (Yankee et al. 1973; Lohrmann et al. 1974). Ideally, HLA-matched platelets should also be ABO-compatible between donor and recipient. When used in the alloimmunized patient, HLA-compatible but ABO-incompatible platelets result in a significant reduction in the recovery of the donor platelets (Duquesnoy et al. 1979). This is not of sufficient magnitude to prohibit the use of ABO-mismatched but otherwise HLA-matched platelets.

Granulocyte Transfusions

Infection remains the leading cause of death in acute leukemia and becomes a major threat to survival with absolute neutrophil counts less than 1000 cells/mm^3 (Bodey 1975). Large numbers of granulocytes estimated to be in the order of 5×10^{10} cells are needed to raise the count from 0 to 2000 cells/mm^3. If the total blood volume of an adult contains 1 to 2×10^{10} granulocytes, then approximately 30 to 40 units of blood would be needed to yield this increment. Further complicating matters is the short (four to seven hours) life of granulocytes in the peripheral circulation.

Three methods are available for procuring granulocytes: continuous-flow centrifugation (CFC), intermittent-flow centrifugation (IFC), and filtration leukapheresis (FL) (Lister and Yankee 1978). The first two methods permit an average four-hour collection from the donor of 1 to 1.5×10^{10} mature functionally intact granulocytes. The third permits collection of 5 to 10×10^{10} granulocytes but the procurement method often results in degranulation of the granulocytes together with production of superoxide radicals, leading to functional abnormalities in in vitro tests and possibly in vivo (Levine and Deisseroth 1978). Granulocytes collected by all methods may be clinically useful. The details of granulocyte procurement have recently been reviewed (Higby and Burnett 1980).

The therapeutic role for neutrophil transfusions remains unclear. Although it appears that survival of neutropenic patients with sepsis given granulocyte transfusions and antibiotics is better than that of similar patients given antibiotics alone, the benefit of these transfusions has only been seen in patients whose granulocyte counts did not recover spontaneously within one to two weeks from the beginning of a septic episode. Those whose counts recovered normally did just as well with antibiotics alone (Levine and Deisseroth 1978). Granulocyte transfusions seem to provide a short-term increment in survival by preventing septic deaths during severe marrow hypoplasia. This is only translated into long-term survival if the bone marrow recovers and control is gained over the neoplastic process by intensive chemotherapy. Criticisms directed at the controlled studies reported (Strauss 1978) have emphasized that (1) small numbers of patients have been studied, usually fewer than 20 per control or transfused group, (2) within each group there is a heterogeneity of underlying diseases, (3) different antibiotic practices are evident even within a single study, and (4) a delay of 48 to 72 hours in beginning granulocyte transfusions preselects a subset of patients potentially resistant to antibiotics. The importance of starting neutrophil transfusions at the time of initial sepsis versus a two- to three-day delay is unknown. Similarly, patients with fever and negative cultures have not been shown to benefit from granulocytes (Alavi et al. 1977). In addition, prophylactic granulocyte transfusions for patients undergoing induction chemotherapy for acute nonlymphocytic leukemia have not been of proved benefit. In a randomized prospective study at the University of California at Los Angeles (Winston, Ho, and Gale 1981) 46 noninfected patients undergoing induction chemotherapy were randomized to receive (25 patients) or not to receive (21 patients) prophylactic granulocyte transfusions when their granulocyte count fell below 500 cells/mm^3. There were no statistically significant differences with respect to frequency of septicemia, remission rates, or survival. Patients receiving granulocyte transfusions had more frequent pulmonary complications (pneumonia, pulmonary edema) and an increased risk for cytomegalovirus infections. Blood component therapy is discussed in more detail with a slightly different perspective in chapter 18.

Protected Environments

Although antibiotic treatment has improved over the past decade, the fatality rate from infection in the patient with acute leukemia remains high, especially if the patient fails to achieve a rapid complete remission. Total protected environments have been developed to attempt to minimize septic death in the neutropenic immunocompromised host. Provisions that have been thought necessary include isolation, air filtration, gastrointestinal and cutaneous decontamination, and "sterile" food and water supplies. While protected environments have theoretic benefits they are extremely expensive to operate from both financial and personnel aspects. Their routine use for high-risk patients should thus be founded on information proving enhanced survival without long-term psychological and physical sequelae.

Available data from six randomized clinical trials demonstrate the ability of protected environments (laminar air-flow rooms plus prophylactic oral nonabsorbable antibiotics) to decrease the incidence of infectious complications during intensive chemotherapy as compared to controls (Pizzo and Levine 1977). Episodes of severe infection have not been totally eliminated because of persistent and resistant organisms. Thus the so-called total protected environment is not totally protective. In attempting to define the relative contributions of filtered air systems, protected environments without prophylactic antibiotics, and prophylactic antibiotics alone, firm conclusions cannot be reached due to small numbers of patients in several trials, the use of historical controls, and variations in antibiotic regimens (Pizzo and Levine 1977). Isolation alone may be of value without prophylactic antibiotics, but only one controlled study suggests this (Yates and Holland 1973).

Twelve clinical trials attempted to answer the question as to whether protected environments or prophylactic antibiotics enhance remission rates and duration. Results are contradictory because of imbalances in the characteristics of control and special treatment groups, small numbers of patients in many of the trials, and variations in remission induction chemotherapy within individual trials (Pizzo and Levine 1977). Of interest is the M. D. Anderson Hospital trial (Rodriguez et al. 1978) demonstrating a significant decrease in fatal infections in patients treated within the protected environment (including prophylactic antibiotics) but not in overall major infections (fatal and nonfatal). In addition, patients within the protected environment had a significantly longer duration of survival from diagnosis but surprisingly, did not have a significantly longer duration of initial remission. The reason for this is unclear. The major criticism of this study is the high early death rate in the group not assigned to the protected environment before an adequate trial of chemotherapy could be given. This suggests that the control and protected environment groups of patients may have been "biologically" unbalanced. Appropriate supportive care of the compromised host is discussed in greater detail in chapter 20.

Bone Marrow Transplantation

Bone marrow transplantation has been pioneered by the Seattle group for the treatment of patients with acute leukemia (Thomas et al. 1977). They reported 3 of 14 long-term (52 to 67+ months) identical twin survivors and 6 of 58 long-term (21 to 63+ months) allogeneic survivors among patients treated with marrow transplants for acute myelogenous leukemia (Sanders and Thomas 1978). Despite the encouraging results, recurrent leukemia during the first two years posttransplantation and infection remain major problems for both syngeneic and allogeneic transplants. Graft-versus-host disease with its attendant problems of skin, hepatic, and gastrointestinal organ dysfunction and failure poses a significant threat for the allogeneic marrow recipient despite major histocompatibility locus matching (Sanders and Thomas 1978). At present, bone marrow transplants are being performed in patients with ANLL in complete remission, with the hope of providing long-term disease-free survival. The rationale underlying this experimental approach takes into account the fact that the remission duration of ANLL is short, the chances for a second durable remission are small, the leukemic cell burden is "minimal" when a complete remission is obtained, and the patient may be in optimal medical condition when in first remission.

Initial information from Seattle regarding a select group of 19 patients transplanted from HLA-identical siblings when in first remission from conventional chemotherapy revealed that 12 patients were in remission more than one year following bone marrow transplantation (Thomas et al. 1979). A Kaplan-Meir plot of survival of these patients showed an apparent plateau of 63%. This study has been sharply criticized, as several investigators have achieved a similar survival in young patients treated with chemotherapy alone (Begg, Bennett, and Cassileth 1980). A prospective trial is now under way to compare the results of chemotherapy with those of bone marrow transplantation.

Summary

Despite higher complete remission rates of 50% to 80% in acute non-lymphocytic leukemia, it is discouraging that the majority of patients relapse within one year of achieving remission. Although median survivals in acute myelogenous leukemia are between one and two years, the 40% to 50% long-term disease-free survival seen in childhood acute lymphatic leukemia has not been achieved. Current investigational efforts are being directed at the development of new antileukemic drugs to prevent the emergence of drug-resistant leukemic clones, at the use of late intensification therapy to eradicate dormant leukemic cells, and at improving supportive care measures for the infected pancytopenic patient through transfusion therapy and protected environments.

References

Alavi, J. B. et al. A randomized clinical trial of granulocyte transfusions for infection in acute leukemia. *N. Engl. J. Med.* 296:706–711, 1977.

Alexander, P., and Powles, R. Immunotherapy of human acute leukaemia. *Clin. Haematol.* 7:275–294, 1978.

Alexson, E., and Brandt, K. D. Acute leukemia after azathioprine treatment of connective tissue disease. *Am. J. Med. Sci.* 273:335–340, 1977.

Arlin, Z. A. et al. Therapeutic role of cell kinetics in leukaemia. *Clin. Haematol.* 7:339–362, 1978.

Begg, C. B.; Bennett, J. M.; and Cassileth, P. A. Marrow transplantation for acute nonlymphoblastic leukemia. Letter to the editor. *N. Engl. J. Med.* 302:408–409, 1980.

Benjamin, R. S.; Wiernik, P. H.; and Bachur, N. R. Adriamycin chemotherapy—efficacy, safety and pharmacologic basis of an intermittent single high-dose schedule. *Cancer* 33:19–27, 1974.

Bennett, J. M. et al. Proposals for the classification of the acute leukemias. French-American-British cooperative group. *Br. J. Haematol.* 33:451–458, 1976.

Bloomfield, C. D., and Brunning, R. D. Acute leukemia as a terminal event in nonleukemia disorders. *Semin. Oncol.* 3:297–317, 1976.

Bodey, G. P. Infections in cancer patients. *Cancer Treat. Rev.* 2:89–128, 1975.

Bodey, G. P. et al. Late intensification for acute leukemia in remission. *JAMA* 235:1021–1025, 1976.

Bodey, G. P., and Rodriguez, V. Approaches to the treatment of acute leukemia and lymphoma in adults. *Semin. Hematol.* 15:221–242, 1978.

Bukowski, R. M. et al. Characteristics of acute leukemia in patients with nonmalignant disease receiving alkylating agent therapy. *Blood* 50(suppl.):185, 1977.

Cadman, E. C.; Capizzi, R. L.; and Bertino, J. R. Acute nonlymphocytic leukemia. A delayed complication of Hodgkin's disease therapy: analysis of 109 cases. *Cancer* 40:1280–1296, 1977.

Casciato, D. A., and Scott, J. L. Acute leukemia following prolonged cytotoxic agent therapy. *Medicine* 58:32–47, 1979.

Cassileth, P. A. et al. Feasibility and efficacy of 5-azacytidine used in the therapy of adult acute nonlymphocytic leukemia. *Cancer Clin. Trials.* 2:339–343, 1979.

Cassileth, P. A., and Katz, M. E. Chemotherapy for adult acute nonlymphocytic leukemia with daunorubicin and cytosine arabinoside. *Cancer Treat. Rep.* 61:1441–1445, 1977.

Clarkson, B. D., and Fried, J. Changing concepts of treatment in acute leukemia. *Med. Clin. North Am.* 55:561–600, 1971.

Cohen, J. R. et al. Subacute myeloid leukemia: clinical review. *Am. J. Med.* 66:959–966, 1979.

Coleman, C. N. et al. Hematologic neoplasia in patients treated for Hodgkin's disease. *N. Engl. J. Med.* 297:1249–1252, 1977.

Collins, A. J. et al. Acute nonlymphocytic leukemia in patients with nodular lymphoma. *Cancer* 40:1748–1754, 1977.

Collins, A. J. et al. Acute promyelocytic leukemia. Management of the coagulopathy during daunorubicin-prednisone remission induction. *Arch. Intern. Med.* 138:1677–1680, 1978.

DeVita, V. T.; Lewis, R. J.; and Rosencweig, M. The chemotherapy of Hodgkin's disease. *Cancer* 42:979–990, 1978.

Duquesnoy, R. J. et al. ABO compatibility and platelet transfusions of alloimmunized thrombocytopenic patients. *Blood* 54:595–599, 1979.

Einhorn, N. Acute leukemia after chemotherapy (melphalan). *Cancer* 41:444–447, 1978.

Embury, S. H. et al. Remission maintenance therapy in acute myelogenous leukemia. *West. J. Med.* 126: 267–272, 1977.

Foon, K. A.; Naeim, F.; and Gale, R. P. Acute myelogenous leukemia: morphologic subclass and response to therapy. *Blood* 52(suppl.):249, 1978.

Foucar, K. et al. Therapy-related leukemia: panmyelosis. *Cancer* 43:1285–1296, 1979.

Freireich, E. J. et al. Therapy of acute myelogenous leukemia. *Cancer* 42:874–882, 1978.

Gale, R. P. Advances in the treatment of acute myelogenous leukemia. *N. Engl. J. Med.* 300:1189–1199, 1979.

Gale, R. P., and Cline, M. J. High remission induction rate in acute myeloid leukaemia. *Lancet* 1:497–499, 1977.

Gaydos, L. A.; Freireich, E. J.; and Mantel, N. The quantitative relation between platelet count and hemorrhage in patients with acute leukemia. *N. Engl. J. Med.* 266:905–909, 1962.

Glucksberg, H. et al. Combination chemotherapy for acute non-lymphoblastic leukemia in adults. *Cancer Treat. Rep.* 59:1131–1137, 1975.

Gralnick, H. R. et al. Classification of acute leukemia. *Ann. Intern. Med.* 87:740–753, 1977.

Gralnick, H. R., and Sultan, C. Acute promyelocytic leukaemia: haemorrhagic manifestation and morphologic criteria. *Br. J. Haematol.* 29:373–376, 1975.

Higby, D. J., and Burnett, D. Granulocyte transfusions: current status. *Blood* 55:2–8, 1980.

Howard, J. E.; Glassberg, A. B.; and Perkins, H. A. Post-transfusion thrombocytopenic purpura: a case report. *Am. J. Hematol.* 1:339–342, 1976.

Issell, B. F. Amsacrine (AMSA). *Cancer Treat. Rev.* 7:73–83, 1980.

Jones, M. E., and Saleem, A. Acute promyelocytic leukemia. *Am. J. Med.* 65:673–677, 1978.

Katz, M. E., and Cassileth, P. A. Hyperbilirubinemia during induction therapy of acute granulocytic leukemia. *Cancer* 40:1390–1392, 1977.

Lawrence, H. J. et al. m-AMSA: a promising new agent in refractory acute leukemia. *Proc. Am. Soc. Clin. Oncol.* 21:438, 1980.

Legha, S. S. et al. 4′-(9-acridinylamino)methanesulfon-m-anisidide (AMSA): a new drug effective in the treatment of adult acute leukemia. *Ann. Intern. Med.* 93:17–21, 1980.

Levine, A. S., and Deisseroth, A. B. Recent developments in the supportive therapy of acute myelogenous leukemia. *Cancer* 42:883–894, 1978.

Lewis, B. J., and DeVita, V. T. Combination therapy of the lymphomas. *Semin. Oncol.* 15:431–457, 1978.

Linman, J. W., and Bagby, G. C. The preleukemic syndrome (hemopoietic dysplasia). *Cancer* 42:854–864, 1978.

Lister, T. A., and Yankee, R. A. Blood component therapy. *Clin. Haematol.* 7:407–423, 1978.

Liu, P. I. et al. Autopsy study of leukemia in atomic bomb survivors, Hiroshima-Nagasaki 1949–1969. *Cancer* 31:1315–1327, 1973.

Lohrmann, H. P. et al. Platelet transfusions, from HLA-compatible unrelated donors to alloimmunized patients. *Ann. Intern. Med.* 80:9–14, 1974.

Manaster, J. et al. Remission maintenance of acute non-lymphoblastic leukemia with BCNU (NSC 409962) and cyclophosphamide (NSC 26271). *Cancer Treat. Rep.* 59:537–545, 1975.

Murphy, S., and Hersh, E. Immunotherapy of leukemia and lymphoma. *Semin. Hematol.* 15:181–203, 1978.

Najean, Y., and Pecking, A. Refractory anemia with excess of blast cells: prognostic factors and effect of treatment with androgens or cytosine arabinoside. Results of a prospective trial in 58 patients. *Cancer* 44:1976–1982, 1979.

Necheles, T. F. The acute leukemias. In *Clinical monographs in hematology,* vol. 1, ed. T. F. Necheles. New York: Stratton Intercontinental, 1979, pp. 8, 19–26.

Peterson, B. A. et al. Rapid remission induction with intensive chemotherapy in adult acute non-lymphocytic leukemia. *Blood* 52(suppl.):269, 1978.

Pizzo, P. A., and Levine, A. S. The utility of protected environment regimens for the compromised host: a critical reassessment. In *Progress in hematology,* vol. 10, ed. E. B. Brown. New York: Grune & Stratton, 1977, pp. 311–332.

Preisler, H. et al. Treatment of AML with cytosine arabinoside and anthracycline. *Proc. Am. Soc. Clin. Oncol.* 19:389, 1978.

Reimer, R. R. et al. Acute leukemia after alkylating agent therapy of ovarian cancer. *N. Engl. J. Med.* 297:177–181, 1977.

Rodriguez, V. et al. Randomized trial of protected environment-prophylactic antibiotics in 145 adults with acute leukemia. *Medicine* 57:253–266, 1978.

Saarni, M., and Linman, J. W. Preleukemia. *Am. J. Med.* 55:38–48, 1973.

Saiki, J. H. et al. 5-Azacytidine in acute leukemia. *Cancer* 42:2111–2114, 1978.

Sanders, J. E., and Thomas, E. D. Bone marrow transplantation for acute leukaemia. *Clin. Haematol.* 7:295–311, 1978.

Sieber, S. M. Cancer chemotherapeutic agents and carcinogenesis. *Cancer Chemother. Rep.* 59:915–918, 1975.

Silvergleid, A. J., and Schrier, S. L. Acute myelogenous leukemia in two patients treated with azathioprine for nonmalignant disease. *Am. J. Med.* 57:885–888, 1974.

Strauss, R. H. Therapeutic neutrophil transfusions. Are controlled studies no longer appropriate? *Am. J. Med.* 65:1001–1006, 1978.

Thomas, E. D. et al. One hundred patients with acute leukemia treated by chemotherapy, total body irradiation and allogeneic marrow transplantation. *Blood* 49:511–533, 1977.

Thomas, E. D. et al. Marrow transplantation for acute nonlymphoblastic leukemia in first remission. *N. Engl. J. Med.* 301:597–599, 1979.

Thompson, I.; Hall, J. C.; and Moloney, W. C. Combination therapy of adult acute myelogenous leukemia. *N. Engl. J. Med.* 273:1302–1307, 1965.

Toland, D. M.; Coltman, C. A.; and Moon, T. E. Second malignancies complicating Hodgkin's disease: the Southwest Oncology Group experience. *Cancer Clin. Trials* 1:27–33, 1978.

Valdivieso, M. et al. Clinical and morphological correlations in acute premyelocytic leukemia. *Med. Pediatr. Oncol.* 1:37–50, 1975.

Van Echo, D. A.; Wiernik, P. H.; and Aisner, J. Reinduction therapy for relapsed adult acute non-lymphocytic leukemia patients. *Proc. Am. Assoc. Cancer Res.* 19:144, 1978.

Vaughan, W. P.; Karp, J. E.; and Burke, P. J. Long chemotherapy-free remissions after single-cycle timed sequential chemotherapy for acute myelocytic leukemia. *Cancer* 45:859–865, 1980.

Vogler, W. R.; Miller, D. S.; and Keller J. W. 5-Azacytidine (NSC 102816): a new drug for the treatment of myeloblastic leukemia. *Blood* 48:331–337, 1976.

Von Hoff, D.; Slavik, M.; and Muggia, F. M. 5-Azacytidine. A new anticancer drug with effectiveness in acute myelogenous leukemia. *Ann. Intern. Med.* 35:237–245, 1976.

Weiss, R. B.; Charles, L. M.; and MacDonald, J. S. m-AMSA: an exciting new drug in the National Cancer Institute drug development program. *Cancer Clin. Trials* 3:203–209, 1980.

Wiernik, P. H. Treatment of acute leukaemia in adults. *Clin. Haematol.* 7:259–273, 1978.

Wiernik, P. H. et al. Randomized clinical comparison of daunorubicin alone and the combination of daunorubicin, cytosine arabinoside, 6-thioguanine and pyrimethamine for the treatment of acute non-lymphocytic leukemia. *Cancer Treat. Rep.* 60:41–53, 1976.

Winston, D. J.; Ho, W. G.; and Gale, R. P. Prophylactic granulocyte transfusions during chemotherapy of acute nonlymphocytic leukemia. *Ann. Intern. Med.* 94:616–622, 1981.

Winton, E. F.; Vogler, W. R.; and Rose, K. L. Phase II study of acridinyl anisidide (m-AMSA) (NSC 249992) in refractory adult leukemia. *Proc. Am. Soc. Clin. Oncol.* 21:437, 1980.

Yankee, R. A. et al. Selection of unrelated compatible platelets donors by lymphocyte HLA matching. *N. Engl. J. Med.* 15:760–764, 1973.

Yates, J. W., and Holland, J. F. A controlled study of isolation and endogenous microbial suppression in acute myelocytic leukemia patients. *Cancer* 32: 1490–1498, 1973.

Young, R. C. et al. Advanced ovarian adenocarcinoma: a prospective trial of melphalan versus combination chemotherapy. *N. Engl. J. Med.* 299:1261–1266, 1978.

Zarrabi, M. H.; Rosner, F.; and Bennett, J. M. Acute leukemia and non-Hodgkin lymphoma. Letter to the editor. *N. Engl. J. Med.* 298:280, 1978.

fifty-three

Chronic Granulocytic Leukemia

PAUL L. SCHULMAN

Chronic granulocytic leukemia is to the clinician a perennially fascinating disease. Its interest lies paradoxically both in its superficial uniformity and in its seemingly unlimited variations. While the majority of patients conform to a classical picture in both presenting features and subsequent course, a substantial number deviate from this pattern in ways ranging from the subtle to the extravagant. So numerous are the variations encountered in clinical practice that chronic granulocytic leukemia constantly has something new to teach even the experienced physician. (Spiers 1977)

Chronic granulocytic leukemia (CGL) was actually the first form of leukemia to be described, and was originally called splenic leukemia based on splenomegaly and marked increase in white cell count. It is part of a spectrum of myeloproliferative syndromes that includes the following:

Polycythemia vera

Agnogenic myeloid metaplasia

Primary thrombocythemia

Dysmyelopoietic syndromes
A. Refractory anemia with excess blasts
B. Chronic myelomonocytic leukemia
C. Idiopathic sideroblastic anemia
D. Paroxysmal nocturnal hemoglobinuria
E. Bone marrow failure with cellular marrow

Chronic granulocytic leukemia
A. Philadelphia chromosome positive
B. Philadelphia chromosome negative

Subacute granulocytic leukemia

Erythroleukemia

Acute myelomonocytic leukemia

Acute myeloblastic leukemia

The cause has still not been found, and few patients have been cured. It is rare in childhood and found in the adult population mainly between the third and sixth decades. All races are affected, and it constitutes approximately 15% to 20% of all adult leukemias in the western world. Approximately 3000 to 4000 cases per year are identified in the United States.

Etiology

Viruses have been implicated in the causation of animal leukemia, but their role in human disease is conjectural. Ionizing radiation is definitely an etiology, first recognized following the introduction of x-ray for diagnostic purposes in 1895. There was a dramatic rise in leukemia in physicians approximating 1.7 times the number of cases found in the general population, and it was soon realized that this increase was primarily due to disease encountered in radiologists. With proper shielding techniques this has virtually been eliminated. The atomic bomb experience in Hiroshima and Nagasaki in 1945 provided evidence for the leukemogenic effect of a single dose of radiation therapy with a latent period of approximately three years and maximum incidence approximately six to seven years following exposure. The risk of developing leukemia was directly related to the distance from the actual site of radiation; people at the hypocenter obviously were at maximal risk, having a 50-fold increase in leukemia. Almost all of the leukemias encountered were granulocytic, approximately two-thirds acute and one-third chronic. Of significance is that offspring of those exposed to radiation did not have an increased incidence. The third series relating radiation to leukemia was encountered in England in patients with ankylosing spondylitis treated by radiation. Following a latent period of six to seven years there was a 13-fold increase, predominantly CGL.

Chemical exposure with leukemogenesis has also been unequivocally related to benzene compounds, and all chemicals capable of causing myelotoxicity are potentially suspect. Despite these data in reference to ionizing radiation and chemical compounds, it is highly unlikely that most cases that develop at random are caused by either. The majority of patients have no abnormal exposure.

There is no well-defined hereditary liability, and children born of mothers with CGL are not affected. In addition, identical twins of affected siblings usually do not develop the disease. Leukemic clusters have been described on numerous occasions, but most of these refer to acute leukemias.

This is a myeloproliferative disorder resulting from the malignant transformation of a pluripotential hematopoietic stem cell and in most instances, examination of the bone marrow reveals a unique marker that is diagnostic of the disease.

Cytogenetics

In 1960, Nowell and Hungerford described a small acrocentric chromosome in leukemic cells in the peripheral blood of two patients with CGL. Later that same year they described five more similar abnormalities and noted that they were all in the G group of chromosomes. The abnormality was named after the city in which it was discovered, Philadelphia. The Philadelphia (Ph^1) chromosome is unique in all of neoplastic disease. This was originally thought to represent a deletion of a portion of the long arm of the twenty-first chromosome, with approximately 40% less DNA on the abnormal chromosome. Subsequent studies revealed that this abnormality was truly a translocation with deletion of a portion of the long arm of the twenty-second chromosome with the translocated material being added to the ninth chromosome (figs. 53.1 and 53.2), or occasionally to second, sixth, seventeenth, or nineteenth. The Ph^1 is found to be present in approximately 90% of patients with typical CGL and is characteristically absent in other myeloproliferative disorders. Of great significance is the fact that the Ph^1 abnormality has been found in erythroid, megakaryocytic, and myeloid cell lines, indicating that it occurs early in the stem cell phase prior to differentiation. It has not been found in the lymphoid or fibroblastic lines. When one of a pair of identical twins developed CGL, only the affected member had the Ph^1, therefore proving this to be an acquired disorder. Until recently the Ph^1 has been found to persist in the bone marrow even during com-

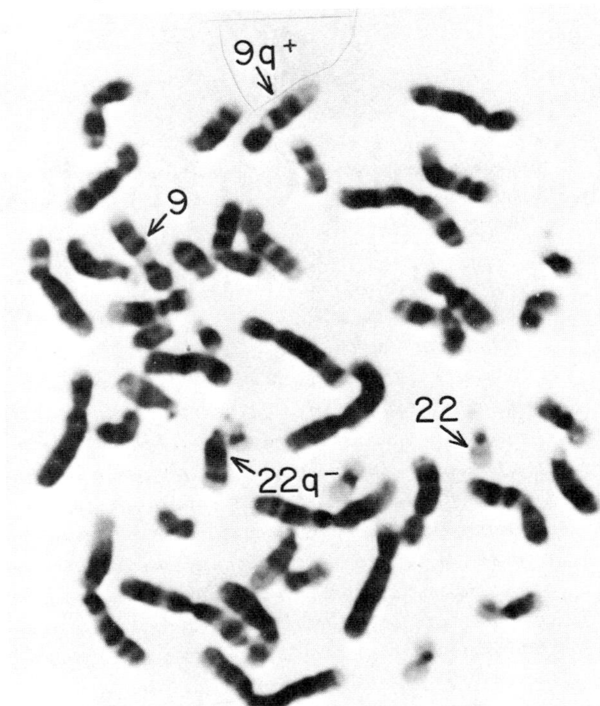

Fig. 53.1. *Metaphase spread of bone marrow cell from patient with chronic granulocytic leukemia. The Ph^1 (22q−) chromosome is shown along with the translocation to chromosome 9 (9q+). Unaffected chromosomes 9 and 22 are also shown. (Photograph courtesy of Dr. W. Roy Breg, Jr., Department of Human Genetics, Yale University School of Medicine.)*

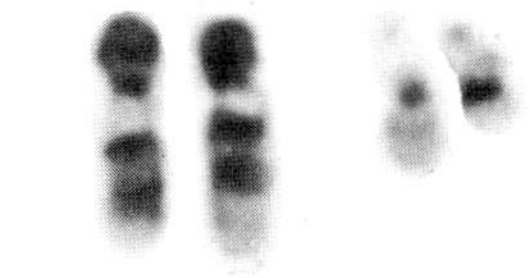

Fig. 53.2. *Enlargement of chromosomes shown in figure 53.1.* Left to right: *chromosome 9, 9q+, 22, 22q−.*

Table 53.1. *Prognosis in Chronic Granulocytic Leukemia*

Philadelphia Chromosome	*Sex Chromosomes*	*Age*	*Prognosis*
Present	45 XO males	All	Good
Present	XY or XX	All	Fair
Absent	XY or XX	Older	Poor
Absent	XY or XX	Infancy	Very poor
Absent or present	Blast transformation	All	Very poor

SOURCES: Compiled from Speed and Lawler 1964; Smith and Johnson 1974; Lawler 1977.

plete hematologic remission. During acute transformation of disease into blast crisis other chromosomal aberrations are often superimposed. Of clinical significance is that patients who are Ph^1-negative often have atypical courses and frequently have a more aggressive form of disease (table 53.1).

Leukemogenesis indicates a change from a normal to a neoplastic state. It is generally thought that damage to a chromosome, for example, from irradiation, produces mitotic abnormalities that can lead to cell death, but occasionally instead can lead to an aberrant growth pattern that may progress to a preleukemic phase of two to six years. Once a disease process becomes established the Ph^1-containing cells persist throughout the disease. Support for the clonal origin came from study of patients heterozygous for the glucose-6-phosphate dehydrogenase (G-6-PD) locus (X-linked). If a tumor is truly unicellular in origin, it is felt that tumor cells should contain only one of the two enzyme types of G-6-PD (A or B). Accordingly, several black women with typical CGL and the heterozygous form of G-6-PD were studied and it was found that both A and B types of enzyme existed in fibroblasts, whereas only A type was found in the red cell and myeloid series. This afforded evidence for the clonal origin of CGL as well as indicating a common stem cell for the erythroid and myeloid precursors.

The prognostic implication of Ph^1-positive chromosomes in CGL is that these patients' median survival is 40 months as opposed to 8 months for Ph^1-negative patients. Mixtures of positive and negative cells have been found in some patients in the chronic phase of disease. There is also a group of patients with acute myeloid leukemia who are found to have the Ph^1 with no prior history of the chronic phase; this situation has been termed the telescoped type of CGL in which the entire chronic phase has been telescoped into a short period of time resulting in acute blast crisis as the presenting manifestation.

Cell Kinetics

Cell kinetic characteristics and the functional status of CGL granulocytes vary greatly and depend on the hematologic status of the patient at the time kinetics are studied. Accordingly, the status of the disease must be known to interpret these measurements properly. Clinical disease is usually divided into three phases: (I) the time of diagnosis or during full-blown relapse, (II) unmaintained remission (after a course of effective therapy), and (III) blast transformation or crisis. During phase I there is a high leukocyte count with infiltration of the marrow and spleen by leukemic cells. At this time many of the kinetic abnormalities could be the result of rather than the cause of increased granulocyte cell mass. The total blood granulocyte pool (TBGP) is 10 to 100 times normal. If only the mature neutrophils are considered, the increase is only 3 to 30 times normal. With diisopropylfluorophosphate (DF ^{32}P) labeling, the granulocyte half-life (T½) in the peripheral blood is 4 to 12 times longer than that of normal polymorphonuclear cells (PMNs) (26 to 89 hours instead of the normal 6 to 7 hours) (Athens et al. 1965). The third abnormality is an increase in the granulocyte turnover rate (GTR). The GTR is increased 2 to 14 times during this phase of CGL. The conclusions, therefore, are that in active CGL with an increased leukocyte count effective production of granulocytes is increased, as is the transit time of granulocytes in the peripheral blood. The prolonged transit time alone is not enough to account for the magnitude of the leukocytosis.

During phase II (remission) the TBGP, the GTR, and T½ return to normal values despite the fact that the Ph^1 persists. Moreover, in remission there is improvement in the function of the neutrophils with improvement in phagocytic activity, migration capacity, and sometimes an increase in the leukocyte alkaline phosphatase to more normal limits.

Other features of phase I are that the PMN abnormalities appear to be due to the increase in TBGP, which apparently alters release of granulocytic cells. Immature cells that are absent from the blood during remission reappear in relapse. Therefore during this chronic phase the increased granulocyte mass causes premature release of immature cells that remain in the blood longer than normal.

In studying the myeloblast at the time of diagnosis, the proliferative activity is generally decreased as indicated by a lower than normal proportion of cells in DNA synthesis. In normal cell populations approximately 40% to 50% are in cycle whereas in active CGL only approximately 20% are in cycle. This slower myeloblastic proliferation occurs only when the white blood cell count (WBC) is higher than 40,000. During unmaintained remission with a near-normal WBC the tritiated thymidine labeling index is approximately 45% (normal). This abnormal proliferative rate is secondary to the increased total granulocyte cell mass, suggesting that myeloblasts are still responsive to the action of some regulatory mechanism.

In phase III (blast transformation) myeloblasts are abundant in the blood and bone marrow with a virtual absence of mature neutrophils. There is an inverse relationship between the percentage of myeloblasts in the marrow and the fraction of cells in DNA synthesis, that is, with 50% blast forms the percent in DNA synthesis is only approximately 5%. Therefore the cells are actually unable to divide and mature, and a large blast population in CGL can be maintained by continuous reentry into cycle of blast forms. This would also explain the lack of activity of cycle-specific drugs.

The development of an agar culture technique that supports growth and differentiation of granulocyte-committed stem cells has made it possible to study humoral regulators of granulopoiesis. This also provides a tool to investigate abnormalities of the white cell compartment in human leukemia. This in vitro system has provided evidence for a regulator of granulopoiesis responsible for the stimulation of colony growth, which is generally known as colony-stimulating factor (CSF). The term CFU-c is used for colony-forming units in culture, and these comprise approximately 0.1% to 1% of the total nucleated cell population of the bone marrow. Morphologically, these are undifferentiated mononuclear cells that are committed to granulocyte or monocyte differentiation; CFU-c are also found in the blood. Recently, qualitative abnormalities have been found in the leukemic state and among these are defects in the growth and maturation capacity of CFU-c.

In vitro studies in the chronic phase of CGL show that in untreated disease (phase I) the colony-forming capacity of bone marrow is either normal or increased, and there is also a greatly increased number of CFU-c present in circulation. A study of 103 patients (Moore 1977) found the incidence of colony-forming cells in the bone marrow increased an average of 15-fold, and circulating CFU-c increased 500-fold. A correlation has been observed between the height of the white count and the total circulating CFU-c. The magnitude of the increase in the granulocyte-committed stem cell compartment is out of proportion to the 5-fold to 20-fold increase in granulocyte production, and therefore would indicate overproduction of committed stem cells from the multipotent stem cell compartment. This may indeed be the underlying defect in CGL.

In addition to the quantitative abnormalities in CFU-c, qualitative abnormalities have been noted in CGL. The concept of inappropriate regulatory control as the major factor in the development of progressive CGL has been reenforced by studies of CSF. Serum and urine levels of CSF can be significantly increased in CGL and in untreated patients with cyclic variations. An inverse relationship has been reported between CSF levels and the height of the white cell count (Gatti et al. 1973), providing evidence for a feedback mechanism. In addition, a marked increase in CSF was noted following removal of white cells by leukapheresis. Normal CSF values are seen after treatment, suggesting that the return to normal hematologic values suppresses formation of CSF.

In addition, in the chronic phase there is a decreased sensitivity of CFU-c to CSF stimulation; however, the sensitivity increases in blastic transformation (Metcalf et al. 1974).

This CSF responsiveness by leukemic cells tends to support the view that CGL remains to some extent under the influence of normal humoral regulatory mechanism. The differences in threshold for stimulation of leukemic versus normal CFU-c, while slight, may actually be of major importance in providing selective growth advantages for leukemic cell lines.

The disease terminates in blast transformation in approximately 80% of cases. This represents the culmination of a process characterized by increasing failure of maturation as immature cells are continually overproduced. This is most frequently associated with a loss of colony formation. Characteristics of the terminal acute phase are not always evident by an increase in myeloblasts, as the promyelocyte or proerythroblast may be the predominant cell. In a minority of cases there is actually a lymphoid morphologic appearance. The onset of a myeloid blastic transformation occurs along with defective cellular maturation in agar culture with a lower threshold for CSF stimulation. This differential sensitivity may partially account for the conversion of CGL to a blastic phase.

Early detection of blast transformation may be possible. The presence of aneuploid metaphases in clinically stable chronic-phase CGL suggests that the processes responsible are at work prior to clinical and hematologic deterioration. In 8 of 103 patients with classic Ph^1-positive CGL there were abnormalities of in vitro growth noted. Of these eight, three were already in blast phase, two died within a week of diagnosis, one had overt blast transformation 16 weeks later, and two had slowly evolving subacute transformation (Moore 1977). Some generalizations concerning early detection of acute leukemia clones in CGL are (1) progressive increase in cluster: colony ratio in the bone marrow or blood (this may precede by several weeks or months actual clinical blast formation), (2) declining incidence in both colony-forming and cluster-forming cells in the marrow and blood, (3) presence of aneuploidy, and (4) qualitative abnormalities. It has been suggested that CGL is actually a preleukemic condition that becomes leukemic only on transformation.

Clinical Features

Signs and symptoms develop insidiously but tend to become continuously and progressively worse over a period of two to six months. Discovery of this disease (with splenomegaly or hematologic abnormality) during a routine examination is uncommon. When this does happen, overt disease usually becomes manifest within a few weeks or months. Occasionally, an unusual increase in the height of the white cell count or an abnormal degree of immaturity may occur in a reactive fashion following an acute hemorrhage or infection, but this may persist longer than expected or recur, and in retrospect may prove to have been an early manifestation of granulocytic leukemia.

Earlier symptoms usually are those of malaise, fatigue, lack of exercise tolerance, pallor, sweating, fever, and weight loss. These are generally associated with some degree of anemia and signs of increased metabolic rate. Aching in the bones may occur as well as fullness in the upper abdomen with early satiety due to hepatosplenomegaly. Later, there may be bleeding in association with platelet abnormalities. Infrequently, prolonged or recurrent infections and, rarely, peripheral vascular insufficiency and priapism may herald the disease. If the disease is long-standing, diffuse demineralization of short bones may occur with osteolytic lesions. With progression, superficial bones become very tender to pressure and aching is noted along marrow-producing bones. Punctate retinal hemorrhages and ecchymoses may be seen. Lymphadenopathy or skin infiltration rarely occur. Destructive bone lesions, orbital chloromas, and soft tissue tumors are usually indicative of the acute stage. The spleen continues to enlarge and may become massive, causing pressure symptomatology or splenic infarction. All of these clinical manifestations respond readily to therapy initially, but generally over a period of one to four years the acute phase develops. Unfortunately, there is still no therapeutic advantage in detecting the disease at an early stage.

Gatti and co-workers (1973) suggest that in addition to overproduction of myeloid cells, there is a failure to clear cells that play a role in the pathogenesis and that the cell separator may be useful therapy. They described a case with cyclic oscillations and remission that lasted a year following leukapheresis. As noted, although this is generally an easy diagnosis and most patients have a rather characteristic course, the variations can be endless. Atypical presentations are usually manifestations of CGL that are no longer pursuing a chronic course and accordingly, the prognostic implications are usually serious. When the blood leukocyte doubling time is approximately 70 days or less, some type of maintenance therapy is probably indicated. Approximately 80% of patients convert to blast crisis, which is usually sudden, fulminating, and fatal within six months (fig. 53.3). There are patients who go into an accelerated phase without actual blast transformation, and their disease follows a more subacute course. Symptoms are directly related to the rise in the white count; therapy is indicated when this occurs as symptoms invariably follow.

A very high WBC with immature cells is a relative emergency. This situation is drastically different from that of chronic lymphatic leukemia. Theologides (1972) has summarized the following unfavorable prognostic clinical features: the absence of Philadelphia chromosome, the presence of increased muramidase in the urine, and detection of fibrosis in the bone marrow. Increasing basophils, a rising leukocyte alkaline phosphatase not resulting from clinical improvement of chemotherapy, appearance of multiple Ph^1 chromosomes or other chromosomal abnormalities, and the development of myelofibrosis, fever, lymphadenopathy, or skin involvement after diagnosis all appear to be unfavorable characteristics and may herald an impending blast transformation. An enlarging spleen associated with thrombocytosis is also a poor prognostic sign.

Laboratory Features

Examination of the blood smear is usually diagnostic, as the peripheral blood resembles bone marrow. Granulocytes in all stages of development are seen in profusion and usually have normal morphology. Myeloblasts and promyelocytes usually do not exceed 10%. There is a progressive rise in the white cell count and a marked degree of eosinophilia or basophilia. One-third or more have thrombocytosis, which may be the presenting feature. A bone marrow examination shows hypercellularity (fig. 53.4) and reveals myeloid: erythroid ratio of 10 to 50:1 (fig. 53.5). The anemia is usually normochromic and normocytic and is due to decreased erythropoiesis. Red cell survival is normal except in patients with massive splenomegaly with red cell sequestration. Serum uric acid may be two to three times normal; it may be exacerbated following therapy, but can be prevented by the use of allopurinol. Leukocyte alkaline phosphatase (LAP) is generally markedly reduced or absent. Approximately 20% of the normal

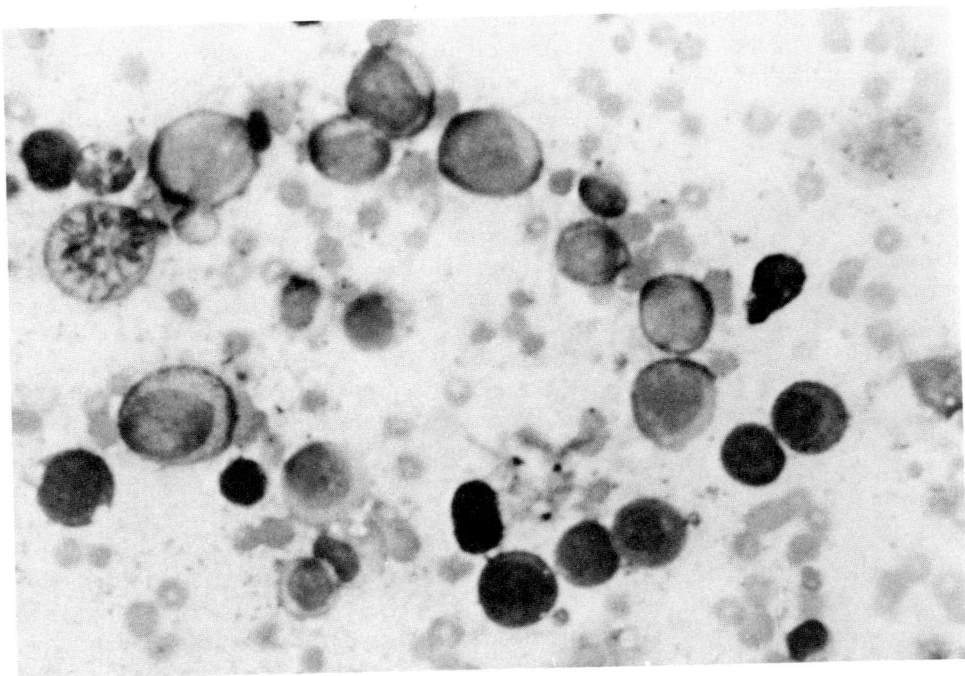

Fig. 53.3. *Bone marrow from CGL in acute blast transformation from the chronic phase.*

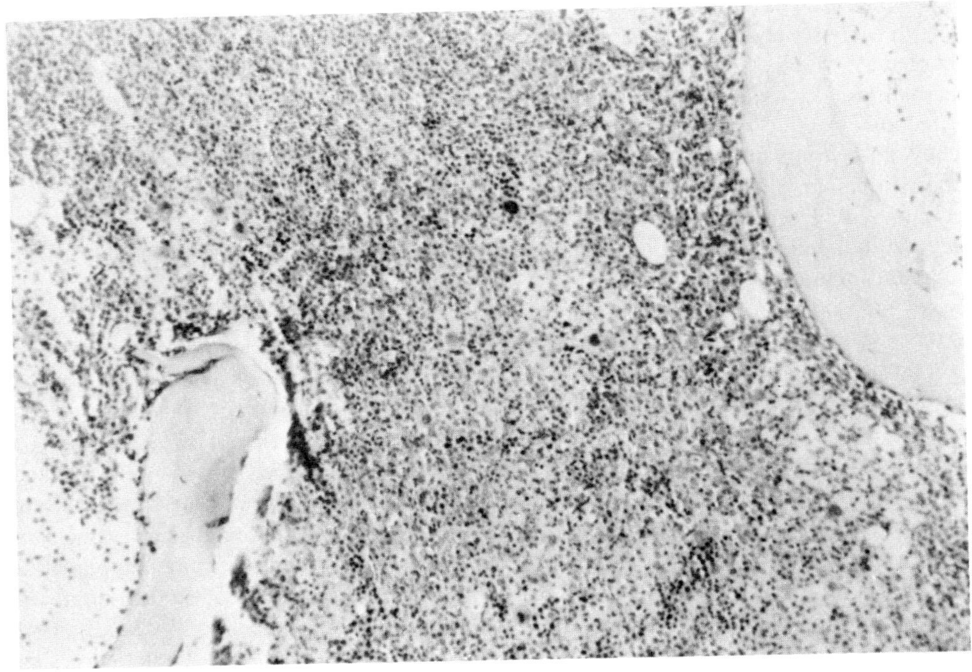

Fig. 53.4. *Bone marrow trephine biopsy showing hypercellularity in patient with chronic-phase CGL.*

mature neutrophils give a positive LAP reaction. During remission the LAP generally returns to normal although the Ph^1 does not, indicating a separate genetic locus for these factors. The serum vitamin B_{12} level is usually elevated in direct proportion to the height of the white cell count in untreated patients, but the level is also three to four times normal in patients who have normal white cell counts during remission.

Therapy

In 1902, radiation therapy was initially used with symptomatic success. Minot, Buckman, and Isaacs (1924) compared treated and untreated cases in a series of 78 patients and found no significant differences in survival. The major benefit of radiation therapy was relief of symptoms as well as alleviation of physical and hematologic abnormalities, with qualitative improvement of survival. For the next 15 years or so the standard therapy was local x-ray therapy to the spleen, long bones, or areas of leukemic infiltration. Total body irradiation was used in 1936, and chromic phosphate ^{32}P was introduced. In 1951, Shimkin, Mettier, and Bierman found no significant improvement in survival, and median survival was 3.1 years. In 1951, busulfan (Myleran) was introduced. In a classic study (British Medical Research Council 1968) of 102 patients comparing radiotherapy to busulfan, it was concluded that splenomegaly could be controlled equally well by either radiation therapy or busulfan, but all other manifestations of disease were better controlled by busulfan. The busulfan-treated group had a median survival of one year longer. The incidence of blast transformation was the same in both groups. Busulfan is the most commonly used drug although other derivatives of nitrogen mustard such as uracil mustard and melphalan are used with equal success. The question of interrupted versus continuous therapy has never been satisfactorily answered.

None of the conventional therapeutic agents or combinations eliminates the Ph^1. Busulfan has profound effects on the platelets and other side effects such as pulmonary fibrosis, skin pigmentation, hypogonadism, and a syndrome with features of Addison's disease, in addition to bone marrow suppression.

Local splenic irradiation is still effective. Hydroxyurea has been used for rapid reduction in blood counts and occasionally, for long-term control of disease. Busulfan, melphalan, hydroxyurea, dibromomannitol, dibromodulcitol, and 6-mercaptopurine produce prompt and almost complete remission in 80% to 90% of cases. In the accelerated or blastic phase there is no good therapy, and as noted, this is a devastating stage of disease. Leukapheresis may be of value in treating impending vascular occlusion by immature cells. Extremely high white cell counts may represent an emer-

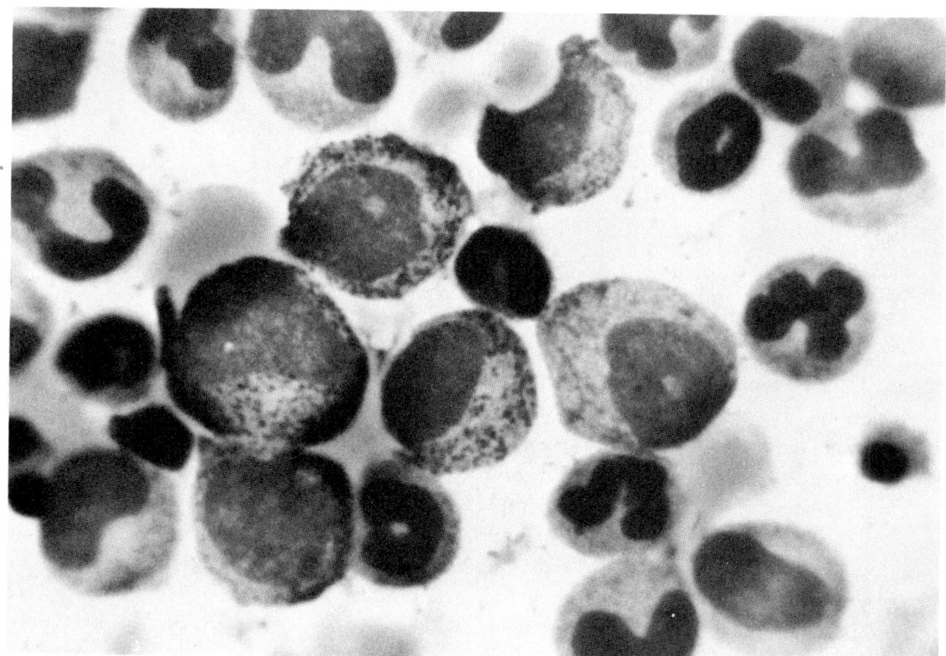

Fig. 53.5. *Wright's stained aspirate of bone marrow from patient with Ph^1-positive CGL.*

gency, since they may cause thrombotic manifestations in cerebral vessels. Accordingly, rapid reduction in white count is highly recommended either by leukapheresis or with chemotherapy, usually with hydroxyurea. Immunotherapy using BCG and mixtures of cultured leukemic cells is being evaluated (Sokal 1977). Splenectomy was previously used only in patients who seemed clinically hypersplenic. Results were disastrous, but there has been a resurgence of interest in this mode of therapy, the rationale being that early in the disease the spleen may be the site in which new clones of abnormal cells develop that can actually disseminate and produce the acute transformation. Accordingly, this has been incorporated into a number of experimental trials combining it with intensive chemotherapy and preoperative splenic irradiation. Of 37 patients, 12 had significant reduction of the Ph^1 clone of cells in the bone marrow, and 7 had complete disappearance of the Ph^1 (Cunningham et al. 1979). This study, although not having changed the type of therapy, was the first to indicate that eradication of Ph^1 is actually possible.

Treatment of the acute blast crisis was advanced following the publication by Canellos and associates (1971) of responses to vincristine and prednisone, which are usually used for acute lymphoblastic leukemia. For many years hematologists have noted lymphoblastic morphology in the terminal phase of known CGL (Boggs 1975). It was subsequently shown that patients whose cells are positive for the enzyme terminal deoxynucleotidyl transferase (TDT) have a much higher response rate to therapy directed against lymphoblastic leukemia (Marks, Baltimore, and McCaffrey 1978). This enzyme is present in 30% of cases of CGL in blast crisis and is found in approximately 95% of patients with untreated lymphoblastic leukemia. It is a DNA polymerase that is present in cortical thymus as well as a subpopulation of bone marrow lymphocytes, and is found only in T cell lymphoblastic lymphomas (McCaffrey 1975). The known B cell disorders such as chronic lymphatic leukemia are TDT-negative. This marker has been used as a predictor of initial responsiveness to vincristine and prednisone in blast phase CGL.

Of considerable interest was the recent report by Fefer and co-workers (1979) of four patients with CGL treated successfully by marrow transplantation from an identical twin. Marrow transplantation in patients in blast crisis of CGL, even with HLA-matched donors, has been disappointing; however, this report regarding the chronic phase of the disease has opened up an entirely new area, suggesting the possibility of successful allogeneic transplant in the chronic phase.

One other possibility is cryopreservation of a patient's bone marrow or blood during the chronic phase of disease. This strategy attempts to turn the clock back when blast crisis develops by repopulating a patient with marrow from the chronic phase (Goldman 1978).

In summary, CGL is a disease well documented and studied for the past 80 to 90 years. The disease can be controlled for a number of years by conventional therapy compatible with good quality survival. It is only recently that enormous amounts of information have been introduced in terms of cell kinetics, cell culture, and cytogenetic studies that have given us the opportunity to attempt aggressive therapy to obliterate the malignant cells with the objective markers of disease.

References

Athens, J. W. et al. Leukokinetic studies. X. Blood granulocyte kinetics in chronic myelocytic leukemia. *J. Clin. Invest.* 44:765–777, 1965.

Boggs, D. R. Hematologic stem cell theory in relation to possible lymphoblastic conversion of chronic myelogenous leukemia. *Blood* 44:449–454, 1975.

British Medical Research Council. Chronic granulocytic leukemia. Comparison of radiotherapy and busulfan therapy. *Br. Med. J.* 1:201–208, 1968.

Canellos, G. P. et al. Hematologic and cytogenetic remission of blastic transformation in chronic granulocytic leukemia. *Blood* 38:671–679, 1971.

Cunningham, I. et al. Results of treatment of Ph^1 + chronic myelogenous leukemia with an intensive treatment regimen (L-5 protocol). *Blood* 53:375–395, 1979.

Fefer, A. et al. Twin-marrow transplantation for chronic granulocytic leukemia. *N. Engl. J. Med.* 300:333–337, 1979.

Gatti, R. A. et al. Cyclic leukocytosis in chronic myelogenous leukemia. New perspectives on pathogenesis and therapy. *Blood* 41:771–782, 1973.

Goldman, J. M. Modern approaches to the management of chronic granulocytic leukemia. *Semin. Hematol.* 15:420–430, 1978.

Lawler, S. D. The cytogenetics of chronic granulocytic leukemia. *Clin. Haematol.* 6:55–75, 1977.

Marks, S. M.; Baltimore, D.; and McCaffrey, R. Terminal transferase and response to vincristine-prednisone in blastic chronic myelogenous leukemia. *N. Engl. J. Med.* 298:812–814, 1978.

McCaffrey, R. Terminal deoxynucleotidyl transferase activity in human leukemic cells and in normal human thymocytes. *N. Engl. J. Med.* 292:775–780, 1975.

Metcalf, D. et al. Responsiveness of human granulocytic leukemic cells to colony-stimulating factor. *Blood* 43:847–859, 1974.

Minot, G. R.; Buckman, T. E.; and Isaacs, R. Chronic myelogenous leukemia: age, incidence, duration, and benefit derived from irradiation. *JAMA* 82:1489–1494, 1924.

Moore, M. A. S. In vitro culture studies in chronic granulocytic leukemia. *Clin. Haematol.* 6:97–112, 1977.

Nowell, P. C., and Hungerford, D. A. Chromosome studies in normal and leukemic human leukocytes. *J. Natl. Cancer Inst.* 25:85–110, 1960.

Shimkin, M. B.; Mettier, S. R.; and Bierman, H. R. Myelocytic leukemia: an analysis of incidence, distribution, and fatality, 1910–1948. *Ann. Intern. Med.* 35:194–212, 1951.

Smith, K. L., and Johnson, W. Classification of chronic myelocytic leukemia in children. *Cancer* 34:670–679, 1974.

Sokal, J. E. Immunotherapy for chronic granulocytic leukaemia. *Clin. Haematol.* 6:129–139, 1977.

Speed, P. E., and Lawler, S. D. Chronic granulocytic leukaemia. The chromosome and the disease. *Lancet* 1:403–408, 1964.

Spiers, A. S. D. The clinical features of chronic granulocytic leukaemia. *Clin. Haematol.* 6:77–95, 1977.

Theologides, A. Unfavorable signs in patients with chronic myelocytic leukemia. *Ann. Intern. Med.* 76:95–99, 1972.

fifty-four

Chronic Lymphocytic Leukemia

W. BRUCE LUNDBERG

Chronic lymphocytic leukemia (CLL) is primarily a disorder of small B lymphocytes resulting in their loss of effective immunologic competence and their gradual accumulation in bone marrow, lymph nodes, spleen, and liver. It afflicts individuals who are in their later decades. It is extremely unusual below the age of 40 years and occurs in men more than twice as often as in women. The illness is often insidious and in more than one-third of patients is diagnosed in the laboratory on a blood count obtained without suspicion of a hematologic problem. Alternatively, the patient may come to the physician complaining of nonpainful adenopathy or left subchondral fullness, and CLL is confirmed on a blood smear. In less than one-third of cases the patient has constitutional symptoms such as fatigue, malaise, anorexia, and weight loss, or complications from infection, bleeding, or organ impairment.

A typical patient might have the following history:

> A recently retired, previously healthy, 66-year-old Connecticut man drives to Florida for a winter vacation. When he departs, he has a mild cough that progresses and is associated with fever when he arrives at his destination.
>
> He seeks help in a hospital emergency room where he is told that in addition to a mild pneumonia he has a generalized increase in lymph nodes, an enlarged spleen, and lymphocytosis. After a week in the hospital on antibiotic therapy he improves and is discharged. He quickly returns home.
>
> On his return the patient feels well again and decides to delay going to the doctor. Two months later he becomes fatigued and is noted to be pale. He consults his physician and a blood count reveals (in addition to the lymphocytosis) severe anemia. Work-up now shows chronic lymphocytic leukemia and autoimmune hemolytic anemia.

Differential Diagnosis

A differential diagnosis of lymphocytosis is the following:

- Lymphocytic leukemoid reaction
- Postinfectious lymphocytosis
- Infectious mononucleosis
- Collagen disease
- Lymphoproliferative diseases
  - ALL—acute lymphocytic leukemia
  - CLL—chronic lymphocytic leukemia
  - LSC—lymphosarcoma cell leukemia
  - HCL—hairy cell leukemia
  - Waldenström's macroglobulinemia
  - Sézary syndrome

The hematologic hallmark is an increase in the absolute number of lymphocytes in the blood. Most authorities require a sustained lymphocytosis of greater than $15,000/mm^3$ to make a definitive diagnosis, which in this setting is not difficult. Diagnosis may be suspected with lymphocytosis of lesser proportions, as is seen more frequently because of the increased use of routine blood counts. Retrospective review of proved cases of CLL often reveals an antecedent increase in the lymphocyte count when it is available. Most cases of unexplained lymphocytosis below 15,000/mm^3 will eventually evolve into diagnosable CLL (Rai et al. 1975). How long this transition takes and with what certainty it will occur are difficult to predict.

Lymphocytic leukemoid reactions are uncommon. They are reported in tuberculosis, carcinoma, and drug reactions. A transient lymphocytosis is also seen in association with viral and *B. pertussis* infections; however, these are most common in children, in whom CLL is not observed. The leukocytosis of infectious mononucleosis can be substantial, and the associated lymphadenopathy and splenomegaly often suggest a malignant process. The characteristic morphology of the mononuclear cells, diagnostic serology, and its predisposition for young adults most often distinguishes mononucleosis from CLL. Patients with collagen disease, especially lupus and rheumatoid arthritis, can demonstrate a mild lymphocytosis and lymphadenopathy. Lymphatic leukemia could be confused with these disorders especially when there is concomitant autoimmune hemolysis or thrombocytopenia, which are seen in both.

It is important to distinguish CLL from other lymphoproliferative conditions. The lymphocyte that circulates in CLL is small (one to two times the size of the red cell) and has a densely clumped nucleus and scanty blue cytoplasm in Wright's stained smears (fig. 54.1). Its nucleus is readily distinguishable from the large open nucleolated nucleus of acute lymphoblastic leukemia. Differentiation of CLL from the leukemic phase of an underlying lymphoma (usually poorly differentiated lymphocytic of the nodular or diffuse types) can be more difficult. Lymphosarcoma cells (LSC) are larger, have more cytoplasm, and looser, more clefted nuclei than the CLL lymphocyte. The peripheral smears of some patients with CLL demonstrate considerable pleomorphism, however (Zacharski and Linman 1969). Many CLL cells can be large and suggest LSC morphologically, but the clinical course cannot be predicted by morphology alone (Peterson et al. 1975). Lymph node biopsy may be required to direct therapy in these cases since the prognosis correlates best with that of the parent lymphoma.

Although hairy cell leukemia (HCL) most often causes pancytopenia, 10% of patients have a significant leukemic phase that can be confused with CLL. Cells in this disease have round and open nuclei and abundant light-staining cytoplasm that streams out in "hairs" in smear preparations. Positive acid phosphatase staining of the cytoplasm, which is tartrate-resistant, will con-

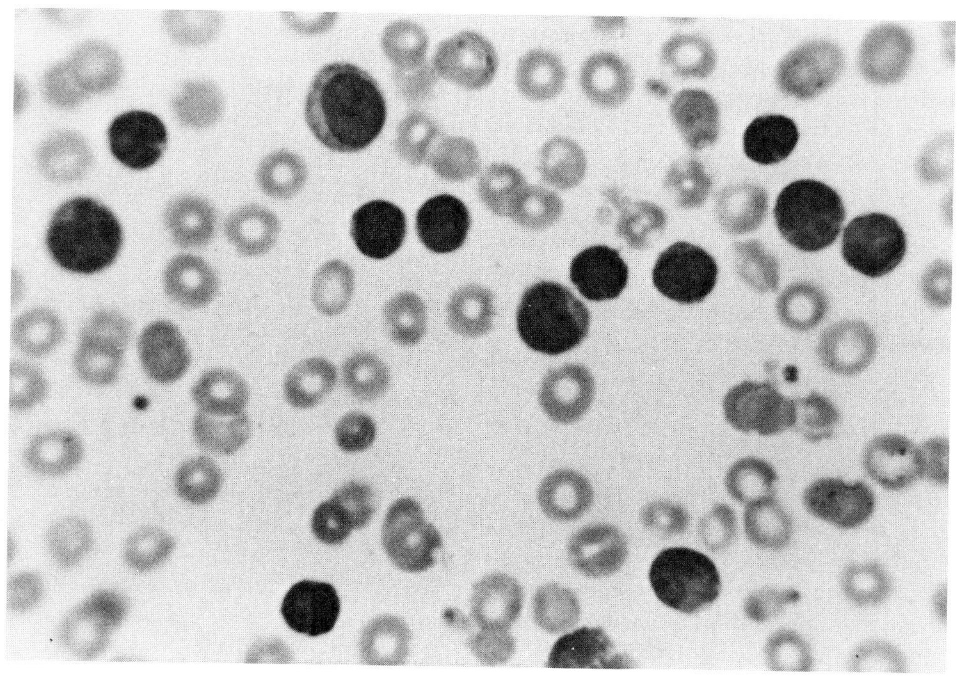

Fig. 54.1. *Wright's stained smear of peripheral blood from patient with typical CLL.*

firm the diagnosis. The cells found in the blood of patients with Waldenström's macroglobulinemia or chronic cold agglutinin disease can be indistinguishable from the CLL lymphocyte, but usually have more plasmacytoid differentiation. In these cases the distinction from CLL is a clinical one, depending on the presence of the IgM monoclonal antibody or high-titer red cell cold agglutinins. The leukemic phase of mycosis fungoides may be associated with a marked leukocytosis. These Sézary T cells have cerebrated nuclei and cytoplasmic inclusions that stain with PAS. The Sézary syndrome is characterized by a diffuse, intensely erythematous, and thick-skinned infiltrate.

Etiology

As with most malignant diseases, factors that dispose to the development of CLL are multiple and not entirely known. There are, however, several noteworthy facts in its epidemiology. There is no association between exposure to ionizing radiation and the disease. Follow-up studies of the Japanese who were survivors of the atomic bomb revealed no increase in incidence (Bizzozero, Johnson, and Ciocco 1966). This finding may be influenced by the spontaneously low incidence of CLL in Orientals (Wells and Law 1960) and the propensity of the Japanese to develop CLL of the T cell subtype (Yodoi 1974). There is, however, no reported increase in CLL in the Caucasian population, in whom CLL is the most common form of leukemia, following exposure to therapeutic ionizing radiation. Although these population differences of occurrence could have an environmental explanation, a genetic influence is further suggested by family studies in which 10% to 20% of patients have a history of lymphoproliferative disease in their families (Fraumeni, Vogel, and DeVita 1969). In addition, studies of families with closely linked cases of CLL have shown uniform morphology and immunology in the affected members (Branda et al. 1978).

Immunology

Because of the availability of circulating leukemic cells, CLL was one of the first diseases in which surface lymphocyte markers were looked for and defined. Many clinical studies had previously shown an association with humoral immunologic abnormalities. Hypogammaglobulinemia or agammaglobulinemia is found in 40% to 50% of patients. Warm autoimmune red cell antibodies are identified in 25% and monoclonal paraproteins in as many as 5%. It is therefore not surprising that in 98% of patients with CLL the leukemic lymphocytes possess B cell surface markers that include receptors for the Fc fragment and the third component of complement and immunoglobulin (most often IgM with or without IgD) (Aisenberg, Bloch, and Long 1973). These surface immunoglobulins are present in quantities smaller than those found on normal B lymphocytes and contain only one class of heavy and one class of light chain (Preud'homme and Seligmann 1972). When a monoclonal serum protein is present it is of the same isotype as the immunoglobulin on the leukemic lymphocytes (Gupta and Good 1980). Both of these findings indicate that CLL is a monoclonal disease. Finally, although the percentage of normal T cells is decreased, absolute T cell number or function is probably not impaired by the disease alone (Davies 1976). Intriguingly, these lymphocyte markers can be used to differentiate CLL lymphocytes from LSC lymphocytes. Lymphosarcoma cells contain more surface immunoglobulin than CLL cells and in contradistinction to CLL, they exhibit capping (Cohen 1978) and fail to bind monkey red blood cells (Gupta and Good 1980).

A small percentage of patients with CLL have lymphocytes that bear surface markers of T cells. They are distinctive clinically, often exhibiting massive splenomegaly without lymphadenopathy (Brouet and Seligmann 1977). They also have neutropenia and the propensity to skin involvement seen with other T lymphoproliferative disorders.

Because IgM and IgD are phylogenetically the most primitive immunoglobulins, and lymphocytes that bind monkey red blood cells are ontogenetically early (Gupta et al. 1976), CLL probably represents a disease of earlier differentiated cells in the developmental lineage of Bursa-equivalent cells (Sweet, Golumb, and Ultmann 1977). The leukemic cells possess deficient amounts of surface immunoglobulin and have defective in vitro responses to nonspecific mitogens (Rubin, Havemann, and Dameshek 1969) and thus do not function normally in host defenses.

Staging the Disease

Because the diagnosis of CLL is usually evident from the blood count alone, initial evaluation is directed at confirming the diagnosis and obtaining certain baseline studies that have prognostic significance. A clinical staging system helps, and is of considerable importance to the patient, as it is from this that the decision of when and how to treat the disease can be made.

Dameshek (1967) observed that symptoms from CLL resulted from displacement and replacement of normal tissues by lymphocyte masses. He proposed that

Table 54.1. *Clinical Staging of Chronic Lymphocytic Leukemia*

Clinical Stage	*Description*	*Median Survival (mo)*
0	Lymphocytosis > 15,000/mm^3 in blood; marrow > 40% lymphocytes	150
I	Lymphocytosis and lymphadenopathy	101
II	Lymphocytosis and hepatomegaly or splenomegaly; lymphadenopathy may or may not be present	70
III	Lymphocytosis with anemia (hgb < 11 g/dl; hct < 33%); lymphadenopathy, hepatomegaly, or splenomegaly may or may not be present	19
IV	Lymphocytosis with thrombocytopenia (platelets < 100,000/mm^3); lymphadenopathy, hepatomegaly, or splenomegaly may or may not be present	19

SOURCE: Modified from Rai et al. 1975.

CLL is a disease of the progressive accumulation of nonfunctioning lymphocytes. As the rate of production of leukemic lymphocytes is not measurably increased (Stryckmans, Debusseher, and Collard 1977) this progressive accumulation appears to result from an extended life span of the cells. Normal lymphocytes circulate through blood, tissues, and lymph nodes and have long and variable life spans—from days to years. Kinetic comparisons of normal and leukemic lymphocytes are therefore difficult to make.

The concept of CLL as a progressive accumulative illness is useful clinically and provides the basis for staging. This system relates the stage (and from it the prognosis) to the total lymphocyte burden and its effect on organ function, especially bone marrow. Staging is particularly useful because of the extremely variable course that patients follow after the diagnosis is made. Some patients will die within the first year while others can live longer than 10 and even as long as 25 years. The accumulative theory explains this marked variation predominantly by differences in the advancement of illness at the time of diagnosis.

There is, however, another important factor that affects the course of patients, that is, the difference in the aggressiveness of the leukemia. Static clinical staging alone does not define this. Galton (1966) suggested that there are two forms of CLL, indolent and aggressive, and that the extreme variability in survival can be explained by this. Staging is useful in each individual, but the clinician must recognize the inherent differences in the pace of disease from one to another. This can be appreciated only by close serial observation.

Rai and co-workers (1975) proposed a staging system that proved to be useful in defining survival when applied retrospectively. This system classifies patients with CLL into five groups (0 to IV) depending on easily defined criteria of lymphadenopathy, hepatosplenomegaly, anemia, and thrombocytopenia (table 54.1). The system has the inherent advantage of relying on data that can easily be obtained clinically. The differences in median survival within stages are impressive except between stages III and IV, and hold up when applied to other reviewed series (Rai et al. 1975). The largest percentage of patients have stage II disease. Those with anemia or thrombocytopenia (stages III and IV) resulting from myelophthisis survive on average less than two years. One must recognize that anemia or thrombocytopenia that results from another cause could lead to inappropriate classification. The individual with CLL in stages II to IV will obviously present variables that may have great prognostic importance, including the presence or absence of hypogammaglobulinemia, nonlymphatic organ involvement, or massive adenopathy. The patient's age and associated medical problems will also influence the course.

Physical and Laboratory Findings

Physical findings are confined initially to the lymph nodes, liver, spleen, and skin. By definition, patients with stage 0 disease have no abnormal physical findings while those with stage I disease have asymptomatic lymphadenopathy alone. This is usually diffuse, although it may be confined to one lymph node group. Some nodes may be minimally enlarged and soft while others may be massive and confluent. Splenomegaly may be minimal or impressive but does not characteristically reach the massive proportions seen with the myeloproliferative syndromes. The spleen may be uncomfortable or painful and inhibit gastric filling, but rarely does it infarct or rupture. Hepatic enlargement closely follows that of the spleen, but liver function is usually not compromised. The skin is involved at some time in almost half the patients. Lesions can be localized or diffuse and a biopsy is required for definitive diagnosis. In addition, these patients can develop skin lesions that are due to complications such as hemorrhagic lesions, steroid-induced purpura, and herpes zoster.

The most important laboratory findings are hematologic. A complete blood count with red cell indices, differential, and numerical platelet count should be obtained. The total leukocyte count, the percentage of lymphocytes and neutrophils, and the morphology of the leukemic cells are all important. Lymphocyte morphology may vary considerably; however, when there is a consistent pattern of large cells with clefted nuclei suggesting LSC leukemia, a lymph node biopsy, which is not necessary in clear-cut CLL, should be performed. Peripheral blood lymphocyte subtyping by surface markers remains a research tool; however, this evaluation is useful in patients with undiagnosed lymphocytosis to confirm monoclonal proliferation. It can also be useful to distinguish CLL from LSC leukemia. The percentage of granulocytes is characteristically depressed, but the absolute granulocyte count is usually adequate to prevent spontaneous infection. Persistent and marked granulocytopenia is an indication of packed marrow or hypersplenism and demands therapeutic intervention.

Some degree of anemia of the normocytic type during the course of CLL is the rule. Microcytic indices, as in other patients, suggest iron deficiency and should prompt a search for gastrointestinal bleeding. Blood in the stool may result from leukemic infiltrate or an intercurrent process such as steroid-induced ulcers or a primary carcinoma. Anemia with macrocytic indices may be the result of vitamin B_{12} or folic acid malabsorption secondary to leukemic involvement of the intestine (Prolla and Kirsner 1964). Malabsorption from superimposed bacterial overgrowth or protozoan infection can also complicate gastrointestinal symptomatology. Macrocytic indices may be the first sign of a compensatory reticulocytosis in response to autoimmune hemolysis.

Ten to twenty percent of patients develop Coombs'-positive IgG warm autoimmune hemolytic anemia (WAHA) at some time (Pirofsky 1976); CLL is more frequently associated with WAHA than any other lymphoproliferative disorder. A direct antiglobulin test should therefore be part of the work-up of the CLL patient with anemia even when the reticulocyte count is not increased, since it can be depressed from marrow infiltration or myelosuppressive therapy.

The platelet count is a sensitive indicator of the degree of underlying marrow involvement or splenic enlargement, and should be followed rather than relying on the less precise smear estimate. During therapy, especially with alkylating agents, the platelet count may be the limiting factor for drug treatment. Severe depression (less than 40,000/mm^3) without anemia or granulocytopenia suggests immunologic platelet destruction. This diagnosis should be considered when adequate numbers of megakaryocytes are found in the bone marrow, but must be distinguished from hypersplenism.

The most common immunologic abnormality is diffuse hypogammaglobulinemia. This results from decreased immunoglobulin production, but it can also be contributed to by protein loss in the bowel in the presence of a gastrointestinal lesion. The diagnosis is suggested by a depression of serum globulin and confirmed by a flattening of the globulin hump on the serum protein electrophoresis. Serum immunoelectrophoresis and quantitative immunoglobulins initially reveal depression of IgA and IgM, and later reduction in IgG levels. An additional finding may be a narrow-based, monoclonal protein spike that is usually IgG. Bence-Jones proteins of the same light chain type can be detected in the presence of a serum paraprotein but not in the quantities usually seen in myelomatosis. The presence of rouleaux in the blood smear will sometimes be a clue to the existence of the paraprotein. Despite these epiphenomena of deranged humoral immunity, delayed hypersensitivity reactions are normal unless the patient has been treated with corticosteroids.

An aspiration and biopsy examination of the bone marrow should be performed in patients with lymphocytosis to confirm the diagnosis of CLL pathologically and to evaluate the extent of replacement of normal hematopoietic tissue. Repeat bone marrow studies may be required to follow the progression of the illness, to decide on the timing of therapy, and to help in the differential diagnosis of cytopenias when they occur. The marrow smear will reveal a generalized increase in the percentage of small lymphocytes intermingled with normal elements and focal areas of complete replacement by lymphocytes (fig. 54.2). The biopsy will characteristically show lymphocytic collections in a nonparatrabecular pattern in a background of diffuse lymphocytosis (Foucar et al. 1979). As the disease progresses the marrow is increasingly replaced by leukemic lymphocytes, and normal hematopoietic elements are crowded out. This myelophthisis causes anemia, thrombocytopenia, and granulocytopenia. A marrow biopsy also can distinguish the well-differentiated lymphocytic infiltrate of CLL from the more immature infiltration seen in association with the leukemic phase (LSC) of non-Hodgkin's lymphoma. In these cases, lymph node biopsy is always preferred to subclassify the lymphoma and thus dictate prognosis and treatment; it is not necessary in uncomplicated CLL.

Renal function is generally not compromised despite the finding of leukemic infiltration of the kidneys in two-thirds of autopsies on patients with CLL (Norris and Weiner 1961). Hydronephrosis resulting from ureteral obstruction by enlarged retroperitoneal lymph nodes or a pelvic mass is most often clinically silent when unilateral. When the BUN is elevated obstructive uropathy must be excluded since it can be treated with local irradiation. Hyperuricemia does not usually result from CLL alone but is seen in elderly patients with other conditions or in association with massive lympholysis resulting from effective therapy.

Pulmonary infiltrates, usually diffuse and nonspecific, develop in one-third of patients with CLL, usually late in their course (Klatte et al. 1963). Hilar adenopathy is not a common finding, but pleural effusions do occur as the result of direct pleural involvement or lymphatic obstruction. These effusions respond to systemic or direct intrapleural therapy. Mediastinal irradiation is generally effective against a chylothorax. Pulmonary manifestations must always be differentiated from intercurrent infectious processes.

Curiously, neurologic disorders from direct leukemic involvement of the central nervous system by CLL are very uncommon. This is true of both parenchymal brain and meningeal infiltration. Neurologic findings should raise the suspicion of an infectious or hemorrhagic process in the nervous system. Leukoencephalopathy develops rarely, but this is a manifestation of the immune defect and not direct leukemic involvement. Skeletal involvement is also uncommon.

Treatment

In view of the variable and often benign nature of this disease (especially when diagnosed at an early stage), the primary decision the physician must make is when, and not how, to treat the patient. This viewpoint is reinforced by the fact that antineoplastic therapy, although capable of ameliorating signs and symptoms of the disease, has not dramatically lengthened the survival. Statistics improved between 1955 and 1964 compared to the preceding 15 years (Zippin et al. 1973); however, further improvements in overall survival have not been forthcoming since the mid-1960s (Huguley 1977). In addition to chemotherapy, earlier diagnosis and the availability of better general medical care have contributed to the improved statistics. Therapeutic nihilism can be overemphasized and treatment begun too late. The median survival of all patients with CLL remains less than five years. Efforts at improved treatment are clearly worthwhile. The disease is responsive to a variety of treatments, and many of its signs and symptoms can be alleviated. The quality, if not the length, of survival of symptomatic patients is improved with antileukemic therapy.

Asymptomatic patients who are started on chemotherapy only after waiting for early signs of disease progression survive as well as those who are treated continuously from the time of diagnosis (Huguley

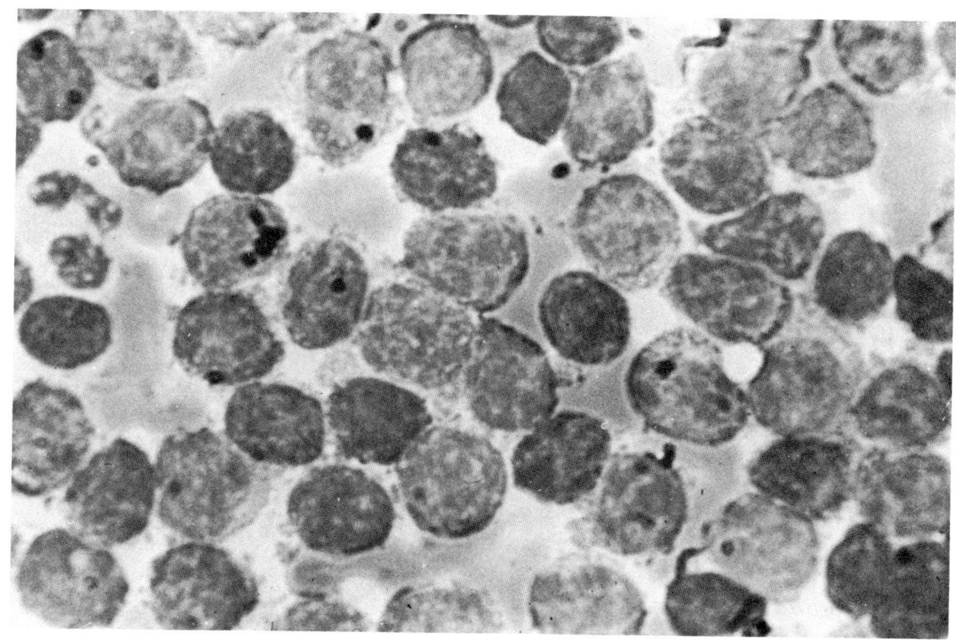

Fig. 54.2. *Wright's stained smear of bone marrow aspirate from patient with CLL.*

1977). These results support the approach of watchful waiting before recommending treatment. There appears to be an important subgroup of patients whose survival is improved by treatment even when it is initiated in stage III or IV disease. This is the group that obtains a complete remission following either chemotherapy (Huguley 1977) or total body irradiation (Johnson 1979). Although this finding closely parallels the results of treatment of other malignant diseases, it must be confirmed in larger numbers of carefully followed and uniformly staged and treated patients. Overaggressive efforts to obtain complete remissions may be detrimental.

After a sufficient period, either long or short, the pace of disease can be determined. Certain clinical features should prompt the initiation of therapy with either local or systemic modalities (Wiltshaw 1977):

1. Symptoms such as weight loss, painful adenopathy, or painful splenomegaly
2. Rapidly increasing lymph node enlargement, or splenomegaly whether symptoms are present or not
3. The presence of acquired autoimmune hemolytic anemia or thrombocytopenia
4. Evidence of progressive impairment in bone marrow function as shown by falling neutrophil or platelet counts, or hemoglobin
5. Bone marrow failure

Constitutional symptoms such as weight loss and marked fatigue require systemic therapy, as will rapidly increasing lymphadenopathy or splenomegaly or evidence of progressive bone marrow impairment. When local lymphocyte accumulations become massive and cause pain, obstruction, or even disfigurement, radiation to the area is usually highly effective. For example, inguinal irradiation can reduce lymphedema of the leg, mediastinal irradiation can resolve a chylothorax, and retroperitoneal irradiation may relieve ureteral obstruction. Radiation therapy to the pharynx or neck is usually effective in reducing obstructing or infected tonsils or cosmetically disfiguring nodes. Skin infiltrates are radiosensitive even with low-energy electron beams. Bone marrow failure requires prompt therapy but is most difficult to treat; blood transfusions are often helpful. Normal marrow stem cells are severely depleted at this stage. Even though leukemic lymphocytes are more sensitive to therapy than normal stem cells, these normal elements are vulnerable because of their depleted numbers and probable increased proliferative rate compared to CLL.

Elevation of the white blood cell count alone is not a sufficient indication for treatment. White cell count elevations of greater than 50,000/mm^3 correlate with disease stages III and IV, and these patients do not live as long as those with lower counts (Phillips et al. 1977). Abrupt changes in white cell count can be seen in association with infections, and it is best to observe the patient closely through these periods as the count often falls again. Two special treatment circumstances are autoimmune hemolysis and thrombocytopenic purpura. These complications require initial control of the destructive processes with steroids prior to initiation of cytotoxic therapy that may shut off the compensatory reticulocytosis or thrombocytosis.

The two most effective classes of drugs for systemic therapy are alkylating agents and corticosteroids. While all alkylating agents have shown some effectiveness, chlorambucil (Leukeran) and cyclophosphamide (Cytoxan, Endoxan) have proved to be the best in CLL. Because of its relatively few side effects chlorambucil is preferred by most clinicians. Objective responses are obtained in approximately two-thirds of the patients (Livingston and Carter 1970). The standard schedule is to give the oral drug daily in a dose of 5 to 10 mg. As the patient responds or shows evidence of hematologic toxicity (predominantly thrombocytopenia) the drug is tapered or stopped. This method is risky if patients are not followed carefully with regular blood counts. Intermittent pulse schedules have been employed more recently (Knospe, Loeb, and Huguley 1974). In theory, the long-lived, slowly proliferating leukemic lymphocyte should be more susceptible to intermittent doses than the normal more rapidly proliferating marrow cells that should recover faster between treatment pulses. Chlorambucil is given over five days in a total cumulative dose of 20 to 30 mg/m^2 every two or three weeks. More total drug can be given in this way with less platelet depression. Whether this will be associated with higher complete remission rates and thus longer survival is not yet clear. Cyclophosphamide may be somewhat less effective than chlorambucil (Kuang et al. 1964) and is cross-resistant with it; however, cyclophosphamide can be used in selected patients with thrombocytopenia because of its relative platelet-sparing effect.

Corticosteroids are lympholytic and result in objective reductions in lymphadenopathy and splenomegaly in about 60% of patients treated (Livingston and Carter 1970). Steroids remain the mainstay of treatment for patients with marrow failure and are the initial choice for those with autoimmune cytopenias. The many debilitating and life-threatening side effects of long-term steroid usage unfortunately quickly outweigh their usefulness. Continuous daily medication should be avoided if at all possible; intermittent dose regimens are preferred.

Unfortunately, there are few useful alternative drug options to alkylating agents or steroids. This is partly because progressive marrow disease and prior drug and radiation toxicity leave the marrow severely compromised. Vincristine (Oncovin), a useful drug in lymphoma that has little marrow toxicity, has limited activity in CLL as a single agent (Livingston and Carter 1970). This also seems to be true of doxorubicin (Adriamycin) (Carter 1975). Bleomycin (Blenoxane), theoretically useful because of its lack of marrow toxicity, has had limited trials in CLL because of its pulmonary toxicity.

Drug combinations have not been extensively used in CLL. Unless survival is clearly improved, an aggressive approach is not indicated. Chlorambucil and prednisone, the two most active agents that have non-overlapping toxicities, are easily combined, resulting in an increased response rate when compared to the use of chlorambucil alone (Han et al. 1973; Sawitsky et al. 1975). More important, the complete remission rate has been increased to 20% with this combination (Knospe, Loeb, and Huguley 1974). Patients who attain a complete remission should live longer as a result.

Total body irradiation (TBI) has been used as a systemic modality in the treatment of CLL. The peculiar radiation sensistivity of the CLL lymphocyte coupled with the systemic nature of the disease from the outset has led radiation oncologists to apply this therapy. A group of patients was treated at the National Cancer Institute with fractionated TBI (Johnson 1979). Thirty-seven of 42 treated with TBI alone attained objective responses and 14 entered complete remission. In the 30 patients with stages III and IV disease median survival was 63 months. This is more than twice that predicted by Rai and co-workers (1975). Some of these patients have also shown a return of depressed immunoglobulin serum levels toward normal, which may represent an improvement of the underlying functional immune defects.

This disease may produce symptoms by progressive lymphocyte accumulation. Lymphocytes can be removed from the body without attempting to decrease their production. In patients with high peripheral counts, cells have been removed efficiently by leukapheresis (Fortuny et al. 1976). If the leukocytosis persists while lymphoid mass is reduced, repeated removal can be accomplished. This apparent mobilization of cells from tissue sites to the blood does occur, since some patients so treated have shown improvement in myelophthisis with increased hemoglobin and platelet counts (Goldfinger and Capostagno 1974). This approach has not yet been shown to be practical for long-term management. That it has not produced more dramatic results raises questions about the basic theories of the cell kinetics in this disease. It has the obvious advantage of no stem cell toxicity.

Local radiation treatments can result in reduction of lymphocytes at distant sites. The mechanism of this "abscopal" effect is not well understood but is probably related to the marked radiosensitivity of leukemic cells as they circulate through radiation portals. Irradiation of the spleen, lymphoid masses, thymus gland, and even extracorporeal blood can result in reduction in lymphoid masses in nonirradiated sites (Richards et al. 1974).

Carefully delivered, low-dose radiation to bulky or painful enlarged spleens usually reduces splenic size and pain. Unfortunately, improvement in anemia or thrombocytopenia in patients irradiated for hypersplenism is rarely accomplished (Byhardt, Brace, and Wiernik 1975). Extreme care must be exercised in irradiating the spleen in CLL since refractory pancytopenia may develop unless low-dose fractions are given with close hematologic monitoring (Richards et al. 1974). In selected patients, splenectomy should be considered. The major problem here is our lack of ability, even with sophisticated radiolabeling studies, to define preoperatively those patients who will have a durable beneficial response to splenectomy. It can be therapeutic in patients with CLL who have refractory autoimmune hemolysis or thrombolysis, in patients with anemia with shortened ^{51}CR red cell survival, and in those with hypersplenism (Adler et al. 1975). Clearly, it is indicated only in highly selected cases and even then it is hard to predict the outcome.

Causes of Death in CLL

Although patients can live for many years with CLL, even in some cases with bulky disease, the illness is progressively debilitating. Some live with their disease for more than 10 years, but the 5-year survival of all patients from the time of diagnosis remains only 50% (Boggs et al. 1966).

Because of the immunodeficiency that accompanies CLL, these patients succumb to overwhelming infections, especially viral and bacterial pneumonias. Infection can be an early manifestation of the illness, at times prompting the diagnosis. At this stage, encapsulated pneumococci and streptococci are common and are usually effectively treated. As the disease progresses, however, serious infections become more frequent and treatment is less successful. As steroid-induced cellular immunodeficiency is added to the existing humoral immune defect in the granulocytopenic patient, the risk of infection from any source becomes overwhelming. Treatment with broad-spectrum antibiotics and even granulocyte transfusions can still be successful, but these serious infections take their toll on the debilitated patient and eventually become untreatable. Prophylaxis against pneumococcus should be given routinely and should be considered in specific clinical situations for other infections. Such measures may include antibiotic prophylaxis for a recurrent cellulitis, viral prophylaxis (amantadine) during epidemics, active immunizations (although the response to antigen is suboptimal), and passive immunization with gammaglobulin (recurrent sinopulmonary infections) or hyperimmune globulin (zoster-immune globulin). Patients with CLL should never be given live vaccines because of the danger of developing active disease such as vaccinia from smallpox vaccine or bovine tuberculosis from BCG.

Patients with CLL have an increased risk of developing second malignancies of any kind (Moertel and Hagedorn 1957). This is true even when compared to a similar elderly control population. These cancers can be pathologically unrelated carcinomas; however, progression of the illness itself to a more malignant lymphoma occurs in 1% to 3% of patients. Interestingly, the change develops in the lymph node phase of disease and not toward a more malignant leukemia. Pathologically, the tumor resembles diffuse histiocytic lymphoma (DHL) developing in a node involved by the well-differentiated lymphocytic infiltrate of CLL (Armitage, Dick, and Corder 1978). This is referred to as Richter's syndrome. Clinically, it is characterized by progressive weight loss, persistent fever, new lymph node masses (especially abdominal), pancytopenia, and at times, a new paraprotein (Long and Aisenberg 1975). The diagnosis is usually established at postmortem examination performed on a patient with an abrupt clinical deterioration after many years of CLL. It has also been made early in the course of CLL, and some of these patients had not received treatment (Armitage, Dick, and Corder 1978). This has led some authors to speculate that the malignant conversion of CLL to DHL is the pathologic equivalent of blastic transformation in chronic myelogenous leukemia, although occurring much less frequently.

It is a curious fact that patients with CLL, even those extensively treated with chemotherapy and radiation, do not have the predisposition to acute leukemic transformation seen in individuals with myeloproliferative disorders. Acute leukemia, especially nonlymphocytic, does occur in patients with CLL, rarely even in those with no prior therapy (McPhedran and Heath 1970; Lawlor et al. 1979). Because of its rareity it probably represents a chance occurrence; however, some cases may also represent pure conversions or different expressions of an abnormality affecting a common stem cell.

Finally, the elderly patient with CLL may die because of the progression of the disease itself or succumb to unrelated supervening medical conditions such as myocardial or cerebral infarction.

References

Adler, S. et al. Splenectomy for hematologic depression in lymphocytic lymphoma and leukemia. *Cancer* 35:521–528, 1975.

Aisenberg, A. C.; Bloch, K. J.; and Long, J. C. Cell-surface immunoglobulins in chronic lymphocytic leukemia and allied disorders. *Am. J. Med.* 55: 184–191, 1973.

Armitage, J. O.; Dick, F. R.; and Corder, M. P. Diffuse histiocytic lymphoma complicating chronic lymphocytic leukemia. *Cancer* 41:422–427, 1978.

Bizzozero, O. J., Jr.; Johnson, K. G.; and Ciocco, A. Radiation-related leukemia in Hiroshima and Nagasaki, 1946–1964. I. Distribution, incidence, and appearance time. *N. Engl. J. Med.* 274:1095–1101, 1966.

Boggs, D. R. et al. Factors influencing the duration of survival of patients with chronic lymphocytic leukemia. *Am. J. Med.* 40:243–254, 1966.

Branda, R. F. et al. Lymphocyte studies in familial chronic lymphatic leukemia. *Am. J. Med.* 64:508–514, 1978.

Brouet, J.-C., and Seligmann, M. Chronic lymphocytic leukaemia as an immunoproliferative disorder. *Clin. Haematol.* 6:169–184, 1977.

Byhardt, R. W.; Brace, K. C.; and Wiernik, P. H. The role of splenic irradiation in chronic lymphocytic leukemia. *Cancer* 35:1621–1625, 1975.

Carter, S. K. Adriamycin—a review. *J. Natl. Cancer Inst.* 55:1265–1274, 1975.

Cohen, H. J. B-cell lymphosarcoma cell leukemia: dynamics of surface membrane immunoglobulin value for differentiation from chronic lymphocytic leukemia. *Ann. Intern. Med.* 88:317–322, 1978.

Dameshek, W. Chronic lymphocytic leukemia—an accumulative disease of immunologically incompetent lymphocytes. *Blood* 29:566–584, 1967.

Davies, S. The variable pattern of circulating lymphocyte subpopulations in chronic lymphocytic leukemia. *N. Engl. J. Med.* 294:1150–1153, 1976.

Fortuny, I. E. et al. The role of continuous flow centrifuge leucapheresis in the management of chronic lymphocytic leukaemia. *Br. J. Haematol.* 32:609–615, 1976.

Foucar, K. et al. Incidence and patterns of bone marrow and blood involvement by lymphoma in relationship to the Lukes-Collins classification. *Blood* 54:1417–1422, 1979.

Fraumeni, J. F., Jr.; Vogel, C. L.; and DeVita, V. T. Familial chronic lymphocytic leukemia. *Ann. Intern. Med.* 71:279–284, 1969.

Galton, D. A. G. The pathogenesis of chronic lymphocytic leukaemia. *Can. Med. Assoc. J.* 94:1005–1010, 1966.

Goldfinger, D., and Capostagno, V. Management of chronic lymphocytic leukemia by long-term leucapheresis. Haemonetics advanced pheresis seminar. Haemonetics Research Institute, Boston, 1974.

Gupta, S. et al. Ontogeny of lymphocyte sub-populations in human fetal liver. *Proc. Natl. Acad. Sci. USA* 73:919–922, 1976.

Gupta, S., and Good, R. A. Markers of human lymphocyte sub-populations in primary immunodeficiency and lymphoproliferative disorders. *Semin. Hematol.* 17:1–29, 1980.

Han, T. et al. Chlorambucil vs. combined chlorambucil-corticosteroid therapy in chronic lymphocytic leukemia. *Cancer* 31:502–508, 1973.

Huguley, C. M., Jr. Treatment of chronic lymphocytic leukemia. *Cancer Treat. Rev.* 4:261–273, 1977.

Johnson, R. E. Treatment of chronic lymphocytic leukemia by total body irradiation alone and combined with chemotherapy. *Int. J. Radiat. Oncol. Biol. Phys.* 5:159–164, 1979.

Klatte, F. C. et al. The pulmonary manifestations and complications of leukemia. *Am. J. Roentgenol.* 89:598–609, 1963.

Knospe, W. H.; Loeb, V., Jr.; and Huguley, C. M., Jr. Bi-weekly chlorambucil treatment of chronic lymphocytic leukemia. *Cancer* 33:555–562, 1974.

Kuang, D. T. et al. Chemotherapy of chronic lymphocytic leukemia. *Arch. Intern. Med.* 114:521–524, 1964.

Lawlor, E. et al. Acute myeloid leukaemia occurring in untreated chronic lymphatic leukaemia. *Br. J. Haematol.* 43:369–373, 1979.

Livingston, R. B., and Carter, S. K. *Single agents in cancer chemotherapy.* New York: IFI/Plenum, 1970.

Long, J. C., and Aisenberg, A. C. Richter's syndrome: a terminal complication of chronic lymphocytic leukemia with distinct clinicopathologic features. *Am. J. Clin. Pathol.* 63:786–795, 1975.

McPhedran, P., and Heath, C. W., Jr. Acute leukemia occurring during chronic lymphocytic leukemia. *Blood* 35:7–11, 1970.

Moertel, C. G., and Hagedorn, A. B. Leukemia or lymphoma and coexistant primary malignant lesions: a review of the literature and a study of 120 cases. *Blood* 12:788–804, 1957.

Norris, H. J., and Weiner, M. The renal lesions in leukemia. *Am. J. Med. Sci.* 241:512–524, 1961.

Peterson, L. C. et al. Morphology of chronic lymphocytic leukemia and its relationship to survival. *Am. J. Med.* 59:316–324, 1975.

Phillips, E. A. et al. Prognostic factors in chronic lymphocytic leukaemia and their implications for therapy. *Clin. Haematol.* 6:203–222, 1977.

Pirofsky, B. Clinical aspects of autoimmune hemolytic anemia. *Semin. Hematol.* 13:251–265, 1976.

Preud'homme, J. L., and Seligmann, M. Surface-bound immunoglobulins as a cell marker in human lymphoproliferative disease. *Blood* 40:777–794, 1972.

Prolla, J. C., and Kirsner, J. B. The gastrointestinal lesions and complications of the leukemias. *Ann. Intern. Med.* 61:1084–1104, 1964.

Rai, K. R. et al. Clinical staging of chronic lymphocytic leukemia. *Blood* 46:219–234, 1975.

Richards, F., II et al. Thymic irradiation: an approach to chronic lymphocytic leukemia. *Am. J. Med.* 57: 862–869, 1974.

Rubin, A. D.; Havemann, K.; and Dameshek, W. Studies in chronic lymphocytic leukemia: further studies of the proliferative abnormality of the blood lymphocyte. *Blood* 33:313–328, 1969.

Sawitsky, A. et al. Comparison of daily and intermittent chlorambucil and prednisone therapy in ALGB study in CLL. *Blood* 46:1039, 1975.

Stryckmans, P. A.; Debusscher, L.; and Collard, E. Cell kinetics in chronic lymphocytic leukaemia (CLL). *Clin. Haematol.* 6:159–167, 1977.

Sweet, D. L., Jr., Golumb, H. M.; and Ultmann, J. E. Chronic lymphocytic leukaemia and its relationship to other lymphoproliferative disorders. *Clin. Haematol.* 6:141–157, 1977.

Wells, R., and Law, K. S. Incidence of leukaemia in Singapore, and rarity of chronic lymphocytic leukaemia in Chinese. *Br. Med. J.* 1:759–763, 1960.

Wiltshaw, E. Chemotherapy in chronic lymphocytic leukaemia. *Clin. Haematol.* 6:223–235, 1977.

Yodoi, J. Two cases of T-cell chronic lymphocytic leukemia in Japan. *N. Engl. J. Med.* 290:572–573, 1974.

Zacharski, L. R., and Linman, J. W. Chronic lymphocytic leukemia vs. chronic lymphosarcoma cell leukemia: analysis of 496 cases. *Am. J. Med.* 47:75–81, 1969.

Zippin, C. et al. Survival in chronic lymphocytic leukemia. *Blood* 42:367–376, 1973.

fifty-five

Lymphomas: An Introduction

DAVID S. FISCHER

Although the recent response to therapy of malignant lymphomas has been most gratifying, there are still problems in etiology, pathology, treatment, diagnosis, and staging. In fact, the subject is in such a state of flux that one can compare it to a game in which the rules keep changing and the players keep switching their names and their positions. For some understanding of where we are going in this field it is necessary to know, at least briefly, where we have been and how we came to where we are.

Historical Development of Hodgkin's Disease

The subject began for all practical purposes with the description by Thomas Hodgkin in January 1832 of the disease that now bears his name. He described the gross pathology of six cases he had personally seen and one case described to him by Robert Carswell (Hodgkin 1832). The case of Carswell was illustrated by water color paintings discovered some 135 years after they had been painted, and republished by Dawson (1968). In a discussion of abdominal tumors, Richard Bright (1838), one of the many outstanding physicians of Guy's Hospital in that remarkable period, included two of Hodgkin's cases for illustration and commented, "There is another form of disease which appears to be of a malignant character, though it varies from the more usual forms of malignant disease; and which has been particularly pointed out by Dr. Hodgkin, as connected with extensive disease of the absorbent glands, more particularly those which accompany the blood vessels."

Nothing more was written on this until Samuel Wilks (1856) described primary and secondary amyloidosis, which he called "lardaceous disease." After describing four variants, he listed a fifth characterized by lymphadenopathy and splenomegaly, describing 10 cases including some from the Gordon Museum of Guy's Hospital Medical School among which were four of Hodgkin's original cases. After completing his manuscript, but before publishing it, Wilks came across Bright's paper and was thereby directed to the earlier publication by Hodgkin, and graciously appended proper credit for the priority. Nine years later, he ensured Hodgkin's immortality by entitling his description of 15 additional patients (Wilks 1865), "Cases of enlargement of the lymphatic glands and spleen, (or Hodgkin's Disease), with remarks."

Although Wilks provided excellent clinical descriptions, the microscopic details were brief. It remained for Langhans (1872) and Greenfield (1878) independently to describe the histopathologic features of the disease for the first time, including large binucleate and multinucleated cells on which the diagnosis depends (fig. 55.1). Kaplan (1972) suggests that these authors deserve the credit for the priority of recognition that erroneously has been given to Sternberg (1898) and Reed (1902) by naming the characteristic cell after them. Reed characterized the disease as a histopathologic entity, but considered it inflammatory in nature.

Since Hodgkin had never examined his original cases microscopically, there had been some doubt as to whether Reed-Sternberg cells were present in the original patients. Remarkably, Fox (1926) was able not only to find three of the original cases in the Gordon Museum, but after 97 years was able to prepare microscopic sections of them. He confirmed the diagnosis of Hodgkin's disease in cases two and four, but thought that case six was a lymphosarcoma or lymphatic leukemia, although he could not be sure.

The first serious attempt at a histopathologic-clinical subclassification of Hodgkin's disease was by Jackson and Parker (1944). They described an infrequent variant with a slow clinical course and few Reed-Sternberg cells but with many lymphocytes, and called it Hodgkin's paragranuloma. They named the majority of typical cases Hodgkin's granuloma and called a small subset of cases, with an aggressive clinical course and an abundance of pleomorphic and anaplastic Reed-Sternberg cells, Hodgkin's sarcoma. Although this classification served for more than 20 years, it was generally unsatisfactory because 90% of the cases were in the granuloma group and correlations with prognosis and response to therapy were poor.

Lukes (1963) described a "new" histologic subtype (although Greenfield had alluded to it 85 years earlier) and called it nodular sclerosing Hodgkin's disease (fig. 55.2), and proposed a six-subgroup classification that included it. This was further developed (Lukes and Butler 1966) and formed the basis of the classification finally adopted by the nomenclature committee at a conference (Milder et al. 1966) cosponsored by the American Cancer Society (ACS) and the National Cancer Institute (NCI) held at Rye, New York, September 13–15, 1965. Hence the classification adopted is known as the Rye classification (Lukes et al. 1966) (fig. 55.3). Some groups (DeVita et al. 1980) further subclassify nodular sclerosis according to a tendency to resemble one of the other three groups.

In a recent review, Byrne (1980) advises continued use of the Rye nomenclature as clinically, although not morphologically, significant. He advises pathologists to use the morphologic criteria originally described by Lukes and Butler (1966) and to translate them to the Rye terminology (table 55.1) in evaluating material from lymph nodes and spleen. When evaluating needle biopsies of bone marrow or liver, the same strict criteria must be used if this is the primary diagnostic material. If the diagnosis of Hodgkin's disease has been firmly established by nodal or splenic material, then Reed-Sternberg cells need not be present to determine that the staging tissues are involved by Hodgkin's

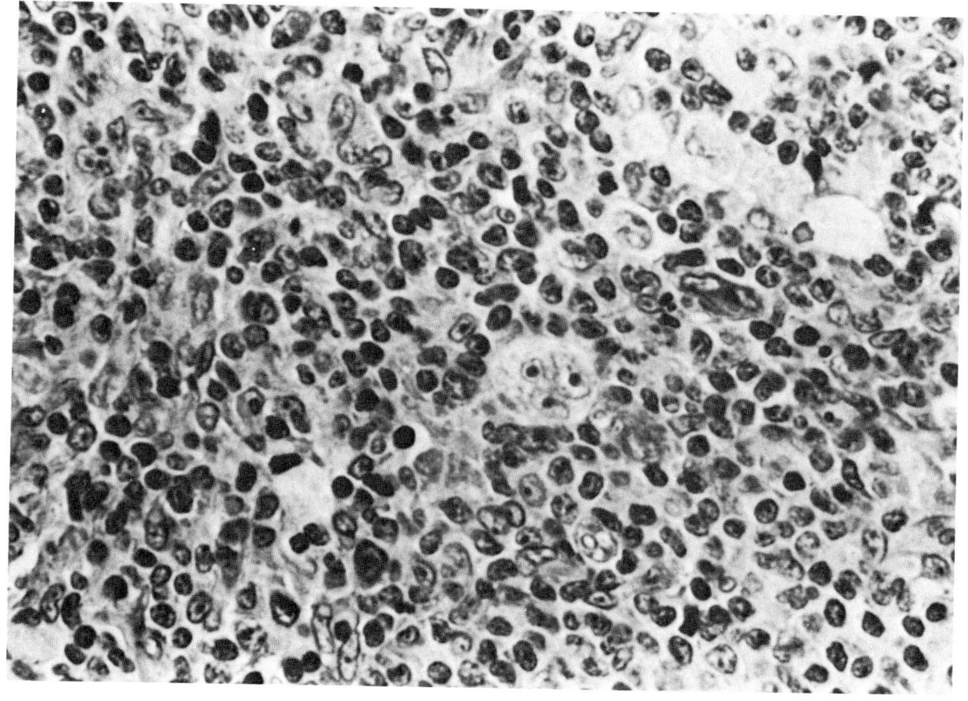

Fig. 55.1. *High-power view of Hodgkin's disease, showing prominent Reed-Sternberg cell in center (×760). (Photograph courtesy of James A. Waldron, M.D., Yale University School of Medicine.)*

Table 55.1. *Rye Histologic Classification of Hodgkin's Disease*

Subtype	*Pattern*	*Description*
Lymphocyte predominance	Diffuse	Abundant lymphocytes; occasional Reed-Sternberg cells; no fibrosis
Mixed cellularity	Diffuse	Moderate lymphocytes, plasma cells, eosinophils, granulocytes; moderate Reed-Sternberg cells; occasional diffuse fibrosis
Lymphocyte depleted	Diffuse	Stromal cells and lymphocytes depleted and replaced by fibrosis; numerous Reed-Sternberg cells
Nodular sclerosis	Nodular	Nodularity due to birefringent collagen bands, dividing areas, moderate lymphocytes, plasma cells, granulocytes, eosinophils; lacunar Reed-Sternberg cells

SOURCE: Modified from Desforges et al. 1979.

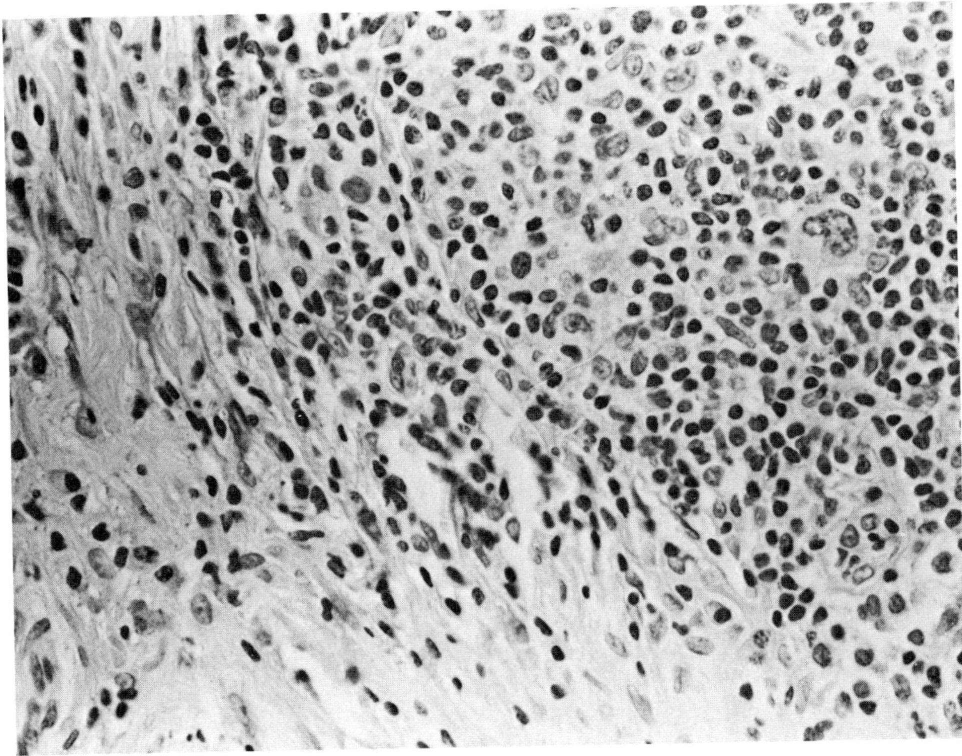

Fig. 55.2. *Medium-power magnification (×475) of lymph node showing nodular sclerosing Hodgkin's disease. Part of a broad collagenous band is seen in the lower left, and a characteristic lacunar cell with a large polypoid nucleus and abundant cytoplasm is seen at upper right. (Photograph courtesy of James A. Waldron, M.D., Yale University School of Medicine.)*

disease. The presence of mononuclear cells with the nuclear features of Reed-Sternberg should be considered diagnostic of involvement. The presence of atypical (reticulum) cells without such nuclear features or the presence of focal fibrosis if present within the cellular milieu observed in Hodgkin's disease should be considered as suggestive of involvement (Byrne 1980).

Staging

With the development of megavoltage radiation therapy and combination chemotherapy, the opportunity for great therapeutic advances was presented. To evaluate and compare treatment modalities in different institutions it was necessary to have agreement not only on histopathologic classification but on extent of disease, and by implication, on prognosis.

The first consensus was achieved at the symposium held at Rye, and hence is called the Rye staging system. It was used for six or more years, and most of the important early papers reported their results according to its guidelines. It is reproduced (Rosenberg 1966) as follows so that early studies and later studies may be compared.

Stage I
: Disease limited to one anatomic region (I_1) or to two contiguous anatomic regions (I_2) on the same side of the diaphragm

Stage II
: Disease in more than two anatomic regions or in two noncontiguous regions on the same side of the diaphragm

Stage III
: Disease on both sides of the diaphragm but not extending beyond the involvement of lymph nodes, spleen, and/or Waldeyer's ring

Stage IV
: Involvement of the bone marrow, lung parenchyma, pleura, liver, bone, skin, kidneys, gastrointestinal tract, or any tissue or organ in addition to lymph nodes, spleen, and/or Waldeyer's ring

Subclassification A for absence or B for presence of otherwise unexplained systemic symptoms: (a) fever, (b) night sweats, and (c) pruritus (later omitted).

By 1971, it was clear that great progress had been made and that there were some deficiencies in the Rye system. Many centers were obtaining more pathologic information by frequently resorting to laparotomy and splenectomy with open liver and sometimes bone marrow biopsy. These pathologic stages (PS) could not be properly compared to clinical stages (CS). Therefore at another symposium cosponsored by ACS and NCI and held at Ann Arbor, Michigan, April 26–28, 1971 (Milder et al. 1971), a revised classification was proposed (Carbone et al. 1971), known as the Ann Arbor staging system:

Stage I
: Involvement of a single lymph node region (I) or of a single extralymphatic organ or site (I_E)

Stage II
: Involvement of two or more lymph node regions on the same side of the diaphragm (II) or localized involvement of extralymphatic organ or site and of one or more lymph node regions on the same side of the diaphragm (II_E)

Stage III
: Involvement of lymph node regions on both sides of the diaphragm (III), which may also be accompanied by localized involvement of

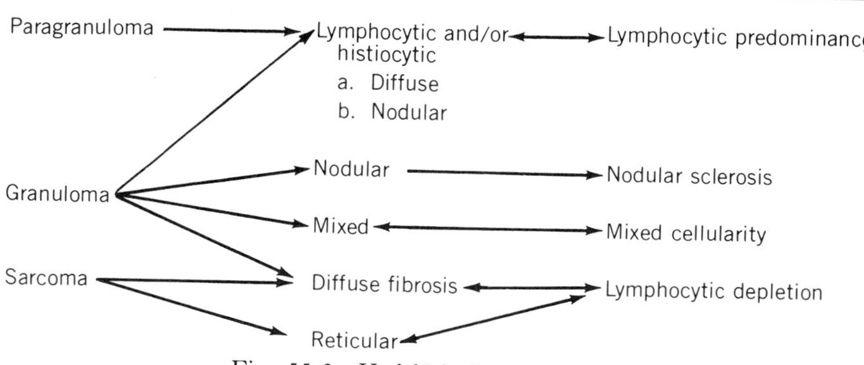

Fig. 55.3. *Hodgkin's disease: comparison of histologic classifications.*

extralymphatic organ or site (III_E), by involvement of the spleen (III_S), or both (III_{SE})

Stage IV

Diffuse or disseminated involvement of one or more extralymphatic organs or tissues with or without associated lymph node enlargement

Subclassification A for absence or B for presence of (a) unexplained weight loss of more than 10% of body weight, (b) unexplained fever above 38° C, and (c) night sweats.

Pathologic staging: designate + for positive; − for negative by biopsy; N for lymph node; H for liver; S for spleen; L for lung; M for marrow; P for pleura; O for bone (osseous); D for skin (dermis).

This also tried to recognize the observation that extralymphatic disease, if localized and related to adjacent lymph node disease, did not adversely affect survival. These patients did as well with treatment compared to patients with disease of the same stage without extralymphatic spread. These patients with contiguous extranodal disease were given the subscript E.

It should be noted that there has been some abuse of this designation. Favorable prognosis was based on the presumption that the extranodal disease was a direct extension into contiguous tissue and could be easily encompassed by a reasonable radiation field. A lung nodule that is not in continuity with hilar or mediastinal nodes is not properly an E, but more likely stage IV. Recently, the value of the E concept has been questioned (Levi and Wiernik 1977). Stage I was modified to involvement of only a single lymph node region (I) or of a single extralymphatic organ or site (I_E). Stage III with involvement of the spleen was designated III_S. Pathologic staging was denoted PS with subscripts to indicate results of biopsies, for example, H+ or H− for liver positive or negative by liver biopsy. Finally, the generalized symptoms were again designated A for absence and B for presence, but pruritus was dropped, and unexplained weight loss of more than 10% of the body weight in the preceding six months was added to the B criteria. The committee emphasized that the CS and PS staging classifications apply *only* to the patient at the time of initial diagnosis and prior to definitive therapy. Bone marrow biopsies must be taken from a clinical or radiographically uninvolved area.

Recently, Desser and co-workers (1977) suggested a division of PS III into subtypes; the upper abdominal involvement was designated III_1 and included involvement of the spleen, splenic nodes, celiac axis nodes, or portal hepatic nodes; lower abdominal involvement, III_2, included disease in paraaortic, iliac, or mesenteric nodes with or without involvement of upper abdominal lymphatic areas. A four-institution study of 130 patients (Golomb et al. 1980) showed better five-year disease-free survival (95% versus 63%, $P < 0.003$) but the same overall salvage survival (100% versus 91%, $P = 0.22$) for the PS III_1 group with radiation therapy plus chemotherapy as compared to radiation therapy alone. The patients with PS III_2 disease had dramatically better five-year disease-free survival (76% versus 32%, $P < 0.001$) and overall five-year survival (84% versus 56%, $P < 0.03$) with the combined modality compared to radiation alone. In view of the increased incidence of second malignancies in patients receiving both modalities compared to either one alone, the authors recommend consideration of extended-mantle radiation therapy alone for PS III_1 disease and chemotherapy alone for PS III_2. Although these results are preliminary and need confirmation, they suggest that valuable information may derive from precise staging and can potentially guide therapy with improved results and less toxicity.

Historical Development of Non-Hodgkin's Lymphoma

Thirteen years after Hodgkin's paper, Virchow (1845) and others independently described the first cases of leukemia. Virchow even defined leukemic and aleukemic forms, and the latter was confused with lymphoid tumors for many years. Finally, Dreschfeld (1892) and Kundrat (1893) independently separated from the aleukemic leukemias a group of lymphoid neoplasms to which Kundrat gave the name lymphosarcoma, and distinguished them from Hodgkin's disease. It was 37 more years until Brill, Baehr, and Rosenthal (1925) described the giant follicle lymphoid hyperplasia that Symmers (1927) independently described, and that was known as Brill-Symmers disease. Subsequently, they both realized that this was a slow-growing malignancy. In 1930, Roulet delineated a group of more aggressive lymphoid tumors he called *retothele sarcome,* which was soon translated into reticulum cell sarcoma. By the early 1940s there was no generally accepted classification of the malignant lymphomas, although that of Gall and Mallory (1942) was the most widely quoted. Most textbooks in the 1950s would accept a listing of the malignant lymphomas as:

Hodgkin's disease

Lymphosarcoma

Reticulum cell sarcoma

Giant follicle lymphoma (Brill-Symmers disease)

The trouble with this and with most of the other classifications was that they did not correlate well with clinical course or response to therapy.

A major advance was made by Rappaport, Winter, and Hicks (1956) when they divided the non-Hodgkin's lymphomas into nodular (fig. 55.4) and diffuse (fig. 55.5) groups and showed that there was a much better prognosis associated with the nodular form. Their second contribution was to reemphasize cytology and show that there was a better survival associated with well-differentiated cell types in contrast to poorly differentiated. In general, these observations were ignored for 10 years until the publication of the following classification in the Armed Forces fascicle (Rappaport 1966):

Nodular	Diffuse
Lymphocytic WD	Lymphocytic WD
Lymphocytic PD	Lymphocytic PD
Mixed H and L	Mixed H and L
Histiocytic	Histiocytic
	Undifferentiated

WD = well-differentiated; PD = poorly differentiated; H and L = histiocytic and lymphocytic; histiocytic may now be called large lymphoid cell; undifferentiated includes both the Burkitt and non-Burkitt types.

Pathologists began to look at it and review their material in terms of the Rappaport classification, which gained great impetus when Dorfman's group (Jones et al. 1973) showed an excellent clinicopathologic correlation in the Stanford University material. Soon the Rappaport classification became widely accepted, especially by cooperative research groups, as it confirmed the correlation between histology and response to therapy. After almost 20 years it seems to hold up fairly well.

During this same period, there has been a revolution in our understanding of the lymphocyte, its subtypes, origins, surface markers, and ability to transform after appropriate stimulation (Gupta and Good 1980; Berard et al. 1978; Kay, Ackerman, and Douglas 1979).

The most successful attempt so far to combine the new knowledge of the role of the lymphocyte in immune

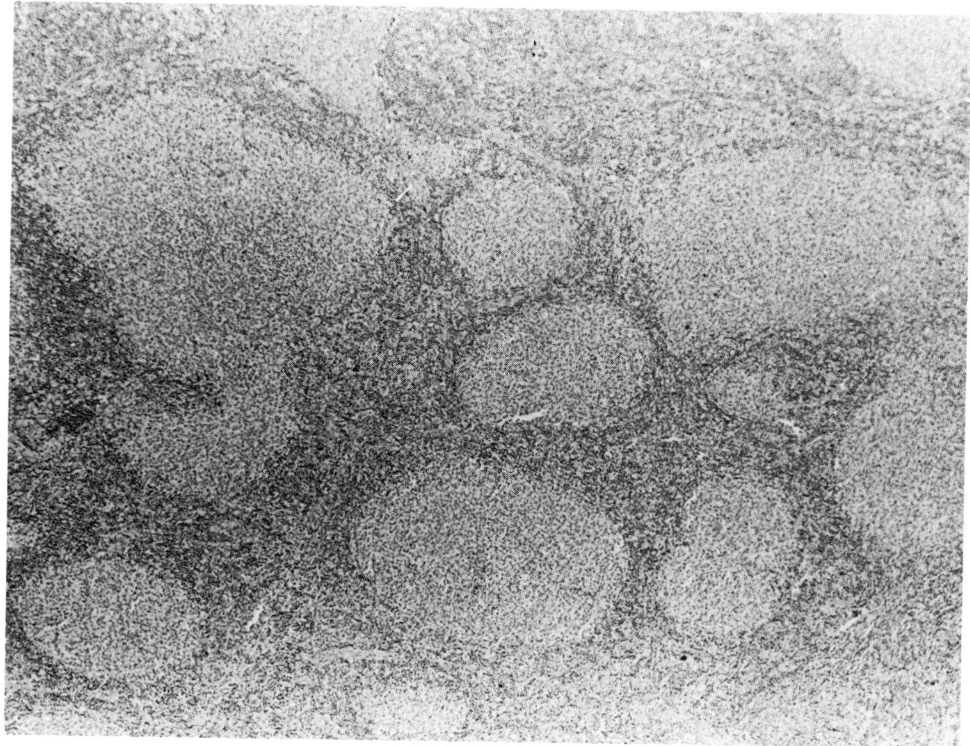

Fig. 55.4. *Low-power (×80) magnification of lymph node showing follicular non-Hodgkin's lymphoma. (Photograph courtesy of James A. Waldron, M.D., Yale University School of Medicine.)*

function with the histopathology of the non-Hodgkin's lymphomas has been by Lukes and Collins (1974, 1975, 1977). Their proposed functional approach is based on T and B lymphocyte systems and lymphocyte transformation.

The classification is as follows, and figure 55.6 compares it to the Rappaport classification (Lukes and Collins 1975; Nathwani et al. 1978).

- Type I
  - U cell (undefined cell) type
- Type II
  - T cell types
  - Mycosis fungoides and Sézary's syndrome
  - Convoluted lymphocyte
  - Immunoblastic sarcoma of T cells
  - Small lymphocyte—CLL—T cell type
- Type III
  - B cell types
  - Small lymphocyte—CLL—B cell type
  - Plasmacytoid lymphocyte
  - Follicular center cell types
    - Small cleaved cell
    - Large cleaved cell
    - Small transformed (noncleaved) cell
    - Large transformed (noncleaved) cell
  - Immunoblastic sarcoma of B cells
  - Hairy cell leukemia
- Type IV
  - Histiocytic diseases

Not fully included in this classification scheme are pediatric cases (Krivit et al. 1977), especially later descriptions of lymphoblastic lymphoma with mediastinal involvement (Nathwani, Kim, and Rappaport 1976; Lichtenstein et al. 1980) and the evolution of some cases of chronic lymphocytic leukemia into diffuse histiocytic lymphoma, so-called Richter's syndrome (Richter 1928; Trump et al. 1980). Also, it is now generally agreed that the large B lymphocyte was being called (incorrectly) a histiocyte. Notwithstanding these deficits, advantages of the Rappaport system are long

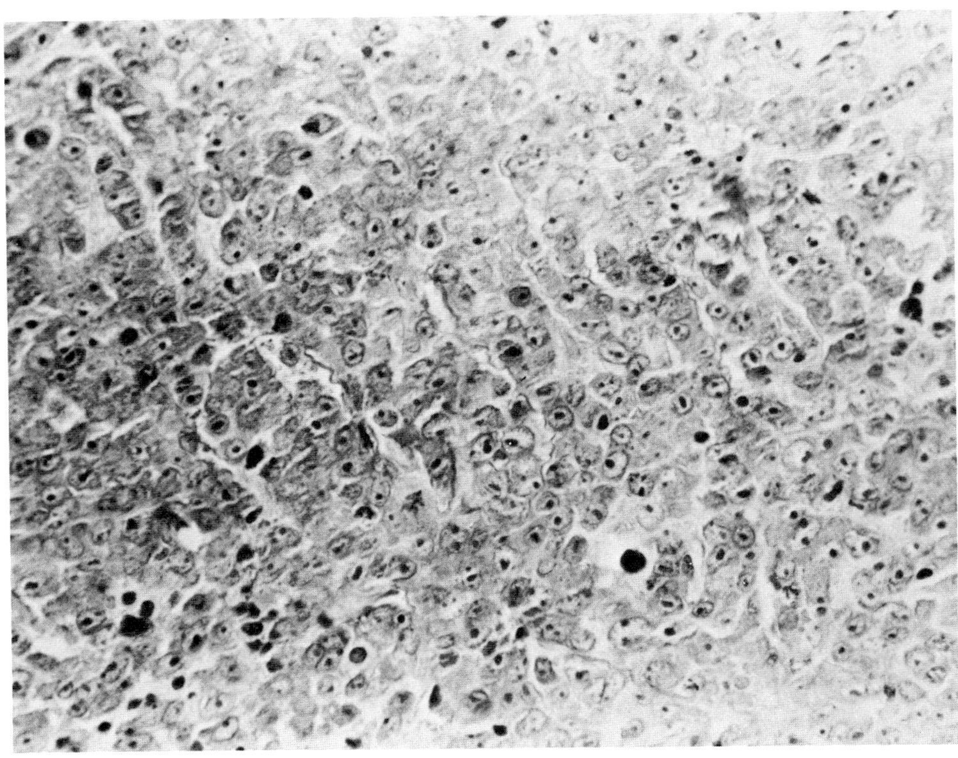

Fig. 55.5. *High-power (×760) magnification of diffuse histiocytic lymphoma showing monomorphic infiltrate of large lymphoid cells with dispersed chromatin and prominent nucleoli. (Photograph courtesy of James A. Waldron, M.D., Yale University School of Medicine.)*

familiarity and its correlation with prognosis in clinical trials. The advantage of the Lukes-Collins system is its compatibility with the growing knowledge of T and B cell function and lymphocyte markers. It may lead to greater understanding of borderline syndromes such as immunoblastic lymphadenopathy that appears to be histologically benign but may be clinically malignant (Lukes and Tindle 1975; Frizzera, Moran, and Rappaport 1975; Pangalis, Moran, and Rappaport 1978), and immunoblastic sarcoma which is histologically and clinically malignant (Michel, Case, and Moinuddin 1979; Lichtenstein 1979).

After many years of effort an international committee (under the cochairmanship of C. W. Berard and R. F. Dorfman, and including H. Rappaport, R. J. Lukes, K. Henry, and K. Lennert) has finally agreed on a working formulation of non-Hodgkin's lymphoma for clinical usage, which it is hoped will replace all prior classifications (Dorfman, Burke, and Berard 1981; Berard et al. 1981). The new formulation is given in table 55.2 and correlated with the Rappaport classification; in this system Burkitt's tumor (Burkitt 1958; Burkitt and O'Conor 1961) figures prominently. As the first form of lymphoma to be associated with the Epstein-Barr virus antibody (Aisenberg 1973; Klein 1975), it may be of viral origin and more susceptible to aggressive therapy both in Africa and in America (Ziegler 1977, 1979, 1981).

Staging of Non-Hodgkin's Lymphomas

Just as our understanding of the pathology of non-Hodgkin's lymphoma (NHL) has lagged behind that of Hodgkin's disease, so too has our staging classification. For want of anything else, we use the Ann Arbor Hodgkin's disease method while waiting for a better staging classification for NHL. In general, however, half the cases of Hodgkin's disease fall into stages I and II and half in stages III and IV, whereas in non-Hodgkin's lymphoma, 75% are stage III or IV at diagnosis. Thus there is less controversy over the need for staging laparotomies as they are rarely necessary in non-Hodgkin's lymphoma. Radiation usually has a primary role only in stage I disease, while chemotherapy is used for stages III and IV disease. The treatment of stage II disease is somewhat controversial, but most medical oncologists favor chemotherapy. Clearly, our concepts and understanding of these diseases are still evolving.

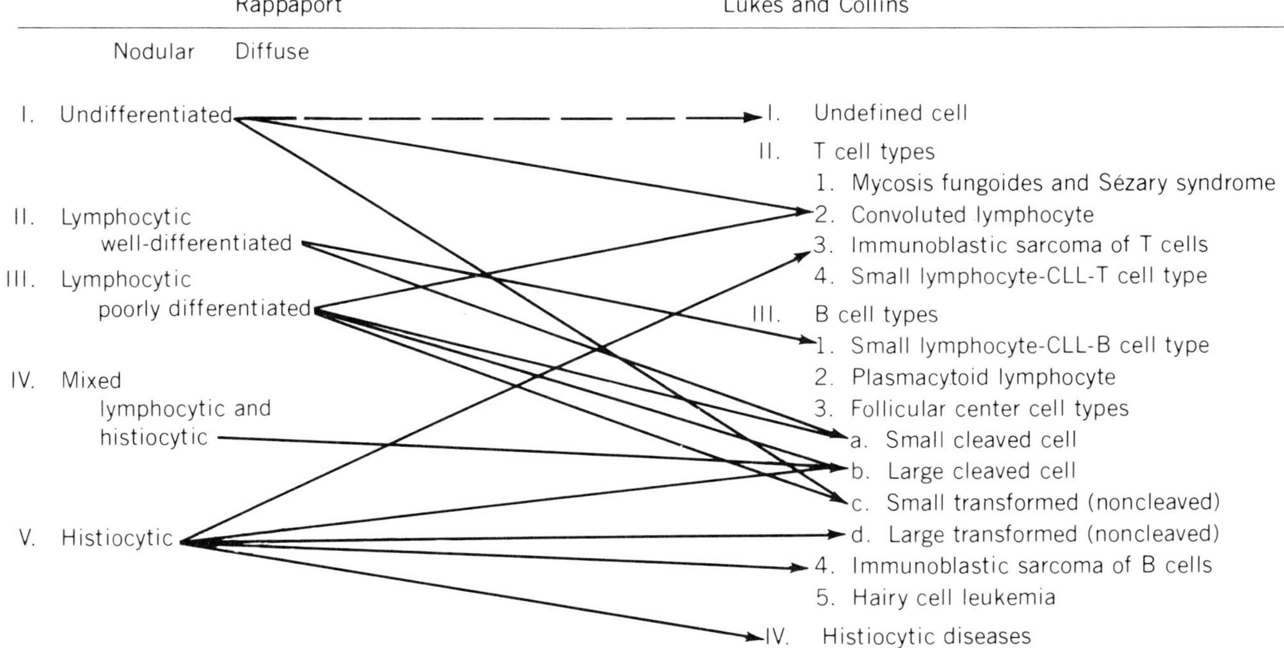

Fig. 55.6. *Comparison of Rappaport and Lukes-Collins classifications. (Modified from Nathwani et al. 1978 and Lukes and Collins 1975.)*

Table 55.2. *A Working Formulation of Non-Hodgkin's Lymphoma for Clinical Use*

Recommendations of an Expert International Panel	*Corresponding Rappaport Classification*
Low Grade	
Malignant lymphoma Small lymphocytic—consistent with chronic lymphocytic leukemia, plasmacytoid	Diffuse well-differentiated lymphoma, chronic lymphocytic leukemia
Malignant lymphoma, follicular Predominantly small cleaved cell—diffuse areas, sclerosis	Nodular, poorly differentiated lymphoma
Mixed, small cleaved, and large cell—diffuse areas, sclerosis	Nodular mixed lymphoma
Intermediate grade	
Malignant lymphoma, follicular Predominantly large cell—diffuse areas, sclerosis	Nodular histiocytic lymphoma
Malignant lymphoma, diffuse Small cleaved cell—sclerosis	Diffuse poorly differentiated lymphoma
Malignant lymphoma, diffuse Mixed, small, and large cell—sclerosis, epitheliod cell component	Diffuse mixed lymphoma
Malignant lymphoma, diffuse Large cell—cleaved cell, noncleaved cell, sclerosis	Diffuse histiocytic lymphoma, large cell lymphoma
High grade	
Malignant lymphoma Large cell, immunoblastic—plasmacytoid, clear cell, polymorphous, epitheliod cell component	Diffuse histiocytic lymphoma, immunoblastic sarcoma
Malignant lymphoma Lymphoblastic—convoluted cell, nonconvoluted cell	Lymphoblastic lymphoma
Malignant lymphoma Small, noncleaved cell—Burkitt's, follicular areas	Diffuse undifferentiated lymphoma, Burkitt's and non-Burkitt's types
Miscellaneous Composite Mycosis fungoides Histiocytic Extramedullary plasmacytoma Unclassifiable Other	

SOURCE: Berard et al. 1981.

References

Aisenberg, A. C. Malignant lymphoma. *N. Engl. J. Med.* 228:883–890; 935–941, 1973.

Berard, C. W. et al. Immunologic aspects and pathology of the malignant lymphomas. *Cancer* 42:911–921, 1978.

Berard, C. W. et al. A multidisciplinary approach to understanding non-Hodgkin's lymphomas. *Ann. Intern. Med.* 94:218–235, 1981.

Bright, R. Observations on abdominal tumors and intumescence. *Guy's Hosp. Rep.* 3:401–460, 1838.

Brill, N. E.; Baehr, G.; and Rosenthal, N. Generalized giant lymph follicle hyperplasia of lymph nodes and spleen. *JAMA* 84:668–671, 1925.

Burkitt, D. A sarcoma involving the jaws in African children. *Br. J. Surg.* 46:218–223, 1958.

Burkitt, D., and O'Conor, G. T. Malignant lymphoma in African children. A clinical syndrome. *Cancer* 14:258–269, 1961.

Byrne, G. E., Jr. Histopathologic diagnosis of Hodgkin's disease. *Semin. Oncol.* 7:103–113, 1980.

Carbone, P. P. et al. Report of the committee on Hodgkin's disease staging classification. *Cancer Res.* 31:1860–1861, 1971.

Dawson, P. J. The original illustrations of Hodgkin's disease. *Arch. Intern. Med.* 121:288–290, 1968.

Desforges, J. F.; Rutherford, C. J.; and Piro, A. Hodgkin's disease. *N. Engl. J. Med.* 301:1212–1222, 1979.

Desser, R. K. et al. Prognostic classification of Hodgkin's disease in pathologic stage III, based on anatomic considerations. *Blood* 49:883–893, 1977.

DeVita, V. T., Jr. et al. Curability of advanced Hodgkin's disease with chemotherapy. *Ann. Intern. Med.* 92:587–595, 1980.

Dorfman, R. F.; Burke, J. S.; and Berard, C. W. A new working formulation of non-Hodgkin's lymphomas: background, recommendations, histological criteria, and relationship to other classifications. In *Advances in malignant lymphomas. Proceedings of the third Bristol Myers symposium on cancer research.* New York: Academic Press, 1981.

Dreschfeld, J. Clinical lecture on acute Hodgkin's (or pseudoleucocythaemia). *Br. Med. J.* 1:893–896, 1892.

Fox, H. Remarks on microscopical preparations made from some of the original tissue described by Thomas Hodgkin, 1832. *Ann. Med. History* 8:370–374, 1926.

Frizzera, G.; Moran, E. M.; and Rappaport, H. Angioimmunoblastic lymphadenopathy: diagnosis and clinical course. *Am. J. Med.* 59:803–818, 1975.

Gall, E. A., and Mallory, T. B. Malignant lymphoma. A clinicopathologic survey of 618 cases. *Am. J. Pathol.* 18:381–429, 1942.

Golomb, H. M. et al. Importance of substaging of stage III Hodgkin's disease. *Semin. Oncol.* 7:136–143, 1980.

Greenfield, W. S. Specimens illustrative of pathology of lymphadenoma and leucocythaemia. *Trans. Pathol. Soc. London* 29:272–304, 1878.

Gupta, S., and Good, R. A. Markers of human lymphocyte subpopulations in primary immunodeficiency and lymphoproliferative disorders. *Semin. Hematol.* 17: 1–29, 1980.

Hodgkin, T. On some morbid appearances of the absorbent glands and spleen. *Medico-Chir. Trans.* 17:68–114, 1832.

Jackson, H., Jr., and Parker, F., Jr. Hodgkin's disease. *N. Engl. J. Med.* 230:1–8; 231:35–44, 1944.

Jones, S. E. et al. Non-Hodgkin's lymphomas. IV. Clinicopathologic correlation in 405 cases. *Cancer* 31: 806–823, 1973.

Kaplan, H. S. *Hodgkin's disease.* Cambridge: Harvard University Press, 1972.

Kay, N. E.; Ackerman, S. K.; and Douglas, S. D. Anatomy of the immune system. *Semin. Hematol.* 16:252–282, 1979.

Klein, G. The Epstein-Barr virus and neoplasia. *N. Engl. J. Med.* 293:1353–1357, 1975.

Krivit, W. et al. Non-Hodgkin's lymphoma in children. *Semin. Oncol.* 4:263–351, 1977.

Kundrat, H. Über Lymphosarkomatosis. *Wien Klin. Wochenschr.* 6:211–234, 1893.

Langhans, T. Das maligne Lymphosarkom. *Virchows Arch. [Pathol. Anat.]* 54:509–537, 1872.

Levi, J. A., and Wiernik, P. H. Limited extranodal Hodgkin's disease: unfavorable prognosis and therapeutic implications. *Am. J. Med.* 63:365–372, 1977.

Lichtenstein, A. Immunoblastic sarcoma. *Cancer* 43: 343–352, 1979.

Lichtenstein, A. K. et al. Primary mediastinal lymphoma in adults. *Am. J. Med.* 68:509–514, 1980.

Lukes, R. J. Relationship of histologic features to clinical stages in Hodgkin's disease. *Am. J. Roentgenol.* 90:944–955, 1963.

Lukes, R. J. et al. Report of the nomenclature committee. *Cancer Res.* 26:1311, 1966.

Lukes, R. J., and Butler, J. J. The pathology and nomenclature of Hodgkin's disease. *Cancer Res.* 26:1063–1081, 1966.

Lukes, R. J., and Collins, R. D. Immunologic characterization of human malignant lymphomas. *Cancer* 34:1488–1503, 1974.

Lukes, R. J., and Collins, R. D. New approaches to the classification of the lymphomata. *Br. J. Cancer* 31:(suppl. 2):1–28, 1975.

Lukes, R. J., and Collins, R. D. Lukes-Collins classification and its significance. *Cancer Treat. Rep.* 61:971–979, 1977.

Lukes, R. J., and Tindle, B. H. Immunoblastic lymphadenopathy: a hyperimmune entity resembling Hodgkin's disease. *N. Engl. J. Med.* 292:1–8, 1975.

Michel, R. P.; Case, B. W.; and Moinuddin, M. Immunoblastic lymphosarcoma: a light, immunofluorescence, and electron microscopic study. *Cancer* 43:224–236, 1979.

Milder, J. W. et al. Obstacles to the control of Hodgkin's disease. *Cancer Res.* 26:1046–1311, 1966.

Milder, J. W. et al. Staging in Hodgkin's disease. *Cancer Res.* 31:1712–1870, 1971.

Nathwani, B. N. et al. Non-Hodgkin's lymphomas: a clinicopathologic study comparing two classifications. *Cancer* 41:303–325, 1978.

Nathwani, B. N.; Kim, H.; and Rappaport, H. Malignant lymphoma, lymphoblastic. *Cancer* 38:964–983, 1976.

Pangalis, G. S.; Moran, E. M.; and Rappaport, H. Blood and bone marrow findings in angioimmunoblastic lymphadenopathy. *Blood* 51:71–83, 1978.

Rappaport, H. Tumors of the hematopoietic system. In *Atlas of tumor pathology,* section 3, fascicle 8. Washington, D.C.: Armed Forces Institute of Pathology, 1966.

Rappaport, H.; Winter, W. J.; and Hicks, E. B. Follicular lymphoma. A reevaluation of its position in the scheme of malignant lymphomas, based on a survey of 253 cases. *Cancer* 9:792–821, 1956.

Reed, D. M. On the pathologic changes in Hodgkin's disease with special reference to its relation to tuberculosis. *Johns Hopkins Hosp. Rep.* 10:133–196, 1902.

Richter, M. N. Generalized reticular cell sarcoma of lymph nodes associated with lymphatic leukemia. *Am. J. Pathol.* 4:285–292, 1928.

Rosenberg, S. Report of the committee on the staging of Hodgkin's disease. *Cancer Res.* 26:1310, 1966.

Roulet, F. Das primare Retothelsarkom der Lymphknoten. *Virchows Arch.* [*Pathol. Anat.*] 277:15–47, 1930.

Sternberg, C. Über eine Eigenartige unter dem Bilde der pseudoleukamie verlaufend Tuberculose des lymphatischen Apparates. *Z. Heilk.* 19:21–90, 1898.

Symmers, D. Follicular lymphadenopathy with splenomegaly. *Arch. Pathol. Lab. Med.* 3:816–820, 1927.

Trump, D. L. et al. Richter's syndrome: diffuse histiocytic lymphoma in patients with chronic lymphocytic leukemia. *Am. J. Med.* 68:539–548, 1980.

Virchow, R. Weisses blut. *Neue Notizen aus dem Geb. der Natur—und Heilkunde (Frorieps neue Notizen)* 36:151–156, 1845.

Wilks, S. Cases of lardaceous disease and some allied affections with remarks. *Guy's Hosp. Rep.* 17(series II:2):103–132, 1856.

Wilks, S. Cases of enlargement of lymphatic glands and spleen (or Hodgkin's Disease), with remarks. *Guy's Hosp. Rep.* 11:56–67, 1865.

Ziegler, J. L. Treatment results of 54 American patients with Burkitt's lymphoma are similar to the African experience. *N. Engl. J. Med.* 297:75–80, 1977.

Ziegler, J. L. Management of Burkitt's lymphoma: an update. *Cancer Treat. Rev.* 6:95–106, 1979.

Ziegler, J. L. Burkitt's lymphoma. *N. Engl. J. Med.* 305:735–745, 1981.

fifty-six

Radiotherapeutic Management of Hodgkin's Disease

LEONARD R. PROSNITZ

The treatment of Hodgkin's disease has become a satisfying endeavor for radiation and medical oncologists. Cure is now possible for most patients with this disease, a remarkable achievement considering that as recently as 15 years ago it was viewed by most physicians as uniformly fatal. Cure is obtained not only in the majority of patients with localized disease, but even in those with far advanced, generalized involvement. These results have been achieved not by the sudden discovery of a "magic bullet" specific for Hodgkin's disease, but by the painstaking application of a complex staging and treatment process, generally by a team of specialists including radiation and medical oncologists, surgeons, and hematopathologists. The phrase multidisciplinary approach sounds almost hackneyed, but is truly essential if optimum results are to be achieved when treating these patients. The radiation therapist and the medical oncologist should participate from the outset in evaluation of the patient and the decision as to optimum treatment. The surgeon's role remains important in staging.

Clinical Evaluation and Staging

Selection of appropriate therapy for patients with Hodgkin's disease is totally dependent on accurate staging. The Ann Arbor classification is the most widely accepted system (Carbone et al. 1971). Particular attention should be paid to the presence or absence of fever, sweats, or weight loss; in a subclassification the absence of these symptoms is designated by A, and their presence by B. Itching and pain after ingestion of alcohol are of interest although not officially considered as B symptoms. If present initially, their reappearance after treatment almost always signifies a relapse. A past history of infectious mononucleosis, tonsillectomy, or contact with an individual with Hodgkin's disease is frequently obtained.

In addition to the usual physical examination, a number of laboratory studies are appropriate:

- Required
  - CBC, platelets
  - BUN, liver function studies, uric acid
  - Chest x-ray
  - Lymphangiogram
  - Bone marrow aspirate and biopsy (for B symptoms and stages III and IV)
- Optional
  - Sedimentation rate
  - Serum copper
  - Liver-spleen scan, bone scan
  - Laparotomy
  - Immunologic testing
  - Gallium scan
  - CT scan
  - Ultrasound
  - Laparoscopy
  - Chest tomograms
  - IVP

Currently, there is some controversy over the merits of lymphangiography and laparotomy. I consider the lymphangiogram to be essential in almost all instances, even if laparotomy is to be done. Many times the lymphangiogram is clearly positive or negative, and in these instances accuracy is 90% or more. At other times the test is equivocal, but still a number of useful purposes are served: (1) suspicious nodes are located for the surgeon to biopsy that are often quite hard to find at laparotomy; (2) the opacified nodes are clearly outlined for the radiotherapist to shape treatment portals; and (3) the size of abdominal nodes may be followed simply with serial abdominal films to gauge response to treatment over a number of months.

Other noninvasive procedures to evaluate abdominal lymph nodes include (1) gallium scanning, (2) CT scanning, and (3) ultrasound. If the tumor picks up gallium the first can be a useful procedure, but the technique is least reliable in detection of abdominal disease, and its accuracy is dependent on the type of scanner that is used. The CT scan and ultrasound show great promise for the future, but experience is limited to date and these have to be considered experimental procedures.

In most patients, laparotomy remains necessary to determine accurately the extent of abdominal disease. Numerous studies have shown that in patients thought to have stage I or II disease on the basis of clinical examination and all laboratory and x-ray studies, 30% will turn out to have unsuspected abdominal disease (Glatstein et al. 1973; Prosnitz, Nuland, and Kligerman 1972). Splenic involvement is particularly difficult to detect clinically.

In our institution and in most others, detection of abdominal involvement that designates stage III Hodgkin's disease results in a substantial alteration in the treatment plan. The National Cancer Institute has suggested relatively uniform treatment plans for clinical stages I and II disease that would not be altered a great deal by laparotomy. In my view, however, such programs carry a greater risk of morbidity than performing the laparotomy and specifically tailoring treatment based on the results.

In patients who clearly have stage IV disease on clinical and laboratory grounds, laparotomy is not generally necessary. I feel that it is still important, however, to determine as accurately as possible the extent of disease since our treatment program for advanced stages entails irradiation of all sites of gross tumor involvement. This determination can usually be accomplished with laparoscopy, which is particularly useful for evaluation of the liver.

It is now apparent that appropriate radiation therapy for early stages of Hodgkin's disease will cure the majority of patients. Figure 56.1 shows the survival and relapse-free survival of 131 patients with stages I and IIA disease treated at Yale since 1969, all of whom underwent staging laparotomy and lymphangiography as part of their initial evaluation. The overall survival is 95% at 5 and 10 years; relapse-free actuarial survival 78% at 5 years and 79% at 10 years. Some relapses do occur between the fifth and tenth years, but only infrequently, and essentially those patients relapse-free at five years may be considered cured.

These results are similar to those obtained at several leading institutions in laparotomy-staged patients. The data from Stanford indicate an overall survival rate of 90%, and a relapse-free survival of 80% in stages IA and IIA disease (Glatstein 1977). The Joint Center for Radiation Therapy at Harvard reported an overall survival rate of 96% at five years and relapse-free survival of 88% (Goodman, Piro, and Hellman 1976). At the Royal Marsden Hospital in London, the relapse-free survival was 80% at five years (Peckham et al. 1975).

These series all consist of patients fully staged with lymphangiography and laparotomy. The extent of staging work-up will alter the composition of the treatment group and therefore the results. In a series of 44 patients with stages IA and IIA disease treated at Yale who were staged with lymphangiography but not laparotomy, relapse-free five-year survival was 53% and overall survival 74% (Prosnitz et al. 1969). Most published series prior to the laparotomy era showed five-year disease-free survivals in the range of 50% to 60%.

In these Yale, Stanford, and Harvard series almost all patients were treated with extended-field radiation therapy—a mantle field covering the lymph nodes above the diaphragm and a separate spade-shaped field to cover the paraaortic nodes and splenic pedicle. In some instances, such as when the lymphangiogram was suspicious despite negative laparotomy, a full inverted Y-field has been used. In a retrospective comparison at our institution, this policy has been associated with considerably fewer relapses than if just a mantle field is used. Two randomized trials from Stanford (Rosenberg and Kaplan 1975; Kaplan 1980) and a national collaborative study (Hutchison 1976) have also shown a lower incidence of relapse in patients treated with extended-field as opposed to involved-field radiotherapy. Survival differences are minimal, presumably because of excellent salvage with multidrug chemotherapy; however, not all patients who relapse are salvaged with chemotherapy, and the additional morbidity associated with this treatment should be avoided whenever possible.

Stages IB and IIB

This is a comparatively rare subgroup of patients about whose management there is considerable controversy but unfortunately, a scarcity of hard data. From 1958 to 1976, there were 173 patients with stage IA and IIA Hodgkin's disease at Yale who received radiation therapy for cure, but during the same time interval there were only 30 with stage IB and IIB disease. Twenty of them underwent staging laparotomy, most of whom then received total nodal irradiation, although a few received somewhat smaller fields. None received chemotherapy as part of initial management. Twelve of the 20 have remained continuously free of disease for periods of 1 to 10 years. The one randomized trial of which we are aware comparing total nodal irradiation alone with total nodal irradiation plus MOPP (mechlorethamine-Oncovin-procarbazine-prednisone) chemotherapy showed no difference either in relapse-free or overall survival (Rosenberg and Kaplan 1975).

Curative Treatment of Stages IIIB and IV Disease

The introduction of combination chemotherapy for advanced Hodgkin's disease by DeVita and colleagues at the National Cancer Institute (NCI) in the mid-1960s constituted a major advance in the treatment of Hodgkin's disease and raised hopes for cure of advanced as well as localized disease. Particularly with the use of radiation in combination with multiple-drug chemotherapy, these hopes are now apparently being realized.

The original DeVita combination—MOPP—is still the most widely used. Other combinations have substituted cytoxan for nitrogen mustard or vinblastine for vincristine with equivalent results. Complete remission has been achieved in 55% to 85% of untreated or previously irradiated patients with advanced disease. Among the complete responders, however, relapses have been fairly common, with a frequency of 35% to 60% (DeVita 1973; McElwain et al. 1973; Frei et al.

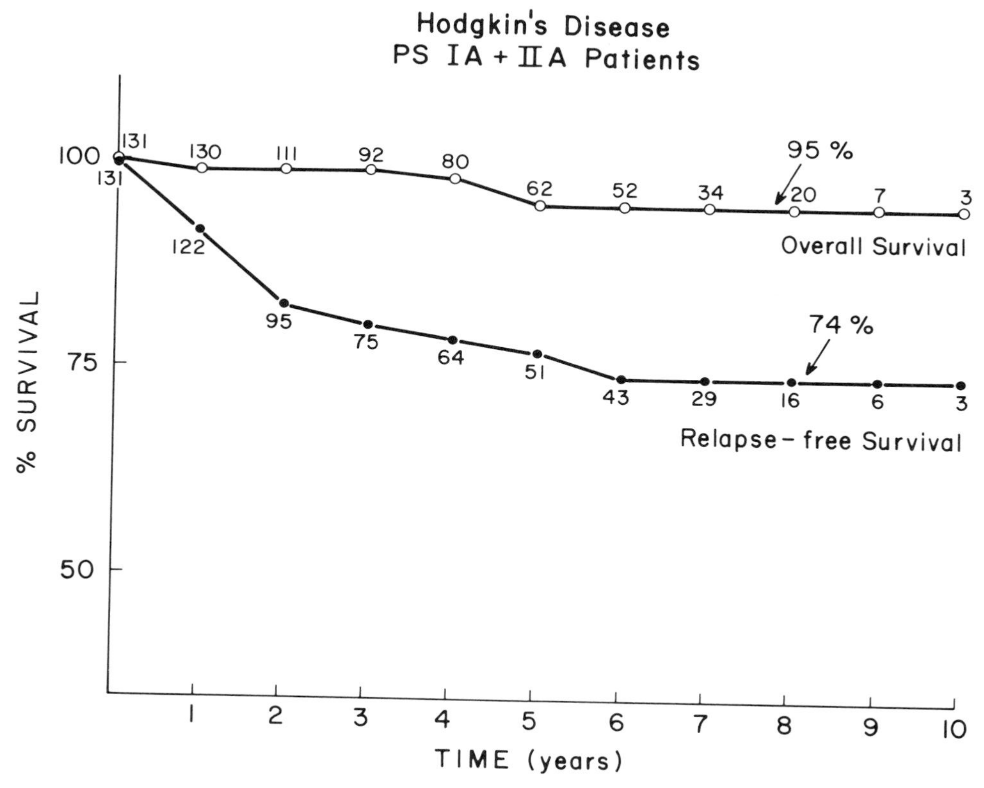

Fig. 56.1. *Relapse-free and overall actuarial survival for patients with stages IA and IIA Hodgkin's disease. (Prosnitz et al. 1980. Reprinted by permission.)*

1973). Nevertheless, many of the original NCI patients have now been followed for periods of up to 10 years with 68% of this particular series remaining in complete remission at five years and few relapses between fifth and tenth years (DeVita et al. 1980).

In an effort to improve the overall treatment for advanced Hodgkin's disease, it seemed logical to add the single most effective agent—radiotherapy. In 1969, we began a program employing five drugs—nitrogen mustard, vincristine, vinblastine, procarbazine, and prednisone—in addition to radiotherapy. It was predicted on theoretical grounds that relapse following chemotherapy would be most likely to occur at sites of gross or clinically apparent disease, since the probability of chemotherapeutic control varies inversely with the number of cells present. This prediction has subsequently been borne out by the Southwest Oncology Group and the NCI, both of which have shown that relapses tend to occur in the sites where the disease was originally located (Frei et al. 1973; Young et al. 1978). Administration of radiation therapy to sites of pretreatment involvement should reduce relapses in these sites.

We reasoned that if cures were to be obtained in advanced disease, chemotherapy obviously would have to be successful in achieving a certain cell kill. Therefore the dose commonly employed when radiation was being used as the single treatment (4000 rad) was not necessary if the radiation was combined with chemotherapy, and lower doses in the range of 1500 to 2000 rad would suffice. Details of the kinetic arguments have been presented previously (Prosnitz et al. 1976).

Lower doses of radiation have the advantage of minimizing bone marrow toxicity, allowing for maximal chemotherapy to be given, and enabling one to treat all areas of pretreatment involvement including parenchymal organs such as lungs or liver, which could never be given doses in the neighborhood of 4000 rad. Our most recent publication on this subject details results in 118 patients with advanced Hodgkin's disease treated with this program from 1969 to 1977 (Farber et al. 1980). Sixty-two patients were previously untreated, and 56 had relapsed following radiotherapy. Ninety-eight of the 118 patients (83%) have entered complete remission; 86 remain in complete remission with a median follow-up of four years.

Survival data are shown in figure 56.2. Overall survival for all patients is 75% at five years; for the complete responders it is 95% at five years. Corresponding relapse-free survival figures are 70% and 90% respectively, since almost all who relapse following chemotherapy and radiation rapidly succumb to their disease. Of the 98 patients who achieved complete remission, only 10 relapsed. This relapse rate appears to be substantially lower than that recorded by other investigators (DeVita et al. 1980).

Several subgroups of patients with a worse prognosis than those with advanced stage of disease as a whole have also been identified. Patients over the age of 40 years have a survival rate of only 50% at five years, compared with 87% for all other patients. Those who have stage IV disease with multiple extranodal sites of involvement have a five-year survival of only 40% compared with others with only a single extranodal site whose five-year survival is 86%.

These rather dramatic results unfortunately have not been achieved without some toxicity secondary to the treatment itself. Acute leukemia has occurred in 3 of 88 long-term survivors, proving fatal for all. Aseptic necrosis of either the femoral or humeral heads or both has occurred in eight patients and has proved to be disabling

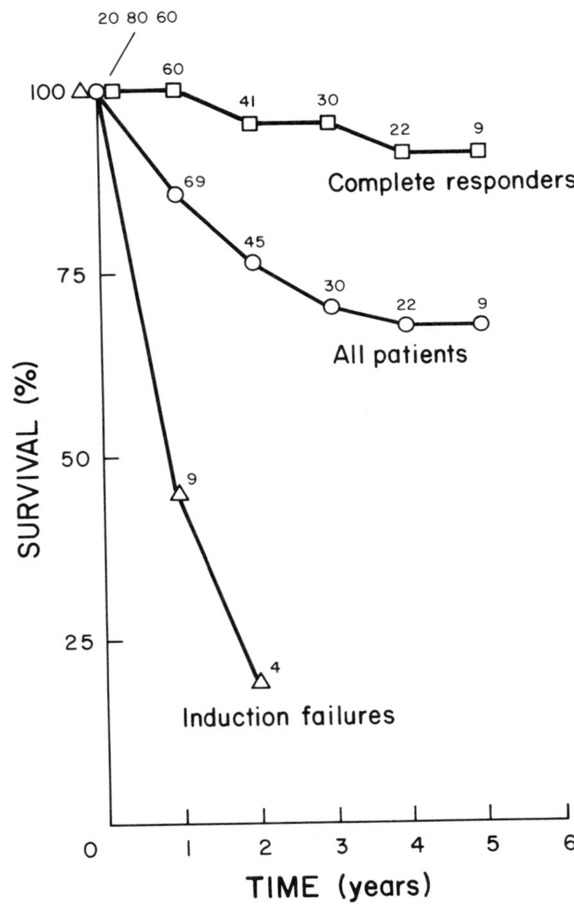

Fig. 56.2. *Actuarial survival of patients treated with combined modality therapy. (Prosnitz et al. 1976. Reprinted by permission.)*

although not life-threatening. In our series, there were two deaths during the induction phases of chemotherapy, both patients dying from overwhelming sepsis, one with pneumococcal sepsis and the other with cryptococcal meningitis.

Hodgkin's Disease of Intermediate Prognosis—Stage IIIA

Following the initial success of radiotherapy in long-term control and cure of stage I and II Hodgkin's disease, attempts were made during the mid-1960s to apply radical radiotherapy techniques to the management of stage IIIA disease. Initially, it was clear that so-called total nodal irradiation (TNI) could be given without prohibitive hematologic toxicity, but fortunately this has not turned out to be a major problem. Stage IIIA is a relatively uncommon subgroup of Hodgkin's disease, comprising about 15% of the total, and it has taken about 10 years in most institutions to accumulate significant data.

Initial expectations were that stage IIIA disease could be cured with the same frequency as IA or IIA disease. This was based largely on the known ability of radiation doses in the range of 4000 rad to achieve local control in a given area 90% to 95% of the time. If there are many areas, however, the probability of control in all is the product of the individual probabilities. For example, if six fields are at risk the theoretical rate of controlling all six ranges from 53% to 74%, depending on whether one uses a 90% or 95% figure for local control in one field. Thus considering only the likelihood of a true recurrence within the radiation field, the odds of success in stage IIIA disease drop considerably from those for stage I or II.

Data now available from several centers concerning results of radiotherapy in IIIA disease are somewhat contradictory. At the Royal Marsden Hospital, in the pre-laparotomy era only 8 of 22 with clinical stage IIIA Hodgkin's disease treated with TNI remain in complete remission. On the other hand, 23 of 30 with pathologic stage IIIA disease treated at the same institution with TNI are in complete remission, although the follow-up on the latter group is much shorter (Peckham et al. 1975).

In a British National Lymphoma investigation (1976) TNI was compared with MOPP chemotherapy in 81 patients with laparotomy-staged IIIA disease randomly allocated between the two treatment arms. Initial complete remission was achieved in 95% of those treated with TNI compared with 74% of those receiving MOPP. Disease-free survival at four years was 71% in the TNI group and 53% in the MOPP group (*P* less than 0.01).

The best results are probably those reported from Stanford (Glatstein 1977). In 31 patients with stage II_SA and III_SA disease (presumably mostly III_SA) treated with TNI only, actuarial disease-free survival was 79% at five years. In a group of 42 patients with stages IIIA and IIIB disease (not further subdivided) treated with TNI and liver irradiation, relapse-free three-year survival was 55% (Rosenberg and Kaplan 1975).

Our own results in stage IIIA disease have been disappointing (Prosnitz et al. 1978). While the overall five-year survival is 80%, relapse-free survival is only 35% (fig. 56.3). The difference is again largely a reflection of the ability of combined chemotherapy and radiation to prolong the survival of relapsing patients. There appears to be an important prognostic difference between patients whose disease was clearly stage IIIA clinically as well as pathologically, and those whose stage became IIIA only after laparotomy. Five-year disease-free survival was much better in the latter (50%) compared with the former (15%).

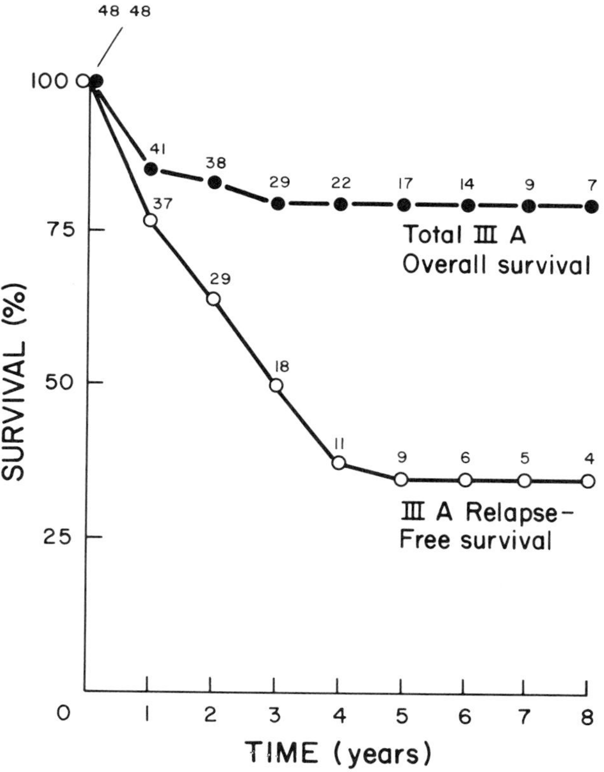

Fig. 56.3. *Overall and relapse-free survival in pathologic stage IIIA Hodgkin's disease following treatment with radiotherapy alone. (Prosnitz et al. 1978. Reprinted by permission.)*

A similar division of patients into different prognostic categories was done by Desser and associates (1977) at the University of Chicago. They found that patients with splenic or splenic hilar node involvement (stage III_1) had a better prognosis than those with para-aortic or pelvic node involvement with or without splenic disease (stage III_2).

The results we have obtained in advanced Hodgkin's disease treated with combined therapy suggest that all clinical stage IIIA disease should be treated with this program, and possibly some patients with only pathologic stage IIIA disease as well. Others claim that chemotherapy alone is appropriate therapy for stage IIIA disease.

Complications of Therapy

The therapeutic gains just described unfortunately have not been realized without some undesirable sequelae. The short-term problems of lymphoma chemotherapy and radiation are well recognized. Some of the long-term problems, however, are less well known.

Radiation Pneumonitis

Symptomatic pneumonitis has been reported with a frequency of 1% to 20%, the incidence varying with what the author chooses to define as pneumonitis, whether prophylactic lung irradiation has been used, and what percentage of patients with large mediastinal masses have been treated. Most cases do not require any specific therapy, but a few will end fatally despite all treatment. One has to be especially careful about pneumonitis when combinations of drugs and irradiation are used, since there may well be an additive effect on normal tissue tolerance.

Radiation Pericarditis

The incidence is directly related to the volume of heart irradiated and the total dose delivered, with a reported frequency from 2% to 13%. Most often it is self-limited, but sometimes surgical intervention is required and again, a few cases may end fatally.

Effects on Fertility

Radiation and chemotherapy both have significant effects on gonadal function, the former being a problem largely in women, the latter in men. If the pelvis is excluded from the radiation field there are no problems. If the pelvis is included, however, in women even with ovarian transposition and subsequent radiation shielding, there is a 50% incidence of permanent sterility and amenorrhea. There may also be significant scatter dose to the testes. Conversely, while chemotherapy may temporarily affect ovarian function, usually this is not permanent, but MOPP chemotherapy has caused permanent sterility in almost all men patients (DeVita 1981).

Bone Changes

Interference with bone growth in the irradiated field is regularly seen in children treated before puberty with doses of 3500 rad or more and may be seen with lower doses as well. In an attempt to avoid such growth problems several centers are now treating early stages of Hodgkin's disease with chemotherapy in combination with low-dose irradiation.

Endocrine Changes

The combination of external beam radiation plus a large iodine load from lymphangiography seems to result in a significant effect on the thyroid gland in many instances, with an incidence of clinical hypothyroidism from 6% to 13% but chemical changes occurring in as many as 40% of patients, principally abnormally high thyroid-stimulating hormone values. Fortunately, this complication is easily correctable with medication.

Secondary Malignancies

This is perhaps the most worrisome complication and seems particularly related to chemotherapy and radiation used together rather than either one alone. Acute leukemia in particular has been observed in approximately 5% of long-term survivors receiving both modalities for Hodgkin's disease.

Non-Hodgkin's Lymphomas

Space does not permit a detailed discussion of the non-Hodgkin's lymphomas, but from the perspective of radiotherapists there are several points worth making. These lymphomas differ from Hodgkin's disease in many important respects. They are a much more heterogeneous group of disorders with distinct clinical behavior patterns related to their histopathology. The non-Hodgkin's lymphomas as a rule tend to be generalized from the outset, and hence appropriate treatment is usually chemotherapy. Local manifestations, however, respond well to radiation, and roughly the same kind of dose-response curve is obtained as in Hodgkin's disease, that is, 4000 rad in four weeks controls disease locally in greater than 90% of instances.

By implication, patients with stage I or II non-Hodgkin's lymphoma should be curable with appropriate doses of radiation therapy.

We have recently analyzed 114 patients with non-Hodgkin's lymphoma, clinical stages I or II, treated with radical radiotherapy alone over the last 15 years (Chen et al. 1979). One-third of these patients had nodular lymphoma, two-thirds diffuse. Fifty percent of those with localized diffuse disease had extranodal involvement compared with 20% of patients with nodular disease; all of these numbers are consistent with reported literature experience. Five-year relapse-free and overall survivals were 83% and 100% respectively for the nodular group and 37% and 59% for the diffuse group. In diffuse stage I disease the relapse-free survival was approximately 50%, and for stage II disease it was 25%.

These results suggest that in patients with localized (stage I) non-Hodgkin's lymphoma the appropriate treatment is radical irradiation. Chemotherapy should be considered for stage II lymphoma, particularly where there is diffuse disease, when the prognosis is not nearly as good. There does not seem to be any benefit from the use of extended-field or total nodal irradiation in the non-Hodgkin's lymphomas as contrasted with Hodgkin's disease. Spread of the former is generally not contiguous, but rather relapses tend to occur at widely disseminated sites.

References

British National Lymphoma Investigation. Initial treatment of stage IIIA Hodgkin's disease: comparison of radiotherapy with combined chemotherapy. *Lancet* 2: 991–995, 1976.

Carbone, P. P. et al. Report of the committee on Hodgkin's disease staging classification. *Cancer Res.* 31:1860–1861, 1971.

Chen, M. G. et al. Results of radiotherapy in control of stage I and II non-Hodgkin's lymphoma. *Cancer* 43:1245–1254, 1979.

Desser, R. K. et al. Prognostic classification of Hodgkin's disease in pathologic stage III, based on anatomical considerations. *Blood* 49:883–893, 1977.

DeVita, V. T., Jr. Combined drug treatment of Hodgkin's disease. *Natl. Cancer Inst. Monogr.* 36:373–379, 1973.

DeVita, V. T., Jr. The consequences of the chemotherapy of Hodgkin's disease. *Cancer* 47:1–13, 1981.

DeVita, V. T., Jr. et al. Curability of advanced Hodgkin's disease with chemotherapy. *Ann. Intern. Med.* 92:587–595, 1980.

Farber, L. R. et al. Curative potential of combined modality therapy for advanced Hodgkin's disease. *Cancer* 46:1509–1517, 1980.

Frei, E., III et al. Combination chemotherapy in advanced Hodgkin's disease. *Ann. Intern. Med.* 79:376–382, 1973.

Glatstein, E. Radiotherapy in Hodgkin's disease. *Cancer* 39:837–842, 1977.

Glatstein, E. et al. Surgical staging of abdominal involvement in unselected patients with Hodgkin's disease. *Radiology* 97:425–432, 1973.

Goodman, R. L.; Piro, A. J.; and Hellman, S. Can pelvic radiation be omitted in patients with pathologic stages IA and IIA Hodgkin's disease? *Cancer* 37:2834–2839, 1976.

Hutchison, G. A. Survival and complications of radiotherapy following involved and extended field therapy of Hodgkin's disease, stages I and II. *Cancer* 38:233–305, 1976.

Kaplan, H. S. *Hodgkin's disease,* 2nd edition. Cambridge: Harvard University Press, 1980.

McElwain, T. J. et al. Combination chemotherapy in advanced and recurrent Hodgkin's disease. *Natl. Cancer Inst. Monogr.* 36:395–402, 1973.

Peckham, M. J. et al. The results of radiotherapy for Hodgkin's disease. *Br. J. Cancer* 32:391–400, 1975.

Prosnitz, L. R. et al. The clinical course of Hodgkin's disease and other malignant lymphomas treated with radical radiation therapy. *Am. J. Roentgenol.* 105: 618–628, 1969.

Prosnitz, L. R. et al. Long-term remissions with combined modality therapy for advanced Hodgkin's disease. *Cancer* 37:2826–2833, 1976.

Prosnitz, L. R. et al. Treatment of stage IIIA Hodgkin's disease: is radiotherapy alone adequate? *Int. J. Radiat. Oncol.* 4:781–787, 1978.

Prosnitz, L. R. et al. Supradiaphragmatic Hodgkin's disease: significance of large mediastinal masses. *Int. J. Radiat. Oncol.* 6:809–813, 1980.

Prosnitz, L. R.; Nuland, S. B.; and Kligerman, M. M. Role of laparotomy and splenectomy in the management of Hodgkin's disease. *Cancer* 29:44–50, 1972.

Rosenberg, S. A., and Kaplan, H. S. The management of stage I, II, and III Hodgkin's disease with combined radiotherapy and chemotherapy. *Cancer* 35:55–63, 1975.

Young, R. C. et al. Patterns of relapse in advanced Hodgkin's disease treated with combination chemotherapy. *Cancer* 42:1001–1007, 1978.

fifty-seven

Chemotherapy of Hodgkin's Disease and the Non-Hodgkin's Lymphomas

CAROL S. PORTLOCK

Chemotherapy plays a major role in the management of patients with lymphoma, and there are many active agents available together with a growing body of evidence demonstrating the potential for cure with drugs alone (table 57.1).

Hodgkin's Disease

The most successful drug program developed thus far has been MOPP (nitrogen mustard, vincristine [Oncovin], procarbazine, and prednisone), used primarily in the treatment of Hodgkin's disease. As first reported by DeVita, Serpick, and Carbone (1970) pathologically documented complete responses were obtained in 81% of patients with stage III or IV disease and the median remission duration was 29 to 42 months. Most important, a 10-year follow-up has shown that relapses from complete remission are rare after four years and that 66% of complete responders remain relapse-free for periods of up to 10 years after discontinuation of all treatment (DeVita et al. 1978). These results have subsequently been confirmed by others, and clearly a "cure" rate of at least 40% to 50% can be achieved with MOPP alone in advanced (stages IIIB and IV) Hodgkin's disease.

Such results require optimal patient management with attention to drug dosage and scheduling, close observation of response, and pathologic documentation of complete remission. A standard course of treatment consists of at least six cycles of MOPP, including two consolidation cycles after restaging. The complete response rate is adversely affected by the presence of B symptoms and prior chemotherapy. Some have reported that sites (bone marrow) and bulk of disease, as well as histology (nodular sclerosis), also adversely influence results. Unlike prior chemotherapy, prior irradiation does not appear to alter the response to MOPP; in one study, patients who had no B symptoms had a superior response rate with 100% achieving complete remission and with no subsequent relapses (DeVita et al. 1978).

Many approaches have been used to improve the complete response rate or remission durability of MOPP. In several prospective studies maintenance chemotherapy has had no significant benefit in prolonging remission duration. Instead, the most important finding has been the completeness of response at the conclusion of treatment, emphasizing the need to restage all patients pathologically and not to discontinue therapy prematurely. Since relapse after MOPP most often occurs in areas of prior disease, particularly lymph nodes (Young et al. 1978), combined chemotherapy with irradiation would seem promising. Unfortunately, to date there are no convincing prospective data to support the hypothesis that the addition of radiation therapy has a significant impact. Several studies are suggestive, however. Using a five-drug regimen and low-dose (2000 rad) irradiation to known disease sites, the Yale group (Prosnitz et al. 1976) has reported a complete response rate of 75%, with less than 10% of patients relapsing. Similarly, alternating MOPP with high-dose (4400 rad) irradiation for patients with stage

Table 57.1. *Approximate Results of Combination Chemotherapy*

	Complete Response Rate (%)	*Five-Year Disease-Free Survival of Complete Responders (%)*	*Five-Year Survival of All Patients (%)*
Hodgkin's disease stages IIIB and IV	81	66	80
Diffuse histiocytic lymphoma stages III and IV	50	95	30–45
Nodular lymphocytic poorly differentiated lymphoma stages III and IV	60–90	25	70
Nodular mixed lymphoma stages III and IV	60–90	80	70

SOURCES: Compiled from DeVita et al. 1978; Anderson et al. 1977; Portlock and Rosenberg 1977, 1979.

IIIB disease (Hoppe et al. 1979) has yielded an 88% complete response rate with less than 10% relapsing thus far. Neither study has a concurrent control of chemotherapy alone, making interpretation of results difficult.

Several drug combinations other than MOPP have been developed as initial or salvage therapy, but none has proved superior. Noncross-resistant combinations containing doxorubicin (Adriamycin) have yielded complete response rates of 25% to 60% in patients failing MOPP (DeVita et al. 1978); in one prospective randomized study, ABVD (doxorubicin [Adriamycin], bleomycin, vinblastine, and dacarbazine) had a comparable complete response rate to MOPP as primary therapy (Bonadonna et al. 1977). Because of such encouraging results, alternating drug regimens of MOPP and a combination containing doxorubicin (MOPP plus ABVD) are now being compared to MOPP alone. There appears to be some benefit of the alternating program in terms of complete response (87% versus 63%, $P = 0.04$) and remission duration (96% versus 65% at three years, $P = 0.09$) (Santoro et al. 1980).

At present there is little experience with MOPP or other drug combinations in early stages of Hodgkin's disease. One study from the British National Lymphoma Investigation (1976) reported a significantly better complete response rate (95% versus 74%) and relapse-free survival (71% versus 53% at two years) for patients with pathologic stage IIIA disease treated with total nodal irradiation as compared to MOPP alone. The National Cancer Institute has reported a 100% complete response rate with no relapses using MOPP alone in patients with stages IIIA and IVA disease (DeVita et al. 1978). Further studies will be necessary to clarify the role of MOPP alone in early disease.

The role of MOPP as an adjunct to the radiation therapy of nodal Hodgkin's disease also remains controversial. In a prospective trial from Stanford (Rosenberg et al. 1978), radiation therapy plus MOPP was significantly better than radiation therapy alone in terms of relapse-free survival (81% versus 60% at eight years); however, this did not translate into a significant improvement in overall survival (85% versus 77% at eight years). The reason for this discrepancy appears to be the ability to salvage and potentially cure patients who relapse following radiation therapy alone (Portlock et al. 1978). Furthermore, not only does combined modality treatment have the additive side effects of both, but as recently reported, there is an apparent increased risk of second malignancies, particularly acute myelogenous leukemia (Coleman et al. 1977).

It is clear that combination chemotherapy offers the potential for cure of patients with advanced (IIIB or IV) Hodgkin's disease. Its role in the treatment of early disease, either as adjuvant or sole primary therapy, remains to be defined. It will be necessary to compare prospectively combined or novel single-modality approaches to standard radiation therapy to assess their relative efficacy and acute and chronic morbidity.

Non-Hodgkin's Lymphomas

As in advanced Hodgkin's disease, combination chemotherapy offers the potential for cure of 40% to 50% of patients with stage III or IV diffuse histiocytic lymphoma (DHL). The pathologically documented complete response rate for DHL is only 40% to 50% rather than 80% as in Hodgkin's disease; in contrast to Hodgkin's disease, relapse from complete remission is rare and usually occurs within the first two years after discontinuing treatment. Several combination chemotherapy programs have been developed for the treatment of advanced DHL. Their relative efficacies must be judged not only by complete response rates, but by remission duration and survival results. Two drug regimens (MOPP or C-MOPP and BACOP)* appear comparable in terms of these measurements in pre-

*C-MOPP: cyclophosphamide, vincristine, procarbazine, and prednisone; BACOP: bleomycin, doxorubicin (Adriamycin), cyclophosphamide, vincristine, and prednisone.

viously untreated patients (Fisher et al. 1977). Both achieve complete response of 40% to 50% with only one relapse among 23 complete responders off therapy for periods of up to eight years. Similar or better complete response rates have been reported with several other drug combinations; however, the complete remissions are not as long. In these instances, results of survival may ultimately be compared to MOPP, C-MOPP, or BACOP. One reason for these differences among combinations is the definition of complete response. If careful restaging is performed one month following completion of all chemotherapy, as many as one-quarter of clinical complete responders will be found to have persistent microscopic disease. If treatment is discontinued prematurely in such patients, occult disease will later be manifested as clinical relapse. Moreover, such a partial remission (clinical complete remission) conveys little if any survival benefit. The median survival of partial responders is usually less than eight months, regardless of the degree of response.

Factors that adversely affect complete remission and thus survival include prior treatment (particularly prior chemotherapy) as well as bulk and sites of extranodal disease (bone marrow, gastrointestinal tract, and meninges) (Strauchen et al. 1978), whereas age, sex, and constitutional symptoms do not. Recently, investigators reported that histologic subgroups of DHL can be identified that correlate with prognosis. Of the aggressive lymphomas, only histiocytic lymphoma (either nodular or diffuse type) has such good results with combination chemotherapy. Few patients with diffuse, mixed lymphocytic and histiocytic lymphoma achieve complete remission or have prolonged survival; those with diffuse, poorly differentiated lymphocytic lymphoma may respond dramatically to treatment, only to relapse later.

Meningeal lymphoma has been reported in up to 25% to 30% of relapsing patients with advanced DHL or diffuse undifferentiated lymphoma. Its development is closely correlated with the presence of bone marrow disease. Whether central nervous system prophylaxis as proposed by Bunn and co-workers (1976) will prove to be of benefit must await studies that take into account the incidence of bone marrow disease and the effectiveness of systemic chemotherapy.

As with Hodgkin's disease, relapse of DHL following chemotherapy usually occurs in previous sites of involvement. Unfortunately, combined programs of chemotherapy and radiation have not shown significant benefit. Because combination chemotherapy results have been so successful in advanced DHL, its role in early disease is beginning to be evaluated. The complete response rate for stage III DHL is at least 80%; therefore one would expect at least comparable results in stage II disease. As reported by Miller and Jones (1979), all 14 patients with stage I or II histiocytic lymphoma achieved complete remission with chemotherapy alone and only 1 has relapsed thus far. Although these results are preliminary, they suggest an important role for chemotherapy alone in early stages of disease.

Unlike advanced diffuse histiocytic lymphoma, the role of combination chemotherapy remains inconclusive in the treatment of advanced indolent lymphomas. Complete remission rates of 60% to 90% have been reported with several combination chemotherapy programs. When tested prospectively, however, combination chemotherapy (CVP: cyclophosphamide, vincristine, and prednisone) was not significantly different from therapy with a single alkylating agent or split-course CVP plus total lymphoid irradiation in terms of complete response (65% to 83%), relapse-free survival (60% at three years), or survival (greater than 80% at five years) (Portlock and Rosenberg 1979). Although it is clear that combination chemotherapy and use of a single alkylating agent are comparable in terms of complete remission rates, what remains to be determined is the impact of either on relapse-free and overall survival. As pointed out by many groups, the complete remissions obtained in advanced indolent lymphomas are generally not durable in spite of prolonged survival. The National Cancer Institute (Anderson et al. 1977) has reported complete response rates of 64% to 77% in patients treated with CVP, MOPP, or C-MOPP. Although no significant differences were noted in the rate of complete remission, the relapse-free survival was significantly better for those with nodular mixed lymphoma (NML) (79% disease-free at 5 years) treated with MOPP or C-MOPP as compared to nodular lymphocytic poorly differentiated lymphoma (NLPD) (median of 16 months) and diffuse lymphocytic well-differentiated lymphoma (DLWD) (median of 23 months) treated with CVP. Nevertheless, actuarial survival for all patients (70% at five years) and for complete responders (more than 80% at five years) was not significantly different when analyzed according to histology. Whether the superior relapse-free survival results for patients with NML will later translate into significantly prolonged survival or cure awaits longer follow-up.

Since most if not all treatment approaches are palliative for stage III or IV indolent lymphomas, it is controversial whether any therapy is required if patients are asymptomatic and clinically well. A retrospective analysis (Portlock and Rosenberg 1979) of 44 such patients who were closely followed without initial therapy revealed that treatment was deferred for a median time of 3 years, and that the median time to need for therapy was significantly shorter for NML (9 months) than for NLPD (32 months) and DLWD (longer than 8 years). For all patients the median survival was 10 years, and there were no significant differences noted according to histology.

Factors that may influence the management of patients with advanced indolent lymphomas include histopathology, sites and pace of disease, constitutional symptoms or other symptoms of disease, potential acute and chronic morbidities of treatment, and the patient's age, general health, and psychological make-up. Whenever systemic therapy is initiated, the intent of treatment should be pathologically documented complete remission and discontinuance of all treatment. In the case of combination chemotherapy, this may require 6 to 18 months of treatment, followed by an additional 2 to 4 months of consolidation therapy. There does not appear to be any significant benefit of maintenance chemotherapy, and unnecessary continuance should be avoided whenever possible.

Approaches to management of patients with lymphoma are evolving rapidly. The role of chemotherapy has proved significant in advanced disease, and its role in early stage disease appears even more promising. Future trials will need to consider the comparative efficacies and toxicities of chemotherapy and radiation, the optimal methods of combining both, and the impact of treatment on survival and its potential for cure.

References

Anderson, T. et al. Combination chemotherapy in non-Hodgkin's lymphoma: results of long-term follow-up. *Cancer Treat. Rep.* 61:1057–1066, 1977.

Bonadonna, G. et al. Combined chemotherapy (MOPP or ABVD)-radiotherapy approach in advanced Hodgkin's disease. *Cancer Treat. Rep.* 61:769–777, 1977.

British National Lymphoma Investigation. Initial treatment of stage IIIA Hodgkin's disease: comparison of radiotherapy with combined chemotherapy. *Lancet* 2: 991–995, 1976.

Bunn, R. A. et al. Central nervous system complications in patients with diffuse histiocytic and undifferentiated lymphoma: leukemia revisited. *Blood* 47:3–10, 1976.

Coleman, C. N. et al. Hematologic neoplasia in patients treated for Hodgkin's disease. *N. Engl. J. Med.* 297:1249–1252, 1977.

DeVita, V. T., Jr. et al. The chemotherapy of Hodgkin's disease: past experiences and future directions. *Cancer* 42: 979–990, 1978.

DeVita, V. T., Jr.; Serpick, A. A.; and Carbone, P. P. Combination chemotherapy in the treatment of advanced Hodgkin's disease. *Ann. Intern. Med.* 73:881–895, 1970.

Fisher, R. I. et al. Prognostic factors for advanced diffuse histiocytic lymphoma following treatment with combination chemotherapy. *Am. J. Med.* 63:177–182, 1977.

Hoppe, R. T. et al. Alternating chemotherapy and irradiation in the treatment of advanced Hodgkin's disease. *Cancer* 43:472–481, 1979.

Miller, T. P., and Jones, S. E. Chemotherapy of localized histiocytic lymphoma. *Lancet* 1:358–360, 1979.

Portlock, C. S. et al. Impact of salvage treatment on initial relapses in patients with Hodgkin's disease, stages I-II. *Blood* 51:825–833, 1978.

Portlock, C. S., and Rosenberg, S. A. Chemotherapy of the non-Hodgkin's lymphomas: the Stanford experience. *Cancer Treat. Rep.* 61:1049–1055, 1977.

Portlock, C. S., and Rosenberg, S. A. No initial therapy for stage III and IV non-Hodgkin's lymphomas of favorable histologic types. *Ann Intern. Med.* 90: 10–13, 1979.

Prosnitz, L. R. et al. Long-term remissions with combined modality therapy for advanced Hodgkin's disease. *Cancer* 37:2826–2833, 1976.

Rosenberg, S. A. et al. Combined modality therapy of Hodgkin's disease: a report on the Stanford trials. *Cancer* 42:991–1000, 1978.

Santoro, A. et al. Noncross-resistant regimens (MOPP and ABVD) vs. MOPP alone in stage IV Hodgkin's disease. *Proc. Am. Soc. Clin. Oncol.* 21:470, 1980.

Strauchen, J. A. et al. Clinical relevance of the histiopathological subclassification of diffuse "histiocytic" lymphoma. *N. Engl. J. Med.* 299:1382–1387, 1978.

Young, R. C. et al. Patterns of relapse in advanced Hodgkin's disease treated with combination chemotherapy. *Cancer* 42:1001–1007, 1978.

fifty-eight

Multiple Myeloma

RICHARD B. WEININGER

The diagnosis of neoplastic disease is most often made by biopsy, with the pathologist having the final word in distinguishing benignity from malignancy. Such is not often the case with myeloma. Rather, the clinician is presented with an array of clinical, laboratory, x-ray, and histologic findings that may encompass myeloma, but that overlap significantly with a variety of non-neoplastic disorders. It is therefore incumbent on the oncologist to establish not only a set of diagnostic criteria but to understand the natural history of myeloma and the benign disorders that may be confused with it. Although it is beyond the scope of this chapter to examine all of these criteria and natural histories in depth, they are briefly reviewed so that the indications for therapy and the therapeutic options follow a logical sequence.

Diagnosis

A patient with myeloma may present a clear clinical picture of multisystem derangement that is dramatic and easy to diagnose. This might include bone pain with fractures and hypercalcemia, serum and urine monoclonal immunoglobulins, anemia, leucopenia, thrombocytopenia, renal insufficiency, spinal cord compression, and bacterial infection. As these features are not present in every patient, a means of investigation must be established that will lead to a correct diagnosis. In so doing, it is helpful to consider the three major effects of malignant plasma cells from which virtually all clinical signs and symptoms arise: invasion of the marrow spaces, production of immunoglobulin and/or immunoglobulin fragments, and lysis of bone.

- Bone destruction:
  - Lytic lesions
  - Osteopenia
  - Hypercalcemia
  - Bone pain or tenderness
  - Normal bones?
- Abnormal protein:
  - Two-thirds of patients have serum spike (greater than 1.5 gm%?)
  - Two-thirds of patients have urine spike (greater than 500 mg/24 hrs)
  - None?
- Plasmacytosis:
  - Presence of clumps or syncytia
  - Absolute number greater than 10%?, 15%?, 20%?
  - Abnormal cytology?

Bone Destruction

Evidence for bone destruction secondary to myeloma may include any or all of the following: bone pain or hypercalcemia not explained by other causes, lytic lesions, pathologic fractures, osteopenia, or tumor masses of bone. Some authors (Kyle and Bayrd 1976) have expressed the belief that myeloma may coexist with normal bone architecture, a point discussed below.

The evaluation of bone involvement by myeloma is for the most part done through skeletal x-rays. Because bone marrow in the adult is confined to the axial skeleton and myeloma cells are found in the marrow spaces, skeletal examination should include the axial components—skull (fig. 58.1), spine, ribs, clavicles, pelvis, and proximal humeri (fig. 58.2) and femurs. In contrast to metastatic carcinoma, the pedicles are rarely involved in myeloma even when there is vertebral body collapse. Since an extensive portion of the skeleton needs to be examined, it would seem to be efficient to employ diphosphonate bone scanning. As opposed to metastases

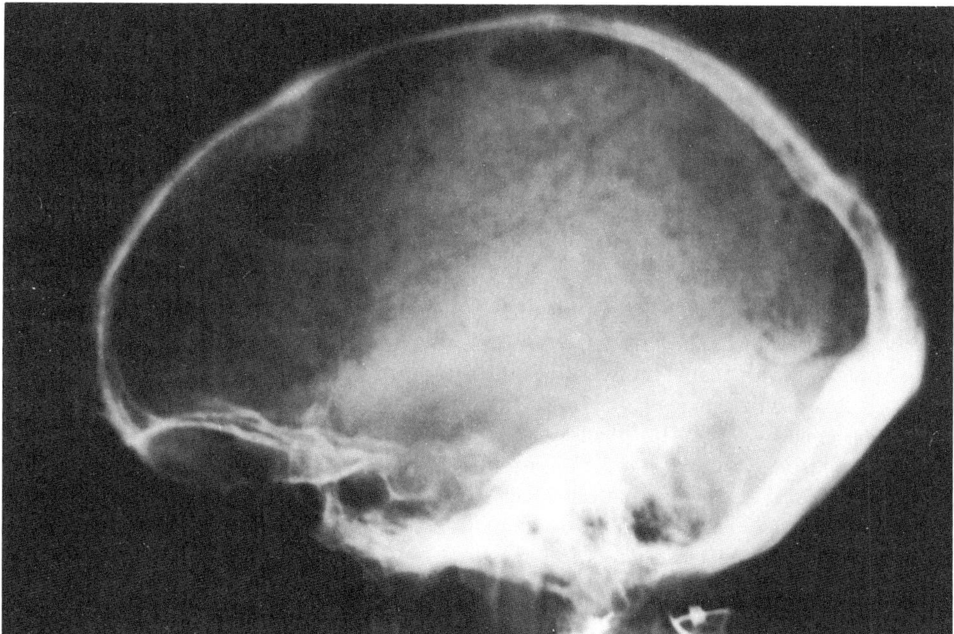

Fig. 58.1. *X-ray of skull from patient with myeloma, showing typical lytic lesions.*

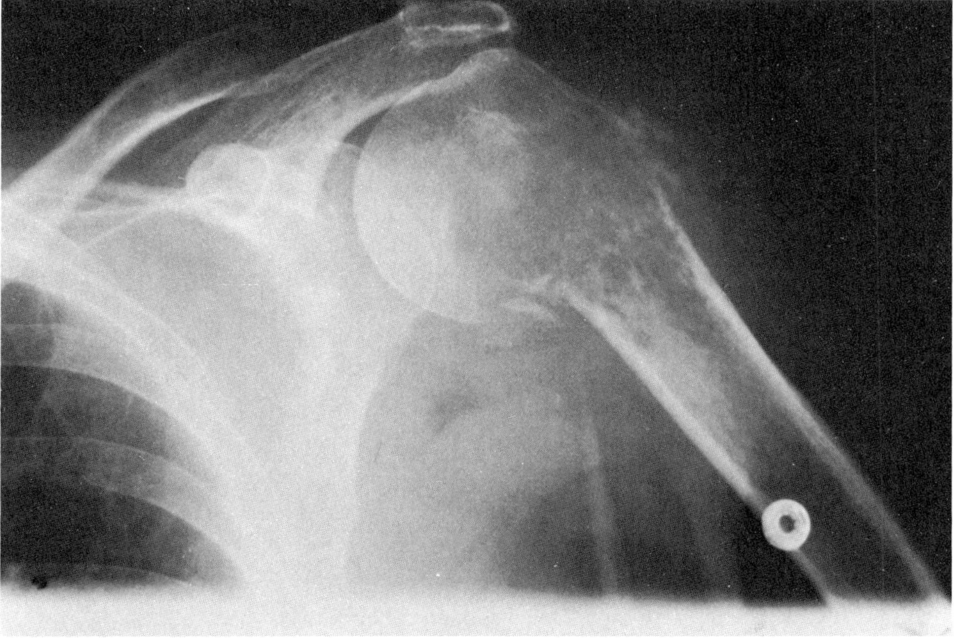

Fig. 58.2. *X-ray of proximal humerus from patient with myeloma showing extensive bone destruction.*

from solid tumors, the bone scan is an insensitive tool for the diagnosis of bone involvement by myeloma (Kyle et al. 1975; Woolfenden et al. 1980). In comparing bone scans with simultaneous skeletal surveys in a series of 17 patients, we detected numerous lesions by x-ray that were read as normal bone by diphosphonate scanning. Conversely, the only lesions found by scan and not by x-ray were those in ribs, a situation more than likely the result of technical difficulties of adequately examining all x-ray facets of ribs rather than an inherent sensitivity of the bone scan (Weininger and Gottschalk, unpublished data). We believe that this discrepancy fits with other concepts of the disease process, for example, a tumor that causes bone lysis but depresses secondary bone formation as witnessed by the normal alkaline phosphatase, absence of sclerotic margins on x-ray, and relative depletion of osteoblasts in histologic sections of myeloma lesions. These findings are indeed to be expected from a tumor that is known to secrete a peptide(s) that activates osteoclasts.

As was shown by Mundy and colleagues (1974), myeloma plasma cells (and other lymphocytic cells) secrete a humoral substance that enhances osteoclast activity and causes release of calcium from bone. It is thought that this osteoclast-activating factor (OAF) is responsible in part for the bone destruction and hypercalcemia seen with myeloma. In fact, the unique susceptibility of hypercalcemia of myeloma to modification by prednisone is probably related to the fact that prednisone in vitro will destroy OAF activity. We must then ask if it is possible for a patient to have well-documented myeloma without abnormalities of bone. Some series in the literature would suggest that as many as 20% of patients will have architecturally normal bones (Kyle and Bayrd 1976). This point seems impossible to resolve, as virtually no patients have had prediagnostic x-rays or bone density studies that could be used for comparison. Therefore I believe one must be cautious when attempting to make the diagnosis of multiple myeloma in a patient whose bone x-rays are apparently normal.

Immunoglobulin Abnormalities

Virtually all patients with myeloma will have a monoclonal immunoglobulin, immunoglobulin fragment (light chain, which is the Bence-Jones protein), or both in their serum and/or urine. The 1% to 2% of myelomas that are nonsecretory will almost always be associated with hypogammaglobulinemia. Since as many as 30% of patients with monoclonal spikes in their serum will have conditions other than myeloma, various discriminating categories have been examined.

The height of the spike has been said by some authors to be a reliable indicator of myeloma, that is, a spike of less than 1.5 or 2 g/dl is more likely to be something else (Ritzman et al. 1975; Bachman 1965; Kyle 1978). Similarly, the presence of Bence-Jones protein (free monoclonal, light chains) in the urine has been equated with a diagnosis of myeloma. Unfortunately, both of these statements present substantial difficulties. There is a wide spread in the height of serum spikes in almost all series of patients with both myeloma and benign gammopathy, so that a value near the median for any individual has little diagnostic value. In the case of Bence-Jones proteinuria, two problems arise: (1) we do not have nearly the experience with urine electrophoresis as we have with serum so the entity of idiopathic or benign Bence-Jones proteinuria is not so well defined as for serum monoclonal spikes, although it clearly exists (Kyle, Maldonado, and Bayrd 1973); (2) determining monoclonality of urinary proteins may not be done accurately (or done at all) in some clinical laboratories, particularly if less than 500 mg in 24 hours is being produced.

It should be noted that when the initial diagnosis of a monoclonal protein is made, both protein electrophoresis (PEP, cellulose acetate) and immunoelectrophoresis (IEP) (fig. 58.3) for typing should be obtained. Follow-up examination should employ the easier, quicker, less expensive PEP, which provides quantitative information about the monoclonal protein that is necessary for long-term monitoring.

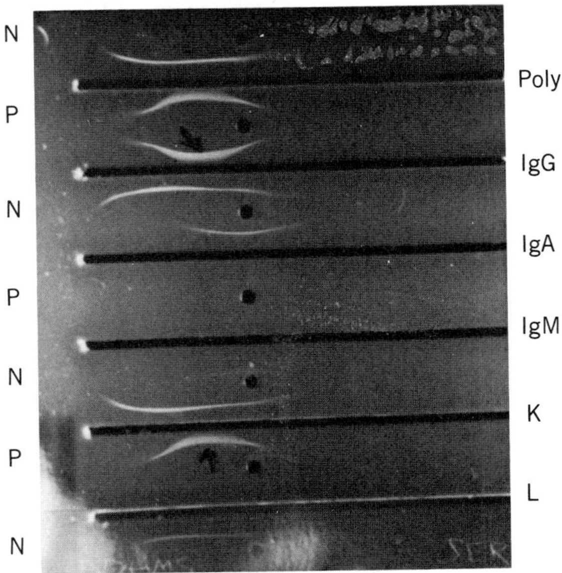

Fig. 58.3. *Serum protein immunoelectrophoresis of patient with IgG Kappa monoclonal gammopathy.*

As mentioned, patients with myeloma who do not have monoclonal serum or urinary proteins will usually have hypogammaglobulinemia. Similarly, those with myeloma who have only Bence-Jones proteinuria (about 30% of all patients with myeloma) will also have hypogammaglobulinemia. Indeed, those with serum spikes alone (about 30% of all patients) or those with serum and urine spikes (about 50%) can be shown to have hypogammaglobulinemia or "depression of background immunoglobulins" (Kyle 1975). This can often be seen on routine PEP, or may be quantitated by immunodiffusion techniques. It should be noted, however, that the level of the background immunoglobulins has not been shown to be prognostic for either survival or infectious episodes.

Thus in evaluating protein abnormalities the presence of a large serum spike, hypogammaglobulinemia of background immunoglobulins, and a significant amount of Bence-Jones proteinuria all lead to the diagnosis of myeloma but are not necessarily diagnostic in any given patient. In questionable cases it is important to follow the height of the serum or urine spike for stability (usually a benign condition) or increase in concentration (usually myeloma) (Kyle 1978). Serial follow-up is best accomplished by doing PEPs every two to three months.

Bone Marrow Abnormalities

The malignant plasma cell in myeloma can be observed in bone marrow (fig. 58.4), although differentiation from normal plasma cells may sometimes present a problem. Normal bone marrow may contain as many as 5% plasma cells, and numerous benign conditions can cause plasmacytosis (i.e., drug reaction, infection, collagen vascular disease, and benign gammopathy). Although there may be a quantitative difference between benign and malignant conditions (some have suggested a 15% to 20% upper limit for benign plasmacytosis), there is a wide variation from one patient to the next that makes this prognosticator less than optimal. In part, the spotty distribution of both normal and malignant plasma cells within the marrow may add to the difficulty in assessing the overall percentage of plasma cells present.

The cytology of the individual plasma cell has also been examined for its diagnostic usefulness. The presence of nucleoli, bizarre cytologic and membrane shapes, and intranuclear and intracytoplasmic deposits (Stavem et al. 1975) all correlate better with malignant rather than benign conditions, although none is absolute. Immunofluorescent and electron microscopic techniques (Graham and Bernier 1975) have also been used to study these cells, and there is suggestive evidence

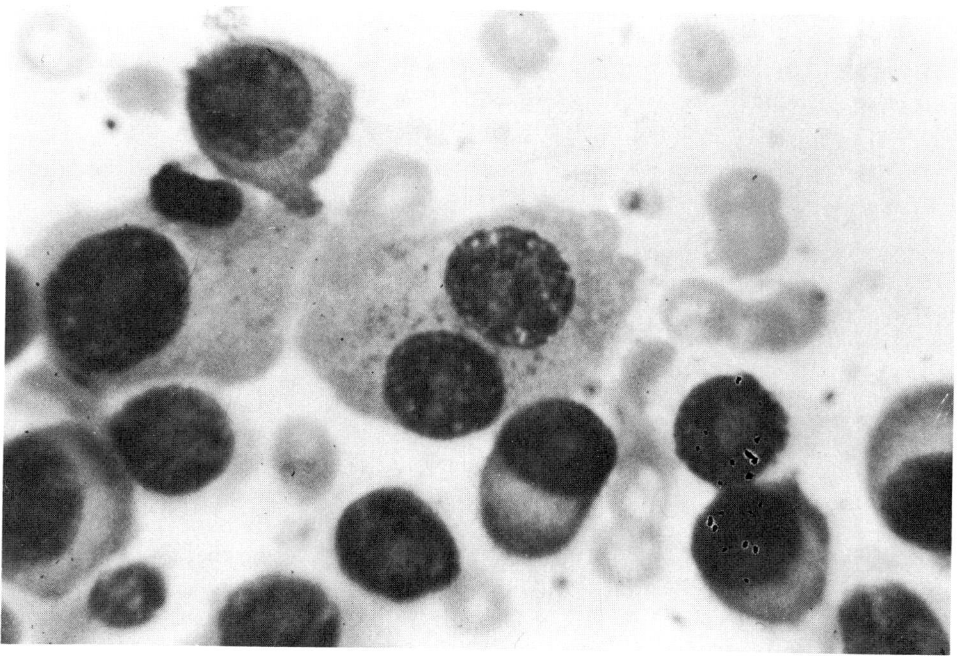

Fig. 58.4. *Bone marrow aspirate from patient with IgG myeloma showing plasma cells and plasmablasts including double nucleated cells.*

that they may be clinically useful. They are expensive and cumbersome, however, have not yet been tried in large numbers of patients, and are often not available.

There is one histologic finding that seems universally to correlate with the diagnosis of myeloma. That is the presence in the marrow of sheets of plasma cells, or syncytia (apparent fusions of cell membranes). When the marrow is thus infiltrated the pathologic diagnosis of myeloma can be made. This picture is often best achieved on bone marrow biopsy.

To summarize the diagnostic dilemma, one may say that a patient with both serum and urine spikes who has lytic bone lesions, low background immunoglobulins, hypercalcemia, and 50% marrow plasmacytosis certainly has myeloma. The presence of sheets of plasma cells establishes the diagnosis beyond doubt. A person with a small serum spike only, normal-appearing bones (or diffuse osteopenia in an elderly patient), and 10% plasma cells that are widely scattered most probably does not. The difficulty arises between the two extremes. It is important to realize that diagnosis will be difficult in a significant number of patients after initial work-up, although it is probably not to their ultimate detriment. Myeloma is not only an incurable disease, there are no data to show that early therapy improves survival. Hence a period of careful follow-up will provide evidence for disease progression if the patient has myeloma and allow ample time for initiation of therapy. The view has been expressed by some that all patients with benign gammopathy are premalignant and will eventually develop clinically evident myeloma; however, there are no data to support this (Norgaard 1971). In fact, follow-up of some patients for over 20 years has failed to show progression to myeloma.

Staging

Staging of disease has played a key role in management, and sometimes cure, of several malignancies, most notably Hodgkin's disease. Because of those successes, various systems have been used to stage virtually all malignancies. Notable exceptions have been the leukemias and myeloma, since they are disseminated at the time of diagnosis and would all therefore be stage IV. About 10 years ago, however, Salmon and colleagues attempted to measure indirectly the number of myeloma cells present in a patient's body by a technique based on the ratio of immunoglobulin produced in in vitro culture to that apparently produced by the tumor in vivo (Salmon and Smith 1970). They derived figures for the number of tumor cells per m^2 for each patient (tumor burden), and purported to show that this number could be correlated with certain clinical features of disease and ultimately with survival. The measurements that were enumerated included the amount of monoclonal serum protein, presence of Bence-Jones proteinuria, degree of renal dysfunction, serum calcium level, estimates of the degree of bone disease, and hematocrit (Durie and Salmon 1975).

This was not the first attempt to correlate outcome with the various clinical characteristics of myeloma. Several authors and multicenter study groups had attempted similar interpretations from either lengthy clinical experience or controlled trials (Snapper and Kahn 1971; Costa, Engle, and Taliente 1969). Salmon's contribution included a correlation with tumor cell number as measured in the in vitro system. Not surprisingly, he reported that most, but not all, patients with advanced clinical disease (high serum spikes, high calcium, advanced bone disease, low hematocrit, high BUN) tended to have high measured tumor cell number and did not fare as well as those without such clinical features. This confirmed clinical observations made a decade or two earlier, but also provided a framework for testing new modes of therapy based on combinations of clinical features. Unfortunately, two major problems have affected the usefulness of such an approach: (1) not all studies agree as to which data are prognostically useful, and (2) although early studies showed improved survival of poor-risk patients with more aggressive multiagent chemotherapy, most recent studies have failed to confirm this.

Therapy

From the time of its initial clinical trials in the 1950s, melphalan (Alkeran) has been standard therapy in myeloma. Initially used in low-dose daily administration (about 2 mg a day), melphalan was soon combined with prednisone to produce median survivals of 18 to 30 months compared to 7 to 10 months for historical controls (Alexanian et al. 1968; Bergsagel et al. 1967; Midwest Cooperative Chemotherapy Group 1964). Although there has never been a direct comparison with untreated patient controls, virtually all workers in the field would agree that melphalan or cyclophosphamide (Cytoxan, Endoxan), which is equally effective as first-line therapy, does indeed prolong survival of treated patients. Perhaps more importantly, it also relieves symptoms such as bone pain, anorexia, fatigue, and weight loss and improves cytopenias, particularly anemia, while causing the monoclonal protein spike to diminish or disappear (figs. 58.5 and 58.6). Only rarely, however, will bone lesions heal or background immunoglobulins return to normal levels.

Spurred by reports of successful therapy of other malignancies using pulsed intermittent chemotherapy, trials with myeloma began in the late 1960s to compare the efficacy of daily melphalan with intermittent higher doses given every four to six weeks (Alexanian et al. 1968; Bergsagel et al. 1967; Hoogstraten et al. 1969). Although there was no difference in survival, pulsed therapy began to gain favor because the total amount of alkylating agent given per day was less. As the first cases of monocytic and myelocytic leukemia following alkylating agent therapy began to be reported at about the same time, intermittent administration became further entrenched as a means of providing the same therapeutic efficacy for less drug and thereby lowering the incidence of alkylating agent-related leukemia (Rosner and Grunwald 1974; Bergsagel et al. 1979).

Over the next decade, from the late 1960s to the present, all drugs known to be active in myeloma—melphalan, cyclophosphamide, vincristine, prednisone, carmustine (BiCNU)—have been used in virtually all possible three-, four-, and five-drug combinations. It is not possible to go into each study here in detail; however, I believe it is fair to say that, at best, combination chemotherapy may provide a small survival advantage (from zero to eight months) for patients with advanced disease at the time of diagnosis (Bergsagel et al. 1979; Harley et al. 1979). This potential advantage needs to be balanced against the increased morbidity of administering greater numbers of drugs. Needless to say, the best results with combination chemotherapy come from an uncontrolled study in which all five of the above drugs were combined in a 35-day repeating cycle (the M-2 protocol) (Case, Lee, and Clarkson 1977). The authors claim a 48-month median survival, surpassing that of controlled trials but similar to another uncontrolled study using daily melphalan alone (Farhangi and Osserman 1973). The major criticism raised about the M-2 study is the lack of early deaths, a feature of virtually all other studies. The implication is therefore that the patients in the M-2 study were in clinically better shape than their counterparts in other studies. Fortunately, the Eastern Cooperative Oncology Group (ECOG) has recently initiated a prospective randomized trial to compare melphalan and prednisone with the M-2 protocol (ECOG #EST-2479).

In addition to determining which drugs to choose in treating myeloma, the length of treatment of patients who have responded favorably to therapy must be established. Spurred by reports of ever increasing incidences of leukemia, recently reported to be 17% after four years of therapy (Bergsagel et al. 1979), Alexanian and colleagues (1978) divided a group of patients who had had good responses to melphalan and prednisone after 12 months to receive either continued therapy or no therapy. They found no difference in survival or time to relapse. Furthermore, relapsing patients off therapy

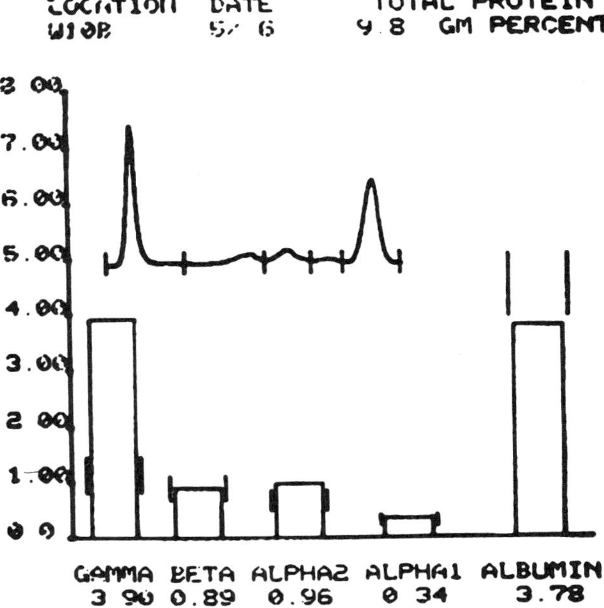

Fig. 58.5. *Serum protein electrophoresis of patient with IgG myeloma at time of diagnosis. Note that the taller spike is that of the myeloma protein.*

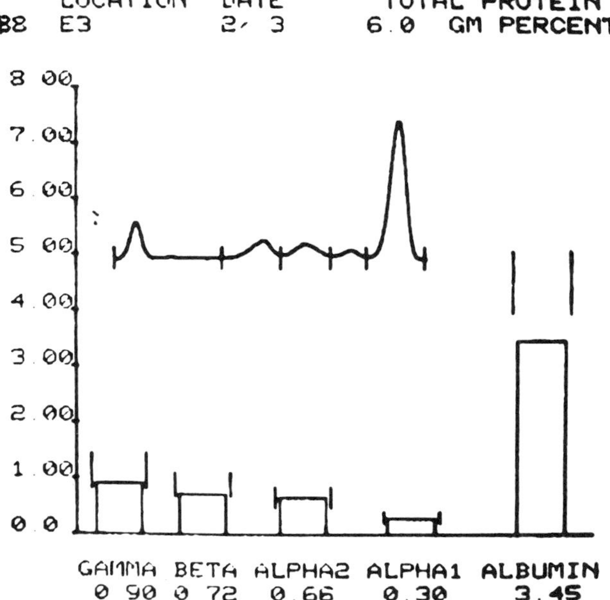

Fig. 58.6. *Same patient as in figure 58.5, shown nine months after beginning therapy. Note the albumin is the predominant peak, and the myeloma protein is now in the normal range.*

could be reinduced 80% of the time, although the second remissions were of shorter duration. These data have been challenged by others who point out that this particular group of patients (the ones receiving no therapy) may have had less advanced disease than their treated counterparts. Early results from other groups have not confirmed Alexanian's, but need to be studied in greater depth because of the obvious desirability of producing the maximum therapeutic effect for the smallest amount of administered alkylating agent.

Finally, the most difficult question to answer is how to treat the patient who has failed initial therapy. There have been several reports of responses to a second or third alkylating agent after failure on a first or second. The usual sequence has been melphalan to cyclophosphamide to carmustine. More recently, doxorubicin (Adriamycin) has been shown to have a 20% to 30% response rate alone, and given in combination with carmustine produced 15% complete and 50% partial responses in melphalan failures when administered every three to four weeks as tolerated (Alberts, Durie, and Salmon 1976). The role for vincristine in relapsing patients has not been well defined (Alexanian et al. 1977).

Recently, hexamethylmelamine, 280 mg/m^2 rather than 200 mg/m^2, has been shown to have a 35% response rate when given with prednisone, although hexamethylmelamine alone at 200 mg/m^2 is virtually without effect (ECOG, unpublished data). High-dose intravenous cyclophosphamide and melphalan have also regained popularity, but results are not yet available. Finally, several centers have used hemibody irradiation in an attempt to salvage a second or third remission, with mixed results. We are beginning such a pilot study now. It should be noted that second remissions, when they occur, are most often partial and rarely exceed six months.

It is appropriate to say that more than anything else, myeloma therapy awaits *new* drugs rather than combinations of old ones.

References

Alberts, D. S.; Durie, B. G. M.; and Salmon, S. E. Doxorubicin/BCNU chemotherapy for multiple myeloma in relapse. *Lancet* 1:926–928, 1976.

Alexanian, R. et al. Melphalan therapy for plasma cell myeloma. *Blood* 31:1–10, 1968.

Alexanian, R. et al. Combination therapy for multiple myeloma. *Cancer* 40:2765–2771, 1977.

Alexanian, R. et al. Unmaintained remissions in multiple myeloma. *Blood* 51:1005–1011, 1978.

Bachmann, R. The diagnostic significance of the serum concentration of pathological proteins (M-components). *Acta Med. Scand.* 178:801–808, 1965.

Bergsagel, D. E. et al. The treatment of multiple myeloma. *Adv. Cancer Res.* 10:311–359, 1967.

Bergsagel, D. E. et al. The chemotherapy of plasma-cell myeloma and the incidence of acute leukemia. *N. Engl. J. Med.* 301:743–748, 1979.

Case, D. C., Jr.; Lee, B. J.; and Clarkson, B. D. Improved survival times in multiple myeloma treated with melphalan, prednisone, cyclophosphamide, vincristine and BCNU. *Am. J. Med.* 63:897–903, 1977.

Costa, G.; Engle, R. L.; and Taliente, P. Criteria for defining risk groups and response to chemotherapy in multiple myeloma. *Proc. Am. Assoc. Cancer Res.* 10:15, 1969.

Durie, B. G. M., and Salmon, S. E. A clinical staging system for multiple myeloma. *Cancer* 36:842–854, 1975.

Farhangi, M., and Osserman, E. F. The treatment of multiple myeloma. *Semin. Hematol.* 10:149–161, 1973.

Graham, R. C., Jr., and Bernier, G. M. The bone marrow in multiple myeloma. *Medicine* 54:225–243, 1975.

Harley, J. B. et al. Improved survival of increased-risk myeloma patients on combined triple alkylating agent therapy: a study of the CALGB. *Blood* 54:13–22, 1979.

Hoogstraten, B. et al. Intermittent melphalan therapy in multiple myeloma. *JAMA* 209:251–253, 1969.

Kyle, R. A. Multiple myeloma: review of 869 cases. *Mayo Clin. Proc.* 50:29–40, 1975.

Kyle, R. A. Monoclonal gammopathy of undetermined significance. *Am. J. Med.* 64:814–826, 1978.

Kyle, R. A. et al. Multiple myeloma bone disease: the comparative effect of sodium fluoride and calcium carbonate or placebo. *N. Engl. J. Med.* 293:1334–1338, 1975.

Kyle, R. A., and Bayrd, E. D. *The monoclonal gammopathies.* Springfield, Ill.: Charles C. Thomas, 1976, p. 106.

Kyle, R. A.; Maldonado, J. E.; and Bayrd, E. D. Idiopathic Bence-Jones proteinuria: a distinct entity? *Am. J. Med.* 55:222–226, 1973.

Midwest Cooperative Chemotherapy Group. Multiple myeloma. *JAMA* 188:741–745, 1964.

Mundy, G. R. et al. Evidence for the secretion of an osteoclast-stimulating factor in myeloma. *N. Engl. J. Med.* 291:1041–1046, 1974.

Nørgaard, O. Three cases of multiple myeloma in which the preclinical asymptomatic phases persisted throughout 15 to 24 years. *Br. J. Cancer* 25:417–422, 1971.

Ritzmann, S. E. et al. Idiopathic (asymptomatic) monoclonal gammopathies. *Arch. Intern. Med.* 135:95–106, 1975.

Rosner, F., and Grunwald, H. Multiple myeloma terminating in acute leukemia. *Am. J. Med.* 57:927–939, 1974.

Salmon, S. E., and Smith, B. A. Immunoglobulin synthesis and total body tumor cell number in IgG multiple myeloma. *J. Clin. Invest.* 49:1114–1121, 1970.

Snapper, I., and Kahn, A. *Myelomatosis: fundamentals and clinical features.* Baltimore: University Park Press, 1971.

Stavem, P. et al. Needle-like crystals in plasma cells in a patient with a plasma cell proliferative disorder. *Scand. J. Haematol.* 14:24–34, 1975.

Woolfenden, J. M. et al. Comparison of bone scintigraphy and radiography in multiple myeloma. *Radiology* 134:723–728, 1980.

fifty-nine

Epidemiology, Etiology, and Detection of Primary Lung Cancer

JOHN L. POOL

The world-wide epidemic of lung cancer is a phenomenon of this century. Until 1930, few physicians ever saw such cancer. Since that time incidence has skyrocketed so that now it causes 100,000 new cases and 90,000 deaths a year in the United States alone (Department of Health, Education and Welfare 1975). The smoking population has also increased; in the Western countries averaging 56 new smokers per 100,000 adult population per year. In the developing countries figures are less exact: lung cancer may be less prevalent, but the more visible oropharyngeal cancers with tobacco smoke and tobacco chewing as known etiologic agents are frequently seen. Cocarcinogens are alcohol, betel nut, and poor dental hygiene (Hoffmann and Wynder 1971; Wynder 1974). The distribution of lung cancer by sex has changed over the last 35 years, the male:female ratio gradually decreasing from 9:1 in favor of men to perhaps 2:1 or 3:1. Meigs (1977) reported from the Connecticut Tumor Registry that in the age group of 35 to 44 years there was a higher absolute numerical figure among women as compared to men. This has been predicted for some time due to the increasing numbers of women smoking cigarettes (Report of the Surgeon General 1980). In 1979, HEW Secretary Califano reported that in the 17- to 18-year-old group, there were more girls smoking than boys: 29% as compared to 19%. It is now predicted that lung cancer may be the major cause of cancer death in women by 1985 (Holleb 1981; Stellman and Stellman 1981).

The emphasis on tobacco smoking as the principal cause of lung cancer is justified thanks to innumerable studies in the laboratory on dogs and mice with the products of tobacco combustion (Wynder and Hecht 1976; Auerbach et al. 1970). Studies with humans also demonstrate a considerable increase in the incidence of cancer among smokers as compared to nonsmokers: 90 out of 100 lung cancer patients will have smoked two packs a day for 20 years (Wynder and Hecht 1976). The statistics of the American Cancer Society show a linear relationship between number of cigarettes smoked and the risk of lung cancer. Wynder (1974) has demonstrated that low-tar cigarettes lower the risk. No risk can be demonstrated when the tar content is 1 mg or 2 mg per cigarette. Discontinuation of smoking gradually returns the risk to that of nonsmokers in about 12 years (Pool, Gray, and Holman 1972).

The disease is seldom apparent before the age of 40 years, although sporadic cases have been identified in individuals as young as 15 years. The peak incidence is at 55 years, as contrasted with breast cancer in which the incidence is still increasing in the ninth decade of life. Tobacco smoking has been implicated as a cause of cancer of the larynx, esophagus, and bladder. Smith (1978) in England and Cahan and colleagues in the United States (1950) have demonstrated a 20% risk of new primary lung cancer or pulmonary metastasis 5 to 10 years after successful operations (Pool 1971). Continued smoking increases this risk. More lung cancer occurs in urban than rural environments, although studies of the Holland Tunnel policemen and the Southern Pacific railroad engineers did not show altered incidence over the population at large. Miners of uranium in Colorado, workers in coke manufacture, and distillers of petroleum have all shown a high incidence of lung cancer that has decreased with improved ventilation in the workplace. Asbestos workers and members of their households *may* develop mesothelioma of pleura, pericardium, or peritoneum. Asbestos workers who smoke have an increased risk, not of mesothelioma, but of lung cancer, which is higher than that of smokers who are not exposed to the inhalation of these mineral fibers (Hoffmann and Wynder 1971).

Identifying Lung Cancer

What can we do to identify the presence and extent of lung cancer? The International Union against Cancer and the American Joint Commission on Cancer Staging and End-Results Reporting have developed a staging system to improve accuracy of diagnosis and comparability of diagnostic and therapeutic measures (Carr 1981). Tumor size and location and the presence of intrathoracic nodal metastases and other metastases are charted as T, N, and M, and combinations provide three stages of increasing tumor burden. In the lung, clinical staging is defined to include history, physical examination, review of al types of chest x-rays, bronchoscopy, neck node biopsy, mediastinoscopy, bone scan, CT scan of brain and thorax, and blood chemistries (especially of liver function), and bone marrow biopsy. Surgical staging includes all of the above plus an exploratory thoracotomy. Pathologic staging includes all of the above plus examination of the resected primary tumor or autopsy (Pool, Gray, and Holman 1972; Pearson et al. 1972).

Before treatment, it is important to verify the diagnosis of cancer (Fontana 1977). Cancer cells can be found 75% of the time by exfoliate cytology (Granlund and Ritts 1976; Martini et al. 1974). Meticulous instruction in coughing and expectorating to secure lower respiratory tract mucus without food contamination is essential, as are prompt fixation and experienced interpretation (Saccomanno et al. 1974).

Surveys of high-risk populations—men over age 45 smoking two packs of cigarettes a day—have yielded 7 cancers per 1000 examinations initially, and 3 per 1000 yearly thereafter. Chest x-rays and fiberoptic bronchoscopy are part of the examination (Woolner et al. 1981). Five-year surgical salvage for asymptomatic cancer approaches 80%, but it is only 8% to 10% after hemoptysis or other respiratory complaints develop (Heitzman, Proto, and Goldwin 1979). Positive sputum cytology in a patient with a negative chest x-ray (Saccomanno et al. 1965) leaves the surgeon in the quandry of not knowing where the cancer is. The malignant cell could come from the nasopharynx, larynx, the trachea, or anywhere in the lower respiratory tract. Careful bronchoscopic exploration of all major branches of both lungs must be carried out. Washings, brushings, and biopsies are mandatory and no thoracotomy can be undertaken until the surgeon exactly identifies the site of malignant cells. This is stage 0 disease, namely, positive cytology and negative chest x-ray short of bronchography (Martini et al. 1974; Melamed et al. 1977).

The work-up needed to identify the extent of a presumed lung cancer is an area of considerable controversy. It goes without saying that operative risk must be determined. Only the surgeon can evaluate what treatment will best meet an individual patient's needs (Ramsey et al. 1969). Some are content with one plane chest tomography and brief bronchoscopic inspection. For another approach, Pearson and co-workers (1972) embarked on an investigative study of presumably operable lung cancer that in addition to conventional films and bronchoscopy included pulmonary angiography and mediastinoscopy. They concluded that patients in whom the hilum seemed to be involved, or the primary lesion was more than 6 cm in diameter, or in whom at bronchoscopy the lesion was within 1 cm of the carina, deserved angiography and mediastinoscopy. At thoracotomy their resectability rate increased from 70% to nearly 90%.

Bronchoscopy, both rigid and flexible, may tell more about disease extent than any x-ray films (Laurer et al. 1979; Zarala 1975; Fontana 1977). Epidermoid cancer may be surrounded by extensive in situ changes, and the location of this pathology influences extent of resection. Intraluminal as opposed to extraluminal blockage can be differentiated. Biopsy of the posterior one-third of a normal appearing main carina will show unsuspected lymphatic permeation by cancer cells in 6% of right lung cancers (Robbins et al. 1979). Transbronchoscopic aspiration biopsy of mediastinal and hilar nodes can identify metastasis (Wang et al. 1981). Because such information is vital to therapeutic decision-making, these procedures are best carried out by the surgeon.

When a coin (solitary round) lesion is found in the parenchyma of the lung, its identification is difficult. Previous films must be reviewed to see if this lesion is new or was present previously. Change in size can indicate rate of growth. The primary lung cancer of low malignancy may change very little in a five-year span, but this is unusual. Benign lesions such as a hamartoma will also enlarge. Too much reliance cannot be placed on rate of growth with regard to identity or prognosis (Pool 1980, 1981; Freant, Joseph, and Adkins 1974). McCormack and Martini (1979), in a study of some 453 resected metastatic deposits, determined that doubling time does not relate to prognosis. Radiographic characteristics of the coin lesion are important. It has been pointed out that a crescent toward the hilum of the lung is suggestive of primary as opposed to metastatic lung cancer and that the S curve of an atelectatic lobe or segment identifies hilar adenopathy concomitant with atelectasis. The lesion's contour is significant. It may be absolutely smooth in granulomas, cysts, and mucous plugs; in cancer it is usually slightly crenulated. The presence of calcium as determined tomographically can identify granuloma only when there is a true central nidus or onion skin periphery. Cancer occurs in scars that may have calcifications eccentric to the shadow (Sindelar et al. 1978). Computerized axial tomography (CAT) helps identify the location and number of lesions within the lung substance (Schaner et al. 1978; Heitzman, Proto, and Goldwin 1979). Definition is not as exact as tomography even when the speed of each slice is under two seconds. Lesions less than a centimeter in diameter such as minute granuloma and subpleural lymph nodes are found but cannot always be differentiated from primary or metastatic cancer. Polygraphic tomography centered at the lesion with slices two millimeters apart can best define structure.

Aspiration Biopsy

A technique for identifying the contents of a coin lesion when exfoliate cytology by sputum, washings, or brushings is unsuccessful is aspiration biopsy (Pool, Gray, and Holman 1972; Sinner 1979). It has been used since 1940 on undiagnosed lung lesions and can be extremely valuable, not only in coin lesions, but in other pulmonary deposits where one wishes histologic proof short of a thoracotomy. This would apply especially to poor-risk patients or those with obvious bone or brain metastasis in whom sputum and bronchoscopic washings have failed to provide such information. The procedure is carried out under fluoroscopic guidance with a thin-walled 19-gauge needle. The incidence of pneumothorax is about 15%, but the need for tube drainage is rare. Hemoptysis may occur but is quite unusual and has seldom been life-threatening. In my own experience with some 400 patients there were no deaths. Two rather large hemoptyses occurred and promptly ceased; there was an incidence of 15% of pneumothorax, about 1% requiring tube drainage. Memorial Sloan-Kettering Cancer Center in New York reported (Smith et al. 1974) in a series of 1800 patients that they had two incidents of cardiac arrest, both responding to prompt cardiopulmonary resuscitations. The etiology of this serious complication was not determined. One must remember, as in many other biopsy procedures, that failure to establish a diagnosis does not mean that cancer is absent. It should also be remembered that in bony hard scars and in granulomas the chance of a positive diagnosis is remote. The procedure is best not carried out if the patient has had contralateral pneumonectomy, has large blebs, or is severely emphysematous.

Lung cancers in general can be diagnosed 85% of the time by the aspiration technique (Sinner 1979; Wang et al. 1981), but success is not as likely in lesions 1.5 cm in diameter or smaller. The method may differentiate some types of metastasis from primary disease, but the sample is usually too small to allow precise pathologic categorization. The decision whether a solitary pulmonary nodule is metastasis or new primary tumor in a patient who has or has had cancer of another organ must be based on excellent histologic information (McCormack and Martini 1979). In fact, in obscure pancreatic cancers only autopsy may disclose the disease. The laws of probability suggest, however, that when the other cancer is in the breast, upper respiratory, or digestive tract, the solitary pulmonic lesion is more likely to be a primary than a secondary growth. When the other cancer is of genitourinary origin, metastasis is a 50-50 chance; in melanoma or sarcoma the pulmonary lesion is almost always metastatic (Cahan et al. 1950).

Radiography

Radiographic studies, principally with tomography, can often define the extent of disease within the lung itself. The CT scan is proving invaluable in identifying direct extension into the chest wall, as occurs with Pancoast tumor, and the extent of involvement within the mediastinum. I have used the esophagram to identify large subcarinal and paratracheal nodes. Opacification of the vena cava and esophagus also helps identification by CT scan of large nodes, although it does not tell what is in that node (Heitzman, Proto, and Goldwin 1979). Another recently devised technique is gallium scan (Cellerino et al. 1973; DeMeester et al. 1976). If picked up by a primary cancer and also by mediastinal tissues, gallium is highly suggestive of mediastinal metastasis and mediastinoscopy or anterior mediastinotomy would then be warranted. If, however, the primary site picked up gallium but the mediastinum did not, the need for mediastinal exploration prior to thoracotomy would be much less. One should remember, however, that if the primary site does not pick up gallium, whether or not the mediastinum does is immaterial because one could not tell whether mediastinal pick-up was due to sarcoidosis, other inflammatory change, or cancer. Such patients require mediastinoscopy.

Scalene lymph nodes are often the first extrathoracic site of nodal cancer, and when a node is palpable in this area, even though it is less than 1 cm in diameter, in a patient with known lung cancer it is likely to contain metastasis; only about 6% of nonpalpable scalene nodes do. Biopsy of nonpalpable scalene nodes is less revealing than mediastinoscopy. Neck node biopsy should be a bilateral procedure because drainage from any lobe of the lung can go to either supraclavicular space through the network of mediastinal lymphatics.

Mediastinoscopy

Mediastinoscopy is indicated when invasion of that area is suspected by location of tumor or enlarged nodes within the hilum, or in the presence of an anaplastic cancer, either large or small cell type, or when radiographic studies cannot explain mediastinal widening (Smith 1978). If thoracotomy has a high risk the procedure may be used, even at the same anesthesia, to make sure that the larger operation will not be in vain. It is also an aid in deciding between palliative and aggressive chemotherapy. Mediastinoscopy allows exploration of the anterior and right-hand surfaces of the trachea to the carina.

The alternative is right or left anterior mediastinotomy, permitting wider exploration of the ipsilateral mediastinal hilum and may be extended to include a limited intrapleural examination. On the left side the subaortic window is exposed, an area not accessible by mediastinoscopy.

The finding of extranodal cancer is a grave prognostic sign and makes the idea of pulmonary resection useless, except as palliation to control hemorrhage or cancer-related lung abscess. The exact site of mediastinal intranodal metastasis is highly important. When only ipsilateral nodes are involved, a salvage rate of 15% at five years is achieved by radical lung resection that includes a careful mediastinal node dissection. More extensive node involvement is best handled by palliative measures (Weiss 1974; Cahan, Watson, and Pool 1951).

Thoracotomy

There are indications and contraindications for thoracotomy for diagnosis of primary lung cancer and for its treatment. Surgery is the main treatment, achieving better results than external or interstitial radiation (Pool, Gray, and Holman 1972). The overall salvage for resectional surgery is 25% or 30% at five years (Ramsey et al. 1969; Weiss 1974). Therefore exploratory thoracotomy will be indicated in patients suspected of having lung cancer when no spread beyond the lung except to ipsilateral mediastinal nodes is evident by studies previously outlined.

The contraindications to exploratory thoracotomy for diagnosis include invasion of the superior vena cava, the presence of vocal cord paralysis, or diaphragmatic paralysis. A rare exception occurs when the phrenic nerve is involved by the primary tumor on a resectable portion of the pericardium. The presence of pleural effusion that is bloody or contains cancer cells (Monif, Stewart, and Block 1976) and invasion of mediastinal tissues, diaphragm, or the vertebrae are in general contraindications to resectional surgery. Liver scanning has not been completely reliable in identifying liver metastases; however, combining ultrasound and isotopic liver scans has made for a higher yield and more accuracy (Wittes and Yeh 1977). Scanning of the brain will usually identify even small metastases (Jacobs, Kinkel, and Vincent 1977). Bone scans are also useful.

In conclusion, it is worthwhile to identify primary lung cancer and to stage it accurately so that no patient is denied the possibility of resectional surgery, currently our only form of definitive therapy (Henschke and Flehinger 1967).

References

Auerbach, O. et al. Effects of cigarette smoking on dogs. II. Pulmonary neoplasms. *Arch. Environ. Health* 21: 754–768, 1970.

Cahan, W. G. et al. Multiple cancers: primary in the lung and other sites. *J. Thorac. Surg.* 20:335–348, 1950.

Cahan, W. G.; Watson, W. L.; and Pool, J. L. Radical pneumonectomy. *J. Thorac. Surg.* 22:449–471, 1951.

Carr, D. T. Diagnosis and staging in lung cancer, 1980. Second World Conference on Lung Cancer. Copenhagen, June 1980. *Excerpta medica*, eds. H. H. Hansen and M. Roth. New York: Excerpta Medica Foundation, 1981.

Cellerino, A. et al. Operative and pathologic survey of 50 cases of peripheral lung tumors scanned with 67 gallium. *Chest* 64:700–705, 1973.

DeMeester, T. R. et al. Gallium 67 scanning for carcinoma of the lung. *J. Thorac. Cardiovasc. Surg.* 72:699–708, 1976.

Department of Health, Education and Welfare, Public Health Service. *The health consequences of smoking 1975*. DHEW Publication No. (CDC) 76-804. Washington, D.C.: U.S. Government Printing Office, 1975.

Fontana, R. S. Early diagnosis of lung cancer. *Am. Rev. Respir. Dis.* 116:399–402, 1977.

Freant, L. J.; Joseph, W. L.; and Adkins, P. C. Scar carcinoma of the lung, fact or fantasy? *Ann. Thorac. Surg.* 17:531–537, 1974.

Granlund, D. U., and Ritts, R. E. Soluble proteins of human bronchogenic carcinoma. *Mayo Clin. Proc.* 51:19–27, 1976.

Heitzman, E. R.; Proto, A. V.; and Goldwin, R. L. The role of computerized tomography in the diagnosis of diseases of the thorax. *JAMA* 241:933–936, 1979.

Henschke, W. K., and Flehinger, B. J. Decision theory in cancer therapy. *Cancer* 20:1819–1826, 1967.

Hoffmann, D., and Wynder, E. L. A study of tobacco carcinogenesis. XI. Tumor initiators, tumor accelerators, and tumor promoting activity of condensate fractions. *Cancer* 27:848–864, 1971.

Holleb, A. I. Smoking: the ticking time-bomb for teenage girls. *CA* 31:44–45, 1981.

Jacobs, L.; Kinkel, W. R.; and Vincent, R. Q. "Silent" brain metastasis from lung carcinoma determined by computerized tomography. *Arch. Neurol.* 34:690–693, 1977.

Laurer, G. L. et al. The usefulness of fiberoptic bronchoscopy in evaluating new pulmonary lesions in the compromised host. *Am. J. Med.* 66:580–585, 1979.

Martini, N. et al. Radiologically occult lung cancer report of 26 cases. *Surg. Clin. North Am.* 54:811–823, 1974.

Martini, N. et al. Prospective study of 445 lung carcinomas with mediastinal lymph node metastases. *J. Thorac. Cardiovasc. Surg.* 80:390–399, 1980.

McCormack, P. M., and Martini, N. The changing role of surgery for pulmonary metastases. *Ann. Thorac. Surg.* 28:139–145, 1979.

Meigs, J. W. Epidemic lung cancer in women (editorial). *JAMA* 238:1055, 1977.

Melamed, M. R. et al. Preliminary report of the lung cancer detection program in New York. *Cancer* 39:369–382, 1977a.

Melamed, M. R. et al. Radiologically occult in situ and incipient invasive epidermoid lung cancer: detection by sputum cytology in a survey of asymptomatic cigarette smokers. *Am. J. Surg. Pathol.* 1:5–16, 1977b.

Monif, G. R. G.; Stewart, B. N.; and Block, A. J. Living cytology: a new diagnostic technique for malignant pleural effusions. *Chest* 69:626–629, 1976.

Pearson, F. G. et al. The role of mediastinoscopy in the selection of treatment for bronchial carcinoma with involvement of superior mediastinal lymph nodes. *J. Thorac. Cardiovasc. Surg.* 64:382–390, 1972.

Pool, J. L. Survival in lung cancer. *N.Y. State J. Med.* 71:2045–2050, 1971.

Pool, J. L. Diagnosing the solitary pulmonary nodule. *Conn. Med.* 44:185–187, 1980.

Pool, J. L. The identification for surgical treatment of pulmonary metastases. *Conn. Med.* 45:407–408, 1981.

Pool, J. L.; Gray, G. F.; and Holman, C. W. Tumors of the lung and trachea. In *Bronchopulmonary diseases and related disorders*, eds. C. W. Holman and C. Muschenheim. New York: Harper and Row, 1972, pp. 785–821.

Ramsey, H. E. et al. The importance of radical lobectomy in lung cancer. *J. Thorac. Cardiovasc. Surg.* 58: 225–230, 1969.

Report of the Surgeon General. *The health consequences of smoking for women*. Washington, D.C.: U.S. Department of Health and Human Services, Public Health Service, 1980.

Robbins, H. M. et al. Biopsy of the main carina. Staging lung cancer with the fiberoptic bronchoscope. *Chest* 75:484–486, 1979.

Saccomanno, G. et al. Cancer of the lung: the cytology of sputum prior to the development of carcinoma. *Acta Cytol. (Baltimore)* 9:413–423, 1965.

Saccomanno, G. et al. Development of carcinoma of the lung as reflected in exfoliated cells. *Cancer* 33:256–279, 1974.

Schaner, E. G. et al. Comparison of computed and whole-lung tomography in detecting pulmonary nodules: a prospective conventional radiologic-pathologic study. *Am. J. Roentgenol.* 131:51–54, 1978.

Sindelar, W. F. et al. Lung tomography in cancer patients: full-lung tomograms in screening for pulmonary metastases. *JAMA* 240:2060–2063, 1978.

Sinner, W. N. Pulmonary neoplasms diagnosed with transthoracic needle biopsy. *Cancer* 43:1533–1540, 1979.

Smith, J. et al. Percutaneous needle aspiration lung biopsy. *Clin. Bull. Memorial Sloan-Kettering Cancer Center* 4:63–68, 1974.

Smith, R. A. The importance of mediastinal lymph node invasion by pulmonary carcinoma in selection of patients for resection. *Ann. Thorac. Surg.* 25:5–11, 1978.

Stellman, S. D., and Stellman, J. M. Women's occupations, smoking and cancer and other diseases. *CA* 31:29–43, 1981.

Wang, K. P. et al. Transbronchial needle aspiration for diagnosis of lung cancer. *Chest* 80:48–50, 1981.

Weiss, W. Operative mortality and five-year survival in patients with bronchogenic carcinoma. *Am. J. Surg.* 128:799–804, 1974.

Wittes, R. E., and Yeh, S. D. J. Indications for liver and brain scans: screening tests for patients with oat cell carcinoma of the lung. *JAMA* 238:506–507, 1977.

Woolner, L. B. et al. Mayo lung project. Evaluation of lung cancer screening through December 1979. *Mayo Clin. Proc.* 56:544–555, 1981.

Wynder, E. L. Towards reducing tobacco-related cancers. *Excerpta Medica International Congress Series #351* 3:138–143, 1974.

Wynder, E. L., and Hecht, S., eds. Lung cancer. *UICC Technical Report Series* 25:48–49, 1976.

Zarala, D. C. Diagnostic fibroptic bronchoscopy: techniques and results of biopsy in 600 patients. *Chest* 68:12–19, 1975.

sixty

Small Cell Cancer of the Lung

DAVID S. FISCHER

Small cell carcinoma of the lung (also called oat cell carcinoma or small cell bronchogenic carcinoma) is the most rapidly growing and metastasizing of the lung cancers. Until recently, survival was short and therapy of minimal value. Advances in chemotherapy have changed the prognosis from dismal to hopeful. The results of therapy are so different that we have segregated the discussion of lung cancer into small cell and non-small cell (or sometimes into the less desirable terms, oat cell and non-oat cell). The current World Health Organization classification (Yesner et al. 1981) is as follows:

Epithelial tumors

1. Squamous cell (epidermoid) carcinoma
   a. Spindle cell (squamous)
2. Small cell carcinoma
   a. Oat cell
   b. Intermediate cell
   c. Combined oat cell
3. Adenocarcinoma
   a. Acinar
   b. Papillary
   c. Bronchiolo-alveolar
   d. Solid carcinoma with mucus
4. Large cell carcinoma
   a. Giant cell
   b. Clear cell
5. Adenosquamous carcinomas
6. Carcinoid tumor
7. Bronchial gland carcinomas
   a. Adenoid cystic
   b. Mucoepidermoid
8. Other

Of the estimated 112,000 Americans (82,000 men, 30,000 women) who developed lung cancer in 1979 (Silverberg 1979), about 97,500 (72,300 men, 25,200 women) will die of it; about 20% of each group will be in the small cell carcinoma subgroup. This is a largely anaplastic tumor of bronchogenic origin and associated with cigarette smoking almost exclusively. It tends to grow very rapidly and to metastasize early. Hence median overall survival without therapy is about 2 months (7 weeks for those with metastases and 14 weeks for those with local disease). For the untreated or surgically treated patient, there is no significant alteration in prognosis associated with age, sex, race, site of primary tumor (main bronchus, hilus, peripheral, or apical), radiologic appearance (solitary or multiple, circumscribed or noncircumscribed), presence or absence of pneumonitis, atelectasis, histologic subtype, or mediastinal invasion (Mountain 1978). There is an increase in survival time for patients with better performance status (Hansen, Dombernowsky, and Hirsch 1978) and the one-third with limited disease (lesion confined to one hemithorax and the ipsilateral scalene nodes) as compared to the two-thirds with extensive disease (those with remaining unresectable tumor including pleural effusion). Sites of metastasis are:

Most common
- Liver
- Bone (and marrow)
- Brain
- Lymph nodes

Less common
- Adrenals
- Pancreas
- Kidneys
- Heart

Diagnosis

The diagnosis is suggested by cough or hemoptysis, or by a chest x-ray with a centrally placed tumor, usually in the hilum or mediastinum but occasionally, peripherally. The tumor has a high growth fraction and is thought to be of APUD (amine precursor uptake and decarboxylation) cell origin. On electron microscopy it frequently exhibits neurosecretory granules.

Diagnostic work-up is directed largely at obtaining histologic confirmation of the disease by the simplest method, such as bronchoscopy, cytology, scalene node biopsy, mediastinoscopy, or bilateral bone marrow aspiration and biopsy. If small cell carcinoma is suspected and cannot be confirmed by other techniques, thoracotomy is a last resort. Once the diagnosis is established, determination of the extent of disease is indicated. Work-up is as follows:

- Liver function tests, especially lactic dehydrogenase (LDH), SGOT, and alkaline phosphatase
- *Liver scan—of questionable reliability when performed alone
- *Liver ultrasound—of questionable reliability when performed alone
- Peritoneoscopically directed liver biopsy (if histiology is needed)
- Bone scan
- X-ray survey of bones that appear abnormal on scan (unreliable if negative)
- Computerized tomographic brain scan
- Whole body gallium scan
- Bone marrow aspiration and biopsy

Normal biochemical liver function study, scan, or ultrasound do not rule out liver involvement, but if all three are normal it is unlikely. A single positive indirect presumptive study would make this more likely, and if all of the studies were abnormal the suspicion of liver disease would be strong. A negative liver or bone marrow biopsy would not rule out metastasis, but a positive histologically characteristic biopsy would make the diagnosis certain. A positive marrow aspiration or biopsy has been documented in 17% to 50% of cases (Hansen, Dombernowsky, and Hirsch 1978). Although bone scan is frequently positive early in the course of disease, lytic bone lesions on x-ray are uncommon.

Treatment

Surgery

Distant metastases certainly contraindicate attempts at surgical resection. Even when disease appears localized it is usually not resectable (Broder, Cohen, and Selawry 1977). In a review of 121 patients at Memorial Sloan-Kettering Hospital in New York City, only nine had resectable disease and none of them survived five years (Martini, Cliffton, and Beattie 1973). A larger study of 159 patients included only two cases of resectable disease but one patient did survive five years (Takita et al. 1973). Autopsy studies show that the majority of those undergoing resection still have residual disease (Mathews et al. 1973). Hence experienced thoracic surgeons are not anxious to attempt to resect small cell carcinoma but reserve surgery primarily for diagnosis. Therapy for many years was primarily radiation and now is chemotherapy with or without radiation.

Radiation Therapy

Although small cell carcinoma is the histologic subtype of lung cancer most sensitive to radiation, radiotherapy alone does not usually improve patient survival (Broder, Cohen, and Selawry 1977) (figs. 60.1 and 60.2), although one study showed slight prolongation compared to placebo (Roswit, Patno, and Rapp 1968). It is used primarily for the control of inoperable limited (regional) disease, for palliation of local complications (superior vena cava syndrome, bronchial obstruction, hemoptysis, and painful metastases), and for the treatment of chemotherapy sanctuaries (brain and spinal cord). With longer survival of patients on chemotherapy there is an increasing incidence of brain metastases. Hence prophylactic cranial irradiation (PCI) is being

*Liver scan and ultrasound together have a much higher degree of reliability.

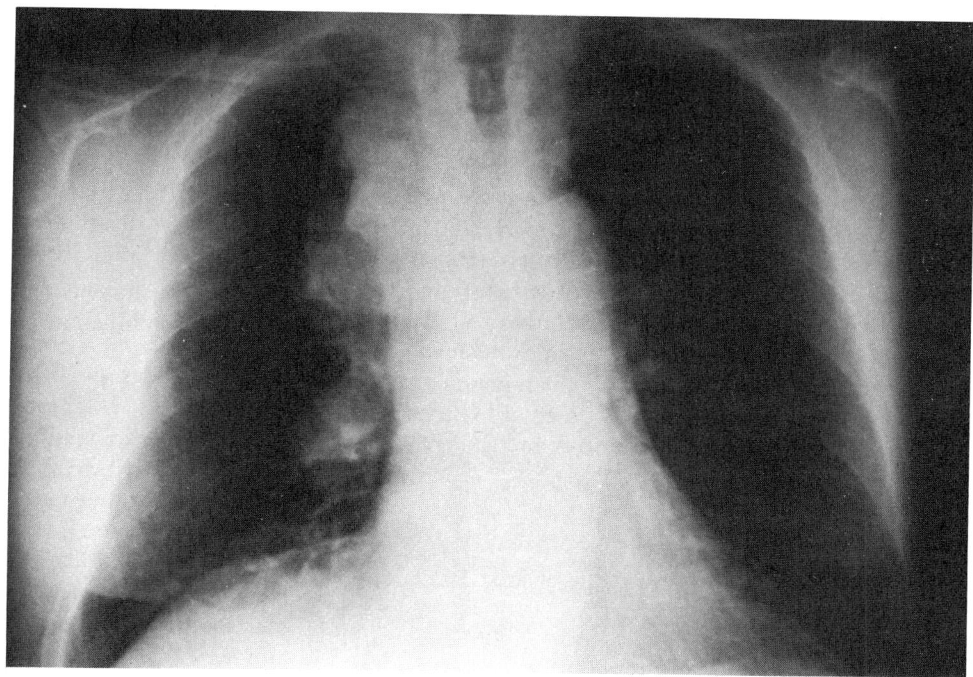

Fig. 60.1. *Chest x-ray of patient with small cell carcinoma of the lung at time of diagnosis showing mass in right upper lobe and hilum. The right scalene node was histologically positive. Extensive work-up showed no other metastasis at that time.*

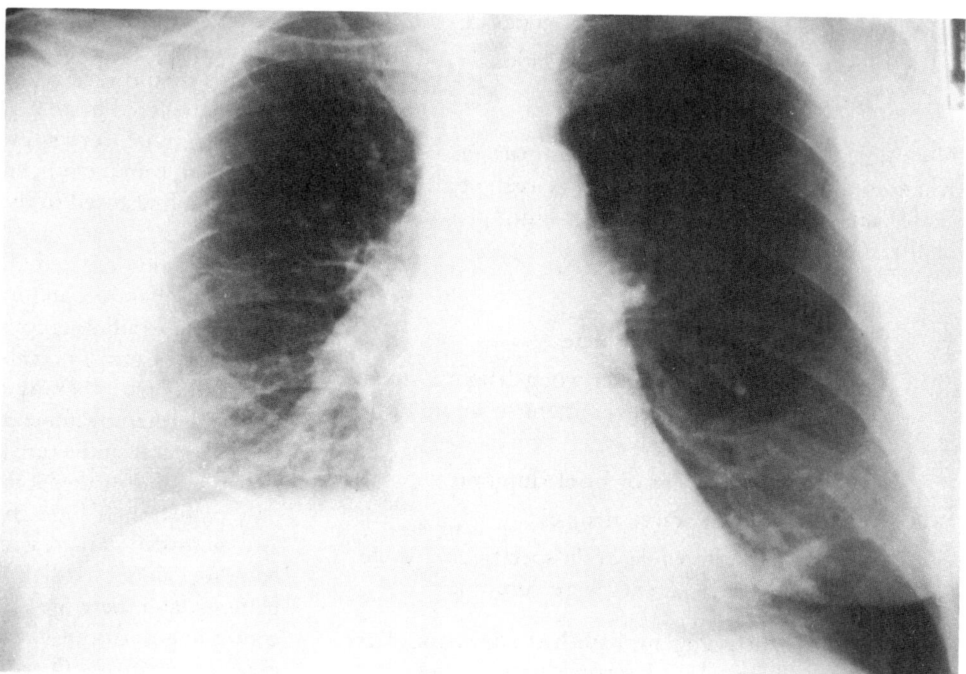

Fig. 60.2. *Same patient as in figure 60.1, following split-course radiation therapy and combination chemotherapy. Although the patient had a good local response, he progressed with brain, liver, and bone metastases, and died shortly thereafter.*

evaluated in those who go into apparent complete remission (Bunn, Nugent, and Matthews 1974). In patients receiving PCI there is a decreased incidence of brain metastases but no change in overall survival. This therapy should not be given until the patient enters complete remission, usually in six weeks. Recent studies have questioned the value of irradiation to the primary tumor in regional limited disease (Hansen et al. 1979), but the issue is unresolved and we give radiation plus chemotherapy. It has already been demonstrated that radiation therapy to the primary tumor and mediastinum in extensive disease does not improve median or long-term survival over that of chemotherapy alone (Weiss 1978; Livingston et al. 1978). Hemibody irradiation is being studied (Fitzpatrick and Rider 1976).

Chemotherapy

Small cell carcinoma is sensitive to at least 10 chemotherapeutic agents:

Cyclophosphamide (Cytoxan)
Doxorubicin (Adriamycin)
Lomustine (CCNU, CeeNU)
Methotrexate (Mexate)
Vincristine (Oncovin)
Procarbazine (Matulane)
Mechlorethamine (Mustargen)
VP-16-213 (investigational) (etoposide)
Hexamethylmelamine (investigational)
Cisplatin (Platinol)

No single agent has a significant impact on survival when used alone, although several (Green et al. 1969) cause marked tumor shrinkage and slight prolongation of life. General responses are:

- Single agents:
  - Responses not complete
  - Responses were better when drug was given on a high-dose intermittent schedule rather than continuously
  - Responses were of brief duration
- Combinations of active drugs:
  - Best results when cycle-specific and cycle non-specific agents were combined

Combinations of active agents have had a dramatic effect in increasing survival and raising hopes of eventual cure.

Prerequisites for effective combination chemotherapy are:

1. Development of optimal time sequence of drug administration
2. Maximum use of individual drugs to achieve highest therapeutic index
3. Use of drugs with different modes of action to prevent early resistance
4. Establishment of the efficacy of each component in the combination

Most regimens are based on the use of an alkylating agent such as cyclophosphamide combined with a minimally myelosuppressive *Vinca* alkaloid such as vincristine. A third drug improves results, usually doxorubicin or methotrexate. Four-drug combinations tend to add a nitrosourea, procarbazine, or an experimental agent such as VP-16-213 (etoposide) or hexamethylmelamine. Complete response rates and survival seem to increase with increasing numbers of drugs up to four, although the increment is smaller with each addition (Bunn et al. 1977). In a compilation of studies, an overall response rate of 60% with a 23% complete response rate was demonstrated in a mixture of limited and extensive disease (Seydel 1978).

Trials of intensive chemotherapy that may result in prolonged leukopenia necessitating hospitalization and antibiotic therapy are in progress. Early reports (Cohen et al. 1977) suggest a higher response rate (90%) and a higher complete response rate (30%) with longer survival, but at the expense of increased toxicity. These patients should receive allopurinol for the first week of therapy to avoid urate nephropathy. Some of the studies in progress are very aggressive and include concepts of induction, reinduction, and early and late intensification along the lines used in the acute leukemias (Livingston 1980).

In a randomized clinical trial the combination of cyclophosphamide and radiotherapy was found to be superior to radiotherapy alone (Host 1973). The response rates and survivals in studies using two or more drugs plus radiotherapy appear to be superior to those with radiotherapy alone or in combination with a single drug. Several studies are attempting to define the role of radiation, and it seems that in extensive disease, this is only palliation of local complications, and is not generally successful in increasing survival compared to chemotherapy alone. Palliation occurs in 50% to 90% of patients, and there are no differences in results between continuous and split-course therapy. In limited disease, excellent results with radiation plus chemotherapy have been reported by several groups (Livingston et al. 1978;

Greco et al. 1979). Some preliminary reports have questioned the necessity of chest radiation (Hansen et al. 1979; Stevens, Einhorn, and Rohn 1979).

A large cooperative study by the Southwest Oncology Group reported on a combination of chemotherapy and radiation (Livingston et al. 1978). Their protocol is close to the approach that we have used for the past few years. Chemotherapy was given on day one with each patient receiving cyclophosphamide, 750 mg/m^2; doxorubicin, 50 mg/m^2; and vincristine, 1 mg total dose for 12 weeks. Cyclophosphamide and doxorubicin were repeated three weeks later and then omitted until radiation therapy was completed. They were resumed at the twelfth week of study and continued at the same dose every three weeks until a total dose of doxorubicin equal to 450 mg/m^2 had been administered. Doxorubicin was then discontinued and cyclophosphamide was increased to 1000 mg/m^2 every four weeks; methotrexate, 30 mg/m^2, was given three weeks after each dose of cyclophosphamide. All drugs were given intravenously by push with appropriate dose reductions for leukopenia and thrombocytopenia.

Radiation of 3000 rad in 10 daily fractions over 2 weeks was administered to the whole brain and the primary tumor, beginning at the sixth week of therapy. Patients with limited disease received an additional 1500 rad over 5 daily fractions to the primary tumor at week 15, with the chemotherapy withheld for 2 weeks. Therapy was discontinued if there was evidence of progression or at two years, whichever was sooner.

There were 250 patients with extensive disease (70%) and 108 with limited disease (30%). Complete regression of tumor was obtained in 14% of those with extensive disease and 41% with limited disease, and complete or partial response in 57% and 75% respectively. Median survival was 26 weeks for patients with extensive disease and 52 weeks for those with limited disease. Response was superior in patients with a better performance status. Those achieving a complete remission had a longer response duration, with one-third having disease-free survival in excess of a year. Toxicity from the combined treatment modalities was no greater than expected from the components given separately: fatal in 3.9% and life-threatening but reversible in 8.4%.

Of particular importance in this study is the improved outlook for patients with limited disease at diagnosis. Fully one-half survive a year from the start of treatment, and long-term disease-free survival appears likely for a small fraction. For patients with extensive disease the addition of radiation to the primary site and whole brain prophylaxis made no impact on the median survival over that expected with combination chemotherapy alone, although the incidence of de novo recurrence in the brain was reduced from 20% to 3%. This reflects failure to appreciably increase the complete response rate. A similar study by the Southeastern group (Krauss et al. 1980) compared patients with limited disease in a randomized protocol using radiation therapy alone or with combination chemotherapy. The median duration of disease-free survival of the patients receiving combination therapy was 27 weeks compared to 9.9 weeks for those treated with radiation alone.

Attempts to improve on these results include the high-dose intensive regimens already mentioned (Cohen et al. 1977) and cyclic regimens of noncross-reactive drugs as primary therapy and consolidative therapy. Such a program (Cohen et al. 1979) is being evaluated now with primary therapy consisting of cyclophosphamide, lomustine, and methotrexate and consolidative therapy with doxorubicin, vincristine, and procarbazine. A similar regimen uses cyclophosphamide, doxorubicin, and vincristine as primary and hexamethylmelamine and etoposide (VP-16-213) for consolidation therapy (Greco et al. 1978). It is hoped that combined modality treatment and better combinations will produce more long-term survivors with less toxicity (Alexander et al. 1977; Holoye et al. 1977). We now have several patients with limited disease who have survived beyond four years without maintenance chemotherapy and who have no evidence of disease. Another patient had extensive disease (brain metastasis) and is alive four years later (figs. 60.3 and 60.4). There is now a registry for such long survivors (Matthews, Rozencweig, and Muggia 1979). Also, immunotherapy and immunochemotherapy are being explored with some early positive results (Israel et al. 1977). In general, however, immunotherapy has so far failed to improve the results of chemotherapy (Aisner and Wiernik 1980).

Complications

The development of facial edema, plethora, prominent neck veins, headache, and difficulty breathing are clues to the superior vena cava syndrome, a dread complication. Other characteristics of superior vena cava obstruction in small cell carcinoma are:

1. It is nearly always associated with right lung tumors.
2. Bronchoscopy (fiberoptic) is indicated if histologic diagnosis is needed.
3. Mediastinoscopy is contraindicated.
4. Indicates nonresectability.

5. Angiography may cause phlebitis or hemorrhage.
6. Combination chemotherapy and radiation are equally effective.

As this is one of the true oncologic emergencies, therapy must be prompt and sometimes must precede histologic and dynamic verification of the diagnosis. We usually give high-dosage steroids and either radiation therapy or aggressive chemotherapy, and occasionally both, depending on the individual circumstances. Chemotherapy appears to be as successful as radiation in the initial treatment (Kane et al. 1976).

Paraneoplastic syndromes are not uncommon with small cell carcinoma. While 17 different tumor products have been associated with it (Richardson et al. 1978) the more common ectopic hormones are ACTH, antidiuretic hormone (ADH), and calcitonin. Therapy is directed primarily at the tumor, but specific and symptomatic therapy is usually necessary for palliation of the hormonal effects.

Brain and leptomeningeal metastases occur in about 25% of patients if they survive long enough. With increasing length of survival, more such metastases are anticipated unless prophylactic cranial irradiation is used, although this does not protect against leptomeningeal metastasis. Intrathecal methotrexate is being considered for prophylaxis and treatment of this complication. If performed too early in the course of chemotherapy, PCI may be self-defeating, as a nidus of residual tumor may again metastasize to the brain and there is no effective therapy after the initial whole brain irradiation (Posner 1977). The hope that chemotherapy with nitrosoureas would prevent or cure brain metastases has not been realized. If PCI has not been given, high-dose steroids and whole brain irradiation may provide some increased disease-free survival. Another hope is that one of the many drugs currently in phase II studies will be more successful (Weiss et al. 1980).

Conclusions

Small cell carcinoma of the lung has become increasingly susceptible to successful treatment. Median survival has increased from 2 to 12 months and there is cautious optimism that our 3- and 4-year survivors who have no evidence of disease may be cured.

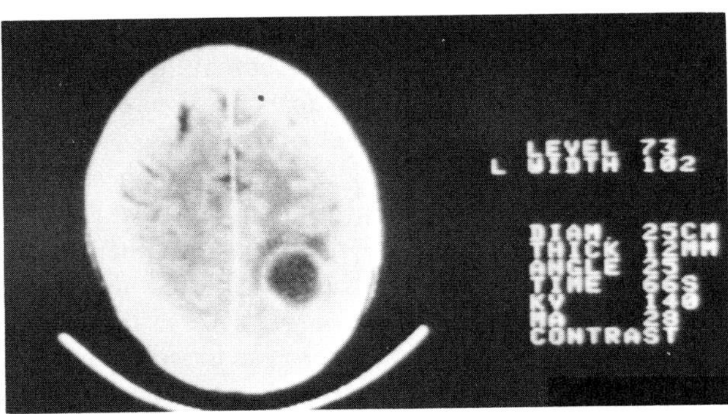

Fig. 60.3. *CT scan of brain of patient with metastasis from small cell carcinoma of the lung.*

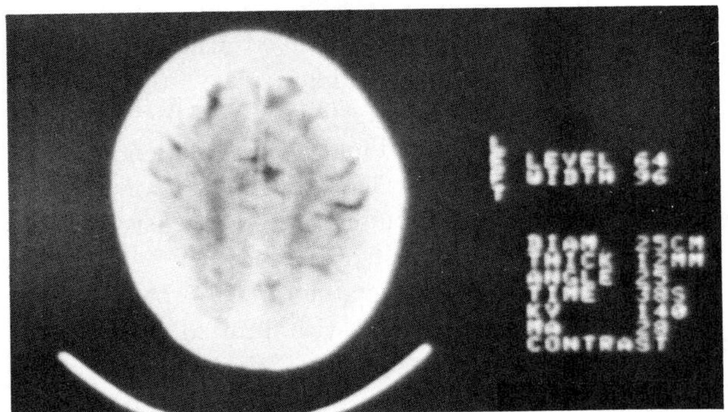

Fig. 60.4. *CT scan of brain of patient from figure 60.3, following radiation therapy and systemic chemotherapy. The patient is alive and free of disease at four years, having had no therapy for the last 30 months.*

References

Aisner, J., and Wiernik, P. H. Chemotherapy versus chemoimmunotherapy for small cell undifferentiated carcinoma of the lung. *Cancer* 46:2543–2549, 1980.

Alexander, M. et al. Combined modality treatment for oat cell carcinoma of the lung: a randomized trial. *Cancer Treat. Rep.* 61:1–6, 1977.

Broder, L. E.; Cohen, M. H.; and Selawry, O. S. Treatment of bronchogenic carcinoma. II. Small cell. *Cancer Treat. Rev.* 4:219–260, 1977.

Bunn, P. A. et al. Advances in small cell bronchogenic carcinoma. *Cancer Treat. Rep.* 61:333–342, 1977.

Bunn, P. A.; Nugent, J. L.; and Matthews, M. J. Central nervous system metastases in small cell bronchogenic carcinoma. *Semin. Oncol.* 5:314–322, 1974.

Cohen, M. H. et al. Intensive chemotherapy of small cell bronchogenic carcinoma. *Cancer Treat. Rep.* 61: 349–354, 1977.

Cohen, M. H. et al. Cyclic alternating combination chemotherapy for small cell bronchogenic carcinoma. *Cancer Treat. Rep.* 63:163–170, 1979.

Fitzpatrick, P. J., and Rider, W. D. Half-body radiotherapy. *Int. J. Radiat. Oncol. Biol. Phys.* 1:197–207, 1976.

Greco, F. A. et al. Therapy of oat cell carcinoma of lung: complete remissions, acceptable complications and improved survival. *Br. Med. J.* 2:10–11, 1978.

Greco, F. A. et al. Small cell cancer. Complete remission and improved survival. *Am. J. Med.* 66:625–630, 1979.

Green, R. A. et al. Alkylating agents in bronchogenic carcinoma. *Am. J. Med.* 46:516–524, 1969.

Hansen, H. H. et al. Chemotherapy versus chemotherapy plus radiotherapy in regional small cell carcinoma of the lung. *Proc. Am. Assoc. Cancer Res.* 20:277, 1979.

Hansen, H. H.; Dombernowski, P.; and Hirsch, F. R. Staging procedures and prognostic features in small cell anaplastic bronchogenic carcinoma. *Semin. Oncol.* 5:280–287, 1978.

Holoye, P. Y. et al. Combination chemotherapy and radiation therapy for small cell carcinoma. *JAMA* 237:1221–1224, 1977.

Host, H. Cyclophosphamide as adjuvant to radiotherapy in the treatment of unresectable bronchogenic carcinoma. *Cancer Treat. Rep.* 4:161–164, 1973.

Israel, L. et al. Immunochemotherapy in 34 cases of oat cell carcinoma of the lung with 19 complete responses. *Cancer Treat. Rep.* 61:343–347, 1977.

Kane, R. C. et al. Superior vena caval obstruction due to small cell anaplastic lung carcinoma. *JAMA* 235:1717–1718, 1976.

Krauss, S. et al. Combined modality treatment of localized small cell lung carcinoma. *Cancer Clin. Trials* 3:297–306, 1980.

Livingston, R. B. Small cell carcinoma of the lung. *Blood* 56:575–584, 1980.

Livingston, R. B. et al. Small cell carcinoma of the lung: combined chemotherapy and radiation. *Ann. Intern. Med.* 88:194–199, 1978.

Martini, M.; Cliffton, E. E.; and Beattie, E. J., Jr. Survival of lung cancer patients vis-a-vis therapy and cell type. *Proc. Seventh Natl. Cancer Conf.* 7:739–742, 1973.

Matthews, M. J. et al. Frequency of residual and metastatic tumor in patients undergoing curative surgical resection for lung cancer. *Cancer Chemother. Rep.* 4:63–67, 1973.

Matthews, M. J.; Rozencweig, M.; and Muggia, F. M. Long-term survivors with small cell carcinoma of the lung (SCCL). *Proc. Am. Soc. Clin. Oncol.* 20:411, 1979.

Mountain, C. F. Clinical biology of small cell carcinoma: relationship to surgical therapy. *Semin. Oncol.* 5:272–279, 1978.

Posner, J. B. Management of central nervous system metastases. *Semin. Oncol.* 4:81–91, 1977.

Richardson, R. L. et al. Tumor products and potential markers in small cell lung cancer. *Semin. Oncol.* 5:253–262, 1978.

Roswit, B.; Patno, M. E.; and Rapp, R. The survival of patients with inoperable lung cancer: a large-scale randomized study of radiation therapy versus placebo. *Radiology* 90:688–697, 1968.

Seydel, H. G. Radiation therapy in small cell lung cancer. *Semin. Oncol.* 5:288–298, 1978.

Silverberg, E. Cancer statistics, 1979. *CA* 29:6–21, 1979.

Stevens, E.; Einhorn, L.; and Rohn, R. Treatment of limited small cell lung cancer. *Proc. Am. Soc. Clin. Oncol.* 20:435, 1979.

Takita, J. et al. Small cell carcinoma of the lung. Clinicopathologic studies. *J. Thorac. Cardiovasc. Surg.* 66:472–477, 1973.

Weiss, R. B. Small cell carcinoma of the lung: therapeutic management. *Ann. Intern. Med.* 88:522–531, 1978.

Weiss, R. B. et al. Treatment of small cell undifferentiated carcinoma of the lung: update of recent results. *Cancer Treat. Rep.* 64:539–548, 1980.

Yesner, R. et al. *Histologic typing of lung tumors, WHO.* Geneva, Switzerland: WHO, 1981.

sixty-one

Chemotherapy of Non-Small Cell Cancer of the Lung

DAVID P. PURPORA

Carcinoma of the lung, with a median survival of three to nine months from diagnosis, represents the most frequent and frustrating problem confronting the clinical chemotherapist. Approximately one-half of all patients with lung cancer have extensive disease when first diagnosed. In those with metastatic disease, surgery has no definitive role and radiation has been limited to a local method to attempt symptomatic palliation. Chemotherapy, the third major form of treating cancer, has been employed with great success in lung cancer only against the small cell type. Over the last 20 years, various cooperative groups have tested a variety of chemotherapeutic agents in thousands of patients with less than impressive results. Nevertheless, some progress has been made, and has followed the sequence set forth and fully developed in other malignant diseases such as childhood leukemia, Hodgkin's disease, diffuse histiocytic lymphoma, nonseminomatous testicular cancer, and limited small cell cancer of bronchogenic origin.

The first step is identification of active single agents reported to have activity in lung cancer: alkylating agents, antitumor antibiotics, plant alkaloids, antimetabolites, nitrosoureas, hydrazine derivatives, and miscellaneous compounds. Commonly used drugs from each class of chemotherapeutic agents are shown in table 61.1 with their reported response rates according to cell type (Selawry 1974).

As can be seen, only a handful of agents produce a significant response, and complete remissions are rare. Thus monochemotherapy cannot be expected to have a significant impact on survival in lung cancer and should be avoided unless used in combination or in sequence with other modalities, namely radiation. Isolated reports claiming impressive gains should be greeted with skepticism, as they usually involve small numbers of patients, often lack controls, and deal with patients with good functional capacity, limited tumor load, and recent radiotherapy to the major involved site. Similarly, criteria for response should be carefully considered; for example, cavitation of a tumor sometimes is interpreted as a therapeutic effect as opposed to a natural sequel of outgrowing its blood supply.

Thus we can characterize the monochemotherapy of lung cancer as follows:

1. Objective responses with the most active agents occur in about 20% to 35% of patients and are rarely complete.
2. Median duration of such responses is three months.
3. Palliation is short-lived and its impact on survival is minimal.

As we have seen in other tumors, it is conceivable that further improvement can be made by means of dose scheduling or by developing rescue techniques that allow escalation of doses. Finally, the legacy of the past 20 years of experience with single-agent chemotherapy has allowed us to proceed to step two in the sequence, which is the identification of active combinations of drugs.

Table 61.1. *Activity of Single Agents in Non-Small Cell Lung Cancer with Response Rates According to Cell Type*

Alkylating Agents	*Epidermoid (%)*	*Adenocarcinoma (%)*	*Large Cell (%)*
Mechlorethamine	33	29	27
Cyclophosphamide	19	17	23
Lomustine (CCNU)	35	23	17
Carmustine (BCNU)	15	0	9
Hexamethylmelamine	12	15	18
Cisplatin	38	15	27
Antibiotics			
Doxorubicin (Adriamycin)	19	15	25
Bleomycin	13	13	?
Mitomycin	?	27	?
Plant derivatives			
Vinblastine	16	12	10
Vincristine	11	9	?
Etoposide (VP-16-213)	10	?	?
Antimetabolites			
Methotrexate	25	32	27
Procarbazine	20	19	18

SOURCE: Modified from Selawry 1974.

Table 61.2. *Polychemotherapy of Bronchogenic Carcinoma*

	Response by Cell Type (%)				*Patient Number by Cell Type*			
Drugs	*Epidermoid*	*Small Cell*	*Adenocarcinoma*	*Large Cell*	*Epidermoid*	*Small Cell*	*Adenocarcinoma*	*Large Cell*
Procarbazine	12	50	0	45	8	2	5	11
Procarbazine + fluorouracil	55	44	83	40	11	9	6	10
PROC + CTX + MTX + VCR								
Simultaneously	39	69	0	0	18	16	3	1*
Sequentially	14	27	0	0	22	11	2	3*
Simultaneously + randomized + nonrandomized	28	62	71	50	46	53	7	19*
CTX + MTX	0	31	6	0	0	30	28	0
CTX + MTX + CCNU	0	57	30	0	0	31	28	0
CTX + MTX								
Median survival (days)		170	135	0				
CTX + MTX + CCNU								
Median survival (days)		250†	240†	0				

SOURCE: Modified from Selawry 1974.

* Includes large cell anaplastic and "other" bronchogenic carcinomas.

†Statistically significant superiority.

Polychemotherapy

The basic principle of combination chemotherapy is to employ drugs that have a convergent effect on the tumor with divergent toxicity to the host (table 61.2). With few exceptions, each component drug should be effective when used alone. Ideally, the combinations of drugs and the sequence in which they are given should be based on cell kinetics to optimize the results. Selawry (1974) is an excellent source of information on early polychemotherapy studies, some of which demonstrated improvement in response rates and survival when compared with the single-agent experience. These studies failed to demonstrate an impact on the majority of patients so treated, however, and other groups studying such regimens in a prospective randomized fashion failed to show clear-cut superiority.

Oncologists have never been accused of being therapeutic nihilists and as a result, combinations of drugs have been tried more extensively than ever before over the last five years in an attempt to complete the sequence alluded to earlier, namely, the identification of regimens that have an impact on survival, first in a minority, and later in a majority of patients so treated. The most important new regimens reported in the last five years are discussed here.

Chahinian and associates (1977) reported on the methotrexate, Adriamycin, cyclophosphamide, CCNU (MACC) regimen for bronchogenic carcinoma that has shown activity and prolongation of survival for all cell types of lung cancer. The initial series reported 41 patients (later this was extended to 83 patients) with an overall response rate of 86.6% for small cell carcinoma and 44% for non-small cell types (Chahinian et al. 1979). As can be seen in figure 61.1, the objective responders had a much better survival than the nonresponders, whose survival was similar to that of the placebo group in the Veterans Administration lung study (Green et al. 1969). The results have been analyzed by major histologic subgroups (Chahinian, personal communication). One can see (fig. 61.2) that the patients with small cell carcinoma did as well on the four-drug MACC program as the group of Israel and associates (1977) on eight drugs, and better than the

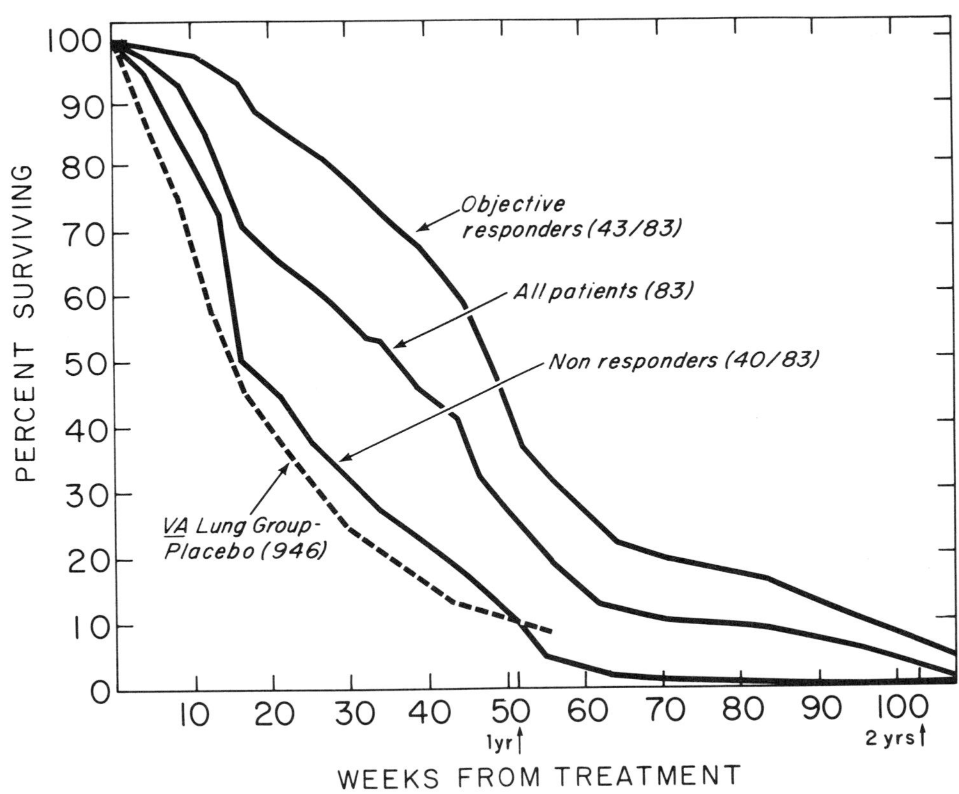

Fig. 61.1. *Comparison of survival of responders, nonresponders, and entire group treated with MACC chemotherapy in contrast with the placebo group in the VA Lung Group study. Numbers of patients are shown in parentheses. (Chahinian et al. 1979. Reprinted by permission.)*

NCI-VA group on MCC (methotrexate, cyclophosphamide, and CCNU) (Hansen et al. 1976) or the VA lung study group on cyclophosphamide or placebo (Green et al. 1969). Combining responders and nonresponders, those with adenocarcinoma treated with MACC (fig. 61.3) did better than the VA lung study cyclophosphamide and placebo groups. The overall response of patients with squamous cell carcinoma to MACC therapy compares favorably to the responders in the BACON regimen (Livingston et al. 1976) and is superior to the VA lung study placebo group (fig. 61.4).

Later, 100 patients with proved advanced and progressing lung cancer were randomized to one of three regimens: MACC alone, MACC and levamisole, or MACC and *C. parvum*. As one can see in table 61.3, there were responses in all cell types and the prolongation of survival in responders was nearly twice that of nonresponders. There is a suggestion that immunotherapy in the form of levamisole may favorably affect survival when added to MACC. Actuarial survival based on extent of disease, response to MACC, and correlation with cell type demonstrates that there is a response to combination chemotherapy in advanced lung cancer. The MACC polychemotherapy is a standard against which subsequent regimens for non-small cell lung cancer can be compared. One word of caution: despite the continued efficacy of the MACC regimen in all types of lung cancer reported by Chahinian and others in over 141 patients, a recent negative report on the combination appeared in the literature (Vogl et al. 1979) demonstrating the difficulties in duplicating results in subsets of patients treated by large cooperative groups in diverse institutions and settings. Only 5 patients out of 43 (12%) responded with partial remissions, and toxicity, particularly hematologic, was prohibitive (Vogl et al. 1979). The authors concluded that the MACC regimen is not superior to single agents, is more toxic, and should not be employed either for advanced disease or as a surgical adjuvant. To the objective observer, this glaring disparity of results only points out the need for continued prospective randomized trials of regimens for all malignancies.

Other commonly used regimens include lomustine plus doxorubicin (Trowbridge et al. 1978), COMB (cyclophosphamide, Oncovin, methyl-CCNU, and bleomycin) (Bodey et al. 1977), CAMP (cyclophosphamide, Adriamycin, methotrexate, and procarbazine) (Bitran et al. 1976, 1978), BACON (bleomycin, Adriamycin, CCNU, Oncovin, and nitrogen mustard) (Livingston et al. 1976), MOCA (methotrexate, Oncovin, cyclophosphamide, and Adriamycin) (Sarna et al. 1977), and AMCOF (Adriamycin, methotrexate, cyclophosphamide, Oncovin, and 5-fluorouracil) (Reynolds and O'Dell 1978). The COMB regimen did not increase survival in squamous cell lung cancer despite a response rate of 33%

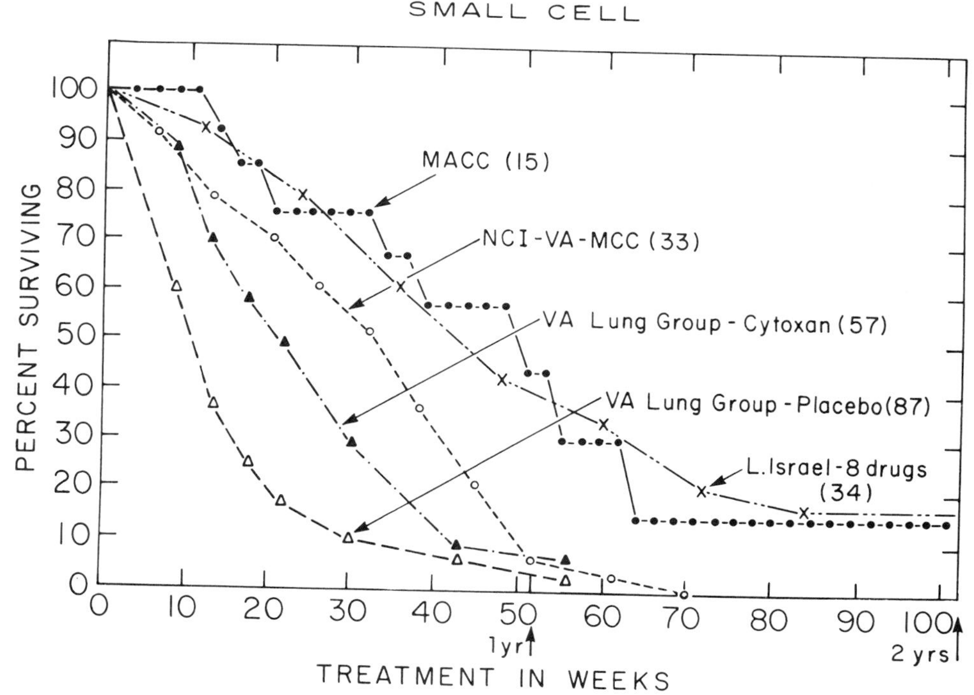

Fig. 61.2. *Comparison of survival curves of patients with small cell carcinoma of the lung treated with various regimens. Numbers of patients are shown in parentheses. (Chahinian, unpublished data. Reprinted by permission.)*

Table 61.3. *Response (CR or PR Greater than 50%) by Cell Type*

Regimen	*Squamous*	*Adenocarcinoma*	*Small Cell*	*Large Cell*
MACC (A)	3 PR/8	(1 CR + 2 PR)/9	(4 CR + 2 PR)/10	1 PR/5
MACC + L (B)	1 PR/5	(1 CR + 2 PR)/8	(2 CR + 1 PR)/8	2 PR/3
MACC +CP (C)	(2 CR + 3 PR)/9	1 CR/10	(2 CR + 1 PR)/6	(1 CR + 2 PR)/8
Totals	(2 CR + 7 PR)/22	(3 CR + 4 PR)/27	(8 CR + 4 PR)/24	(1 CR +5 PR)/16

SOURCE: Chahinian 1978.

NOTES: Overall objective response rate was 38%, and 34% in cell types other than small cell. Median actuarial survival for all patients was 29 weeks (A = 28, B = 31, C =27), for responders was 39 weeks (A = 34, B = 39, C = 43), and for nonresponders was 22 weeks (A = 16, B = 23, C = 17). L = levamisole, CP = *C. parvum*.

(Livingston et al. 1976), and in a more recent study the response rate was 5% and was not superior to cyclophosphamide alone (Bodey et al. 1977). The BACON program produced a 42% response rate in squamous cell carcinoma with a median survival time (MST) of 20 weeks (Livingston et al. 1976).

Three other drug combinations are comparable to MACC: CAMP, MOCA, and AMCOF. Therapy with CAMP produced a response rate of 48% with a MST of eight months (Bitran et al. 1976). It was started only one to two weeks after radiotherapy to the lung in most patients, however, which obscures the impact of chemotherapy on survival. The MACC regimen was implemented only after local or distant failure; MOCA treatment produced an overall response of 29% in patients with non-small cell cancer with a similar impact on survival (Sarna et al. 1977). The AMCOF regimen was compared in a randomized fashion to cyclophosphamide alone and COMF (cyclophosphamide, Oncovin, methotrexate, and 5-fluorouracil). Median survival was three months with cyclophosphamide, six months with COMF, and 14 months with AMCOF (fig. 61.5). The median survival of those with adenocarcinoma or epidermoid carcinoma treated with cyclophosphamide was 3 months, 6 months for COMF, and 15.5 for AMCOF (Reynolds and O'Dell 1978). In this

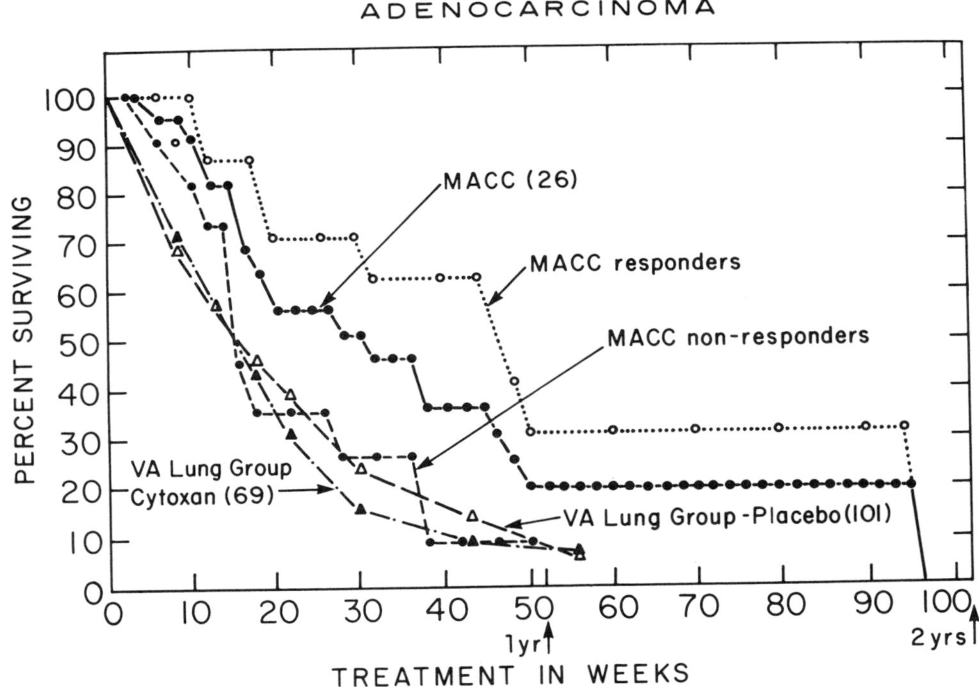

Fig. 61.3. *Comparison of survival of responders, nonresponders, and entire group with adenocarcimona of the lung treated with MACC chemotherapy in contrast with the placebo and cyclophosphamide groups of the VA Lung Group study. Numbers of patients shown in parentheses. (Chahinian, unpublished data. Reprinted by permission.)*

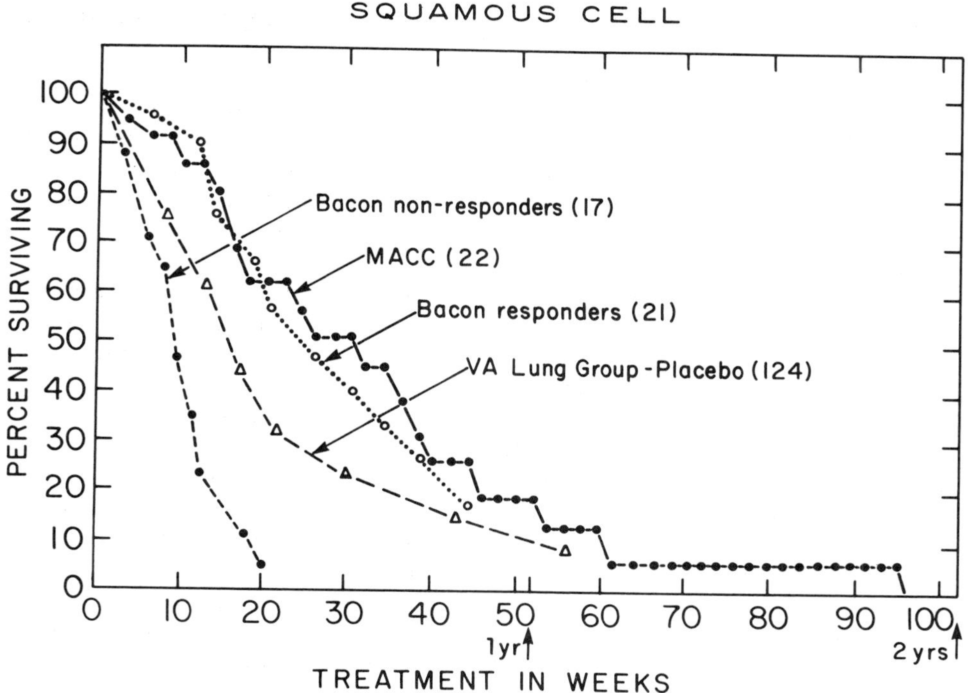

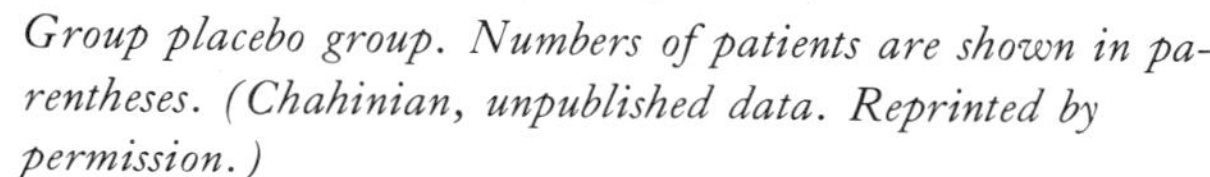

Fig. 61.4. *Survival of patients with squamous cell carcinoma of the lung, treated with MACC in contrast with responders and nonresponders to BACON chemotherapy and the VA Lung Group placebo group. Numbers of patients are shown in parentheses. (Chahinian, unpublished data. Reprinted by permission.)*

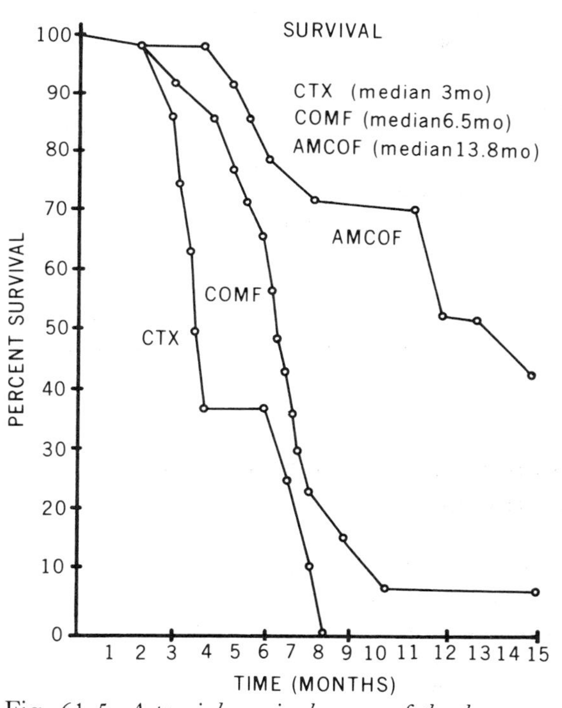

Fig. 61.5. *Actuarial survival curves of the three groups (CTX, COMF, and AMCOF) showing the superior survival with AMCOF. Median survivals were 3 months for CTX, 6 months for COMF, and 14 months for AMCOF. (Reynolds and O'Dell 1978. Reprinted by permission.)*

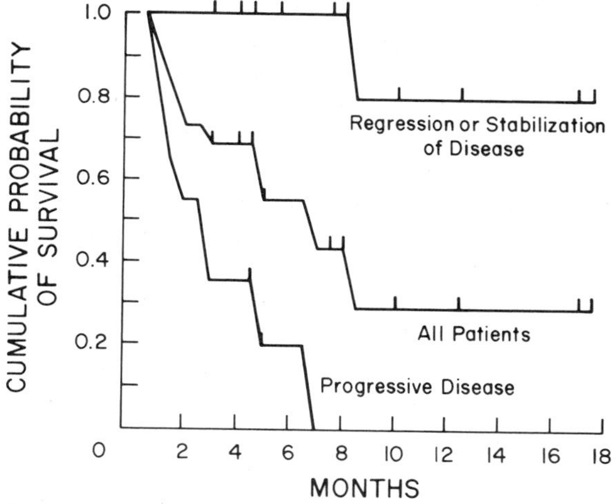

Fig. 61.6. *Life-table analysis of survival for patients with adenocarcinoma of the lung treated with the FAM regimen. (Schein et al. 1978. Reprinted by permission.)*

study, radiation was given to primary and bulky tumor sites.

Recently, two studies using doxorubicin and mitomycin in combination have reported a favorable effect on the survival of patients with advanced adenocarcinoma of the lung. The first of these (Samson et al. 1978) is the MAC regimen (mitomycin, Adriamycin, and cyclophosphamide) in which 25% of the patients achieved an objective response and had a median survival of 39 weeks, whereas nonresponders lived only 17 weeks.

The second combination, reported by Schein and co-workers (1979), used 5-fluorouracil, Adriamycin, and mitomycin (FAM) in 25 patients with unresectable primary adenocarcinoma of the lung. Nine of 25 patients (36%) treated with FAM had an objective response (1 CR, 8 PR) with a median response duration of 7 months. Median survival for the entire series was 6.5 months, whereas the projected median survival for responders is 11.5 months (fig. 61.6).

More recently, cisplatin-based regimens have been reported to possess activity in non-small cell bronchogenic carcinoma. Gralla and associates (1979) reported on a protocol using high-dose cisplatin with mannitol-induced diuresis combined with cyclophosphamide and doxorubicin. An overall partial response rate of 28% was observed, including a 38% response rate in patients with good performance status, with a median survival of 16 months in responders. Eagan and co-workers (1979) reported a 38% response rate when cisplatin was given by infusion together with doxorubicin and cyclophosphamide given by intravenous push. A 43% response rate was reported by Casper and associates (1979) using the combination of vindesine plus cisplatin. A follow-up (Itri et al. 1981; Gralla et al. 1981) compared cisplatin at a dose of 120 mg/m^2 to 60 mg/m^2 and found the same response rate but longer remission and survival duration at the higher dose. Adding bleomycin, cyclophosphamide, or doxorubicin plus cyclophosphamide increased the toxicity but not the response or survival duration. Satisfactory results were also observed with vinblastine in combination with cisplatin (Bitran, Desser, and Shapiro 1981).

Finally, cisplatin and VP-16-213 combination chemotherapy in non-small cell bronchogenic carcinoma was reported to produce a 47% response rate in 17 patients with epidermoid carcinoma; two responses were complete. One of two patients with adenocarcinoma had a partial response (Longeval et al. 1980).

Adjuvant Chemotherapy

As we have seen in recent years, chemotherapy can be effective in a variety of tumors in delaying the appearance of metastases following surgical removal of bulky disease. The results in breast cancer demonstrate the efficacy of combination chemotherapy in eradicating subclinical micrometastases permitting prolonged disease-free survival and in some cases, cure. Only in the small cell variety has combination chemotherapy demonstrated such a benefit for lung cancer. Theoretically, for a regimen to be effective in the adjuvant setting it must produce remissions in patients with metastatic disease 50% of the time. Thus the adjuvant trials in lung cancer using single agents (Crosbie et al. 1966) were probably doomed to failure due to the low order of drug efficacy. There have been numerous prospective randomized clinical trials involving over 3000 patients with lung cancer using mechlorethamine, cyclophosphamide, and vinblastine, each of which was unsuccessful in prolonging disease-free survival (Slack 1970; Higgins 1972; Curreri 1962).

At the time of this writing, no reports have appeared in the literature showing a benefit for early application of combination chemotherapy following apparently curative resection. The enthusiasm for prospective randomized trials to test this hypothesis has been dimmed because of the lack of regimens effective in a majority of patients with metastatic non-small cell lung cancer. Also, the concept of treating these patients with combination chemotherapy following so-called debulking procedures has not been explored with any vigor. It remains for the large cooperative groups to test various regimens in the adjuvant setting in high-risk patients. The resistance of lung cancer to any one form of therapy suggests that only an intensive combined modality approach with surgery, radiotherapy, chemotherapy, and perhaps immunotherapy will yield the desired results, namely, prolonged disease-free survival.

Combination Chemotherapy and Radiotherapy

Except for small cell bronchogenic carcinoma, results of radiotherapy combined with single agents have been disappointing. Prospective randomized studies involving over 2000 patients treated with radiotherapy (RT) alone versus RT plus single-agent therapy, either mechlorethamine or other alkylating agents, have failed to demonstrate any real benefit (Bergsagel et al. 1972; Broyet et al. 1968; Palmer et al. 1978).

Cooperative groups are currently evaluating the two modalities in non-small cell carcinoma using intensive combinations of drugs. The progress seen in the small cell variety of lung cancer may eventually be achieved in the other cell types.

Clearly, we now have chemotherapeutic regimens that can provide significant palliation resulting in improvement of performance status as well as survival in up to 40% of patients so treated. Further progress requires the introduction of new agents and combinations that are mutually noncross-resistant. Just as we have seen for lymphoma and small cell lung cancer, radiation can be used for consolidation and to treat bulky disease. Studies are ongoing to test combination chemotherapy with and without radiation in patients suitable for resection of the primary tumor where the risk of relapse and subsequent death is greater than 50% within five years. The final step in the sequence—long-term disease-free survival—should be achieved in a substantial number of patients.

References

Bergsagel, D. E. et al. Lung cancer: clinical trial of radiotherapy alone vs. RT plus cyclophosphamide. *Cancer* 30:621–627, 1972.

Bitran, J. D. et al. Cyclophosphamide, Adriamycin, methotrexate and procarbazine (CAMP)—effective four-drug combination chemotherapy for metastatic non-oat cell bronchogenic carcinoma. *Cancer Treat. Rep.* 60:1225–1230, 1976.

Bitran, J. D. et al. Metastatic non-oat cell carcinoma—therapy. I. CTX, Adriamycin, MTX and procarbazine (CAMP). *JAMA* 240:2743–2746, 1978.

Bitran, J. D.; Desser, R. K.; and Shapiro, C. M. Velban and cisplatin in the treatment of refractory stage III_{m1} non-small cell bronchogenic carcinoma (NSBC). *Proc. Am. Soc. Clin. Oncol.* 22:501, 1981.

Bodey, G. P. et al. Therapy of advanced squamous carcinoma of the lung. Cyclophosphamide versus COMB. *Cancer* 39:1026–1031, 1977.

Broyet, D. et al. Results of a trial of radiotherapy and chemotherapy in bronchopulmonary cancer. *Eur. J. Cancer* 4:437–445, 1968.

Casper, E. S. et al. Vindesine (DVA) and cis-dichlorodiammineplatinum (II) (DDP) combination chemotherapy in non-small cell lung cancer. *Proc. Am. Soc. Clin. Oncol.* 20:336, 1979.

Chahinian, P. A. Personal communication of unpublished data, 1981.

Chahinian, P. A. et al. Chemotherapy only (MACC) vs chemotherapy and levamisole or *Corynebacterium parvum* (CP) in advanced lung cancer. A randomized trial. *Abstracts of Chemotherapy Foundation Symposium* 4:55–57, 1980.

Chahinian, P. A. et al. Chemotherapy for bronchogenic carcinoma. *JAMA* 237:2392–2396, 1977.

Chahinian, P. A. et al. MACC (methotrexate, Adriamycin, cyclophosphamide and CCNU) in advanced lung cancer. *Cancer* 43:1590–1597, 1979.

Crosbie, W. A. et al. A controlled trial of vinblastine sulfate in the treatment of cancer of the lung. *Br. J. Dis. Chest* 60:28–35, 1966.

Curreri, A. Nitrogen mustard as an adjuvant to pulmonary resection in the treatment of carcinoma of the lung. *Cancer Chemother. Rep.* 16:123–124, 1962.

Eagan, R. T. et al. Phase II study of cyclophosphamide, Adriamycin and cis-dichlorodiammineplatinum II by infusion in patients with adenocarcinoma and large cell carcinoma of the lung. *Cancer Treat. Rep.* 63:1589–1591, 1979.

Gralla, R. J. et al. Cis-dichlorodiammineplatinum (II) in non-small cell carcinoma of the lung. *Cancer Treat. Rep.* 63:1585–1588, 1979.

Gralla, R. J. et al. Cisplatin and vindesine combination chemotherapy for advanced carcinoma of the lung: a randomized trial investigating two dosage schedules. *Ann. Intern. Med.* 95:414–420, 1981.

Green, R. A. et al. Alkylating agents in bronchogenic carcinoma. *Am. J. Med.* 46:516–525, 1969.

Hansen, H. H. et al. Combination chemotherapy of advanced lung cancer: a randomized trial. *Cancer* 38:2201–2207, 1976.

Higgins, G. The use of chemotherapy as an adjuvant to surgery for bronchogenic carcinoma. *Cancer* 30: 1383–1387, 1972.

Israel, L. et al. Immunochemotherapy in 34 cases of oat cell carcinoma of the lung with 19 complete responses. *Cancer Treat. Rep.* 61:343–347, 1977.

Itri, L. M. et al. Vindesine with cisplatin in non-small cell lung cancer (NSCLC): the influence on survival and the effect of adding conventional agents. *Proc. Am. Soc. Clin. Oncol.* 22:521, 1981.

Livingston, R. B. et al. BACON (bleomycin, Adriamycin, CCNU, Oncovin and nitrogen mustard) in squamous lung cancer. Experience in 50 patients. *Cancer* 37:1237–1242, 1976.

Longeval, E. et al. Cisplatin (CDDP)–VP-16-213 combination chemotherapy in non-small cell (NSC) bronchogenic carcinoma: phase I-II clinical trial. *Proc. Am. Soc. Clin. Oncol.* 21:368, 1980.

Palmer, R. L. et al. Comparison of low-dose radiation therapy alone or combined with procarbazine for unresectable epidermoid carcinoma of the lung, stage T3, N1, N2 or M1. *Cancer* 42:424–428, 1978.

Reynolds, R. D., and O'Dell, S. Combination modality therapy in lung cancer. *Cancer* 42:385–389, 1978.

Samson, M. K. et al. Mitomycin-C in advanced adenocarcinoma and large cell carcinoma of the lung. *Cancer Treat. Rep.* 62:163–165, 1978.

Sarna, G. P. et al. Chemoimmunotherapy of bronchogenic carcinoma. *Proc. Am. Assoc. Cancer Res.* 18:89, 1977.

Schein, P. et al. FAM chemotherapy for adenocarcinoma of the lung. In *Mitomicin C—current status and new developments*, eds. K. Carter and S. T. Crooke. New York: Academic Press, 1979, pp. 140–141.

Selawry, O. S. The role of chemotherapy in lung cancer. *Semin. Oncol.* 1:259–272, 1974.

Slack, N. D. Bronchogenic carcinoma: nitrogen mustard as a surgical adjuvant and factors influencing survival. *Cancer* 25:987–1002, 1970.

Trowbridge, C. et al. CCNU-Adriamycin therapy in bronchogenic carcinoma. *Cancer* 41:1704–1709, 1978.

Vogl, S. E. et al. MACC chemotherapy for adenocarcinoma and epidermoid carcinoma of the lung. *Cancer* 44:864–868, 1979.

sixty-two

The Role of Radiation Therapy in Lung Cancer

DANIEL S. KAPP

The magnitude of the problem of lung cancer management is emphasized by the fact that during the past 25 years over 2500 patients with primary lung cancer have been seen at the Yale–New Haven Hospital and the affiliated West Haven Veterans Administration Hospital, with over 1800 of these patients referred for radiation therapy. As has been the finding in other institutions, approximately 50% of these patients had evidence of distant metastases at the time of first examination and of the remainder only 50% had operable tumors. Of patients able to undergo thoracotomy and attempted curative resection, only 25% to 35% survived five years. The majority therefore require additional treatment, and for many of them radiation therapy is considered.

This modality can be used with curative, palliative, or prophylactic intent. Radiation therapy to achieve cure can be given alone or as preoperative or postoperative treatment. It may be indicated on an emergency basis for alleviation of superior vena caval obstruction, spinal cord compression, obstructive pneumonitis, or gross hemoptysis. Treatments can effectively ameliorate cough, pain, dyspnea, and other symptoms often associated with advanced lung cancer. Prophylactic irradiation of possible sanctuary sites such as the brain may be indicated in small cell disease. The use of adjuvant immunotherapy with radiation therapy in unresectable, limited, non-small cell lung cancers is an experimental treatment.

Radiation Therapy with Curative Intent

Radiation Therapy Alone

Numerous thoracotomy and autopsy studies have demonstrated the ability of radiation therapy to effectively sterilize sites of lung cancer in approximately 30% to 50% of patients adequately treated (table 62.1). It was initially unclear, however, whether this resulted in any improvement in the survival of patients with inoperable disease over what would be expected from a placebo-treated group. To answer this question a randomized multiple institution VA Hospital study was undertaken (Roswit, Patno, and Rapp 1968). The majority of the patients had previously untreated lung cancer and were randomized to radiation therapy alone (308 patients) compared to a lactose tablet placebo (246 patients). The group receiving radiation therapy showed a statistically significant increased survival rate. The results were not extremely dramatic, probably because most of the patients had fairly advanced disease at the time of randomization.

The superiority of surgery compared to radiation therapy for unresectable squamous cell carcinomas was indicated in a study by Morrison and co-workers (1963). Fifty-eight patients with biopsy-proved disease were randomized between radiation therapy and surgery and a 30% four-year survival rate was obtained for those patients treated with surgery as opposed to a 6% survival rate for those treated with radiation therapy. For patients with anaplastic carcinomas, overall four-year survival

Table 62.1. *Local Sterilization of Lung Cancer by Radiation Therapy*

Reference	*Number of Patients*	*Dose Range*	*% Local Control (Surgery or Autopsy)*
Bromley and Szur 1955	66	3700–6000 rad/4.5–7 wks	47
Lawton et al. 1966	20	5925 rad (avg)/5–6 wks	40
Manfredi et al. 1966	16	4000–4600 rad/4 wks	31
Bloedorn 1966	82	5500–6000 rad/5.5–6 wks	33 primary site 77 regional node
Rissanen et al. 1968	60	4800–6250 rad/5–8 wks	30
Shields et al. 1970	77	3000–6000 rad/4–6 wks	27
Abadir and Muggia 1975	21	4000–6000 rad/4–6 wks	38
Eisert, Cox, and Komaki 1976	197	1200–2000 ret	34*
		< 1450 ret	27
		> 1450 ret	51

*Clinical or autopsy findings.

Table 62.2. *Radical Radiotherapy in Inoperable and Unresectable Bronchogenic Carcinoma*

Institution	*Number of Patients*	*One-Year Survival (%)*	*Five-Year Survival (%)*
Duke University	347	40	6
Stanford University	284	30	6
Hammersmith Hospital	513	36	6
Columbia University (unresectable at thoracotomy)	103	59	9
Columbia University (clinically inoperable)	150	40	3
Ellis Fischel Hospital	277	30	6
Mayo Clinic	188	37	3
Mount Sinai Hospital	141	57	10
Biopsy only	53	—	11
Incomplete resection	21	—	24
A. Maxwell Evans Clinic*	141	57	10
Vanderbilt Hospital†	203	—	6

SOURCE: Modified from Lee 1974.
*Coy and Kennelly 1980.
†Aristizabel and Caldwell 1976.

rates were approximately 10% in each group with no significant difference between the treatment modalities. Patient selection plays a significant role in determining the outcome of any series. Smart (1966) studied patients with relatively early lung cancer and surgically resectable lesions who were treated with radiation therapy alone. The five-year survival rate was 22.5%, which is similar to that obtained in many of the surgical series in the literature (Stanford et al. 1976). Unfortunately, the results of most series where radical radiation therapy was employed in inoperable and unresectable disease showed significantly lower survival rates of between 3% and 10% (table 62.2).

Nonetheless, radiation therapy cures for unresectable lung cancer do occur and long-term results warrant the prompt institution of treatment in appropriate patients. The following case illustrates the techniques employed in radical treatment.

> A 54-year-old woman complained of hoarseness and shortness of breath. Physical examination revealed a fixed left vocal cord, and a chest x-ray revealed a left hilar mass and a paralyzed left hemidiaphragm (fig. 62.1A). Bronchoscopy and mediastinoscopy were negative, and on exploratory thoracotomy a mass was noted in the left hilar area that invaded the pericardium, aorta, and left phrenic nerve. Biopsy of this mass revealed a poorly differentiated carcinoma, and subsequent metastatic work-up was negative. The patient received 4500 rad in 15 fractions over 32 days to the tumor and the mediastinal region. An anterior-posterior treatment portal was initially employed (fig. 62.1B), and a cone-down field was used for the final portion of radiation therapy (fig. 62.1C). The patient remains free of any evidence of recurrence of disease now more than seven years after the completion of therapy. Chest x-rays six years after cessation of treatment indicated no evidence of active disease (fig. 62.1D).

In contrast to the usual experience with non-small cell carcinomas of the lung, small cell anaplastic carcinomas have often been shown to respond quite dramatically and rapidly to radiation therapy. Excellent local control rates have been achieved when sufficiently high doses have been given (Choi and Carey 1976). This fact, coupled with the finding of high incidence of distant metastases in small cell disease, suggested the initial use of radiation therapy rather than surgery. A study under the auspices of the Medical Research Council of Great Britain compared radiation versus surgery in clinically limited small cell carcinomas of the bronchus (Fox and Scadding 1973). The patients were randomized to receive either surgery (71 patients) or radical radiation therapy (73 patients). Although the one-year survival rates were approximately 22% in each group, there were statistically significant improved 5- and 10-year survivals in those treated with radiation therapy as compared to surgery (table 62.3). The median survival for those receiving radiation therapy was significantly increased compared to surgically treated patients (300 days versus 199 days).

Chemotherapy is playing an increasingly important role in the management of small cell carcinoma of the lung. Nonetheless, five-year cures have been produced in patients with limited disease treated with radiation therapy alone. A representative case is as follows.

> A 61-year-old woman complained of hemoptysis and dyspnea on exertion. Physical examination was negative but chest x-ray revealed a right hilar mass. Bronchoscopy revealed a mass in the right main stem bronchus, biopsy of which was consistent with small cell carcinoma. Metastatic work-up was negative, and the patient received radical radiation therapy consisting of 3600 rad in 16 fractions over 28 days to the mediastinum and right hilum. The AP-PA opposed fields were used, and subsequent treatment employed lateral fields with a dose of 1800 rad in 6 fractions over 9 days. The patient remains free of any evidence of carcinoma now six years after completion of radiation therapy. Her most recent chest x-ray shows no evidence of active disease.

It is necessary to mention the possible complications of radiation therapy. Numerous technical and pretreatment factors will influence the incidence and severity of side effects: radiation field size, dose per treatment, total treatment time, and total treatment dose. Other lung diseases and prior or subsequent chemotherapy may enhance any radiation-induced damage. The acute complications of irradiation, including cough, dysphagia, esophagitis, and loss of appetite, are usually transitory, beginning during the second week of treatment and resolving within one to two weeks after therapy is completed. It is important that patients are made aware of such possible side effects so that they do not confuse them with the symptoms of progressive disease. Delayed or chronic side effects, including radiation pneumonitis, pericarditis, and myelitis, can occasionally be severe but are rarely life threatening if appropriate attention to normal tissue tolerance is observed. With careful attention to keeping radiation volumes as small as clinically justified, long-term morbidity will be minimal.

Preoperative Radiation Therapy

The fact that a relatively small percentage of patients were cured with either radiation or surgery alone raised hopes that perhaps the combination of radiation therapy followed by surgery would produce dramatically improved results. A large randomized prospective study was undertaken by the Veterans Administration Hospital system to test this hypothesis (Warram 1975). Patients with operable lesions were randomized between immediate surgery and preoperative radiation followed by surgery. The group treated with surgery alone had a 16% five-year survival, which was not statistically dif-

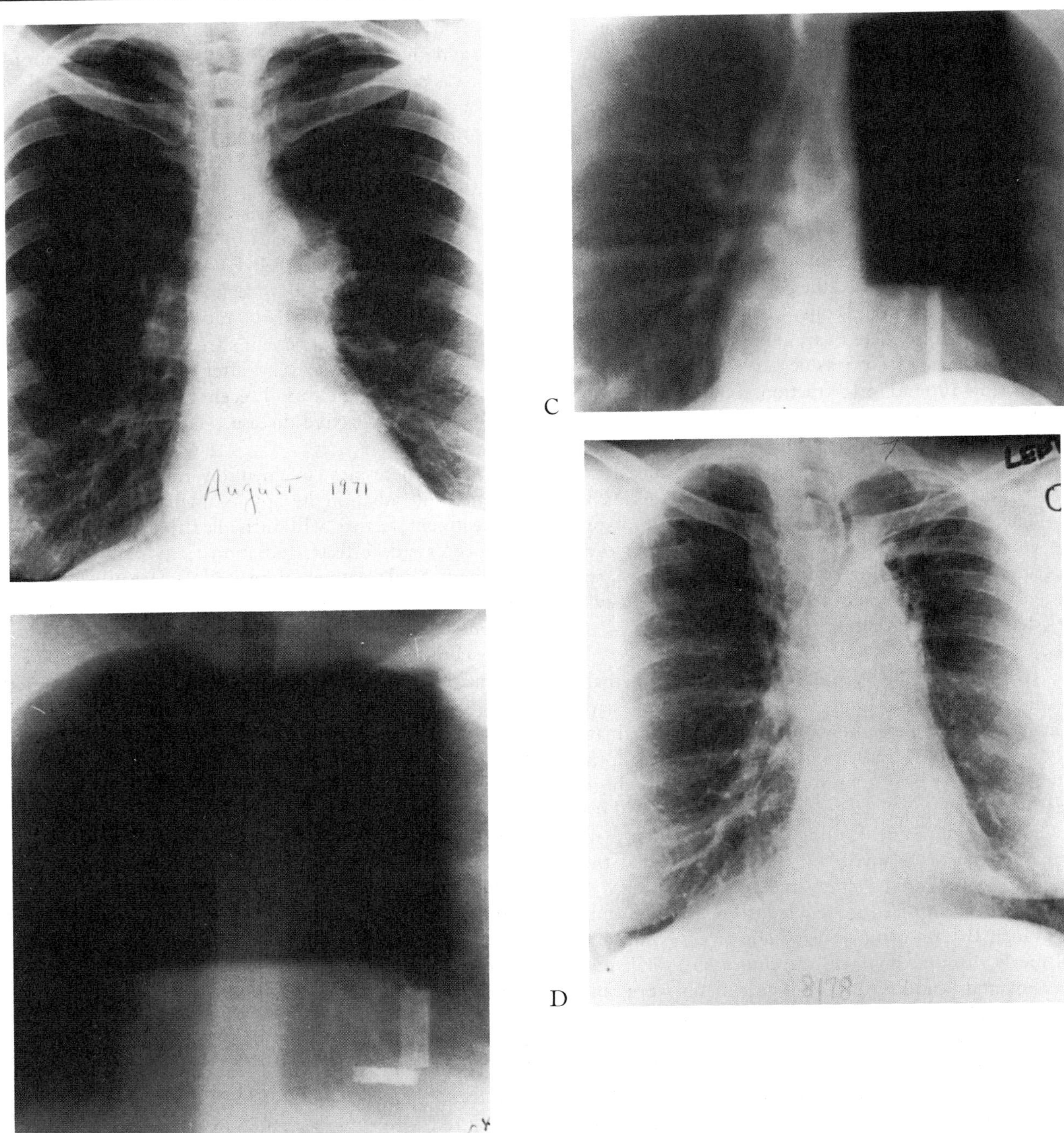

Fig. 62.1. *Curative radiation therapy for inoperable lung cancer.* A, *Pretreatment chest xiray demonstrating the left hilar mass and elevated left hemidiaphragm.* B, *Anterior/posterior opposed radiation therapy treatment portal.* C, *Radiation therapy treatment portal for boost field (total tumor dose 4500 rad, 15 fractions, 32 days).* D, *Chest x-ray six years after completion of radiation therapy.*

Table 62.3. *Radiation Therapy versus Surgery in Small Cell Carcinoma of the Bronchus*

Treatment	*Survival Rates (%)*			*Mean Survival (days)*
	1-Year	*5-Year*	*10-Year*	
Surgery	21	1	0	199*
Irradiation	22	4	4	300*

SOURCE: Modified from Fox and Scadding 1973.
$^{*}P \leqslant 0.04$.

ferent from the results produced by the combination (14%). Similar recurrence patterns were seen for both groups. For patients with initially inoperable disease (mediastinal or supraclavicular nodal involvement, chest wall invasion, or encroachment of tumor on the carina) who underwent surgery after radiation therapy, the five-year survival was 8%, which was not statistically different than for patients with similar disease who received radiation therapy alone (6%). The rates are similar to those of other published series for patients with inoperable lung cancer treated with radiation therapy alone (table 62.2).

Even though the Veterans Administration Hospital study did not demonstrate any survival benefits for preoperative radiation therapy, other studies including those by Paulson (1975) have demonstrated some value of this treatment for patients with carcinomas involving the superior pulmonary sulcus (the so-called Pancoast tumors). Such tumors give rise to characteristic symptom patterns because of their location in the superior pulmonary sulcus adjacent to the first thoracic and eighth cervical nerve roots, the subclavian vessels, the sympathetic chain, and the stellate ganglion. Often the ribs or vertebrae are involved by direct extension of tumor, and the patient may have severe pain in the distribution of the first thoracic and cervical nerve roots. There may also be an associated Horner's syndrome due to the involvement of the sympathetic chain and stellate ganglia. Paulson has reviewed the results from 92 patients with primary carcinoma involving the superior sulcus, 61 of whom completed the combined preoperative radiation therapy and surgery. Excluding the two operative deaths, the 5-year survival of the remaining patients was 35%, the 10-year survival rate 29%. Pancoast tumors are frequently treated with a combination of surgery and radiation therapy; their treatment is illustrated by the following case.

The patient, a 54-year-old man, presented with a three-month history of right shoulder pain. Chest x-ray revealed a right upper lobe mass and erosion of the second rib (fig. 62.2A). Metastatic work-up and bronchoscopy were negative. The patient underwent preoperative radiation therapy to a dose of 3000 rad in 10 fractions over a 14-day period delivered to the mediastinum and right upper lobe (fig. 62.2B). Some tumor regression was noted (fig. 62.2C), and approximately one month later the patient underwent a right upper lobectomy with resection of the ribs, which revealed necrotic epidermoid carcinoma with rib invasion and positive hilar node. Because there was noted invasion of the tumor into the soft tissues of the neck, the patient received additional postoperative radiation therapy to this region marked by metallic clips (fig. 62.2D). The patient remains alive and well for more than four years after completion of treatment.

Occasionally, a patient has an extensive local tumor that the surgeons feel may be marginally resectable. In such selected cases preoperative radiation therapy *may* play some role in overall management although this has not been established in any randomized prospective series (Sherman et al. 1978).

Postoperative Radiation Therapy

With the development of megavoltage techniques in the early 1960s, routine postoperative radiation therapy following potentially curative surgical resection became more widely employed. Paterson and Russell (1962) studied 202 patients with histologically proved lung cancer who were randomized to pneumonectomy or pneumonectomy plus radiation therapy. Irradiation was delivered with a newly developed 4-meV linear accelerator using relatively small fields covering the residual hilum and adjacent mediastium. Approximately 20% of patients failed to receive the proposed dose of 4500 rad. No significant difference in three-year survival rates was noted between patients treated with surgery alone or postoperative irradiation (36% versus 33%). A suggestion of improved survival was noted for those with anaplastic tumors (25% receiving surgery alone versus 35% with surgery plus radiation). There were several problems with this study. The fields employed were relatively small, and experience with the equipment was limited at the initiation of the study. If

Table 62.4. *Postoperative Radiation Therapy in Patients with Positive Lymph Nodes*

Reference	*Five-Year Survival Rate*	
	No Irradiation (No./%)	*With Irradiation (No./%)*
Kirsh et al. 1971	0/12–0%	7/36–19%
Green et al. 1975	1/30–3%	23/66–35%

one stratifies the results according to years of patient entry into this study, one sees a considerable range of survivors for the combination treatment, with a three-year survival rate for patients treated in 1955 of 9.1%, while for those treated in 1958 (when presumably more experience with the equipment had accrued) it was 45%. In addition, no attempt was made to assess survival figures according to local tumor extent or nodal status.

Two subsequent studies have demonstrated improvement in survival with the use of postoperative radiation therapy for selected patients with positive mediastinal or hilar nodes. In a retrospective review by Kirsh and associates (1971) of 231 patients with lung cancer, 48 were found to have positive lymph nodes at the time of gross resection of tumor. Thirty-six received postoperative irradiation (5000 to 5500 rad), while 12 received no additional treatment. A significant difference in the five-year survival rate for those who received the postoperative therapy was seen (19% versus 0%). The difference was most dramatic for patients with tumors of squamous cell histologies.

Similarly, the retrospective review by Green and colleagues (1975) demonstrated the advantage of postoperative radiation therapy in patients with positive nodes. Two hundred and nineteen patients with resectable lung cancer were retrospectively grouped into those with and without nodal metastases. One hundred and twenty-five patients received postoperative irradiation with tumor doses ranging from 3000 to 6000 rad. Their five-year survival was 31% compared to 16% in those receiving surgery alone. The difference was most marked in patients who had positive nodes: 3% five-year survival for those treated with surgery alone, as opposed to 35% for combined therapy (table 62.4). Similar survival rates were obtained for patients with either hilar or mediastinal nodes. A recent study (Choi et al. 1980) lends supportive evidence for this, particularly for patients with adenocarcinomas. Therefore considerable evidence suggests a possible role for postoperative

A

B

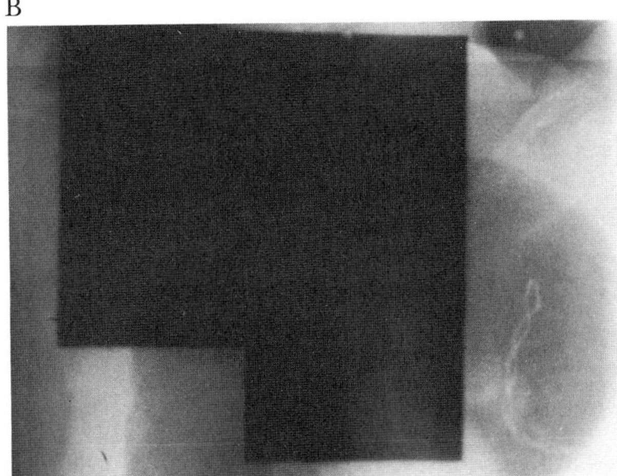

Fig. 62.2. *Combined radiation therapy and surgery in the treatment of Pancoast tumors.* A, *Initial chest x-ray illustrating the right upper lobe mass and erosion of the second rib.* B, *Preoperative radiation therapy anterior/posterior treatment portal.* C, *Repeat chest x-ray after completion of initial radiation therapy.* D, *Postoperative radiation therapy treatment boost field (2700 rad, 12 fractions, 15 days).*

radiation therapy in selected patients who at the time of gross tumor resection are noted to have positive mediastinal or hilar nodal involvement.

Palliative Radiation Therapy

Superior Vena Caval Obstruction

Several emergency situations can develop in patients with lung cancer that require prompt radiotherapeutic intervention. Development of superior vena caval obstruction (SVCO) often can be the initial event. The syndrome occurs in about 3% to 4% of all these patients, and 75% to 80% of the obstructions are due to lung cancer (Perez et al. 1978). In recent years, only 5% of SVCO was from benign causes, although in the past up to 40% was due to syphilitic aortic aneurysm or tuberculous mediastinitis (Schechter 1954). The syndrome is produced by extrinsic compression of the superior vena cava and associated tributaries or by the development of intracaval thrombosis. The patient may have distension of the veins of the thorax or neck, edema or plethora of the face, tachypnea, or cyanosis. Chest x-ray most often demonstrates a mass involving the superior mediastinum and/or the right hilum, but it may appear normal. Superior vena cavagram or scan can be obtained to demonstrate the site of obstruction (Lokich and Goodman 1975).

Management consists of *prompt* irradiation to the mediastinum, hilum, and any adjacent pulmonary lesions employing either a rapid high-dose per fraction schedule or conventionally fractionated radiation. Supportive therapy is individual, and when necessary should include oxygen, diuretics, steriods, and anticoagulants.

No proved benefit has been demonstrated for the concurrent use of chemotherapy for SVCO caused by bronchogenic carcinoma. This is one of the few situations in the practice of radiation therapy in which institution of treatment is based on clinical findings alone, and it should not be delayed pending histologic diagnosis or extensive metastatic work-up. The risk of possible massive hemorrhage or respiratory compromise following surgical manipulation in regions of dilated veins and edematous tissue has been stressed. As subsequent management will be dependent on the tumor histopathology, however, a tissue diagnosis should be obtained once the patient has stabilized and the increased venous pressure has abated.

C

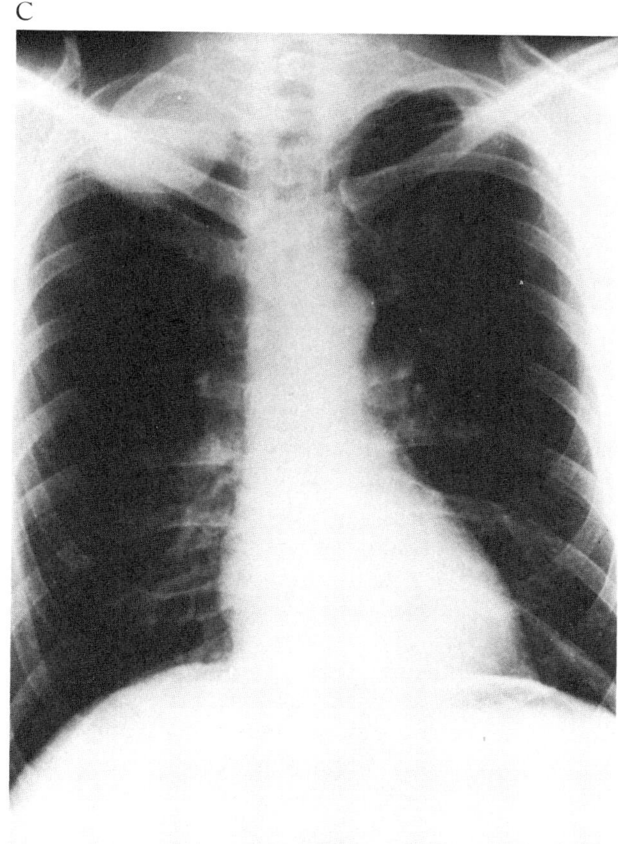

D

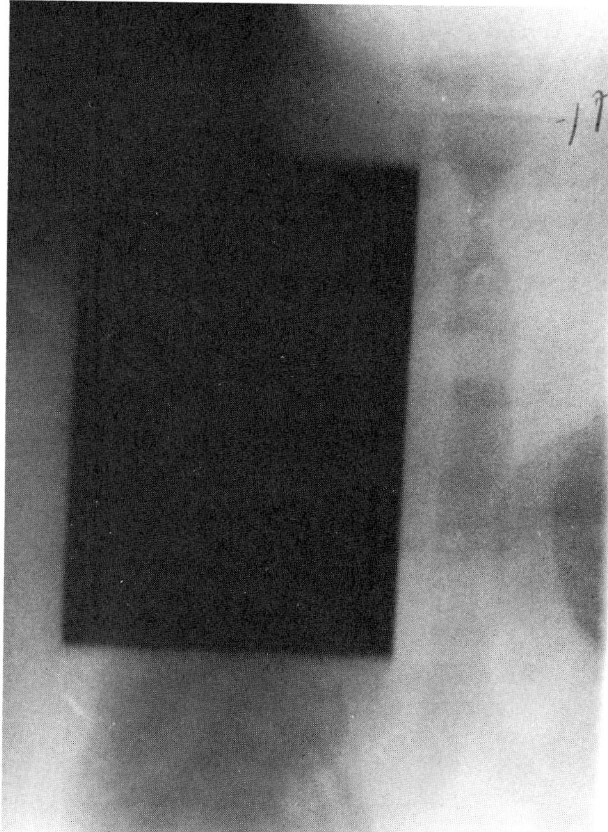

The response to radiation therapy in these patients is often dramatic, with excellent or good symptomatic response reported in 70% to 90% of the patients within one week of the start of therapy (Perez et al. 1978; Davenport et al. 1978). More rapid high-dose per fraction courses are thought by some to produce especially prompt relief of symptoms (Rubin et al. 1963), but the ultimate outcome of treatment appears to be the same as with conventional fractionation provided sufficient total dose is delivered. Although in most cases the management of SVCO is palliative in intent, the existence of superior vena caval obstruction does not per se preclude curative radiation therapy. Indeed, a small percentage of patients will be long-term survivors following appropriate, prompt radiation intervention (Perez et al. 1978).

Spinal Cord Compression

A second problem requiring prompt treatment that often develops in patients with lung cancer is spinal cord compression secondary to epidural metastases. Bruckman and Bloomer (1978) have recently reviewed the occurrence of this complication and report that bronchogenic carcinoma represents the most common primary tumor site. The symptoms include pain and progressive motor dysfunction, paresthesias, sensory loss, and loss of sphincter control. Immediate diagnostic work-up is imperative and should include spine films since bony abnormalities are seen in more than 66% of the cases. A lumbar myelogram should be performed, and if a complete block is noted a cisternal dye injection should be obtained to delineate its extent. Cerebrospinal fluid should also be obtained at the time of the myelogram for cytology, cell count, and chemistries. The most common location for epidural metastases from lung cancer is the thoracic spine.

In Bruckman and Bloomer's review, radiation therapy alone was recommended in patients who had minimal or slowly progressive symptoms, incomplete block by myelogram, or metastases to the cauda equina. The authors recommended concomitant high-dose steroids. For patients with rapidly progressive or acutely severe neurologic deficits, those in whom the primary site of disease remains unknown, those with high cervical cord compression, or patients failing to respond to radiation therapy, their recommendation was for initial decompressive laminectomy to be followed by postoperative radiation therapy. The response to treatment was dependent on the severity and rapidity of onset of motor dysfunction, with the best results from treatment being obtained in patients with less severe dysfunction and slow onset of symptoms. The recovery rates were best for posterior lesions and worse for anterior lesions; more favorable responses were noted in the upper thoracic than in the lower thoracic spine areas. Only 14% of patients treated were reported to have a satisfactory response (defined as sphincter control and ability to walk without assistance for three or more months) to treatment.

Considerable controversy exists as to the role of decompressive laminectomy in the treatment of these patients. Gilbert and co-workers (1978) strongly advocate the use of radiation therapy alone in most situations. A recent review of 235 patients seen at Memorial Sloan-Kettering Cancer Center was undertaken. The patients were grouped into those receiving surgery and postoperative irradiation versus those who received radiation therapy alone. In the later years of the study, most were placed on concurrent high-dose steroids. The majority of patients in this series had pain that was usually local or radicular. For those whose primary disease was bronchogenic carcinoma, the majority of epidural metastases were in the thoracic spine. The blocks demonstrated on myelogram were usually at the site of the vertebral body involved by the tumor, and the majority of tumors were anterior to the spinal cord. The radiation portal was that of a single posterior field encompassing at least one or two vertebral bodies above and below the level of the block. There was a wide variation in the dosage and fractionation schedules, with emphasis on initiating therapy with several high-dose per fraction treatments. The addition of laminectomy prior to irradiation was demonstrated retrospectively to have no benefit to patients with epidural metastases from lung cancer. The authors felt that the procedure was indicated only when the diagnosis of the primary tumor was in doubt, when relapse occurred in a previously irradiated area, or when the symptoms progressed during radiation therapy.

A conflicting result, however, has been reported by Brady and associates (1975) in their review of 133 patients with metastatic spinal cord tumors. Their reported response rate was 61% for patients treated by surgical decompression followed by radiation therapy, which was superior to that obtained for patients treated with surgery alone (29%) or with irradiation alone (47%). They concluded that the combination was most likely to yield the best result. It therefore remains unclear as to the role of surgical decompression, particularly for those less radiosensitive tumors such as the non-small cell bronchogenic carcinomas, or for patients with rapidly progressive paralysis. The optimal fractionation schedule and steroid dose remain to be further defined.

Brain Metastases

Brain metastases occur in 20% to 40% of patients with carcinoma of the lung. Often, prompt therapeutic intervention is required to relieve life-threatening symptoms caused by increased intracranial pressure. Brain metastasis occurs most frequently in small cell carcinoma of the lung and least often in patients with squamous cell disease. In a review by Deeley and Edwards (1968) 24% of patients had no other metastatic disease outside of the brain. A single focus of metastasis may occur approximately 10% of the time. Prompt intervention with radiation therapy is felt by many to be the treatment of choice, and the concomitant use of high-dose steroids may be beneficial. The role of surgery remains controversial. Montana, Meacham, and Caldwell (1972) found no difference in survival between patients treated with craniotomy and radiation therapy versus those treated with irradiation alone. It is felt by some neurosurgeons that surgical removal of the lesion is the treatment of choice if one is relatively certain that a solitary metastasis exists and if there is no evidence of disease spread outside the central nervous system. In addition, surgery is in order if there is uncertainty in diagnosis of metastasis versus a primary tumor.

Radiation therapy of symptomatic brain metastases results in palliation in approximately 80% of the cases with an occasional long-term survivor noted. Chu and Hilaris (1961) reviewed 218 patients with intracranial metastases, 34% of whom had lung cancer. Initial signs and symptoms included headache, dizziness, nausea and vomiting, incontinence, visual changes, changes in mentation, and seizures. Physical examination demonstrated papilledema, hemiparesis, hemiplegia, paresthesias, central nervous system palsies, cerebellar signs, and coma. The patients were treated with whole brain irradiation with opposing lateral fields, with doses on the order of 3000 rad in three weeks. The treatment was well tolerated, with 83% having symptomatic responses lasting one month or longer. Those treated with doses of more than 2750 rad had significantly longer remissions.

Of 88 patients with clinically diagnosed brain metastases treated by radiation (Deeley and Edwards 1968), significant palliation was obtained in 48%. Those with squamous cell lung cancers had the best response. Survival rates for patients who completed therapy were 14% at one year and 4% at three years.

Hazra and co-workers (1972) reviewed the results at Johns Hopkins University in 55 patients with brain metastases treated with a variety of modalities including radiation therapy, steroids, and surgery. In this retrospective nonrandomized study the most significant improvement and the longest survivals were obtained in patients treated primarily with radiation therapy. Although steroids often produced short-term improvement, the average survival in patients treated with steroids alone was in the order of 9 weeks in comparison to 27.8 weeks for those treated with radiation therapy.

The optimal treatment schedule for palliation remains unclear. Hendrickson (1977) has reported the response rate of over 1000 patients with brain metastases, 62% of whom had lung cancer as the primary site. Varying fractionation schedules from 2000 rad in one week to 4000 rad in four weeks were used but steroids and chemotherapy were not controlled. Eighty percent to 90% of the patients treated had partial or complete improvement of symptoms, and no significant differences in response rates among the treatment schedules could be delineated. It was felt that the higher doses in the shorter times were slightly superior both in the promptness and duration of symptomatic relief.

As mentioned, one occasionally obtains long-term disease control in patients treated for brain metastases in lung cancer, particularly if the brain is the only site of metastatic spread. One such case is presented.

> The patient is a 64-year-old woman, who presented in January 1974 with hoarseness and progressive cough. Local cord paralysis was noted, and a chest x-ray revealed a large left hilar mass with mediastinal involvement. Exploratory thoracotomy revealed a large tumor mass wrapped around the aorta. Histopathology revealed a small cell carcinoma. Metastatic work-up including brain scan was negative (fig. 62.3A). The patient was treated with a split-course radiation therapy technique with excellent response obtained, except for some subsequent radiation fibrosis and pneumonitis. The patient did well until June 1975 when she developed loss of balance, and a brain scan (fig. 62.3B) revealed a right parieto-occipital metastasis which was aggressively treated with radiation therapy. Post-treatment brain scan returned to normal (fig. 62.3C). The patient remained free of disease for two and one-half years when she developed an adenocarcinoma of the

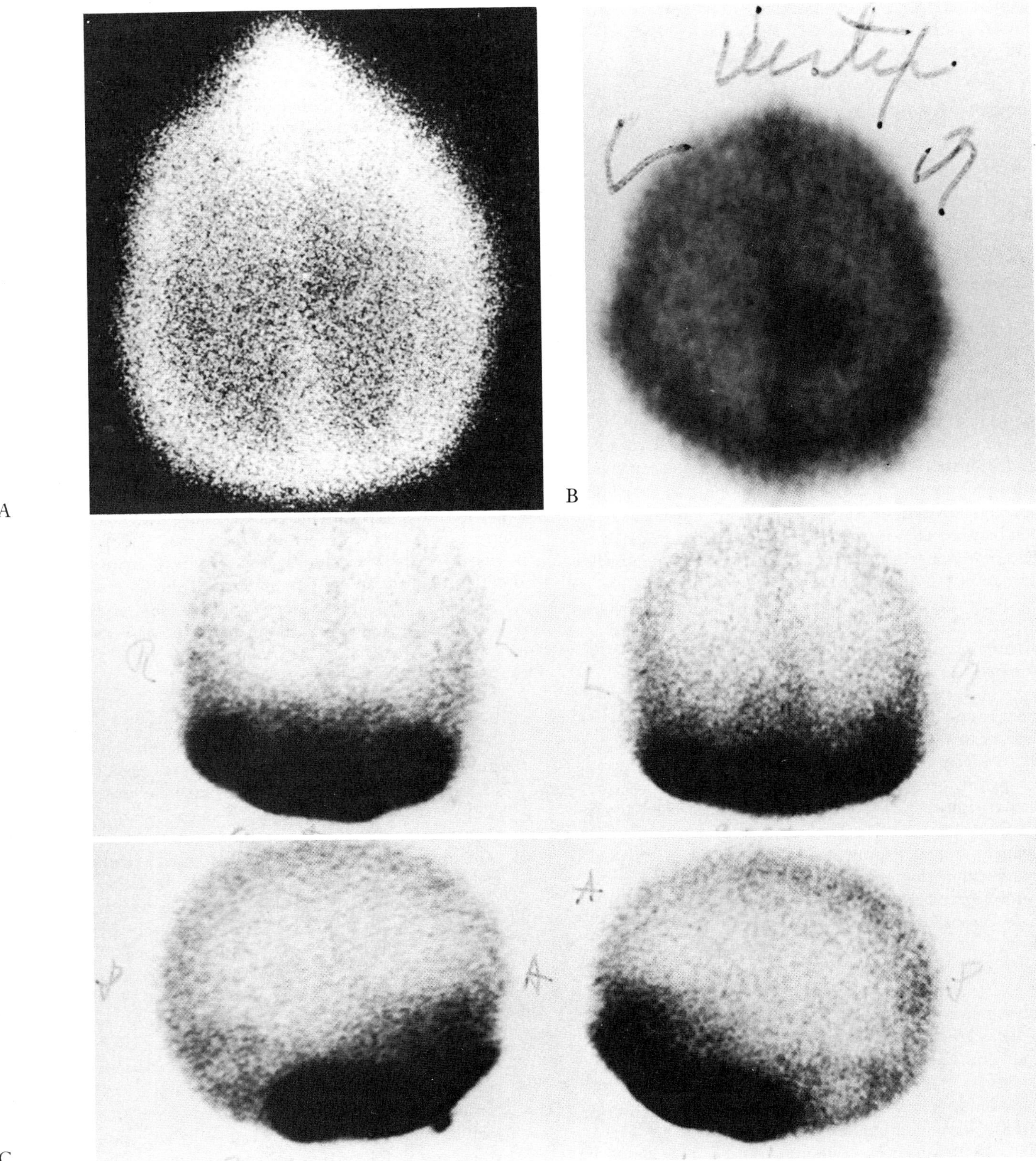

Fig. 62.3. *Long-term local control of lung cancer metastatic to brain.* A, *Normal brain scan obtained at the time of initial evaluation in January 1974.* B, *Brain scan in June 1975 revealing the right parietal-occipital metastasis.* C, *Brain scan five months after completion of radiation therapy (total dose 4150 rad) showing excellent tumor response.*

Table 62.5. *Palliative Radiation Therapy in Management of Lung Cancer*

Symptom	*Improved (%)*	*No Change (%)*	*Worse (%)*
Hemoptysis	75–95	5–25	—
Cough	50–75	29–40	3
Pain	60–72	24–40	4

SOURCES: Line and Deeley 1971; Schultz 1966; Garland and Sisson 1956.

gallbladder and subsequently died from widespread intraabdominal adenocarcinoma. Autopsy, however, revealed no evidence for residual small cell carcinoma, even in the lung or in the brain regions.

Palliation of Other Symptoms

Radiation therapy is useful in the palliation of symptoms including hemoptysis, cough, and bone pain secondary to metastatic disease. Several studies have demonstrated that between 60% and 90% of patients have symptomatic improvement following radiation therapy (table 62.5).

Small Cell Carcinoma

Intrathoracic Disease

There are some exciting recent developments concerning chemotherapy in the treatment of small cell carcinoma of the lung (see chapter 60). Such tumors can also respond promptly to radiation therapy, and in the small percentage that are localized at diagnosis, the treatment can be curative (Matthews et al. 1980). Although its role in this era of multiagent chemotherapy is questioned by some, radiation doses of between 4000 and 5000 rad have been shown to produce local control in 80% to 90% of patients treated (Choi and Carey 1976) and occasional cures have been obtained. Only one instance of five-year survival has been reported to the best of my knowledge following chemotherapy alone for small cell carcinoma of the lung (Matthews et al. 1980). When radiation therapy is used with curative intent it is important that relatively high doses be employed. Low doses, even in conjunction with chemotherapy, have not been shown to be effective (Alexander et al. 1977). One recent study (McMahon et al. 1979) compared low-dose radiation (3000 rad) with intermediate doses (4000 to 4500 rad) delivered to the primary tumor site and mediastinum in conjunction with chemotherapy. Increased median survival time and increased duration of local intrathoracic control was seen in patients treated with the higher radiation doses whether they had limited or extensive disease.

Prophylactic Brain Irradiation

When used prophylactically against possible micrometastases, lower doses, such as 3000 rad in 10 treatments, have proved to be efficacious in suppressing the occurrence of clinical disease in the irradiated sites. Bunn, Nugent, and Matthews (1978) have reviewed the high frequency of brain metastases reported in small cell carcinomas of the lung and noted their occurrence in 30% of 740 patients studied at autopsy. Three randomized trials have been reviewed using prophylactic cranial irradiation, and all demonstrated the statistically significant ability of radiation therapy to decrease the number of central nervous system relapses. Combining these studies, the incidence of relapses with brain disease in the prophylactically irradiated group of 103 patients was 6% compared to 28% of the 127 patients who were not so treated. Prolongation of survival, however, has not yet been achieved. This probably awaits the development of more effective chemotherapeutic agents to control the disease at other sites. Nonetheless, we now have at our disposal, with relatively benign therapy, the ability to prevent the often quite incapacitating effects of cranial metastases. Therefore prophylactic cranial irradiation should be employed in any study situation once disease at the other sites has been brought into remission.

At Yale our current protocol employs multiple-agent chemotherapy with doxorubicin, cyclophosphamide, vincristine, and etoposide (VP-16-213). The last drug when used alone reportedly showed an overall response rate of 44% in patients with small cell carcinoma of the lung (Eagan et al. 1976). Patients with limited disease confined to one hemithorax, mediastinum, and supraclavicular region receive split-course radiation therapy (total dose 5400 rad) in addition to the polychemotherapy. Patients with advanced disease receive radiation therapy optionally to symptomatic sites of disease or in emergency situations. Prophylactic whole brain irradiation is employed in all patients who have obtained complete remissions following systemic chemotherapy.

References

Abadir, R., and Muggia, F. M. Irradiated lung cancer. An autopsy analysis of spread pattern. *Radiology* 114:427–430, 1975.

Alexander, M. et al. Combined modality treatment for oat cell carcinoma of the lung: a randomized trial. *Cancer Treat. Rep.* 61:1–6, 1977.

Aristizabal, S. A., and Caldwell, W. L. Radical irradiation with the split-course technique in carcinoma of the lung. *Cancer* 37:2630–2635, 1976.

Bloedorn, F. G. Rationale and benefit of preoperative irradiation in lung cancer. *JAMA* 196:340–341, 1966.

Brady, L. W. et al. The treatment of metastatic disease of the nervous system by radiation therapy. In *Tumors of the nervous system,* ed. H. G. Seydel. New York: John Wiley & Sons, 1975.

Bromley, L. L., and Szur, L. Combined radiotherapy and resection for carcinoma of the bronchus: experiences with 66 patients. *Lancet* 2:937–941, 1955.

Bruckman, J. E., and Bloomer, W. D. Management of spinal cord compression. *Semin. Oncol.* 5:135–140, 1978.

Bunn, P. A.; Nugent, J. L.; and Matthews, M. J. Central nervous system metastases in small cell bronchogenic carcinoma. *Semin. Oncol.* 5:314–322, 1978.

Choi, N. C. H. et al. Basis for new strategies in postoperative radiotherapy of bronchogenic carcinoma. *Int. J. Radiat. Oncol. Biol. Phys.* 6:31–35, 1980.

Choi, N. C. H., and Carey, R. W. Small cell anaplastic carcinoma of the lung. Reappraisal of current management. *Cancer* 37:2651–2657, 1976.

Chu, F. C. H., and Hilaris, B. B. Value of radiation therapy in the management of intracranial metastases. *Cancer* 14:577–581, 1961.

Coy, P., and Kennelly, G. M. The role of curative radiotherapy in treatment of lung cancer. *Cancer* 45:698–702, 1980.

Davenport, D. et al. Radiation therapy in the treatment of superior vena caval obstruction. *Cancer* 42:2600–2603, 1978.

Deeley, T. J., and Edwards, J. M. R. Radiotherapy in the management of cerebral secondaries from bronchial carcinoma. *Lancet* 1:1209–1213, 1968.

Eagan, R. T. et al. VP-16-213 versus polychemotherapy in patients with advanced small cell cancer. *Cancer Treat. Rep.* 60:949–951, 1976.

Eisert, D. R.; Cox, J. D.; and Komaki, R. Irradiation for bronchial carcinoma: reasons for failure. I. Analysis of local control as function of dose, time, and fractionation. *Cancer* 37:2665–2670, 1976.

Fox, W., and Scadding, J. G. Medical Research Council comparative trial of surgery and radiotherapy for primary treatment of small celled or oat celled carcinoma of bronchus. *Lancet* 1:63–65, 1973.

Garland, L. H., and Sisson, M. A. The results of radiation of bronchial cancer. *Radiology* 67:48–62, 1956.

Gilbert, R. W. et al. Epidural spinal cord compression from metastatic tumor: diagnosis and treatment. *Ann. Neurol.* 3:40–51, 1978.

Green, N. et al. Postresection irradiation for primary lung cancer. *Radiology* 116:405–407, 1975.

Hazra, T. et al. Management of cerebral metastasis from bronchogenic carcinoma. *Johns Hopkins Med. J.* 130:377–383, 1972.

Hendrickson, F. R. The optimum schedule for palliative radiotherapy for metastatic brain cancer. *Int. J. Radiat. Oncol.* 2:165–168, 1977.

Kirsh, M. et al. Treatment of bronchogenic carcinoma with mediastinal metastases. *Ann. Thorac. Surg.* 12:11–21, 1971.

Lawton, R. L. et al. Preoperative irradiation in the treatment of clinically operable lung cancer. *J. Thorac. Cardiovasc. Surg.* 51:745–750, 1966.

Lee, R. E. Radiotherapy of bronchogenic carcinoma. *Semin. Oncol.* 1:245–252, 1974.

Line, D., and Deeley, T. J. Palliative therapy. In *Carcinoma of the bronchus,* ed. T. J. Deeley. New York: Appleton-Century-Crofts, 1971.

Lokich, J. J., and Goodman, R. Superior vena cava syndrome. *JAMA* 231:58–61, 1975.

Manfredi, F. et al. Preoperative irradiation in bronchogenic carcinoma. *Am. Rev. Respir. Dis.* 94:584–588, 1966.

Matthews, M. J. et al. Long-term survivors with small cell carcinoma of the lung. *Eur. J. Cancer* 16:527–531, 1980.

McMahon, L. J. et al. Patterns of relapse in patients with small cell carcinoma of the lung treated with Adriamycin-cyclophosphamide chemotherapy and radiation therapy. *Cancer Treat. Rep.* 63:359–362, 1979.

Montana, G. S.; Meacham, W. F.; and Caldwell, W. L. Brain irradiation for metastatic disease of lung origin. *Cancer* 29:1477–1480, 1972.

Morrison, R. et al. The treatment of carcinoma of the bronchus. A clinical trial to compare surgery and supervoltage radiotherapy. *Lancet* 1:683–684, 1963.

Paterson, R., and Russell, M. H. Clinical trials in malignant disease. IV. Lung cancer. Value of post-operative radiotherapy. *Clin. Radiol.* 13:141–144, 1962.

Paulson, D. L. Carcinomas in the superior pulmonary sulcus. *J. Thorac. Cardiovasc. Surg.* 70:1095–1104, 1975.

Perez, C. et al. Management of superior vena cava syndrome. *Semin. Oncol.* 5:123–134, 1978.

Rissanen, P. M. et al. Autopsy findings in lung cancer treated with megavoltage radiotherapy. *Acta Radiol. Ther. Stockh.* 7:433–442, 1968.

Roswit, B.; Patno, M. E.; and Rapp, R. The survival of patients with inoperable lung cancer: a large-scale randomized study of radiation therapy versus placebo. *Radiology* 90:688–697, 1968.

Rubin, P. et al. Superior vena caval syndrome. Slow low-dose versus rapid high-dose schedules. *Radiology* 81:388–401, 1963.

Schechter, M. M. The superior vena cava syndrome. *Am. J. Med. Sci.* 227:46–56, 1954.

Schultz, M. D. Bronchogenic carcinoma stages III and IV. Palliation by radiotherapy. *JAMA* 196:33–34, 1966.

Sherman, D. M. et al. An aggressive approach to marginally resectable lung cancer. *Cancer* 41:2040–2045, 1978.

Shields, T. W. et al. Preoperative x-ray therapy as adjuvant in the treatment of bronchogenic carcinoma. *J. Thorac. Cardiovasc. Surg.* 59:49–61, 1970.

Smart, J. Can lung cancer be cured by irradiation alone? *JAMA* 195:16–17, 1966.

Stanford, W. et al. Results of treatment of primary carcinoma of the lung. Analysis of 3,000 cases. *J. Thorac. Cardiovasc. Surg.* 72:441–449, 1976.

Warram, J. Preoperative irradiation of cancer of the lung: final report of a therapeutic trial. *Cancer* 36:914–925, 1975.

sixty-three

Soft Tissue and Bone Sarcomas

IVAN S. LOWENTHAL
DAVID S. FISCHER

Soft tissue sarcomas are of mesenchymal origin and can occur in any of the nonvisceral connective tissues. These, along with the primary bone tumors, Ewing's sarcoma, and osteogenic sarcoma, account for about 1% of all malignant tumors in adults and for about 7% in children. They include a variety of types (fig. 63.1) in which several histopathologic patterns may be present simultaneously. Therefore diagnosis is dependent on the amount of tissue studied and its dominant features. Accordingly, for therapeutic purposes they are often considered as one group. Although the response rate to chemotherapy has been fairly consistent for the various types, clinical values that appear to have prognostic significance include histopathologic grade, tumor size, and pathologic type (Suit, Russell, and Martin 1975). These should be taken into account in evaluating chemotherapy trials. A review of the subject has recently been published (Sears et al. 1981).

Childhood Sarcomas

The treatment of sarcomas in children was one of the first examples of the multimodal approach to cancer therapy. Since radical surgery and radiation therapy or conservative surgery and radiation therapy give equivalent local control and survival, the use of radiation therapy in the treatment of the primary tumor has permitted surgery aimed at conservation of function (Dritschilo et al. 1978). This combination treatment has not improved survival, however, because many sarcomas are high-grade, high-stage lesions with occult distant metastases at the time of diagnosis. Therefore chemotherapy has been incorporated into primary treatment before there is clinical evidence of systemic disease.

Chemotherapy has been demonstrated to be active in macrometastatic tumors, which is the basis for its use against microscopic, clinically occult disease. Vincristine, cyclophosphamide, dactinomycin, and/or doxorubicin—single agents with activity against sarcomas in children—have been most frequently used in combination in multimodal approaches.

Rhabdomyosarcoma

In multidisciplinary protocols for therapy of embryonal rhabdomyosarcoma, surgical reduction of tumor volume is usually the first step in achievement of a tumor-free state. Radiation therapy administered postoperatively is more successful in eradicating localized microscopic foci than gross disease. Combination chemotherapy is then used to treat occult distant metastases. This approach has resulted in a marked increase in tumor-free survival. Ghavimi and co-workers (1975) report that 100% of children with embryonal rhabdomyosarcoma stages I and II and 67% with stage III disease are alive disease-free up to 42 months. This compares to the approximately 20% survival rate of patients treated previously with surgery and/or radiation therapy alone.

Similar results have been reported by the Children's Cancer Study Group (CCSG) (Raney, Schnaufer, and Donaldson 1974). A control group of children whose tumors were completely resected received radiation therapy but no chemotherapy; 57% developed local recurrence or metastases compared to only 18% of those who also received chemotherapy.

Donaldson and associates (1973) reported on 19 patients with head and neck rhabdomyosarcoma who underwent surgical biopsy alone followed by aggressive radiation therapy and chemotherapy. Seventy-four percent were alive without recurrence from two to seven years at the time of the report.

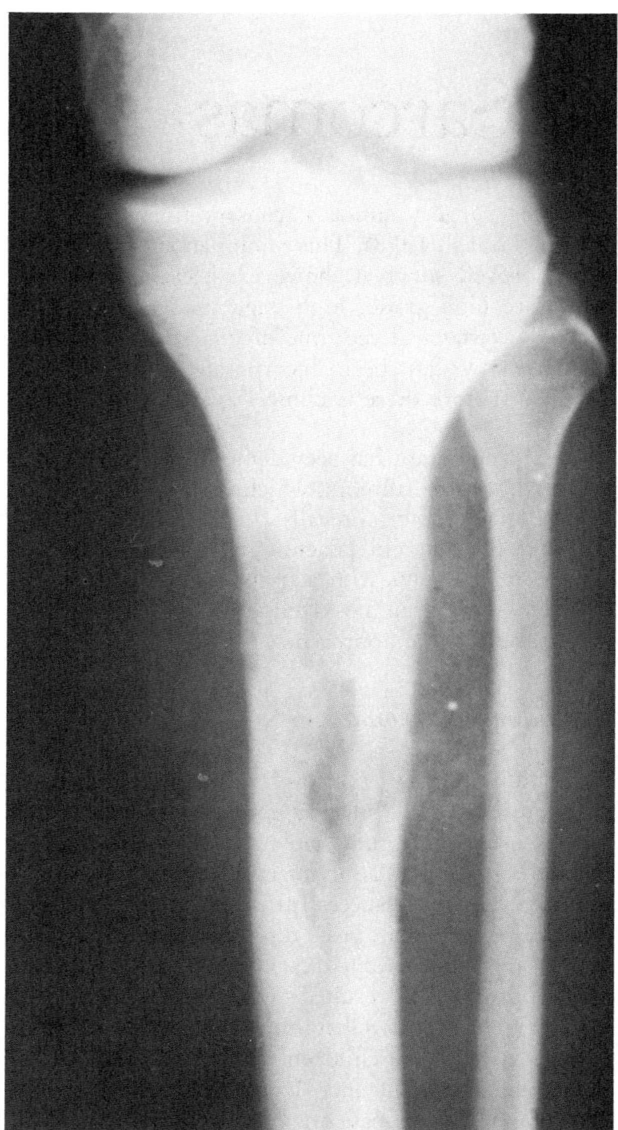

Fig. 63.1. *X-ray of tibia involved by fibrosarcoma of bone.*

More recently, the Intergroup Rhabdomyosarcoma Study has reported two-year relapse-free survival rates of 83% and 72% for localized and regional disease, respectively, treated after resection with vincristine, dactinomycin (Actinomycin D), and cyclophosphamide (VAC) combination chemotherapy with and without radiation therapy (Tefft 1979). They have shown that postoperative irradiation is unnecessary when VAC is administered for two years to patients with localized disease. In addition, in more advanced disease where there is incomplete resection or biopsy alone is performed, radiation therapy is as effective at doses of 3500 to 4000 rad as at 5000 to 6000 rad when patients also receive adjuvant chemotherapy.

Ewing's Sarcoma

A similar approach to the treatment of Ewing's sarcoma has resulted in marked improvement in survival. After local treatment with surgery only or with radiation therapy the five-year survival is less than 15%. The intergroup Ewing's Sarcoma Study has enrolled 264 children with a reported three-year survival for all patients of 56% (Tefft 1979). The most efficacious adjuvant chemotherapy after radiotherapy was a combination of VAC plus doxorubicin, with 74% of patients disease-free at two years. In another study of the adjuvant therapy of Ewing's sarcoma, a European group reported 50% of patients disease-free at three years after treatment with vincristine, cyclophosphamide, doxorubicin, and procarbazine for 18 months following radiation therapy (Le Mevel et al. 1979). Presently, a more intensive chemotherapy protocol is being evaluated by this group aimed at eliminating early relapses that occur primarily in the first two years.

Osteosarcoma

Osteogenic sarcoma occurs predominantly in children and young adults. Previously, the only agents with limited activity in this disease were the alkylating agents with which response rates up to 20% were reported. In the early 1970s, doxorubicin was found to be effective in 30% to 40% of patients. At about the same time, high-dose methotrexate-citrovorum factor (CF) programs demonstrated a similar response rate when methotrexate was administered every three weeks. With careful monitoring, large doses of methotrexate with CF rescue could be given on a weekly basis and this program has produced an objective response in over 80% of patients with overt osteogenic sarcoma (Frei et al. 1978). Recently, cisplatin has been reported to be effective, even in patients previously treated with chemotherapy (Ochs et al. 1978).

As in rhabdomyosarcoma and Ewing's sarcoma, the rationale for adjuvant chemotherapy in most cases of osteosarcoma is that it is microscopically disseminated at the time of diagnosis. This is shown by the development of pulmonary metastases in 80% of untreated patients soon after amputation (Frei et al. 1978). Also, as is true in most instances, chemotherapy is more effective against minimal disease than against large tumors, and to achieve cure virtually all malignant cells must be destroyed.

The use of adjuvant chemotherapy has improved the previous disease-free survival from 20% in untreated patients to 50% at three years when methotrexate and vincristine are used as adjuvant therapy, and to 70% when doxorubicin is added. Late relapses are infrequent with either combination. The Mayo Clinic recently reported an improvement in survival even in patients who received no postoperative adjuvant chemotherapy. For patients accrued between 1972 and 1974, the three-year survival had become 50%, compared to the 20% to 25% noted previously for untreated patients (Taylor et al. 1978). Although this change has not been reported by other institutions conducting trials in osteogenic sarcoma, it does call into question the use of historical controls. It is possible that prognostic variables such as age, histology, and size and location of tumor as well as the use of newer, more sensitive diagnostic techniques such as the lung CT scan and better surgery have played a role in the results obtained with adjuvant chemotherapy. A preliminary report of a prospective randomized study of high-dose methotrexate adjuvant therapy versus postoperative observation alone reveals 52% of patients disease-free at two years with no significant difference between groups (Edmonson et al. 1980).

In patients who relapse after receiving adjuvant chemotherapy it has been shown that the time to development of metastatic disease may be delayed and the number of metastases decreased (Jaffe et al. 1978). This, together with the increasing effectiveness of systemic therapy, has led to treatment programs of curative intent for patients whose disease relapses. These involve combined chemotherapy and surgery for resectable pulmonary metastases. Therapy is initiated with one or the other depending on the clinical situation.

Thoracotomy may precede chemotherapy when metastases are solitary and occur after a prolonged disease-free interval, usually greater than a year. Alternatively, chemotherapy will precede surgery if metastases occur early or are diffuse, making the presence of nonvisible deposits of tumor in the lung likely and resection impractical. In such instances thoracotomy is performed to remove residual disease after chemotherapy, which may be continued postoperatively.

In the instance of late solitary metastases that are less likely to be associated with subclinical disease, Rosen and colleagues (1978) report that 70% of patients are alive and free of disease at a median follow-up of three years, although some have been followed for five years disease-free. Some patients who relapsed after initial thoracotomy and chemotherapy underwent repeat thoracotomy and chemotherapy and continue disease-free. Fewer patients survived who initially had early or diffuse metastases presumably representing more rapidly growing tumors or tumors that demonstrated less response to previous adjuvant chemotherapy. Even in this circumstance, however, 12 of 31 patients remain disease-free with a median follow-up of 19 months from the start of chemotherapy (Rosen et al. 1978).

The results with adjuvant therapy of primary and metastatic osteogenic sarcoma show that chemotherapy is effective in controlling, and in some instances eradicating, both micrometastatic and macrometastatic disease. In particular, it has been shown that metastatic bone lesions could be effectively treated with chemotherapy (Rosen et al. 1979). This has led to the use of chemotherapy before primary surgery to allow earlier treatment of occult disease, which primarily effects survival, and determination of the dose of chemotherapy necessary to achieve a response to be used postoperatively as adjuvant therapy. In addition, it allows time for development of an endoprosthesis for subsequent en bloc resection of tumor, thus avoiding amputation.

These authors (Rosen et al. 1979) have reported on the use of preoperative as well as postoperative chemotherapy in the treatment of primary osteogenic sarcoma using a combination of high-dose methotrexate-CF, vincristine, doxorubicin, and cyclophosphamide. The four-year survival for the group receiving adjuvant chemotherapy alone is 52% versus 77% for patients receiving preoperative and postoperative chemotherapy. They feel that a predominant reason for this better result is the ability to escalate the methotrexate dose up to 20 gm until a tumor response is obtained, and thus an effective dose is determined for use as adjuvant therapy following surgery. More recently, bleomycin and dactinomycin have been incorporated into the treatment regimen, but the follow-up of patients so treated is too short to adequately determine the effect of this combination on survival.

Newer approaches to the adjuvant therapy of osteogenic sarcoma appear promising. New chemotherapy combinations now being tested include doxorubicin and cisplatin. In one preliminary report of patients treated with this combination, 10 of 11 remain disease-free with a mean time on study of 21 months (Ettinger et al. 1979).

Another approach is the use of Coumadin to inter-

Table 63.1. *Single-Drug Therapy with Adriamycin in Metastatic Sarcomas: Cumulative Literature Survey*

Diagnosis	*Number of Patients*	*Number of Responses*	*Response Rate (%)*
Soft tissue sarcomas			
Rhabdomyosarcoma	79	21	27
Fibrosarcoma and neurofibrosarcoma	38	9	24
Leiomyosarcoma	37	12	32
Synovial cell carcinoma	22	7	32
Liposarcoma	19	6	32
Angiosarcoma	16	7	44
Undifferentiated sarcoma	16	3	19
Unspecified and miscellaneous	130	31	24
Total	357	96	27
Bone sarcomas			
Osteogenic sarcoma	81	18	22
Ewing's sarcoma	63	27	37
Chondrosarcoma	17	1	6
Total	161	46	29
All sarcomas	518	142	27

SOURCE: Gottlieb et al. 1975.

fere with tumor cell emboli lodging in capillary beds. Hoover and colleagues (1978) have reported 56% survival after five to eight years in nine patients begun on Coumadin therapy before primary surgery. In addition, experimental studies have shown a greater effect of chemotherapy when combined with an anticoagulant, so this may be optimal treatment.

Adult Sarcomas

Whereas VAC combination chemotherapy gives an approximately 45% response rate in childhood soft tissue sarcomas, responses in adult sarcomas are probably less than 20% (Pinedo and Kenis 1977), and were even lower prior to the advent of doxorubicin. This agent has produced significant improvement; alone, it is reported to give a response rate of 30% in previously treated patients (table 63.1) (Gottlieb et al. 1975), which is increased to 45% in previously untreated patients (Benjamin, Wiernik, and Bachur 1974). Also, patients treated with at least 60 mg/m^2 every three weeks respond better than those receiving a lower dose (O'Bryan et al. 1977). The overall response rate of doxorubicin alone or in combination in Southwest Oncology Group studies was 46% (table 63.2) (Gottlieb et al. 1975).

In animal studies doxorubicin has been shown to have an increased effectiveness without increased toxicity when combined with dacarbazine (DTIC) (Griswold, Laster, and Schable 1973). The response rate of adult soft tissue sarcomas to this combination is 47% (Pinedo and Kenis 1977), which is similar to doxorubicin alone, although the duration of remission is reported to be increased (Gottlieb 1974). Omura and Blessing (1978) reported a randomized trial of doxorubicin versus the same dose of doxorubicin plus dacarbazine and found no difference in the response rate (28%) or duration of response (five months) in uterine sarcomas.

One of the most effective regimens in the treatment of adult soft tissue sarcomas is a combination of cyclophosphamide, vincristine, doxorubicin, and dacarbazine. In 136 evaluable patients, 14% showed a complete response and 43% a partial response resulting in an overall response rate of 55% (table 63.3) (Gottlieb et al. 1975). Of the various histologic types, only chondrosarcoma failed to respond. The response rate for

Table 63.2. *Results of Southwest Oncology Group and M.D. Anderson Sarcoma Studies with Adriamycin Alone and in Combination (1971–74)*

Diagnosis	Number of Patients*			Response Rate† (%)
	Evaluable	With CR	With PR	
Angiosarcoma	35	3	17	57
Chondrosarcoma	29	1	4	17
Ewing's sarcoma	15	2	2	27
Fibrosarcoma	90	9	37	51
Leiomyosarcoma	147	14	60	50
Liposarcoma	71	7	28	49
Mesothelioma	36	3	9	33
Neurofibrosarcoma	50	7	15	44
Osteogenic sarcoma	87	5	23	32
Rhabdomyosarcoma	69	13	25	55
Synovial cell sarcoma	25	4	10	56
Undifferentiated sarcoma	76	9	27	47
Total	730	77	257	46

SOURCE: Gottlieb et al. 1975.
*CR = complete response, PR = partial response.
†Overall CR rate = 11%.

liposarcoma was somewhat less than for other histologic diagnoses.

Because of the results obtained with doxorubicin and combinations containing doxorubicin in the treatment of metastatic soft tissue sarcoma, similar schedules are being tested in the adjuvant therapy of patients at high risk for recurrence and in combination with radiation therapy where less than radical surgery is performed. Rosenberg and associates (1978) treated patients with adjuvant doxorubicin and cyclophosphamide or chemoimmunotherapy following either radical or limited surgery and radiation therapy. There have been only 5 recurrences in 49 patients, with no difference between groups, and both have a prolonged disease-free interval and improved survival compared to historical controls. Thus adjuvant therapy appears to have delayed or prevented dissemination of tumor cells. Antman and co-workers (1980) reported on 17 patients primarily treated with surgery, radiation therapy, or a combination who received adjuvant chemotherapy with cyclophosphamide, doxorubicin and dacarbazine for one year. Survival at 18 months (minimum follow-up for study patients) was 55% for historical controls (patients matched for stage and histology) and 95% for study patients. Seventy-nine percent of the latter were continuously disease-free. Thus chemotherapy appears promising as an adjunct to surgery or radiation therapy

Table 63.3. *Response According to Diagnosis after Therapy with Cyclophosphamide, Vincristine, Doxorubicin, and Dacarbazine*

Diagnosis	Number of Patients		Response Rate (%)
	Evaluable	With CR/PR*	
Angiosarcoma	5	0/4	80
Chondrosarcoma	6	0/2	33
Ewing's sarcoma	1	0/0	0
Fibrosarcoma	23	4/9	57
Leiomyosarcoma	28	2/17	68
Liposarcoma	10	1/5	60
Mesothelioma	6	0/2	33
Neurofibrosarcoma	13	3/5	62
Osteogenic sarcoma	11	1/2	27
Rhabdomyosarcoma	15	6/4	67
Synovial cell sarcoma	3	0/2	67
Undifferentiated sarcoma	15	2/4	40
Total	136	19/56	55

SOURCE: Gottlieb et al. 1975.
*CR = complete response; PR = partial response.

in the multimodal approach to soft tissue sarcomas in adults. Although they are somewhat less responsive to chemotherapy than childhood soft tissue sarcomas, survival appears to be improving with fewer recurrences even in patients who have had limited surgery, possibly because of the increased use of doxorubicin in combination chemotherapy.

Kaposi's Sarcoma

The syndrome of "Idiopathic Multiple Hemorrhagic Sarcoma" was first described by Moricz Kaposi (1872), a dermatologist who was also the first to describe and name xeroderma pigmentosa (Mann 1974). As originally described, it is a neoplastic condition of elderly East European men characterized by multiple skin and subcutaneous tumors that grow slowly. It is believed to start in the mid-dermis and extend upward with interweaving bands of spindle cells and vascular structures embedded in a network of reticular and collagen fibers, sometimes with lymphocytic infiltration. The vascular component may appear as cleft spaces between the spindle cells or as delicate capillaries (Safai and Good 1981). The histology in lymph nodes and viscera is similar. The condition was generally considered to be rare and exotic and relatively chronic although ultimately fatal.

Interest in the disease has been rekindled by the observations that the disease is common in central and south Africa (Dutz and Stout 1960; Ackerman and Murray 1963), that it afflicts infants and children of both sexes, that its distribution parallels that of Burkitt's lymphoma, that it is lymphopathic in these youngsters, and that it may be rapidly lethal. Just as Burkitt's lymphoma is associated with the Epstein-Barr virus (Klein 1975), tissue culture cell lines of Kaposi's sarcoma have demonstrated herpes-type viruses on electron microscopy studies (Giraldo, Beth, and Haguenau 1972), and antibodies to cytomegalovirus have been found in the serum of patients with this disease (Giraldo, Beth, and Henle 1978) in Africa, Europe, and the United States.

Clinical Features

European and American patients with Kaposi's sarcoma have generally been from central and eastern Europe and northern Italy. Most have been men (10:1) between the ages of 50 and 70. Their lesions usually present as dark blue to reddish-purple round or oval macules, plaques, or nodules, usually on the extremities, especially the toes (fig. 63.2) or the feet (fig. 63.3), but may appear anywhere in the skin or mucous membranes. Occasionally, lymph nodes or visceral organs may be involved. Edema of the lower extremities may precede or follow the appearance of the tumor, and the lesions may coalesce to form large masses that may erode, ulcerate, or fungate. When the disease is confined to the skin, it is usually slow and indolent and compatible with long survival (8 to 13 years) with or without therapy. When it presents in organs other than the skin or metastasizes to lymph nodes and viscera, the clinical course is much more aggressive and a fatal outcome may supervene in months to a few years. A tentative clinical classification is given in table 63.4.

The African form of the disease usually presents in infants and children and seldom after the age of 40. It involves lymphoid tissues primarily and may spread to viscera with hepatosplenomegaly, lung, and large and small bowel lesions.

Immunology

There is accumulating evidence to suggest that Kaposi's sarcoma is associated with reduced immunity. Several cases have been reported in patients immunosuppressed for the receipt of renal transplants (Myers et al. 1974; Hardy et al. 1976), in patients with multiple myeloma (Mazzaferri and Penn 1968), in a patient with temporal arteritis receiving corticosteroids (Leung, Fam, and Osaba 1981), and in patients with systemic lupus (Klein, Pereira, and Kantor 1974). Of particular inter-

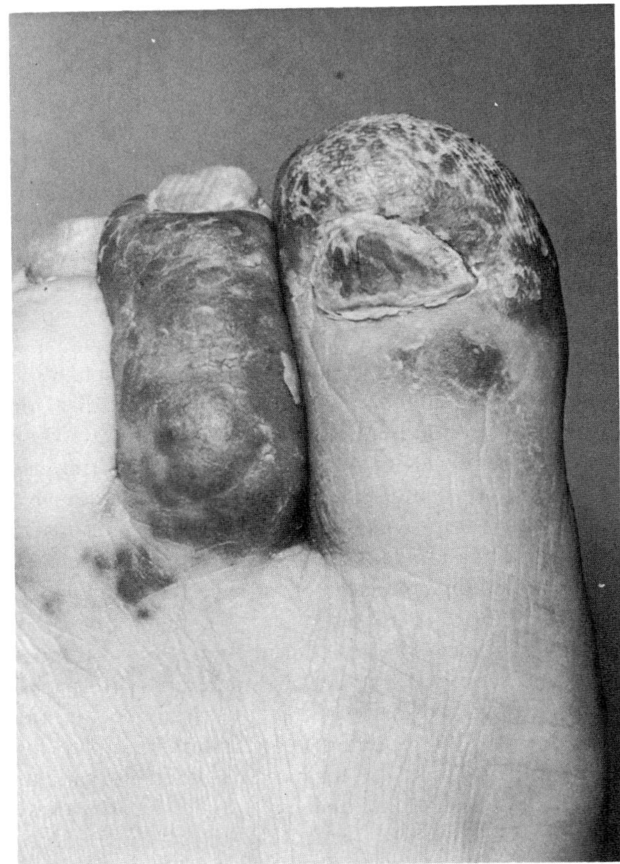

Fig. 63.2. *Left toes of patient with Kaposi's sarcoma.*

Table 63.4. *Clinical Classification of Kaposi's Sarcoma*

Clinical Type	*Behavior*	*Age*	*Bone Involvement*	*Lymph Node Involvement*	*Predominant Skin Lesions*
Nodular	Indolent	> 40	Rare	Rare	Nodule, plaque
Florid	Locally aggressive	> 40	Often	Rare	Fungating, exophytic
Infiltrative	Locally aggressive	> 40	Always	Rare	Diffuse infiltration
Lymphadenopathic	Disseminated aggressive	< 40	Rare	Always	Rare

SOURCE: Modified from Safai and Good 1981.

est is the high incidence of patients with Kaposi's sarcoma who have a second malignancy (37%), especially lymphoma (58%) (Safai et al. 1980).

Recently an intriguing report of a possible association of Kaposi's sarcoma with *pneumocystis carinii* in homosexual men has been published (Center for Disease Control 1981a, 1981b). In a 30-month period, 26 homosexual men (20 in New York City and 6 in California) ranging in age from 26 to 51 years, were found to have the characteristic histopathologic lesion in skin, lymph nodes, or other organs, and eight died. In the following two months, 26 additional cases were reported. Eight patients had pneumonia and six had biopsy confirmation of *pneumocystis carinii*. Of the 12 who had serologic tests for cytomegalovirus (CMV), all were positive; of the 3 in whom urine, blood, or lung were cultured, all yielded CMV growth. One can only speculate why these presumably healthy young men were afflicted with diseases usually seen only in those who are severely immunosuppressed. It is not clear whether the tumor, infection, or immunosuppression was primary.

Radiation therapy has been standard treatment for many years. It is usually effective in producing remissions of long duration in small- and moderate-sized lesions. In a group of 60 patients, a 93% response rate was noted (Lo et al. 1980). Its effectiveness is inversely related to the size and duration of the tumor (Duncan 1977). To handle the larger lesions, six to eight weekly total skin electron beam treatments have been employed

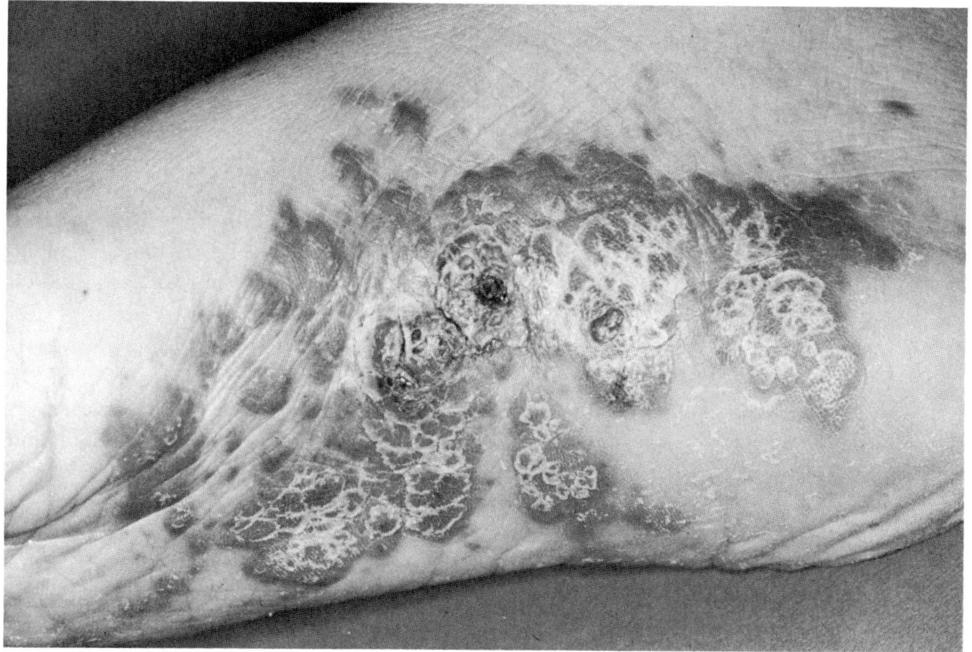

Fig. 63.3. *Sole of foot of patient with Kaposi's sarcoma.*

in 20 patients with an overall response rate of 100% and a complete remission rate of 85% lasting 10 to 92 months (Nisce, Safai, and Poussin-Rosillo 1981).

Chemotherapy has been moderately successful, using a variety of single agents. Objective responses were seen in 9 of 21 patients (43%) treated with carmustine (BCNU) and in 6 of 10 treated with bleomycin (Vogel et al. 1973b). At present, vinblastine seems to be the most popular systemic single agent, with many reports of small series with 75% to 90% response rates (Klein et al. 1980; Tucker and Winkelmann 1976), and many of them of long duration (Solan, Greenwald, and Silvay 1981). Intralesional vincristine has also been reported to be effective (Odom and Goette 1978). Responses have been reported with dacarbazine (Vogel et al. 1973a), cyclophosphamide and dactinomycin (Vogel et al. 1971), and the combination of dactinomycin and vincristine (Vogel et al. 1973c). Undoubtedly, many additional drugs will be used, both alone and in combination, in attempts to achieve long-term control with chemotherapy or multimodal treatment.

References

Ackerman, L. V., and Murray, J. F., eds. *Symposium on Kaposi's sarcoma*. New York: Hafner Publishing Co., 1963.

Antman, K. et al. Effective adjuvant chemotherapy of localized soft tissue sarcoma. *Proc. Am. Assoc. Cancer Res.* 21:141, 1980.

Benjamin, R. S.; Wiernik, P. H.; and Bachur, N. R. Adriamycin chemotherapy—efficacy, safety, and pharmacologic basis of an intermittent single high-dosage schedule. *Cancer* 33:19–27, 1974.

Center for Disease Control. Follow-up on Kaposi's sarcoma and pneumocystis pneumonia. *Morbidity and Mortality Weekly Report* 30:409–411, 1981a.

Center for Disease Control. Kaposi's sarcoma and pneumocystis pneumonia among homosexual men—New York City and California. *Morbidity and Mortality Weekly Report* 30:305–308, 1981b.

Donaldson, S. S. et al. Rhabdomyosarcoma of head and neck in children. Combination treatment by surgery, irradiation, and chemotherapy. *Cancer* 31:26–35, 1973.

Dritschilo, A. et al. The role of radiation therapy in the treatment of soft tissue sarcomas of childhood. *Cancer* 42:1192–1203, 1978.

Duncan, J. T. K. Radiotherapy in the management of Kaposi's sarcoma in Nigeria. *Clin. Radiol.* 28:503–509, 1977.

Dutz, W., and Stout, A. P. Kaposi's sarcoma in infants and children. *Cancer* 13:684–694, 1960.

Edmonson, J. H. et al. Postsurgical treatment of primary osteosarcoma of bone—comparison of high-dose methotrexate vs. observation: preliminary report. *Proc. Am. Soc. Clin. Oncol.* 21:476, 1980.

Ettinger, L. J. et al. Adriamycin (ADR) and cis-diamminedichloroplatinum (DDP) as adjuvant therapy in primary osteosarcoma (OS). *Proc. Am. Soc. Clin. Oncol.* 20:438, 1979.

Frei, E., III et al. Adjuvant chemotherapy of osteogenic sarcoma: progress and perspectives. *J. Natl. Cancer Inst.* 60:3–10, 1978.

Ghavimi, F. et al. Multidisciplinary treatment of embryonal rhabdomyosarcoma in children. *Cancer* 35: 677–686, 1975.

Giraldo, G.; Beth, E.; and Huguenau, F. Herpes-type virus particles in tissue culture of Kaposi's sarcoma from different geographic regions. *J. Natl. Cancer Inst.* 49:1509–1526, 1972.

Giraldo, G.; Beth, E.; and Henle, W. Antibody patterns to herpesviruses in Kaposi's sarcoma. II. Serologic association of American Kaposi's sarcoma with cytomegalovirus. *Int. J. Cancer* 22:126–131, 1978.

Gottlieb, J. A. Proceedings: combination chemotherapy for metastatic sarcoma. *Cancer Chemother. Rep.* 58: 265–270, 1974.

Gottlieb, J. A. et al. Adriamycin used alone and in combination for soft tissue and bony sarcomas. *Cancer Chemother. Rep.* 6:271–282, 1975.

Griswold, D. P.; Laster, W. R., Jr.; and Schable, F. M., Jr. Therapeutic potentiation by Adriamycin and 5-(3,3-dimethyl-1-triazeno)-imidazole-4-carboxamide against B16 melanoma, C3H breast carcinoma, Lewis lung carcinoma and leukemia L1210. *Proc. Am. Assoc. Cancer Res.* 14:15, 1973.

Hardy, M. A. et al. De novo Kaposi's sarcoma in renal transplantation: case report and brief review. *Cancer* 38:144–148, 1976.

Hoover, H. C., Jr. et al. Osteosarcoma: improved survival with anticoagulation and amputation. *Cancer* 41:2475–2480, 1978.

Jaffe, N. et al. High-dose methotrexate in osteogenic sarcoma: a 5-year experience. *Cancer Treat. Rep.* 62:259–264, 1978.

Kaposi, M. Idiopathisches multiples Pigmentsarkom der haut. *Arch. Dermatol. Syph.* 4:265–273, 1872.

Klein, E. et al. Treatment of Kaposi's sarcoma with vinblastine. *Cancer* 45:427–431, 1980.

Klein, G. The Epstein-Barr virus and neoplasia. *N. Engl. J. Med.* 293:1353–1357, 1975.

Klein, M. D.; Pereira, F. A.; and Kantor, I. Kaposi's sarcoma complicating systemic lupus erythematosus treated with immunosuppression. *Arch. Dermatol.* 110:602–604, 1974.

Le Mevel, B. et al. Five-year survival of Ewing's sarcoma patients treated by radiotherapy and adjuvant chemotherapy. In *Adjuvant therapy of cancer,* vol. 2, eds. S. E. Jones and S. E. Salmon. New York: Grune & Stratton, 1979, pp. 403–408.

Leung, F.; Fam, A. G.; and Osaba, D. Kaposi's sarcoma complicating corticosteroid therapy for temporal arteritis. *Am. J. Med.* 71:320–322, 1981.

Lo, T. C. M. et al. Radiotherapy for Kaposi's sarcoma. *Cancer* 45:684–687, 1980.

Mann, S. G. Kaposi's sarcoma, experience with ten cases. *Am. J. Radiol.* 121:793–800, 1974.

Mazzaferri, E. L., and Penn, G. M. Kaposi's sarcoma associated with multiple myeloma. Report of a patient and review of the literature. *Arch. Intern. Med.* 122:521–525, 1968.

Myers, B. D. et al. Kaposi's sarcoma in kidney transplant recipients. *Arch. Intern. Med.* 133:307–311, 1974.

Nisce, L. A.; Safai, B.; and Poussin-Rosillo, H. Once weekly total and subtotal skin electron beam therapy for Kaposi's sarcoma. *Cancer* 47:640–644, 1981.

O'Bryan, R. et al. Dose-response evaluation of Adriamycin in human neoplasia. *Cancer* 39:1940–1948, 1977.

Ochs, J. J. et al. Cis-dichlorodiammineplatinum (II) in advanced osteogenic sarcoma. *Cancer Treat. Rep.* 62:239–245, 1978.

Odom, R. B., and Goette, D. K. Treatment of cutaneous Kaposi's sarcoma with intralesional vincristine. *Arch. Dermatol.* 114:1693–1694, 1978.

Omura, G. A., and Blessing, J. A. Chemotherapy of stage III, IV and recurrent uterine sarcomas: a randomized trial of Adriamycin (AD) versus AD + dimethyl triazeno imidazole carboxamide (DTIC). *Proc. Am. Assoc. Cancer Res.* 19:26, 1978.

Pinedo, H. M., and Kenis, Y. Chemotherapy of advanced soft tissue sarcomas in adults. *Cancer Treat. Rev.* 4:67–86, 1977.

Raney, R. B., Jr.; Schnaufer, L.; and Donaldson, M. H. Soft tissue sarcoma in childhood. *Semin. Oncol.* 1:57–64, 1974.

Rosen, G. et al. Chemotherapy and thoracotomy for metastatic osteogenic sarcoma. A model for adjuvant chemotherapy and the rationale for the timing of thoracic surgery. *Cancer* 41:841–849, 1978.

Rosen, G. et al. Primary osteogenic sarcoma: the rationale for preoperative chemotherapy and delayed surgery. *Cancer* 43:2163–2177, 1979.

Rosenberg, S. A. et al. Prospective randomized evaluation of the role of limb-sparing surgery, radiation therapy, and adjuvant chemoimmunotherapy in the treatment of adult soft tissue sarcomas. *Surgery* 84:62–69, 1978.

Safai, B. et al. Association of Kaposi's sarcoma with second primary malignancy. *Cancer* 45:1472–1479, 1980.

Safai, B., and Good, R. A. Kaposi's sarcoma: a review and recent developments. *CA* 31:2–12, 1981.

Sears, H. F. et al. Soft tissue sarcomas. *Semin. Oncol.* 8:129–237, 1981.

Solan, A. J.; Greenwald, E. S.; and Silvay, O. Long-term complete remissions of Kaposi's sarcoma with vinblastine therapy. *Cancer* 47:637–639, 1981.

Suit, H. D.; Russell, W. O.; and Martin, R. G. Sarcoma of soft tissue: clinical and histopathologic parameters and response to treatment. *Cancer* 35:1478–1483, 1975.

Taylor, W. F. et al. Trends and variability in survival from osteosarcoma. *Mayo Clin. Proc.* 53:695–700, 1978.

Tefft, M. Cooperative group studies of pediatric bone and soft tissue sarcoma: present status and future direction. In *Adjuvant therapy of cancer,* vol. 2, eds. S. E. Jones and S. E. Salmon. New York: Grune & Stratton, 1979, pp. 393–402.

Tucker, S. B., and Winkelmann, R. K. Treatment of Kaposi's sarcoma with vinblastine. *Arch. Dermatol.* 112:958–961, 1976.

Vogel, C. L. et al. Treatment of Kaposi's sarcoma with actinomycin D and cyclophosphamide: results of a randomized clinical trial. *Int. J. Cancer* 8:136–143, 1971.

Vogel, C. L. et al. Effective treatment of Kaposi's sarcoma with 5-(3,3-dimethyl-1-triazeno) imidazole-4-carboxamide (NSC 45388). *Cancer Chemother. Rep.* 57:65–71, 1973a.

Vogel, C. L. et al. Phase II clinical trials of BCNU (NSC-409962) and bleomycin (NSC-125066) in the treatment of Kaposi's sarcoma. *Cancer Chemother. Rep.* 57:325–333, 1973b.

Vogel, C. L. et al. Treatment of Kaposi's sarcoma with a combination of actinomycin D and vincristine: results of a randomized clinical trial. *Cancer* 31:1382–1391, 1973c.

sixty-four

Melanoma

JOHN M. KIRKWOOD

Melanoma is a cancer that has fascinated more physicians and terrified more patients than most others. The following brief review of new knowledge of its biology and new approaches to its therapy may allay the confusion that has developed around this tumor.

Incidence and Epidemiology

The incidence of melanoma has risen fairly consistently during the past few generations in this country and in a wide range of other nations. This increase is paralleled by a growing mortality rate, with melanoma now the cause of 2.5% of fatal malignant disease. It arises from pigment cells, or melanocytes, which may occur dispersed in the skin at the dermoepidermal junction, or in nevi (moles) in the junction, epidermis, or dermis. Melanoma is infrequent in blacks and more common in fair-skinned individuals who freckle. It may arise more in nevi than homogenously pigmented skin, but nevi are common, numbering approximately 16 per adult, while melanoma is comparatively rare. Epidemiology as well as its topography on the body surface argue for a major causal role of sun exposure (UV). While melanoma may arise in the pigment cells of the eye, mucosae, or meninges, cutaneous melanoma far outnumbers these other types.

A significant premalignant potential is generally recognized in nevi of (1) congenital origin, (2) the B-K hereditary syndrome of atypical nevi and multiple primary melanoma (Clark et al. 1978), (3) lentigo maligna, and (4) all nevi of individuals with a prior history of melanoma. Surveillance for suspicious change in nevi is warranted in these situations, and possibly also when nevi occur on the palms, soles, and mucosal surfaces, especially of blacks. Simple excision of lentigo maligna and congenital, atypical, or otherwise suspicious nevi is a rational approach to melanoma prophylaxis.

Prognosis

The biology of the primary lesion provides a second possible avenue of therapy, for we now recognize two phases in the development of most melanomas: (1) a radial phase of growth, wherein malignant cells are distributed centrifugally through the junction with little tendency to vertical invasion downward into the dermis, or upward into the epidermis; and (2) a vertical phase of invasion in which there is more likely to be ulceration with upward invasion from the junction, or distant dissemination through deep lymphatic or hematogenous vascular channels (Clark et al. 1969, 1975).

Our new appreciation of the prognostic implications of the tumor's behavior has led to the widespread adoption of two systems of microstaging. One, called the Breslow system, uses millimeter depth of the primary melanoma as recorded from an ocular micrometer on a conventional microscope, and has been shown to offer the most accurate prediction now known of risk for recurrence and death from tumor (table 64.1). The

Table 64.1. *Risk of Melanoma Relapse and Death at Two to Five Years According to Depth of Primary Lesion*

mm Breslow Depth	*Relapse at 2 to 5 Years (%)*
≤ 0.76*	10
0.77–1.50	15–30
1.51–3.99	30–55
≥ 4.0	55–85

SOURCES: Breslow et al. 1978; Balch et al. 1979.

*Without significant evidence of regression, according to Breslow et al. 1978, Balch et al. 1979, and others.

second, the Clark system, determines invasion by levels: level I is confined in situ to the junction and epidermis; level II lesions are confined to the papillary dermis without expanding this layer; level III tumors fill and expand the papillary dermis; level IV lesions invade the reticular dermis; and level V lesions invade the subcutaneous region. The Clark system predated the Breslow system in its acceptance by pathologists and is still often the only microstage available to the clinician. Recent multifactorial analyses of their independent prognostic value, however, suggest that the effectiveness of the Breslow system far exceeds that of all other indices, including those that appear independently to influence prognosis, such as lymph node invasion, Clark level, pigmentation, and ulceration of the primary tumor (Balch et al. 1978, 1979). The risk of recurrence in melanomas of the extremities appears to be a linear function of the depth of the primary (Breslow et al. 1978). Factors that from time to time have been independently found to have prognostic importance to retrospective analyses, including sex, age, site, and tumor morphology, appear less important when examined in multifactorial fashion.

Surgical Treatment

The surgical approach is predicated on the experience of nearly 80 years in which it has become customary to excise primary melanoma with wide margins of 4 to 5 cm down to fascia, using a graft to cover the defect. The need for wide margins (4 to 5 cm in all directions) has often been compromised in primary lesions of the face, and newer techniques of flap rotation may sometimes allow for coverage of truncal resections without a conventional graft. Yet the major opportunity for cure occurs on initial operation. Less radical techniques, dispensing with standard margins for thin primary lesions, will require lengthy large trials to establish equivalent therapeutic benefits (Breslow 1979).

A major surgical question has been raised regarding the role of prophylactic lymphadenectomy in patients who have no clinical evidence of lymph node metastasis at diagnosis, especially in the case of primary tumor of an extremity where lymphatic drainage is obvious and accessible. Two large randomized prospective comparative trials have suggested that there is no benefit from prophylactic lymphadenectomy in reduction or delay of recurrence or in prolongation of life (Veronesi et al. 1977; Sim et al. 1978). Application of the Breslow microstaging system to a retrospective study at the University of Alabama has suggested benefit to a subgroup of patients with primary melanomas of Breslow level 0.76 to 3.99 mm (Balch et al. 1979). This is reasonable in the context of the previously reviewed biology of the primary tumor and its apparent stepwise evolution through phases of radial and vertical spread. Patients with thin tumors less than 0.76 mm have a small enough risk of recurrence and a low enough yield of tumor-involved nodes at surgery that it has made little sense to subject them to lymph node dissection except under special circumstances (Cohen et al. 1977; Gromet, Epstein, and Blois 1978). Patients with primary tumor thickness greater than 4 mm have such a high risk of dissemination that removal of lymph nodes may often be done in the presence of microscopic distant metastatic disease. Thus it may only be in the circumstance of intermediate-depth tumors that elective lymphadenectomy is beneficial. Accurate staging and determination of prognosis are still at times sufficient grounds for lymph node dissection, and it is reasonable to pursue surgical staging for these purposes in adjuvant trials.

Adjuvant Treatment

Once the primary surgery with or without lymphadenectomy has been performed, the previously cited prognostic factors are used to determine ranges of risk for recurrence and for possible adjuvant therapy. It has conventionally been accepted that patients with Clark levels IV and V melanoma or Breslow thickness over 1.50 mm are at high risk of recurrence, and that they may reasonably participate in therapeutic trials to alter the expected outcome. Clark level III is in a borderline zone, as are Breslow thicknesses of 0.76 to 1.50 mm where the risk of recurrence is moderate but low enough that it may be difficult to establish any benefit from therapy.

Adjuvant therapy for high-risk melanoma may include two programs. First, there may be presurgical and intraoperative use of drugs or immunologic stimulants to reduce tumor burden and augment the patient's immune resistance to the tumor. One such randomized prospective trial at Yale involves intraoperative perfusion of the affected extremity with chemotherapy with dacarbazine (DTIC) preceded by intralymphatic administration of a nonspecific immune stimulant (methanol-extracted residue [MER] of bacillus Calmette-Guerin [BCG] after lymphangiogram in patients who are randomized to immunotherapy. Patients who receive immunotherapy are subsequently treated with monthly intradermal BCG for 12 months following surgery. Pilot trials using intralesional or perilesional BCG are promising.

The second approach has been suggested by observations of the pigment systems of individuals with this disease. The malignant disease of melanocytes that we call melanoma is paradoxically associated with the appearance of spontaneous depigmentation and loss of pigment cells in a significant number of patients (fig. 64.1). This has been observed in 25% to 30% of those examined carefully with UV (Wood's) lamps (Lerner and Nordlund 1978). Examination of the pigment cell system in the eye has further revealed parallel development of abnormalities of the choroid and uveal tract of individuals with some cutaneous depigmenting disorders (Albert, Nordlund, and Lerner 1979). These findings suggest that a careful prospective examination of the pigment system as a whole will reveal biologically and prognostically important correlations. We have observed an association between atypical (protracted or spontaneously remitting) course of melanoma and the occurrence of depigmentation. As it has been known that therapeutic depigmentation may be achieved in patients with idiopathic depigmentation in the common disease called vitiligo (seen in approximately 1% of the population), we are testing whether it is possible to improve the prognosis of individuals with high-risk melanoma with the use of topical depigmenting agents.

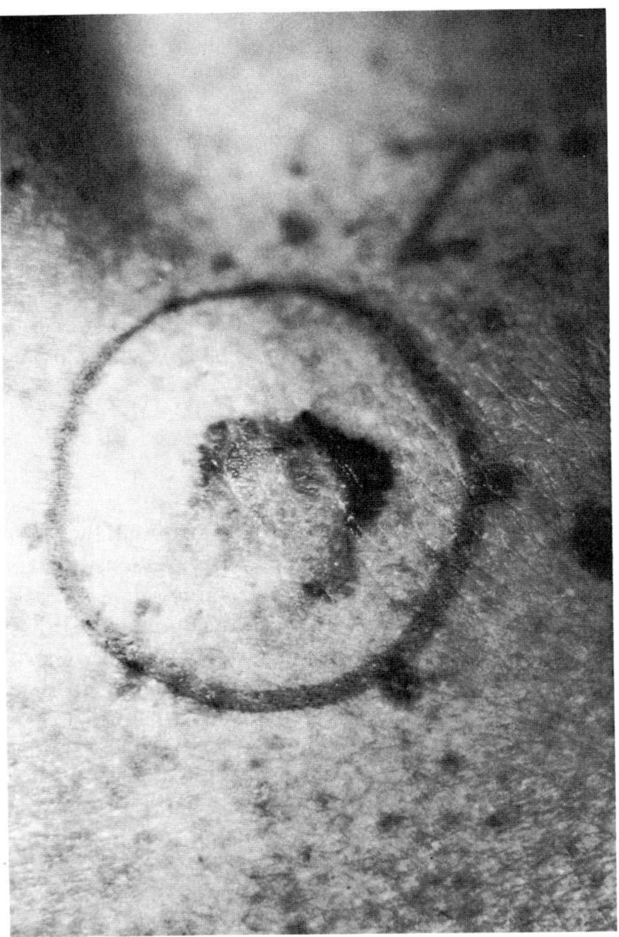

Fig. 64.1. *Superficial spreading melanoma with typical regression, loss of pigmentation, and central deep invasion.*

Adjuvant postoperative therapy has been attempted in numerous previous trials invalidated by complete omission of controls or by use of improper controls (Seigler et al. 1979; Eilber et al. 1976). Thus it has been impossible to derive any compelling conclusions of therapeutic benefit from published experiences. A recent trial (Wood et al. 1978) has suggested that decarbazine and BCG administered systemically may be more effective than either agent alone, although this trial unfortunately omitted a control arm of surgery only. The World Health Organization has undertaken a comparative adjuvant trial of BCG, dacarbazine, both, or neither, and accrued sufficient patients over the past several years showing no differences to date. We are presently testing whether depigmentation therapy or chemoimmunotherapy (dacarbazine-BCG) is significantly more effective than observation alone for moderate-risk and high-risk patients after excision of all primary and nodal disease in patients stratified for Breslow depth and stage.

The use of commercial BCG of strains other than Tice, Pasteur, and Connaught cannot now be justified on the basis of trials against human or experimental melanoma. Commercially available BCG used for tuberculosis prophylaxis has exhibited no significant clinical antitumor prophylactic effects in any published trials. It has been even suggested that under certain circumstances BCG may enhance tumor growth in experimental animals and humans. Close laboratory monitoring of immune function, particularly against the patient's own tumor, is reasonable in all forms of immunotherapy as none can yet be said to have been established in standard practice.

Table 64.2. *Activity of Single Drugs against Melanoma: Series of More than 20 Patients with Objective Response > 10%*

Drug	Response (%)	Number of Evaluable Patients
Dacarbazine (DTIC)	23.4	1088
Triethylenethiophosphoramide	20.8	24
TEPA	18.8	16
Dibromodulcitol	16.7	18
Methotrexate	15.4	13
Melphalan	16.7	24
Carmustine	17.1	140
Vincristine	11.5	26
TIC mustard	11.5	26
Cyclophosphamide	12.5	32
Cytarabine	11.1	27

SOURCE: Modified from Bellet et al. 1979.

Therapy of Advanced Disease

Systemic Therapy

Drug therapy of inoperable melanoma has often been frustrating; indeed, there are many medical oncologists who either do not medically treat metastatic disease or resort directly to agents in phase I or II trials. The benefit from drugs in patients who do respond to therapy can often be gratifying, with median duration of responses to agents such as dacarbazine or nitrosoureas as long as five to seven months. The statistical fact that only one in four or five patients may respond favorably to standard single-agent chemotherapy (table 64.2) is now potentially overcome by methods developed for screening tumors for drug sensitivity. Much as antimicrobial therapy can now be predicated on reliable in vitro sensitivity tests, it is possible that we may employ similar tests for melanoma in the future (Salmon et al. 1978; Marsh and Kirkwood 1980).

The Eastern Cooperative Oncology Group is piloting a number of agents through an evolving phase II trial that has previously examined chlorozotocin, zinostatin, and different schedules of semustine (methyl-CCNU). It is currently comparing the most effective schedule of semustine (150 mg/m^2/three weeks) to methyl-GAG and dibromodulcitol. Phase II studies of dibromodulcitol, a hexitol alkylating agent with moderate myelosuppressive and gastrointestinal toxicity, have been spurred on by evidence that this agent has significant activity against melanoma in patients who have previously failed decarbazine and a nitrosourea (Bellet et al. 1978). The Yale melanoma unit has not, unfortunately, confirmed this level of activity. Combinations of agents have shown a wide range of activities and statistically have generally failed to exceed the activity of dacarbazine by any meaningful margin. A regimen of vinblastine, bleomycin, and cisplatin (VBP) appears to have reached median durations of survival in advanced disease of more than 27 weeks (Nathanson, Kaufman, and Carey 1981). As such, and with the ability to remit visceral disease completely, this regimen deserves further study. Appropriately stratified randomized trials compairng dacarbazine to VBP will provide useful information in the next few years.

Interferons of several types have opened one of the newest avenues for phase I-II treatment of metastatic melanoma. The melanoma unit at Yale was chosen as one of several sites for evaluating antitumor effects of leukocyte interferon purchased by the American Cancer Society (ACS). There is as yet no clinical evidence for its antitumor efficacy in human melanoma. Studies in tissue culture with human melanoma as well as tests against mouse melanoma indicate that it may inhibit the division of tumor cells. More interesting is the fact that it may do so in a novel fashion, inhibiting cells that are in the resting phase where few other anticancer drugs have any effect. If early clinical studies now in progress indicate that interferon has any significant effect against human melanoma, it will be immediately relevant to combine it with other chemotherapeutic agents such as dacarbazine and dibromodulcitol, or semustine. Interferon has potent effects on the immune system and is an immunotherapeutic agent in its own right. Its effect on tumor-specific and nonspecific immunity is being examined in patients treated during the ACS trial.

Other phase II studies now active at our institution include an evaluation of high-dose antiestrogen therapy (tamoxifen, 100 mg/m^2/day) in metastatic melanoma. This is based on pilot data that estrogen receptors and progesterone receptors frequently exist in the cytosol of human melanoma cells.

Radiotherapy

Radiotherapy given in conventional fractionation has exhibited variable effects against advanced melanoma. New methods of delivery have been developed, including high-dose fractionation (600 rad weekly), that have improved the response rate of soft tissue disease (Habermalz and Fischer 1976). While there may be somewhat increased toxicity from this program when applied to visceral disease, especially of the brain, it promises to control previously insurmountable problems with CNS metastasis (Vlock et al., in press). Radiotherapy programs are being developed for the adjuvant treatment of areas at extremely high risk for relapse, such as the site of resected regional soft tissue disease and late isolated brain recurrence. These may add much to palliation, and with better systemic therapy, offer a prospect of improved cure rates.

In summary, melanoma is a tumor of increasing incidence and unknown etiology. Several adjuvant programs including chemotherapy, immunotherapy, and combinations of the two are currently under evaluation as well as programs directed against the pigment cell more specifically. It is not settled which is best, or whether there is any significant benefit from operative lymph node removal in patients without clinical evidence of lymph node involvement. Adequate primary surgery is the most important part of a curative approach to melanoma. Multidisciplinary approaches are likely to be most beneficial for melanoma patients in the future.

References

Albert, D. M.; Nordlund, J. J.; and Lerner, A. B. Occular abnormalities occurring with vitiligo. *Ophthalmology* 86:1145–1158, 1979.

Balch, C. M. et al. A multifactorial analysis of melanoma prognostic histopathological features comparing Clark's and Breslow's staging methods. *Ann. Surg.* 188:732–742, 1978.

Balch, C. M. et al. Tumor thickness as a guide to surgical management of clinical stage I melanoma patients. *Cancer* 43:883–888, 1979.

Bellet, R. E. et al. Chemotherapy of metastatic malignant melanoma. In *Human malignant melanoma,* eds. W. H. Clark, Jr.; L. I. Goldman; and M. J. Mastrangelo. New York: Grune & Stratton, 1979.

Breslow, A. Prognostic factors in the treatment of cutaneous melanoma. *J. Cutan. Pathol.* 6:208–212, 1979.

Breslow, A. et al. Stage I melanoma of the limbs: assessment of prognosis by levels of invasion and maximum thickness. *Tumori* 64:273–284, 1978.

Clark, W. H. et al. The histogenesis and biologic behavior of primary human malignant melanoma of the skin. *Cancer Res.* 29:705–727, 1969.

Clark, W. H. et al. The developmental biology of primary human malignant melanoma. *Semin. Oncol.* 2:83–103, 1975.

Clark, W. H. et al. Origin of familial malignant melanoma from heritable melanocytic lesions. The BK mole syndrome. *Arch. Dermatol.* 114:732–738, 1978.

Cohen, M. H. et al. Prognostic factors in patients undergoing lymphadenectomy for malignant melanoma. *Ann. Surg.* 186:635–642, 1977.

Eilber, F. R. et al. Adjuvant immunotherapy with BCG in treatment of regional node metastasis from malignant melanoma. *N. Engl. J. Med.* 294:237–240, 1976.

Gromet, M.; Epstein, W. L.; and Blois, M. J. The regressing thin melanoma: a distinctive lesion with metastatic potential. *Cancer* 42:2282–2292, 1978.

Habermalz, H. J., and Fischer, J. J. Radiation therapy of malignant melanoma, experience with high individual treatment doses. *Cancer* 38:2258–2262, 1976.

Lerner, A., and Nordlund, J. Vitiligo—what is it? Is it important? *JAMA* 239:1183–1187, 1978.

Marsh, J. C., and Kirkwood, J. M. In vivo drug sensitivity of clonogenic human melanoma cells. *Proc. Am. Assoc. Cancer Res.* 21:279, 1980.

Nathanson, L.; Kaufman, S. D.; and Carey, R. W. Vinblastine, infusion bleomycin, and cis-dichloro-diammine-platinum chemotherapy in metastatic melanoma. *Cancer* 48:1290–1294, 1981.

Salmon, S. E. et al. Quantitation of differential sensitivity of human tumor stem cells to anticancer drugs. *N. Engl. J. Med.* 298:1321–1327, 1978.

Seigler, H. F. et al. Specific active immunotherapy for melanoma. *Ann. Surg.* 190:366–373, 1979.

Sim, F. H. et al. A prospective randomized study of the efficacy of routine elective lymphadenectomy in management of malignant melanoma. *Cancer* 41:948–956, 1978.

Veronesi, U. et al. Inefficacy of immediate node dissection in stage I melanoma of the limbs. *N. Engl. J. Med.* 297:627–630, 1977.

Vlock, D. R. et al. High dose fraction radiation therapy for intracranial metastases of malignant melanoma: a comparison with low dose fraction therapy. *Cancer,* in press.

Wood, W. C. et al. Randomized trial of adjuvant therapy for "high-risk" primary malignant melanoma. *Surgery* 83:677–681, 1978.

sixty-five

Primary Brain Tumors

LEONARD R. FARBER

Primary brain tumors are the second most common childhood neoplasm, and in adults they are more common than Hodgkin's disease. Eleven thousand new cases are diagnosed annually in the United States, and primary brain tumors account for 9000 deaths a year. The malignant gliomas comprise well over half of these, with glioblastoma multiforme showing the highest incidence.

Pathology

Brain tumors may arise in the cerebrum as an astrocytoma, oligodendroglioma, or glioblastoma multiforme. In the cerebellum, the most common tumors seen are the medulloblastoma and the cerebellar astrocytoma. The former can spread supratentorially. In the brain stem, ependymomas and gliomas are found. Three-quarters of ependymomas arise below the tentorium, most commonly in or about the fourth ventricle. Calcification is frequently seen in these tumors. Brain stem gliomas occur especially in the pons.

The pathologic grading of gliomas has been clearly defined (Kernohan et al. 1949) and takes into consideration cellularity, mitoses, presence or absence of multiform cells, endothelial proliferation, and necrosis. In grades I and II disease there is a minimal degree of cellularity and few, if any, mitoses present. In grade III gliomas histologic examination reveals increased cellularity, multiform cells, and the presence of mitoses. Grade IV malignant tumors are characterized histologically by the same findings as in grade III, plus endothelial proliferation and necrosis. So-called benign tumors of the dura (meningiomas) and nerves (neuromas) may rarely become malignant and be seen as meningeal or neurosarcomas. Neuroectodermal and mesenchymal tumors may combine in the form of malignant gliosarcomas.

Diagnosis

Symptoms at the time of diagnosis include headache (33%), seizures (19%), personality changes (12%), motor deficits (9%), speech deficits (6%), visual deficits (4.5%), and sensory deficits (4%) (Walker 1975).

General symptoms depend on the production of increased intracranial pressure associated with obstructive hydrocephalus, edema, and generalized dysfunction of the cerebral cortex. As mentioned, headache is the most common symptom; those that change in character, are recurrent, and are worse in the morning or awaken the patient at night are most suggestive of a primary brain tumor. Mental changes are often subtle and gradual in onset and may take any form. Generalized convulsions and papilledema are frequently seen. Focal symptoms may take the form of focal seizures, visual loss, hearing impairment, speech disturbances, and motor or sensory deficits.

The diagnosis of primary brain tumors has been advanced dramatically in recent years with the advent of computerized axial tomography (CT). As seen on CT, intracranial tumors may displace normal brain structures, produce cerebral edema, may contain calcifications, and if malignant, usually enhance when contrast is given. Angiography is performed for confirmation, and for neurosurgical localization to aid in resection.

Treatment

Medical Management

Medical management consists primarily of corticosteroids to reduce the edema surrounding the tumor. They almost always improve general symptoms such as headache and mental changes, and although somewhat less beneficial against specific clinical symptoms, they still may reduce seizure frequency and activity and improve ataxia and weakness. A usual starting dose of dexamethasone (Decadron) is 16 mg a day, 4 mg every six hours; or prednisone, 25 mg every six hours. Larger doses can be given. It has been found that where lesser doses are ineffective, or after initially being effective they become less so because of regrowth of tumor, increases in the dose may achieve significant palliation. Anticonvulsants are frequently used, relying on phenytoin (diphenylhydantoin) (Dilantin) or phenobarbital for long-term seizure control. Recurrence of seizures occurring late after primary therapy and when adequate levels of anticonvulsants are present usually indicates recurrence and regrowth of tumor and should be thoroughly investigated.

Surgical Management

Surgery has been the mainstay of treatment for nearly the last half century (Goldsmith and Carter 1974) for the following reasons: (1) it establishes the diagnosis, (2) it provides symptomatic therapy, especially by reducing intracranial pressure, (3) it removes tumor bulk as a form of anticancer treatment, (4) it permits time for other anticancer therapy (radiation and chemotherapy) to be delivered, which usually requires a minimum of one to two months, (5) by removing tumor bulk surgery *may* convert remaining tumor cells from a nonproliferating to rapidly proliferating state in which they may be more sensitive to both radiation and chemotherapy (Hoskins et al. 1975), and (6) in the case of benign tumors (i.e., grade I astrocytomas or meningiomas), complete removal may result in cure or long-term control.

Tumors of the frontal and temporal lobe lend themselves to far more complete removal than do those in the parietal lobe, deep-seated cortical tumors, and brain stem tumors. Many neurologic series in the literature document that only patients (with glioblastoma multiforme) whose tumors have been extensively resected survive more than one year (Goldsmith and Carter 1974).

Radiation Therapy

Radiation therapy has been routinely given following surgery for the treatment of primary brain tumors for many years. The best survivals in all series in the literature have been seen with doses in excess of 5000 rad, and usually closer to 6000 rad, total dose. Four to five thousand rad are given to the whole brain, with the remaining one to two thousand rad being given in cone-down fashion to the site of bulk tumor (Marsa et al. 1975; Sheline 1977).

There are several tumor types in which the value of radiation therapy following surgery is clearly shown. In the case of well-differentiated astrocytomas, if the tumors can be totally resected there is a high (over 90%) chance of cure. Incomplete resection alone rarely results in cure. When incomplete resection has been followed by irradiation, from 25% to 50% of patients may be expected to be alive 5 to 10 years after treatment has been completed (Sheline 1977). Astrocytomas can be seen in association with oliogodendrogliomas (so-called mixed tumors), and patients' survival following radiation approximates 40% to 50% at 10 years. These tumors are commonly seen in the 25- to 50-year age group. Deep-seated cerebral gliomas are rare tumors that are seen in the pediatric age group. Frequently they are treated without biopsy or are biopsied only and cannot be removed because of their involvement of vital structures. Radiation therapy, using 4000 rad whole brain irradiation followed by 1500 to 2000 rad cone-down to the site of the primary tumor, has resulted in overall survival of 50% of children at the 10-year mark (Marsa et al. 1975). Perhaps the most frequently seen childhood tumors are medulloblastomas in which surgery followed by craniospinal axis irradiation (because of the high incidence of cerebrospinal fluid seeding) has resulted in a 30% to 50% long-term survival rate (Bloom 1977). Brain stem gliomas are often incompletely removed, and the survival rate following similar treatment is less than that of medulloblastoma. Cerebellar astrocytomas occur in a somewhat older age group than medulloblastomas and have a much better survival rate, approximating 70% in some series. Ependymomas and spinal cord gliomas are also seen in the pediatric age group. While some centers treat all ependymomas with craniospinal irradiation, others give local radiation only to low-grade tumors, reserving radiation to the craniospinal axis for those high-grade ependymomas from which there is a significant chance (approximately 20% to 30%) of cerebrospinal fluid seeding (Mork and Loken 1977). The malignant gliomas (malignant astrocytomas, grade III gliomas, and grade IV glioblastoma multiforme) have very poor survival rates in spite of aggressive radiation therapy. The value of irradiation has been clearly denoted in both grades of malignant gliomas. In grade III gliomas, five-year survival of 2% has been improved to 16% with whole brain radiation therapy. In the grade IV glioblastoma multiforme, while one-year survival has been improved from under 10% to 20% or more with radiation as opposed to resection alone, five-year survival still is negligible whether radiation is given or not (Marsa et al. 1975; Sheline 1977).

Chemotherapy

Chemotherapy has been used in the treatment of primary brain tumors for nearly 20 years, but recently significant advances have been made. The blood-brain barrier has proved far less insurmountable than has the refractoriness of many malignant tumors to the agents currently in use. In all instances of treatment it is difficult to judge the response especially with the concurrent use of corticosteroids. The CT scan should define the response to chemotherapy with the greatest precision, but few, if any, series in the literature have used this procedure in a prospective manner.

Single-agent chemotherapy has used a wide variety of agents; the most effective seem to be the nitrosoureas (carmustine, lomustine, and semustine). Procarbazine (Matulane), etoposide (VP-16), cisplatin, and vincristine are others that are felt to be active in the treatment of malignant gliomas and that are readily available. It is felt by most chemotherapists that alkylating agents, most antimetabolites, and doxorubicin are ineffective in the treatment of primary brain tumors in doses and by methods of administration that are standard for treatment of other solid tumors.

Combined Modality Treatment

Before detailing the results reported in controlled studies for treatment of malignant gliomas, a significant perspective has been established by the findings of a series reported from the Kaiser Permanente Group in Los Angeles (Gilbert et al. 1979). They were concerned that patient selection would affect the results of treatment. Their conclusions were that greater than 40% of patients with malignant glioma were not treated, usually because of a poor functional state, a grade IV tumor, parietal lobe location of the tumor, and age greater than 60 years. Radiation therapy and chemotherapy following surgery benefited those who had a good postoperative status and who were under 60 years of age. Treatment with presently available modalities (radiation therapy and nitrosoureas) was not worthwhile for patients who had poor functional status following surgery. Patients with a good functional status and with grade III nonparietal tumors were long-term survivors.

The Brain Tumor Study Group, a multiinstitution organization sponsored by the National Cancer Institute, has been studying the effects of postoperative radiation therapy and chemotherapy for the past decade (Walker et al. 1978). This study included more than 300 patients, and their criteria for eligibility were that maximal surgery was performed, a pathologic review was done, and there was an estimated survival of two months. Patients were divided into four groups: (1) supportive care without further treatment; (2) carmustine (BCNU) chemotherapy, 80 mg/m^2 intravenously daily for three days every six to eight weeks; (3) 4000 rad whole brain irradiation followed by cone-down; and (4) carmustine and radiation therapy. The groups were well matched for age, histology, and corticosteroid use, but unfortunately, the carmustine group had a higher proportion of patients with parietal lesions and who had subtotal resection only. They found, as did others, that the following correlated with poor survival: age, surgical biopsy only, and parietal location. The median survival for patients given supportive care only was 17 weeks, those given carmustine 25 weeks, the patients receiving radiation therapy 37.5 weeks, and those receiving carmustine and irradiation 40.5 weeks. Of great interest was that at 12 months following treatment patients receiving combined treatment had a 32% survival compared to 24% in the radiation therapy group. At 18 months this is even more striking, where 19% of those receiving combined treatment survived, as opposed to only 4% of patients given radiation therapy only.

A second Brain Tumor Study Group investigation comparing radiation therapy, radiation therapy and carmustine, semustine (methyl-CCNU), and radiation therapy and semustine has been reported (Walker and Strike 1976). The median survival is as follows: radiation alone—37 weeks, radiation plus carmustine—52 weeks, semustine alone—27 weeks, and radiation plus semustine—43 weeks. Median survival of only patients treated adequately (those who completed irradiation and one cycle of chemotherapy and survived longer than two months following surgery) is as follows: radiation therapy—40 weeks, radiation plus carmustine—62 weeks, semustine—33 weeks, and radiation plus semustine—50 weeks. The group receiving radiation plus carmustine had a median survival in excess of one year and of great importance was that 25% were alive at two years.

The findings of these studies can be summarized: (1) extensive resection of gliomas followed by radiation has lengthened survival from 12 to 36 weeks, and (2) the addition of nitrosoureas (carmustine or semustine) has further extended median survival to 48 weeks. Combined modality therapy (surgery plus irradiation plus chemotherapy) has resulted in 20% to 25% of patients surviving more than two years. These studies are highlighted by large numbers of patients and by their multiinstitutional nature.

The benefit of chemotherapy was described in another report (Solero et al. 1979) that achieved a 42-week median survival with radiation alone, similar to the results previously noted. When surgery was followed by radiation plus carmustine, a 52-week median survival was noted. Surgery followed by radiation plus lomustine (CCNU) resulted in a 64-week median survival, with 15% two-year survival. At Memorial Sloan-Kettering Cancer Center, lomustine, procarbazine, and vincristine have been used following surgery and radiation therapy. A median survival of 63 weeks has been found, with 44% of patients alive at 18 months (Shapiro and Young 1976).

While many series in the literature are reported as showing no difference between irradiation alone and irradiation plus nitrosoureas with or without other drugs, nearly all of them suffer from small numbers of patients, retrospective controls, and lack of stratification for the important prognostic variables mentioned earlier (Brisman et al. 1976; Seiler et al. 1978; Reagan et al. 1976). The single largest studies from the Brain Tumor Study Group showed definite benefit from combined modality therapy, and the standard by which other therapies should be measured seems to be radiation therapy and carmustine following maximal surgical removal of tumor. It seems clear that combination therapy, including maximal surgery if possible, 5500 to 6000 rad irradiation given postoperatively, and carmustine or possibly other nitrosoureas as well can result in nearly one-fourth of patients with this disease alive at two years. There is clear-cut palliation gain for the majority doomed to relapse and ultimately die of their disease, so treatment of this type should be offered to nearly all those who achieve a reasonable functional status following maximal surgical removal of tumor. Newer combinations of drugs, better means of delivering irradiation, and earlier means of detection (which should be greatly augmented by the use of CT scan) may improve these survival figures.

One possible means of doing so is with the use of hypoxic-cell radiosensitizers such as metronidazole (Flagyl) and similar compounds. The theory behind their use is that the center of the tumor is necrotic, and hypoxic radioresistant cells are located centrally. These electron-affinitive agents can sensitize previously hypoxic cells to radiation therapy by a process of reoxygenation. In the single randomized study reported (Urtasun et al. 1976), the median survival of the group given radiation plus metronidazole was double that of the group given irradiation alone. The side effects of the high doses required include peripheral neuropathy and seizures, and therefore widespread use must be cautioned against. These drugs remain investigational for this purpose; however, they offer promise for improved survival of patients with malignant gliomas and other primary brain tumors that are treated with irradiation.

References

Bloom, H. J. G. Medulloblastoma: prognosis and prospects. *Int. J. Radiat. Oncol. Biol. Phys.* 2:1031–1033, 1977.

Brisman, R. et al. Adjuvant nitrosourea therapy for glioblastoma. *Arch. Neurol.* 33:745–750, 1976.

Gilbert, H. et al. Combined therapy in malignant gliomas: further insights. In *Adjuvant therapy of cancer,* vol. 2, eds. S. E. Jones and S. E. Salmon. New York: Grune & Stratton, 1979, pp. 455–463.

Goldsmith, M. A., and Carter, S. K. Glioblastoma multiforme—a review of therapy. *Cancer Treat. Rev.* 1: 153–165, 1974.

Hoskins, T. et al. Chemotherapeutic implications of growth fraction and cell cycle time in glioblastomas. *J. Neurosurg.* 43:127–135, 1975.

Kernohan, J. et al. Symposium on new and simplified concept of gliomas: simplified classifications of gliomas. *Proc. Staff Meet. Mayo Clin.* 24:71–75, 1949.

Marsa, G. W. et al. Megavoltage irradiation in the treatment of glioma of the brain and spinal cord. *Cancer* 36:1681–1689, 1975.

Mork, S. J., and Loken, A. C. Ependymoma, a follow-up study of 101 cases. *Cancer* 40:907–915, 1977.

Reagan, T. J. et al. Controlled study of CCNU and radiation therapy in malignant astrocytoma. *J. Neurosurg.* 44:186–190, 1976.

Seiler, R. W. et al. Radiotherapy combined with procarbazine, bleomycin and CCNU in the treatment of high-grade supratentorial astrocytomas. *J. Neurosurg.* 48:861–865, 1978.

Shapiro, W. R., and Young, D. F. Chemotherapy of malignant glioma with CCNU alone and CCNU combined with vincristine sulfate and procarbazine hydrochloride. *Trans. Am. Neurol. Assoc.* 101:217–220, 1976.

Sheline, G. E. Radiation therapy of brain tumors. *Cancer* 39:873–881, 1977.

Solero, C. L. et al. Controlled study with BCNU vs. CCNU as adjunctive therapy following surgery plus radiotherapy for glioblastoma multiforme. *Cancer Clin. Trials* 2:43–48, 1979.

Urtasun, R. et al. Radiation and high-dose metronidazole in supratentorial glioblastoma. *N. Engl. J. Med.* 294:1364–1367, 1976.

Walker, M. D. Malignant brain tumors—a synopsis. *CA* 25:114–120, 1975.

Walker, M. D. et al. Evaluation of BCNU and/or radiotherapy in the treatment of anaplastic gliomas. *J. Neurosurg.* 49:333–343, 1978.

Walker, M. D., and Strike, T. A. An evaluation of methyl-CCNU, BCNU and radiotherapy in the treatment of malignant glioma. *Proc. Am. Assoc. Cancer Res.* 17:163, 1976.

sixty-six

Chemotherapy of Head and Neck Cancer

JOSEPH R. BERTINO
CHARLES D. KOWAL

Head and neck cancer refers to a group of tumors that include cancer of the lips, tongue, oral cavity, tonsils, sinuses, larynx, hypopharynx, and nasopharynx. Except for disease of basal cell origin (skin) and a small number of sarcomas, these tumors are usually of epidermoid (squamous) origin. They comprise about 6% of all cancer, but because of the concomitant difficulties in treatment and rehabilitation they cause suffering and difficulties out of proportion to their incidence. Many patients with this disease succumb to the local effects of tumor on the respiratory or upper digestive tract.

Etiology

Tobacco (chewing and smoking) in the United States and ethanol abuse play important roles in causation of these tumors (Williams and Horn 1977). Direct evidence for tobacco involvement is seen in India, where betel nut and tobacco chewing gives rise to a high incidence of buccal cell carcinoma. The mechanism whereby tobacco and alcohol affect incidence remains unknown. One possibility that has been explored in the laboratory is that ethanol causes an increase in the metabolic activation of tobacco smoke carcinogens. Results of some work in Syrian hamsters seem to indicate that chronic alcohol consumption increases sensitivity of cheek pouch to the effects of low doses of certain carcinogens (Freedman and Shklar 1978).

In Algeria, Tunisia, and southeast Asia, especially China, there are large numbers of cases of nasopharyngeal carcinoma. Attempts to find an environmental factor have not as yet been successful. These patients have been found, however, to have significant amounts of Epstein-Barr virus (EBV) antibodies in their serum (de-Thé and Geser 1974), whereas those with squamous cell carcinomas do not. Moreover, there is some evidence that a high percentage of the long-term survivors with nasopharyngeal cancer no longer have antibodies (IgA) against the EBV antigens. The prognostic value of EBV serologic tests, especially IgA antibodies, in this patient population is presently under study.

Classification and Grading

Squamous cell carcinomas of the head and neck are usually classified according to the following characteristics:

1. Well-differentiated—characterized by cells showing well-defined keratinization and pearl formation.
2. Moderately well-differentiated—these cells have less keratin and pearl formation, have more frequent mitosis, and there is less cellular uniformity.
3. Poorly differentiated—cells lack keratin formation, show frequent mitosis; intercellular bridges

characteristic of squamous cell origin can be demonstrated.

Prognosis

Prognosis depends on several factors including degree of differentiation of the tumor, size and location of primary disease, and spread to lymph nodes or to distal sites. Staging systems that attempt to take into account tumor locations and spread are used, such as the International Union Against Cancer (Union Internationale Contre le Cancer) (UICC) guidelines. Although the N classification that refers to cervical node status is uniform for all head and neck primaries, the T or primary tumor classification depends on size, *or,* in circumstances where size is not easily measured, the areas involved. The following example is given for cancer of the oral cavity.

A. Primary lesion
- T_{IS} — carcinoma in situ
- T_1 — tumor 2 cm or less in diameter
- T_2 — tumor 2 to 4 cm in diameter
- T_3 — tumor greater than 4 cm in diameter
- T_4 — tumor greater than 4 cm in diameter with invasion of antrum, base of tongue, pterygoid muscle

B. Cervical nodes
- N_0 — no clinically positive nodes
- N_1 — single node, homolateral, less than 3 cm in diameter
- N_2 — single node, homolateral, 3 to 6 cm in diameter, or multiple nodes, none greater than 6 cm in diameter
- N_3 — massive homolateral nodes, bilateral or contralateral nodes

C. Distant metastasis
- M_0 — no known metastasis
- M_1 — distant metastasis present

For simplification, the TNM staging is usually converted to a I to IV grouping:

Stage I — $T_1\ N_0\ M_0$
Stage II — $T_2\ N_0\ M_0$
Stage III — $T_3\ N_0\ M_0$
T_1 or T_2 or $T_3\ N_1\ M_0$
Stage IV — $T_4\ N_0$ or $N_1\ M_0$
Any T N_2 or $N_3\ M_0$
Any T any N M_1

Treatment

Surgery

Early stage disease (T_1 to T_2), especially in the lip, anterior tongue, and oral cavity, is usually treated by surgery if good cosmesis can be expected. Improved surgical techniques have permitted the treatment of most early lesions without functional disfigurement and have the advantage over radiation therapy, which causes long-lasting xerostomia and altered taste. Some of these procedures using new prostheses appear to be able to restore speech even after laryngectomy. Larger lesions (T_3 to T_4) are in general best handled by combinations of surgery and irradiation, and at Yale the latter is usually given postoperatively. Lymph node involvement, even in so-called favorable sites, decreases five-year survival rates markedly, and various combination approaches using chemotherapy with surgery and radiation therapy are being attempted. In addition to the different sites, stages, and degrees of differentiation that determine treatment and prognosis, other important factors must be considered. For example, malnutrition is commonly encountered either secondary to poor diet and ethanol abuse or to the direct effects of the tumor on the upper digestive tract. Age, mental status, and the patient's ability to cooperate and tolerate formidable surgical procedures or prolonged irradiation are also important. Thus despite the need for carefully controlled stratified studies, treatment must be individualized.

Radiation Therapy

Radiation therapy is employed in combination with surgery for many larger lesions, and is the treatment of choice for most nasopharyngeal and glottic primary tumors (Fletcher and Jesse 1977; Lindberg and Fletcher 1978). It also appears to be an effective method of eradicating microscopic disease in the neck in certain patients (Lindberg and Fletcher 1978). Although improved surgical and radiotherapeutic techniques have led to improved five-year survival rates, local or metastatic recurrence continues to be the major problem in patients with advanced disease. One area of drug research that may improve local failure rates involves hypoxic-cell sensitizers used with irradiation, since it is believed that hypoxic tumor cells are not killed by currently employed radiation techniques.

Chemotherapy

Several effective agents against head and neck cancer have been developed including methotrexate, cisplatin,

Table 66.1. *Activity of Single-Agent Chemotherapy*

Drug	*Number of Patients*	*Overall Response Rate (%)*
Methotrexate	232	38
Cisplatin	100	32
Bleomycin	298	21
5-Fluorouracil	118	15
Hydroxyurea	18	39
Cyclophosphamide	77	36
Vinblastine	35	29
Cytarabine	49	9
Doxorubicin	34	23

SOURCES: Adapted from Bertino, Boston, and Capizzi 1975; Carter 1977; Taylor 1979.

and bleomycin (table 66.1). Other agents have also shown some activity.

Methotrexate (MTX) is the most studied drug in this disease, and response rates have been reported between 20% and 60%. There is some suggestion that the site of the primary tumor is important; this plus the dosage schedules employed explain in a large measure these variable responses (Bertino, Boston, and Capizzi 1975). As a single agent, we believe high-dose weekly MTX with leucovorin (LV) rescue gives the highest response rates, and if patients are monitored carefully (serum MTX and creatinine levels), is the least toxic. Unfortunately, if patients with recurrent or advanced disease are treated with MTX, despite the high response rate, duration of response is usually short (median two to four months). The reasons for this rapid onset of resistance to both conventional MTX and the high-dose regimens are not known. A recent cooperative clinical trial compared weekly intravenous MTX with biweekly MTX plus LV, and biweekly MTX, LV, cyclophosphamide, and cytarabine in advanced disease (DeConti and Schoenfeld 1981). Response rates were not different among the arms, but response duration and survival were significantly superior in the MTX alone group.

Recent studies have shown that cisplatin is also highly effective, and response rates of 30% have been reported. The use of this drug in elderly patients, who often have borderline renal function, is difficult, since the drug is nephrotoxic.

A third well-studied drug is bleomycin. Response rates of 20% to 30% have been recorded, and well-differentiated tumors have shown encouraging response. Again, duration of response has been short (two to three months).

Other drugs that have been reported to have some activity in head and neck cancer are hydroxyurea, cytarabine, 5-fluorouracil, cyclophosphamide, doxorubicin, and the *Vinca* alkaloids.

Intraarterial Chemotherapy

The ability to deliver drugs directly to the tumor through cannulation has the advantage of achieving high tumor concentration with lower systemic concentrations. Various techniques have been used in this regard including low-dose continuous intraarterial perfusion (a dose too low to cause systemic effects but with local tumor activity), high-dose intraarterial administration with systemic rescue (e.g., MTX with systemic LV rescue), or the use of drugs that are metabolized in the systemic circulation of liver—nitrogen mustard, dichloromethotrexate (Cleveland et al. 1969), and 5-fluorouracil (5-FU). In general, because of the complications of catheter placement in elderly patients, and with earlier reports of only marginal advantage in intraarterial use for most drugs (Nervi et al. 1970, 1978), this practice has largely been abandoned in most centers. This is perhaps unfortunate, because good studies comparing responses to similar tumors in a controlled manner to systemic versus intraarterial therapy are lacking. Some recent studies, however, appear to be reviving the interest in this form of therapy, and have reported high rates of response with intraarterial delivery of such drugs as bleomycin (Inuyama 1978; Turrisi et al. 1978), cisplatin, or mitomycin (Inuyama 1979).

Combination Chemotherapy

The inability of single-agent therapy to result in complete remissions and the short duration of partial responses produced are compelling arguments for the development of combination chemotherapy regimens. Several drug combinations have been studied, but for the most part these studies suffer from the lack of suitable single-agent controls and proper stratification. Despite these reservations, some recent reports of combinations appear to be encouraging for the treatment of advanced disease (table 66.2). Cisplatin plus bleomycin, or these drugs plus methotrexate has produced greater than 50% response rates (Randolph et al. 1978; Kaplan et al. 1979). A timed, kinetically based protocol using vincristine, bleomycin, methotrexate, 5-FU, and leucovorin also has produced a high response rate (Price et al. 1978). We also reported that the use of sequential methotrexate followed by 5-FU produces a response rate of 86%, in addition to 20% complete responses (Pitman et al. 1980). Our impression is that the duration of response will also be prolonged over that expected from single-agent therapy; however, additional follow-up is required.

Table 66.2. *Some Drug Combinations Used to Treat Advanced Disease*

Reference	*Treatment Program*	*Response (%)*	*Number of Patients*
Randolph et al. 1978	Cisplatin plus bleomycin	71	15
Kaplan et al. 1979	Cisplatin, bleomycin, MTX	63	46
Shaw et al. 1980	MTX, 5-FU, vincristine, bleomycin, leucovorin rescue	75	76
Pitman et al. 1980	MTX followed by 5-FU plus leucovorin rescue	86	21

Combined Modality Therapy

The use of chemotherapy together with irradiation and surgery is an attractive approach to further improve treatment results. Issues that must be addressed are (1) the timing of chemotherapy in relation to surgery and radiation therapy, (2) the drugs to be used, and (3) the duration of therapy. It seems clear that following irradiation or surgery, chemotherapy is less effective than in patients who have not had these treatments. Chemotherapy following these modalities makes the most sense, however, since at this point microscopic disease that persists could be most sensitive to these agents (Taylor, Bytell, and Sisson 1979). At the present time we are leaning toward the split approach, that is, chemotherapy before and following surgery or irradiation. Such a trial is justified only if effective chemotherapy programs are developed and if the studies are properly controlled.

Hyperthermia

Hyperthermia, either alone or in combination with drugs or radiation therapy, has great potential; use of this modality is being vigorously pursued in several centers. An initial trial of focused ultrasound hyperthermia to treat patients with refractory head and neck tumors (in collaboration with Dr. P. Lele of the Massachusetts Institute of Technology) has been encouraging. A high response rate (88%) without any significant toxicity has resulted from relatively short exposures (20 minutes) to modest hyperthermia (42° to 43° C) (Lele et al. 1980).

References

Bertino, J. R.; Boston, B.; and Capizzi, R. L. The role of chemotherapy in the management of cancer of head and neck: a review. *Cancer* 36:752–758, 1975.

Carter, S. K. The chemotherapy of head and neck cancer. *Semin. Oncol.* 4:413–424, 1977.

Cleveland, J. C. et al. Arterial infusion of dichloromethotrexate in cancer of the head and neck—a clinical pharmacology study. In *Current topics in surgery research,* eds. G. D. Zuidema and D. B. Kinner. New York: Academic Press, 1969, pp. 113–120.

DeConti, R. C., and Schoenfeld, D. A randomized prospective comparison of intermittent methotrexate, methotrexate with leucovorin, and a methotrexate combination in head and neck cancer. *Cancer* 48:1061–1072, 1981.

de-Thé, G., and Geser, A. Nasopharyngeal carcinoma: recent studies and outlook for a viral etiology. *Cancer Res.* 34:1196–1206, 1974.

Fletcher, G. H., and Jesse, R. H. The place of irradiation in the management of the primary lesion in head and neck cancer. *Cancer* 39:862–867, 1977.

Freedman, A., and Shklar, G. Alcohol and hamster buccal pouch carcinogenesis. *Oral Surg.* 46:794–805, 1978.

Inuyama, Y. Bleomycin treatment of head and neck carcinoma in Japan. In *Bleomycin, current status and new developments,* eds. S. K. Carter, S. T. Crooke, and H. Umezawa. New York: Academic Press, 1978.

Inuyama, Y. Mitomycin treatment for head and neck cancer in Japan. In *Mitomycin C, current status and new developments,* eds. S. K. Carter, and S. T. Crooke. New York: Academic Press, 1979.

Kaplan, B. H. et al. Chemotherapy of advanced cancer of the head and neck with methotrexate, bleomycin and cis-diamminedichloroplatinum in combination. *Proc. Am. Soc. Clin. Oncol.* 20:384, 1979.

Lele, P. P. et al. Treatment of advanced squamous cell cancers of the head and neck region by local hyperthermia by focused ultrasound. Presented at the International Head and Neck Oncology Research Conference, September 8–10, 1980, Rosslyn, Va.

Lindberg, R. D., and Fletcher, G. H. The role of irradiation in the management of head and neck cancer: analysis of results and causes of failure. *Tumor* 64:313–325, 1978.

Nervi, C. et al. A reappraisal of intra-arterial chemotherapy. *Cancer* 26:577–582, 1970.

Nervi, C. et al. The relevance of tumor size and cell kinetics as predictors of radiation response in head and neck cancer. *Cancer* 41:900–906, 1978.

Pitman, S. W. et al. Sequential methotrexate–5-fluorouracil: a highly active drug combination in advanced squamous cell carcinoma of the head and neck. *Proc. Am. Soc. Clin. Oncol.* 21:473, 1980.

Price, L. A. et al. Improved results in combination chemotherapy of head and neck cancer using a kinetically based approach: a randomized study with and without Adriamycin. *Oncology* 35:26–28, 1978.

Randolph, V. L. et al. Combination therapy for advanced head and neck cancer: induction of remissions with diamminedichloroplatinum (II), bleomycin and radiation therapy. *Cancer* 41:460–467, 1978.

Shaw, H. J. et al. Prospects for improved survival in head and neck cancer using a kinetically based adjuvant chemotherapy protocol. Presented at the International Head and Neck Oncology Research Conference, September 8–10, 1980, Rosslyn, Va.

Taylor, S. G., IV. *Head and neck cancer. The current approach to diagnosis and treatment*. Syracuse, New York: Bristol Laboratories, 1979.

Taylor S. G., IV; Bytell, D.E.; and Sisson, G. A. Adjuvant chemoimmunotherapy in head and neck cancer. In *Recent results in cancer research*. New York: Springer-Verlag, 1979.

Turrisi, A. T. T., III et al. The role of bleomycin in the treatment of advanced head and neck cancer. In *Bleomycin, current status and new developments*, eds. S. K. Carter, S. T. Crooke, and H. Umezawa. New York: Academic Press, 1978.

Williams, R. R., and Horn, J. W. Association of cancer sites with tobacco and alcohol consumption and socioeconomic status of patients: interview study from the Third National Cancer Survey. *J. Natl. Cancer Inst.* 58:525–547, 1977.

sixty-seven

Endocrine Tumors

JOHN C. MARSH

Tumors of endocrine organs present special problems since they may be functional and thereby contribute to morbidity by overproduction of hormones of the parent gland. Such tumors may be histologically and clinically benign or they may be aggressively malignant with metastasis and death. Some of the malignant tumors are relatively undifferentiated and are not functional, that is, they do not produce sufficient hormone to be clinically important from the standpoint of endocrine effects. Some endocrine tumors are quite rare and the malignant ones are often even more so, so that one physician's or institution's experience may be sparse. This may be particularly true in the area of chemotherapy. This chapter is concerned with malignant endocrine tumors only.

Carcinoma of the Thyroid

Pathophysiology

Cancers of the thyroid are estimated to account for 1% of all cancers and about 0.4% of cancer deaths. They are rarely functional, but when a tumor does produce hormone it is usually of the follicular histologic type. Thyroid cancer occurs more commonly in women, with an approximate 3:1 woman:man ratio. The papillary histologic type is the most frequent (60% to 70%), with follicular next (about 30%), followed by anaplastic (including spindle and giant cell) and medullary, noteworthy for its production of calcitonin. The anaplastic variety may contain elements of papillary and follicular cancer, but its prognosis is substantially worse than for well-differentiated types.

It has been estimated that 15% to 20% of solitary thyroid nodules are malignant, whereas only about 0.01% to 0.1% cases of thyrotoxicosis are associated with thyroid cancer (Vander et al. 1968). Such solitary nodules are even more likely to be malignant in children and men. The etiology is unknown, although incidence is increased following thymus irradiation, head and neck radiotherapy, as in Hodgkin's disease, and after total body irradiation. The use of iodine 131 as therapy for benign thyroid diseases is reported not to be associated with an excess risk of thyroid cancer (Holm et al. 1980). Prolonged thyroid-stimulating hormone (TSH) stimulation in hypothyroidism has also been reported to result in thyroid cancer.

Diagnosis

Papillary and follicular cancers are commonly solitary nodules while the anaplastic variety are more often associated with pressure symptoms such as dysphagia, dyspnea, hoarseness, pain, and increasing size of the gland. Diagnostic tests include radioisotopic scanning of the thyroid (a so-called cold nodule being somewhat more suggestive of cancer), neck x-rays with barium swallow (looking for dense paratracheal calcifications suggestive of medullary carcinoma, or fine hazy calcifications suggestive of the papillary or follicular varieties), indirect laryngoscopy to evaluate the vocal cords, ultrasonography to differentiate cystic from solid lesions, chest film, and bone scan. Thyroid function tests are usually normal and of little diagnostic value. Radioactive iodine (RAI) uptake can be seen with functioning metastases of the follicular type of carcinoma.

Papillary Cancer

Papillary thyroid cancer is usually slow-growing and metastasizes to local lymph nodes and more rarely, to distant sites such as mediastinal nodes and lungs. Young patients do better than older ones. The five-year survival in one series was 82%, with surgery (total thyroidectomy) the usual treatment. Even patients who die have a fairly long survival, the average being eight years in one series (Silverberg et al. 1970). Some institutions recommend removal of all paratracheal lymph nodes at the time of thyroidectomy, and if these are positive to proceed to radical neck dissection. When elective radical neck dissections are done in patients with clinically negative node involvement in the neck, even though microscopic disease may be found about 50% of the time, there does not seem to be an improvement in survival (Hutter et al. 1970). If neck nodes are clinically involved, dissection seems to be beneficial. Postoperative external irradiation appears to benefit patients with definite or probable residual tumor left after operation (Simpson and Carruthers 1978).

Papillary thyroid cancer may be mixed with the follicular variety and the prognosis is then somewhat worse, approaching that of the follicular type.

Gross tumor masses may respond to external irradiation, but may regress very slowly. In the Toronto series the interval to maximum regression was 2 to 14 months with a mean of 8 months (Simpson and Carruthers 1978). Combined external beam irradiation and radioiodine may be useful in treating distant metastases or inoperable primary tumors, although the papillary variety tends to take up RAI less avidly than the follicular type. The response rate to RAI in metastatic papillary carcinoma was high in young patients at Memorial Sloan-Kettering Cancer Center (six of six) but low in older patients (Leeper 1972). Exogenous thyroid administration sufficient to suppress TSH is also recommended, both after primary therapy and as part of the treatment of metastases.

Follicular Cancer

Follicular carcinoma is usually avid in taking up RAI and is a somewhat more aggressive tumor with a mean survival of about three years in those who die of their disease. It tends to involve bones more often than the papillary type does. Surgery is the treatment of choice, and once again postoperative radiotherapy with both external beam and RAI has been reported to add to the efficacy of long-term control (Simpson and Carruthers 1978). Survival depends on tumor differentiation, being about 90% with the well-differentiated type and 60% for the poorly differentiated type. Older patients with metastatic disease have been reported to be more sensitive to RAI than younger ones in the Memorial Sloan-Kettering Cancer Center experience, but the numbers of the latter are small (Leeper 1972). Thyroid suppression is again recommended.

Medullary Cancer

Medullary carcinoma is solid, somewhat slow-growing, involves local structures and regional nodes, and contains amyloid as well as calcium deposits. It produces calcitonin. The 10-year survival is about 40% (Woolner et al. 1968). This is probably the least common kind of thyroid cancer.

Anaplastic Cancer

Anaplastic carcinoma of either small or large cell type is usually beyond local control by the time of surgery. The large cell tumor is refractory to radiotherapy and RAI, but the small cell variety may respond to external irradiation. Survival is usually a matter of a few months.

Chemotherapy

Chemotherapy is reserved for patients with metastatic disease, and virtually all those with anaplastic thyroid cancer should be treated. Those with papillary or follicular carcinoma rarely require it, but on occasion are candidates if RAI, thyroid suppression, and local irradiation have failed. Doxorubicin is the best known agent, being reported to have response rates from 35% to 55% when used alone (Gottlieb and Hill 1974, 1975; Bonnadonna et al. 1975; Shimaoka and Reyes 1976). Cisplatin also has some activity (three of six patients responding) (Shimaoka and Reyes 1976), and a current cooperative group protocol is comparing the results of doxorubicin alone and in combination with cisplatin. To date there is no difference between the regimens with respect to response rate (20%) or survival, although one arm appears to be giving more complete responses. Median survival in this study is about five months, with one-year survival of 30%. These data are incomplete and the study continues.

In the experience of Gottlieb and Hill (1974), responding cell types were medullary, papillary-follicular, and anaplastic. Nonresponders had a median survival of 4 months and responders of over 11 months.

Adrenocortical Carcinoma

Pathophysiology

Cancer of the adrenal cortex is rare, with an estimated incidence of two cases per million. The female:male ratio is approximately 2:1, and the median age is 35 to 40 years. Tumors may be characterized as functioning or nonfunctioning, depending on whether or not they produce an excess of adrenal cortical hormones. The two-thirds of cases that are functioning may have Cushing's syndrome, precocious puberty, the adrenogenital syndrome (with virilization or feminization), or more rarely, evidence of hypersecretion of aldosterone with hypertension and hypokalemic alkalosis. The most common steroid abnormality is increased excretion of urinary 17-ketosteroids, but increases in 17-hydroxycorticoids are also common, and urinary estrogens may be elevated. Serum cortisol may also be elevated, and urinary aldosterone may be increased.

Nonfunctioning adrenal tumors tend not to manifest themselves early but to be present when first examined as large masses that have already grown to involve local structures or metastasized; their cure rate is therefore somewhat less. Abdominal mass, pain, backache, and fever are common symptoms. Some patients with nonfunctioning tumors may excrete increased levels of hormonally inactive precursors such as pregnenolone metabolites that may serve as markers (Richie and Gittes 1980).

Growth of the tumor locally can cause invasion or obstruction of the kidney with hematuria. Local and regional node involvement and peritoneal spread are common, with local spread in 65% of one series (Hutter and Kayhoe 1966a). The lung was involved in 53% and the liver in 44%. Distant nodes (supraclavicular, hilar, and axillary) were found in 11%, with bone and brain involvement being less common.

The primary site is usually more often on the left, although there was no difference between sides in the series of Hutter and Kayhoe (1966a).

A staging system has been advocated that is based on tumor size, node involvement, and metastases. Stage 1 is a tumor less than 5 cm with no regional or distant involvement; stage 2 is greater than 5 cm; stage 3 has local invasion or regional node involvement; and stage 4 has distant metastases. Younger patients and women tend to have lower stages of disease.

Radiologic diagnosis may come from calcification in the adrenal area or displacement of a kidney downward as demonstrated by intravenous pyelogram. Retroperitoneal air insufflation is no longer necessary or advisable since the newer techniques of CT scanning and ultrasonography have both become quite useful and more accurate. Angiography can help in distinguishing adrenal from upper pole kidney lesions in doubtful cases. Steroid precursors with iodine 131 have also been useful in demonstrating increased uptake by primary tumor and localizing metastases.

Treatment

The treatment of choice, as with most cancers, is surgical removal. Since the average size at surgery is about 10 cm, en bloc dissection with removal of neighboring structures such as kidney, spleen, and part of the pancreas is often necessary. Patients with low-stage tumors (stage 1 or 2) do well; five of six in one series were alive at five years (Sullivan, Boileau, and Hodges 1978). Unfortunately, only 6 of 28 patients in this series had low-stage disease. Median survival for patients with stage 3 disease in this series was about two years, and only three months for those with stage 4 disease. Recurrence can occur as long as 12 years after diagnosis and primary surgery.

Although radiation therapy has not been shown to have a role in producing cure or improving surgical results, good palliation, particularly for bone metastases, has been reported when 3000 to 4000 rad were given over two to three weeks (Percarpio and Knowlton 1976).

Treatment of surgically incurable disease revolves largely around the use of o,p'DDD (mitotane, Lysodren). In 1948, when it was being evaluated as an insecticide, it was found that feeding this compound to dogs caused adrenal hemorrhage and atrophy. It was subsequently put to clinical trial in adrenal cancer. A direct cytotoxic effect on adrenal mitochondria has been described, as has inhibition of normal or neoplastic steroid production. When the clinical results of several large trials are pooled the response rates in terms of a decrease of at least 30% in elevated urinary steroid levels are 70% to 85%, whereas the objective tumor response is 34% to 61%. While nonfunctioning tumors may respond, the rate is somewhat lower (20%) than in functioning tumors (35%) although the difference was not significant (Hutter and Kayhoe 1966b). A more recent series (Lubitz, Freeman, and Okun 1973) has a higher response rate than that of Hutter and Kayhoe, attributed to earlier recognition of the disease and beginning of chemotherapy. Responders live longer than nonresponders, with the mean duration of response being about 10 months in each series. The prognosis and response rate are somewhat better in women. Nonresponders lived an average of two months. There have been several long-term (4.5 to 10 years) survivors reported with chemotherapy (Richie and Gittes 1980).

The excessive hormone production can also be treated with metyrapone or aminoglutethimide, but when used alone these agents do little for the basic problem (Schein 1972).

Major problems attending the use of mitotane are gastrointestinal symptoms that are usually dose-limiting, and central nervous system effects such as lethargy, somnolence, dizziness, or vertigo. Skin rash and liver function abnormalities are much less common. Steroid replacement is often required. The gastrointestinal effects reportedly are overcome with the concurrent use of cellulose acetylphthalate in Cushing's disease (Luton et al. 1979). Whether this will be useful in adrenal cancer remains to be seen. Plasma levels of mitotane may be measureable many months after cessation of therapy (Hogan et al. 1978).

Nonfunctioning tumors have been given special emphasis in the literature. In one series (Lewinsky et al. 1974) they comprised about 15% of the total cases and were thought to be capable of making steroids, albeit not able to make excess active hormones such as cortisol, sex hormones, or aldosterone, perhaps due to specific enzyme defects not present in functioning tumors and accounting for the accumulation of cholesterol in some of them. Two-thirds of the patients died within the first year. One patient had a brief response to combination chemotherapy with cyclophosphamide, vincristine, methotrexate, and 5-fluorouracil.

In another series (Hogan et al. 1980) anaplastic carcinomas were contrasted to well-differentiated ones, which were twice as common. The anaplastic variety was more common in men, had a worse prognosis (5 months versus 40 months median survival), was not associated with overproduction of hormones, and were refractory to mitotane. They also were associated with skin metastases in contrast to the well-differentiated tumors. It was suggested that anaplastic tumors should not be treated with mitotane since such attempts were doomed to failure, but that other agents or combinations be used. This seems to be a reasonable approach, as mitotane may well be less soluble in such tumors than in the well-differentiated variety, and several months may be lost waiting for a response.

Adriamycin is currently being evaluated by the Eastern Cooperative Oncology Group (ECOG) in patients with mitotane-resistant or nonfunctioning tumors. Recently, four patients have been reported to respond to cisplatin with responses lasting four to nine months. They were either refractory to or no longer responsive to mitotane (Tattersall et al. 1980). At least three of these had poorly differentiated tumors.

Malignant Pheochromocytoma

Pathophysiology

Pheochromocytoma is a relatively uncommon catecholamine-secreting tumor arising from the adrenal medulla or paraganglionic tissue such as the organ of Zuckerkandl. Only about 7% to 15% are malignant, and these are often slow-growing. In one series of 100 cases (Melicow 1977), only 7 were malignant; 2 of 83 arising from the adrenal were malignant; as were 5 of 17 of those having their origin in extra-adrenal tissue. The distribution of metastatic lesions based both on autopsied and nonautopsied cases (41 total) was bone (44%), liver (37%), lymph nodes (37%), lungs (27%), and central nervous system (10%) (Schonebeck 1969).

Clinical manifestations include hypertension (about 1% of hypertensive patients or less are estimated to have pheochromocytomas), seizures, headache, sweating, and syncope. Nonfunctioning tumors occur in about one-sixth of all patients with pheochromocytoma and are likely to be malignant. Urinary catecholamine and vanillylmandelic acid measurements are useful in diagnosis and in following the course of the disease.

Treatment

Control of catecholamine-related symptoms is more effective than antitumor therapy in patients with inoperable or metastatic tumors. Because the tumor is often slow-growing, the most significant palliation is often with adrenergic blocking agents. Phenoxybenzamine, the alpha-adrenergic receptor blocking agent, is used at a dose of 20 to 60 mg/day and is useful for control of hypertension and sweating. Propranolol, the beta-blocker, is given usually at a dose of 80 to 160 mg/day. We have observed a patient with inoperable, slowly growing tumor maintained very well on this combination for more than five years.

Surgery is the treatment of choice for both benign and malignant pheochromocytomas, and it may even be appropriate to debulk slowly growing incurable disease.

Radiotherapy is said to be relatively ineffective, perhaps because of hypoxia due to the effect of catecholamines (Drasin 1978). It has not been shown to be effective as primary or as surgical adjuvant therapy but is said to be palliative when given to lymph nodes or bone metastases in doses of 4000 rad.

Results with cytotoxic chemotherapy are anecdotal. Drasin (1978) collected six cases from the literature and mentioned one of his own. Among drugs that seem to have activity are cyclophosphamide and doxorubicin. Vincristine and methotrexate, each used in combination with cyclophosphamide in one patient, were ineffective. The rarity of this tumor makes it unlikely that more information will be forthcoming soon.

Because of activity in islet cell tumors and malignant carcinoids (tumors that, like the adrenal medulla, are derived from neural crest) streptozocin has been used in at least two cases of malignant pheochromocytoma (Hamilton et al. 1977). Unfortunately, neither patient responded.

Islet Cell Carcinoma

Pathophysiology

Islet cell tumors (benign and malignant) of the pancreas are estimated to occur with a frequency of about one in 100,000. They are capable of hypersecretion of insulin (B cells), glucagon (A cells), or gastrin (D cells). Serotonin, ACTH, secretin, and a hypercalcemic factor have also been described as products of islet cell tumors, with characteristic clinical syndromes (Schein et al. 1973).

Between 10% and 25% of islet cell tumors are malignant (Schein 1972; Service et al. 1976). Ninety percent of the functioning tumors secrete excessive amounts of insulin, either alone (75%) or in combination with glucagon or gastrin (Broder and Carter 1973). Rarely, they secrete gastrin alone. About 20% of malignant islet cell tumors are nonfunctioning.

These carcinomas occur in adults, with a median age of 52 years. Men and women are equally affected, with no particular racial predilection in this country. Fasting hypoglycemia is the predominant clinical symptom, with a small number demonstrating the Zollinger-Ellison syndrome secondary to gastrin hypersecretion. This includes intractable peptic ulceration, gastric acid hypersecretion, and diarrhea. An abdominal mass is relatively rare in functioning tumors but more common in the nonfunctioning ones. Because these tumors are usually in the body or tail of the pancreas, jaundice is rare at diagnosis. Insulin values are generally elevated and some patients have an increased amount of "big" insulin or proinsulin.

At the time of diagnosis 90% of patients with both functioning and nonfunctioning tumors have liver metastases. Local extension into the peritoneum and abdominal nodes is also seen in 5% to 10%, with no bone and lung involvement (Broder and Carter 1973). At autopsy, these latter organs sometimes (5% to 10%) show evidence of disease, but liver involvement is universal.

Treatment

In an old series (Howard et al. 1950) the median survival of 22 patients untreated with systemic measures was less than a year. In the 52 patients of Broder and Carter (1973) treated with streptozocin, the median survival from onset of symptoms was 38 months, from diagnosis 30 months, and from treatment 17 months. Patients' sex and tumor status (functioning versus nonfunctioning) played no significant role. Responders lived a median of 42 months from diagnosis while nonresponders lived a median of 17 months, a significant difference. The response rate was 64% for biochemical measurements and 52% for measureable disease.

In a more recent series of 81 patients from a cooperative study (Moertel, Hanley, and Johnson 1980) the median projected survivals from treatment in two groups was 16.5 and 26 months, corresponding to streptozocin without and with 5-FU, respectively. In the Broder and Carter series, survival ranged up to 19 years. These are relatively slowly growing tumors whose prognosis has been enhanced by improvements in hormone assays, antihormonal therapy, and anticancer treatment.

Palliation of the hypoglycemia, which is almost invariably present, includes parenteral glucose, dietary adjustment of carbohydrate intake, and the diuretic diazoxide. It inhibits insulin release and through beta-adrenergic stimulation increases hepatic gluconeogenesis and decreases use of peripheral glucose. Edema from renal sodium retention, hypertension, gastric irritation, hyperuricemia, and hirsutism may complicate its use (Schein 1972). It has no antitumor effect. The oral dose is 100 to 1000 mg daily in divided doses. A thiazide diuretic may be necessary to counteract sodium retention.

Clearly, streptozocin (described in detail in chapter 23 on nitrosoureas) is the keystone drug in malignant islet cell tumors. As mentioned, there is a significant response rate and beneficial effect on survival. Its diabetogenic effect was first noted in animals and exploited clinically in 1968. It can produce dramatic resolution of hypoglycemia. A current patient of mine is an elderly woman with metastatic disease who required a constant intravenous infusion of glucose. After the first few days of streptozocin this was no longer necessary, and she is now into her third year of treatment with an excellent partial response. Response rates vary from 34% (Moertel, Hanley, and Johnson 1980) to 52% (Broder and Carter 1973). Toxicity includes nausea and vomiting acutely, which are almost universal. With a five-day program this tends to become less each day although it may resume again with the next course. Renal toxicity, defined by proteinuria, can occur in up to half the patients and more severe toxicity in about 20%. Fatal renal toxicity occurred in 11% of the National Cancer Institute (NCI) series (Broder and Carter

1973). Liver function abnormalities occurred in 27%, and hematologic toxicity, usually anemia, in 20%.

Some activity occurs with 5-FU when used alone. Three of 12 patients in the NCI series had previously responded to 5-FU before being treated with streptozocin. The recent ECOG controlled trial has shown a superiority of 5-FU plus streptozocin to streptozocin alone (Moertel, Hanley, and Johnson 1980) in terms of response rate (63% versus 36%), complete response rate (33% versus 12%), and projected median survival (outlined above). New studies are evaluating the effects of doxorubicin combined with streptozocin, and of chlorozotocin.

Carcinoid Tumors

Pathophysiology

Carcinoid tumors occur in endodermally derived tissue and in teratomas. Eighty-five percent to 90% occur in the gastrointestinal tract, the remainder being largely from the lung (10% to 14%) and a very few arising in the ovary (Godwin 1975). Within the gastrointestinal tract, the appendix accounts for about 30% of tumors and the ileum and rectum both about 20%, with tumors arising from other parts of the small intestine, colon, and stomach far less frequently (Godwin 1975; Zahariai et al. 1975). Carcinoid tumors are the most common neoplasms of the appendix and ileum. Marks (1979) has reviewed a large series and compared it with the literature.

It has been claimed that the usual assessment of malignancy by histologic criteria is not reliable and that invasion and distant spread are much more accurate indicators of prognosis. In the Memorial Sloan-Kettering Cancer Center experience, the 60% of patients with gastrointestinal carcinoids that were still intramural had an 85% five-year survival, while those whose tumors had invaded to the serosa or beyond had a 5% five-year survival. The former group tended to be asymptomatic while about 90% with the invasive variety had symptoms (Zahariai 1975). Tumors of the appendix are usually benign by these criteria, being discovered at surgery for appendicitis or other causes; those of the ileum and colon are more often invasive. Surgery is the definitive therapy and results depend largely on the degree of invasiveness. Most patients with pulmonary carcinoids do well; five-year survivals in the literature range from 40% to 95% (Godwin 1975).

About 10% of patients have the carcinoid syndrome. In tumors of the gastrointestinal tract this is nearly always associated with liver metastases, while tumors derived from the lung and ovary need not be, presumably because of the access of serotonin to the systemic circulation in the latter situations, or with liver metastases (Schein 1972). Serotonin is thought to be responsible for the symptoms of diarrhea, abdominal pain, and malabsorption. The excretion of 5-hydroxyindoleacetic acid (5-HIAA) in the urine can be a useful tumor marker. The symptoms may at times be ameliorated by antidiarrheal therapy, but at times may require peripheral antagonists of serotonin such as cyproheptadine or methysergide. Parachlorophenylalanine is sometimes used successfully to inhibit the synthesis of serotonin, although allergies manifested by eosinophilia and pulmonary infiltrates may develop, and eosinophilia is said to be an indication that the drug should be stopped (Schein 1972). Mental changes and dizziness may also occur.

The flush of the carcinoid syndrome has been attributed to bradykinin, formed by the interaction of the tumor product, kallikrein, with a plasma protein. Phenothiazines and steroids have sometimes been helpful in relieving this distressing symptom.

Treatment

Antitumor agents that have been used with some success include 5-FU and streptozocin (Moertel et al. 1971; Moertel 1975).

Mengel and Shaffer (1973) have also described responses to the single agents melphalan, cyclophosphamide, and methotrexate, or to a combination of the last two. Because of the lack of myelotoxicity of streptozocin, it has been combined with agents such as 5-FU or cyclophosphamide without dose reduction of the last two agents. These combinations were tested in a recent ECOG study (Moertel and Hanley 1979). The response rate for the entire group of patients with carcinoids from any source was 33% with 5-FU and streptozocin and 26% for cyclophosphamide and streptozocin. Responses were better for tumors of the small intestine (41% overall) than for those from the lung (12%) or unknown primary site (17%). Response durations were for a median of about seven months. Median survival times from the time of diagnosis for all patients with respect to the tumor site were: small bowel, 29.3 months; lung, 14.9 months; colon, 10.1 months; and unknown origin, 8 months. There was a reasonably good correlation between response of urinary 5-HIAA excretion and objective tumor response. Patients with the carcinoid syndrome (75% of the total) had a somewhat higher response rate (31%) than those who did not

(24%). As is usually the case, patients with better initial performance status had better response rates.

A current study in progress has shown that doxorubicin is also active in this disease. It is not clear at the present time which drugs, either singly or in combination, are best, but it is encouraging that several of them have been shown to be active. Clearly, this is a promising area for careful multiinstitutional cooperative studies.

Invasive Thymoma

Pathophysiology

While thymomas are not strictly speaking endocrine tumors, they have been associated with a variety of syndromes such as myasthenia gravis, red cell aplasia, and lupus erythematosus, which may implicate humoral factors secreted by these tumors. They are composed of various mixtures of epithelial and lymphoid cells. Their malignancy or benignity can usually not be discerned by histologic appearance but must be determined by the extent to which they are locally invasive or metastatic.

Treatment

Treatment has typically been surgery, often combined with radiotherapy. Operation alone is usually curative in noninvasive tumors, and five-year survival ranges between 80% and 100% (Evans et al. 1980). For invasive tumors, however, the corresponding figures are 23% to 54%. Age under 25 years, predominance of epithelial cells in the tumor, and the presence of symptoms indicating invasion are factors that tend to worsen the prognosis (Boston 1976). The role of radiation therapy is not clear, but certainly its use has been associated with some long-term survivals. Preoperative irradiation has been used to reduce the mass of some bulky tumors, but it is probably used most commonly postoperatively following diagnosis and whatever surgery can be accomplished.

Metastatic sites include regional lymph nodes, liver, pleura, lungs (by either direct extension or hematogenous spread), paraaortic nodes, and even kidney (Boston 1976; Evans et al. 1980). Single agents reported to have activity in metastases include cisplatin (Talley et al. 1973), doxorubicin (Boston 1976), and maytansine (Jaffrey, Denefrio, and Chahinian 1980). Combinations that have been reportedly active include the Yale Hodgkin's disease regimen (nitrogen mustard, vincristine, procarbazine, and vinblastine) (Boston 1976) and COPP (cyclophosphamide, vincristine [Oncovin], prednisone, and procarbazine) (Evans et al. 1980). The latter was administered prior to radiation therapy in four patients in whom the diagnosis had been made by biopsy, with partial regressions in each. Three of the patients were disease-free at 34, 33, and 3 months after completion of treatment, one of them having resection of residual tumor. Another died of pneumonitis, possibly radiation-induced, without evidence of tumor at autopsy. A fifth patient, treated for recurrent metastatic disease three years after incomplete resection and possible control by steroids during that time, had stabilization during COPP treatment with no clear regression, and rapid progression when treatment was stopped.

It would seem that drugs useful in lymphoma may produce clear benefit in thymoma, and further clinical trials are in order.

References

Bonnadonna, G. et al. Adriamycin (NSC 123127) studies at the *Instituto Nazionale*. *Cancer Chemother. Rep.* 6:231–246, 1975.

Boston, B. Chemotherapy of invasive thymoma. *Cancer* 38:49–52, 1976.

Broder, L. E., and Carter, S. K. Pancreatic islet cell carcinoma. I. Clinical features of 52 patients. II. Results of therapy with streptozotocin in 52 patients. *Ann. Intern. Med.* 79:101–107, 108–118, 1973.

Drasin, H. Treatment of malignant pheochromocytoma. *West. J. Med.* 128:106–111, 1978.

Evans, W. K. et al. Combination chemotherapy in invasive thymoma. Role of COPP. *Cancer* 46:1523–1527, 1980.

Godwin, J. D., II. Carcinoid tumors. An analysis of 2837 cases. *Cancer* 36:560–569, 1975.

Gottlieb, J. A., and Hill, C. S., Jr. Chemotherapy of thyroid cancer with Adriamycin. *N. Engl. J. Med.* 290:193–197, 1974.

Gottlieb, J. A., and Hill, C. S., Jr. Adriamycin (NSC 123127) therapy in thyroid carcinoma. *Cancer Chemother. Rep.* 6:283–296, 1975.

Hamilton, B. P. M. et al. Attempted treatment of inoperable pheochromocytoma with streptozotocin. *Arch. Intern. Med.* 137:762–765, 1977.

Hogan, T. F. et al. o,p′-DDD (mitotane) therapy of adrenal cortical carcinoma. *Cancer* 42:2177–2181, 1978.

Hogan, T. F. et al. A clinical and pathological study of adrenocortical carcinoma. *Cancer* 45:2880–2883, 1980.

Holm, L.-E et al. Malignant thyroid tumors after iodine 131 therapy. *N. Engl. J. Med.* 313:188–191, 1980.

Howard, J. M. et al. Collective review: hyperinsulinism and islet cell tumors of the pancreas with 398 recorded tumors. *Int. Abstr. Surg.* 90:417–455, 1950.

Hutter, A. M., Jr., and Kayhoe, D. E. Adrenal cortical carcinoma. Clinical features of 138 patients. *Am. J. Med.* 41:572–580, 1966a.

Hutter, A. M., Jr., and Kayhoe, D. E. Adrenal cortical carcinoma. Results of treatment of o,p′DDD in 138 patients. *Am. J. Med.* 41:581–592, 1966b.

Hutter, R. V. P. et al. Elective radical neck dissection: an assessment of its use in the management of papillary thyroid cancer. *Cancer* 20:87–93, 1970.

Jaffrey, I. S.; Denefrio, J. M.; and Chahinian, P. Response to maytansine in a patient with malignant thymoma. *Cancer Treat. Rep.* 64:193–194, 1980.

Leeper, R. D. Medical management of thyroid cancer. *Clin. Bull. Memorial Sloan-Kettering Cancer Center* 2:3–6, 1972.

Lewinsky, B. S. et al. The clinical and pathologic features of "non-hormonal" adrenocortical tumors. *Cancer* 33:778–790, 1974.

Lubitz, J. A.; Freeman, L.; and Okun, R. Mitotane use in inoperable adrenal cortical carcinoma. *JAMA* 223:1109–1112, 1973.

Luton, J. P. et al. Treatment of Cushing's disease by o,p′DDD. *N. Engl. J. Med.* 300:459–464, 1979.

Marks, C. *Carcinoid tumors: a clinicopathologic study.* Boston: G. K. Hall & Co., 1979.

Melicow, M. One hundred cases of pheochromocytoma (107 tumors) at Columbia-Presbyterian Medical Center, 1926–1976. *Cancer* 40:1987–2004, 1977.

Mengel, C. E., and Shaffer, R. D. The carcinoid syndrome. In *Cancer medicine,* eds. J. F. Holland and E. Frei III. Philadelphia: Lea & Febiger, 1973, pp. 1584–1594.

Moertel, C. G. Clinical management of advanced gastrointestinal cancer. *Cancer* 36:675–682, 1975.

Moertel, C. G. et al. Phase II study of streptozotocin (NSC 85998) in the treatment of advanced gastrointestinal cancer. *Cancer Chemother. Rep.* 55:303–307, 1971.

Moertel, C. G., and Hanley, J. A. Combination chemotherapy trials in metastatic carcinoid tumor and the malignant carcinoid syndrome. *Cancer Clin. Trials* 2:327–334, 1979.

Moertel, C. G.; Hanley, J. A.; and Johnson, J. A. Streptozotocin alone compared with streptozotocin plus fluorouracil in the treatment of advanced islet cell carcinoma. *N. Engl. J. Med.* 303:1189–1194, 1980.

Percarpio, B., and Knowlton, A. H. Radiation therapy of adrenal cortical carcinoma. *Acta Radiol. Ther.* 15:288–292, 1976.

Richie, J. P., and Gittes, R. F. Carcinoma of the adrenal cortex. *Cancer* 45:1957–1964, 1980.

Schein, P. S. Chemotherapeutic management of the hormone-secreting endocrine malignancies. *Cancer* 30:1616–1626, 1972.

Schein, P. S. et al. Islet cell tumors: current concepts and management. *Ann. Intern. Med.* 79:239–257, 1973.

Schonebeck, J. Malignant pheochromocytoma. *Scand. J. Urol. Nephrol.* 3:64–68, 1969.

Service, F. J. et al. Insulinoma. Clinical and diagnostic features of 60 consecutive cases. *Mayo Clin. Proc.* 51:417–429, 1976.

Shimaoka, K., and Reyes, J. Chemotherapy of thyroid carcinoma. In *Thyroid research,* eds. J. Robbins and I. E. Braverman. Amsterdam: Excerpta Medica, 1976, pp. 586–589.

Silverberg, S. G. et al. Fatal carcinoma of the thyroid: histology, metastases, and causes of death. *Cancer* 25:792–802, 1970.

Simpson, W. J., and Carruthers, J. S. The role of external radiation in the management of papillary and follicular thyroid cancer. *Am. J. Surg.* 136:457–460, 1978.

Sullivan, M.; Boileau, M.; and Hodges, C. V. Adrenal cortical carcinoma. *J. Urol.* 120:660–665, 1978.

Talley, R. W. et al. Clinical evaluation of toxic effects of cis-diamminedichloroplatinum (NSC 119875). Phase I clinical study. *Cancer Chemother. Rep.* 57:465–471, 1973.

Tattersall, M. H. N. et al. Cis-platinum treatment of metastatic adrenal carcinoma. *Med. J. Aust.* 1:419–421, 1980.

Vander, J. B. et al. Significance of nontoxic thyroid nodules: final report of 15-year study of incidence of thyroid malignancy. *Ann. Intern. Med.* 69:537–540, 1968.

Woolner, L. B. et al. Thyroid carcinoma: general considerations and follow-up data on 1181 cases. In *Thyroid neoplasia,* eds. S. Young and D. R. Inman. New York: Academic Press, 1968, pp. 51–79.

Zahariai, Y. M. et al. Carcinoid tumors of the gastrointestinal tract. *Cancer* 35:588–591, 1975.

sixty-eight

Solid Tumors in Children

SUE MCINTOSH

Malignant tumors constitute a major cause of morbidity and fatality in the young (Altman and Schwartz 1978; Sutow, Vietti, and Fernbach 1977). In decreasing order of frequency, the most common solid neoplasms in children and adolescents are: central nervous system tumors, lymphomas, Wilms' tumor (nephroblastoma), neuroblastoma, bone tumors, and soft tissue sarcomas.

Many of these tumors, particularly if they are localized, are potentially curable. Their management is often best designed by cooperative efforts of specialists in pediatric surgery, radiation therapy, and pediatric oncology. Since the patients, in particular young children and infants, are in crucial phases of physical and emotional growth and development, management of their cancers must be approached with two principles in mind: first, control, and hopefully cure, of the malignancy, and second, treatment with a minimum of toxicity (acute, subacute, and chronic), particularly with regard to skeletal growth and maturation, fertility, oncogenesis, and cosmetic integrity. The increasing effectiveness of combined treatment modalities has provided the incentive to minimize long-term effects of all types of therapies and still maintain a high likelihood of tumor control.

The care of acute and chronic illness in a child requires care of the family. Education of parents and young patients is essential. It is important to alleviate the parents' guilt and provide encouragement for maintenance of discipline and a realistic approach to the physical and emotional aspects of the child's illness. All children should be told the basic nature and treatment of the cancer in a simple, gentle fashion, with acknowledgement that therapy may be difficult. Drawings are useful in these explanations. Since guilt and fear of separation are often troublesome, the child should be told that the disease is not a consequence of misbehavior and that members of the family and the medical staff will always be available. Adolescents and older children deserve more detail. They as well as their parents need to understand that there are many types of cancers and to share the hope that with their cooperation their disease may be cured.

Tumors of the Central Nervous System

These are likely to be primary tumors of the brain or spinal cord rather than metastases from another site. One important exception is neuroblastoma, which tends to invade the dura and the epidural space from bone metastases. The major types of brain tumors in children include astrocytoma of the cerebrum or cerebellum, glioblastoma multiforme, craniopharyngioma, ependymoblastoma, and medulloblastoma.

Cerebral tumors produce symptoms of increased intracranial pressure and focal neurologic deficits. Craniopharyngiomas and pituitary tumors may produce hormonal abnormalities such as hypopituitarism or deficits in visual field examinations. Ependymoblastomas and medulloblastomas often prevent free flow of cerebrospinal fluid and may produce hydrocephalus in infants and increased intracranial pressure in older children. Ataxia and vomiting are predominant symptoms of medulloblastoma and cerebellar tumors.

Diagnosis suspected on clinical examination can be confirmed by radiographic contrast studies with computerized cranial tomography or angiography. Prior to surgical biopsy, placement of a ventriculoperitoneal shunt may be necessary to correct obstructive hydrocephalus and maximize the safety of the procedure. Biopsy is mandatory for all accessible tumors. In some instances, such as medulloblastoma, improved neurosurgical techniques using the operating microscope have improved the chances of subtotal or total excision of gross tumor.

Surgical extirpation is the management of choice for slowly growing tumors such as cystic astrocytoma or ependymoblastoma. The primary or secondary therapy for incompletely resected tumors is radiotherapy (Sheline 1977). Total doses required for tumor control are often in the range of 5000 to 6000 rad delivered over five to six weeks. Midline tumors of the cerebellum, in particular medulloblastoma, are likely to seed meninges of the spinal cord with "drop" metastases. Accordingly, the field of irradiation should cover the entire craniospinal axis. Adjuvant chemotherapy is still in its infancy (Van Eys and Cangir 1978). In selected tumors (for example, medulloblastoma) success with adjuvant chemotherapy has been suggested by some preliminary reports (Venes et al. 1979). Other possible adjuncts to radiotherapy that are still in the stages of research development include radiosensitizers and immunotherapy.

Lymphomas

Hodgkin's Disease

Hodgkin's disease, one of the more chronically developing malignancies, is primarily a tumor of adolescence (Shah et al. 1976). Although any lymphoma can appear in any group of lymph nodes, the areas most commonly affected initially are the cervical or supraclavicular nodes and the anterior mediastinum. Adenopathy evolves slowly and generally is discovered when the nodes reach a size of 2 cm or more. They tend to be rubbery or firm to palpation and frequently are matted to neighboring nodes. An anterior mediastinal mass may accompany cervical or supraclavicular adenopathy but occasionally it is the only site of tumor involvement. Large chest tumors may produce a nagging cough, chest pain, swelling of the neck and head because of venous obstruction, or persistence of respiratory symptoms following a respiratory infection.

A biopsy of enlarged nodes is warranted whenever serious concern exists regarding the presence of a lymphoma. If a mediastinal mass is present (fig. 68.1), the biopsy should be obtained from a palpably enlarged supraclavicular or cervical node, a minor procedure compared to thoracotomy. If such a node is not available and the chest must be entered, the procedure should be limited to a biopsy of the tumor. A complete resection should not be attempted as this can jeopardize the patient's life unnecessarily, since lymphomas can be controlled or cured with radiotherapy or chemotherapy.

Once the diagnosis is made the patient must be evaluated thoroughly for extent of disease. Noninvasive techniques include the following: documentation or history of pruritus, jaundice, weight loss, fevers, or night sweats; full chest tomography to determine the extent of lymphadenopathy, hilar and mediastinal masses, extension into the lung parenchyma, or the presence of pleural disease; liver enzyme levels, erythrocyte sedimentation rate; copper level; bipedal lymphangiography; bone marrow biopsy; and gallium scan. Further selective studies (x-rays, bone scan, and so on) are dictated by the findings in these tests.

In selected cases in which the mode of therapy is certain, as in stage IV disease, laparoscopy with percutaneous liver biopsies may be the procedure of choice for surgical staging. In most patients, however, full staging laparotomies may well be required to determine the presence of microscopic disease in the abdomen (Annotation 1978; Jenkin et al. 1979). In individuals with chest involvement there is a 30% likelihood that subclinical microscopic disease below the diaphragm will be discovered by a thorough staging laparotomy and splenectomy. In preparation for splenectomy, pneumococcal vaccine is advised as soon as the diagnosis of Hodgkin's disease has been made.

Traditionally, patients with stage I or IIA disease (no systemic symptoms, restricted to one side of the diaphragm) have been treated with radiation therapy to extended fields. The dose for control of active lymphoma approximates 4500 rad and is delivered over a period of several weeks. Cure can be expected in about 90% of patients with stage I and about 80% with stage IIA disease (Hellman et al. 1978). Side effects that may occur from this dose to a large thoracic field in growing children include the following: cessation or slowing of skeletal growth, fibrosis and atrophy of muscles, hypothyroidism and thyroid tumors, carotid artery stenosis, pulmonary fibrosis, and constrictive pericarditis (D'Angio 1978). Radiotherapy to an abdominal field may produce infertility and slowing of spinal growth.

Disseminated disease (stage IIIB or IV) dictates primary therapy with combination chemotherapy, with or without adjuvant radiotherapy (Lange et al. 1978; Prosnitz et al. 1976). Chemotherapy in children and adolescents generally has the same acute and subacute side effects as it does in adults. Young patients with Hodgkin's disease have a high chance—approximately 80%—of obtaining complete remission with the use of combinations of agents; however, chemotherapy induces infertility in most males and in about half of females. Secondary amenorrhea during treatment is a frequent occurrence. In addition, radiotherapy and chemotherapy, particularly in combination, are carcinogenic in themselves, producing a risk of 1% to 5% of developing a secondary malignancy—acute myelogenous leukemia, musculoskeletal tumors, or non-Hodgkin's lymphomas.

In children particularly, the advantages of different therapies for Hodgkin's disease must be balanced against the risks regarding growth and development. Localized disease can be cured in 75% to 90% of patients treated with irradiation, and preliminary reports suggest that a high percentage can also be cured with chemotherapy. More limited use of radiotherapy and more liberal administration of chemotherapy may obviate many of the chronic toxicities associated with the former, but may also be expected to produce a slight increase in the risk of secondary malignancies.

Non-Hodgkin's Lymphomas

Non-Hodgkin's lymphomas (NHL) in children are a particularly aggressive group of lymphomas that tend to disseminate early, metastasizing to other nodes, the bone marrow, and the central nervous system. Unlike Hodgkin's disease, non-Hodgkin's lymphomas are rapidly growing tumors and require expeditious evaluation and institution of therapy.

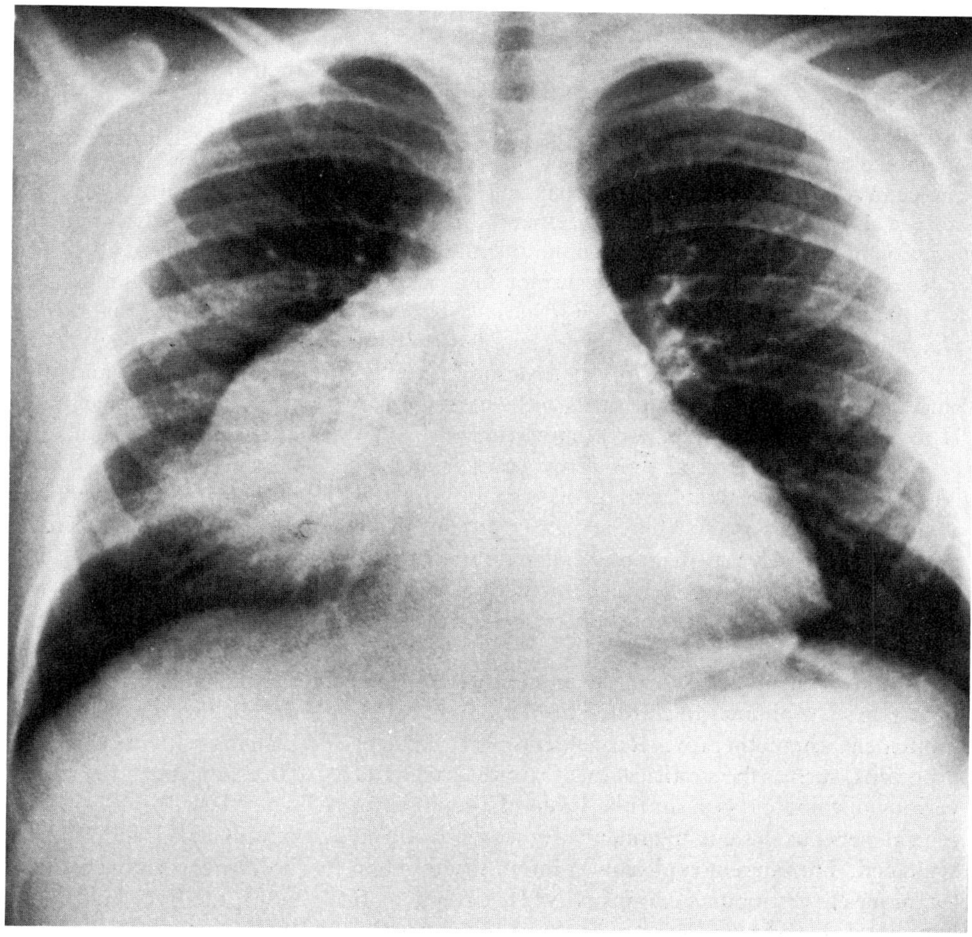

Fig. 68.1. *Chest radiograph of an adolescent with a large mediastinal mass due to Hodgkin's disease. Differential diagnosis includes non-Hodgkin's lymphoma, acute leukemia, and teratoma.*

The lymphocytic types, most of which are histologically diffuse rather than nodular, have a propensity to occur in the preadolescent and adolescent age groups. Particularly in the young man, they occur as a rapidly enlarging mediastinal mass and may produce increasing respiratory distress from tracheal or tracheobronchial compression. Acute airway compromise represents a medical emergency in which therapy (irradiation or corticosteroids) may need to be instituted before a definitive biopsy can be performed.

Performance of lymph node biopsy and nonsurgical evaluation for extent of disease are similar to those described for Hodgkin's disease. Examination of the bone marrow and cerebrospinal fluid is of strategic importance because of the tendency of these lymphomas to spread to the marrow and meninges. Leukemic transformation is common, and marrow involvement of as much as 25% may indicate the need for treating the patient on an antileukemia regimen. Staging laparotomy is restricted to those rare pediatric patients with a nodular histologic pattern.

Since most NHLs in children are histologically diffuse (lymphocytic 80%, histiocytic 20%), intensive chemotherapy with multiple drugs is the treatment of choice (Wollner, Exerby, and Lieberman 1979; Weinstein et al. 1979). Although the ingredients and administration of these programs vary among institutions, the most effective drugs for reducing tumor bulk rapidly and maintaining remission are high-dose cyclophosphamide, corticosteroids, vincristine, and doxorubicin (Adriamycin), although additional drugs may be included. With this approach, patients with true stage I or II disease have a high likelihood (approximately 90%) of sustained complete remission of two years or longer. More than half of patients with mediastinal tumors will attain long remissions. Most pediatric patients have disseminated disease at diagnosis and will attain complete remission with aggressive chemotherapy, but still have a substantial rate of disease recurrence and eventual fatality.

Only recently has long-term control of non-Hodgkin's lymphomas in children been successful with multiagent chemotherapy. Refinements of treatment programs, such as the stratification of clinical stages and various histologic types, and the value of prophylactic central nervous system treatment are currently being evaluated. The current explosion in immunopathologic techniques to distinguish origins of NHL from T or B lymphocytes, their various predispositions to marrow and meningeal metastasis, and the hope for development of specific immunotherapies should provide the oncologist with effective, specific methods of control.

Wilms' Tumor

Wilms' tumor, a malignancy intrinsic to the kidney, is the most common abdominal neoplasm in young children and infants. It is believed to originate in microscopic hamartomatous or nephroblastomatous rests in the developing kidney. Its greatest incidence is among children under four years of age, and it is rarely seen in those over eight years. Children with Wilms' tumor have an enlarging abdominal mass (fig. 68.2), sometimes associated with abdominal pain, lassitude, and anorexia, and perhaps hematuria or hypertension. The tumor grows extremely rapidly and becomes centrally necrotic, providing a site of hemorrhage. Therefore it is not unusual for a patient to have anemia at the time of diagnosis because of blood loss into the tumor. Since these tumors are extremely friable and likely to rupture into the abdominal cavity, it is wise for abdominal palpations to be limited to those necessary to establish their dimensions.

When an abdominal mass is discovered in an infant or a child, a rapid, efficient evaluation is mandatory. Following physical examination and an accurate blood pressure assessment, the most useful diagnostic tests are urinalysis and an intravenous pyelogram (IVP). Definition of an intrinsic renal mass can usually be made on IVP, which shows a large mass usually located in the upper pole of one kidney, causing severe distortion of the calyceal system and inferior displacement of the collecting system and ureter. As part of the IVP, an early film of the vascular phase of the contrast material will often enable the radiologist to note the vascular nature of the mass and to look for metastases in the liver and in other parts of the abdomen. Other radiologic studies such as arteriography, inferior venocavagram, and selective retrograde studies may be useful in selected patients but in general are not necessary. A preoperative chest x-ray will establish the presence or absence of metastatic pulmonary lesions. Their presence, however, should not influence management of the primary abdominal tumor, because with appropriate therapy even patients with metastatic Wilms' tumor may be cured (Breslow et al. 1978).

Usual sites of metastases are the neighboring lymph nodes, abdominal cavity (particularly if there has been preoperative or intraoperative rupture of the capsule), the liver, and the lungs. Rarely, the tumor may metastasize to cortical bone or the central nervous system.

Because this is potentially a highly curable malignancy it is imperative that surgery, radiotherapy, and chemotherapy be performed by experienced individuals.

Treatment

Surgery

There is extensive experience with operative management of Wilms' tumor. Dissection and removal may be extremely difficult, and spillage into the abdominal cavity may occur even in the most experienced hands. A large transabdominal incision is made to facilitate removal of the tumor in toto without spillage. The renal vein is clamped before manipulation of the malignancy. Following resection, lymph nodes at the hilum of the kidney and the paraaortic region are examined by sight or palpation, and enlarged nodes are removed for histologic examination. The opposite kidney and the liver are palpated carefully for smaller tumors or nodules. The wound is closed with full-thickness wire sutures so that chemotherapy and radiotherapy can be instituted during the postoperative period without risk of wound dehiscence.

Pathologic evaluation of the resected Wilms' tumor is of increasing importance in determining therapy. The presence of tubular structures and abortive glomeruli are signs of the tumor's attempt to differentiate into normal renal tissue, and they indicate a favorable histologic picture. Absence of these structures and the presence of a highly sarcomatous mesenchymal histology are indicative of an unfavorable prognosis. Such disease is treatable and sometimes curable, but not as highly curable as that with favorable histology (Beckwith and Palmer 1978). The pathologist is also instrumental in determining, by examination of multiple sections of the tumor, whether there is invasion through or into the surrounding capsule. Tumor thrombus extending into the renal vein is not unusual (fig. 68.3).

Chemotherapy

Prior to the advent of effective chemotherapeutic agents, Wilms' tumor was cured in only about 25% of young children, mostly infants, by surgical resection and/or radiotherapy. The availability of dactinomycin and later vincristine and other agents has converted the majority of these children to potentially curable candidates for treatment (D'Angio et al. 1976). Much of the knowledge of effective therapeutic regimens has been derived from the national Wilms' tumor studies.

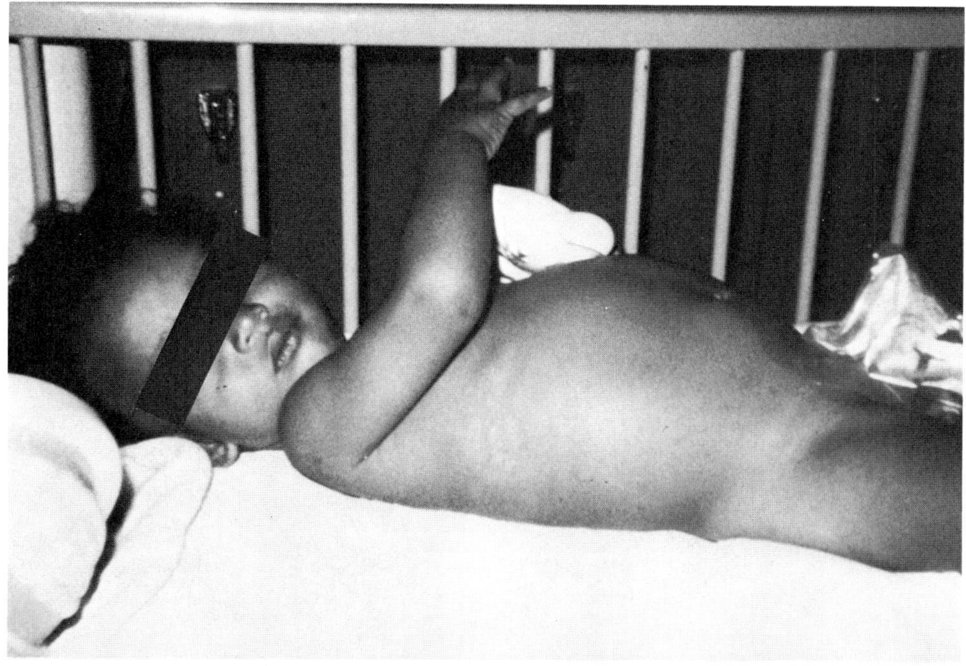

Fig. 68.2. *Large abdominal mass in a young child with Wilms' tumor. Differential diagnosis includes neuroblastoma, rhabdomyosarcoma, and non-Hodgkin's lymphoma.*

Dactinomycin and vincristine used in combination are highly effective in reducing gross metastases or preventing the growth of microscopic metastases. Both drugs should be used with great caution in infants, since they are extremely toxic to children under one year of age. Dactinomycin may be started in the immediate postoperative period and is given in a five-day course, 15 μg/kg/day, every six weeks to three months. Vincristine is instituted as soon as bowel function has been established and may be given weekly or in combination with the courses of dactinomycin. The dose, 1.5 mg/m^2, should not exceed 2 mg in any individual. Common side effects from dactinomycin are alopecia, anorexia, mucosal ulceration, bone marrow depression, diarrhea, and synergistic toxicity with radiotherapy. Particularly when used with radiotherapy the drug infrequently can cause hepatitis. The usual toxicities of vincristine include neuropathy, irritability, constipation, alopecia, and occasionally, severe bowel dysfunction with ileus. Both drugs are given intravenously, and both may cause severe excoriation of the subcutaneous tissues if extravasated.

Other drugs that have been used with variable success are doxorubicin (Adriamycin) and cyclophosphamide. Inclusion of one or both of these agents should be considered for the patient with an unfavorable histology or with metastatic disease at the time of diagnosis.

Adjuvant chemotherapy following removal of the tumor is continued for 6 to 15 months. This approach is curative in 90% of children with a relatively small, well-contained, completely resected Wilms' tumor with favorable histology. Large tumors or those with local extension require the addition of radiotherapy, and the majority of these patients with histologically favorable disease are curable.

Radiotherapy

Wilms' tumors are relatively radiosensitive, but radiation therapy is not a definitive modality in itself. In situations where the child is young, the tumor is of favorable histology, and the mass is relatively small, completely encapsulated, and resected without spillage, radiotherapy is not necessary. For most other patients, however, the radiotherapist should be consulted with regard to treating the area formerly occupied by the tumor or, if abdominal spillage or rupture has occurred, the areas of spillage. The optimal dose fractionation is uncertain, particularly with the concomitant use of radiosynergistic drugs such as dactinomycin and doxorubicin. Traditionally, 3000 to 4000 rad have been administered—doses that cause growth delays in the bony skeleton and musculocutaneous changes. Lower doses may be as effective, particularly with the use of multiple chemotherapeutic agents.

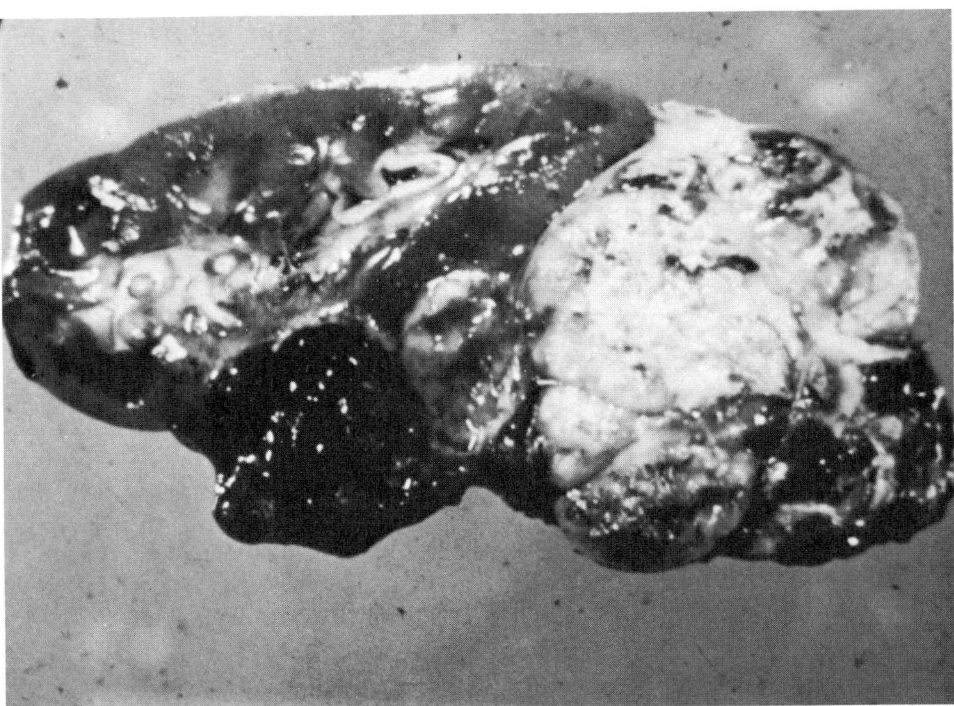

Fig. 68.3. *Cut surgical specimen showing a large Wilms' tumor with extension into the renal vein.*

Bilateral Wilms' Tumor

In 5% to 10% of cases Wilms' tumor will be present in both kidneys. The excretory urogram is of strategic importance in evaluation of the contralateral kidney. The child with bilateral tumors presents the management team with a dilemma for management and a choice of several options:

1. Removal of the kidney containing the larger tumor, followed by combination chemotherapy to shrink the contralateral tumor, followed by surgical resection of the smaller contralateral tumor or tumors. This approach is most successful if the contralateral tumor is in the pole of the kidney and therefore accessible to surgical resection.
2. Removal of the kidney containing the larger tumor, followed by irradiation and chemotherapy with no attempt to resect the contralateral tumor. This approach may be necessary if there are multiple tumors or tumorlets in the contralateral kidney that are not accessible to surgical resection.
3. Limited biopsy of the larger tumor without an attempt at resection, followed by reduction of all tumor masses with chemotherapy with or without radiotherapy, followed by resection of both tumors with an attempt to preserve normal renal tissue on both sides.
4. Autotransplantation, in which both kidneys are removed. The kidney containing the smaller tumor is kept viable and the tumors dissected free of normal renal parenchyma. That kidney is then reimplanted.
5. Bilateral nephrectomies followed by dialysis, chemotherapy, and radiotherapy, after which the patient who is cured of disease becomes a candidate for renal transplantation (Ragab et al. 1972).

Mesoblastic Nephroma

Mesoblastic nephroma is a nonmalignant, hamartomatous, intrinsic renal tumor of infancy. Its signs and symptoms are identical to those of Wilms' tumor and may be found in the neonate. Pathology is of crucial importance in this instance, because mesoblastic nephroma can be clearly differentiated from Wilms' tumor histologically. Since this is a nonmalignant lesion, and since chemotherapy and radiotherapy are highly toxic to neonates and young infants, it is imperative that the distinction be made before further therapy is instituted. Mesoblastic nephroma requires only surgical resection and regular examinations of the patient thereafter.

Neuroblastoma

Neuroblastoma, like Wilms' tumor, is a malignancy of infants and young children. Ganglioneuroblastoma may occur as a malignant paraspinal mass in older individuals. The most likely sites of origin of neuroblastoma are the adrenal medulla, which is likely to produce a large abdominal mass and to metastasize before discovery, and the paraspinal sympathetic ganglia. A small number of patients have disseminated disease at initial examination, and the primary site is unknown.

Neuroblastoma is a highly immunogenic and neurohormonal tumor. Tumor-specific antibodies, cytotoxic lymphocytes, and blocking antibodies can be found in the patient's blood. In most instances, catecholamine metabolites—particularly homovanillic acid, vanillyl mandelic acid (VMA), and dopamine—are detectable in the urine and may be used to follow tumor activity.

The young infant under one year of age has the best prognosis. Many infants have localized disease that is well controlled with surgical resection or relatively small doses of radiotherapy. Even with certain types of metastases—liver, spleen, skin, and limited amounts to the bone marrow—long-term control may be effected in the majority by removal of the primary tumor or by irradiation of large tumors. Chemotherapy has little to offer as an adjunct to therapy in this age group. The remarkable incidence of long-term survival or spontaneous cure among infants may well be immunologically mediated.

The older infant and child, however, have a more malignant process. If the neuroblastoma is localized (primarily those occurring in the paraspinal regions), potential cure is possible (Castleberry 1979). Unfortunately, many older patients have metastatic disease at the time of diagnosis. Although many chemotherapeutic drugs, notably cyclophosphamide, have produced temporary disappearance of disease, and with combination chemotherapy these remissions have lasted one year or longer, the majority eventually succumb to progressive disease (Finklestein et al. 1979).

Because neuroblastoma tends to metastasize to the central nervous system and to cortical bone and lymph nodes, many of the complications of progressive disease are crippling and painful. A common neurologic complication, particularly of paraspinal tumors, is spinal cord compression by epidural tumor extension of the paraspinal mass. The child with paraparesis or bladder or bowel dysfunction should have a myelogram performed without delay to delineate the extent of epidural tumor. The compression may be relieved by surgical laminectomy and tumor resection, or in selected cases, by radiotherapy and corticosteroids. Increased intracranial pressure is likely to result from plaques of tumor growing from skull metastases into the epidural space and the dura mater. The treatment of choice is whole brain irradiation. Periorbital edema, blue discoloration, and proptosis are frequent from involvement of the orbital lamina and soft tissues by tumor metastases and can usually be well controlled with local radiotherapy.

Cortical bone metastases are often extensive, producing inability to move or walk, pathologic fractures, and severe pain. Although local radiotherapy may be useful to control intractable pain in a small area, diffuse pain is best controlled by chemotherapeutic agents and regular narcotics. The terminal stages of disseminated neuroblastoma often evolve over many months and challenge medical and parental caretakers to provide supportive and palliative care for the dying child and the family.

Bone and Soft Tissue Sarcomas

The predominant pediatric bone tumors occur in older children and adolescents in whom Ewing's tumor and osteogenic sarcoma are the most common (Mankin 1979; Glicksman, Maurer, and Vietti 1979). Both produce pain and are more likely to develop in the metaphysis of long bones.

Ewing's Tumor

Ewing's tumor, a malignancy of vascular origin, may resemble osteomyelitis in its clinical and radiologic appearance. An adequate biopsy is necessary to establish the diagnosis. Since this tumor is histologically one of the small round cell types it must be differentiated from neuroblastoma and rhabdomyosarcoma in pediatric patients. Its pattern of metastasis is to the bony skeleton, lungs, nodes, and nervous system; therefore evaluation should include bone x-rays and scan and full-chest tomography.

Local control usually can be adequately accomplished in relatively small tumors with high doses of radiotherapy to the entire bone in which the tumor has arisen (Graham-Pole 1979). In two instances amputation or resection should be seriously considered: (1) if the primary tumor is large, or (2) if curative doses of radiotherapy in a growing child will cause marked discrepancies of the affected limb when full growth is reached. Chemotherapy with combined drugs including cyclophosphamide, vincristine, dactinomycin, and perhaps doxorubicin is mandatory adjuvant therapy to treat disseminated microscopic disease, which is presumed present in most patients at the time of diagnosis (Chan et al. 1979).

Other aspects of therapeutic management still under study are the roles of central nervous system prophylaxis and preventive lung irradiation.

Osteogenic Sarcoma

A highly aggressive bone-forming malignancy, osteogenic sarcoma occurs in the adolescent and young adult population. Local therapy requires resection in toto or amputation. In selected patients with smaller tumors, en bloc resection followed by allograft bone transplantation has produced a functional limb (Razek et al. 1977). Osteosarcoma tends to metastasize to the lungs and musculoskeletal system; evaluation of the patient at diagnosis is similar to that described for Ewing's tumor.

The adjuvant therapy of osteogenic sarcoma is controversial (Glicksman, Mauer, and Vietti 1979). A paucity of firm data exists because of lack of simultaneous control or comparative treatment groups. In the opinion of some (Taylor et al. 1978), the natural history of osteosarcoma has changed dramatically in the past 30 years, so that with early recognition and treatment of the primary tumor, long-term survival is improved with amputation alone. In the opinion of others (Jaffe and Frei 1976) based on historical control statistics, adjuvant chemotherapy has been instrumental in increasing survival rates. The chemotherapeutic agents most widely recommended include doxorubicin, high-dose methotrexate with folinic acid rescue, cyclophosphamide, and vincristine. Immunotherapy has also been used.

Even including patients who have metastatic disease at the time of diagnosis or who develop metastases within a few weeks, over half sustain complete remissions of two years or longer with any of these regimens.

Rhabdomyosarcoma

Rhabdomyosarcoma is a highly malignant neoplasm of embryonic muscle, and is the most common soft tissue sarcoma in the pediatric age group. Its differentiation from other sarcomas and embryonal carcinomas may require electron microscopy.

Rhabdomyosarcoma most commonly arises in the orbit, nasopharynx, pelvis (bladder, prostate, uterus, or spermatic cord), and extremities, but may occur in any location. This neoplasm has a propensity for local, lymphatic, and hematogenous invasion. With combined modalities of treatment, however, the majority of children without metastases can be cured (Razek 1977).

Surgical removal of the primary tumor is the treatment of choice for local control if it is relatively small and accessible. Many are not resectable, however, because of local extension or because of their anatomic inaccessibility. Radiotherapy in doses of 5000 to 6000 rad over five to six weeks to a wide local field produces tumor necrosis (Dritschilo et al. 1978). The combined use of dactinomycin, cyclophosphamide, vincristine, and doxorubicin successfully prevents metastatic tumor growth in the majority of patients.

Both radiotherapy and chemotherapy have been extensively employed to shrink large rhabdomyosarcomas so that surgical resection can be accomplished. This is of particular importance in pelvic tumors in which definitive obliteration of the primary mass need not necessarily require pelvic exenteration (Ortega 1979).

Conclusion

The majority of malignant tumors in infants, children, and adolescents are curable through skilled cooperative management by the pediatric surgeon, radiotherapist, and chemotherapist. Options of therapy must consider the chronic effects of treatment as well as the curability of the neoplasm in the rapidly developing young patient. Education and emotional support of both child and family are important.

References

Altman, A. J., and Schwartz, A. D. *Malignant diseases of infancy, childhood, and adolescence*. Philadelphia: W. B. Saunders, 1978.

Annotation. Staging laparotomy for Hodgkin's disease—reassessment. *Lancet* 2:875–879, 1978.

Beckwith, J. B., and Palmer, N. F. Histopathology and prognosis of Wilms' tumor. *Cancer* 41:1937–1944, 1978.

Breslow, N. E. et al. Wilms' tumor: prognostic factors for patients without metastases at diagnosis. *Cancer* 41:1577–1589, 1978.

Castleberry, R. P. et al. Management of localized thoracic neuroblastoma. *Med. Pediatr. Oncol.* 7:153–161, 1979.

Chan, R. C. et al. Management and results of localized Ewing's sarcoma. *Cancer* 43:1001–1006, 1979.

D'Angio, G. J. Complications of treatment encountered in lymphoma-leukemia long-term survivors. *Cancer* 42:1015–1025, 1978.

D'Angio, G. J. et al. The treatment of Wilms' tumor. *Cancer* 28:633–646, 1976.

Dritschilo, A. et al. The role of radiation therapy in the treatment of soft tissue sarcomas of childhood. *Cancer* 42:1192–1203, 1978.

Finklestein, J. Z. et al. Multiagent chemotherapy for children with metastatic neuroblastoma. *Med. Pediatr. Oncol.* 6:179–188, 1979.

Glicksman, A. S.; Maurer, H. M.; and Vietti, T. J. Overview of conference on sarcomas of soft tissue and bone in childhood. *Med. Pediatr. Oncol.* 7:55–67, 1979.

Graham-Pole, J. Ewing sarcoma: treatment with high-dose radiation and adjuvant chemotherapy. *Med. Pediatr. Oncol.* 7:1–8, 1979.

Hellman, S. et al. The place of radiation therapy in the treatment of Hodgkin's disease. *Cancer* 42:971–978, 1978.

Jaffe, N., and Frei, E., III. Osteogenic sarcoma: advances in treatment. *CA* 26:351–359, 1976.

Jenkin, D. et al. Hodgkin's disease in children: treatment with low-dose radiation and MOPP without staging laparotomy. *Cancer* 44:80–86, 1979.

Lange, B. et al. Treatment of advanced Hodgkin's disease in pediatric patients. *Cancer* 42:1141–1145, 1978.

Mankin, H. J. Current concepts in cancer: advances in diagnosis and treatment of bone tumors. *N. Engl. J. Med.* 300:543–544, 1979.

Ortega, J. A. A therapeutic approach to childhood pelvic rhabdomyosarcoma without pelvic exenteration. *J. Pediatr.* 94:205–209, 1979.

Prosnitz, L. R. et al. Long-term remissions with combined modality therapy for advanced Hodgkin's disease. *Cancer* 37:2826–2833, 1976.

Ragab, A. H. et al Bilateral Wilms' tumor. *Cancer* 30:983–988, 1972.

Razek, A. A. et al. Combined treatment modalities of rhabdomyosarcoma in children. *Cancer* 39:2415–2421, 1977.

Shah, N. K. et al. Hodgkin's disease in children. *Med. Pediatr. Oncol.* 2:87–90, 1976.

Sheline, G. E. Radiation therapy of brain tumors. *Cancer* 39:873–881, 1977.

Sutow, W. W.; Vietti, T. J.; and Fernbach, D. J. *Clinical pediatric oncology*. St. Louis: C. V. Mosby, 1977.

Taylor, W. F. et al. Trends and variability in survival from osteosarcoma. *Mayo Clin. Proc.* 53:695–700, 1978.

Van Eys, J., and Cangir, A. Chemotherapy for childhood brain tumors. *J. Pediatr.* 93:544–546, 1978.

Venes, J. L. et al. Chemotherapy as an adjunct in the initial management of cerebellar medulloblastomas. *J. Neurosurg.* 50:721–724, 1979.

Weinstein, H. J. et al. Improved prognosis for patients with mediastinal lymphoblastic lymphoma. *Blood* 53:687–694, 1979.

Wollner, N.; Exerby, P. R.; and Lieberman, P. H. Non-Hodgkin's lymphoma in children. *Cancer* 44:1990–1999, 1979.

sixty-nine

Cancer of Unknown Primary

DAVID S. FISCHER

Although cancer of unknown primary origin is always a perplexing problem, it need not be a totally discouraging one any more. Therapy is available based on histology, site of involvement, age, and extent of tumor spread.

The incidence of unknown primary cancer varies in different series with estimates of 0.5% (Didolkar et al. 1977), 2.3% (Johnson et al. 1964), 3% (Holmes and Fouts 1970), 3% (Lleander et al. 1972), 6.7% (Stewart et al. 1979), and 10% (Moertel et al. 1972). Overall, in an unselected series, approximately 3% of malignancies will be from an unknown primary site at the time of initial therapy. This concept is important because some authors confine the definition to autopsy review (Holmes and Fouts 1970). I have previously defined the cancer of unknown primary as

> *a cancer whose primary site is unknown at the time when the therapeutic decision must be made. It is presumed of course, that an adequate work-up has been performed before such a decision is to be made, but it is clear that such a work-up cannot be endless and cannot be conducted without regard to the patient's comfort, well-being and both the patient's and society's financial and medical assets which are necessarily limited (Fischer 1975).*

Incidence figures will also be determined, even under the present definition, by the fastidiousness or intellectual integrity of the physician in regard to the quality of evidence and precision of diagnosis. For example, if a physician designates a squamous cell carcinoma found in a cervical lymph node from an unknown primary site as head and neck cancer, the statistics would then reflect this diagnosis and not "unknown primary." Similarly, a physician may sign a death certificate as metastatic adenocarcinoma found in the liver with no known primary site as pancreatic carcinoma because the barium enema and gastrointestinal series were negative, and Moertel and co-workers (1972) had shown that this was the most common primary site in this circumstance. There may be less anxiety associated with making a precise organ-related diagnosis even without proof than with admitting one's inability to make an etiologic diagnosis. Death certificates are probably one of the largest sources of error.

In cases that are correctly signed out as unknown primary but later found by autopsy or other information to be of a specific site, a problem develops when they are correctly entered in the tumor registry computer by primary site because the unknown primary circuit is erased. Hence a later search for cases of unknown origin in such a computerized registry may be unrewarding. Several years ago, Dr. Barbara Christine, then director of the Connecticut Tumor Registry, did a computer search of cases of unknown primary in that registry and found almost none. A review of the same years at the Hospital of St. Raphael in New Haven, Connecticut, turned up 198 cases originally coded as unknown primary in their manual file tumor registry, which is then reported to the Connecticut Tumor Registry. When the unknown primary diagnosis was corrected by sub-

Table 69.1. *Histology of Unknown Primary Cancers by Percentage*

Type	*Fischer 1975*	*Johnson et al. 1964*	*Lleander et al. 1972*	*Didolkar et al. 1977*	*Holmes and Fouts 1970*
Adenocarcinoma	32.2	43	40	40.5	32.2
Undifferentiated carcinoma	24.4	38	16	33.5	15.9
Epidermoid carcinoma	6.6	8	4	14.5	10.1
Carcinoma (not otherwise specified)	10.0	0	16	0	17.2
Undifferentiated malignancy	15.5	0	16	11.1	13.7
No tissue diagnosis	4.4	0	8	0	0
Other	6.6	11	0	0.4	9.8
Total number of cases	90	185	25	254	686

sequent information, the Hospital of St. Raphael registry kept the original entry and a notation was made that the file had been transferred to the new diagnostic category. Thus the problem of the unknown primary could be studied and the evolution of knowledge of the case followed to elucidate the site of origin when it was finally found. Undoubtedly, a computer could be programmed to retain the original entry and cross-reference it to the corrected diagnosis, and it is hoped that tumor registries will do this.

Histology

Both the prognosis and therapy of cancer of unknown primary (CUP) depend to a considerable extent on histology. Reports in the literature designate three major categories. One group is confined to cervical node metastases (Jesse et al. 1973; Devine 1978; Jesse and Neff 1966; Barrie, Knapper, and Strong 1970; Fried et al. 1975; MacComb 1974; Comess et al. 1957; France and Lucas 1963) that are squamous cell or epidermoid carcinoma in more than 90% of cases, with a few being adenocarcinoma or melanoma. Another group is confined to adenocarcinomas by the authors' definition (Moertel et al. 1972; Snyder et al. 1979; Stewart et al. 1979; Valentine et al. 1979; Woods et al. 1980) so that 100% of cases are some form of adenocarcinoma. The broadest studies include all histologic types and some in which only the fact of malignancy is established (Fischer 1975; Johnson et al. 1964; Lleander et al. 1972; Didolkar et al. 1977; Holmes and Fouts 1970). The distribution of histologic types in these broad reports is summarized in table 69.1. In general, 40% are adenocarcinoma, about 25% are undifferentiated or anaplastic carcinoma, about 10% are epidermoid carcinoma, and about 25% are malignancies that cannot be more precisely categorized. It is important for the clinician to work closely with the pathologist and review the histology, as lymphomas, germ cell tumors, ovarian, prostatic, and breast carcinomas have a better prognosis with specific therapy now available.

Sites

The initial discovery of the unknown primary carcinoma may arise from a palpable mass, usually a lymph node and more rarely, an abdominal or skin tumor; it may show up on a chest x-ray, bone x-ray or scan, liver or brain scan; or it may be detected microscopically in the evaluation of pleural, peritoneal, or spinal fluid, or bone marrow aspiration or biopsy. The distribution of presenting sites in a few unrestricted series is given in table 69.2. These incidence figures probably understate the frequency of cervical lymph node involvement either because (1) those cases are admitted to an ear, nose, and throat or head and neck service and are reported separately; or (2) their site of origin is determined with a higher frequency than some others and they are then eliminated from the reported series because the primary is no longer unknown (Holmes and Fouts 1970) or because the work-up is relatively well known (Osteen et al. 1978).

Metastases to Lymph Nodes

Lymph node groups that are more easily palpated include cervical, supraclavicular, axillary, and inguinal nodes. Of these, the cervical nodes are most frequently affected by metastases, and these have the most favorable

Table 69.2. *Sites of Unknown Primary Cancer by Percentage*

Primary Site	*Johnson et al. 1964*	*Holmes and Fouts 1970*	*Didolkar et al. 1977**
Lymph nodes	23	18.8	49.2
Bone	21	15.7	20.9
Liver	18	10.5	12.2
Lungs, pleura	14	15.4	39.0
Intraabdominal	11	18.3	11.4
Skin	7	1.6	11.4
Brain, CNS	6	8.9	0
Generalized	0	9.2	0
Total number of cases	185	617	254

*Multiple sites were frequently involved.

prognosis. Depending on the series, the primary site is identified in about one-third of cases and will be from the head and neck area in about 60% and from below the clavicle in the other 40% (Krementz et al. 1977). Supraclavicular node metastases are less common and have a much worse prognosis. In the series of Jesse and associates (1973) 26 of 210 patients had supraclavicular node disease and few survived very long. Except for thyroid, the source of the metastases was below the clavicle. Common sources of lymph node metastases, in approximate order of frequency in autopsy series, are:

Cervical Nodes	Supraclavicular Nodes
Nasopharynx	Thyroid
Tonsil	Lung
Thyroid	Breast
Larynx	Esophagus
Tongue	Stomach
Hypopharynx	Pancreas
Lung	Colon
Esophagus	Prostate
Stomach	
Pancreas	
Colon	
Prostate	

Work-up and management of cervical node CUP was formerly considered straightforward (Barrie, Knapper, and Strong 1970; Jesse and Neff 1966; Fried et al. 1975; MacComb 1974). After visual inspection, needle, incisional, or excisional biopsy was performed by a technique that would not compromise a later radical neck dissection. If the primary site still remained obscure, indirect and direct laryngoscopy and nasopharyngoscopy were performed. Many patients had blind biopsies of the nasopharynx and base of the tongue. Recently, Devine (1978) argued strongly against blind biopsies of the nasopharynx or aerodigestive tract because the yield was almost nil and the procedure obscured the area for later examination and diagnosis. He also indicated a reluctance to perform needle biopsies in small and mobile nodes and restricted this procedure to large fixed nodes. These always had a poor prognosis and were rarely if ever amenable to radical neck dissection. The advice of Martin and Morfit (1944) is recalled:

> *Before incising or excising a cervical tumor for diagnosis, the surgeon should ask himself what he will do if the histologic report indicates that cancer is present. If he feels competent to treat the patient for cancer, well and good; if, on the other hand, he proposes to refer the patient with cancer elsewhere for treatment, then he should, in all fairness to the patient, refer him for diagnosis also, without doing a preliminary incisional biopsy.*

The therapeutic approach to cervical node CUP must be individualized. Nevertheless, the guidelines suggested by Marchetta and colleagues (1963) seem as relevant now as they were then. Surgery, usually a neck dissection, is indicated if the neck mass is clinically operable, is located in the cervical area, and is grade I or II histologically. Contraindications to surgery are (1) a large, fixed mass, (2) a supraclavicular mass, (3) a mass over the mastoid area, and (4) anaplastic carcinoma. These are treated with radiation.

In general, patients with single mobile cervical masses of keratinizing squamous carcinoma and adenocarcinoma should have a neck dissection. Adenocarcinoma in the supraclavicular area is treated with irradiation. In the past, postoperative radiation therapy was given routinely when lesions involving several nodes were resected. Irradiation of 5000 to 7000 rad after neck dissection directed at a possible primary lesion and extending from the nasopharynx to the clavicle can be debilitating, however, and the resulting dry mouth and throat may be almost intolerable. Techniques that spare the larynx, hypopharynx, or nasopharynx are recommended (Jesse et al. 1973). Radiation therapy remains the treatment of choice for inoperable lesions.

Axillary lymph node CUP in women usually represents an occult mammary carcinoma. Westbrook and Gallager (1971) reviewed 18 such cases with special attention to mammography and thermography, and found that even careful pathologic examination may miss the primary lesion. There is a high incidence of histologically early disease (intraductal carcinoma) in these cases. Prognosis is as good as or better than it is for palpable breast cancer with axillary metastases.

In a larger study from the same institution (Copeland and McBride 1973), 60 cases of axillary node CUP were reviewed but the 18 just reported were eliminated from the study. Of the 42 cases reported, 23 were men. Only nine primary sites were eventually found. Survivals were relatively good with eight patients alive from 2 to 10 years at the time of the report, and two who died were free of malignancy at postmortem examination. With the greater availability and experience with mammography, xerography, thermography, and ultrasound of the breast, fewer cases of axillary CUP are anticipated. Following are sources of axillary and inguinal CUP from the larger literature in approximate order of frequency in autopsy series:

Axillary	Inguinal
Breast	Cervix
Lung	Uterus
Stomach	Ovary
Pharynx	Rectum
Melanoma	Anus
Ovary	Prostate
Sarcoma	Melanoma

Inguinal lymph node CUP may be from several primary sites. It is becoming relatively uncommon as better diagnostic methods of evaluating the pelvis are available. Ovarian primaries are being detected by ultrasound and cul-de-sac puncture and the presence of estrogen and progesterone receptors in the biopsy specimen. Prostatic tumors that are not detectable by physical examination are frequently diagnosed by transrectal needle biopsy or by the presence of elevated titers of acid phosphatase, whether tartrate-resistant or labile, and antigenically detectable by radioimmunoassay. Colonic lesions not seen by sigmoidoscopy and barium enema are detected by fiberoptic colonoscopy and are suspected in the presence of high titers of carcinoembryonic antigen (CEA).

Diagnostic techniques for all sites of lymph nodal CUP is improving. Premelanosomes in the cytoplasm of tumor cells may be detected by electron microscopy (EM) and distinguish amelanotic melanoma from anaplastic carcinoma, a frequently recurring problem. Immature tumor cells of the reticuloendothelial system can often be recognized with greater accuracy by their fine structural characteristics as revealed by EM. Histochemical studies sometimes help differentiate a cell of origin. Readily available special stains include mucin, PAS, iron stains for hemosiderin to distinguish it from melanin, and reticulin stains for connective tissue or lymphoid tumors.

Metastases to Other Sites

The lung is the most common target of blood-borne metastases. Diagnosis of pulmonary metastases is much easier than determining their source, particularly the solitary pulmonary nodule, as it may be a primary or metastatic malignancy, a granuloma, benign tumor, mycotic infection, or other lesion. Diagnosis is sometimes achieved with sputum cytology, bronchoscopy (rigid or fiberoptic) with brush biopsy or transbronchial biopsy, fluoroscopically directed percutaneous needle biopsy of lung or pleura, scalene node biopsy, or open lung biopsy. Pleural fluid cytology is sometimes diagnostic but less frequently than malignant ascites fluid cytology. The more common sources of metastases to the lung and pleura are listed as follows in approximate order of frequency in autopsy series:

To: Lung	To: Pleura
From: Breast	From: Breast
Colon	Lung
Other lung	Skin
Pancreas	Stomach
Ovary	Colon
Prostate	Cervix

Table 69.3. *Source of Carcinoma of Unknown Primary by Percentage*

Primary Site	*Nystrom et al. 1977*	*Didolkar et al. 1977*	*Moertel et al. 1972*	*Habermalz et al. 1972*
Pancreas	20	6.5	38	3
Lung	18	40.3	2	15.6
Liver, gallbladder	11	2.6	19	0
Colorectal	10	3.9	12	1.2
Gastric	8	6.5	12	3
Renal	6	5.2	5	0
Ovary	4	3.9	0	0
Prostate	3	0	2	1.8
Adrenal	1	2.6	5	0
Head and neck	2	1.3	0	70.6
Breast	3	0	5	1.8
Others	17	27.2	2	0.5
Total number of cases	152	77	42	167

To: Lung *(continued)*
From: Stomach
Skin
Uterus
Bladder
Kidney
Testis

The lung as a source rather than a target of CUP is the most common (Didolkar et al. 1977) primary site depending on the series and its composition (table 69.3). One study (Nystrom et al. 1977) was from a general medical oncology service and specifically excluded squamous cell carcinoma and restricted the series to adenocarcinoma or undifferentiated carcinoma. Another (Didolkar et al. 1977) was primarily from a surgical service but the patients had a minority of high and midcervical lymph node lesions and few of them were associated with a clear etiologic diagnosis at autopsy. A third report (Moertel et al. 1972) was restricted to adenocarcinoma on a gastroenterology service and would be expected to have few cases of lung cancer. Further data (Habermalz et al. 1972) are a summation of several series of cervical node metastases, and the relatively high incidence of the lung as a source reflects involvement of supraclavicular and lower cervical nodes.

Lung malignancies frequently metastasize by way of arterial circulation and from there can go to any organ of the body, most frequently to the brain (fig. 69.1), liver, bone, and another lung site.

Bone is the second most common site for blood-borne metastases. These are usually osteolytic although breast and prostate metastases are commonly osteoblastic (as are other sites on occasion). The diagnosis can be made by x-ray or bone scan; the scan is more sensitive but the x-ray is more precise. Common sources of bone metastases are:

Breast	Uterus
Prostate	Colon
Lung	Skin
Kidney	Testis
Bladder	Cervix

Liver is the third most common site of metastases of CUP in a general series and the most common site in a study confined to adenocarcinoma (Moertel et al. 1972). The diagnosis is suspected on physical examination by the finding of hepatomegaly and circumstantial evidence accrued with liver function tests (especially alkaline phosphatase, 5′-nucleotidase, lactic dehydrogenase (LDH), and bilirubin), liver scan and ultrasound, or hepatic arteriography. The definitive diagnosis must be established histologically by percutaneous needle biopsy or by open biopsy. The source of metastases to the liver and peritoneum in descending order of frequency from a large autopsy series (Howe and Maniatis 1950) is as follows:

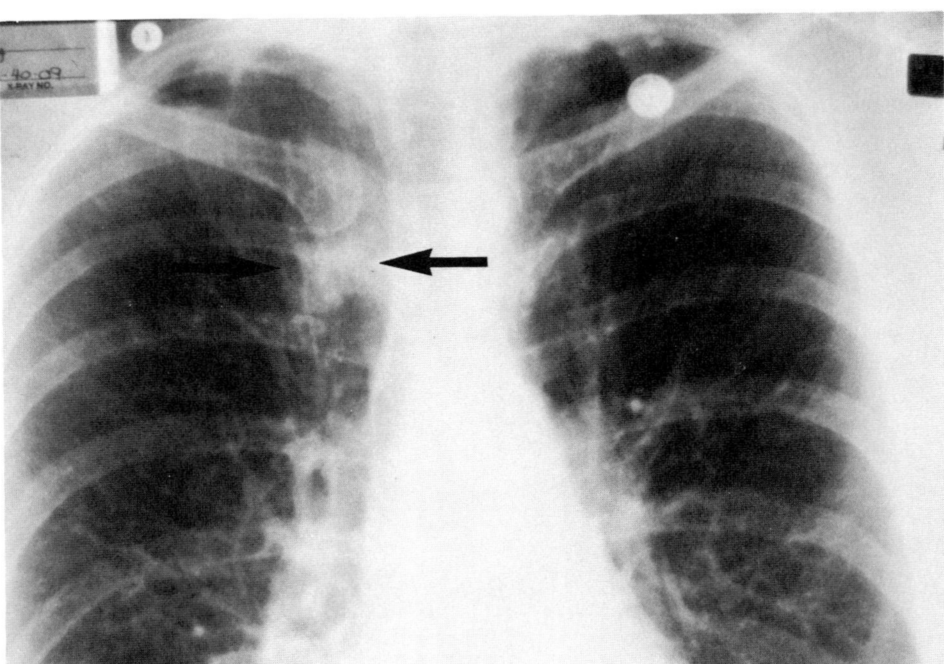

A

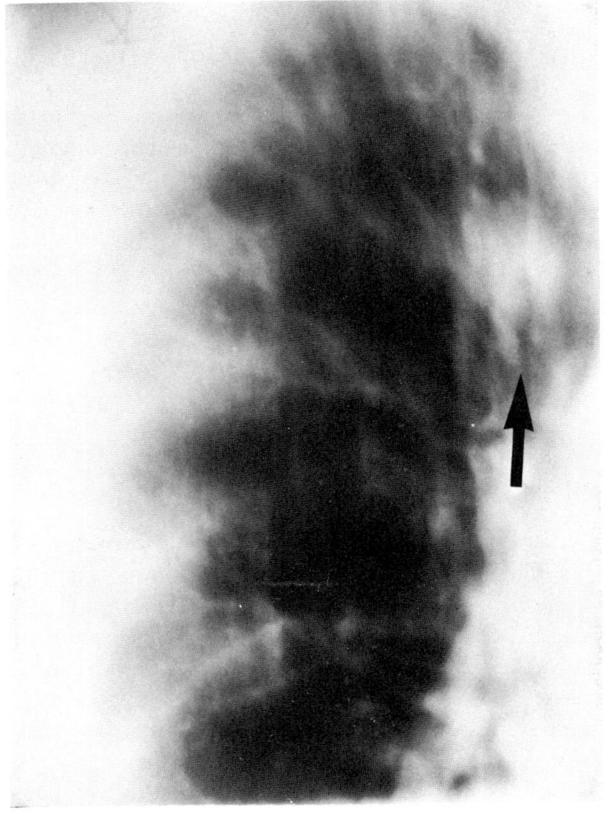

B

Fig. 69.1. *This patient presented with seizures and was found on CT scan of the brain to have multiple tumors. Search for a primary was extensive after the plain chest film,* A, *was read as negative. A tomogram of the chest,* B, *finally showed the primary lesion* (arrow). *Review of the original plain film,* A, *showed that the tumor was present* (arrows).

To: Liver	To: Peritoneum
From: Colon	From: Ovary
Breast	Colon
Pancreas	Pancreas
Lung	Stomach
Stomach	Breast
Ovary	Cervix
Gallbladder	Bladder
Bladder	Uterus
Uterus	Gallbladder
Bile ducts	
Prostate	
Skin	
Kidney	
Cervix	
Esophagus	
Testis	

Brain metastases are most often from lung, breast, or melanoma. The occasional colon, gastric, pancreatic, testicular, or prostatic brain metastasis is usually a secondary from a previous lung or liver metastasis.

Diagnostic Work-up

The traditional wisdom of medicine is that precise diagnosis leads to more selective treatment and a better therapeutic result. In conformity with this outlook, Krementz and Cerise (1970) emphasized the importance of a thorough search for the primary cancer. This was to include a careful history and physical examination (including pelvic, rectal, proctoscopic, and ENT examinations), stool and urine for occult blood, CBC and liver profile, and routine chest x-ray. These were to be supplemented with intravenous pyelograms, gastrointestinal series and barium enemas, cytologic examinations of abnormal exudates or body fluids, and appropriate radionuclear scans of the liver, brain, and bones and when indicated, endoscopy of the colon, stomach, esophagus, larynx, nasopharynx, tracheobronchial tree, and urinary bladder.

Recently, several groups have done a cost-benefit analysis of this aggressive work-up and have questioned its efficacy. Osteen and colleagues (1978) reviewed the charts of 67 patients to evaluate the effectiveness of some common diagnostic studies used to identify the primary sources of systemic metastases. The results were surprisingly poor. No diagnosis or the wrong diagnosis was made in 29 of the 67 cases. In the absence of symptoms referable to the system examined, radiologic contrast studies were not helpful. When there was little evidence of metastatic disease elsewhere, the bone scan was a valuable procedure for finding occult metastases. The liver scan was much less useful. The least helpful study was gray-scale ultrasound. Needle biopsy was a remarkably ineffective method for obtaining tissue and did little more than add confusion and delay. They concluded that in the light of present ineffective current therapy for most metastatic solid tumors (pancreas, colon, and lung), a limited work-up will produce almost identical results to one that is more elaborate and costly.

Nystrom and co-workers (1979) reviewed the records of 266 patients with metastatic nonsquamous cell carcinoma of unknown origin who underwent upper and lower gastrointestinal contrast studies, IVPs, and chest x-rays for location of a primary cancer site. Of the 129 identified, only 22 were verified antemortem, whereas autopsy showed 25 cases with false positive examination results. The patients did not have many of the commonly occurring tumors such as breast, colon, and prostate. When the primary was finally found, the metastatic pattern displayed at initial diagnosis was frequently atypical for the site from which it originated. For example, in proved cases of lung cancer there was a paucity of metastatic bone disease (4%) and a large proportion of women patients. Conversely, patients with pancreatic and liver cancer had an unusually high incidence of metastatic bone disease (30%), and those with prostatic cancers had an unusually low incidence of bone metastases (25%) but a surprisingly high proportion of lung (75%) and liver (50%) involvement. Since these tumors do not follow usual patterns, contrast roentgenographic studies that are costly, uncomfortable, of low yield, and often misleading, should be limited to cases with specific organ dysfunction.

The most vigorous dissent from the consensus that thorough work-up leads to better treatment comes from Australia (Stewart et al. 1979). Of 1300 patients referred to a medical oncology unit, 87 (6.7%) had CUP after history, physical examination, and chest x-ray were completed. After extensive investigations, only eight primary tumor sites were identified by nonsurgical techniques. In 2 patients primary diagnosis was established at laparotomy, and in a further 13 clinical follow-up eventually led to recognition of the primary tumor site before death. Only eight patients had tumors that were responsive to presently available systemic treatment (four ovarian, two prostatic, and two germ cell tumors). They concluded that in general, early precise diagnosis does not significantly influence the outcome and survival of this group of patients. They

Table 69.4. *Survival of Cancer of Unknown Primary*

Reference	*Types*	*Median (months)*	*Range (months)*
Snyder et al. 1979	Adenocarcinoma	2	0.5–78
Osteen et al. 1978	Cervical excluded	3	1 –25
Johnson et al. 1964	All types	9.3	1 –60+
Lleander et al. 1972	Cervical excluded	?	3 –37+
Valentine et al. 1979	Adenocarcinoma	7+	?
Woods et al. 1980	Adenocarcinoma	3.8	1.5–16.5
Didolkar et al. 1977	All types	9	1 –215
Stewart et al. 1979	Adenocarcinoma	3.5	1 –28
Copeland and McBride 1973	Axillary nodes	16	1 –120
Krementz et al. 1977	Cervical nodes	35	

Table 69.5. *Therapy of Unknown Primary Carcinoma*

	Poor Risk Over Age 60	*Good Risk Under Age 60*
Regimen A		
5-Fluorouracil	300 mg/m^2	400 mg/m^2
Methotrexate	20 mg/m^2	30 mg/m^2
Cyclophosphamide	600 mg/m^2	800 mg/m^2
Regimen B		
5-Fluorouracil	300 mg/m^2	400 mg/m^2
Methotrexate	20 mg/m^2	30 mg/m^2
Doxorubicin	30 mg/m^2	40 mg/m^2

NOTE: All drugs are given intravenously on day 1 and repeated on day 22.

recommended that efforts should be directed at excluding the possibility of a treatable primary tumor by a few simple investigations such as acid phosphatase, alpha-fetoprotein, beta-human chorionic gonadotropin, imaging of pelvic organs, and measurement of estrogen receptors.

Treatment

It is clear from the literature that patients with CUP in the high or midcervical nodes have a relatively good median survival of three years or so compared to the dismal three to four months associated with adenocarcinomas or nonsquamous cell carcinomas (table 69.4).

To try to improve the prognosis, in 1976 we began a prospective randomized trial of two chemotherapy regimens (table 69.5). We had difficulty with participation in the arm with doxorubicin because of its high cost and our inability to obtain independent funding. Although the numbers in that arm are small, preliminary analysis suggests that the agent does not yield superior results (Fischer and Markham 1981).

Earlier reports of chemotherapy using 5-fluorouracil alone gave a 6.2% complete response (CR) rate in a group of 65 patients (Johnson et al. 1964), and a 16% response rate in 88 patients with a median duration of response of four months (Moertel et al. 1972) in adenocarcinomas. No conclusions can be drawn from another study (Lleander et al. 1972) in which 10 different drug regimens were used to treat 25 patients with noncervical node CUP.

Intravenous combination chemotherapy was given to 14 patients (Valentine et al. 1979) consisting of cyclophosphamide, 400 mg/m^2; doxorubicin, 40 mg/m^2; and 5-fluorouracil, 500 mg/m^2 and repeated every 21 days with appropriate dose modifications. Two patients (14%) obtained objective response, and after failing this therapy one patient responded to a regimen of vinblastine, 15 mg and bleomycin, 15 units given intravenously every four weeks. An additional four patients showed subjective improvement and objective stability on the three-drug regimen. The median survival of the entire group was more than 7 months and for the responders it was more than 15 months at the time of the report. This is clearly superior to earlier reports.

In a randomized study of two combination chemotherapy regimens (Wood et al. 1980), 25 patients were given intravenous DM (doxorubicin, 50 mg/m^2 on days 1, 22, and 43; and mitomycin, 20 mg/m^2 on days 1 and 43) and compared to a group given intravenous CMF (cyclophosphamide, 500 mg/m^2; methotrexate, 40 mg/m^2; and 5-fluorouracil, 600 mg/m^2) on day 1 and then every 21 days. The DM group had nine responses (36%) with one CR and eight partial (PR), and a median survival of 4.5 months; the CMF group had one PR (4.5%) and a median survival of 1.75 months. The authors have since treated 16 additional patients with DM with six PRs (37.5%).

As we make progress in developing new and better chemotherapy drugs and learn to use them with an improved therapeutic index in a variety of known tumors (ovary, testis, breast, Hodgkin's disease, gestational trophoblastic tumors, and so on), one would hope that similar progress will occur with cancers of unknown primary site.

References

Barrie, J. R.; Knapper, W. H.; and Strong, E. W. Cervical nodal metastases of unknown origin. *Am. J. Surg.* 120:466–470, 1970.

Comess, M. H. et al. Cervical metastasis from occult carcinoma. *Surg. Gynecol. Obstet.* 104:607–617, 1957.

Copeland, E. M., and McBride, C. M. Axillary metastases from unknown primary sites. *Ann. Surg.* 178:25–27, 1973.

Devine, K. D. Cancer in the neck without obvious source. *Mayo Clin. Proc.* 53:644–650, 1978.

Didolkar, M. S. et al. Metastatic carcinomas from occult primary tumors. A study of 254 patients. *Ann. Surg.* 186:625–630, 1977.

Fischer, D. S. Management of cancer of unknown primary. *Conn. Med.* 39:205–208, 1975.

Fischer, D. S. and Markham, L. L. Survival after therapy for carcinoma of unknown primary (CUP). *Proc. Am. Soc. Clin. Oncol.* 22:389, 1981.

France, C. J., and Lucas, R. The management and prognosis of metastatic neoplasms of the neck with an unknown primary. *Am. J. Surg.* 106:835–839, 1963.

Fried, M. P. et al. Cervical metastases from an unknown primary. *Ann. Otol. Rhinol. Laryngol.* 84:152–157, 1975.

Habermalz, H. et al. Halslymphknotenmetastasen bei unbekanntem Primärtumor: Ausgangsort, Therapie, Prognose. *Strahlentherapie* 144:267–275, 1972.

Holmes, F. F., and Fouts, T. L. Metastatic cancer of unknown primary site. *Cancer* 26:816–820, 1970.

Howe, E. R., and Maniatis, W. R. Malignancies and their spread; an analysis of 1300 primary malignancies from 6500 consecutive autopsies at Hartford Hospital, 1925–1950. *Hartford Hosp. Bull.* 5:3–26, 1950.

Jesse, R. H. et al. Cervical lymph node metastasis: unknown primary cancer. *Cancer* 31:854–859, 1973.

Jesse, R. H., and Neff, L. E. Metastatic carcinoma in cervical nodes with an unknown primary lesion. *Am. J. Surg.* 112:547–553, 1966.

Johnson, R. O. et al. Response of primary unknown cancer to treatment with 5-fluorouracil (NSC 19893). *Cancer Chemother. Rep.* 38:63–64, 1964.

Krementz, E. T. et al. Metastases of undetermined source. *CA* 27:289–299, 1977.

Krementz, E. T., and Cerise, E. J. Metastatic lesions of undetermined source. *Hosp. Med.* 6:91–112, 1970.

Lleander, V. C. et al. Chemotherapy in the management of metastatic cancer of unknown primary site. *Oncology* 26:265–270, 1972.

MacComb, W. S. Metastatic cervical nodes of unknown primary origin. *CA* 24:229–232, 1974.

Marchetta, F. C. et al. Carcinoma of the neck. *Am. J. Surg.* 106:974–979, 1963.

Martin, H., and Morfit, H. M. Cervical lymph node metastasis as the first symptom of cancer. *Surg. Gynecol. Obstet.* 78:133–159, 1944.

Moertel, C. G. et al. Treatment of the patient with adenocarcinoma of unknown origin. *Cancer* 30:1469–1472, 1972.

Nystrom, J. S. et al. Metastatic and histologic presentations in unknown primary cancer. *Semin. Oncol.* 4:53–58, 1977.

Nystrom, J. S. et al. Identifying the primary site in metastatic cancer of unknown origin. *JAMA* 241:381–383, 1979.

Osteen, R. T. et al. In pursuit of the unknown primary. *Am. J. Surg.* 135:494–498, 1978.

Snyder, R. D. et al. Adenocarcinoma of unknown primary site: a clinicopathological study. *Med. Pediatr. Oncol.* 6:289–294, 1979.

Stewart, J. F. et al. Unknown primary adenocarcinoma: incidence of overinvestigation and natural history. *Br. Med. J.* 1:1530–1533, 1979.

Valentine, J. et al. Combination chemotherapy for adenocarcinoma of unknown primary origin. *Cancer Clin. Trials* 2:265–268, 1979.

Westbrook, K. C., and Gallager, H. S. Breast carcinoma presenting as an axillary mass. *Am. J. Surg.* 122:607–611, 1971.

Woods, R. L. et al. Metastatic adenocarcinomas of unknown primary site. *N. Engl. J. Med.* 303:87–89, 1980.

index

C

D

E

N

O

P

T